Large Animal Clinical Procedures *for* Veterinary Technicians

Large Animal Clinical Procedures
for Veterinary Technicians

Third Edition

Kristin Holtgrew-Bohling, DVM

Owner, Town & Country Veterinary Clinic, PC
Auburn, Nebraska

ELSEVIER

ELSEVIER

3251 Riverport Lane
St. Louis, Missouri 63043

LARGE ANIMAL CLINICAL PROCEDURES FOR VETERINARY
TECHNICIANS, THIRD EDITION   ISBN: 978-0-323-34113-4

Notices

Knowledge and best practice in this field are constantly changing. As new research and experience broaden our understanding, changes in research methods, professional practices, or medical treatment may become necessary.

Practitioners and researchers must always rely on their own experience and knowledge in evaluating and using any information, methods, compounds, or experiments described herein. In using such information or methods, they should be mindful of their own safety and the safety of others, including parties for whom they have a professional responsibility.

With respect to any drug or pharmaceutical products identified, readers are advised to check the most current information provided (i) on procedures featured or (ii) by the manufacturer of each product to be administered, to verify the recommended dose or formula, the method and duration of administration, and contraindications. It is the responsibility of practitioners, relying on their own experience and knowledge of their patients, to make diagnoses, to determine dosages and the best treatment for each individual patient, and to take all appropriate safety precautions.

To the fullest extent of the law, neither the Publisher nor the authors, contributors, or editors assume any liability for any injury and/or damage to persons or property as a matter of products liability, negligence, or otherwise or from any use or operation of any methods, products, instructions, or ideas contained in the material herein.

Previous editions copyrighted 2012 and 2006.

ISBN: 978-0-323-34113-4

Content Strategist: Shelly Stringer
Associate Content Development Specialist: Katie Gutierrez
Publishing Services Manager: Catherine Albright-Jackson
Senior Project Manager: Doug Turner
Book Designer: Ashley Miner

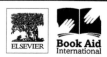

Working together
to grow libraries in
developing countries

www.elsevier.com • www.bookaid.org

To the professors in the Professional Program in Veterinary Medicine at the University of Nebraska–Lincoln and Dr. Mike Speece of Town & Country Veterinary Clinic in Auburn, Nebraska.

The appreciation I have for your dedication and investment in my career as a veterinarian is inspiring. The level of education and mentorship you have shown me is second to none. Your commitment to my success will never be forgotten.

Acknowledgments

Thank you to Dad, for your support throughout the years; to Mom, for being my best friend; and to Bob, for the time and support you have shown me with everything. To Brett and Trever: live your dreams—no matter how big or small, they are yours.

I would like to recognize the veterinarians, veterinary technicians, and veterinary assistants with whom I have had the privilege of working and learning. I couldn't have done this without you!

Thank you to Dr. Gregg Hanzlicek, Dr. Brett Andrews, and Dr. Noel Johnson for giving me such great opportunities, believing in me, teaching me so much valuable information, and providing guidance in my career.

Thank you to Dr. Michael Cooper for your guidance and wisdom. You are an excellent teacher.

Thank you to Dr. Joni Brunssen for being such a great mentor, friend, and boss. Your work ethic and determination are an inspiration.

Thank you to the students in the Veterinary Technician Program at Vatterott College from 2005 to the present. Your continued dedication to this field was a major factor in my decision to write this textbook.

Thank you, Shelly Stringer and the staff at Elsevier, for believing in me and helping me so much along the way.

Thank you, Bailey, Harley, and Cupcake, for your patience with photographs.

Thank you to the many breed associations and livestock support companies for supplying valuable information and photographs for future veterinary technician students.

Thank you, Bob, Brett, and Trever, for allowing me time and providing me support. I love you!

Thank you to my family, friends, and neighbors for all of your encouragement and support during this project.

Thank you to Grandma Kay and Grandma Holtgrew for believing in me all of these years!

Thank you to Kim and Ron Holtgrew, owners of Holtgrew Farm and Trucking, for assisting me with so many great photographs. I love you, Mom and Dad.

Thank you to Ashley and Jon, owners of Zeisler Dairy and Zeisler Charolais, for all of the photographs.

Thank you to Willie Bohling for allowing me to photograph your livestock.

Kristin Holtgrew-Bohling, DVM

Having grown up in a rural community of Nebraska, I thought that everyone understood where their food came from. However, when I moved to Omaha, Nebraska, for my veterinary technician externship, I realized that this was not the case. When I started teaching veterinary technicians about large animal medicine, I noticed that their questions more often related to why decisions were made and why practices were recommended and less often to the procedures themselves. The third edition of *Large Animal Clinical Procedures for Veterinary Technicians* covers the basic elements of the livestock industry to help students relate the principles and practices of agriculture in the veterinary community with the care of large animals.

All the information from the second edition has been updated, and I have added two new chapters, "Livestock Nutrition" and "Diagnostic Imaging." I have also added more details about clinical pathology, equipment boxes, and new online chapters covering the poultry industry. So after much thought and careful consideration, I have created a textbook that will help students understand the "big picture" as it relates to large animal medicine, with helpful study tools, as well as a quick reference for those technicians working in the industry on a daily basis.

This textbook is designed to help students obtain the basic information needed to succeed in the large animal field, and it offers students and instructors a comprehensive look at the roles and responsibilities of veterinary technicians.

ORGANIZATION

Deciding how to organize a textbook of this scope was difficult, but after reviewing all of the information multiple times, I realized that the best approach would be to begin with a general overview of large animal production. Starting with production will help students understand why they are asked to learn about the large animal procedures found later in the textbook. Then I decided to cover the topics that are the cornerstone of the large animal industry: reproduction and nutrition. Much of the information on reproduction and nutrition is the same for all species, so covering it at the beginning helps instructors save time and allows them to emphasize the differences among species when discussing the chapters about individual species. The next section of the book covers the everyday responsibilities of a veterinary technician in large animal practice. Students can then read about equine, bovine, ovine, caprine, camelids, and porcine species in separate sections, each of which includes four chapters that examine husbandry, clinical procedures, surgery, and disease.

EVOLVE WEBSITE

On the Evolve website, students and faculty can access photographs of large animal instruments commonly used with large animals, as well as all the illustrations from the book. The Evolve site also contains four supplemental chapters on poultry. These chapters discuss husbandry, clinical procedures, surgical procedures, and diseases common to poultry. Instructors can also use the available Test Banks and PowerPoint lecture outlines. These outlines will help instructors find supplemental materials and design projects for students that will enrich their classroom experience, with the goal of getting their students to ask, Why?, because the students who do tend to stand out and succeed in their careers.

Kristin Holtgrew-Bohling, DVM

Contents

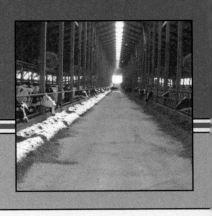

1

The Importance of Livestock

OUTLINE

LEARNING OBJECTIVES

After reading this chapter, you will be able to

- List and explain the functions of livestock
- Describe the economic importance of livestock
- Describe the size and scope of the large animal industry
- Describe the normal cycle that exists within the dairy industry
- Describe the structure within the meat industry
- Describe the basic components of the fiber industry

KEY TERMS

Artificial insemination
Backgrounding
By-products
Calving interval
Claw
Clip
Creep feeders
Commercial farming
Commodity
Connecting air
Dry lot

Farrowing
Farrow to finish
Free stall barn
Freshening
Grid
Milk replacer
Milk tubes
Milking unit
Nursery
Order buyers
Parlor

Pasture
Quality grade
Slivers
Streak canal
Suspension cup
Teat cup assembly
Thermal neutral zone
Vertical integration
Yield grade

KEY ABBREVIATIONS

USDA: United States Department of Agriculture
TNZ: Thermal neutral zone

THE IMPORTANCE OF LIVESTOCK FOR THE WORLD

Agriculture is one of the oldest sciences and one of the most important. Without a firm understanding of agriculture, all humans would struggle to find enough food, shelter, and clothing to survive. The main reason for maintaining our animal agricultural populations is to provide a nutritious and desirable form of food for human consumption. Only approximately 11% of the world's land area is suitable for production of foods that can be directly consumed by humans. Approximately 75% of energy intake consumed by ruminants and 30% consumed by nonruminants is from waste materials that cannot be consumed directly by the human population. With world food production already inadequately able to provide balanced diets for people of the world, it is important that we continue to use livestock (Fig. 1-1).

Supplies of protein are particularly scarce and costly for the populations of most developing countries. The World Health Organization has reported that hunger and related malnutrition are the greatest threats to the world's public health. The United Nations Food and Agriculture Organization estimates that nearly 870 million people of the 7.2 billion people in the world, or 1 in 8, were suffering from chronic undernourishment in 2010 to 2012. Almost all the hungry people live in developing countries, representing 15% of the population of developing counties. An estimated 7,615,360 will die of starvation in 2015 (http://www.worldhunger.org/).

The malthusian theory is that the world population increase will outpace increases in the means of providing food. For example, in terms of the global population crisis, in the time it takes you to read this sentence, 24 people will be added to the earth's population; within an hour, the number will reach 12,000; by the day's end, the number will be 288,000; and in 48 hours the human population growth will be enough to fill a city the size of San Francisco. The world population will jump from 7 billion to 9 billion by 2050. Farmers will need to double food production by then to keep pace.

Providing food to meet caloric intake is not enough. Adequate protein is also required for normal body function. Protein is needed for growth, maturation, pregnancy, lactation, and recovery from disease. It has been well established that nutritionally animal proteins are superior to vegetable proteins for humans. The superiority results primarily from the better balance of amino acids in animal products.

THE IMPORTANCE OF LIVESTOCK IN THE UNITED STATES

The United States is the world's largest exporter of agricultural products. In 2013, agricultural exports were valued at $140.9 billion, a new record. Farmer and rancher families comprised less than 1% of the U.S. population but produced approximately 22% of the meat, 32% of the fluid milk, 29% of the eggs, and 41% of the poultry products of the world. According to the 2012 United States Department of Agriculture (USDA) agricultural census, the total value of agricultural products sold from farms in the United States was $394.6 billion, a record high. This value is 33% higher than that of 2007. The value of the livestock and livestock products themselves that were sold in 2007 was $153 billion. The percentage of livestock products sold from farms in the United States constitutes 51.7% of the total market value of agricultural products sold in 2007.

Livestock producers also create income for the United States and stimulate the economy with the purchase of goods to raise livestock. According to the USDA 2012 agriculture census, producers spent $351.8 billion on production expenses in 2012, an increase of 10.4% since 2011. Of those production expenses, 16% was spent on feed, and 11.3% was spent on the purchase or lease of livestock. Jobs created from agriculture should not be overlooked when evaluating the importance of agriculture to our economy. Approximately one in every six jobs in private employment is related to agriculture. These statistics alone are the reason some economists believe that agriculture is the foundation of our economy (Figs. 1-2 to 1-4).

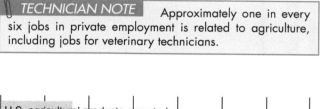

TECHNICIAN NOTE   Approximately one in every six jobs in private employment is related to agriculture, including jobs for veterinary technicians.

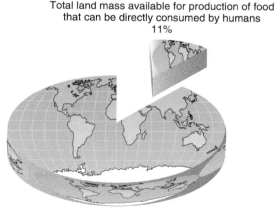

Total land mass available for production of food that can be directly consumed by humans
11%

Total land mass available for production of food that cannot be used for direct human consumption
89%

FIGURE 1-1 World food consumption by category.

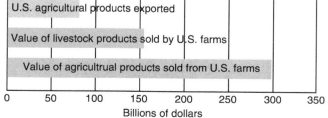

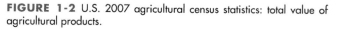

U.S. agricultural products exported

Value of livestock products sold by U.S. farms

Value of agricultrual products sold from U.S. farms

| 0 | 50 | 100 | 150 | 200 | 250 | 300 | 350 |

Billions of dollars

FIGURE 1-2 U.S. 2007 agricultural census statistics: total value of agricultural products.

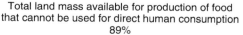

Animal agriculture is used to stabilize farm incomes by providing other areas of income for farmers and ranchers. It also allows farmers and ranchers to save on shipping costs of bulky feeds by concentrating them into the form of meat through the use of livestock.

Clothing is supplied through agriculture with the production of wool, mohair, and cashmere. Wool markets have been gradually declining in United States for several years now because of the use of synthetic fibers, although there is still an economic market for the product. Leather used in shoes, belts, gloves, and clothes constitutes 5% to 10% of the market value of livestock animals.

By-products are any animal products other than meat. These products contribute significantly to U.S. society. Examples of by-products include organs, fat, bones, and various glands. Examples of products made with by-products include candy, house insulation, gum, sandpaper, wallpaper, ice cream, fertilizers, canned meats, buttons, perfumes, glue, camera film, lanolin, gelatin desserts, marshmallows, dice, piano keys, toothbrushes, cosmetics, rug padding, waxes, soap lubricants, printing ink, candles, and upholstering materials for furniture. By-products are also used as feeds for other animals. Another major use of by-products includes medications, such as insulin, cortisone, epinephrine, thrombin, rennet, heparin, and corticotropin. Not only do livestock contribute to medications, but they also supply a research model for scientists to study human and animal health (Fig. 1-5).

Livestock are also doing their part to "go green." Sixty-four percent of the U.S. land mass is used for the production of livestock: 36% for grazing and 28% for production of hay and other forage crops and grain. Livestock help conserve soil and soil fertility in the land on which these livestock feeds are grown. Livestock manure is applied to these areas to replenish nutrients in the soil used by plants for growth (Fig. 1-6). Organic agriculture is becoming a huge part of U.S. agricultural production, and livestock help play a role in conservation of our natural resources.

The traditional use of livestock as a power source has come and gone in U.S. society. However, with continued research into more effective ways to produce power, scientists have discovered the use of methane gas, produced from fecal material, as a power source. Several large feedlots in the United States have built biogas plants. These plants use methane gas as a form of energy. Fuel for electricity, cooking, and heating needs of an average U.S. farm could be supplied by the manure of about 40 cows. The cost of energy contributes

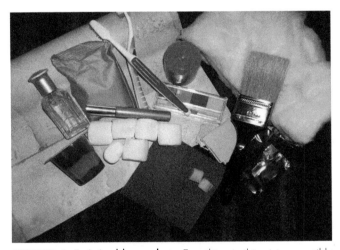

FIGURE 1-5 Animal by-products. Everything in this picture possibly can be made from animal by-products: the rug everything is sitting on, perfume, gelatin, marshmallows, sandpaper, pudding, gum, paintbrush, candy, insulation, wallpaper, toothbrushes, ink in the print cartridge, and cosmetics.

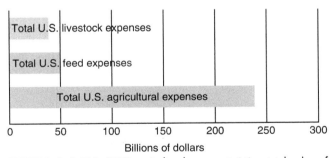

Total U.S. livestock expenses

Total U.S. feed expenses

Total U.S. agricultural expenses

0   50   100   150   200   250   300
Billions of dollars

FIGURE 1-3 U.S. 2007 agricultural census statistics: total value of agricultural expenses.

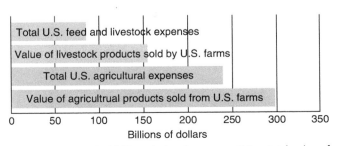

Total U.S. feed and livestock expenses

Value of livestock products sold by U.S. farms

Total U.S. agricultural expenses

Value of agricultrual products sold from U.S. farms

0   50   100   150   200   250   300   350
Billions of dollars

FIGURE 1-4 U.S. 2007 agricultural census statistics: total value of products and expenses.

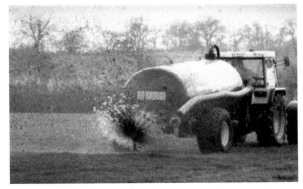

FIGURE 1-6 Manure spreaders. Manure spreaders are used to spread manure across land. This helps replace valuable nutrients used by plants. (From Pritchard G, Dennis I, Waddilove J: Biosecurity: reducing disease risks to pig breeding herds. *In Pract* 27:230-237, 2005; Jackson PGG, Cockcroft PD: *Handbook of pig medicine*, St. Louis, 2007, Saunders.)

largely to the average cost of food supplied to grocery stores. This trend is extremely realistic in view of the increases in energy costs and jumps in grocery prices in recent history.

Recreation is another benefit that can be attributed to the use of livestock in the United States. There are an estimated 9.2 million horses in the United States, and their owners annually spend an estimated $102 billion on these horses annually. This fact not only contributes to their economic importance but also signifies the importance of horses as a recreational hobby. More people attend horse races annually than see minor or major league baseball games or attend automobile races (Fig. 1-7). Horses are not the only animals used as a form of recreation. Not only is horse racing a large industry, but also recreational riding, rodeo, western riding, English riding, dressage, and jumping all make up a large part of this industry. If you have ever visited a county or state fair, you have seen people enjoying the exhibition of livestock as well.

U.S. LIVESTOCK TRENDS

Table 1-1 lists the 10 leading states for livestock and livestock production *commodity* cash receipts for several livestock categories.

Many of the trends that exist within the livestock industry are created because of consumer demand for certain products. The U.S. population's lifestyle and eating habits significantly affect production, processing, and marketing of meat products. Current research also plays a role in the production of U.S. meat products.

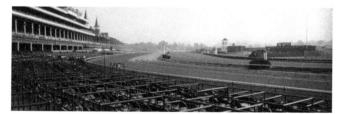

FIGURE 1-7 Churchill Downs, home to one of the biggest horse races in the United States, the Kentucky Derby.

Legislation and consumer perspective are important trends in livestock production. Livestock producers are aware of the impact that consumers have on the value of their livestock. Producers sometimes make adjustments to procedures used on farms to allow for a more positive consumer perspective.

> **TECHNICIAN NOTE**   Consumer views and preferences often influence livestock production. A major trend that is currently sweeping the livestock industry is the increased awareness of animal welfare. For example, pain control is becoming the standard for procedures such as dehorning and castration. Livestock producers understand the impact that consumers have on the industry, and livestock welfare is therefore becoming more and more important to the producer.

Since the 1980s, we have seen a gradual decline in small farming and ranching operations and an increase in the number of livestock raised each year. This trend is indicative of the gradual conversion to *commercial farming* operations. Commercial farming operations are larger in scale, and this allows lower per unit cost of production. This industry is a business; lower per unit costs of production allow for larger profits.

Research is also a major component of the livestock industry. With an increasing population we must find better, more economical ways to raise livestock to continue feeding the world's population. The two major areas of research in livestock production are reproduction and nutrition. Reproduction and nutrition are the cornerstones of the industry.

Livestock producers are placing emphasis on livestock health. Currently, producers lose 15% to 20% of their income as a result of parasites, toxins, and disease. Only 10% of all livestock producers are currently using effective disease prevention practices. Veterinary technicians must do

TABLE 1-1	Leading States in Livestock and Livestock Production Commodity Cash Receipts					
RANK	LEADING STATES IN CASH RECEIPTS FROM LIVESTOCK	BEEF CATTLE AND CALVES	SWINE	DAIRY PRODUCTS	SHEEP AND LAMBS	WOOL
1	Texas	Texas	Iowa	California	Texas	Texas
2	Iowa	Nebraska	Minnesota	Wisconsin	California	Wyoming
3	California	Kansas	North Carolina	New York	Colorado	Montana
4	Nebraska	Iowa	Illinois	Idaho	Wyoming	California
5	Kansas	Colorado	Indiana	Pennsylvania	Utah	Colorado
6	Wisconsin	Oklahoma	Missouri	Texas	South Dakota	South Dakota
7	Minnesota	California	Oklahoma	Minnesota	Idaho	Utah
8	North Carolina	South Dakota	Nebraska	Michigan	Montana	Idaho
9	Oklahoma	Missouri	Ohio	New Mexico	Oregon	Iowa
10	Georgia	New Mexico	Kansas	Washington	Iowa	Oregon

From U.S. Department of Agriculture Economic Research Service, 2014, <http://www.ers.usda.gov/> (Accessed 16.02.2015.)

their part to communicate these losses to their clients (when appropriate). Performing quality client education will help producers to understand these losses and what they can do to prevent them.

> **TECHNICIAN NOTE** Producers currently lose 15% to 20% of their income as a result of parasites, toxins, and disease. Preventive medicine needs to become more prominent in today's veterinary practice, and we must start with good client education.

THE IMPORTANCE OF VETERINARY MEDICINE WITHIN THE LIVESTOCK INDUSTRY

As a veterinary technician it is your job to provide quality veterinary care to sick or injured animals, but as a technician in the large animal industry it is also important for you to help the veterinarian maintain a safe food supply for the world. Livestock must be healthy to undergo the harvest process. Some livestock diseases and parasites are zoonotic and can be contracted through the consumption of meat. Other livestock diseases could devastate livestock production and leave the world's population to starve. In fact, some government officials are concerned about biologic welfare attacks that are centered on the destruction of agriculture.

Economically speaking, livestock production profit margins are small. Poor husbandry and health management practices can cause loss of profits and, if prolonged, even bankruptcy. Producers should try to minimize diseases and stress. Prevention of diseases and stress will help reduce poor performance. Veterinary technicians must keep in mind that the large animal industry is a business. The goal of the livestock producer is to produce the most product, of the highest quality, at the lowest cost.

> **TECHNICIAN NOTE** The goal of the livestock producer is to produce the most product, of the highest quality, at the lowest cost.

Veterinary technicians must have a thorough understanding of livestock production systems to understand and assist in medical treatments. The rest of this chapter focuses on giving a brief overview of each production system so that technicians will be better able to understand the principles and practice of large animal veterinary medicine. This is a brief overview of these systems. You can purchase several books on each industry, and some people receive doctorate degrees just focusing on this type of information. So these systems are much more complicated than as presented here. However, this overview should help you understand the basic principles used to make decisions that take place in veterinary medicine.

> **TECHNICIAN NOTE** Veterinary technicians must have a thorough understanding of livestock production systems to understand and assist with medical treatments.

THE DAIRY INDUSTRY

DAIRY HOUSING

The type of housing used for dairy production can vary greatly. The most common type of dairy housing used into today's industry is the *free stall barn*. Free stall barns are loose housing systems (Fig. 1-8). The cows are able to move anywhere they wish throughout the pen (Fig. 1-9). These systems typically have resting areas for the cows to lie down. Advantages to free stall barns include cleaner environments, less bedding expense, greater ease of parlor use, fewer space requirements, fewer teat and udder injuries, and greater ease of use. Some dairy cattle are housed in dry

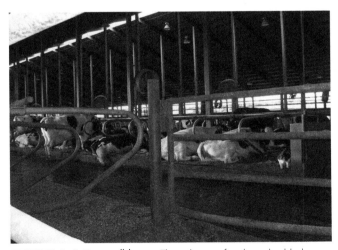

FIGURE 1-8 Free stall barns. These barns often have bedded areas where the cows can lie down. This dairy actually has water beds for the cows to lie on.

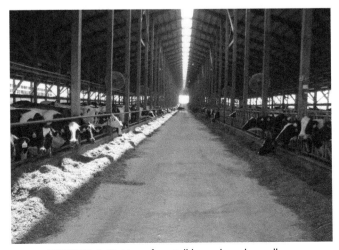

FIGURE 1-9 Many free stall barns have long alleys.

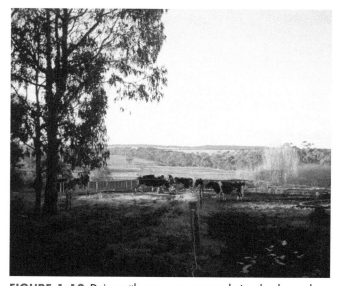

FIGURE 1-10 Dairy cattle graze on pasture during the day and are brought to the parlor for milking. This picture is of a dairy in Timboon, Victoria, Australia.

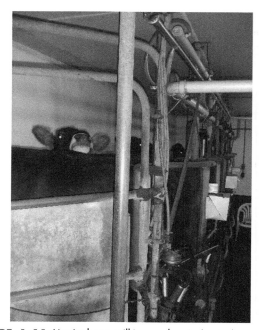

FIGURE 1-11 Herringbone milking parlor. In herringbone milking parlor, each cow stands at an angle to the pit, like the fingers on a herringbone necklace. (Courtesy Zeisler Dairy, Butte, Nebraska.)

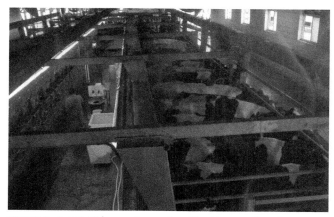

FIGURE 1-12 Side-opening parlors like this one allow the cows to stand parallel to each other.

lots or pastures and are brought inside only for milking in the parlor (Fig. 1-10).

THE PARLOR

The parlor is a separate area where the cows are milked. It usually has a pit where the producer stands during the milking process. The cows are above the producer, thus allowing easy access to the udder. There are four types of milking parlors:

- Herringbone
- Polygon
- Side opening
- Rotary or carousel

The most common milking parlor in use today is the herringbone (Fig. 1-11). Common sizes are 4 and 10. For example, a double-4 parlor holds 4 cows on each side. This allows for 8 cows to be milked at a time. Some herringbone parlors allow only individuals in and out. The cows stand at an angle to the pit. The cows enter and leave as groups. Polygon milking parlors are much like herringbones, but they have more than 2 sides.

Side-opening parlors are arranged so that cows stand parallel to each other (Fig. 1-12). These types of parlors can be designed in several ways. Side-opening parlors allow small groups to enter and exit.

Rotary milking parlors are arranged so that cows enter onto a turning platform that rotates slowly. The major advantage is that a large number of cows can be milked in a small space. Costs typically are high for this type of parlor, and usually two or more people are required to operate it. The cows are milked as they ride on the platform.

Dairies that use a parlor also have a holding pen. It is an area that is used to confine the cows before milking. Cows should not be left in the holding area for more than 2 hours because of stress, which can lead to decreased milk production.

THE MILKING UNIT

The milking unit is the piece of equipment that is applied to the cow's teats (Fig. 1-13). The *milking unit* consists of four parts: the *teat cup assembly,* the claw or suspension cup, connecting air, and milk tubes. The teat cup assembly is a steel shell with a liner that fits over the cow's teats. The liner is called an inflation. The inflation squeezes and relaxes on the teat, thereby causing milk to flow through the system. The claw or suspension cup connects the teat cup assembly to the connecting air tubes.

MILKING PROCEDURE

Each time the cows or heifers enter the barn, they undergo the same procedure. The teats of each cow or heifer are washed using chlorine or iodine. Obtaining milk from the udder should be done as cleanly as possible; you should milk

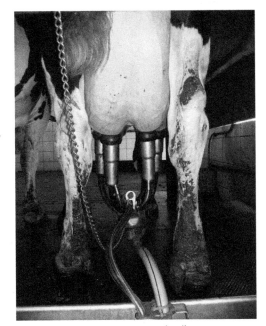

FIGURE 1-13 A typical milking unit.

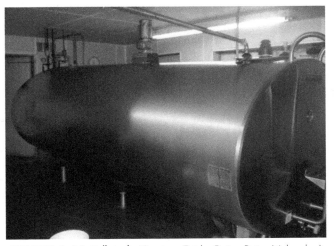

FIGURE 1-14 Bulk tank. (Courtesy Zeisler Dairy, Butte, Nebraska.)

only teats that are clean, dry, and free of dirt and debris. Your hands also should be clean and dry. Usually, only the teats are washed in preparation for milking because of the risk of causing mastitis by washing the entire udder before milking. If the entire udder is washed, the water and contaminants (e.g., caked feces, mud, urine) flow with gravity down the sides of the udder and off the teat ends. Each teat should then be towel dried with a paper towel.

> **TECHNICIAN NOTE** Do *not* wash the entire udder when preparing a cow or heifer for the milking procedure or for milk collection.

Two or three squirts of milk from each quarter are removed to stimulate milk letdown and evaluate the milk for abnormal qualities, such as those that occur with mastitis. During milking, the teat orifice *(streak canal)* must open, which provides a route for bacteria to ascend up into the mammary gland. This is the route by which virtually all septic mastitis occurs. Mastitis does not occur by seeding of the mammary gland through the blood, as is commonly believed. Because the teat orifice cannot be completely sterilized, it is important to keep contamination of the area around the orifice as low as possible, especially while the orifice is open.

> **TECHNICIAN NOTE** During the milking process, you should strip each teat and evaluate the milk for evidence of mastitis.

Milking should be done in a clean, dry, stress-free environment. Milk letdown requires the pituitary hormone oxytocin. Epinephrine, which is released as part of the

stress response, counteracts the effects of oxytocin. Loud noises, barking dogs, and unfamiliar personnel all may reduce milk letdown. One minute after milk letdown is stimulated, the milking unit should be attached. Once milking has decreased significantly or ceased, the milking unit can be removed. The vacuum to the claw should be shut off, and a finger can be used to break the seal by pushing on the top of the liner with your finger. Some milking units automatically drop off when the milk flow decreases to a set point. All four cups should be removed at once. The procedure should end with the post dip. Most often the post dip contains chlorine, iodine, chlorhexidine, or cetyl pyridine chloride. The post dip helps to keep the teats soft and is used to provide some residual germicidal action during this period when the teat orifice is open and susceptible to bacterial entry. The teat orifice closes gradually over 1 to 2 hours after the milking process, but newer research suggests it may take much longer than this for the orifice to close.

Cows that are sick, have mastitis, or have just freshened should be milked separately from the cows that are producing milk for sale. Cows with these conditions may have higher levels of somatic cells that can affect milk profitability as well as the quality of the milk.

THE BULK TANK

Once the cows are milked, the milk travels to the milk house, where the milk is cooled, filtered, and stored. This is often the location of the bulk tank. A bulk tank is a large stainless steel tank where milk is cooled and stored (Fig. 1-14).

THE LACTATION CYCLE

The dairy cycle is the same for both the goat and the cow. The cycle consists of four phases: phase one, phase two, phase three, and phase four, also known as the dry phase (Fig. 1-15).

Phase One/Freshening

The lactation cycle begins with phase one. It starts with *freshening* ("calving" or "kidding"), depending on the species. Parturition triggers milk production. Milk production levels

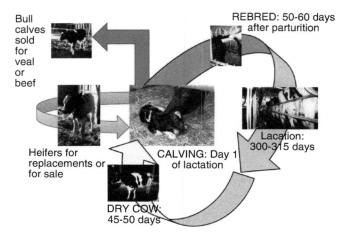

FIGURE 1-15 The dairy cycle.

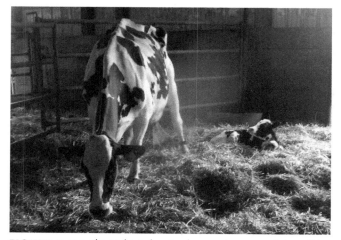

FIGURE 1-16 This Holstein has just begun phase one of the milking phase with the birth of her new calf.

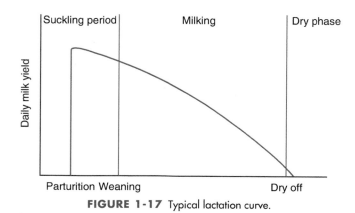

FIGURE 1-17 Typical lactation curve.

climb rapidly. The butterfat level of the milk produced starts out high and then decreases. The female's feed intake increases but lags behind the high demand for rapidly increasing milk production. This often leads to a decrease in body weight during this time. Metabolic and infectious diseases are common during this stage of milk production. Some of the diseases commonly seen during this stage of lactation include milk fever, left and right displaced abomasums, ketosis, metritis, mastitis, and retained placentas. Phase one lasts 10 to 12 weeks and ends when the female reaches peak milk production. Cows typically are rebred around 50 to 60 days after calving, which ensures a 12- to 13-month *calving interval.* A large percentage of dairy cattle will be bred using *artificial insemination.*

After parturition, the calf or kid is removed from the female within a few hours (Fig. 1-16). This helps shorten the adjustment period when the calf or kid is removed. Calves or kids are bottle-fed colostrum for a few days and are then transitioned to *milk replacer.* Most bull calves (male calves) can be sold for meat production. Heifer calves (female calves) also can be sold for meat production, or they can be retained as replacement heifers, which will enter their own

lactation cycle around the age of 3 years. Goats follow a similar pattern.

Phase Two

Reaching peak milk production signifies the change from phase one to phase two. Phase two includes weeks 12 to 24 of lactation. The cow's feed intake can now match her production levels, and she will begin to regain some of her weight and perhaps surpass her calving weight. The goal of phase two is to maintain peak milk production levels for as long as possible, thus allowing for increased profits. Figure 1-17 shows a typical lactation curve for a dairy cow. The graph represents important reference points during the lactation cycle and how milk production typically correlates with them.

Phase Three

Phase three of milk production is characteristic of a gradual decline in milk production that lasts from week 24 of the lactation cycle to dry off (when milking is stopped). This is the longest phase of milk production. The cow's dry matter consumption decreases as her milk production declines.

Phase Four

Phase four of milk production, also known as the dry phase, consists of the last 6 to 8 weeks before parturition. It is an important phase of the milk cycle because many management decisions influence the next lactation cycle. Females typically need to be dry for a period of 45 to 60 days. During the dry period, females should be provided good nutrition, which will ensure proper body score condition before calving or kidding.

> **TECHNICIAN NOTE**   Proper body score conditions during phase four can help prevent disease in phase one of the following lactation cycle.

Three management practices can be used to stop lactation. Producers can just stop milking, they can not milk out the cow thoroughly, or they can milk every other day. When the cow enters the dry phase, producers should perform a preventive treatment for mastitis, which includes a dry cow mastitis treatment and a teat dip. The udder should be observed closely for abnormal swelling for a period of 2 to 3 weeks.

All females will not follow this exact protocol and will have varied days of lactation. When producers compare records from different females, they adjust all the female records to a 305-day lactation cycle, with 45 to 60 days in the dry phase. Reasons for standardizing records to compare females include the following: (1) variability in how many times per day a female was milked, which can vary from farm to farm; (2) the time of the year the cows calved (cows tend to produce less milk when they calve in the summer); and (3) the usually lower milk production of first-calf heifers compared with mature cows. The adjusted records can be used to determine when a cow/doe should be culled from the herd or the type of genetic improvements for which producers may want to select.

Cows typically produce 6 to 7 gallons of milk per day. When you take into account the lactation cycle, it results on average in 2305 gallons per cow per year or approximately 19,825 pounds of milk per year. One gallon of milk weighs about 8.6 pounds. Goats typically produce on average 1853 pounds of milk per year; this is around 281 gallons per year or 1 to 2 gallons of milk per day. In most dairies, not all females freshen at the same time. By dividing the herd into groups that will freshen around the same time, producers can spread income and resources throughout the year.

MILK PROCESSING

Most of the milk that is being sold enters the processing plant. Milk undergoes a four-step process before it is sold to the consumer. First, the milk goes through a tri-process separator, which separates, standardizes, and clarifies the milk through centrifugal force. Then the milk is pasteurized. Pasteurization is a process of promptly heating and cooling the milk to remove bacteria without influencing the flavor or nutritional value of the milk. After pasteurization, the milk is homogenized to break down the fat globules, thus preventing creaming. Finally, the milk can be fortified, for example, by adding vitamins. There has been much talk about the consumption of raw milk. Many diseases can be transmitted to people through the consumption of raw milk, and as a technician you may be asked about raw milk consumption.

PRODUCTS

The most common animal associated with milk production is the cow. However, goats and, more recently, sheep also produce milk for human consumption. The United States produces more than $21 billion in milk each year. About 86% of the milk is sold through farmer milk marketing cooperatives. The rest is sold to private firms, used on the farm, or sold directly to consumers.

Milk products that are produced from bovine origin can be classified into two categories: grade A and grade B. Of the milk marketed in the United States, 96% is processed for use in fluid products, cheese, butter, and frozen dairy products. Grade A milk is produced on farms that have met certified standards. These standards exist through the Grade "A" Pasteurized Milk Ordinance developed by the Public Health Service. The ordinance is recognized as the national standard for milk production. The following regulations apply to grade A milk production.

- Raw milk must be cooled to 45° F or less within 2 hours after milking.
- The blended temperature after subsequent milking should not exceed 50° F.
- Milk cannot exceed a bacterial count of 100,000 per milliliter before it is mixed with milk from other producers.
- After the milk from several producers has been mixed together, the bacterial count cannot exceed 300,000 per milliliter before it is pasteurized.
- Milk cannot exceed 750,000 somatic cells per milliliter.
- No antibiotics must be detectable in the milk.

Grade A milk products are milk products eligible for fluid use. Products include whole milk (3.25% milk fat), low-fat milk (0.5% to 2.0% milk fat), skim milk (<0.5% milk fat), coffee cream, whipping cream, half and half, and sour cream. Approximately 36% of the milk produced in the United States is used for fluid milk consumption.

Grade B milk, also known as manufacturing milk, is produced under conditions that are less strict than those established for grade A milk production. Grade B products must meet standards found in the "Milk for Manufacturing Purposes and its Production and Processing, Recommended Requirements" from the USDA. Some of the most important standards include the following:

- Bacterial count less than 500,000 per milliliter
- Somatic cell counts less than 750,000 per milliliter
- No drug residues present in the milk

Grade B products can be mixed with surpluses of grade A products to produce cheese, butter, and powdered milk. Approximately 30% of the milk produced is used to make cheese; 20% of the milk sold in the United States is used for production of butter; 10% is used for frozen products such as ice cream and sherbet; and approximately 4% is used for production of evaporated and condensed milk, evaporated and condensed buttermilk, dried whole milk, dry skim milk, dry cream, dry whey, lactose, and yogurt. When milk is priced, it is classified into four groups. Class I is used for liquid milk consumption, flavored milk, and eggnog. Class II is used for ice cream, yogurt, cottage cheese, and cream. Class III is used for most cheeses. Class IV is used for butter and any milk product that is dried.

TRENDS

Grade A milk usually is priced higher than grade B milk. This is one reason for the shift in production within the United States from grade B to grade A production. For every dollar invested into a dairy, return usually is between 6% and 9%; however, a large investment is needed to begin a dairy operation.

Yearly trends in the dairy industry include milk product consumption peaking in May and being the lowest in November, with fluid milk consumption at its lowest level in June. The price for milk also varies throughout the year, with the highest prices in October, November, and December. The lowest prices are paid in May and June.

The common trend in milk and milk product consumption over the past few years has shown a gradual decline. Cheese is the only product that has shown a steady increase in per capita consumption. The trend most likely reflects the use of substitute products such as margarine.

The location of dairy production within the United States has also shifted. The major production of dairy products used to be in the Midwest, but this has shifted to the Southwest. Reasons for the shift include a large population base. Milk produced in highly populated areas has lower shipping costs. The climate is favorable, allowing the cows to remain in their *thermal neutral zone* (TNZ). Cattle can use energy that would have been used for maintaining body temperature to increase production. The Southwest typically has more favorable attitudes toward economic growth, although some shift in the industry back to the Midwest has occurred because of the inability to meet environmental regulations. Control of runoff manure is a major concern. Proper handling of manure requires large areas of land that are not available in the Southwest because of the population density but are available in the Midwest.

Dairy products are not an important import or export market for the United States; less than 2% of dairy product is imported, and only approximately 1% is exported.

THE BEEF INDUSTRY

Figure 1-18 shows the typical movement of cattle through the beef industry. The beef industry is generally divided into four production systems: seed stock or purebred breeders, cow/calf producers, stocker feeders, and feedlots. Although the lines can be blurred and often are, if you have a general understanding of this particular system you will be able to understand the majority of industry practices.

SEED STOCK PRODUCERS

Seed stock producers or purebred breeders raise cattle for sale to cow/calf producers or other seed stock producers. The cattle raised are used as replacement heifers or bulls to improve genetics within the commercial cow/calf herd. Seed stock producers are largely responsible for genetic advancement within the beef industry. Many of these producers are involved in showing calves and may have a history of traveling or have special requirements. The yearly cycle for a seed stock producer is similar to that of a cow/calf producer.

COW/CALF PRODUCERS

Cow/calf producers raise calves for sale to feedlots. Producers breed cows and heifers to produce calves that can be sold into feedlots. These types of production systems are often found in areas of the United States where land cannot be used for crop production. Most cow/calf producers are located in the western range states and the upper Great Plains (Fig. 1-19). Most cows and heifers are bred to calve in the spring, but fall calving does take place in the United States. Calves born in the spring are weaned in the fall. Calves that are sold in the fall are sold as feeder calves. These calves enter a feedlot or become stocker feeders.

Calves are sold per pound or price per hundred pounds.

> **TECHNICIAN NOTE** Calves are sold per pound or price per hundred pounds.

The USDA uses cattle grading to report market prices for feeder calves. The grading system is intended for use in cattle younger than 36 months but can be used to describe stock cows for market reporting purposes. Factors that are used to determine grades of feeder calves include thriftiness, frame size, and thickness. There are 10 grades of feeder calves. These grades use a combination of frame score and thickness to classify the calves. Frame scores are large, medium, and small. Numbers that correlate with muscle mass run from 1 to 3. Number 1 classification is the thickest, has the heaviest muscle, and the highest proportion of beef breeding. Number 3 has the least amount of these traits.

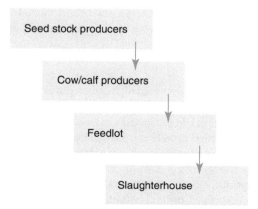

FIGURE 1-18 The flow of cattle though the beef industry.

Seed stock producers
↓
Cow/calf producers
↓
Feedlot
↓
Slaughterhouse

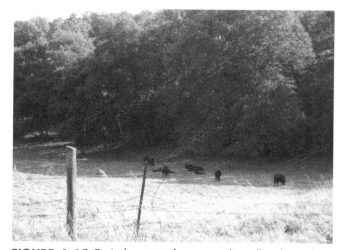

FIGURE 1-19 Typical pastures have natural windbreaks, such as trees, or human-made windbreaks, such as fences.

STOCKER FEEDERS

Calves may go directly to the feedlot. However, some producers choose to take lighter-weight calves and put them in a stocker feeder program. Stocker feeders are producers who take the calves and place them on a high-roughage diet through the winter. This practice, known as *backgrounding,* is an intermediate stage that is sometimes used in cattle production and begins after weaning and ends upon placement in a feedlot. These calves are sold around 1 year of age and are referred to as yearling feeders when they finally enter the feedlot.

Ownership during this phase of production may be retained by the cow/calf producer, or ownership may change.

FEEDLOTS

The feedlot is the last stage of meat production before harvest. Calves may enter the feedlot directly from the cow/calf producer or from stocker feeders. Some cow/calf producers have contracts with feedlots, so the calves are purchased directly from the cow/calf producer. Other calves are purchased at livestock auctions. Several feedlot owners will contract with order buyers or employ a buyer. Order buyers are people who travel to auctions in an effort to find calves that meet the requirements of feedlot owners. The order buyer purchases these calves for the feedlot producers.

There are two types of feedlots: commercial producers and farmer feeders. Commercial producers have the capability to raise 1000 or more head of cattle. Most often, the feeds are purchased rather than grown by the producers. Farmer feeders are producers who raise fewer than 1000 head. These producers often use feeds they have grown as a crop. Producers do this in hopes the cattle will pay out more than if the grain had just been marketed at harvest.

There also two types of feeding systems: intermediate finishing and deferred finishing. Intermediate finishing involves purchasing feeder calves and immediately transitioning them to a high-concentrate diet with small amounts of roughage. This produces a quicker finish than deferred finishing. Steer calves are fed for approximately 275 days and heifer calves for approximately 230 days. This system is used because steer calves gain weight 10% faster than heifers and are 10% to 15% more efficient in converting feed to gain. If yearling calves are purchased and immediately finished, the process for steers takes approximately 275 days and for heifers approximately 30 days. This system works well for heavier-weight calves. Calves typically are fed for a period of 4 to 7 months and are then marketed to the slaughterhouse. Because most of the cows in the United States calve in the spring and are weaned in the fall, feeder calves enter the feedlot from October to November and leave in April or May.

Deferred finishing is effective for lighter-weight calves, which are purchased in the fall or are fed roughage through the winter. These calves are essentially the same as stocker feeders, except ownership does not change when they are placed on a finishing ration. Some feedlots place calves in a finishing program in the spring, with the calves finishing 120 to 150 days later. Others feed calves on *pasture* through the summer for 90 to 120 days and then finish them in the feedlot during the fall for about 90 to 120 days.

Throughout the beef production process, cattle most commonly are marketed by the pound. However, cattle can be marketed on a *grid.* Purchasing cattle on a grid is a system of selling cattle based on their attributes or lack of attributes. It takes into account not only weight but also other factors such as quality grade and yield grade. The feedlot producers want to produce cattle with a live weight of 1000 to 1250 pounds for steers and 900 to 1050 pounds for heifers and prefer the cattle grade "choice." Because of the quality of meat, the ability to gain weight, and the behavior of cattle, the beef industry severely discourages certain types of cattle; this includes bulls. Most packinghouses dock producers for sending a pregnant heifer to market.

Packinghouses use slaughter grades to certify cattle sold on contract and report pricing. Classification can be accomplished through *quality grade* and *yield grade.* Quality grades are based on the amount and distribution of finish on the animal, the fullness and firmness of muscling, and maturity. The quality grades for slaughter cattle are prime, choice, select, standard, commercial, utility, cutter, and canner.

The yield grade is influenced by carcass weight, rib eye area, thickness of fat over the rib eye area, and amount of kidney, pelvic, and heart fat. Yield grades are 1, 2, 3, 4, and 5. Yield grade 5 includes animals with the highest level of fat coverage.

BEEF HOUSING AND EQUIPMENT

Seed stock producers and cow/calf producers often use similar types of housing for their cattle. These types of operations require the least amount of housing. Cows often are maintained on pasture from spring through fall. During the winter months, cows can be kept on pastures as well, with minimal housing. Shelter during the winter can include windbreaks, loafing sheds, or natural shelters such as trees. Cows are often moved into dry lots or smaller pastures during the calving seasons for closer observation. During calving, open-front calving barns can be used to provide shelter. Producers should make sure that they have separate areas for weaned calves, bulls, heifers, and cows. Types of feeding systems used include the pasture itself, hay bale feeders, feed bunks, portable feed bunks, and *creep feeders.* Creep feeders are used to feed calves before weaning without having to worry about adult cows gaining access to the feed.

Feedlot housing often uses a dry lot. The three types of dry lot housing are feeding barn and lot (Fig. 1-20), open barn

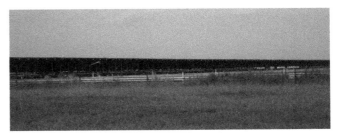

FIGURE 1-20 Feeding barn and lot.

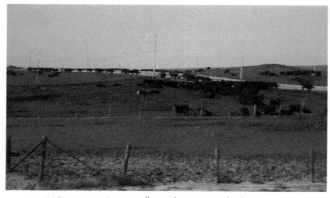

FIGURE 1-21 Feedlot with an open dry lot system.

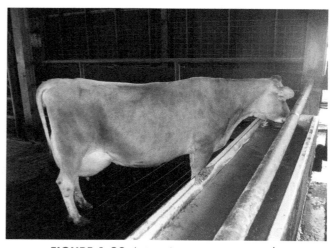

FIGURE 1-23 Automatic concrete water trough.

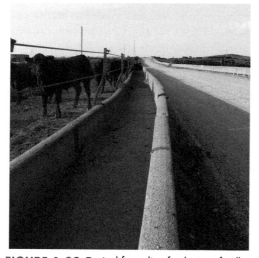

FIGURE 1-22 Typical fence line feeder in a feedlot.

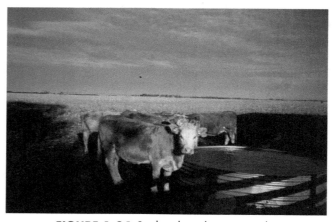

FIGURE 1-24 Stock tank used to water cattle.

and dry lot, and open dry lot (Fig. 1-21). The difference between the feeding barn and lot and the open barn and dry lot is the location of the feeding. In the feeding barn and dry lot system, cattle are fed inside the barn. In the open barn and dry lot system, cattle are fed using fence line feeders (Fig. 1-22). The open dry lot system does not use a barn but does use windbreaks or natural shelters.

Use of confinement housing within the commercial feedlot industry has increased. Two types of confinement housing are used in the feedlot industry: cold and warm confinement barns. Cold confinement barns have the same temperature as the outside environment. Warm confinement barns are insulated and warmer than the outside temperature during the winter. However, research has shown no increases in production that substantiate the use of these types of systems.

Watering systems for cattle often include automatic water troughs, concrete water troughs (Fig. 1-23), and water tanks (Fig. 1-24).

Fresh water should always be offered and should not be allowed to freeze during the winter months. To prevent water troughs from freezing, a continuous flow of water or heated or frost-free hydrants can be used.

Other types of equipment include sunshades, mineral feeders, and back rubbers used to treat parasites. Another valuable tool is an autogate, which consists of metal poles anchored into the ground with a large pit underneath. Most cattle will not cross over these poles, but they allow the producer to drive across. If a traditional gate were used, the driver would need to get out of the vehicle to open the gate.

TRENDS

Trends in the beef industry include fewer small operations and larger commercial operations. This trend likely is the result of the lower unit production costs, increased use of contracts, and retained ownership of cattle through the finishing process. Most of the large commercial cattle feedlots are located in Texas, Kansas, Nebraska, and Oklahoma.

THE PORK INDUSTRY

The four types of pork production systems are *farrowing*, growing or nursery, finishing, and farrow to finish, in which all phases of production are accomplished on one farm. Some farms are farrow to finish, in which the entire operation is

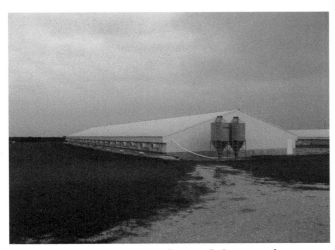

FIGURE 1-25 Environmentally controlled swine confinement.

performed within one or just a few buildings. Other producers work with only one level of production or with a combination of levels and have one or several buildings. The farrowing operation involves breeding, gestation, and farrowing. Sows or gilts raised on the farrowing operation are bred, maintained through gestation, and farrowed out. Piglets are born weighing 3 to 4 pounds and are weaned from the mother at 3 to 8 weeks of age. The piglets often weigh approximately 10 to 25 pounds at weaning.

Piglets are often sold or moved on contract to the growing or nursery facility. Piglets remain in the nursery for approximately 4 to 10 weeks. When they reach 40 to 60 pounds, they are moved to the finishing facility, where they are fed out until they reach market weight of approximately 220 to 260 pounds. Pigs gain an average of 1.4 to 1.8 pounds per day. With these high average daily gains, the time from breeding to market is approximately 9 to 10 months. Time from farrowing until market usually is 5 to 6 months.

Most pigs are marketed by directly selling them to the processor, although some still are marketed through live auction. Some pigs are sold on the basis of weight. Some hogs sold directly to the processor are sold on carcass merit, which means that premium prices are paid for pigs with low amounts of fat and high amounts of muscle. The USDA has established a grading system for swine. The system is based on carcass quality and yield of four lean cuts: ham, loin, picnic shoulder, and Boston butt. Barrows and gilts are graded as U.S. number 1, U.S. number 2, U.S. number 3, U.S. number 4, and U.S. utility. Slaughter sow grades are U.S. number 1, U.S. number 2, U.S. number 3, medium, and cull. Feeder pigs are graded as U.S. number 1, U.S. number 2, U.S. number 3, U.S. number 4, U.S. utility, and U.S. cull.

PORK HOUSING AND EQUIPMENT

The kinds of swine facilities have changed significantly over the years. In the 1970s, swine commonly were housed on pastures or in dry lots. In today's industry, most swine are raised in confinement (Fig. 1-25). The shift in swine housing is the result of several factors, the most significant being more

commercial swine producers and fewer small farm operations. Other factors include more specialization within the stages of swine production, reduced labor requirements, and better control of the macroenvironment, including temperature and humidity, which creates fewer stresses on the animal and allows it to remain in its TNZ. Another aspect of confinement rearing is the ability to provide animals with a cleaner environment in which to live. Sanitation of these types of housing is extremely important in preventing disease.

> **TECHNICIAN NOTE** Most swine in the United States are raised in confinement housing.

Many of the confinement-type housing units are now operated as all-in/all-out facilities. This means that all the animals that enter the confinement together must leave together. This is a great strategy for minimizing disease spread. Another aspect of preventing disease transmission in these types of housing systems is the shower-in/shower-out practice. This type of protocol requires workers, veterinarians, salespersons, and anyone else entering the facility to take a shower and dress in clothing provided by the producer before they enter the facility. This approach decreases the risk that people could serve as fomites for diseases. Before exiting the facility, the opposite occurs; visitors are asked to remove the clothing provided and shower again before leaving the facility. This allows the facility to remain as closed as possible, thus preventing the spread of disease.

Gestation housing can be performed on a pasture or in confinement. Sows and gilts kept in confinement are often kept in gestation crates. Sows and gilts remain in the crates 24 hours per day until about a week before farrowing, when they are moved into the farrowing facility. In 2007, several states banned the use of gestation crates in response to concern from animal rights activists. Other forms of housing during gestation that are used now include free access gestation stalls, which are similar to free stall housing in the dairy industry, and group pen housing. Most pigs are kept in climate-controlled houses. During farrowing, the sow or gilt is kept in a crate to prevent her from injuring the piglets when she lies down. Death by crushing is one of the most common causes of death in newborn piglets. Good producers make quite an effort to provide an environment that is clean, dry, and comfortable for both the sow or gilt and the piglets. Before farrowing, sows and gilts are commonly kept in gestation crates.

Once sows and gilts are close to farrowing, they are moved into the farrowing house. Most farrowing houses are confinement based because of the warmer temperatures needed by piglets. These facilities should be warm, draft free, and dry. Farrowing usually is performed in crates or pens (Fig. 1-26). If pens are used, producers should not house more than three sows together and must provide a pig brooder. A pig brooder is an area of the pen, often the corner, that allows the piglets an area to lie down under a heat lamp, away from the

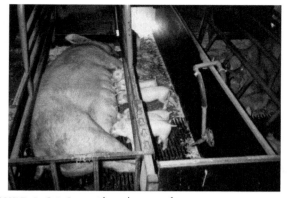

FIGURE 1-26 Sow with piglets in a farrowing crate. (Courtesy D. Chennells. From Jackson PGG, Cockcroft PD: *Handbook of pig medicine*, St. Louis, 2007, Saunders.)

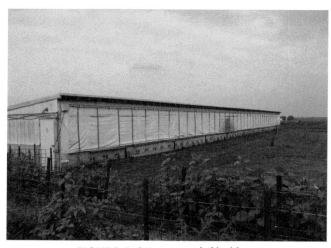

FIGURE 1-27 Apron-sided building.

mother. In a farrowing, crate areas flanking the crate are kept at higher temperatures to maintain the appropriate TNZ for the piglets.

After the piglets are weaned, they are moved into a nursery. Nurseries should be kept clean and dry to help prevent disease. After weaning, the pigs weigh 40 to 60 pounds and are placed together with pigs of similar age, size, and sex. The animals drink from automatic waterers that ensure a constant supply of clean water. Feed is supplied from automatic feeders into J-feeders, where the animals obtain all the feed they want. Housing from nursery to finishing is similar, except for adjusting space requirements as the pigs grow or reducing the number of pigs per pen.

Each of these housing systems can include solid floors, partially slatted floors, and slatted floors. Solid floors require more labor for cleaning. Slatted floors are more labor friendly and use a liquid manure system.

Although pigs are not commonly housed on dirt in today's industry, some producers use this method of housing. One of the common misconceptions about pigs is that they are dirty. The basis of this misconception comes from a pig's desire to wallow in the mud. Pigs perform this behavior because it helps keep them cool in hot weather and also helps keep parasites off them. Pigs actually are clean if given the room; pigs will use only a certain part of their pens to drop wastes and will keep the rest of their area clean.

Maintaining the appropriate temperature within swine facilities is important for health and production. In confinement housing, producers use heaters to increase the temperature of hog confinements. During the summer when producers need to cool swine, they can use ventilation and sprinkler systems.

Ventilation is also extremely important for the health and productivity of swine. Some facilities use fans, open-front buildings, and apron-sided buildings (Fig. 1-27). Ventilation is important in the winter for controlling moisture and odor and in the summer for temperature control. Ventilation is always necessary to control the level of toxic gases and odors produced from manure.

Waste management is an important aspect of livestock production. To dispose of manure and odor, waste from finishing pens is flushed into ponds called lagoons. In the lagoons, bacteria help break down the waste materials into a slurry, which does not have as bad an odor as untreated manure.

The waste material is periodically pumped from the lagoons and is spread on pastures or cropland as fertilizer. The lagoon content provides a means of disposing of the manure but also supplies a high-quality, organic fertilizer for crops.

TRENDS

Trends within the swine industry include movement from small farming operations to commercial contracts and vertical integration. In vertical integration, the company that produces the animal also owns the packing plant that slaughters the animal for market. Other trends in the industry include multiyear marketing. In multiyear marketing, a producer contracts with a packer to deliver a specific number of hogs to the plant each year. The hogs usually are required to be of certain quality, and producers receive a premium for the higher quality. This type of marketing provides the producer with a place to market the hogs, as well as a reward for the higher quality, and the packer is guaranteed a supply of pork.

THE MUTTON/CHEVRON INDUSTRY

Four systems of raising sheep are used in the United States: fall lambs, early spring lambs, late spring lambs, and accelerated lambing. Some of the lambs born from the systems may enter a feedlot.

Fall lambs are born before December 25. This system must use a breed of sheep that breeds out of season. Some of those breeds include Rambouillet, Merino, Dorset, Corridedale, and Tunis. These lambs are marketed from early spring to June. The lambs usually weigh between 35 and 60 pounds. In some areas, lambs are sold at 50 to 90 days of age. These lambs, called hothouse lambs, are sold into a specialty market popular in New York City and Boston. Another specialty market for these lambs is Easter lambs, which enter this market weighing between 20 and 40 pounds.

Early spring lambs are born in January and February. The lambs are marketed before the end of June, with better prices expected during this time of year. Breeding in this system usually takes place by August 1. Because of the time of year, good housing for the lambs and a good parasite control program are recommended.

Late spring lambs are born in March, April, and May. Most lambs are fed roughage before they are marketed; the system requires few concentrates. This system allows producers to place lambs on the feeder lamb market if they prefer to finish them. This type of system requires a high-quality parasite control program. Lambs often are worth less at finish as a result of seasonal price changes.

Accelerated lambing is a system that produces three lamb crops in 2 years. This system also requires the use of breeds that breed out of season. The lambs often are finished in a feedlot system and are weaned early. This system requires increased breeding management and labor. Feedlot lambs are purchased at weaning and can be grazed or fed in a feedlot until finished.

MUTTON/CHEVRON HOUSING AND EQUIPMENT

Expensive housing for sheep is not necessary. Most often, pasture and lambing barns are used. This type of system is similar to that used by cow/calf producers. Some producers do use confinement housing for sheep; however, the economics of this practice have not yet been proven. Predators tend to be the biggest challenge associated with sheep housing. Predator prevention can include the use of guard animals such as dogs or llamas.

THE PACKINGHOUSE

The slaughter process consists of eight generalized steps: stunning, hoisting, sticking, skinning, dressing-halving, cooling, grading, and aging. Stunning refers to the act of rendering the animal unconscious. Several methods are used, the most common being a captive bolt gun. The captive bolt gun operates by projecting a metal cylinder into the frontal lobe of the brain. An animal with a destroyed frontal lobe of the brain no longer has any conscious nervous activity. Other methods include carbon dioxide and electrical shock.

The animal is hoisted by the back legs to a rail system; then the jugular veins and carotid arteries are severed. Sticking is performed at this point in the slaughter process to ensure good blood drainage from the quality meat cuts over the loin of the animal. Blood drainage is necessary for consumer acceptance. It ensures the proper meat coloration expected by the consumer. The carcass is then dehaired and the hide is removed. The carcass is eviscerated, by removing all of the internal organs for inspection. The carcass is cut in halfway down the spinal column; then it is cooled, graded, and aged.

THE FIBER INDUSTRY

The fiber industry includes animals raised for fiber, although in the United States these animals are often also used for meat production, except for llamas and alpaca. Animals are often raised on pasture with little labor or expense, other than nutrition and medical attention.

WOOL

Wool production in the United States has gradually declined, although sheep production has remained steady since 2004. The decline in sheep production can be attributed to low wool prices resulting from the manufacture of synthetic fibers. In the United States, wool production is considered a by-product of the sheep industry, with less emphasis placed on wool production and more emphasis placed on meat production. Much of the wool produced in the United States is of lower quality than wool produced in other countries. Wool produced in the United States commonly is urine stained or contains vegetable residue. These characteristics lower the value of the wool. It is important to market the wool properly rolled (flesh side out), tied (paper twine only), and stored in a dry place. Wool should never be stored in plastic bags. Wool from different ages of sheep and of different colors should be separated.

The value of wool depends on the grade of wool and the amount of clean wool that can be produced from grease wool (wool before it has been cleaned). Grades are based mainly on the diameter, length, and density of the fiber.

The three systems of grading wool currently used are the micron system, the numerical count (USDA system), and the American system. The micron system is used internationally and measures the diameter of the wool fiber. The USDA system has 16 grades. Each grade equates with the number of hanks (1 hank is 560 yards long) of yarn that can be spun from 1 pound of wool top. Wool top is wool that has been partially processed. The American system has 7 grades. Wool is placed into a grade based on the diameter of the fiber.

Wool also can be classified by its use within the fiber industry. Apparel wool is used to make cloth. It is subdivided into two categories: worsted and woolen classes. Longer fibers are used to produce strong yarn and are classified as worsted. Shorter fibers are used for weaker yarn and are classified as woolen. Carpet wool is used for making carpets. Carpet wool is coarser than apparel wool.

After wool and mohair are sheared and graded, they are marketed through wool pools, warehouse operators, or cooperatives, or they are sold directly to wool mills. Wool prices vary throughout the year. The highest price for wool typically is seen in May, although prices remain high from May to July and peak again in October. The lowest prices are seen in January, February, August, September, November, and December.

Sheep typically are sheared in early spring and, if accelerated lambing is used, again in late summer. Most of the shearing is performed by custom shearers.

MOHAIR

Goat fiber, called mohair, can be marketed. More than 95% of the mohair in the United States is produced in Texas. Mohair can be sold by the pound, sold by the clip (the fiber produced from one shearing), or marketed through a grading system. The grading system for mohair is similar to that of sheep wool. The fibers are graded on fineness. Kids produce the finest fiber, and bucks and old weathers (castrated male goats) produce the coarsest fiber.

LLAMA AND ALPACA FIBER

Llamas typically are sheared annually. Llamas have a dual-fiber coat; they have a fine covering, but it is intermingled with long guard hairs. These long, stiff guard fibers can be left in if the wool is going to be used for carpet or rugs, but they must be removed before knitting or weaving with the fiber. Alpacas also are sheared annually. They produce between 5 and 8 pounds of fleece per year. The fiber is often used in the production of fine textiles. Llama and alpaca fibers do not contain lanolin, so they do not have to be processed before use.

FIBER PROCESSING

Wool processing consists of washing (scouring) the wool to remove grease (unrefined lanolin), vegetable matter, and other impurities. The fibers are squeezed and dried. Then the wool is blended. Several batches of the wool are mixed together to unify the fiber. Carding can be performed, in which the wool is rolled into narrow ropes or strands of fiber called *slivers*. Wool that is coarse or has a short fiber length can be twisted into a ball. This process is called "roving," and the fiber is sold as wool or yarn. Spinning machines twist the roving into yarns of a wide variety of qualities, including strength, firmness, size, and ply. If fabric is being made, the yarn is woven or knitted into a fabric. Quality control tests are performed, and any chemical finishes are applied. Dyeing of the fibers can be done at any stage of the fiber production process.

FIBER HOUSING AND EQUIPMENT

Housing for animals raised for fiber is similar to the housing used by cow/calf producers and that used for sheep and goat meat production.

THE HORSE INDUSTRY

The horse industry primarily centers on the use of horses as recreational pets. Horses are kept for personal use or as backyard pets, purely for personal enjoyment. Horses also are kept for performance events. These horses are used for performing in rodeos, western shows, and English shows.

An entire textbook could be written just on the different types of performance events in which horses are used. The industry is complex, and it is important for veterinary technicians to understand that horses have a wide range of jobs and levels at which they are asked to perform. For veterinary technicians who have an interest in working in practices with a high equine patient load, it would be wise to become familiar with these events and the types of movements these horses encounter. This knowledge will better help you to perform the basic physical and lameness examinations, as well as to take histories and communicate with your clients.

HORSE HOUSING AND EQUIPMENT

Horses can be kept in a variety of housing types, such as stalls, dry lots, and pasture. They can give birth in any of these situations. Horse housing and equipment are discussed under hospital management in Chapter 5.

CASE STUDY

Dr. Cooper, the doctor you are currently working for, is called out on a farm call to evaluate Mrs. Kettler's nonambulatory cow. When the doctor arrives, he diagnoses the cow with a broken leg. The doctor gives Mrs. Kettler an estimated cost for the fracture repair. He estimates the cost to be $2000. In the current economic market, the cow/calf producer knows the estimated value of the cow is $800. What decision do you think the cow/calf operator will make?

CASE STUDY

Feedlot owner Mr. Holtgrew has made an appointment for his 1250-pound steer, which is coughing and has nasal discharge. When Dr. Brunssen arrives at the farm, she diagnoses the steer with a bacterial respiratory infection. The veterinarian is going to prescribe antibiotics. What consideration for the patient should the veterinarian make in her choice of antibiotic?

SUGGESTED READING

Campbell JR, Kenealy MD, Campbell KL: *Animal sciences: the biology care and production of domestic animals*, ed 4, New York, 2003, McGraw-Hill.

Gillespie JR, Flanders FB: *Modern livestock and poultry*, ed 8, Clifton Park, NY, 2010, Delmar Cengage Learning.

Herren RV: *The science of animal agriculture*, ed 2, Albany, NY, 2006, Delmar Thomson Learning.

Senger PL: *Pathways to pregnancy and parturition*, ed 2, Pullman, Wash, 2005, Current Conceptions.

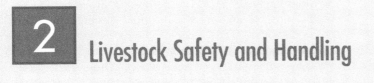

2 Livestock Safety and Handling

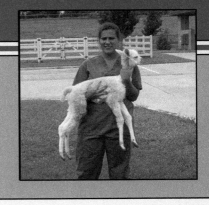

LEARNING OBJECTIVES

After reading this chapter, you will be able to

- Understand potential risks that exist with the practice of large animal veterinary medicine
- Tie multiple types of knots to ensure an effective set of tools for large animal restraint
- Understand the basic natural instincts of each large animal species
- Understand the importance of protecting yourself, veterinary personnel, and clients while handling patients
- Apply common methods of large animal restraint safely, efficiently, and effectively

KEY TERMS

Alleyway	Fetlock	Posting
Augers	Half hitch	Power takeoffs
Backstop	Halter	Restraint
Bight	Hanking	Squeeze
Biosecurity	Herd	Stanchions
Bovine	Hitches	Standing part of a rope
Bucks	Hog snare	Stocks
Bull	Hydraulics	Suspensory ligament
Calves	Knots	Tail gate
Camelid	Lead rope	Tail jack
Casting	Loop	Tailing
Cattle prod	Nose band	Throw
Chain shank	Nose lead	Tub
Chemical restraint	Nose ring	Twitches
Chestnut	Palpation gate	Whipping
Chute	Physical restraint	Working chute
Cria	Point of balance	
End of a rope	Poll	

KEY ABBREVIATIONS

OSHA: Occupational Safety and Health Administration
PTO: Power takeoff

SAFETY IN THE LARGE ANIMAL VETERINARY PRACTICE

Agriculture is one of the most dangerous occupations in the United States. Approximately 1,854,000 full-time workers were employed in production agriculture in the United States in 2012. In 2012, 374 farmers and farm workers died of a work-related injury, resulting in a fatality rate of 20.2 deaths per 100,000 workers. Tractor overturns were the leading cause of death for these farmers and farm workers. On average, 63 fatal injuries and 12,500 nonfatal injuries and illnesses in farmers and farm workers involve animals each year. Human error is a major reason for these accidents. Being tired, not paying attention, and using poor judgment are frequent causes of life-threatening accidents. The livestock themselves do not constitute the only area where safety precautions should be considered; chemical safety, environmental safety, animal disease, grain handling, building problems, and fire safety should also be considered.

Chemical safety is extremely important. Some of the drugs used in the livestock industry could cause a pregnant employee to abort after absorption of the drug through the skin. Some drugs can be fatal if they are injected accidentally into a human instead of the intended animal. Veterinary technicians should always read the labels of the chemicals or drugs they are handling. Technicians should store and handle the drugs according to the label or package insert. Veterinary technicians should follow Occupational Safety and Health Administration (OSHA) standards when working in any veterinary practice.

Environmental safety is important. Technicians should not handle livestock in unfavorable weather conditions without appropriate protection. Lightning and inclement weather can be deadly.

Wearing clothing appropriate for the weather is important. The proper attire can help prevent heat stroke. During warm weather, wearing lightweight, light-colored cotton is recommended. Khaki pants are lighter than denim pants, and they keep technicians cooler in extremely warm weather. Sweating in the warm weather can cause dehydration. Technicians should consume water periodically throughout the day to prevent dehydration. In cold weather, layers of clothes, long underwear, warm socks, a hat, insulated boots, and gloves are recommended. If you layer your clothes, you can always remove a layer if you become warm. Personnel who handle livestock should not wear jewelry.

TECHNICIAN NOTE Personnel who handle livestock should not wear jewelry.

Animal disease is another area of concern for technicians. Several diseases and parasites of the livestock industry have zoonotic potential. Precautions should be taken when there is a risk for exposure to these types of diseases. Disease prevention is important not only for zoonotic disease but also for *biosecurity* (Fig. 2-1). Technicians should wear masks, disposable gowns, disposable shoe covers, and disposable gloves and should use disinfectant footbaths to help prevent disease transmission.

Grain handling can be dangerous for the technician or producer. Avoid wearing loose clothing around *augers* and *power takeoffs (PTOs)*. People who drive grain/livestock trucks cannot see all areas around the semitruck and trailer and may not be able to see you (Fig. 2-2). The grain itself can be dangerous; when piled, it can develop air pockets that are almost impossible to get out of if a person falls into them.

Buildings with cement floors can become slick when wet and cause you to fall. If buildings are not maintained, jagged edges of metal or wood can cut veterinary personnel, producers, or livestock. Equipment can provide areas for damage to fingers and hands if they become caught between the metal and the animal.

Steps to prevent fire should be considered. Hay burns quickly when ignited and can destroy entire barns in minutes. Malfunctioning equipment as well as lightning and human error can be sources of fire.

ROPES

ROPE CARE

Ropes are valuable pieces of equipment in the large animal industry. Ropes can be used for *casting, halters,* and leg restraint.

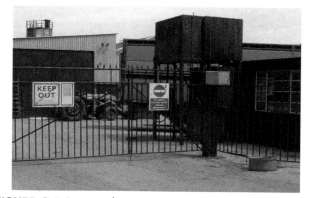

FIGURE 2-1 Perimeter fences and gates should be clearly signed. (From Jackson PGG, Cockcroft PD: *Handbook of pig medicine,* St. Louis, 2007, Saunders.)

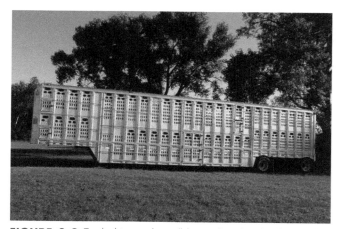

FIGURE 2-2 Truck drivers who pull livestock trailers (cattle pots) like this one have blind spots and may not see you. It is important to pay attention when you are working around any type of equipment. (Courtesy Holtgrew Farms and Trucking, Stuart, Nebraska.)

Ropes should be inspected before use. If the ropes are manufactured, such as *lead ropes,* the metal clasps should be inspected for rust and free-moving pieces. Ropes that are dirty or have kinks, stress points, tears, or frayed ends should be repaired or removed from use in the veterinary clinic. The four main ways to fix fraying at the *end of a rope* are (1) melting the end of the rope with fire (nylon ropes), (2) tying an overhand knot in the end of the rope, (3) coating the end of the rope with a stop-fray product, and (4) whipping (Fig. 2-3). Faulty ropes can cause serious injuries to veterinary personnel, clients, and the animals. Ropes should be cleaned with warm water. Detergent should not be used on a rope because it deteriorates the fibers and results in a weaker rope, thus shortening the life span of the rope.

> **TECHNICIAN NOTE** Ropes should be washed only in water; detergents shorten the life span of ropes.

WHIPPING

Whipping can be used to stop fraying at the end of a rope. You will need a smaller cord to wrap around the rope (Fig. 2-4, *A*). It is better to have more cord than not enough. Fold the cord in half. Lay the cord on the rope, with the connected end of the cord on the end of the rope (Fig. 2-4, *B*). Then, pick up one strand of the cord and pull it toward

the top of the rope so that the shorter end of the cord is approximately ½ inch longer than the area of fraying you would like to cover. While holding the cord in place, take the long end of the cord and wrap it around the short end of

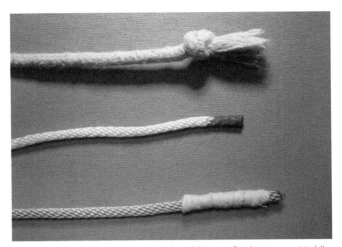

FIGURE 2-3 *Top,* Tying an overhand knot to finish a rope. *Middle,* Special coating to finish a rope. *Bottom,* Whipping. (From Sheldon CC, Sonsthagen T, Topel JA: *Animal restraint for veterinary professionals,* St. Louis, 2006, Mosby.)

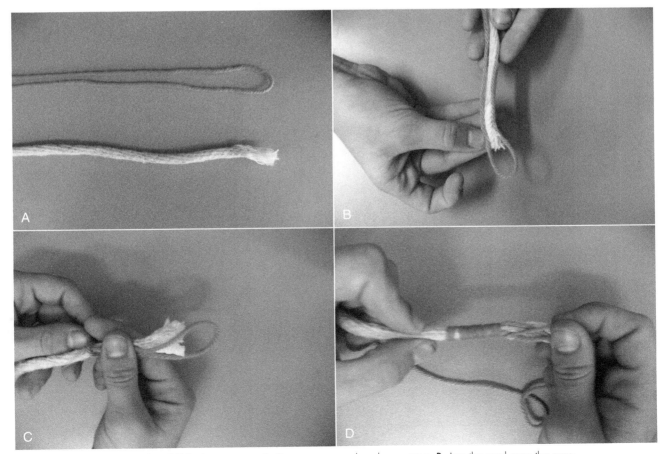

FIGURE 2-4 Whipping process. **A,** Line up your cord and your rope. **B,** Lay the cord over the rope. **C,** Begin to wrap the cord around the rope at the end away from the bight. **D,** Rope that is halfway finished.

Continued

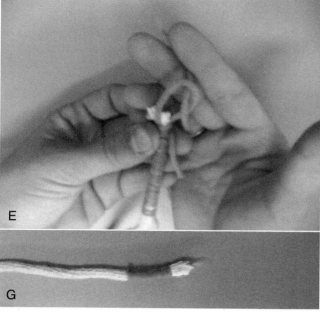

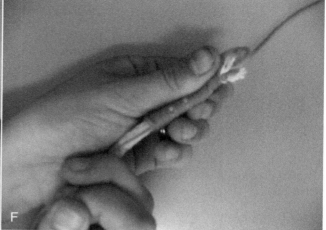

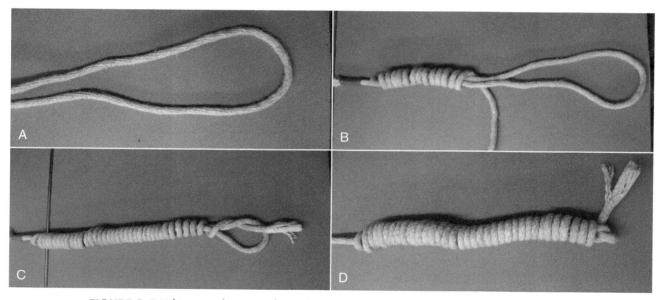

FIGURE 2-4, CONT'D E, Pull the end of the cord through the bight. **F,** Take the loose end on the cord and pull. This will hide the bight and finish the rope. **G,** Rope that has been whipped.

FIGURE 2-5 Whipping technique can be used to store ropes, except a cord is not used. **A,** Fold your rope. **B,** Start wrapping the rope over itself. **C,** Pull the end of the rope through the bight. **D,** Do not pull the loose end of the rope all the way through; pull just enough to secure the rope in place.

the cord and rope while working toward the end of the rope (Fig. 2-4, *C* and *D*). Once the cord is wrapped completely around the end of the rope up to the bighted end, pass the cord through the loop and pull tight (Fig. 2-4, *E*). Then take the ½ inch of cord on the other end and pull it. This secures the whipping and hides the loop (Fig. 2-4, *F* and *G*). Clip the extra strands of cord from each end of the whipping, and you are finished. Whipping can also be used to store or hang ropes. The only difference is that you are just whipping around the single strand of cord instead of two ropes.

The rope will be finished in the same way except you do not pull your loop all the way under, just enough to keep it from untying (Fig. 2-5).

HANKING

When ropes are stored, they can be stored using "hanking." Hanking works well for long lengths of ropes and electrical cords. Make a loop in one end of the rope (Fig. 2-6, *A*). While holding the loop with one hand, reach through the loop and pull the long end of the rope (Fig. 2-6, *B*). Pull the long end

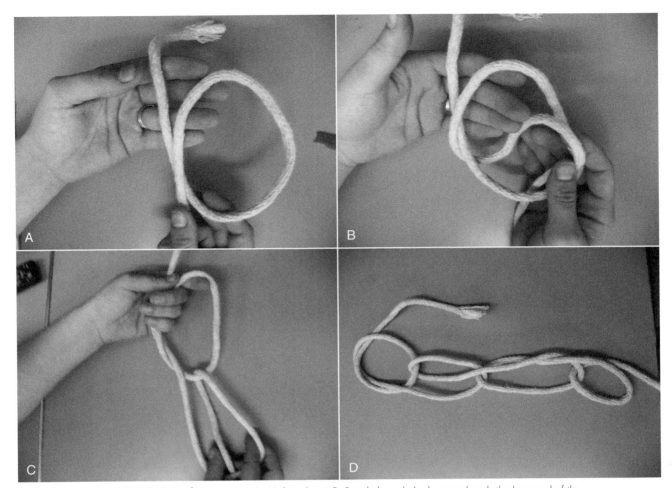

FIGURE 2-6 Hanking process. **A,** Make a loop. **B,** Reach through the loop and grab the long end of the rope. **C,** Pull only enough of the long end of the rope through to create a new loop. **D,** Continue until the rope is completely hanked.

through the original loop just enough to create another loop (Fig. 2-6, *C*). Repeat the process until the entire rope is chained together. Once the last of the rope has been chained, place the end of the rope through the last loop and tighten (Fig. 2-6, *D*). To unravel, remove the end from the last loop and pull. It should unravel easily. If it does not, try pulling on the other end of the rope.

KNOTS AND HITCHES

Knots are an "intertwining of one or two ropes in which the pressure of the standing part of the rope alone prevents it from slipping." *Hitches* are a temporary fastening of a rope to a hook, post, or other object, with the rope arranged so that the standing part forces the end against the object with sufficient pressure to prevent slipping.

The *standing part of a rope* is the longer strand of rope and is usually attached to an animal. The end is the shorter strand of the rope; this is the strand often manipulated. A *bight* is a sharp bend in the rope. A *loop* or *half hitch* is a complete circle formed in the rope. Loops can open toward you or

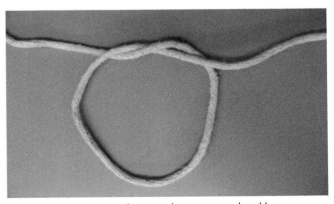

FIGURE 2-7 Throw used to create overhand knot.

away from you. In a *throw*, one rope is wrapped around another to make part of a knot.

OVERHAND KNOT

To form an overhand knot, make a half hitch, and then bring the end through the resulting loop (Fig. 2-7).

SQUARE KNOT

Fold over a few inches of one rope and create a loop with it (Fig. 2-8, *A*). Pass the second rope behind the first just above your fingers, which should be holding the loop in place. Then feed the ends of the second rope back through the loop and pull both ropes in opposite directions (Fig. 2-8, *B* to *E*).

SURGEON'S KNOT

The surgeon's knot begins with two throws. Once the two throws are complete, proceed as if you were finishing a square knot (Fig. 2-9).

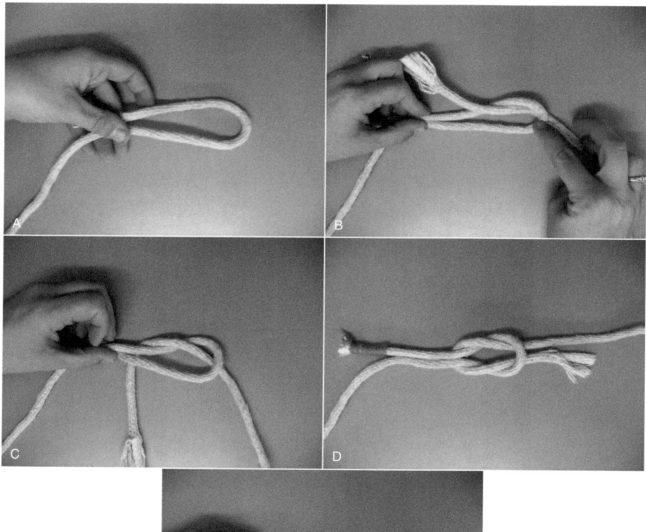

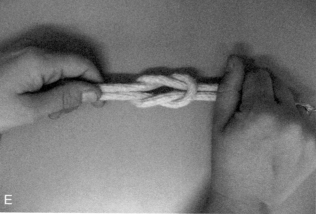

FIGURE 2-8 How to make a square knot. **A,** Make a bight. **B,** Slide the unbighted rope end through the bight. **C,** Pass the unbighted rope over the bighted rope. **D,** Bring the unbighted rope around and through the bight. **E,** Pull on both sides of the rope to create the knot. Pull tight, and the ropes will be connected.

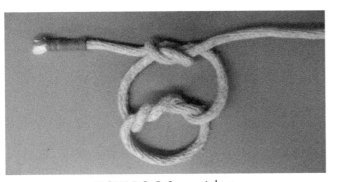

FIGURE 2-9 Surgeon's knot.

REEFER'S KNOT

Begin by making one throw (Fig. 2-10, *A*). Then make a bight in one end of the rope. Fold the bight back over the other end of the rope (Fig. 2-10, *B*). Take the unbighted end and wrap over the bight and through the hole between the first throw and the bighted end (Fig. 2-10, *C*). Pass the rope through the hole (Fig. 2-10, *D*). Then pull the two ropes in opposite directions (Fig. 2-10, *E*). To untie, pull the loose end of the bight. The knot should unravel easily.

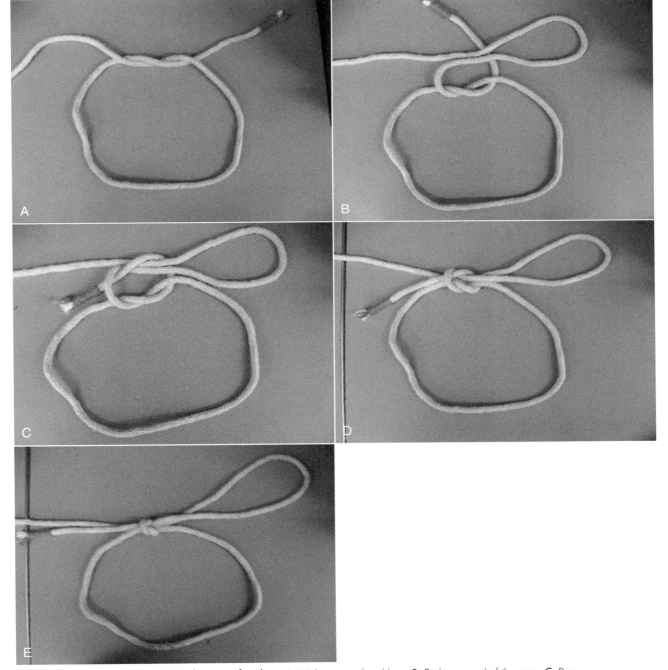

FIGURE 2-10 Making a reefer's knot. **A,** Make an overhand knot. **B,** Bight one end of the rope. **C,** Pass the other end of the rope around the bight. **D,** Take the end of the rope and pass it through the hole. **E,** Pull tight for a finished reefer's knot.

TOM FOOL'S KNOT (DOUBLE BOWLINE KNOT)

The tom fool's knot can be used to tie two legs of an animal together. Both sides of the tom fool's knot are adjustable, thus making it easy to accommodate any size leg. Begin by finding the middle of the rope. Hold your hands approximately 12 inches apart. First create a small loop in the rope. Hold this loop with your left hand. Then create a second loop in your right hand (Fig. 2-11, *A*). Look down at the top of the rope; one of the loops should be toward you, and the other loop should be away from you in reference to the piece of rope connecting the two loops (Fig. 2-11, *B*). Now pass the two loops over each other (Fig. 2-11, *C*). Then take your left index finger and reach underneath the loops and pull the opposite loop to the left. At the same time, take your right index finger over the loops and pull the opposite loop to the right (Fig. 2-11, *D* to *F*). To test the loop, pull both loose ends (Fig. 2-11, *G*). To adjust the size of each loop, just pull on the loops. You can secure the loops to a specific size by tying a square knot over the top of the tom thumb's knot.

QUICK-RELEASE KNOT

The lead rope can be used to tie the animal's head to a secure object, although this is rarely necessary and may have disastrous consequences if the horse panics and tries to run away. For most veterinary procedures, tying the animal does not justify the risks involved. If tying the head is necessary, use only a modified slip knot that can be released in an emergency, and allow the animal enough slack to allow some movement of its head and neck. The less ability the horse has to move its head, the more likely it will resist. In addition, a horse should never be tied with a chain over its nose or in its mouth. Never leave a tied horse unattended. Be sure that whatever object the animal is tied to will not break and be dragged by the animal if it breaks free. Horses and cattle can sometimes react to loud noises or movements, and this creates a dangerous situation. Quick-release knots allow the veterinary technician easily to approach the animal from the side, pull on the end of the rope, and release the animal from wherever it is tied.

First start by passing the rope around the post or object to which you would like to tie the rope. Some people prefer to pass the rope around the post twice. Make a loop in the end of the rope that is not attached to the animal. Hold the loop in your left hand. Hold the loose end of the rope in your right hand (Fig. 2-12, *A*). Lay the loop over the loose end of the rope in your right hand (Fig. 2-12, *B*). Work close to the post to ensure the least amount of slack. Reach though the loop with your thumb and finger on the right hand grasping the loop from under the rope attached to the animal (Fig. 2-12, *C* and *D*). Pull the loop in your thumb and finger to the right and the end attached to the animal to your left (Fig. 2-12, *E*). Some horses are very intelligent and have figured out how to untie themselves by grasping the end not attached to them. Some people slip the end of the rope through the loop to ensure that the horse does not escape. However, remember you must remove the end before pulling, or it will not release. To ensure that you have tied the knot correctly, pull on the loose end of the rope—it should untie easily. If excess amounts of lead rope are hanging from the knot, you can hank the end of the rope to keep it off the ground. You should practice tying this knot from the other side of the horse to make sure that you can do it both ways. It can become confusing, so practice will help avoid awkwardness in front of a client. Also practice tying to horizontal and vertical bars.

> **TECHNICIAN NOTE**   Horses and livestock should always be tied with a quick-release knot.

SHEET BEND

A sheet bend is used to tie two ropes together. Begin by making a bight in one of your ropes (Fig. 2-13, *A*). Then slide the end of the other rope underneath the bight (Fig. 2-13, *B*). Pick up the end of the rope and pass it over one side of the bight. Then bring the rope under the bight and back over through the bight (Fig. 2-13, *C*). Place the end under the first strand that is still inside the bight and bring it up over the side of the bight (Fig. 2-13, *D*). Pull both ends in opposite directions (Fig. 2-13, *E*).

BOWLINE

Bowlines are used to create a loop that can easily be placed around the animal's neck. They are nonslip and are safe for this use. Begin by making a circle in the rope (Fig. 2-14, *A*). The circle should be the size of loop you want when finished. Hold your fingers on the long end of the rope and drop the shorter end that will make up your loop. At the level of your fingers, make a small loop (Fig. 2-14, *B* and *C*). Grab the end you just dropped, and pull it through your loop, (Fig. 2-14, *D*). Place the end behind the cross made by your loop, and bring the end back through your loop (Fig. 2-14, *E*). Now tighten the knot (Fig. 2-14, *F* and *G*).

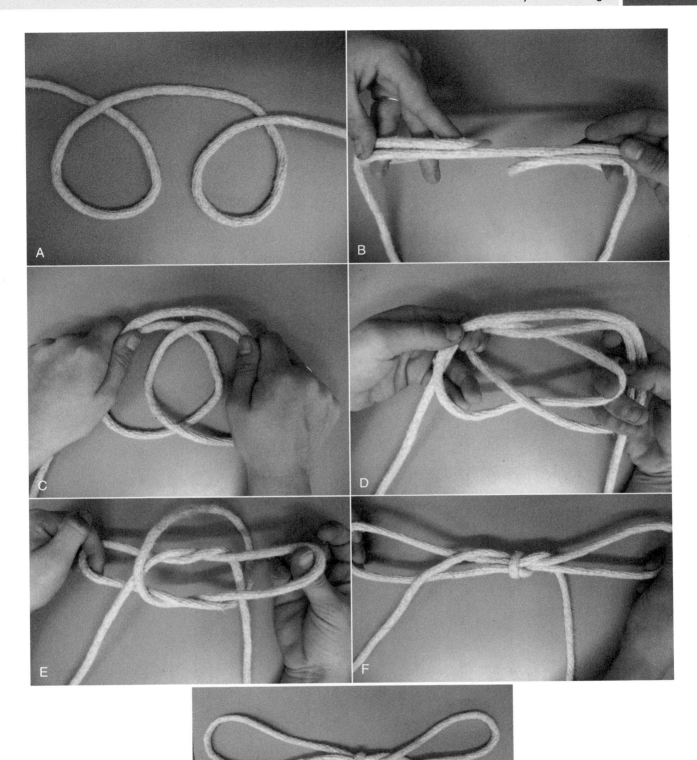

FIGURE 2-11 Making a tom fool's knot. **A,** Make two loops. **B,** Make sure one loop is away from you and one loop is toward you. **C,** Lay the loops over each other. **D,** Reach through the loop and pick up the ropes with the opposite hand. **E,** Pull each rope in opposite directions. **F,** Completed tom fool's knot. **G,** Pull on the loose ends to release the knot.

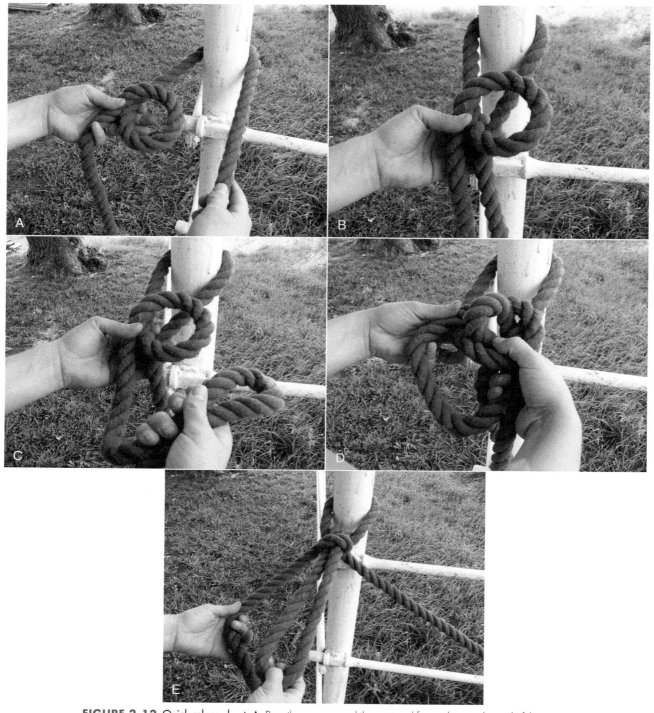

FIGURE 2-12 Quick-release knot. **A,** Pass the rope around the post and form a loop in the end of the rope not connected to the animal. **B,** Place the loop over the end of the rope connected to the animal. **C,** Create a bight in the end of the rope that also has the loop. **D,** Pass the bight behind the loop and the end of the rope connected to the animal. **E,** Pull the bight up through the loop and tighten.

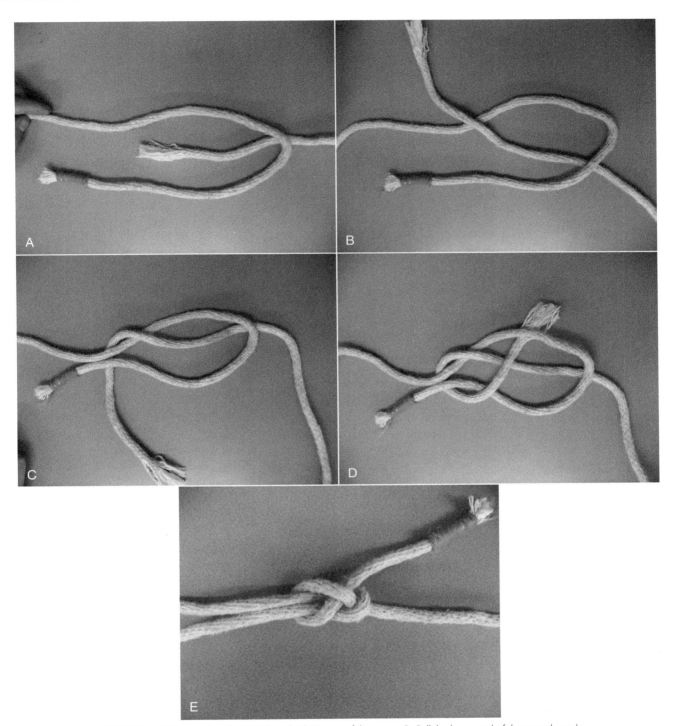

FIGURE 2-13 Sheet bend. **A,** Make a bight in one of the ropes. **B,** Pull the loose end of the rope through the bight. **C,** Pass the loose end of the rope over one side of the bight. **D,** Pull the loose end under the bight and bring it back under itself. **E,** Pull tight for a completed sheet bend.

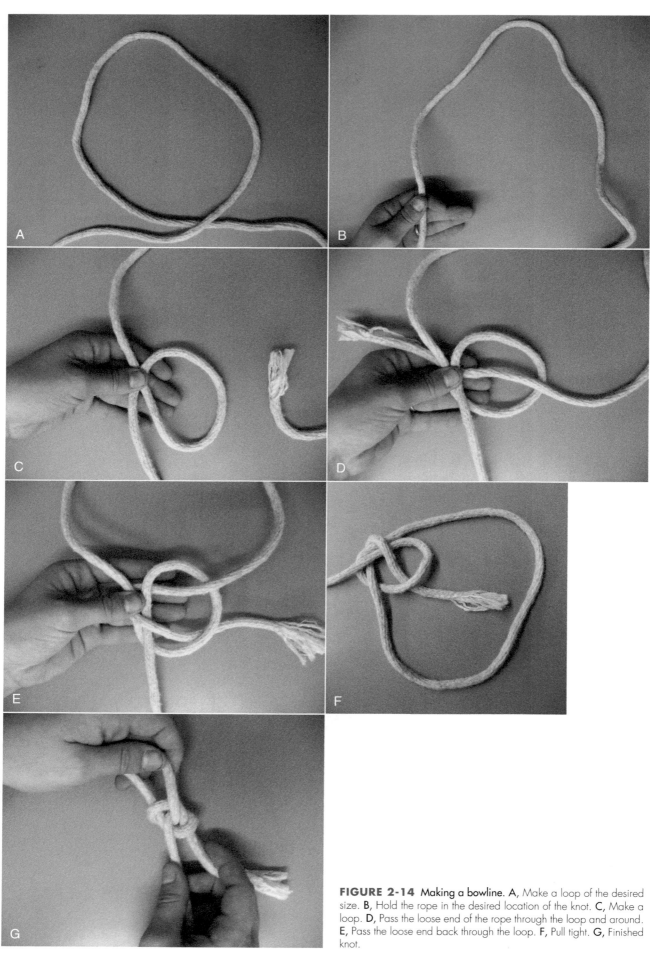

FIGURE 2-14 Making a bowline. **A,** Make a loop of the desired size. **B,** Hold the rope in the desired location of the knot. **C,** Make a loop. **D,** Pass the loose end of the rope through the loop and around. **E,** Pass the loose end back through the loop. **F,** Pull tight. **G,** Finished knot.

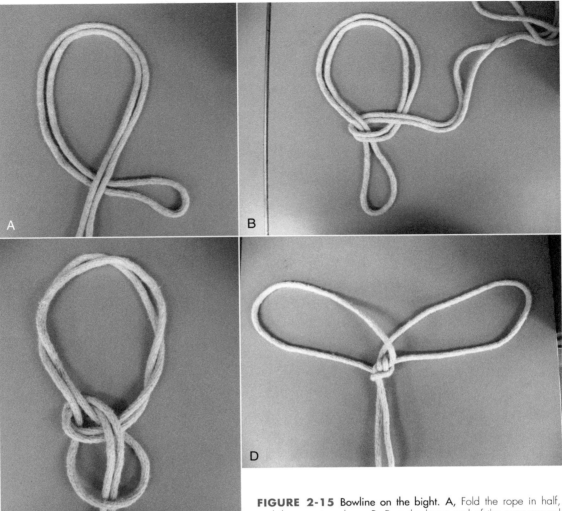

FIGURE 2-15 Bowline on the bight. **A,** Fold the rope in half, and then create a loop. **B,** Pass the loose end of the rope around the bight. **C,** Pass the loose ends of the rope through the bight. **D,** Pull tight on the two large loops to complete the knot.

BOWLINE ON THE BIGHT

A bowline on the bight can be used to restrain an animal's legs and neck. Begin by folding your rope completely in half. From here on out, pretend that it is just one rope. You will never separate the two strands. Make a loop of the desired size (Fig. 2-15, *A*). Then hold your thumb over the crossed portion of the ropes in the loop. Take the loose strands and wrap them around your thumb (Fig. 2-15, *B*). Once around both sides of the ropes, push the ropes back through the hole made by the placement of your thumb. Then place the strands through the loop (Fig. 2-15, *C*). Pull on the large loops to tighten the rope (Fig. 2-15, *D*).

HALF HITCH

Start by placing your rope around a post or leg. Bring the strand around and under. Pull up on this end of the rope. Drop down to the next hitch. Bring the strand around, but this time lay the loose end over the rope. This type of hitch is often used to tie in a surgical patient (Fig. 2-16).

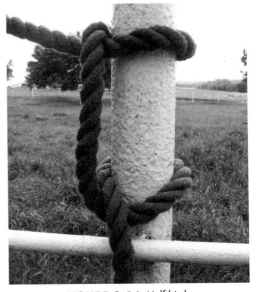

FIGURE 2-16 Half hitch.

CLOVE HITCH

Start as if you were making a tom fool's knot. Hold one loop in each hand. Overlap the loops, although you must place the two strands of rope that are on opposite sides together. The main rope will look like it is crossing both strands. Place both loops in this position over the post you would like to tie to, and pull the loose ends (Fig. 2-17).

TAIL TIE

The tail tie can be used to hold the tail out of the way during veterinary procedures. A tail rope should never be tied to an immovable object. The tail rope is not a substitute for the hindquarters; if an animal demonstrates that it cannot provide any support of its own rear body weight, the animal should not be left dangling by a tail rope. The tail tie is performed just beyond the end of the last coccygeal vertebra (Fig. 2-18).

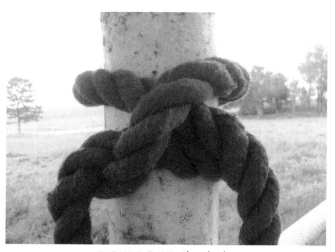

FIGURE 2-17 Clove hitch.

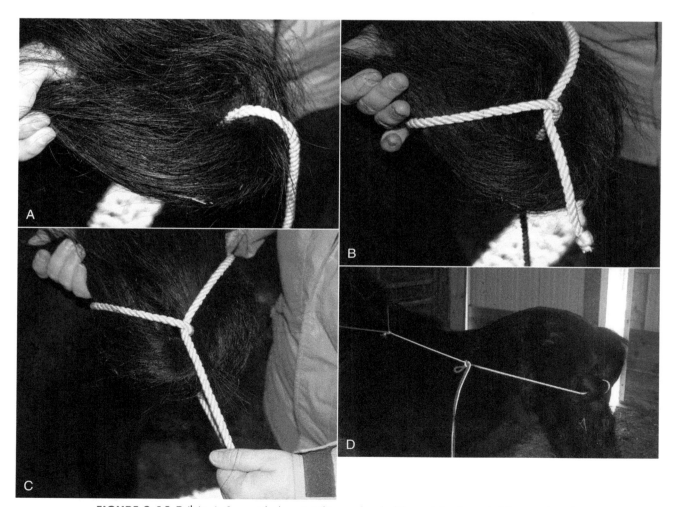

FIGURE 2-18 Tail tie. **A,** Support the horse's tail in your hand while you bring the end of the rope through the bight. **B,** Pass the end of the rope around the bight so that it ends up on top. Bring the end under the rope until it is looped around the horse's tail. **C,** Tighten by pulling the short and long ends together. **D,** Tie the long portion of the rope to one of the horse's front legs or the neck by using a bowline knot. (From Sheldon CC, Sonsthagen T, Topel JA: *Animal restraint for veterinary professionals,* St. Louis, 2006, Mosby.)

> **TECHNICIAN NOTE**   Tail ties should never be tied to immovable objects.

No part of the vertebral column should be included in the tie; only the tail hairs are incorporated into the knot. Gather all the hair and fold it over the rope. Hold the hair together with your right hand. Bring the short end of the rope underneath the tail. Make a bight in the short end of the rope. Hold the bight with your thumb and forefinger. Slide the bight over the tail, one strand on the top and one strand on the bottom. There should be a loop where your thumb and forefinger are located. Pass the short end of the rope up through the loop. Take the two loose ends of the rope and pull in opposite directions.

TEMPORARY ROPE HALTER

Begin by tying a bowline in a long rope and passing it over the horse's head. The rope can also be placed around the neck and then a bowline can be tied. Be careful to ensure that the knot is *not* a slip knot (Fig. 2-19, *A*). Then create a bight in the rope and pass it through the rope already encircling the horse's neck (Fig. 2-19, *B*). Pass the bight over the horse's nose (Fig. 2-19, *C* and *D*).

RESTRAINT

Restraint is the term used to imply control of an animal, and it may be necessary for medical and nonmedical procedures. The two types of animal restraint are physical restraint and chemical restraint. Sometimes both must be used to accomplish a procedure. *Physical restraint* refers to methods that are applied to the animal with or without use of special equipment. *Chemical restraint* refers to the use of pharmaceuticals to alter the animal's mental or physical abilities.

Restraint is more of an art than a science. Skilled restrainers know the behavior and nature of the species with which they work. This level of savvy takes time to acquire and is often best learned by watching experienced personnel. Good restraint involves understanding the natural instincts of each species being handled, being able to read an individual's temperament, and recognizing the extent of handling and training that an individual has (or has not) received. Each animal is an individual, and each has a different background. A method of restraint that is totally effective for one animal may be completely ineffective for another. Avoid a cookie-cutter approach in which all animals are treated similarly. Be flexible. When the selected

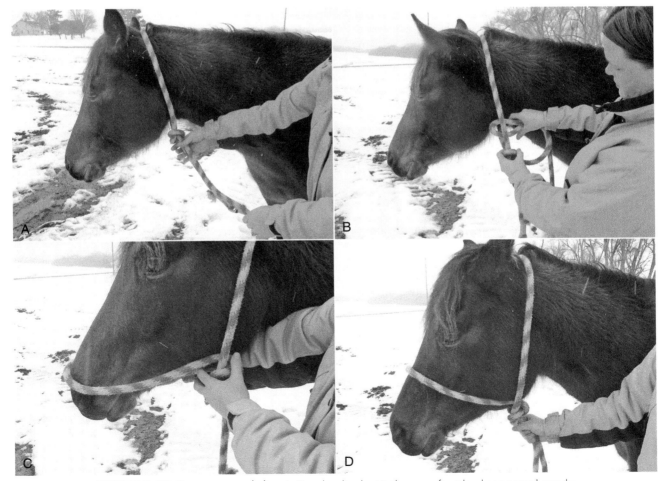

FIGURE 2-19 Temporary rope halter. **A,** Tie a bowline knot in the rope after it has been passed over the horse's neck. **B,** Create a bight in the rope and pass it through the rope over the horse's head. **C,** Pass the bight over the nose. **D,** Finished temporary rope halter.

method of restraint is not working, go to plan B. Realize that you cannot force restraint on an animal that is intent on not accepting it, especially when the animal outweighs and outmuscles you many times over.

> **TECHNICIAN NOTE**   Learning good restraint takes time. Watching experienced personnel is an excellent way to learn animal restraint.

> **TECHNICIAN NOTE**   You must outthink an animal that outweighs you. Remember if one approach does not work, try another.

Be sure to plan ahead for the procedure. Few things are more frustrating than struggling to have an animal properly restrained, only to realize that a piece of equipment is out of reach or is not working properly. Veterinary technicians should always familiarize themselves with the facility before beginning a procedure. You must understand the flow of the *alleyways,* where the animals will be coming from and where they are being asked to go. Technicians should also become familiar with the proper operation of all equipment. Each *working chute,* although similar in design, will have differences, and it is essential to become familiar with those differences before handling the livestock. The safety of the personnel and the animals requires this understanding. Although in theory all livestock equipment would be in tip-top shape, in reality the facilities available on some farms are in various states of repair and disrepair, and some small "backyard" farms may not have any special facilities at all. The ability to improvise, and remain safe, is essential.

> **TECHNICIAN NOTE**   Before beginning any type of restraint, familiarize yourself with the equipment.

Animals should be protected from dangers such as sharp objects, hooks, buckets, loose boards, and light fixtures in case the animals rear, kick, or throw the head or body. Do not risk serious lacerations or fractures from restraint for an otherwise simple procedure. Survey the area for potential hazards before beginning a procedure. The best prevention is to take the animal to an area without potential hazards or

remove the hazards where possible. Patience is a virtue, and your virtue will be tested. Some procedures simply cannot be done safely on certain individuals in certain situations.

Take good care of your personal safety. Avoid getting into a position or place from which you cannot leave quickly, such as a stall corner or between the animal and a fence or wall. In addition, do not be afraid to speak up if you are uncomfortable with a given situation or not up to the task. Your safety is of the utmost importance.

Another consideration is the possibility of professional liability lawsuits. The veterinarian is recognized legally as an expert and is responsible for anticipating the responses of his or her patients to veterinary procedures. Sometimes the veterinarian's choice of restraint is influenced by this consideration and may even lead to the veterinarian's refusal to perform certain procedures. The safety of the animal and the safety of the people handling the animal must be not only legal but also ethical.

> **TECHNICIAN NOTE**   The safety of the animal and the safety of the people handling the animal must be not only legal but also ethical.

Finally, realize that any form of restraint can become abusive. Applying a restraint method improperly or for too long can cross the line of humane restraint. Use the *least* amount of restraint necessary to do the job *safely,* and do not apply the restraint any longer than necessary.

> **TECHNICIAN NOTE**   Use the least amount of restraint necessary to do the job safely, and do not apply the restraint any longer than necessary.

COVERING THE EYES

Covering the eyes is a time-honored method that can be applied to one or both of the animal's eyes. Sometimes the animal will be submissive if it cannot see the area being worked on during a procedure. Covering the eye on the same side as the procedure is the most common method but often is applied incorrectly. Placing the hand completely over the animal's eye to force it shut usually is unnecessary and often is met with resistance (Fig. 2-20, *A*). All that is necessary is to block the animal's view of the procedure by using an open hand like a curtain but allowing the animal to keep its eye open (Fig. 2-20, *B*).

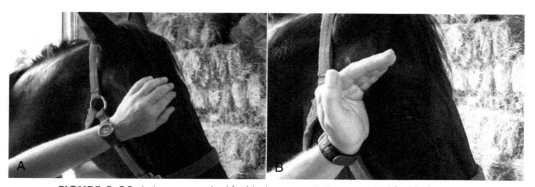

FIGURE 2-20 A, Improper method for blocking view. **B,** Proper method for blocking view.

Some animals respond favorably to blindfolding (Fig. 2-21). These individuals and situations must be carefully selected because not all animals accept a blindfold. Blindfolding is usually done by placing a towel over both eyes and tucking it underneath the halter. The blindfold should be easily removable and quickly accessible by the handler in case the animal panics.

PHYSICAL RESTRAINT OF HORSES

Much of horses' behavior relates to their being prey animals. When horses are placed in a frightening situation, their natural instinct is to run away. Sometimes this instinct is so strong that they injure themselves in their effort to flee. Few horses become aggressive in a frightening situation, but they can become so. Precautions must be taken with these individuals. In addition, horses are *herd* animals, and another strong natural instinct they have is to resist attempts to separate them from others in their group.

Halter and Lead Rope

The horse's head should always be attended. Control of the head usually enables control of the horse. For most procedures, the person "on the head" stands on the same side as the person performing the procedure and has the greatest responsibility for restraint of the animal and the safety of his or her co-worker. The reason for standing on the same side as the person performing the procedure is that if pain or fear is perceived by the horse, its natural instinct is to move away from that stimulus, and a person at the horse's head who is on the opposite side from the person performing the procedure will be run over or stepped on.

One of the most basic acts of horsemanship is placing a halter and lead rope. It is also the first step in gaining control of a horse's head, which is the key to controlling the horse.

The horse should be approached from its left side; avoid standing directly in front of the horse. The reason a horse is approached from the left side is that most horses are trained to handle from the left and are therefore most accustomed to this approach (Fig. 2-22). It is good practice to stand in front of the horse's shoulder, but behind the ears. This position helps to avoid being struck with a front foot if the horse strikes at the handler. Usually, the halter is placed first, and then the lead rope is attached to the halter. In some horses, the lead rope must be placed around the neck first for initial control while the halter is being placed (see Fig. 2-22; Fig. 2-23, *A*). However, you may place the halter and lead rope while they are attached to each other. The halter has a small loop (the *nose band*), which is placed around the nose, and a larger loop (the *crown strap*), which is placed over and behind the ears (Fig. 2-23, *B*). Buckles or snaps are used to open and close the loops (Fig. 2-23, *C*). As a courtesy to the horse, try not to drag the halter over the eyes and ears. Rather, spread the halter apart to avoid the eyes, and lift or unbuckle the halter to avoid the ears. Once the halter is positioned and the buckles or snaps are secured, the lead rope is attached (Fig. 2-23, *D* and *E*).

Once placed, the halter and lead rope can be used to lead the horse. The horse should not be led by grasping the halter. If the horse moves its head up or away, the operator may lose his or her grip, and if the horse bolts or runs, the operator risks being dragged and seriously hurt. Use the lead rope to lead the horse. Hold the lead away from any buckles or chains, and *never* coil the lead around the fingers, hand, or arm. If the horse bolts or runs, coiled rope may tighten around body parts, and serious injury or death may result. Do not let the lead rope drag on the ground because the horse may step on the rope or the handler may become tangled in the rope, with resulting injury

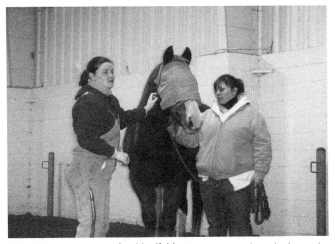

FIGURE 2-21 Use of a blindfold. Notice it is only tucked into the halter for easy removal in case the horse panics.

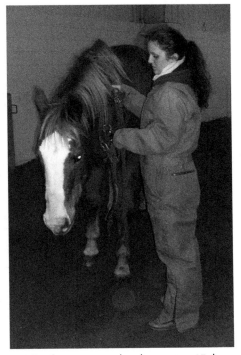

FIGURE 2-22 Always approach a horse at a 45-degree angle to the shoulder.

(Fig. 2-24). One must be very careful when handling young, inexperienced horses because sudden movements or loud noises can startle them and create a very dangerous situation quickly.

Sometimes a buddy system approach—taking a second horse along—is helpful if the horse must be taken away from the group. Horses are naturally suspicious and respond best to a calm, deliberate approach. Using voice and touch in a calm manner helps to gain their trust. Good horse handlers typically maintain vocal and physical contact with the animals they are handling. Approaches to the horse usually are best made at a 45-degree angle to the shoulder, rather than from behind. Initial hand contact with the neck or withers makes a good introduction before you move on to other areas of the horse's body. Horses traditionally are handled primarily from their left side (the "near" side). Unless the horse has not been handled, it most likely will be accustomed to a left-sided approach. Be careful when working in the horse's visual blind spots (Fig. 2-25). Because of the location

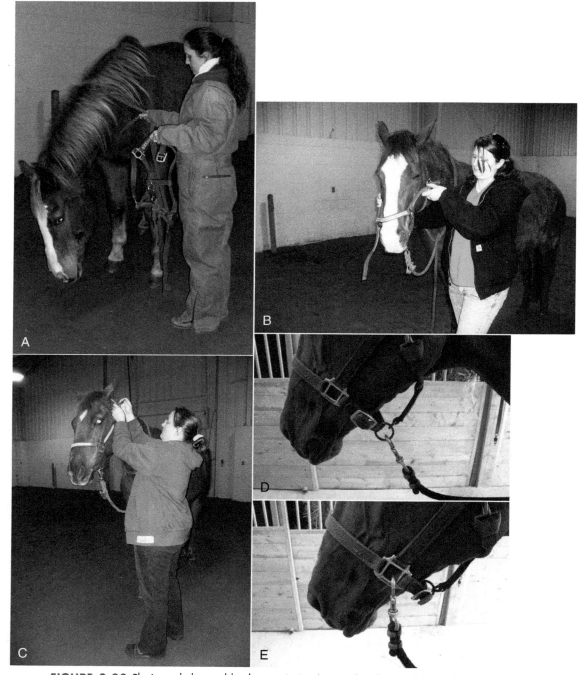

FIGURE 2-23 Placing a halter and lead rope. **A,** Lead rope placed around the neck to obtain initial control of the horse. **B,** Placement of the nose band over the nose. **C,** Securing the buckle of the crown strap. **D,** Attachment of the lead rope to the halter. **E,** Alternative attachment of the lead rope to the halter.

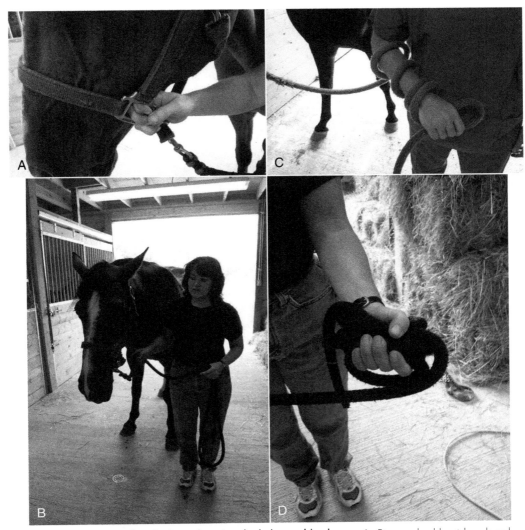

FIGURE 2-24 Leading the horse by using the halter and lead rope. **A,** Fingers should not be placed through the buckles or snaps of the halter. **B,** Proper hold of the lead rope. **C,** Improper coiling of the lead rope around the arm. **D,** Improper coiling of the lead rope around the hand.

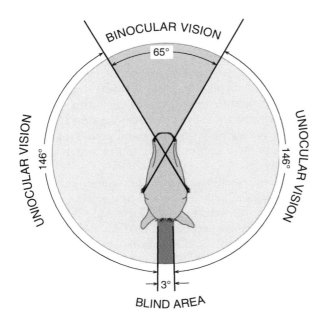

FIGURE 2-25 Great care should be taken when working in the horse's visual blind spots. (From Maggs C, Miller P, Ofri R: *Slatter's fundamentals of veterinary ophthalmology,* ed 5, St. Louis, 2013, Saunders.)

of their eyes, horses cannot see directly behind their hindquarters, directly in front of the tip of their nose, directly between the eyes in the forehead, and the area directly above the head and between the ears. If you must work in these areas, avoid unannounced or rapid movements. Avoid working in these areas unless you are protected by a barrier or mechanical device.

Horses may strike with the front legs or kick with the hindlegs in response to pain or fear. Horses may also throw their heads violently, causing injury. In some cases horses will bite. Even a normally "good horse" may display these responses when in pain or fear. Assume that all horses are capable of these responses when they are placed in certain situations.

To lead the horse, walk purposefully in the intended direction and do not look back at the horse. Some horses resent being held tightly by the lead rope, and giving the rope some slack may encourage the horse to follow the handler. Most horses respond best when the handler walks to the side of the head or neck. Avoid walking far in front of the horse, where control of the horse is minimal.

When controlling the horse's head for a procedure, the person on the head should realize that his or her first responsibility is the co-worker's safety. If the horse becomes fractious, the best practice usually is to move the horse's hindquarters away from the clinician. This is done not by moving the hind end of the horse directly but by moving the horse's head; the hindquarters usually move opposite to head movement. In other words, turning the horse's head to the left usually causes the hindquarters to move to the right, and vice versa. This is often counterintuitive to the person handling the horse. Most people who are new to horse restraint often push the horse away from them with the halter and lead rope. Because you should always be handling the horse from the same side as the doctor, this action will throw the hind end of the horse directly at your assistant or, worse, your doctor. The best thing for you to do is pull the horse toward you. This will result in the horse's moving its rear end away from the people with whom you are working.

> **TECHNICIAN NOTE** When multiple people are working on a horse, it is important that you all stand on the same side. Then if the horse acts up you can pull the horse toward you, and it will move its hind end away from the people with whom you are working. This action will help to keep everyone safe.

Lead ropes are made from many materials (e.g., nylon, leather, hemp, cotton) and have two basic designs: with or without a chain. Without a chain, the rope serves only as a lead; the addition of a chain provides possibilities for several degrees of physical restraint. Using the chain portion of a lead to restrain foals, as described later, is not appropriate.

> **TECHNICIAN NOTE** Using chain leads to restrain foals is not appropriate.

Chain shanks or lead shanks can be purchased with varying lengths of chain and thicknesses of chain links. When a simple lead rope does not provide enough control, the chain portion of a chain shank can be placed over the nose, under the nose, or in the mouth for increasing restraint. To use the chain in this fashion, the halter must have side rings to slide the chain through and fasten the chain snap. Placing the chain over the nose is a mild form of restraint. The chain is passed (1) through the left ring of the nosepiece and over the nose to attach to the right nosepiece ring (Fig. 2-26, *A*), (2) through the right nosepiece ring and continuing to the right upper ring (Fig. 2-26, *B*), or (3) through the right nosepiece ring and continuing under the halter to attach to the large nosepiece ring between the mandibles (Fig. 2-26, *C*). Care should be taken to cross the chain over the halter nose band so that the nose band can act as a protective interface between the chain and the horse's skin (Fig. 2-26, *D*). A light, quick snap of the lead usually gets the horse's attention.

Placing the chain under the chin is not recommended. Many horses throw their heads or rear to avoid pressure from a chin shank, with possible injury to themselves (Fig. 2-27). Some horses respond only to this placement, however, and extreme caution should be used if this approach is going to be tried.

The chain can also be placed in the mouth as the next level of restraint. The chain can be placed in two basic positions. It can be positioned like a mouth bit (Fig. 2-28), although the links of the chain tend to pinch the tongue and cheeks when pressure is applied, thus causing many horses to resist any pressure on the lead. The other location is between the maxillary gums and the upper mucosal surface of the lip (Fig. 2-29).

Elevating a Leg

Elevating a leg is a mild form of restraint that is basically intended to discourage a horse from moving around or kicking, as occurs when trying to place leg bandages, taking radiographs, or clipping hair. Leg elevation is not as useful for painful procedures, but it can be combined with other forms of restraint for increased effect. Elevating legs is also a common procedure for cleaning and examining the feet and legs. It is also a key component of a thorough lameness examination.

Before leg elevation, the horse should be standing "square," that is, all four legs should be directly underneath the horse, with the weight evenly distributed. It is physically difficult for any horse to pick a leg up if it is standing with its legs sprawled or is balanced awkwardly.

As with other horse-handling procedures, contact with the horse is helpful in communicating intentions. To elevate a forelimb, place one hand on the withers or shoulder area, and run the other hand slowly down the back side of the

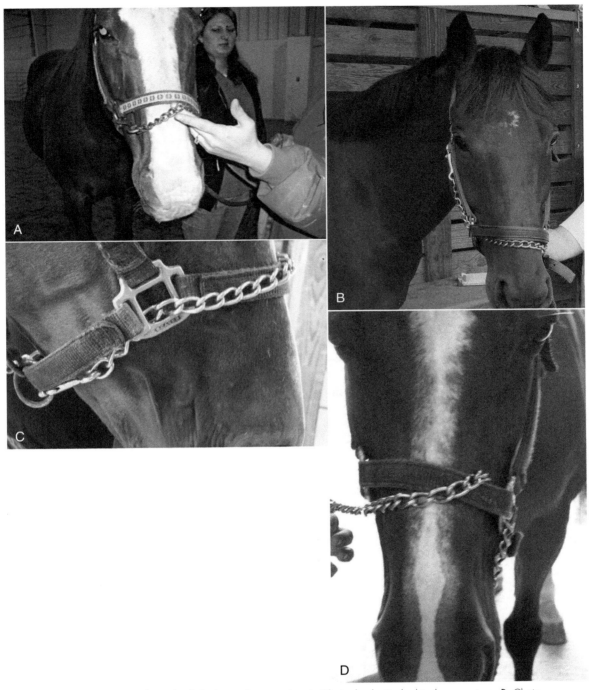

FIGURE 2-26 Chain shank for increasing restraint. **A,** Chain shank attached to the nosepiece. **B,** Chain shank attached to the right upper ring. **C,** Chain shank attached between the mandibles. **D,** Chain should cross the nosepiece to provide some protection for the horse. (**B,** From Bassett JM, McCurnin DM: *McCurnin's clinical textbook for veterinary technicians,* ed 7, St. Louis, 2010, Saunders.)

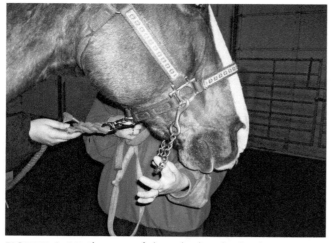

FIGURE 2-27 Placement of chain shank under the chin. When the loose end of the rope is pulled tight and the fingers are removed, the chain shank can be used as a form of head restraint.

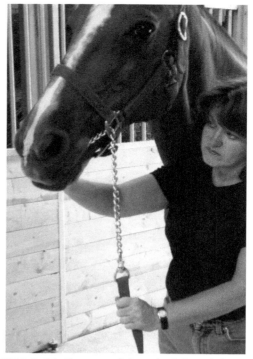

FIGURE 2-28 Placement of chain shank through the mouth.

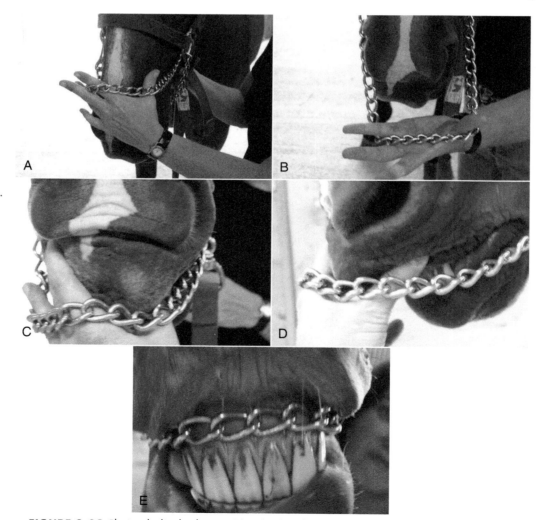

FIGURE 2-29 Placing the lip shank. **A,** Holding the chain for placement of the lip shank. **B,** Slack is given to the chain. **C,** Elevating the upper lip to position the chain. **D,** Elevating the upper lip to position the chain. **E,** Proper position of the chain against the upper gum. Note that the chain lies flat against the gums.

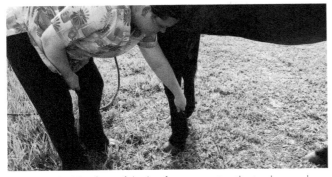

FIGURE 2-30 Lifting of the leg from squeezing the tendons and *suspensory ligament* of the palmar surface of the leg.

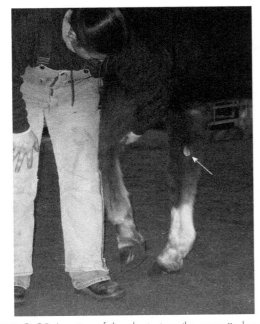

FIGURE 2-31 Location of the chestnut on the opposite leg *(arrow)*. Squeezing the chestnut.

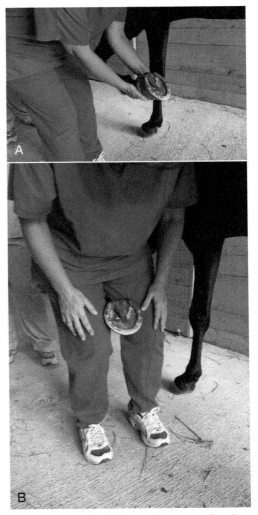

FIGURE 2-32 A, The forelimb can be supported with one hand. B, The forelimb can be supported between the thighs to free up the hands.

leg to be lifted. Once at the level of the carpus, it is advised to scratch or massage the inside of the carpus. Some horses are trained to lift their feet to this stimulus. If this does not work, continue sliding until you reach the digital tendons. When the sliding hand reaches the digital tendons, a gentle *squeeze* of the tendons usually results in lifting of the leg (Fig. 2-30). If squeezing alone does not work, try pressing your shoulder into the horse's shoulder to shift its weight onto the opposite forelimb. Once the weight has shifted, the horse will be more inclined to elevate the leg. If these methods fail to work, try gently squeezing the *chestnut* of the limb you want lifted (Figs. 2-31 and 2-32). If you are lifting a front leg to discourage a horse from kicking with a hindleg, lift the forelimb on the same side as the "threatening" hindlimb. Working on the same side is not only safer, but also usually more effective.

To elevate a hindlimb, face the rear of the horse and maintain contact with one hand on the horse's hindquarters.

Slide the other hand down the leg to the digital tendons, and squeeze the tendons. As with the forelimb, you can use your shoulder to apply pressure onto the horse's hip. This pressure can help the horse shift its weight to the opposite hindlimb and encourage lifting the leg.

Once a leg has been lifted, it can be held with the hands or cradled in the lap or thigh area, depending on the procedure to be performed. Do not support the leg so well that you become a substitute leg for the horse, thus allowing it to kick or move at your expense, or rest so hard on your legs that muscle fatigue or bruising occurs. Horses tend to resist having their legs pulled away from the median plane (abduction) and stand better when a leg is held as close to its normal position as possible directly underneath it (Fig. 2-33).

Tail Restraint

Tail restraint is effective for foals and small ponies but not for adults. Grasp the tail near its base, and elevate it straight up

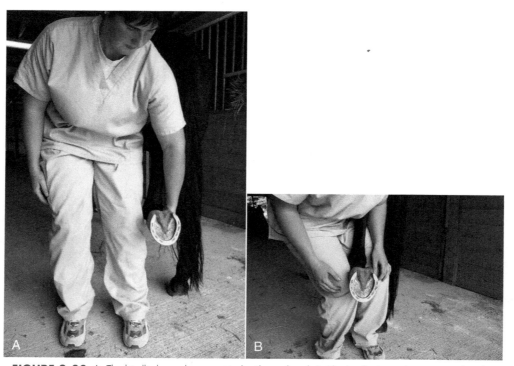

FIGURE 2-33 **A,** The hindlimb can be supported with one hand. **B,** The hindlimb can be supported on the thighs to free up the hands.

and slightly over the back. At the same time, use the other arm to encircle the shoulders or base of the neck. Be aware that many foals have a tendency to rear when restrained; therefore, the restrainer should keep his or her head out of the area immediately above the head and neck to avoid being struck.

When working with any horse's hind end, it is important to stay as close as possible to the horse or out of kicking distance.

The tail of a horse is considerably more substantial than the tail of a cow; it is strong enough to be used to move, lift, or support the hindquarters. Horses with neurologic or musculoskeletal diseases may need assistance to stand or remain standing, and horses recovering from anesthesia may need assistance standing. The tail tie can be helpful in these situations because it provides a safe means of securing a rope to the horse's tail. The rope then can be placed over a supporting beam or through a pulley or block and tackle, where it can be positioned for support.

Another example of using the tail for restraint includes pulling it to the side and forcing the horse to shift its weight to the leg on that side. This can be helpful in some situations, but realize if the horse really wants to pick up that foot it will and use it as a weapon if it believes the stimulus warrants such a reaction. This technique can be used with adults, but again realize that it does not stop them from kicking if they want to kick.

Twitches

Twitches are among the oldest and most commonly used methods of restraint. The reason that twitches work has

been debated for many years. Some people believe that twitches divert the horse's attention by creating pain that exceeds that of less painful procedures being performed elsewhere on the body; others believe that acupressure points are activated, causing release of natural endorphins in the brain. Whatever the mechanism, the effectiveness of twitches cannot be argued.

The two classifications of twitches are natural and mechanical. Natural twitches are applied with the hands directly on the horse; no special equipment is required. Mechanical twitches are human-made devices that are placed directly on the horse. Twitches of any type are *not* appropriate for foals.

Natural twitches are the shoulder (skin) twitch, the ear twitch, and the lip twitch. The shoulder twitch ("shoulder roll" or "skin twitch") is actually applied to the skin over the lateral aspect of the neck. This skin is loose and can be picked up with the fingers and pinched firmly (Fig. 2-34, *A*). For added effect, the skin can be picked up with all the fingers and rolled like a motorcycle accelerator; this can be done with one or both hands (Fig. 2-35, *B*). This twitch is a mild form of restraint and loses its effectiveness after a few minutes. If the shoulder twitch is applied tightly for long, some horses swell locally after the hold is released, and a welt results. Such welts disappear within 24 hours with no special treatment and are not a physical problem, but they may give the client a bad impression.

The ear twitch is very effective for some horses, but others vehemently resist it. To apply this twitch, do not grab the ear directly; this may startle the horse. Rather, place your hand on the neck and slide it to the base of the ear. Slowly grasp the base of the ear, squeeze it, and rotate the ear slightly, again like a motorcycle accelerator (Fig. 2-35). Like the shoulder twitch, the ear twitch loses its effectiveness in a short period. Grasping at the base of the ear, not in the middle or tip, is important. Realize that the cartilage of the ear pinna can be broken, resulting in permanent deformity, and the nerves to the pinna can be damaged. Therefore, if the horse elevates its head or rears, it is best to let go and try another approach (Fig. 2-36). When considering the application of an ear twitch, it is wise to obtain the client's or veterinarian's approval.

> *TECHNICIAN NOTE*   Permanent deformity of the pinna can result from ear twitching. Care should be taken to avoid any damage to the nerves and cartilage of the ear.

> *TECHNICIAN NOTE*   Before performing an ear twitch, you should always ask the owner or veterinarian for permission.

Biting the horse's ear is still accepted in some parts of the country as a restraint method, but it is not commonly accepted and is not recommended for use by medical professionals.

The upper lip can be twitched with either hand. The lip can simply be grasped, squeezed, and jiggled back and forth if necessary. Grabbing a lip may be enough restraint for many horses. For more force application to the upper lip, mechanical twitches are necessary.

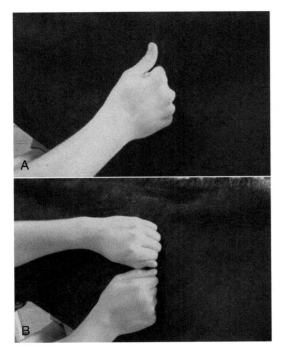

FIGURE 2-34 Shoulder twitch. **A,** The skin is grasped and pinched firmly. **B,** The skin is grasped and rolled.

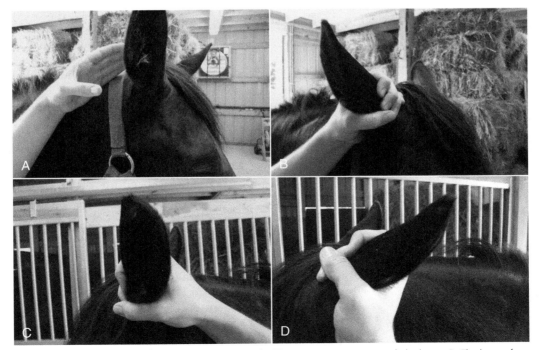

FIGURE 2-35 Ear twitch. **A,** The ear is approached by maintaining contact with the horse. **B,** The base of the ear is grasped. **C,** The ear is squeezed. **D,** The ear can be rotated for added effect.

Mechanical twitches can be homemade or commercially bought (Fig. 2-37). They are designed to "pinch" the upper lip. The traditional twitch is constructed from a wooden handle with a rope or chain loop attached to one end. To place the twitch, first control the twitch handle with a hand or tuck it under an armpit while placing the twitch loop; otherwise, the handle is free to swing and hit the handler and/or the horse and cause injury. The upper lip is grasped with the hand, and the loop is transferred from the hand to the lip by sliding the loop over the fingers (Fig. 2-38, *A*). Once the lip has been placed through the loop, the twitch handle is rotated to twist the loop firmly around the lip. The handle should be rotated as if it were being rolled up the nose toward the ears, not downward toward the lower lip. Avoid occluding the nostrils while placing the twitch; horses cannot mouth breathe and tend to panic when the nostrils are blocked (Fig. 2-38, *B* to *F*). By twisting the handle, the loop can be tightened or loosened for varying degrees of control. Care should always be taken to control the twitch during use. Letting go

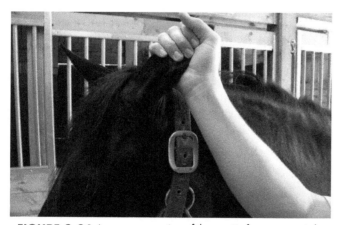

FIGURE 2-36 Improper grasping of the ear tip for an ear twitch.

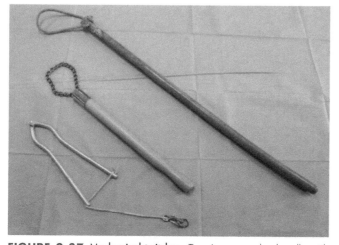

FIGURE 2-37 Mechanical twitches. *Top,* Long wooden handle with a rope loop. *Middle,* Short wooden handle with a chain loop. *Bottom,* Aluminum humane twitch.

of this type of twitch quickly can result in spinning and hitting someone and causing serious injury.

The twitch handle comes in various lengths; however, the shorter the handle, the closer the operator will be to the front feet and the less useful the twitch will be if the horse rears. Many horse handlers prefer a twitch handle 30 to 40 inches long.

The other type of mechanical twitch is called the "humane twitch." It consists of two handles that function as a scissors-type "clamp" on the nose. Pressure is controlled by opening or closing the arms of the clamp. This type of twitch usually is made of aluminum and has a string with a clip attached to it so that it can be "self-retaining" by clipping it to the halter. In reality, the humane twitch is limited in usefulness. The arms are short (12 inches), and maintaining a grip on the device is difficult if the horse elevates its head. When it is applied as a self-retaining twitch, the string tends to loosen. If the horse swings its head, the handles become a potential weapon, injuring the horse or the handler. The humane twitch is used in some situations but is ineffective and potentially harmful in others (Fig. 2-39).

After the twitch is in place, one person should hold the twitch handle and the lead rope, with care taken not to wrap the lead around the handle or any part of the hand or arm (Fig. 2-40). The twitch does not replace the lead rope. The person on the head still has primary responsibility for control of the horse and the safety of co-workers. The pressure of a chain twitch is adjusted by twisting the twitch handle to tighten or loosen the chain. The pressure of a humane twitch is adjusted by squeezing the handles. Apply only enough pressure with the twitch to accomplish the procedure and only as long as necessary. Sometimes jiggling the twitch helps to get the horse's attention without having to crank down tightly on the twitch. In addition, be aware that the upper lip can become numb after prolonged application, and bleeding from the nose is possible. When the lip turns blue and cool to the touch, the twitch has usually lost its effectiveness and should be loosened or removed.

Stocks

Stocks are rectangular enclosures made of wood or metal (Fig. 2-41). They are designed to confine the horse to a small area with restricted movement, usually only 2 feet of lateral movement and 1 to 2 feet of front-to-back movement. Because of the varying sizes of horses, stocks may be adjustable for the width and length of the patient. The side panels or rails of the stocks usually adjust to allow access to the body parts being worked on by the veterinary personnel. Horse stocks typically are open above (i.e., they have no ceiling).

Horse stocks and cattle stocks or chutes have different constructions. Cattle chutes are purposely designed to squeeze the cow's neck firmly and sometimes have panels that can be used to squeeze the cow's body firmly. Horses cannot tolerate this type of tight, rigid confinement and typically violently resist it. Therefore, horses should never be placed in cattle chutes.

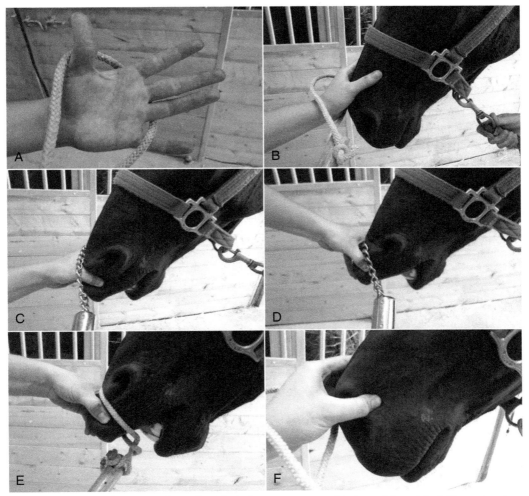

FIGURE 2-38 Placing a mechanical twitch. **A,** Proper positioning of the loop of the twitch. **B,** Place a hand on the nose and slide it toward the upper lip. **C,** Grasp the upper lip and elevate it slightly. **D,** Elevate the hand and wrist to help transfer the loop from the hand over the lip. **E,** Transfer the loop onto the upper lip. **F,** Avoid blocking the nostrils while placing the twitch.

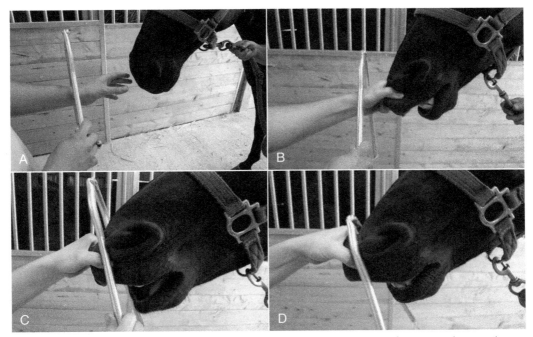

FIGURE 2-39 Placing a humane twitch. **A,** Approach to place the humane twitch. **B,** Grasp the upper lip. **C,** Proper placement of *the* humane twitch, with the lip within the straight portion of the twitch arms. **D,** Improper placement of the humane twitch, with the lip within the rounded portion of the twitch arms.

Stocks are not necessary for all procedures. They are most often used to protect the clinician from being kicked when working on the hindquarters. Stocks are also useful for standing surgical procedures during which the horse must be prevented from wandering. Horses are naturally suspicious of stocks and may need to be tranquilized before they are led into the stocks. Some horses may vehemently resist entering or staying in stocks, so stocks are not suitable or safe for every patient. Good judgment must be used. When young horses are being handled and resistance to stocks is observed, it can be extremely useful to encourage these young horses to walk completely through the stocks on several occasions before the gates are closed. This approach is often appreciated by clients and makes things go much faster

in the future because the horse did not have a bad experience. These situations can also become very dangerous, and so patience is a virtue.

Stocks usually have two gates, one at each end. Both gates are opened, and the handler leads the horse through the rear gate into the stocks. Once the horse has cleared the rear gate and the handler has cleared the front gate, an assistant quietly closes the rear gate. The handler or assistant closes the front gate. If there are four gates, as in Figure 2-42, the top rear gate should be closed first, then the bottom rear gate, followed by the top front gate and finally the bottom front gate. When releasing the horse from the stocks, the front bottom should be opened first to prevent a horse from jumping out of the stocks, followed by the top front. Any adjustments to the side rails then can be made, if necessary, although it is generally best to have

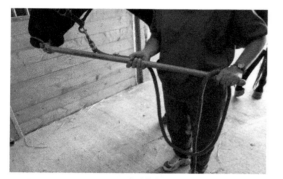

FIGURE 2-40 Proper way to hold the twitch. The lead rope is not wrapped around the twitch handle. Mechanical twitches should *never* be applied to foals and should never be applied to the ears. Twitching the lower lip is possible but not advisable because many horses rear or throw their heads in response.

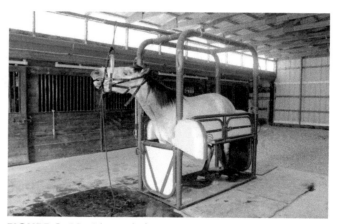

FIGURE 2-42 When multiple gates are present on stocks, it is important to close gates in a systematic fashion to avoid injury. When removing a horse from the stocks, it is important to open the bottom gate first; this helps prevent a horse from trying to jump out.

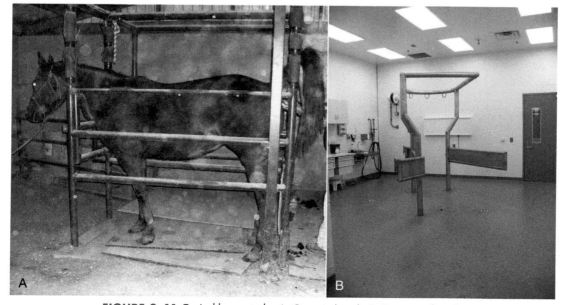

FIGURE 2-41 Typical horse stocks. **A,** Occupied stock. **B,** Unoccupied stock.

made the adjustments before the horse entered because the noise and movement may startle the horse. Occasionally, it may be dangerous for the handler to walk through the stocks with the horse. If sedation of the horse is not effective or feasible, the handler can remain outside the stocks and carefully try to guide the horse through the gates.

Temporary makeshift "stocks" can be made on the farm by stacking straw or hay bales to prevent personnel from being kicked or to limit a horse's motion.

Horses should *never* be left unattended while they are confined in any type of stocks.

Restraint of Foals

Capturing and restraining foals always begin with catching and controlling the mare. Foals naturally follow their dams, so leading the mare essentially results in leading the foal. Having assistants walk calmly behind the pair encourages the foal to move forward and stay close to the mare. Older foals may be accustomed to a halter and lead rope but naturally want to follow and be near the mare.

Controlling the mare is important for the safety of personnel because some mares may be aggressive in attempting to protect their foals. Therefore, someone should always be responsible for restraining the mare. In general, mares become more resistant as the distance between them and the foal increases. The best results with the mare usually come when she is allowed to be as close as possible to the foal and is able to see and hear what is happening. Sometimes the mare must be sedated to assist working safely on the foal.

Once the mare is controlled and the foal is in the desired enclosure (e.g., stall, paddock), approach the foal slowly from the side. Touching the foal on the neck or withers simulates the natural approach of the mare, but human touch is seldom appreciated at this age, and most foals instinctively try to escape by bolting forward, rearing, kicking, or "hitting reverse." Therefore, once you make contact, it should be quick and purposeful. To restrain a foal properly, place one arm around the foal's shoulders or base of the neck; control the hind end by placing your arm around the hindquarters or by using a tail hold with the hand (Figs. 2-43 and 2-44). The restrainer should avoid putting his or her head directly above the head or neck of the foal because many foals rear or throw their heads in an effort to resist being held.

Try not to oversupport a foal's body weight. Foals have a tendency to sag toward the ground when this is done.

For procedures that must be performed with the foal in lateral recumbency on the ground, the foal should be sedated first and then gently laid on the ground by lifting the foal's body up and over. Unsedated foals should not be thrown to the ground unless sedating them first is medically contraindicated or impossible to accomplish. Once a foal is on the ground, three people can provide ideal restraint. One person keeps pressure on the foal's neck to keep it from struggling to rise; this person may use hand pressure or gentle pressure by kneeling along the crest of the neck (never the

ventral aspect of the neck, which could obstruct breathing). Another restrainer is responsible for the front legs, by using the hands to grasp each leg just above the carpus of the front limbs. The third restrainer grasps both hindlimbs just above the tarsus. Grasping the legs below the carpus or tarsus runs the risk of growth plate fractures of the lower leg if the foal struggles. If additional control of the lower legs is required, the restrainers can straddle the lower legs and secure them between their own legs while keeping their hold above the carpus or tarsus.

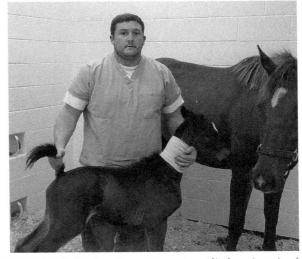

FIGURE 2-43 The handler *must* move in swiftly from the side of the foal, capture the tail first, and sweep the arm under the neck of the foal. At the same time, the mare handler must move the mare to a safe location. (From Bassert JM, McCurnin DM: *McCurnin's clinical textbook for veterinary technicians,* ed 7, St. Louis, 2010, Saunders.)

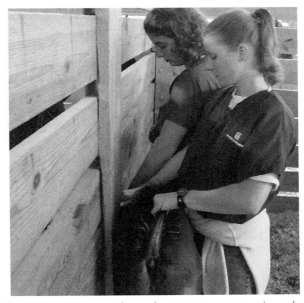

FIGURE 2-44 Two people may be necessary to capture larger foals. The first person enters from the rear, and the second comes around behind the mare and grabs the foal under the neck. The foal is then moved toward a solid wall for support. (From Bassert JM, McCurnin DM: *McCurnin's clinical textbook for veterinary technicians,* ed 7, St. Louis, 2010, Saunders.)

If it is necessary to have a foal stand when it is lying down, one can run fingers briskly up the spine, starting at the tail and moving toward the head. This simulates licking of the foal by the mare and almost always encourages the foal to stand.

CHEMICAL RESTRAINT OF HORSES

A summary of drugs used for sedation in horses can be found in Chapter 10.

PHYSICAL RESTRAINT OF CATTLE

Cattle show different behaviors according to their breed, sex, and age. Breed usually determines the destiny of cattle by classifying them as either a beef breed or a dairy breed. Beef and dairy cattle life cycles, husbandry, and handling are dramatically different. Before entering the feedlot, beef animals are largely maintained in open range or field settings and are only occasionally handled by humans. They do not often develop trust in humans and therefore resist handling and restraint. They are very suspicious of enclosures such as pens and *chutes*. Dairy animals, especially females, are handled more frequently because of periodic milking. Therefore, dairy cows tend to be easier to handle than their beef cattle counterparts.

Because of the size and strength of these animals, they should not be underestimated; even an apparently docile individual can become exceedingly dangerous to handle in some circumstances. *Bulls* of all breeds typically are unpredictable and aggressive and should never be trusted; "never turn your back on a bull" is good advice. Dairy bulls, in particular, are regarded as some of the most dangerous domestic animals to handle and restrain. Cows with *calves* are often aggressive in an effort to protect their calves and can inflict serious injury. The herding instinct is strong in cattle. When they are completely separated from others, as is necessary for some procedures, they may struggle violently to rejoin the herd. Some cattle will even try going over or through fences or other objects that stand in their way of rejoining the herd. Cattle tend to remain calmer when they can see other cattle.

Most veterinary procedures on cattle require two stages of animal handling. First, the individual must be separated from the herd; and second, the individual must be restrained appropriately for the procedure.

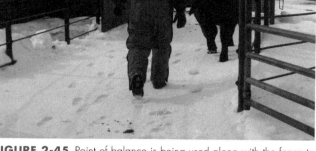

FIGURE 2-45 Point of balance is being used along with the fence to move the cow into the tub. (From Sheldon CC, Sonsthagen T, Topel JA: *Animal restraint for veterinary professionals*, St. Louis, 2006, Mosby.)

Moving and Herding

Each farm presents a unique layout of fences, pastures, barns, and facilities for separating individuals from the herd. The usual method of separation begins with driving a group of cattle containing one or more desired individuals into a smaller working area, such as a corral or pen.

Herding cattle must be done as calmly as possible. Cattle should not be made to move any faster than a walk. The shoulder area is critical to moving cattle; if approached from behind the shoulder, cattle generally move forward (Fig. 2-45).

If approached from in front of the shoulder, they tend to move backward. The shoulder is referred to as the *point of balance* for this species. Loud noises and rapid motions should be avoided. Once a group of cattle is suspicious of a situation, it can be difficult to gain control. Similarly, when moving groups of cattle toward enclosures and through gates, it is wise to keep unfamiliar vehicles, equipment, and personnel out of sight and quiet. Asking the farmer if assistance in herding the cattle is necessary, and, if so, how the famer wants to go about it is good practice; do not assume that help is needed or wanted.

After the cattle have been moved into a smaller pen, there will sometimes be a *tub* that crowds the animals up toward the alleyway (Fig. 2-46). Other designs may implement a Bud box. A Bud box is a dead-end pen that takes advantage of cattle's natural instinct that, when blocked, they want to return to where they came from and they want to go around things when they feel pressure from them (Fig. 2-47). Once the cattle have entered the alleyway, they often are reluctant to move forward unless they perceive that they will have a way out of it (Fig. 2-48).

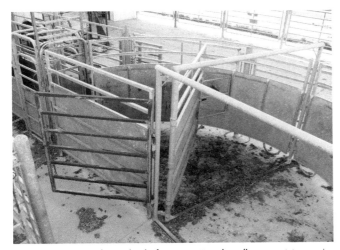

FIGURE 2-46 The "tub" before *entering* the alleyway. Notice the movable wall that can be pushed forward to crowd the animals toward the alleyway.

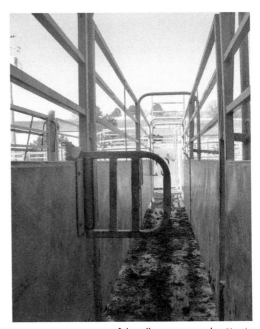

FIGURE 2-48 Appearance of the alleyway to cattle. Shadows in the *alleyway* are one of the reasons cattle do not like to move freely through alleyways. Also, notice the appearance of a dead end. Cattle typically do not travel through areas that appear to have a dead end.

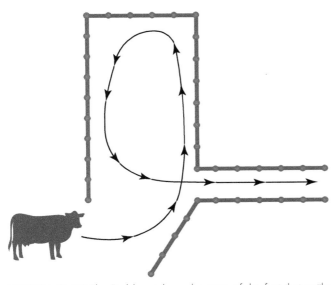

FIGURE 2-47 The Bud box takes advantage of the fact that cattle want to move back the way from which they came.

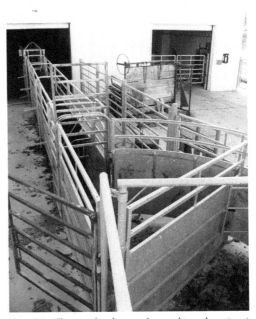

FIGURE 2-49 Alleyway leading to the working chute just inside the building.

The alleyway is a narrow walkway designed so that cattle must walk through it in single file. The alleyway typically leads to a working chute, which provides head and body restraint for one animal at a time (Fig. 2-49). A single animal enters the working chute and is restrained there while procedures are performed. Afterward, the animal is either released back to the herd or separated from the herd; the latter is usually called sorting off.

Some alleyways contain *backstops*. Backstops are springloaded panels that can be pushed forward as the animal moves through the chute and then pop back into place once the animal is past the chute (Fig. 2-50).

Backstops do not allow the animal to back all the way down the alley after it has been moved forward. Backing down the alley is a common behavior seen in cattle being handled within the alleyway. When backstops are not available, some people use steel or wood posts inserted behind the cattle to prevent backing behavior in the alleyway.

Tailing is used to encourage cattle to move forward. The middle of the tail is grasped and twisted forward to one side or the other, over the back and off the midline (Fig. 2-51). Firm pressure is applied, but excessive pressure can fracture

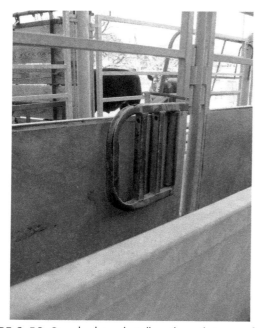

FIGURE 2-50 Open backstop that allows the cattle to move forward.

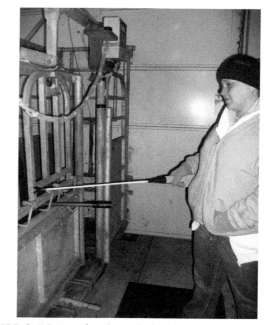

FIGURE 2-52 Use of cattle prods should be reserved for encouraging animals to move when other methods have failed. The prods should be used judiciously and briefly and applied only to areas with sufficient muscle mass.

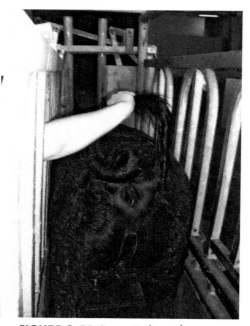

FIGURE 2-51 Proper "tailing" of a steer.

the tail. This maneuver creates some discomfort, and the usual response of the cow is to walk forward, away from the pressure. Again, do not stand directly behind the animal while tailing it. You must also be extremely careful not to break the tails of the animals you are trying to encourage to move.

Use of electric *cattle prods* is reserved for encouraging animals to move when other methods have failed. These devices should be used judiciously and briefly, and they should be applied only to body areas with sufficient muscle mass (Fig. 2-52). They should never be applied to the head. Sometimes just the noise of the activated prod provides enough

encouragement to move an animal without actually applying the prod to the animal.

> **TECHNICIAN NOTE**   Use of electric cattle prods should be reserved for use only after other methods have failed.

Chute Restraint

At the end of the alleyway you will find a cattle chute. The animal is encouraged to enter the chute by giving the impression that it can walk all the way through it. As the animal tries to walk forward out of the chute, however, the end of the chute has a mechanism, called the head catch, which traps the neck between two vertical bars (Fig. 2-53). The bars close down to a width that neither the head nor shoulders can fit through, thereby greatly limiting the ability of the animal to move forward or backward. However, the head and neck can move up and down and from side to side (Figs. 2-54 and 2-55). When handling cattle in chutes, it is extremely important to remember that the head can become a dangerous weapon, and you should always be aware of their ability to use it that way.

> **TECHNICIAN NOTE**   Cattle are encouraged to enter the chute by giving them the impression that they can walk all the way through it. This is achieved by keeping the head gate open as they enter the chute.

This restraint presents great danger to personnel and to the animal because throwing the head violently is the animal's primary method of defense. Until and unless the head

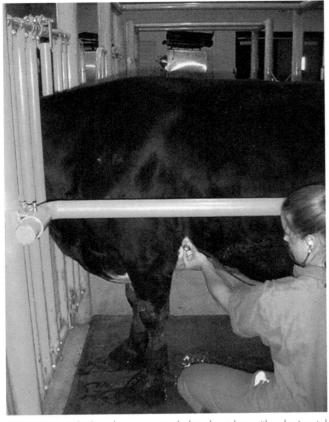

FIGURE 2-53 *Stanchions* are simple head catches with a horizontal single bar on the sides and an open rear area. (From Sheldon CC, Sonsthagen T, Topel JA: *Animal restraint for veterinary professionals*, St. Louis, 2006, Mosby.)

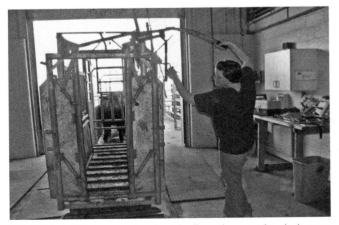

FIGURE 2-54 An open head catch allows the animal to think it can walk completely through the chute.

is fully restrained, the operator should never place his or her body in a position to be struck by the animal's head because the power of a head strike can result in severe personal injury.

> 🖋 *TECHNICIAN NOTE* Until the animal's head is fully restrained, the operator should never place his or her body in a position to be struck. The power of a head strike can cause severe personal injury.

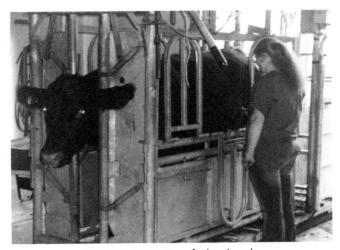

FIGURE 2-55 Use of a head catch.

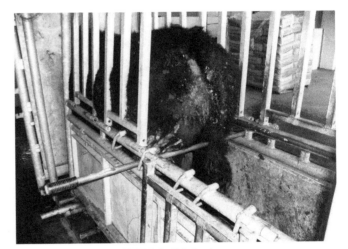

FIGURE 2-56 Posting up.

The method of applying the head catch bars depends on the chute design. Some chutes have self-closing head catch mechanisms that are activated by the animal's shoulders as it tries to walk through the chute; others must be closed manually. Handlers must be aware of the metal levers attached to the chute because sometimes the levers are triggered to move by tremendous speed and force, thus inflicting personal injury. Another type of chute is the hydraulic chute. All the moving parts for these types of chutes are operated by *hydraulics;* the head catch, *tail gate,* squeeze, and chute width all can be adjusted by the pull of a lever.

If the chute operator misses the head and the animal is allowed to escape, extra time is needed, and unnecessary stress is placed on the animal. Keep in mind that stress predisposes the animal to disease and decreases the animal's performance. Therefore, technicians should practice and become adept at catching. Once the animal is captured in the chute, you may see *posting* used to keep the animal forward in the chute (Fig. 2-56). Once the head is caught, cattle often pull back and brace their head against the head catch. "Posting up" cattle helps keep the animal forward and is beneficial when performing procedures on the head. Care should be taken always to hold the post with two hands, to ensure good control (Fig. 2-57). If the animal backs up during placement, it can throw the post and cause serious injury to personnel. The post should be placed so that it has little ability to move and is secured on both sides of the chute. When placing the

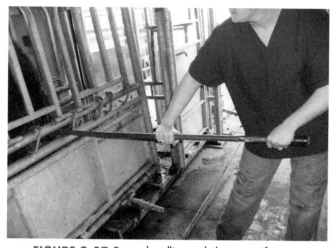

FIGURE 2-57 Proper handling and placement of a post.

bar, remember to stand behind the bar so you are behind the animal and *not* beside it. This is important because if the animal decides to back up during placement of the bar and you are in the wrong place, the animal will push on the bar, which can trap you between the bar and the chute. So always stay behind the animal behind the bar.

> **TECHNICIAN NOTE**   Always stay behind the animal, behind the bar!

> **TECHNICIAN NOTE**   Stress predisposes an animal to disease and decreases an animal's performance.

In addition to the head catch, working chutes may have adjustable side panels that close inward to touch the sides of the animal (squeeze chute), greatly limiting the ability of the body to move laterally. The side panels have bars that can be removed or folded down to allow access to the part of the body being worked on by the veterinary personnel. Only one drop-down side panel should ever be opened at one time, to prevent leg injuries if the animal is caught in the open panels (Fig. 2-58). The head catch is always applied first, and then

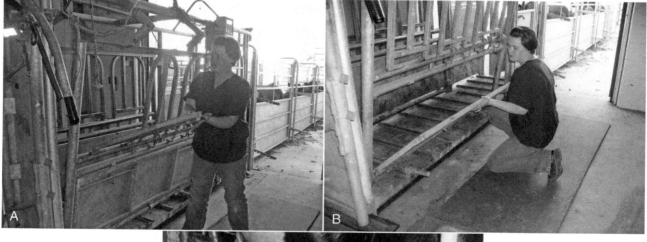

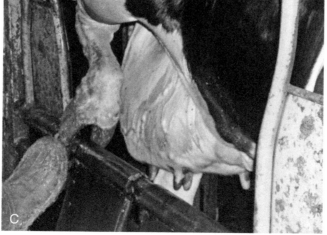

FIGURE 2-58 A, Side panels that can fold down to allow access to the animal. **B,** Another type of drop-down panel often used for semen collection, leg examinations, and urine collection. **C,** Example of a foot caught within a chute.

the squeeze is applied. To release the animal, the head gate is released and then the squeeze is released. A rear gate, if present, is not opened until the animal has exited the chute and materials are ready for the next animal. If the exit procedure is not performed in this order, the cattle often will back up in the chute. They then need to be encouraged to move forward again, and this wastes precious time when dealing with large herds.

Many of the chutes used for cattle also have a *palpation gate*/cage (Fig. 2-59). The palpation cage allows the producer or veterinarian access to the posterior half of the animal. Care should be taken when handling palpation gates. If latches do not work appropriately or if they are opened at the wrong time, they can swing open and allow the cattle to escape or cause serious injury to personnel.

Squeeze chutes and head catches designed for adult cattle are not suitable for use on calves or other large animal species. Chutes for use on these specific animals are available on the market for purchase. Careful attention must be given if an animal collapses or goes down in a working chute. The design of some chutes may occlude the trachea or blood flow to the head or may cause serious injury to the legs if they become wedged in the bars or rails. Some chutes have the ability to open an entire side (Fig. 2-60). This feature is helpful when animals collapse and are unable to gain their footing.

Other concerns that should be addressed when working cattle in a chute include the ability of an animal to injure a leg, which occurs most often when cattle are not being handled calmly. Personnel should have only one hand inside the chute, except with palpation cage use. Following this policy will help ensure the personnel some ability to release themselves if a limb were to become wedged in the chute.

Head Restraint

Head restraint may be applied to cooperative animals that have been trained to lead via halter. However, most individuals must be placed in a chute first before a halter can be applied. Once the animal's body is secured within the working chute and head catch, further restraint of the head may be desired. When applying head restraint, stay an arm's length away from the animal's head and avoid being in a position where you may be struck by any part of the head.

Rope cattle halters are perhaps the safest method of head restraint. Cattle halters are used to control the head by tying or securing the head to an immovable object by using a rope attached to the halter. However, unlike horses, few cattle are accustomed to being led by halter and lead rope; therefore, leading seldom is possible. Cattle halters typically are made of one continuous piece of rope, with a "slip" portion that allows adjustment for individual animals. The halter has two loops: a smaller loop designed to fit around the nose (nose loop or nose band) and a larger loop that goes across the *poll,* behind the ears (crown loop or head stall). The crown loop is loosened and placed first, and then it is passed over and behind the ears. When placing the crown loop it is important to toss it over the ears and catch the rope behind the poll and ears. This technique prevents you from having your fingers smashed between the animal's head and the chute because cattle typically tend to pull back and brace themselves against the head gate during this procedure.

> **TECHNICIAN NOTE**   Toss the halter over the ears of your bovine patients to avoid smashing your fingers.

The nose loop is placed at a level approximately halfway between the eyes and the nostrils. Finally, the free end of the rope is pulled to take up slack and tighten the halter. Once positioned, the halter should not be on or near the eyes, nor should the nose loop be so low that nostril breathing is occluded (Fig. 2-61).

> **TECHNICIAN NOTE**   When placing a halter, ensure the halter does not occlude breathing or scratch the animal's eyes.

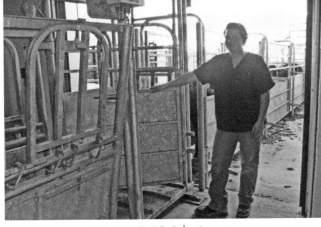

FIGURE 2-59 Palpation gate.

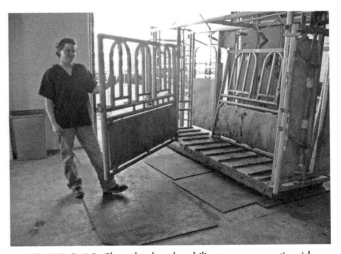

FIGURE 2-60 Chute that has the ability to open an entire side.

The free end of the rope may be used to pull or tie the head in position for the desired procedure.

Nose leads (cattle "nose tongs") are another method of head restraint. They apply blunt, pinching pressure to the nasal septum that creates discomfort and makes the animal reluctant to move. Nose tongs are not to be used as the only head restraint; they may be used to supplement a halter or head catch. Nose tongs usually have a rope attached to the handles; the rope can be used to pull or tie the head to either side for procedures. To apply the nose lead, it is helpful to take advantage of the animal's curiosity. Open the jaws of the tongs, go slowly toward the animal's nose, slip one ball tip into one nostril (Fig. 2-62, *A*), and then position the other ball tip in the other nostril and close the handles. This should be done as one rapid, smooth motion. When the handles are closed, slack is taken out of the attached rope (Fig. 2-62, *B*), which then can be used to handle and secure the instrument (Fig. 2-62, *C*). This device must be used carefully. If the animal falls or resists violently, the nasal septum may be torn. It is best not to tie nose tongs to an immovable object; however, if the rope must be tied, a quick-release knot should be used and closely attended. Nose tongs are not intended for use on calves.

> **TECHNICIAN NOTE**   Nose tongs should *never* be used as the only form of head restraint.

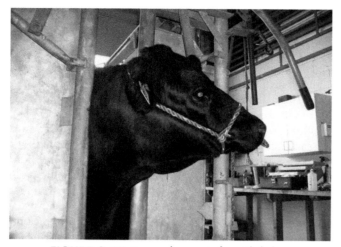

FIGURE 2-61 Proper placement of a cattle halter.

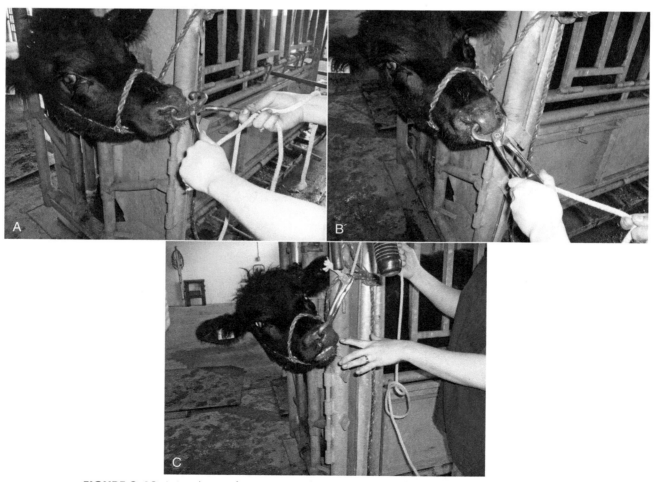

FIGURE 2-62 A, Introduction of nose tongs into the nose. **B,** Closing of nose tongs within each nasal cavity. **C,** Added restraint and control of the head through nose tongs.

Nose rings are placed through the nasal septum and are often used in bulls (Fig. 2-63). Ropes or poles can be attached to the nose ring for additional control of the head, but, as with nose leads, the nasal septum can be torn. Nose rings should not be used to tie the head for head restraint.

Tail Restraint

The tail of cattle is not as strong as the tail of the horse; the vertebrae are much smaller and are easily broken. The tail is never used to move or lift a recumbent cow. However, the tail may be used for restraint for short periods of time through the use of a tail hold *(tail jack)*. The tail hold is used to supplement other forms of restraint and may discourage (but not prevent) kicking.

The handler should stand behind the cow, but off to one side to avoid being kicked. The tail hold is applied by using both hands to grasp the tail close to its base, in the proximal third of the tail. The tail is lifted directly up and over the back, and constant pressure is applied toward the head while keeping the tail on the midline (Fig. 2-64).

Tying the tail out of the way is sometimes necessary for cleanliness during some procedures, but it is not used for restraint of the animal. The tail tie for cattle is performed similar to the tail tie for the horse, by using the hair of the switch to fold over twine, roll gauze, or narrow rope. Care must be taken not to incorporate the tail's vertebrae into the tie. The tail should be secured only to the animal itself (as in horses), rather than to an immovable object. The tail can be tied around the neck or over the back and around the opposite upper forelimb (Fig. 2-65).

Leg Restraint

Cattle are as capable as horses of delivering hard, fast kicks with the hindlegs "Cow kicking" refers to the common tendency of cattle to swing the kicking leg forward, then laterally, then out behind them. The handler can be struck with a hindleg kick even when he or she is standing by the animal's shoulder. It is a common misconception that cattle cannot

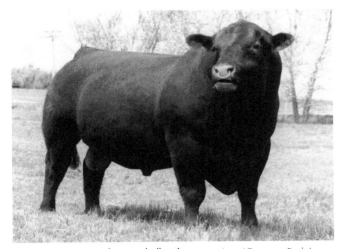

FIGURE 2-63 Red Angus bull with a nose ring. (Courtesy Red Angus Association of America, Denton, Texas.)

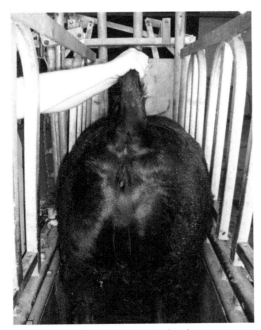

FIGURE 2-64 Tail jack.

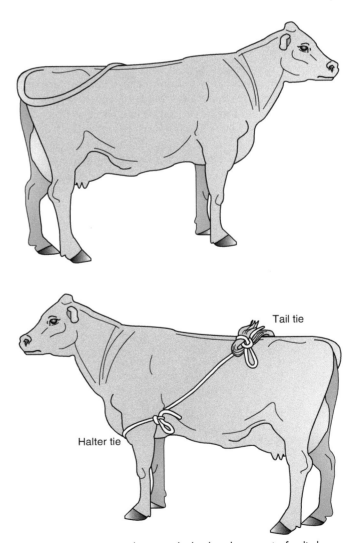

Tail tie

Halter tie

FIGURE 2-65 Tail tie over the back to the opposite forelimb.

simply kick straight behind (like a horse) or kick with both hindlegs at the same time.

Hobbles (sometimes called hobbles) are devices designed to prevent kicking. Various commercial and homemade devices are available to fasten to the hindlegs, either around the pasterns or over the common calcaneal tendons just above the hocks. Milking hobbles are popular among dairy farmers. They consist of two U-shaped metal bands connected by a chain that passes across the front of the hindlimbs (Fig. 2-66). The metal bands are placed over the common calcaneal tendons by holding a band in each hand and reaching across the front of the rear legs to apply the first metal band to the opposite rear leg. The band for the near leg is then quickly placed (Fig. 2-67). The handler should be prepared to move quickly if the cow kicks during placement of the bands.

Another method of discouraging kicking is use of pressure on the flank. This is most often done with a flank rope. A rope (with an eye on one end) is passed over the body of the animal just cranial to the udder (females) or the prepuce (males), encircling the body. The free end is passed through the eye and is pulled tightly to place pressure on the flanks (Fig. 2-68). Be careful not to place the rope directly on the udder or prepuce.

Another method to prevent kicking that uses the same concept of pressure on the abdomen is the anti-kick bar (Fig. 2-69).

Lifting legs is necessary to examine feet and trim hooves. Cattle seldom stand still to allow these procedures to be done. The animal should first be restrained in a chute or other appropriate manner. Occasionally, an animal may allow the leg to be lifted by hand, but most animals need the leg elevated with the use of ropes (Fig. 2-70). For lifting a front leg, a rope with an eye on one end is used to form a loop or double loop around the leg at or just above the *fetlock* area. The free end is then passed over the back of the animal or over a top rail of the chute for leverage as it is pulled to elevate the leg.

The rope should not be tied but rather held by an assistant so that the rope can be immediately released if the animal goes down. A second rope may be added if the leg needs to be pulled laterally after it is elevated.

The hindlegs must be extended and lifted to the rear of the animal. This requires a beam, pulley, or hook above and slightly behind the animal for leverage (Fig. 2-71). The rope is passed around the fetlock or hock and tightened; then the free end is passed over a beam or through a pulley or hook

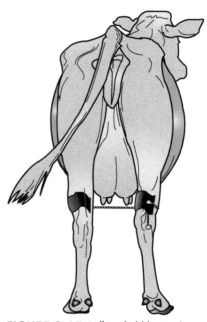

FIGURE 2-67 Milking hobbles in place.

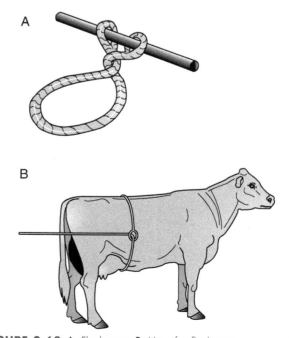

FIGURE 2-68 A, Flank rope. **B,** Use of a flank rope on a cow in a cattle chute. (From McCurnin DM, Bassert JM: *Clinical textbook for veterinary technicians,* ed 6, St. Louis, 2006, Saunders.)

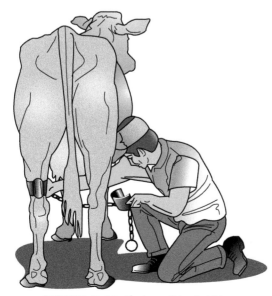

FIGURE 2-66 Placing milking hobbles.

behind and above the animal. Pulling on the free end elevates and extends the leg caudally.

Another method for restraining feet is a tilt table. A tilt table looks just like a regular chute, but, unlike a regular chute, the animal can be turned onto its side once it is restrained, which allows easy access to the animal's feet and legs. Small tilt tables are available for calves and small ruminants. Tilt

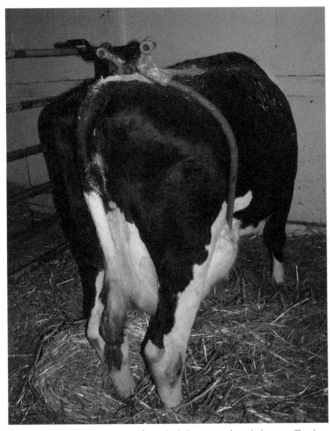

FIGURE 2-69 Placement of anti-kick bar over the abdomen. The bar can be tightened after it is in place. (From Sheldon CC, Sonsthagen T, Topel JA: *Animal restraint for veterinary professionals*, St. Louis, 2006, Mosby.)

tables provide secure strapping for the body, head, and legs. Sedation is sometimes required to "table" the animal (Fig. 2-72). If lateral recumbency is anticipated to last longer than 30 minutes, it is advisable to withhold food and water from the animal for several hours to reduce the risk of bloat and regurgitation.

Casting

Casting is a method of forcing an animal to the ground, usually with ropes. Unlike casting horses, casting cattle is relatively simple, performed by using ropes to apply firm, constant pressure to sensitive points on the body. The animal responds by lying down, usually with little struggling (Fig. 2-73). Once the animal is down, its legs may be tied if necessary for the procedure. Several configurations of casting "harnesses" have been described. It is important not to trap the udder, prepuce, or scrotum in the body ropes. Control of the head should be gained before any method of casting is applied (Fig. 2-74).

Recumbent ruminants are susceptible to bloat of the rumen or reticulum. Risk of bloat can be minimized by placing the animal in sternal recumbency, although this position is seldom feasible for most procedures that require casting. If lateral recumbency is required, right lateral recumbency is preferred; this positions the rumen uppermost, where it can be observed for signs of bloat. All efforts should be made to minimize the time an animal lies in any recumbent position.

> **TECHNICIAN NOTE** If possible, place cattle in right lateral recumbency to monitor for signs of bloat.

Recumbent Animals

Cattle usually stand up when a human enters their immediate area. Occasionally, an animal may not rise or may have physical conditions that make it reluctant to rise. If the animal must be placed onto its feet and the animal is capable, the handler should stand along the backside of the animal, never between

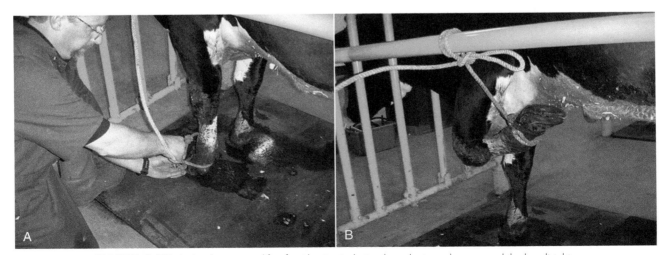

FIGURE 2-70 A, Another way to lift a front leg in stocks involves placing a loop around the leg distal to the fetlock. **B,** The rope is tied around the stock bar with a quick-release knot. (From Sheldon CC, Sonsthagen T, Topel JA: *Animal restraint for veterinary professionals*, St. Louis, 2006, Mosby.)

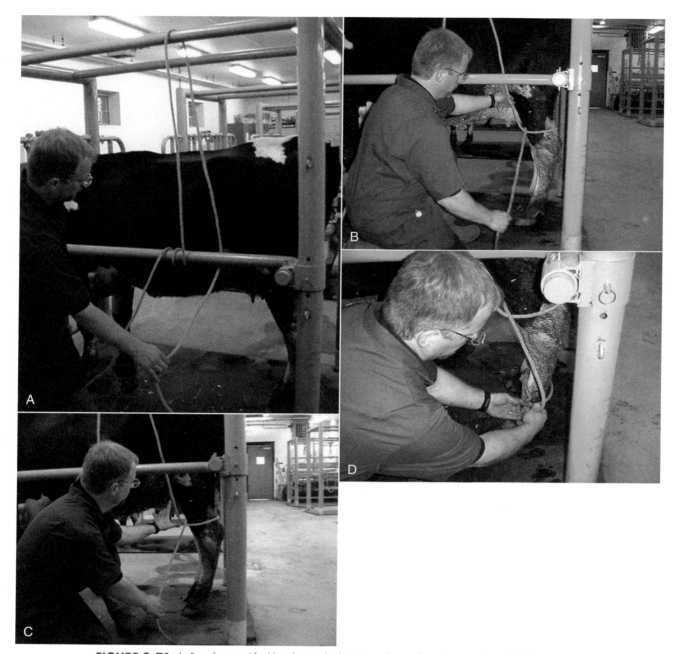

FIGURE 2-71 A, Rear feet are lifted by placing the lariat over the top bar, by using the end of the rope on the outside of the chute to place a half hitch around the side bar. **B,** With the other end of the rope, place a half hitch above the hock so that the end comes out on the lateral side. **C,** Never sit when doing this procedure. Kneel with one knee up so that you can fall back out of the way if the cow kicks. **D,** Form a loop and hook it into the honda distal to the dewclaw.

the legs or by the head. The back, rib, or thigh area can be tapped, slapped, or poked with the hand or a blunt item, such as a stick, or gently rocked back and forth with the foot. The handler may also thrust his or her knees into the animal's back and rib area. More severe instruments, such as a whip or electric cattle prod, should be reserved for cases where standing is absolutely necessary for assessment or treatment of serious or life-threatening situations and are best used by experienced personnel. Again, the animal's physical capability to stand should be determined before these devices are used.

> **TECHNICIAN NOTE**   When working with a recumbent animal, always work along the animal's spine to prevent being kicked.

Calf Restraint

Young calves are naturally curious and usually are easy to catch and restrain if the dam is not present. If a calf is with its dam, the calf will follow its mother into barns or small pens, but it also will use her as a shield to avoid capture. Separating the

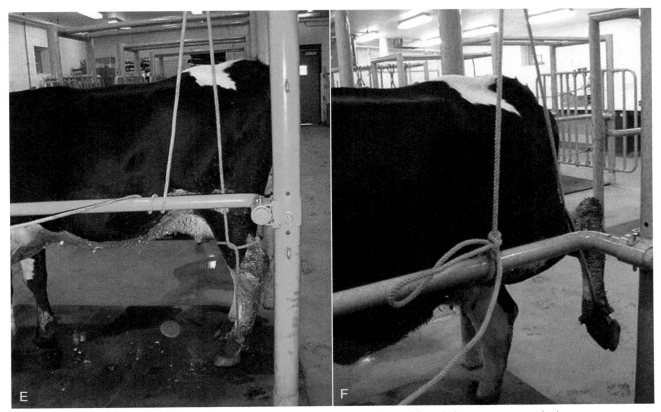

FIGURE 2-71, cont'd E, Pull on the rope that is wrapped around the side bar to start raising the leg. F, When the leg is lifted to the desired height (usually the hock above or level with the stifle), secure the rope by using a quick-release knot to prevent injury if the cow falls. (From Sheldon CC, Sonsthagen T, Topel JA: *Animal restraint for veterinary professionals*, St. Louis, 2006, Mosby.)

pair for the procedure or restraining the cow may be necessary. Be aware of the cow's protective instincts in these situations; a cow may become aggressive in attempts to protect her young.

To hold or guide a calf, place one arm around the front of the neck or chest. Wrap the other arm behind the hindquarters or grasp the base of the tail if more control is necessary. If a calf must be placed into lateral recumbency, it can be placed on the ground by "flanking." Standing alongside and facing the calf, reach both arms across the calf's back, down the side of the body, then under the calf's body to grasp the legs nearest to you. Then lift the calf off the ground and allow it to slide down your legs to the ground. Do not throw the calf to the ground; use your legs to ease the descent (Fig. 2-75). Once the calf is down, you can quickly place one knee over the neck and one over the back to keep the calf down while the procedure is performed (do not place your entire body weight on the calf, and do not occlude the trachea). Often, the legs are secured with rope loops above the pasterns that are tied with a quick-release knot; the procedure determines which legs need to be tied.

PHYSICAL RESTRAINT OF SHEEP

Sheep are timid animals. They do not seem to enjoy being stroked or petted. They are easily frightened but seldom respond with aggression. Any aggression is displayed as head butting or stomping of the front feet. When sheep are frightened, their usual response is to flee, and they may cause serious injury to themselves in their efforts to escape. They may even exhaust themselves to the point of collapse or hyperthermia trying to get away from perceived danger. Therefore, unlike other large animal species for which the handler is exposed to significant risk of injury when catching and restraining them, the primary concern when attempting to catch and restrain sheep is injuring the sheep themselves.

Moving and Herding

Like cattle operations, some sheep operations have a similar setup of alleyways and chutes. The only differences are the size and type of chutes used. Sheep have extremely strong flocking instincts and tend to behave as a group. When one sheep becomes nervous or fearful, the entire flock tends to follow suit; therefore, it may be impossible to gain any control once the flock is upset. Using a calm, quiet, patient approach is essential with these animals. Animal handling in this type of facility is similar to handling of cattle.

Individual Sheep Handling and Restraint

When an individual sheep needs to be restrained for a procedure, doing so often is easier without the use of a chute.

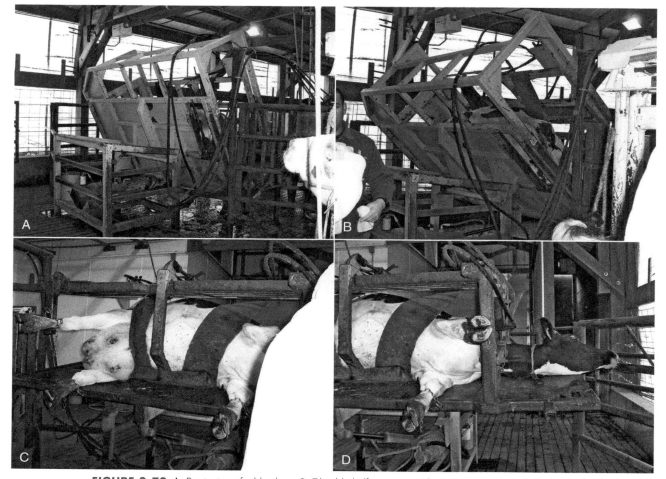

FIGURE 2-72 A, Beginning of table tilting. **B,** Tilt table halfway on its side. **C,** Proper restraint being used on a tilt table. **D,** Notice placement of the belts and the way the legs are secured.

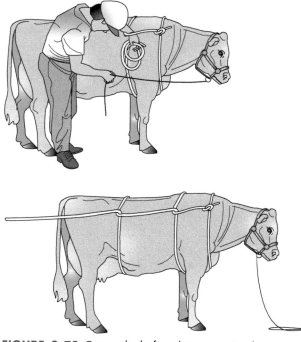

FIGURE 2-73 One method of applying a casting harness. Pulling caudally on the free end forces the animal to lie down.

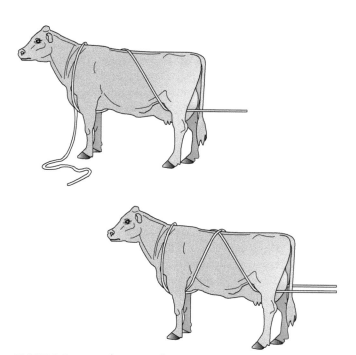

FIGURE 2-74 Burley casting harness. Pulling on the two free ends of the rope forces the cow to lie down.

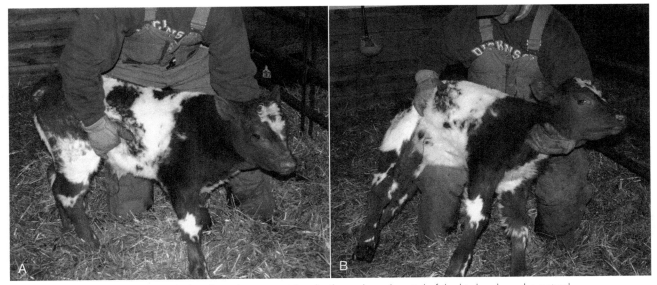

FIGURE 2-75 A, A calf can be supported under the neck, and control of the hind end can be gained with the other hand. **B,** If you are unable to grab the leg closest to you, grasp the flank of the calf and ease it to the ground using this method. (From Sheldon CC, Sonsthagen T, Topel JA: *Animal restraint for veterinary professionals,* St. Louis, 2006, Mosby.)

When catching sheep, several points are key. Individual sheep need to be separated from the flock. This is often accomplished by first driving the flock into an enclosure or pen and then cornering a single sheep against a fence or wall, where it can be handled. Hurdles (small, handheld wooden panels or sections of fence) are useful for limiting escape routes when trying to isolate an animal against a wall or in a corner. The sheep may try to flee by going through the fence or climbing along the fence or wall; therefore, these structures must be carefully chosen to minimize the risk of injury to the animal. Not much force is required to fracture the legs or vertebrae, so catching sheep by grabbing its legs or throwing it to the ground should be avoided. Another common tendency to avoid is catching sheep by grabbing the wool; this can easily pull out the wool and bruise or rip the skin, which is fragile. Grabbing by the horns (when present) must be done with care to avoid breaking them.

Sheep are held by circling the neck with one arm and placing the other arm around the rump. The rear end may also be controlled by placing an arm over the back to grasp the skinfold of the lower flank (Fig. 2-76).

Many procedures can be done by simply backing the sheep into a corner, straddling the animal between the handler's legs, and squeezing the sheep's shoulders firmly between the handler's legs (Fig. 2-77). The head or neck can be controlled in this position.

Procedures such as examination of the hooves, shearing, and vaccination require immobilizing the animal with a technique known as "setting up" the sheep. This method essentially sits the sheep down on its rump. Because the animal's feet do not have contact with the ground, the animal cannot struggle and basically becomes submissive to the handler. There are several methods of setting up sheep. The restraint is applied by standing to the side of the sheep, with

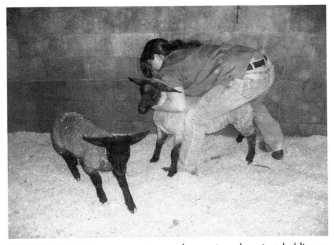

FIGURE 2-76 Proper capture and restraint when just holding a sheep for a procedure. Notice the excitement of the other lamb because of the presence of a human.

one hand under the neck and the other reaching across the back to grasp either the flank skinfold or the upper portion of the opposite hindleg or by reaching back under the abdomen to grasp the upper hindleg on the same side as the handler (Fig. 2-78). Once the hold is secured, the head is turned to face the rump, the sheep is lifted slightly off the ground, and the animal is set down (not thrown) on its buttocks on the ground in front of the handler (Fig. 2-79). The sheep is supported in a tilted-back sitting position against the legs of the handler, similar to a recliner. In this position, the handler's hands are free to perform procedures or restrain the front legs (Fig. 2-80). The animal can be lowered from this position into lateral or dorsal recumbency if necessary.

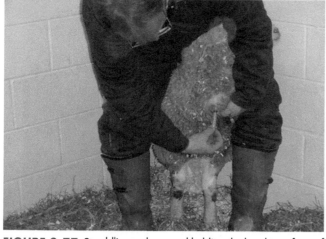

FIGURE 2-77 Straddling a sheep and holding the head as a form of restraint. (From Sheldon CC, Sonsthagen T, Topel JA: *Animal restraint for veterinary professionals*, St. Louis, 2006, Mosby.)

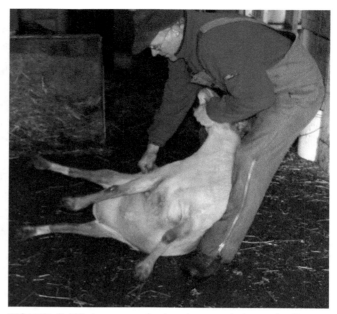

FIGURE 2-79 As you step back with your right leg and pull up on the flank, the sheep is thrown off balance, and you can pull it to a sitting position. (From Sheldon CC, Sonsthagen T, Topel JA: *Animal restraint for veterinary professionals*, St. Louis, 2006, Mosby.)

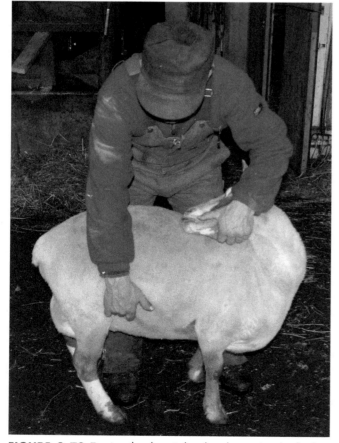

FIGURE 2-78 Turning the sheep's head and grasping the flank in preparation to set the sheep. (From Sheldon CC, Sonsthagen T, Topel JA: *Animal restraint for veterinary professionals*, St. Louis, 2006, Mosby.)

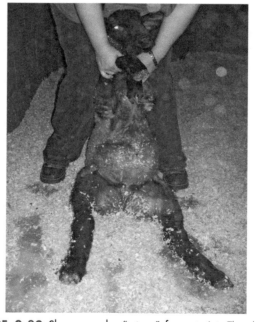

FIGURE 2-80 Sheep may be "set up" for restraint. The sheep is in proper position on its rump. Note the reclined position of the sheep against the handler's legs.

Another type of restraint is the shepherd's crook. Shepherd's crooks are properly applied around a hindleg, at the level of the hock or above. Placing the crook below the hock risks fracturing the leg. Once the hindleg is caught, the handler quickly moves in to grasp the sheep as described earlier. The crook may cause trauma if it is placed around the neck because it is not intended for this location.

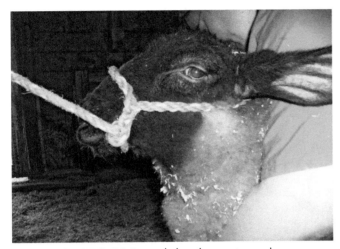

FIGURE 2-81 Proper halter placement on a sheep.

Halters are also another form of restraint. Most sheep are not halter broken and will not walk on halter, but a halter can be useful for gaining head control or tying an animal. The halter is similar to that of a cattle halter but smaller (Fig. 2-81).

Lamb Restraint

Small lambs are carried by placing one hand under the body and between the forelimbs to support the sternum and the other hand around the neck (Fig. 2-82).

Castration and tail docking are performed at an early age, usually in the first to second week of life. For these procedures, the lamb is restrained in dorsal recumbency with its back in the handler's lap or against the handler's body. The head is placed against the handler's body, and the right limbs are held (above the fetlock) by the right hand; the left limbs are held by the left hand.

PHYSICAL RESTRAINT OF GOATS

Although similar in size to sheep, goats are entirely different in temperament and behavior. Goats are gregarious and seem to enjoy the company of other species of animals.

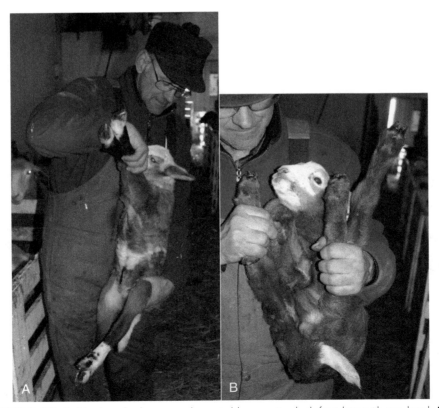

FIGURE 2-82 A, Newborn lambs are easily carried by grasping both front legs with one hand. **B,** Tilt the lamb back to expose its tail and scrotum. (From Sheldon CC, Sonsthagen T, Topel JA: *Animal restraint for veterinary professionals,* St. Louis, 2006, Mosby.)

They are inquisitive and often respond to human touch and affection (Fig. 2-83).

Goats may show aggression, usually in the form of head butting. This behavior is usually preceded by raising of the hair on the spine, stamping of the front feet, and making a characteristic sneezing or snorting noise. Head butting can cause significant personal injury, regardless of whether horns are present. *Bucks* (intact male goats) may be especially aggressive during the breeding season.

> **TECHNICIAN NOTE**   Goats are gregarious.

Moving and Herding

Goats do not have the same flocking instinct as sheep and show more of a tendency toward independent behavior. If herded like sheep or cattle, the group often fragments and scatters. Goats form a social hierarchy within a group, and dominant males and females can be identified. If the dominant goat in the group can be identified, leading that individual to the desired location often causes the others to follow. Goats are not commonly handled in alleyway and chute systems.

Head Restraint

Goats can be restrained by the beard, if present. One hand is used to grasp the beard while the other arm is placed around the neck to control the head. The beard can be handled firmly and can even be used to lead the goat, but it should not be used to apply unnecessary force or punishment (Fig. 2-84). Horns, if present, can be used for head restraint. Horns should be held near their base. Rough handling by the horns often is resented. Goats resent being held by the ears, and owners consider ear restraint to be abusive. Goats can also be placed in lateral recumbency by using the method shown in Figure 2-85.

Goats can be handled with chains, which provide a convenient way to hold onto the animal (Fig. 2-86).

Leg Restraint

Front legs are elevated by grasping the leg at the fetlock and lifting it so that it bends at the knee. The leg can be held in one hand or rested on the handler's knee. Rear legs are also lifted by the fetlock and brought out slightly behind the goat (Fig. 2-87). Legs should always be lifted to a comfortable position for the goat; otherwise, the goat will resist.

Kid Restraint

Small kids usually are held in the lap for procedures such as dehorning (Fig. 2-88). The kid is placed in sternal recumbency on the handler's lap by folding its front legs beneath it. The handler's forearms are placed on the kid's back and pressed down to keep the kid from rising. The hands can be used to control the head. Kids may also be held in dorsal recumbency in the lap or against the handler's legs, the same way as for lambs.

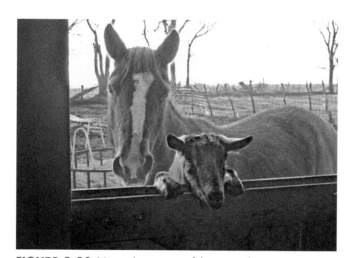

FIGURE 2-83 Notice the curiosity of this goat when someone enters the barn.

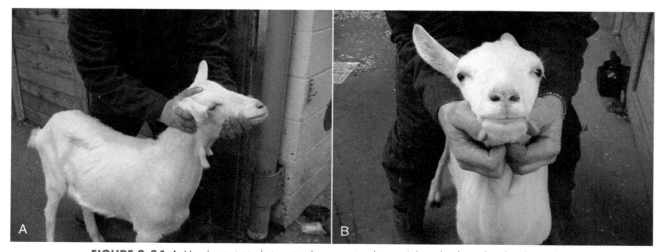

FIGURE 2-84 **A,** Head restraint technique involves grasping the goat's beard with one hand and encircling its neck with your other hand to stabilize its head. **B,** Use of the mandible as a form of head restraint. (From Sheldon CC, Sonsthagen T, Topel JA: *Animal restraint for veterinary professionals,* St. Louis, 2006, Mosby.)

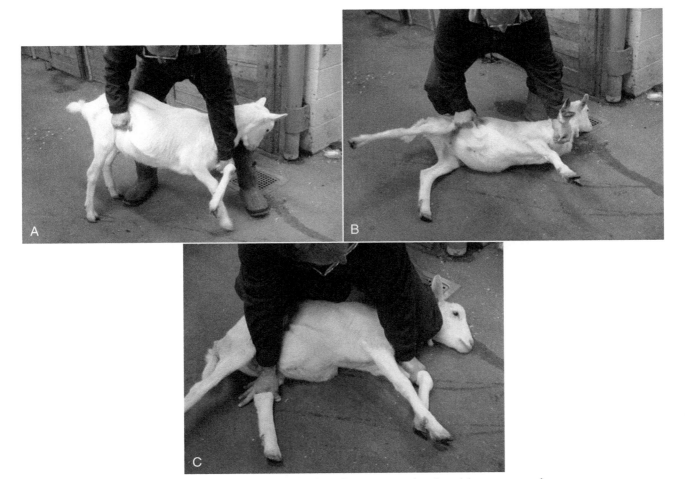

FIGURE 2-85 A, Reach over the goat's back, and grasp its near front leg while you use your forearm to control its head and neck. **B,** Raise its back legs by grasping its flank and lifting. **C,** Gently and carefully put the goat down onto the ground. Once the goat is down, firmly hold all four legs, and gently press your knee on the goat's neck to keep the animal recumbent. (From Sheldon CC, Sonsthagen T, Topel JA: *Animal restraint for veterinary professionals,* St. Louis, 2006, Mosby.)

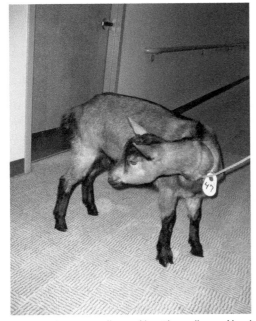

FIGURE 2-86 This goat walks readily with a collar and leash. Notice the ease of identification with neck tags.

PHYSICAL RESTRAINT OF CAMELIDS

Camelid restraint typically is a combination of equine and *bovine* (cattle) restraint methods. Although camelids are generally gentle, some can be aggressive or spit regurgitated stomach contents at humans when annoyed.

> **TECHNICIAN NOTE** Camelids spit regurgitated stomach contents at humans when they are annoyed.

With simple observation of the camelid's ears and tail, the technician can gather an idea about the animal's state of mind. A relaxed camelid holds its ears up. The ears are slightly rotated forward. The tail lies flat against the rectum. Camelids that are annoyed hold their ears back to the neck and when extremely annoyed hold them down on the neck. As they become more and more annoyed, the tail lifts off the rectum and into the air, sometimes even directly out from the body. Male camelids do not tend to be more aggressive than female camelids, as with other species of livestock, although orphan or bottle-raised male camelids can be extremely dangerous.

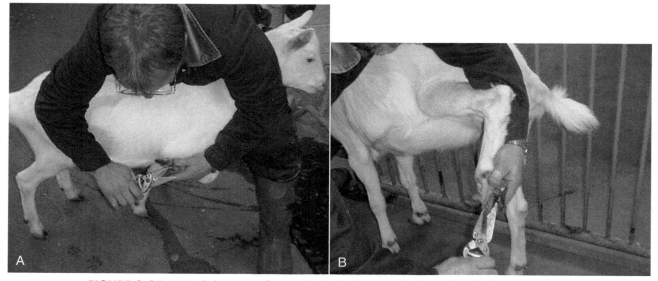

FIGURE 2-87 A, Forelimb restraint of a goat. **B,** Hindlimb restraint of a goat. (From Sheldon CC, Sonsthagen T, Topel JA: *Animal restraint for veterinary professionals,* St. Louis, 2006, Mosby.)

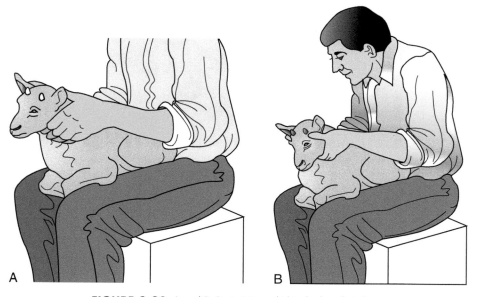

FIGURE 2-88 A and **B,** Restraining a kid in the handler's legs.

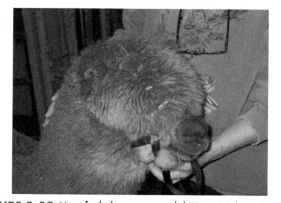

FIGURE 2-89 Use of a halter on a camelid. (From Niehaus A: Dental disease in llamas and alpacas. *Vet Clin North Am Food Animal Pract* 25:281-293, 2009.)

Some camelids are trained to walk on a halter and can be restrained in the same manner as a horse (Fig. 2-89). Halter placement on camelids should be performed as illustrated in Figures 2-90 to 2-92.

If biting is a problem, a muzzle can be placed over the halter to prevent biting. Otherwise, the restrainer can direct the head away from the personnel working on the animal to prevent their being bitten or being spat on. A towel can also be laid across the muzzle of the animal to prevent the handlers from being spat on.

When restraining a camelid, you can restrain the head of the animal as if you were restraining a dog (Figs. 2-93 and 2-94). Place one arm under the jaw and pull the head toward you; with your other hand you can push down on the shoulders or hold the tail up. Another approach is to form a

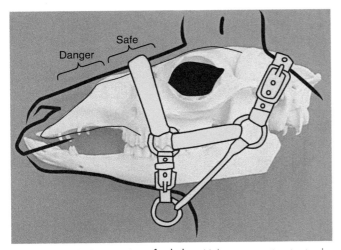

FIGURE 2-90 Construction of a halter. Halter construction is simple, but fitting a halter correctly is a complex procedure. (From Cebra C, Anderson D, Tibary A, et al, editors: *Llama and alpaca care: medicine, surgery, reproduction, nutrition, and herd health,* St. Louis, 2014, Saunders.)

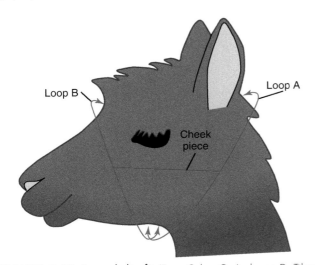

FIGURE 2-91 Proper halter fit. (From Cebra C, Anderson D, Tibary A, et al, editors: *Llama and alpaca care: medicine, surgery, reproduction, nutrition, and herd health,* St. Louis, 2014, Saunders.)

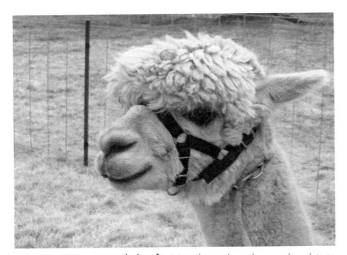

FIGURE 2-92 Proper halter fit. Note how close the noseband is to the eye. (From Cebra C, Anderson D, Tibary A, et al, editors: *Llama and alpaca care: medicine, surgery, reproduction, nutrition, and herd health,* St. Louis, 2014, Saunders.)

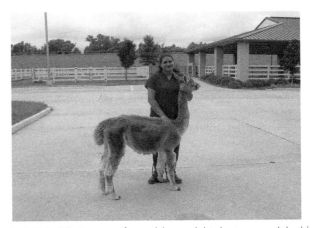

FIGURE 2-93 Restraint of an adult camelid is best accomplished by holding the head and neck close to the handler's chest while the other hand rests on the animal's shoulders with slight pressure. (From Bassert JM, McCurnin DM: *McCurnin's clinical textbook for veterinary technicians,* ed 7, St. Louis, 2010, Saunders.)

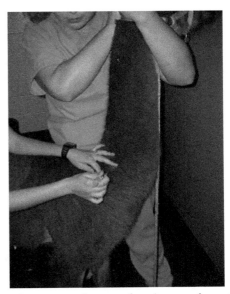

FIGURE 2-94 Two people can perform this type of restraint to allow more access to the neck. (From Jones M, Boileau M: Camelid herd health. *Vet Clin North Am Food Animal Pract* 25:254-263, 2009.)

bracelet around the camelid's head; this allows the camelid to keep its balance, which helps the animal to stand still during procedures (Fig. 2-95). Camelids can also be restrained in sternal recumbency (Fig. 2-96).

Most camelids are accustomed to being handled from the left. Direct eye contact should be avoided because camelids perceive this as danger. Contact with their ears also should be avoided.

Stocks and chutes can be used with camelids. The procedure is the same; however, if using a chute, do not place excessive squeeze on the animals because they will most likely lie down (Figs. 2-97 to 2-99). Tilt tables can be used for shearing (Fig. 2-100).

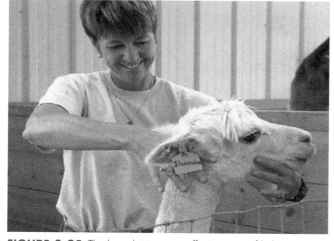

FIGURE 2-95 The bracelet is a very effective way of helping an animal remain in balance and therefore still. It is *not* a hold but a technique for using the head to keep the body in balance. (From Cebra C, Anderson D, Tibary A, et al, editors: *Llama and alpaca care: medicine, surgery, reproduction, nutrition, and herd health*, St. Louis, 2014, Saunders.)

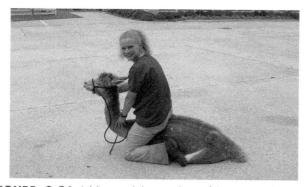

FIGURE 2-96 Adult camelids can be safely restrained in sternal recumbency or the cushed position. (From Bassert JM, McCurnin DM: *McCurnin's clinical textbook for veterinary technicians*, ed 7, St. Louis, 2010, Saunders.)

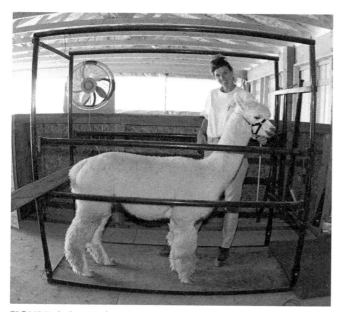

FIGURE 2-97 Stocks are commonly used for camelid restraint, but a combination of equine stocks and cattle procedures is used. (From Cebra C, Anderson D, Tibary A, et al, editors: *Llama and alpaca care: medicine, surgery, reproduction, nutrition, and herd health*, St. Louis, 2014, Saunders.)

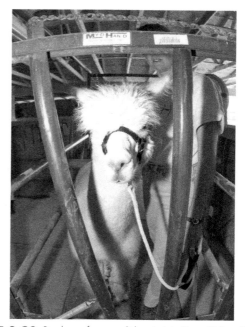

FIGURE 2-98 Stock use for camelid restraint. (From Cebra C, Anderson D, Tibary A, et al, editors: *Llama and alpaca care: medicine, surgery, reproduction, nutrition, and herd health*, St. Louis, 2014, Saunders.)

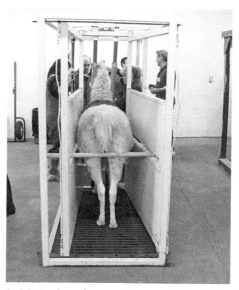

FIGURE 2-99 Stock use for camelid restraint. (From Cebra C, Anderson D, Tibary A, et al, editors: *Llama and alpaca care: medicine, surgery, reproduction, nutrition, and herd health*, St. Louis, 2014, Saunders.)

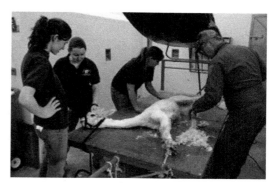

FIGURE 2-100 Use of a tilt table as a form of restraint.

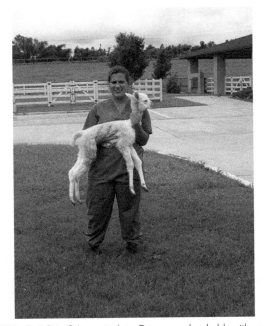

FIGURE 2-101 *Cria restraint.* Crias can be held with one arm around the chest and the other arm supporting the abdomen in front of the rear legs. (From Bassert JM, McCurnin DM: *McCurnin's clinical textbook for veterinary technicians,* ed 7, St. Louis, 2010, Saunders.)

Cria Restraint

Cria (baby camelid) heads can be restrained like adult heads. Your other arm should support the abdomen as the animal is held (Fig. 2-101).

PHYSICAL RESTRAINT OF SWINE

The method used to handle swine is determined largely by the age and size of an animal and the nature of the procedure to be performed. Swine have been described as stubborn but smart animals. They do not have a strong herd instinct, but they do prefer being with other pigs rather than being alone. Pigs are very vocal animals that express fear, panic, and stress by squealing and screaming. As with many species, when one animal in a group becomes fearful or distressed, the other members of the group tend to follow suit; therefore, it is wise for you to be calm.

Pigs are not athletic animals, but that does not mean they are slow. Smaller pigs especially can be quite agile and difficult to catch. Their legs are relatively thin and somewhat easily fractured; catching them or tying them by the legs must be done carefully.

Pigs may be aggressive; biting is their only real defense. Their teeth are sharp, and their jaws are powerful. It is very important to understand that an aggressive pig not only will stand its ground but also often will go after the object of its anger. It is a good idea to define the best "escape route" from a pen before entering it. Sows with litters are especially protective and should be approached with care, especially in an enclosed area. Boars with tusks should also be respected.

Swine are easily stressed by environmental heat. If they are further stressed by handling or other frightening situations, they can quickly become hyperthermic ("heat stroke"). Signs of heat stroke include dyspnea and open-mouth breathing, tail twitching, reluctance to move, muscle tremors, rigidity, and elevated rectal temperature. Because hyperthermia can be rapidly fatal, emergency efforts to cool swine are indicated when heat stroke is observed. Care should be taken when handling swine on hot, humid days.

Pigs dominate each other by biting the top of the neck. Handlers can take advantage of this behavior by pressing down with the hands or tapping with a cane on the top of the neck or back. Exerting this dominance before handling the pig often makes the handling easier.

Catching and Moving Swine

Moving and driving swine from behind in an open area are difficult because the pigs tend to pick their own direction to move. Instead, it is best to limit their choices; pigs respect solid barriers and tend to move away from them. Handheld wooden or plastic panels, called "hurdles," "pig boards," or "hog panels," are often used to separate and direct pigs in an open area (Fig. 2-102). Swine handlers usually carry lightweight canes that are used to tap on the animal when they wish to move it. Tapping on the hindquarters encourages the animal to move forward, and tapping with the cane on a shoulder helps move the pig to the right or left. When the hurdle and cane are used in combination, the animal usually can be successfully moved. Pigs can also be encouraged to move with the use of stick (Fig. 2-103).

Blindfolding a pig causes it to walk backward. A towel or bucket can be loosely placed or held over the head and a cane used to tap and direct the pig while it walks backward to the desired location. Tugging on the tail to either side can also be used to guide the direction of the pig.

Standing Restraint

The most common form of individual restraint is the *hog snare*. A snare consists of a pipe sleeve and a rope or cable that runs through it. The cable is looped on one end, and the other end is held in the operator's hand. The loop is tightened or loosened by pulling on the free end, like a noose. The loop is loosened, and the pig is approached. When the pig opens its mouth, the loop is quickly slid into the mouth and tightened to form a circle around the snout and upper jaw (maxilla), with the sleeve drawn tightly down on the top of the snout. Never use the snare on the bottom jaw (mandible) because it

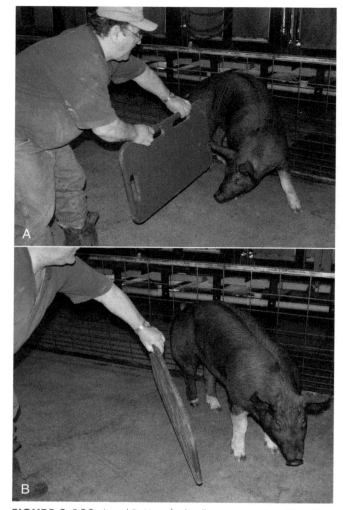

FIGURE 2-102 A and **B,** Use of a hurdle to move swine. (From Sheldon CC, Sonsthagen T, Topel JA: *Animal restraint for veterinary professionals,* St. Louis, 2006, Mosby.)

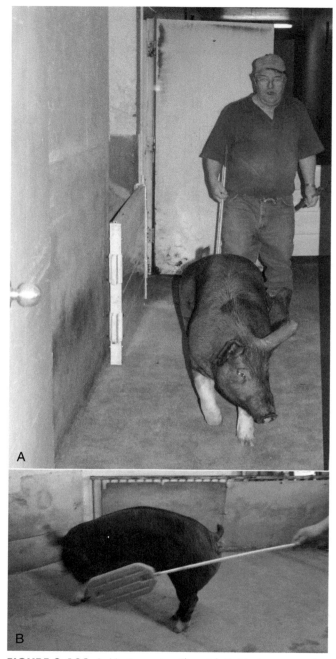

FIGURE 2-103 A, Moving a pig with a stick. **B,** Moving a pig with a paddle. (From Sheldon CC, Sonsthagen T, Topel JA: *Animal restraint for veterinary professionals,* St. Louis, 2006, Mosby.)

can easily be dislocated or removed. The snare should be used only on the maxilla. The operator should stand directly in front of the pig (Fig. 2-104). The natural response of the pig is to lean backward away from the snare; if the snare is not firmly in position, the pig can easily escape. When the hog snare is secured properly, minor procedures such as injections and blood samples can be performed. This form of restraint is for use on mature animals and never for use on piglets. It should not be kept tightened for long periods of time, generally less than 20 to 30 minutes. When used on boars with tusks, the loop should be placed behind the tusks. The snare should not be too high so that it irritates the eyes or too low in that it occludes breathing. Any signs of cyanosis should prompt removal of the snare. Snares can be obtained commercially or homemade from 1-inch pipe and a cable or rope.

> **TECHNICIAN NOTE**   Hog snares are a common form of restraint for adult swine but should not be used on piglets.

A similar form of restraint is the snubbing rope (Fig. 2-105). A rope with an eye at one end is used to form a simple loop. The handler can approach the pig from behind or from the front. The rope loop is dangled in front of the snout. When the mouth is opened, the loop is placed through the mouth and quickly tightened, and the handler stands in front of the pig for control. As with the hog snare, the natural reaction of the pig is to lean backward. The rope can be tied to a solid object if desired.

Both the hog snare and snubbing rope cause vocalization by the pig, and the squealing typically continues until the pig is

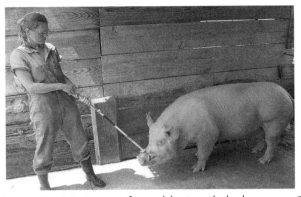

FIGURE 2-104 Capture of an adult pig with the hog snare. The handler approaches from the side of the pig and carefully loops the snare over the upper jaw just in front of the cheek teeth. After the snare is tightened, the pig obviously resents it and resists by pulling back against the snare. This allows the handler to brace against the pig and hold it steady for examination or sample collection. (From Bassert JM, McCurnin DM: *McCurnin's clinical textbook for veterinary technicians*, ed 7, St. Louis, 2010, Saunders.)

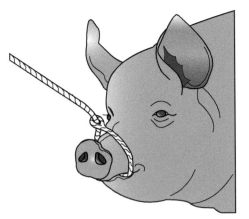

FIGURE 2-105 Snubbing rope.

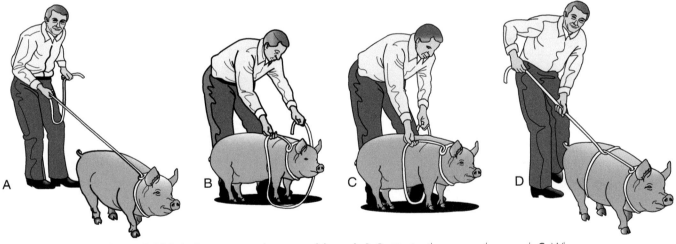

FIGURE 2-106 **A,** Passing a rope loop around the neck. **B,** Positioning the rope on the ground. **C,** When the pig steps through the rope, a half hitch is made in the rope. **D,** Rope harness in position and snugged down for restraint.

released. Pigs can produce extremely loud squeals and screams when they are restrained. Many pig farmers use earplugs, for good reason. Long-term exposure to this noise can damage hearing. Animals that have repeated experience with these forms of restraint can become adept at avoiding them.

> 📎 **TECHNICIAN NOTE**   Because of the squeals, it is advisable to wear earplugs if you will be working with swine on a regular basis.

A rope harness can be made for pigs. A rope with an eye is used to form a simple loop that is passed over the neck (Fig. 2-106, *A*). The free end of the rope is loosely placed on the ground just in front of the pig, and the handler stands behind the pig to encourage it to move forward (Fig. 2-106, *B*). When the pig steps forward through the loop, the handler passes the free end under the rope to form a half hitch that circles the pig's body (Fig. 2-106, *C*). The rope is drawn tightly (Fig. 2-106, *D*). The handler should be prepared for the pig to move quickly and unpredictably during the process of placing the harness.

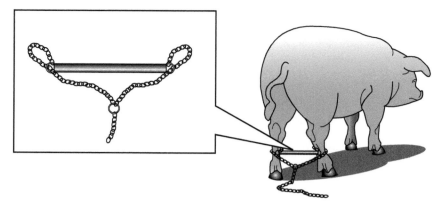

FIGURE 2-107 Placement of hobbles on the rear legs.

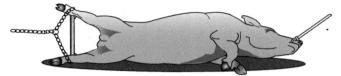

FIGURE 2-108 Casting restraint using hindleg hobbles.

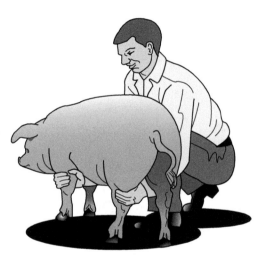

FIGURE 2-109 Casting is possible by hand.

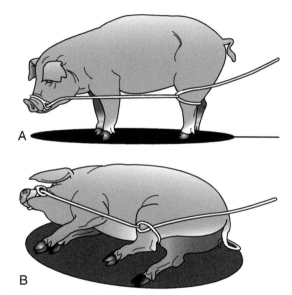

FIGURE 2-110 A, Placing a snubbing rope around a hindleg for casting. **B,** Pulling the snubbing rope produces recumbency.

Hindleg hobbles can be used to restrain an animal. The head is controlled with snout restraint, and the hobbles are placed around the hindlegs (Fig. 2-107). Standing behind the pig and pulling on the center rope pull the legs backward. The pig eventually loses balance and falls on its side. The hobbles can be left in place for the procedure (Fig. 2-108).

Casting and Trough Restraint

Before casting a pig, its head should be controlled with some form of snout restraint (hog snare or snubbing rope). The method used to cast the pig depends largely on the size of the animal. Smaller pigs can be manually cast by standing on the side of the pig and reaching under the pig's body to grasp the far side legs. Pulling the legs toward the handler causes the pig to fall to the ground, away from the handler (Fig. 2-109). Be sure the "landing area" is covered with something soft. Once the animal is down, the legs can be hobbled or tied.

A simple method of rope casting uses a snubbing rope as the casting rope. The snubbing rope is placed, and the free rope is used to circle a hindleg above the hock on the side opposite the desired direction of the fall (i.e., circle the left hindleg to produce right lateral recumbency) (Fig. 2-110, A). Pulling on the rope from behind the pig draws the nose back toward the leg, with resulting loss of balance and a fall to the ground (Fig. 2-110, B).

Some farms have crates, chutes, and head catches designed especially for swine. As an encouragement for pigs to enter these devices, the animals should be able to see clearly through the devices, and the device openings should look large enough for the pigs to fit through. Most of the head-catching devices are opened and closed by handheld levers.

Restraining V-troughs are economical restraining devices for smaller swine. Often they are portable and can be placed on tabletops or against fences or walls. The animal is lifted and placed on its back in the trough for most procedures, but

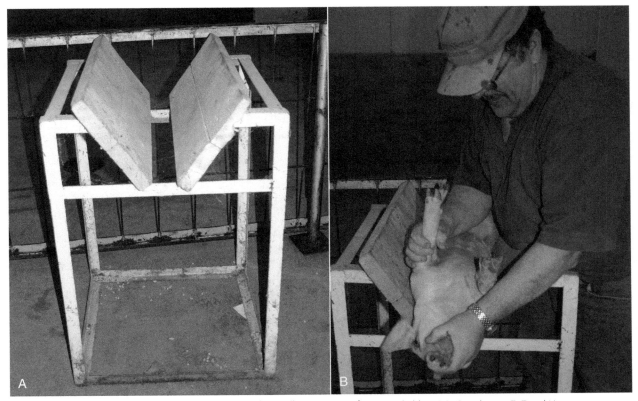

FIGURE 2-111 A and B, Restraint of a small pig in a trough. (From Sheldon CC, Sonsthagen T, Topel JA: *Animal restraint for veterinary professionals*, St. Louis, 2006, Mosby.)

the trough can be tilted from side to side to achieve more lateral positions if desired. Assistants can hold the animal's legs for the procedure, or the legs can be easily tied by looping a rope around one leg, passing it under the trough, and looping it around the opposite leg. Both front and back legs may be tied. The trough can be inclined according to the needs of the procedure (Fig. 2-111).

Restraint of Piglets
Baby pigs should be handled gently but firmly. They should not be chased unnecessarily and should not be caught or lifted by the ears. Piglets should not be lifted by the tail. Squealing piglets tend to upset the sow and other piglets,

so usually it is best to take the piglets to a separate room for procedures.

A very young piglet can be caught by grasping one or both hindlegs in one hand and lifting with the other hand under the body. Once the piglet is off the ground, release the leg and place that hand on top of the shoulders to secure the body firmly (Fig. 2-112). The piglet can also be held under the handler's arms.

Many procedures on piglets weighing up to 20 to 30 pounds are performed with the animal suspended by the back legs and its back supported against the handler's body or thighs. This position is commonly used for many procedures (Fig. 2-113).

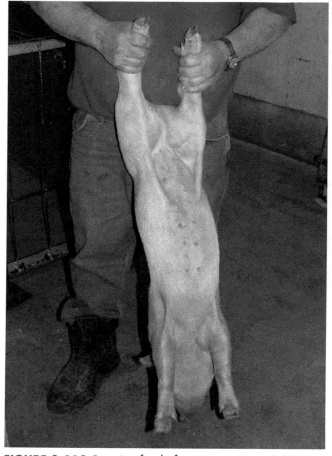

FIGURE 2-112 Restraint of piglet for castration. (From Sheldon CC, Sonsthagen T, Topel JA: *Animal restraint for veterinary professionals*, St. Louis, 2006, Mosby.)

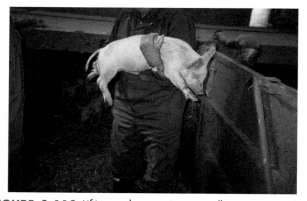

FIGURE 2-113 Lifting and supporting a small pig. (From Jackson PGG, Cockcroft PD: *Handbook of pig medicine*, St. Louis, 2007, Saunders.)

CASE STUDY

You arrive at Mrs. Volker's breeding farms. The client raises approximately 30 Arabian foals each year. She has informed you that there is a foal with a deep puncture wound in the pasture north of her house. She is unable to catch the foal and separate it from its mother. She asks you and the veterinarian to help her. What should you do?

CASE STUDY

You will be assisting in the treatment of a cow with cancer of the eye. Dr. Speece has asked you to bring the animal into the chute and prepare it for a physical examination. What path will the animal most likely take to enter the chute? What will you do to make entry into the chute less stressful on the cow and less frustrating for you? Once the animal is in the chute, how will you restrain it? If the animal resists restraint, what will you do? Will you leave the animal unattended to retrieve the veterinarian for the procedure?

SUGGESTED READING

Ball MA: Restraint techniques, *The Horse* Sept:34-37, 1995.

Bassert JM, Thomas JA, editors: *McCurnin's clinical textbook for veterinary technicians*, ed 8, St. Louis, 2013, Saunders.

French DD, Tully TN: Restraint and handling of animals. In Bassert JM, Thomas JA, editors: *McCurnin's clinical textbook for veterinary technicians*, ed 8, St. Louis, 2013, Saunders.

Fubini SL, Ducharme NG: *Farm animal surgery*, St. Louis, 2004, Saunders.

Gillespie JR, Flanders FB: *Modern livestock and poultry*, ed 8, Clifton Park, NY, 2010, Delmar Cengage Learning.

Pugh DG: *Sheep and goat medicine*, St. Louis, 2002, Saunders.

Sheldon CC, Sonsthagen T, Topel JA: *Animal restraint for veterinary professionals*, St. Louis, 2006, Mosby.

Sirois M: *Principals and practice of veterinary technology*, ed 3, St. Louis, 2011, Mosby.

Smith MC, Sherman DM: *Goat medicine*, Baltimore, 1994, Williams & Wilkins.

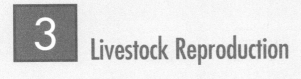

3 Livestock Reproduction

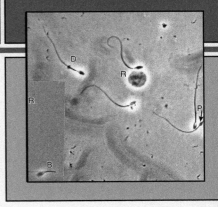

OUTLINE

LEARNING OBJECTIVES

After reading this chapter, you will be able to

- Demonstrate understanding of the normal course of events in the reproductive process
- Exhibit a knowledge of common selection methods used in large animal species
- Demonstrate understanding of the importance of selecting superior livestock to be used in breeding programs
- Understand and describe the components of a male reproductive examination
- Understand the process of synchronization, the categories of drugs that can be used, and the advantages of using these procedures
- Describe the importance of estrous cycle determination and how it can be achieved
- Understand the importance of artificial insemination and embryo transfer
- Describe different breeding systems
- Understand the normal course of parturition and how to address dystocia

KEY TERMS

Artificial insemination
Calf crop
Cesarean section
Chorionic gonadotropin
Crossbreeding
Dystocia
Electroejaculation
Embryo transfer
Estimated breeding value
Estimated progeny differences
Estrus synchronization
External preputial ring
Fetotomy
Flushing
Genetics

Gomer
Grade
Grading up
Hand mating
Harem
Heat detection
Heterosis
Inbreeding
Individual breeding
Linebreeding
Live cover
Lordosis
Mutation
Outcrossing
Paraphimosis

Parturition
Pedigree
Pen mating
Penile paralysis
Phimosis
Priapism
Purebreeding
Sheath
Sidewinder
Standing heat
Stillbirth
Superovulation
Teaser
Traction
Vasectomized

AI: Artificial insemination
AV: Artificial vagina
BCS: Body condition score
BSE: Breeding soundness examination
CASA: Computer-assisted semen analysis
CL: Corpus luteum
DSO: Daily sperm output
EBV: Estimated breeding value
eCG: Equine chorionic gonadotropin

EPD: Estimated progeny difference
FSH: Follicle-stimulating hormone
GnRH: Gonadotropin-releasing hormone
LH: Luteinizing hormone
PAG: Pregnancy-associated glycoprotein
$PGF_{2\alpha}$: Prostaglandin $F_{2\alpha}$
PSPB: Pregnancy-specific protein
SC: Scrotal circumference
TSW: Total scrotal width

THE IMPORTANCE OF REPRODUCTION

Reproductive efficiency is absolutely essential for the success of any livestock operation. In any large animal industry, extreme economic losses will often result if reproduction does not occur efficiently or poor decisions are made. The ultimate goal of the large animal industry is the delivery of live neonates. To produce a live neonate while being economically profitable, the following must occur:
- Selection of superior animals for breeding
- Successful breeding, usually accomplished with estrous cycle determination and reproductive examinations
- Successful conception using multiple breeding systems, *embryo transfer, artificial insemination (AI),* and *live cover*
- Successful implantation, which can be confirmed with use of pregnancy detection
- Successful gestation
Successful parturition, with addressing of any problems, such as dystocia, at the time of parturition.

> **TECHNICIAN NOTE** The ultimate goal of the large animal industry from a reproductive perspective is to deliver a live neonate.

SELECTION

Selection of livestock is extremely important because the animals that are chosen to breed will be the livestock that pass *genetics* to future generations. Care should be taken when choosing which animals should be bred. In general, more emphasis is placed on the selection of males for breeding than females. This is because males contribute a higher percentage of genetics to the herd than females.

> **TECHNICIAN NOTE** In general, more emphasis is placed on the selection of males for breeding than females.

Think about the following. Two *cows* are bred to the same *bull.* Each cow will have one calf. Of the two calves, the bull will contribute 50% of the entire genetic *calf crop.*

Each individual cow will only contribute 25% of the genetics to the entire calf crop. It would be rare to see a calf crop of two. Imagine the percentages if there were 100 cows. The bull still is contributing 50% of the genetics, but each individual cow is only contributing 0.5% of the genetics to the total calf crop. Other aspects of this management practice are the cost and amount of time needed to select superior females in a harem breeding system, which is most often used by livestock producers. In a *harem* breeding system, one male is used to breed several females. Several ways to evaluate the benefits of breeding a particular animal include the following:
- Estimated progeny differences (EPDs)
- Estimated breeding values
- Pedigrees
- Conformation

ESTIMATED PROGENY DIFFERENCES

Estimated progeny differences (EPDs) are used to predict the characteristics of offspring before they are born. EPDs are often used in cattle. Some sheep producers and goat producers have tried to collect this type of data but have met with some resistance from within the industry. EPD data collection has been started for some breeds of horses, not in the United States but in England within the Thoroughbred industry. EPDs are available only for males. Males can provide more statistical dependability because of the greater number of offspring produced by males compared with females, and the increased amount of genetic material supplied to the herd by the males makes these data more important.

When preparing EPD data, information is collected on the offspring produced from the male for which the EPDs are being developed. For example, birth weight, weaning weight, yearling weight, carcass data, ultrasound data, fertility, and scrotal circumference can be collected from the bull's offspring. Scrotal circumference correlates with the amount of sperm-producing tissue and usually is a good indication of sperm production. The EPDs listed in Table 3-1 are not the only EPDs that can be measured; these are just a few of the most common. EPDs vary depending on the breed, and EPDs cannot be compared among breeds.

TABLE 3-1	Example Estimated Progeny Differences for Two Bulls from the Same Breed*								
BULL NAME	**BW† ACC**	**WW‡ ACC**	**YW§ ACC**	**YH‖ ACC**	**SC¶ ACC**	**CEM# ACC**	**MILK** ACC**	**MARB†† ACC**	**FAT‡‡ ACC**
VT Pride	+4.4	+40	+60	+0.5	−0.62	+8	+20	+0.15	+0.026
	0.42	0.30	0.21	0.16	0.18	0.14	0.26	0.14	0.14
Wyatt's Boy	+1.3	+36	+76	+0	−0.55	+7	+16	+0.08	−0.023
	0.98	0.97	0.96	0.96	0.96	0.93	0.96	0.87	0.85

ACC, Accuracy.
*These are hypothetical examples. You must consult each individual breed to define estimated progeny difference information.
†BW (birth weight; expressed in pounds) is a predictor of a sire's ability to transmit birth weight to his progeny compared with that of other sires.
‡WW (weaning weight; expressed in pounds) is a predictor of a sire's ability to transmit weaning growth to his progeny compared with that of other sires.
§YW (yearling weight; expressed in pounds) is a predictor of a sire's ability to transmit yearling growth to his progeny compared with that of other sires.
‖YH (yearling height; expressed in inches) is a predictor of a sire's ability to transmit yearling height compared with that of other sires.
¶SC (scrotal circumference; expressed in centimeters) is a predictor of the difference in transmitting ability for scrotal size compared with that of other sires.
#CEM (calving ease maternal; expressed as a difference in percentage of unassisted births) predicts the average ease with which a sire's daughters will calve as first-calf heifers when compared with daughters of other sires. A higher value indicates greater calving ease in first-calf daughters.
**MILK (maternal milk) is a predictor of a sire's genetic merit for milk and mothering ability as expressed in his daughters compared with daughters of other sires. It is the part of a calf's weaning weight attributed to milk and mothering ability.
††MARB (marbling) is expressed as a fraction of the difference in the U.S. Department of Agriculture's marbling score of a sire's progeny compared with progeny of other sires.
‡‡FAT (fat thickness; expressed in inches) is a predictor of the difference in external fat thickness at the twelfth rib (as measured between the twelfth and thirteenth ribs) of a sire's progeny compared with progeny of other sires.

> **TECHNICIAN NOTE** Estimated progeny differences cannot be compared among breeds.

Therefore, you can use EPDs only to compare two Angus bulls. EPDs would not be useful in comparing an Angus bull and a Hereford bull.

This information is statistically evaluated, and each bull receives a number for each characteristic. The number will have a + or − associated with it. The number then can be used to compare two different bulls. For example, if the VT Pride bull has a +4.4 for birth weight and Wyatt's Boy has a +1.3, you could expect calves born to VT Pride to weight 3 pounds more than calves born to Wyatt's Boy (+4.3 − +1.3 = +3). Of course, these numbers are averages, and bulls must be randomly mated to cows to expect these types of results. The units for each characteristic vary, so producers and veterinary professionals should understand the units associated with each EPD.

The bull's female offspring can contribute data on milk production and mothering ability. The information provided by EPDs can help a producer decide which of the bulls would be the best for his or her production system.

When looking at EPDs, the individual producer's production system, amount of labor, and feed availability will contribute greatly to the producer's choices.

Each EPD has an accuracy number associated with its value. The accuracy number (ACC) gives the producer an indication of the actual accuracy of the EPD. An accuracy close to 1.0 indicates higher reliability. Accuracy is affected by the number of progeny and ancestral records included in the analysis. The more progeny available for data collection, the greater the accuracy of the EPD will be (see Table 3-1).

ESTIMATED BREEDING VALUES

Estimated breeding values (EBVs) are often used in the swine and cattle industry to determine the value of a breeding between two animals before the breeding takes place. The concept is the application of *genetic principles* to *performance records*. Producers often assess the performance of the animal being evaluated for breeding. Essentially, the data used are similar to those collected in EPDs, but the degree of heritability of these traits is applied. For example, certain traits have a higher potential to be inherited than others. Thus, with knowledge of the potential heritability, the overall value of the animals being bred can be estimated by looking at which superior traits the animals have and how likely those traits are to be inherited.

Breeders can use EBVs to predict the outcome of a specific mating. By simply averaging the EBVs of the parents, the genetic merit (value) of the progeny can be determined. Think of the following situation. A boar has an EBV of −6.0 days and a sow has an EBV of −2.0 days for reaching 90 kg. When these two animals are mated, on average the offspring will take 4 days less (−6 + −2 = −8; −8 ÷ 2 = −4) to reach 90 kg than the progeny of other boars and sows with the breed average.

You must consider all the data and understand the value and units as well as the accuracy of these numbers, just as for EPDs, for them to be valuable.

PEDIGREE

Pedigree is also used in determining which male or female should be bred. When decisions are made based on pedigree, producers often evaluate the performance of the animal as well. For example, if a producer were looking to breed a horse that would produce a colt adept at racing, the producer could want to evaluate the performance record of the animal in the pedigree of that stud. Finding that the stud had Seattle

Slew and Dash for Cash in his history could indicate that the foal produced from the mating would have speed and be good at racing. The concept can be considered as follows: Would you expect Michael Jordan's son or my son to be better at basketball? My son is short, and neither of his parents have any basketball skills. The concept does not always work but is one of the bases used to select animals for breeding. This approach is often used in the horse industry. Pedigrees can also be used to select a type of breeding. These systems include *inbreeding, linebreeding, crossbreeding, purebreeding, outcrossing,* and *grading up.*

Breeding Systems
Inbreeding
Inbreeding is the mating of two animals that are closely related.

Linebreeding
Linebreeding is the mating of several generations of offspring to particular animals or their descendants.

Crossbreeding
Crossbreeding is the mating of sires of one breed to dams of another. An example of crossbreeding is the breeding of Angus and Hereford cattle. In this mating, the result is a *black baldy* or *black brockle face calf.* Crossbreeding is used to increase *heterosis,* in which offspring inherit traits from both breeds and are more genetically diverse, thus allowing for increases in performance.

Purebreeding
Purebreeding is the mating of two animals from the same breed. Most often, these animals are registered with their purebred association. In some species, a purebred animal is more valuable than a crossbred or *grade* animal. Grade animals are animals that are not registered with an association. Grade animals do not have specific lineage, and producers often do not know the actual breed of the animals. An example of purebreeding is breeding a registered Quarter horse to a registered Quarter horse.

Outcrossing
Outcrossing is the practice of breeding of animals from different families within the same breed, for example, breeding a horse from a Two Eyed Jack line to a horse from a Smart Little Lena line.

Grading Up
Grading up is the practice of breeding a grade animal to a purebred animal.

CONFORMATION
Animals are also selected based on conformation. For example, cryptorchidism is a genetic condition. Animals that are born cryptorchid unilaterally or bilaterally should not be selected for breeding. Producers also should consider other conformation traits. For example, a 45-degree angle to the

shoulder is considered ideal in the horse. When choosing to breed a horse, the sire and the dam should be as close as possible to perfect conformation. Breeders should always look to improve the breed, and good conformation should be included in the selection process. Each breed and species will have a different set of conformation criteria considered ideal, and producers should be familiar with these characteristics before selecting the appropriate animals to breed.

REPRODUCTIVE ANATOMY

FEMALE ANATOMY
The female anatomy consists of the broad ligaments, ovaries, oviducts, uterus, cervix, vagina, vestibule, and vulva. The purpose of the broad ligaments is to support the reproductive tract in the abdomen. The ovaries are responsible for developing follicles that produce the oocytes. An ovarian bursa is present in ruminants and surrounds the ovary. The ovary consists of a medulla and cortex. In almost all species, the medulla is centrally located and the cortex surrounds the medulla. However, in mares this is the exact opposite, and for this reason mares are able to ovulate only on the ventral border of the ovary because this is the only surface where the cortex can reach the surface at what is known as the ovulation fossa.

The oviducts connect the ovaries to the uterus. The oviduct consists of three parts: infundibulum, ampulla, and isthmus. In most species fertilization, takes place in the infundibulum. The female camelid and horse have a papilla at the uterotubal junction that allows passage of only fertilized eggs into the uterus. The uterus is responsible for housing the fetus during pregnancy, and its inner lining is known as the endometrium.

The cervix connects the vagina and uterus. It is under hormonal influence and is able to close and open during these hormonal influences to ensure that sperm are able to gain access to the reproductive tract and during pregnancy keep foreign material out of the uterus. In ruminants and swine, the cervix has numerous rings that run transversely through the cervix. However, mares' cervical rings are larger and run longitudinally. The vagina connects the cervix to the vestibule. The vestibule contains the suburethral diverticulum, which is the urethral opening present in cows and sows. The vulva is the name of the external genitalia (Fig. 3-1).

MALE ANATOMY
The male anatomy consists of the scrotum, testicles, epididymis, vas deferens, accessory sex glands, penis, and prepuce. The scrotum houses the testicles and is responsible for keeping the testicles thermoregulated, which is important for spermatogenesis. The testicles are responsible for spermatogenesis and are made up of seminiferous tubules. The epididymis connects the testicles and the spermatic cord, and it is responsible for sperm maturation, storage, and transport. The three sections of the epididymis are the head, body, and tail. The tail faces caudally in stallions and camelids. In ruminants

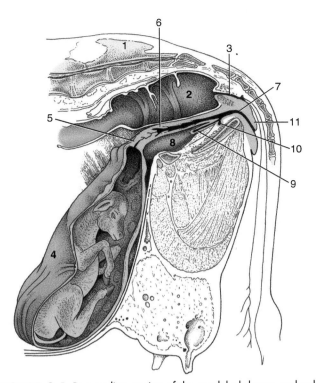

FIGURE 3-1 Paramedian section of the caudal abdomen and pelvis of a pregnant cow. The section is not quite vertical because it cuts through the vertebral canal and an obturator foramen. Note the large placentomes. *1,* Sacrum; *2,* rectum; *3,* anal canal; *4,* uterus; *5,* cervix; *6,* vagina; *7,* vestibule; *8,* bladder; *9,* urethra; *10,* suburethral diverticulum; *11,* vulva. (From Dyce KM, Wensing CJG: *Textbook of veterinary anatomy,* ed 4, St. Louis, 2010, Saunders.)

the tail faces ventrally, and in swine it faces dorsally. The vas deferens connects the urethra to the spermatic cord.

The accessory sex glands include the vesicular glands, prostate gland, and bulbourethral or Cowper's gland. Large animals have all these glands, with the exception of the camelid, which does not have vesicular glands. The accessory sex glands are responsible for producing seminal fluids. The penis is the copulatory organ, and its shape and structure vary considerably. The horse penis is vascular and telescoping in nature. Semen is forced into the cervix by urethral pulses, and loss of semen is avoided through the engorgement of the corona glandis. Ruminants and camelids have a sigmoid flexure. Small ruminants have a urethral process. Boars and camelids have a corkscrew penis. The prepuce is the tissue in which the penis is housed (Fig. 3-2).

REPRODUCTIVE PHYSIOLOGY

FEMALE REPRODUCTIVE PHYSIOLOGY

Veterinary technicians should be familiar with the estrous cycle of all species. All livestock species follow similar estrous behavior, with slight differences in the hours between each landmark within the estrous cycle. Estrous cycle data are discussed in these sections of this book on each species.

The estrous cycle has four phases: *proestrus, estrus, metaestrus,* and *diestrus.* Anestrus in livestock can be seen in seasonally polyestrous species and only in polyestrous species during pregnancy. Table 3-2 contains an overview of female reproductive hormones.

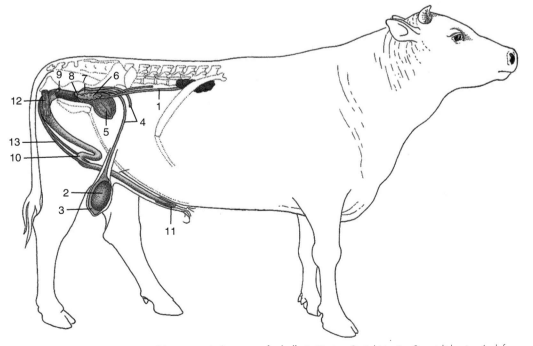

FIGURE 3-2 Disposition of the urogenital organs of a bull. *1,* Ureter; *2,* right testis; *3,* epididymis; *4,* deferent duct; *5,* bladder; *6,* vesicular gland; *7,* ampulla of deferent duct; *8,* body of prostate; *9,* bulbourethral gland; *10,* sigmoid flexure of penis; *11,* glans penis; *12,* ischiocavernosus; *13,* retractor penis. (From Dyce KM, Wensing CJG: *Textbook of veterinary anatomy,* ed 4, St. Louis, 2010, Saunders.)

TABLE 3-2	Female Reproductive Hormones		
HORMONE	**SOURCE**	**FEMALE TARGET TISSUE**	**FEMALE PRIMARY ACTION**
Gonadotropin-releasing hormone (GnRH)	Hypothalamus	Anterior pituitary	Releases FSH and LH from anterior pituitary gland
Luteinizing hormone (LH)	Anterior pituitary	Ovary (cells of theca interna and luteal cells)	Stimulates ovulation, corpus luteum formation, and progesterone secretion
Follicle-stimulating hormone (FSH)	Anterior pituitary	Ovary (granulosa cells)	Promotes follicular development and estradiol synthesis
Estradiol (E_2)	Granulosa cells of follicle	Hypothalamus, entire reproductive tract, mammary gland	Affects sexual behavior, GnRH, elevated secretory activity of entire tract; enhances uterine motility
Progesterone (P_4)	Corpus luteum	Uterine endometrium, mammary gland, myometrium, hypothalamus	Promotes endometrial secretion, inhibits GnRH release, inhibits reproductive behavior, promotes maintenance of pregnancy
Prostaglandin $F_{2\alpha}$ ($PGF_{2\alpha}$)	Uterine endometrium	Corpus luteum, uterine myometrium, ovulatory follicles	Affects luteolysis, promotes uterine tone and contraction, causing ovulation

TECHNICIAN NOTE A thorough understanding of hormones, their actions in the body, and their role in the estrous cycle will help technicians to understand hormone therapies used in veterinary medicine more clearly and improve client education.

Estrous Cycle and Hormone Involvement
Proestrus

Proestrus begins with a decline in progesterone level, which results because the animal has just undergone a surge of prostaglandin $F_{2\alpha}$ ($PGF_{2\alpha}$) in diestrus. The prostaglandin causes lysis of the corpus luteum, which results in the decrease in progesterone. Progesterone blocks gonadotropin-releasing hormone (GnRH), which then blocks follicle-stimulating hormone (FSH) and luteinizing hormone (LH). When the progesterone level decreases at the beginning of proestrus, the block is removed. By unblocking GnRH, FSH production begins. FSH causes the development of follicles on the ovary and with it the development of follicular fluid, which results in increasing estrogen.

Estrus

Once estrogen reaches a specific blood level in the body, it triggers the release of LH, which in turn triggers ovulation. The follicle ruptures, and the egg is released from the follicle. The egg travels down the tube to the infundibulum where, if the animal has been bred, fertilization of the egg will take place.

Metaestrus

Because the follicle has been ruptured, the estrogen levels in the body decrease in response to the absence of the follicular fluid. The follicle becomes the corpus luteum, and production of progesterone begins. Metaestrus is the transition from estrogen as the predominant hormone to progesterone as the predominant hormone.

Diestrus

Progesterone continues to be produced until the end of gestation if the animal is pregnant. If pregnancy does not take place, the body triggers a prostaglandin surge of $PGF_{2\alpha}$. The prostaglandin causes lysis of the corpus luteum, and progesterone begins to decline, which results in the transition from diestrus to proestrus (Figs. 3-3 and 3-4).

Manipulation of the female reproductive tract can be achieved through the use of synthetic and naturally occurring drugs. Table 3-3 shows some of the drugs available to manipulate the female reproductive system, their trade names, the drugs they mimic, and the functions of these drugs in large animal medicine.

MALE REPRODUCTIVE PHYSIOLOGY

Spermatogenesis is the process of making sperm that takes place in the seminiferous tubules of the testis. FSH and LH regulate sperm production (Table 3-4). FSH and LH are released from the anterior pituitary, where FSH stimulates the sperm production in the testicles and LH stimulates the production of testosterone. Testosterone is needed for the spermatogonia to develop into sperm. The sperm begin as germ cells (spermatogonia) deep to the lumen of the seminiferous tubules and go through several divisions before becoming sperm. The three phases of spermatogenesis are the proliferation, meiotic, and differentiation phases. During the proliferation phase, several cellular divisions take place. Some of these cells revert back to primitive cell types, so there is always a continuous supply of stem cells from which more sperm can be made. This process is known as stem cell renewal. The second phase of spermatogenesis is the meiotic phase; this is when genetic diversity occurs and ensures that no two sperm are identical. The third phase of spermatogenesis is differentiation, the phase in which the sperm obtains a head, midpiece, and flagella. The sperm are then released into the lumen of the seminiferous tubules. After release into

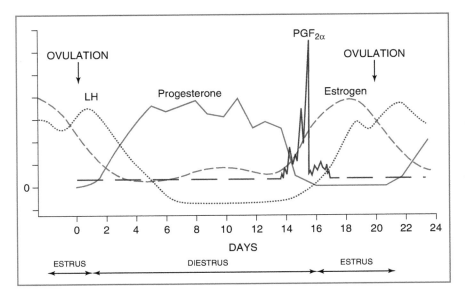

FIGURE 3-3 The equine estrous cycle. Estrus is 4 to 7 days long, and luteinizing hormone (LH) peaks after ovulation. Diestrus begins approximately 2 days after ovulation. Progesterone is high throughout a 14- to 15-day diestrus. If a pregnancy signal is not secreted by the early embryo by day 14 to 16, prostaglandin $F_{2\alpha}$ ($PGF_{2\alpha}$) is released from the uterus, goes to the corpus luteum, and causes luteolysis (luteal death). The cycle then starts over. (From Pinto CRF, Eilts BE, Paccamonti DL: Animal reproduction. In Bassert JM, McCurnin DM, editors: *McCurnin's clinical textbook for veterinary technicians*, ed 7, St. Louis, 2010, Saunders, p 382.)

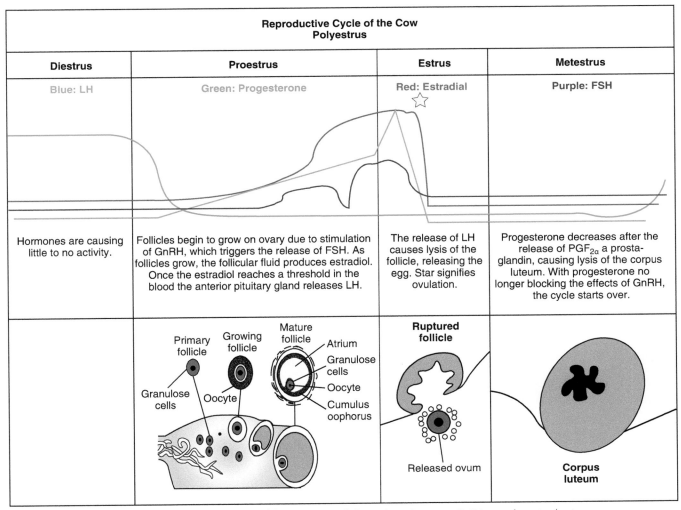

Reproductive Cycle of the Cow **Polyestrus**			
Diestrus	**Proestrus**	**Estrus**	**Metestrus**
Blue: LH	Green: Progesterone	Red: Estradial	Purple: FSH
Hormones are causing little to no activity.	Follicles begin to grow on ovary due to stimulation of GnRH, which triggers the release of FSH. As follicles grow, the follicular fluid produces estradiol. Once the estradiol reaches a threshold in the blood the anterior pituitary gland releases LH.	The release of LH causes lysis of the follicle, releasing the egg. Star signifies ovulation.	Progesterone decreases after the release of $PGF_{2\alpha}$ a prostaglandin, causing lysis of the corpus luteum. With progesterone no longer blocking the effects of GnRH, the cycle starts over.

FIGURE 3-4 Reproductive cycle of the cow. *FSH*, Follicle-stimulating hormone; *GnRH*, gonadotropin-releasing hormone; *LH*, luteinizing hormone; $PGF_{2\alpha}$, prostaglandin $F_{2\alpha}$.

TABLE 3-3	Drugs Used to Manipulate the Female Reproductive System		
DRUG	**LABELED PRODUCTS**	**FUNCTION**	**USES**
Gonadorelin	Cystorelin Factrel Fertagyl	Causes release of FSH and LH	Synchronization of estrus Treatment of cystic ovaries
Chorionic gonadotropin (human [hCG] or equine [eCG])	Follutein P.G. 600 Chorulon APL Generics	Mimics LH with limited FSH activity	Treatment of cystic ovaries
FSH-P	FSH-P	FSH	Superovulation
Estrogens	Estradiol cypionate (ECP) Implants Generics	Estrogen	Treatment of persistent corpus luteum, retained placenta, and pyometrium Induction of estrus in horses Improvement of weight gain in beef cattle
Altrenogest	Regu-Mate	Progesterone	Suppression of estrus in mares
Progesterone	CIDR-vaginal implant	Progesterone	Synchronization
Melengestrol acetate	MGA	Progesterone	Synchronization or increased feed efficiency
Norgestomet + estradiol valerate	Norgestomet	Progesterone + estrogen	Synchronization of estrus in beef cattle and nonlactating dairy cows
Dinoprost tromethamine	Lutalyse AmTech ProstaMate In-Synch	Prostaglandin	Estrus synchronization and abortion in cattle Induction of parturition in swine Timing of estrus in mares
Fenprostalene	Bovilene	Prostaglandin	Induction of abortion in feedlot heifers Synchronization of estrus in beef and nonlactating dairy cows
Fluprostenol	Equimate	Prostaglandin	Estrus synchronization in cycling mares Establishment of estrus cycles in anestrus mares Induction of parturition in mares Treatment of lactational anestrus Facilitation of foal-heat breeding
Cloprostenol sodium	Estrumate	Prostaglandin	Treatment of luteal cysts, mummified fetuses, termination of pregnancy, and estrus synchronization

CIDR, Controlled internal drug release; *FSH,* follicle-stimulating hormone; *LH,* luteinizing hormone.

TABLE 3-4	Male Reproductive Hormones		
HORMONE	**SOURCE**	**MALE TARGET TISSUE**	**MALE PRIMARY ACTION**
Gonadotropin-releasing hormone (GnRH)	Hypothalamus	Anterior pituitary	Releases FSH and LH from anterior pituitary gland
Luteinizing hormone (LH)	Anterior pituitary	Testis (interstitial cells of Leydig)	Stimulates testosterone production
Follicle-stimulating hormone (FSH)	Anterior pituitary	Testis (Sertoli cells)	Affects Sertoli cell function
Estradiol (E_2)	Sertoli cells of the testis	Brain Inhibits long bone growth	Affects sexual behavior
Prostaglandin $F_{2\alpha}$ ($PGF_{2\alpha}$)	Vesicular glands	Epididymis	Affects metabolic activity of spermatozoa, causes epididymal contractions
Testosterone (T)	Interstitial cells of Leydig	Accessory sex glands tunica dartos of scrotum, seminiferous epithelium, and skeletal muscle	Anabolic growth promotes spermatogenesis, promotes secretion of accessory sex glands

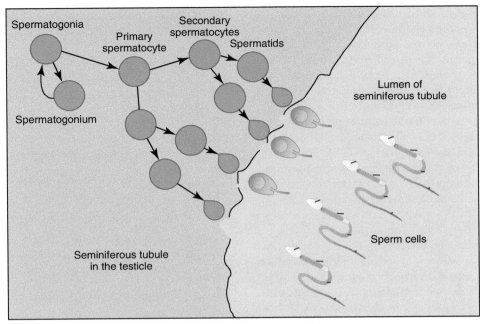

FIGURE 3-5 Spermatogenesis.

the seminiferous tubules, the sperm are transported to the epididymis, where they continue to mature and are stored until ejaculation (Fig. 3-5).

FEMALE BREEDING SOUNDNESS EXAMINATION

Some diseases of the female reproductive tract are unrelated to breeding and reproduction and require diagnostic procedures and medical or surgical treatment. However, most female reproductive system procedures are performed on breeding animals, with the ultimate goal being delivery of a live neonate. To produce a live neonate, the following must occur in any species:

- Successful breeding: In any female, successful breeding is required, and many diseases or reproductive tract abnormalities can prevent this. Mares do not always readily accept the male. In addition, timing of insemination (natural or artificial) must correspond to the time of ovulation, which may be difficult to determine. Therefore, a thorough understanding of each species reproductive cycle is important. The source of the semen may not be at the same location as the female, thus requiring that the semen be shipped to the female or that the female be shipped to the male's farm for breeding.
- Successful conception.
- Successful implantation: Sometimes the egg fails to implant. The period from conception to implantation is prolonged in horses; implantation begins approximately on day 35. Embryonic losses are high during the time before implantation.
- Successful gestation: Several diseases can cause reproductive failure. Poor nutrition can also contribute to gestation problems.
- Successful parturition: The placenta begins to separate early during the delivery process, so the neonate is

deprived of this oxygen source. Careful observation of females during parturition is important. In mares, foals rarely survive dystocias that last more than 1 hour.

The neonatal period is very delicate, and care must be taken to monitor neonates closely for illness or injury. Veterinary medicine is often involved in the reproductive process for all species, and depending on the breeding industry, species, and purpose of the offspring, it can be a tricky and expensive business.

> **TECHNICIAN NOTE**   Veterinary medicine is often involved in the reproductive process for all species, and depending on the breeding industry, species, and purpose of the offspring, it can be a tricky and expensive business.

FEMALE REPRODUCTIVE EXAMINATION

Although, in most livestock species a female reproductive examination does not take place on every female, it is common for a reproductive examination to be performed on mares before the breeding season. However, if problems arise or a female is important, a reproductive examination may be performed in other species.

When beginning the female reproductive examination, it is important to obtain a thorough history, including facts about prior fertility, pregnancies, estrous cycle information, illness, injuries, and current and previous medications. A standard physical examination is performed, followed by an external genital examination. It is important to wrap the tail and allow the veterinarian the best view of the perineum possible. The perineum should be cleaned with warm soap and water, and the vulva should be examined. The labia should meet firmly and evenly and have a slope of less than 10 degrees, with two thirds of the vulvar cleft below the ischial arch. Poor vaginal and labial conformation can result in urovagina, ascending endometritis, or the need for a Caslick procedure as a result of windsucking.

Next, a vaginal speculum is placed, and the veterinarian examines the vaginal vault. Often, rectal palpation and ultrasound examination of the ovaries, uterus, and cervix are performed. The veterinarian is looking for proper location, size, and tone of the uterus. Uterine culture and possibly endometrial (uterine) biopsy may also be performed during a female breeding soundness examination (BSE). The results of the examination allow the veterinarian to assess fertility, identify potential conditions that could interfere with successful breeding, and diagnose venereal diseases.

UTERINE CULTURE

The most common cause of infertility in the mare is uterine infection with bacteria. Mares with uterine infection generally have difficulty conceiving and supporting a pregnancy. Unlike in other domestic species, in horses uterine infections are usually clinically "silent," with minimal or no external signs, such as vulvar discharge or irritation. Systemic illness with signs of septicemia and fever also is unusual. Most infections are fairly superficial in the uterine lining, and the bacteria do not gain entry into the bloodstream in significant numbers (the notable exception is uterine infection after foaling; after foaling, the separation of the placenta exposes many blood vessels in the uterine wall, and bacteria can gain ready entrance into the bloodstream). Therefore, the only clue that a mare may have uterine infection is repeated unsuccessful breeding, either failing to conceive or conceiving and losing the embryo early in pregnancy. These issues usually prompt the client to call a veterinarian.

> **TECHNICIAN NOTE** Uterine infections in horses are usually clinically "silent," with minimal or no external signs.

Performing a uterine culture can confirm the presence or absence of uterine infection (Box 3-1). Sensitivity testing can also be performed to guide proper antibiotic therapy. Some breeders perform uterine culture in mares routinely at the beginning of the breeding season so that early treatment of "dirty" mares can be pursued.

A uterine culturette is used to obtain the culture. Culturettes are commercially available and are generally approximately 24 to 30 inches in length. They consist of an outer protective plastic sleeve and an inner cotton-tipped swab. Most have a guarded tip, which is a "trap door" cap that prevents contamination of the swab as it is passes through the vulva, vagina, and cervix. Once the culturette is in the uterus, the veterinarian presses forward on the swab, and the tip opens to let the swab tip through it.

Samples can help identify organisms such as *Streptococcus zooepidemicus* and *Escherichia coli*. These organisms are commonly isolated from mares that have presented with endometritis. Organisms that may also be identified include *Klebsiella pneumoniae, Pseudomonas aeruginosa* and *Taylorella equigenitalis,* which can be transmitted venereally.

| **BOX 3-1** | Uterine Culture |

Equipment
- Sterile obstetrical sleeve or sterile rectal sleeve
- Vaginal speculum and light source
- Sterile water-soluble lubricant (K-Y Jelly)
- Uterine culturette
- Culture medium or transport tube

Procedure
The mare is restrained, and the tail is held or tied away from the perineum. The perineal/vulvar area is prepared routinely. The veterinarian may pass the culturette either manually, with the hand in a sterile plastic sleeve, or visually through a vaginal speculum. The uterine culturette is passed through the cervix and is used to swab the lining of the uterus. Once the culturette is withdrawn, the cotton swab tip is collected and used for standard bacterial culture procedures. To avoid contaminating the swab, the guarded tip can be cut off or held out of the way. The cotton tip is commonly broken or cut free from the culturette stick and is placed into a sterile glass tube or culture medium for transport to the laboratory. If transportation to the laboratory is delayed, the swab may dry out, killing the bacteria. Adding a small amount of sterile saline solution to the swab and refrigeration may delay drying.

Analysis of the sample commonly includes an air-dried smear for Gram staining, as well as culture plating on blood agar and a gram-negative culture medium. Plates are incubated at 37° C (98.6° F) and are checked daily for growth. Some practitioners request quantification (number of bacterial colonies) in addition to bacterial identification.

UTERINE INFUSION

Infusion is a method of delivering liquids into the uterus (Box 3-2). Indications for the procedure include the following:
- Treatment of uterine infection, in which antibiotics are diluted in a sterile solution (e.g., sterile saline or lactated Ringer's solution) and infused into the uterus; can be repeated daily for several days
- Routine flushing (lavage) of the uterus after an abortion or after foaling
- "Postbreeding" infusion to prepare the uterus to receive an embryo

The volume of liquid infused depends on the underlying reason for the infusion. It may range from less than 100 mL for inseminations to several gallons in the case of postfoaling lavage. For uterine lavage, the goal is to remove debris and exudates from the uterus; therefore, the fluids are usually removed by siphon or internal massage. For administration of antibiotics and for insemination, the goal is keep the infused material in the uterus. Mares often attempt to expel the infused material by assuming a urination stance and straining. If the infusion is intended to stay in the uterus, the mare should not be allowed to assume this position. Walking the mare briskly for several minutes after uterine infusion may help prevent this from occurring.

BOX 3-2 Uterine Infusion

Equipment
- Sterile obstetrical sleeve or sterile rectal sleeve
- Vaginal speculum and light source
- Sterile water-soluble lubricant
- Disposable uterine infusion pipette
- Fluid line (standard intravenous, arthroscopy, or bell intravenous)
- Sterile 60-mL syringes
- Infusion fluids

Procedure
The mare is restrained, and the tail is held or tied away from the perineum. The perineal/vulvar area is prepared routinely. The veterinarian gives the infusion by passing a uterine infusion pipette (or a fluid line) through the cervix into the uterus, similar to the procedure used for artificial insemination. Infusion pipettes may be passed either manually, with the hand in a sterile plastic sleeve, or visually through a vaginal speculum. Once the pipette or fluid line is in position, the fluids are delivered by attaching either a syringe or fluid line connected to the infusion fluids. Gravity flow or pressurized flow may be used. Immediately following the infusion, the mare is walked briskly for several minutes if the infused material is intended to remain in the uterus.

BOX 3-3 Endometrial Biopsy

Equipment
- Sterile obstetrical sleeve
- Sterile water-soluble lubricant
- Sterile uterine biopsy forceps

Procedure
The mare is restrained, and the tail is held or tied away from the perineum. The perineal/vulvar area is prepared routinely. This is a two-step procedure. First, the veterinarian places the biopsy forceps through the vagina and cervix into the uterus. The hand is then withdrawn from the vagina and reinserted into the rectum. Second, with one hand in the rectum and the other hand controlling the biopsy instrument handles, the veterinarian positions the instrument against the uterine wall, and the tissue sample is obtained. The mare may experience temporary discomfort when the sample is snipped. The instrument is then withdrawn, and the tissue sample is placed in the proper fixative. No special aftercare is required.

ENDOMETRIAL (UTERINE) BIOPSY

Biopsy of the lining of the uterus is performed to evaluate the histologic condition of the endometrium, usually as part of an assessment of a mare's fertility (Box 3-3). The endometrium contains the endometrial glands, which support and nourish the embryo. The endometrium is also the site for implantation and development of the placenta. Uterine infections, trauma from foaling, and aging may cause abnormalities such as atrophy of the endometrial glands, fibrosis around the glands, and inflammation, which can interfere with the mare's ability to support pregnancy. Biopsy allows a histopathologist to examine the condition of the endometrium and assess the probability of the mare's being able to support a pregnancy. The histopathologist usually assigns a grade of 1, 2, or 3 to the specimen, with grade 1 representing a normal or minimally abnormal specimen, grade 2 representing mild to moderate disease, and grade 3 representing severe or irreversible disease. Figure 3-6 shows the technique used for endometrial biopsy in alpacas.

TECHNICIAN NOTE Uterine biopsies are graded as 1, 2, or 3. A grade of 1 suggests a normal or minimally abnormal specimen.

The endometrial biopsy is only one piece of information used to evaluate fertility; it is not the only criterion used to assure or condemn a mare's future as a breeding animal. Some mares with grade 1 uteruses cannot maintain a pregnancy; similarly, mares with grade 3 uteruses have been successfully bred. The biopsy is only part of the puzzle and is best used as a management tool for breeding.

The biopsy is obtained with 70-cm long (≈28 inches) stainless steel uterine biopsy forceps (Fig. 3-7). The forceps should be sterilized. The forceps have alligator jaws and can obtain a tissue sample approximately 1.5 mm long and 4 mm wide. It may be necessary to use a small syringe needle to retrieve the sample carefully from the forceps jaws. Once retrieved, the sample is placed in a liquid fixative. The technician should consult the laboratory for the preferred method of fixation. Common fixatives include Bouin's fixative, 10% buffered formalin, and 70% alcohol. Samples should not sit in Bouin's fixative for more than 24 hours.

TECHNICIAN NOTE Bouin's fixative is commonly used for biopsy samples. It consists of 10% buffered formalin and 70% alcohol.

HEIFER DEVELOPMENT

With increasing knowledge about proper heifer development, more and more emphasis is being placed on properly raising these females to ensure the best chance of reproductive success. The objective of producers is to develop enough heifers to ensure the future profitability of the herd. The heifers must reach puberty and be cycling regularly at the start of the breeding season. There are five phases of heifer development:
- Sire selection
- Preweaning management
- Heifer selection at weaning
- Weaning to breeding
- Gestation through parturition and rebreeding

Sire selection is considered previously in this chapter, and discussion of this topic continues in the next section of the chapter, on BSEs. When breeding heifers, it is important to select sires using the previously discussed options for selection

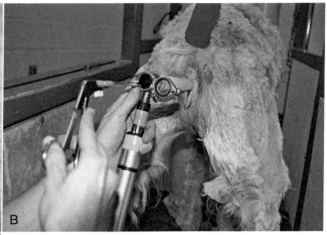

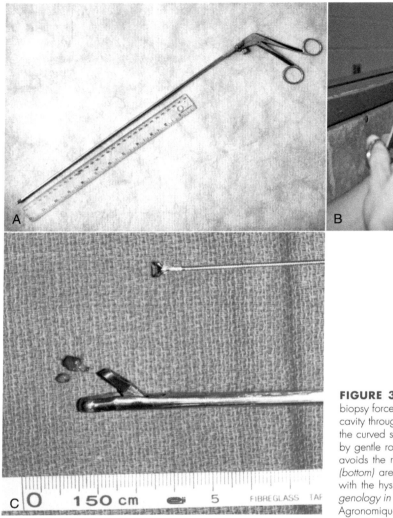

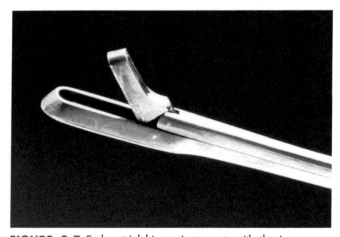

FIGURE 3-6 Endometrial biopsy technique in alpacas. **A,** Turrell rectal biopsy forceps. **B,** The instrument is guided through the cervix into the uterine cavity through a sigmoidoscope and positioned at the base of the left horn; the curved shape of the basket helps both with catheterization of the cervix by gentle rotation of the instrument and placement at the desired level and avoids the risk of biting into the intrauterine septum. **C,** Samples obtained *(bottom)* are significantly larger and more diagnostic than those obtained with the hysteroscopy technique *(top)*. (From Tibary A, Anoaussi A: *Theriogenology in Camelidae,* ed 2, Rabat, Morocco, 1997, Actes Edition, Institut Agronomique et Vétérinaire Hassan II.)

FIGURE 3-7 Endometrial biopsy instrument, with the jaws open. (From Bassert JM, McCurnin DM, editors: *McCurnin's clinical textbook for veterinary technicians,* ed 7, St. Louis, 2010, Saunders.)

and by keeping in mind that low birth weights are important for these young heifers.

Preweaning management involves keeping cows in the herd that will potentially mother the heifers to be kept as replacements in good condition and healthy so they can raise a

healthy calf. It is important to tag calves when they are born to identify their dam as well as their age and any problems that are identified during development. Because puberty is affected by age, it can be important to select heifers that are older as replacements. Puberty of heifers is influenced by age, weight, and breed, so good nutrition is an important factor in development.

Heifer selection at weaning is influenced by many factors, but the first step is to select the oldest heifers in the group and ensure they are between 450 and 600 pounds. These heifers should be in good BCS, body condition score. Because many of the heifers the producer selects will not reach puberty by the time breeding is to occur, it is important for producers to select an extra 10% to 50% of what they expect to keep. Producers will want the heifers to reach 60% to 65% of their expected mature cow weight by breeding. Depending on the amount of time the producer has before their selected breeding date, calves may need to gain weight at a rate of 1 to 1.5 pounds per day.

From weaning to breeding, heifers should be gaining sufficient weight to reach 60% to 65% of their expected mature cow weight. The producers should also select their estimated breeding date, and this date should ideally be 3 to 4 weeks before their cow herd. This is important because the producer will be able to watch these heifers more closely during calving because they will not be calving with the cow herd, and it will allow those heifers another month to accomplish uterine involution and rebreed the subsequent year because they will be joining the mature cow herd at that time. There is considerable evidence showing that first calf heifers tend to take longer to recycle after their first calf. This also allows their calves 3 to 4 more weeks of development and gives them more time to gain weight and be the size of the other calves in the mature cow herd. During this time, it is recommended to have the veterinarian perform body condition scoring, reproductive tract scoring, and pelvic measurements on these heifers. These data can give the producer more information about the likelihood that these heifers will obtain their breeding date goal, as well as information about calving ease.

From gestation through rebreeding, it is important to provide optimal nutrition to these heifers because they will still be growing and asked to breed back in time to join the mature cow herd the following year.

MALE BREEDING SOUNDNESS EXAMINATION

Owners must continually evaluate the reproductive performance of breeding males in the herd. The primary goal of a BSE is to evaluate the current state of fertility of an individual, with the realization that many factors can affect fertility. Animals with fertility problems often are candidates for culling because they would result in an economic loss. The BSE is only one piece of information used in formulating a farm's breeding management program.

The BSE usually is performed just before the *breeding season*. Fertility is assumed only for the time of the examination. In addition to a general health evaluation, the examination emphasizes the physical ability to breed females (especially eyes, legs, and feet). Examination of the *external genitalia*, sperm analysis, and a rectal examination of the internal *accessory sex glands* may be done. The accessory sex glands are evaluated for symmetry, size, consistency, and sensitivity.

It is important to evaluate previous medical records that may be available for the male during a BSE. Scrotal circumference should be compared with previous measurements and changes evaluated as part of their BSE. The producer should be asked about the success of the animal if he has been used for breeding previously. Information such as the pregnancy rate, number of females mated, diseases, illnesses, and nutrition should be obtained.

A basic physical examination should be performed during each BSE, with particular attention to paid vision and conformation. Males must be able to see females in heat, as well as be able to navigate efficiently. Conformation abnormalities or lameness can affect his breeding success.

Examination of the external genitalia must be done carefully to prevent injury to the examiner. Most males tend to resent handling of the genital areas. All males should be

| BOX 3-4 | Potential Damage to the Penis |

Penile paralysis: Inability to retract the penis into the prepuce as a result of nerve or muscle (retractor penis muscle) disease

Phimosis: Inability to extend the penis from the prepuce, usually from excessive swelling of the prepuce that prevents the penis from exiting

Paraphimosis: Inability to retract the penis back into the prepuce, usually from excessive swelling of the prepuce and/or penis

Priapism: Prolonged erection unrelated to sexual desire, usually resulting from failure of the blood to exit the erectile tissue of the glans penis; swelling of prepuce and penis develops within hours and results in paraphimosis in addition to priapism

approached with caution and adequately restrained. The examiner is safest when the clinician is positioned next to the animal's chest. Standing next to the hindquarters should be avoided if possible; even heavily tranquilized animals can kick with the hindlimbs. To evaluate the penis, it must be extended from the *prepuce*. Some males allow manual extension in which the clinician inserts a gloved hand into the prepuce and gently grasps the penis; however, this is uncommon. Most males must be tranquilized to relax the *retractor penis muscle* and allow the penis to extend. Rarely, after tranquilization, the penis remains extended for a prolonged period; this is more likely to occur when *phenothiazine-based tranquilizers* are used. Regardless of the drugs used, veterinary attention should be sought if penile extension persists for longer than 2 hours. Prolonged extension interferes with venous and lymphatic drainage of the prepuce and penis, and the result is the rapid development of severe edema. Permanent damage to the penis (*penile paralysis, paraphimosis,* external trauma, *priapism*) may result if treatment is not instituted promptly (Box 3-4).

> **TECHNICIAN NOTE** Prolonged penile extension is more likely with the use of phenothiazine-based tranquilizers.

The following parameters are evaluated during a male breeding examination.

PREPUCE AND PENIS

The prepuce is commonly referred to as the *sheath* in large animals. The ability to extend the penis, extension of the penis in a straight line, and skin lesions of the prepuce or *glans penis* should be evaluated (Fig. 3-8). The penis and prepuce are susceptible to a variety of benign and malignant tumors, parasitic lesions (habronemiasis), and other growths (Fig. 3-9). These lesions have no typical appearance; any abnormality should arouse suspicion and is best evaluated by a veterinarian. Visualization of the penis of bulls is usually done during the semen collection procedure. Rams are set up on their rump. The *external preputial ring* is pushed caudally and down toward the

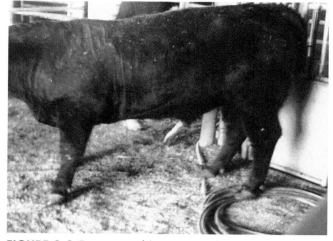

FIGURE 3-8 Examination of the prepuce and penis is a component of the reproductive examination.

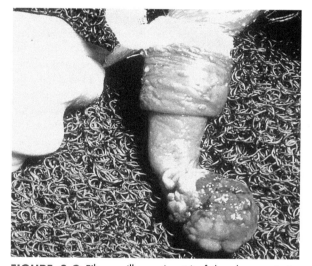

FIGURE 3-9 Fibropapillomas (warts) of the glans penis in a bull. (From Bassert JM, McCurnin DM, editors: *McCurnin's clinical textbook for veterinary technicians*, ed 7, St. Louis, 2010, Saunders, p 1087.)

abdomen to reveal the glans penis, which is gently grasped with a gauze square and pulled into extension. Horses should be examined during penile cleaning.

SCROTUM AND TESTICLES

The shape, size, and consistency of the scrotum and testicles should be evaluated. The skin should be evaluated for dermatitis. The presence of two testicles should be confirmed, as well as their ability to move within the scrotum. Ultrasound can also be used to evaluate the spermatic tissue density and consistency.

MEASUREMENT OF SCROTAL CIRCUMFERENCE

Many factors such as age, breed, and time of year can affect the scrotal circumference. Scrotal circumference is correlated with sperm production, ovulation, and age of puberty of females. Scrotal measuring tapes can be commercially obtained. In

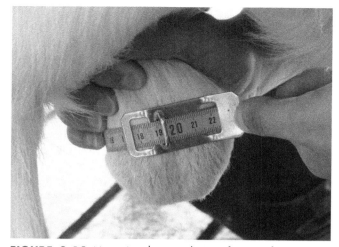

FIGURE 3-10 Measuring the scrotal circumference of a ram. The procedure is the same for bucks. The tape measure should slightly indent the skin, and the examiner should firmly push the testicles into the scrotum with the free hand. Care should be taken to read the measurement at the correct location on the measuring tape. (From Pugh DG: *Sheep and goat medicine*, ed 2, St. Louis, 2011, Saunders.)

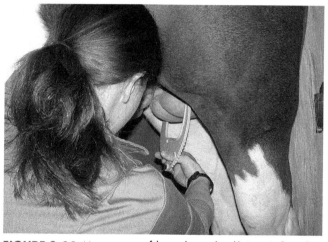

FIGURE 3-11 Measurement of the total scrotal width (TSW) of a stallion using calipers. The testes are pushed ventrally into the scrotal sac, and TSW is measured across the widest point. (From Samper JC: *Equine breeding management and artificial insemination*, ed 2, St. Louis, 2009, Saunders.)

ruminants, the measurement is made by pulling the testicles fully into the scrotal sacs and measuring snugly around the largest circumference point (Figs. 3-10 and 3-11). Normal scrotal circumference measurements in each species can be found in their specific reproductive chapters. In stallions and boars, the scrotal width is determined. An expected daily sperm output (DSO) can be estimate from testicular measurements in stallions.

BREEDING BEHAVIOR

Demonstrating breeding behavior is not always possible at the time of veterinary examination. Owners often must make these observations under natural conditions. The libido and mounting behavior of the male are observed. Intromission into the vagina and ejaculation should be confirmed (Fig. 3-12).

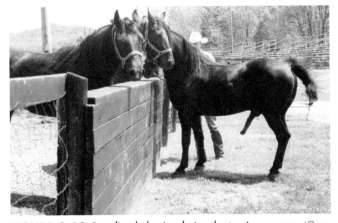

FIGURE 3-12 Breeding behavior during the teasing process. (Courtesy Kim Myers.)

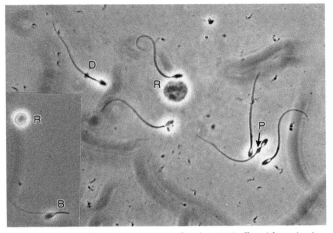

FIGURE 3-13 Equine spermatozoa fixed in 2% buffered formol saline solution and examined on a wet mount slide preparation under oil immersion using a phase-contrast microscope. Morphologic defects of these sperm include distal protoplasmic droplets (D), reversed or bent tails (B), proximal cytoplasmic droplets (P), and round spermatogenic cells (R). (From Blanchard TL, Varner DD, Bretzlaff KN: Testicular degeneration in large animals: identification and treatment. *Vet Med* 86:537-542, 1991.)

SCREENING FOR VENEREAL DISEASE

Samples may be collected during the BSE to identify the presence of venereal diseases further. Screening for these diseases includes uterine cultures or special collection techniques. Diseases and pathogens that may be screened for include *Tritrichomonas foetus, Campylobacter* species, *Taylorella equigenitalis, Pseudomonas aeruginosa, Klebsiella pneumoniae,* equine viral arteritis virus, classic swine fever, leptospirosis, porcine reproductive and respiratory syndrome (PRRS), pseudorabies, and *Brucella ovis.*

SEMEN ANALYSIS

Semen is collected using the procedures described in the following section. After collection, care must be taken to prevent temperature shock of the sperm, which can drastically affect the results of the semen evaluation. All surfaces contacted by the semen must be kept within the appropriate temperature range, from the semen collection container to the slides and microscope stage. This may require some planning, especially in cold climates. The collection bottle is taken rapidly to the laboratory for analysis. The container should not be shaken. It should be kept warm (37° C [98.6° F]) in an incubator or water bath and protected from ultraviolet light until it can be analyzed, which should be as soon as possible. However, if using a water bath to keep the semen warm, it is important to remember not to get water on the semen. Semen analysis is performed on the gel-free fraction of the ejaculate, which contains the majority of the spermatozoa. Many good references on semen analysis that detail the laboratory procedures and the normal and abnormal parameters are available (Fig. 3-13, Box 3-5, and Table 3-5). Specific semen analysis parameters can be found in the chapters on specific species.

SEMEN COLLECTION

Semen may be collected for the following purposes:
- BSE, to determine the quality and quantity of sperm as part of the fertility evaluation
- Evaluation of diseases of the male reproductive tract
- Collection and preparation of semen for AI

Semen collection is accomplished by different methods in different species. When collecting semen, it is important to keep in mind the three sperm fractions. They include the pre-sperm fraction, which is discharged first. This is a very thin secretion, and its purpose is to clean the urethra before ejaculation. The sperm-rich fraction, which is the second fraction, and is more milky; this fraction contains the spermatozoa. The third fraction, the gel fraction, is a gelatinous substance that flushes out sperm that may be left in the urethra after the second fraction has been expelled. The three primary ways to collect semen are *electroejaculation,* use of an artificial vagina (AV), and natural stimulation. No matter which way the semen is obtained, it is important to keep the semen protected and prevent it from cold shock during collection, this helps ensure you can get good sample analysis otherwise estimates of the animals true potential may be wrong, including things like DSO, daily sperm output. Therefore, a collection cup with insulation is recommended. Box 3-6 provides a list of materials needed for electroejaculation.

ELECTROEJACULATION

Electroejaculation is the use of an electroejaculator, a device that emits a mild electrical current that causes erection and ejaculation to occur (Fig. 3-14). Electroejaculation devices vary depending on the species for which they are intended. Probes are available in different sizes. A 19 × 3.5–cm probe is often used for small ruminants. A 6.5- to 7.5-cm diameter probe is often used for bulls weighing less than 2000 pounds. A 9-cm diameter probe is often used for bulls weighing more than 2000 pounds.

The prostate of the male is massaged for approximately 1 minute, and then the probe is inserted with the electrodes facing ventrally. Intermittent electrical stimulation is applied by turning a knob on the electroejaculator box and increasing the levels of stimulation with time. Stimulation should

BOX 3-5 | Semen Analysis

Gross appearance: White, opaque (resembles skim milk). It is free of blood.

Volume (mL): Usually measured by gradations on collection bottle. This is not reliable for ejaculates collected with electroejaculation.

Sperm motility: Estimate of number of sperm showing progressive forward motility. A drop of raw semen is placed on a slide and observed under x10; the sperm is observed for a wave motion.

Grading is subjective:
- Very good: whirling
- Good: slow whirls
- Fair: no whirls
- Poor: little to no motion

Individual sperm motility: The same slide used for sperm motility is covered with a cover slip and evaluated at x40. The individual sperm are assessed subjectively for motility to the nearest 5% to 10%. If the sperm concentration is too high to evaluate, the sperm can be diluted in prewarmed phosphate-buffered saline (PBS) or 2.9% sodium citrate solution to make individual sperm more readily visible.

Sperm concentration: Can be performed electronically with computer-assisted semen analysis (CASA), densimeters, or NucleoCounters (New Brunswick, supplied in North America by Eppendorf, Enfield, Conn.) or manually with a hemocytometer. These values may not be reliable from samples collected by electroejaculation. When the hemocytometer is used, the raw semen is diluted 1:100 in formalin buffer solution. The sperm are counted in the central grid of both chambers of the hemocytometer. The average of the fields is taken, and that equals the semen concentration in 10^6/mL.

Total number of sperm: Multiply volume (mL) by sperm concentration. In stallions, two samples are collected 1 hour apart, and the second sample is used for determining this measurement. Fertile stallions contain more than 1.1 billion normal motile spermatozoa.

Sperm morphology: Light microscope at x1000 magnification is used to examine air-dried, stained smears.

Live sperm percentage: Gathered by using the eosin/nigrosin stain. Only live sperm uptake the stain, and the percentage of live sperm can be determined by counting both the live and dead sperm.

pH: Measured by pH meter. pH paper lacks precision.

Sperm morphology: A drop of semen is mixed with a stain (Hancock, eosin/nigrin), and a smear is prepared and air dried. The sample is examined under the oil immersion lens, and 100 cells are counted. Each cell is classified either as normal or as having a primary or secondary abnormality. Primary abnormalities arise from the testes, whereas secondary abnormalities arise from the epididymis. Abaxial attachment of the midpieces is normal in boars and stallions. Phase contrast microscopy can also be used.

TABLE 3-5 | Semen Analysis

MORPHOLOGY	ABNORMALITY (PRIMARY OR SECONDARY)	MORPHOLOGY	ABNORMALITY (PRIMARY OR SECONDARY)
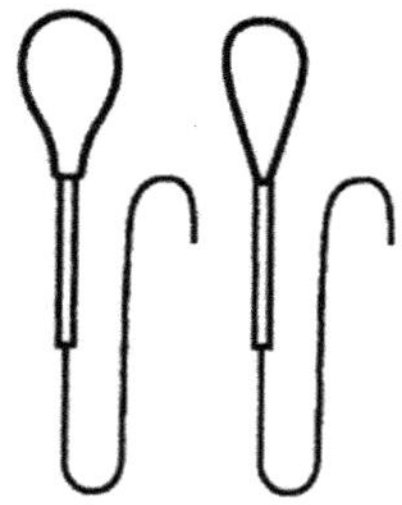	Pyriform head (primary)	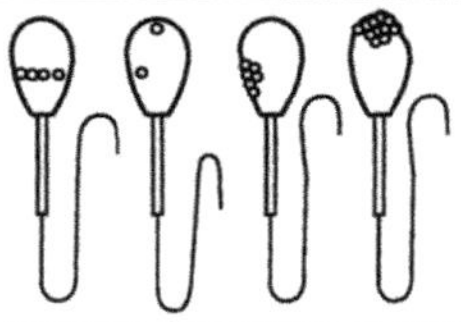	Vacules/craters (primary)
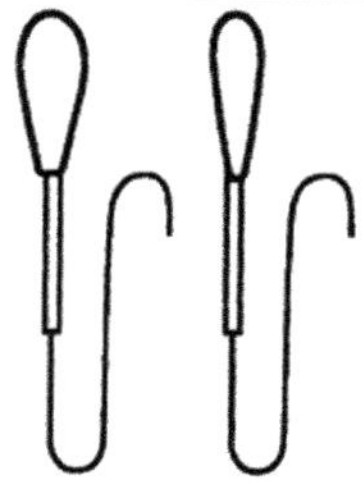	Tapered head (primary)	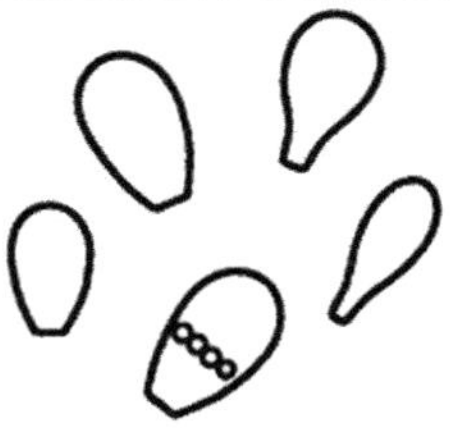	Detached heads (secondary)
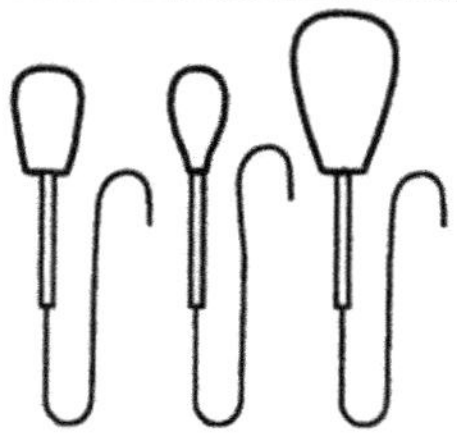	Microcephalic and macrocephalic sperm (primary)	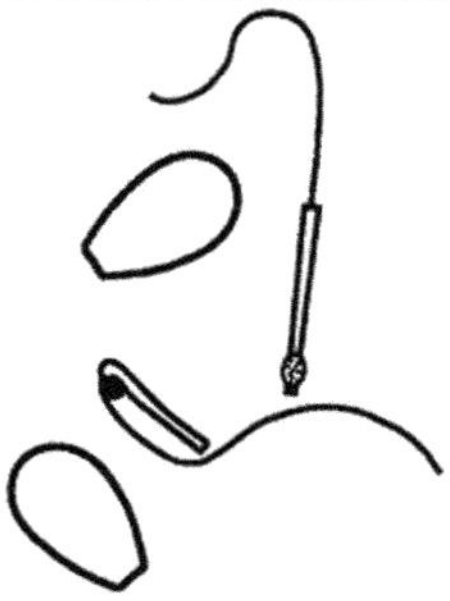	Decapitated defect (secondary)

Continued

TABLE 3-5 | Semen Analysis—cont'd

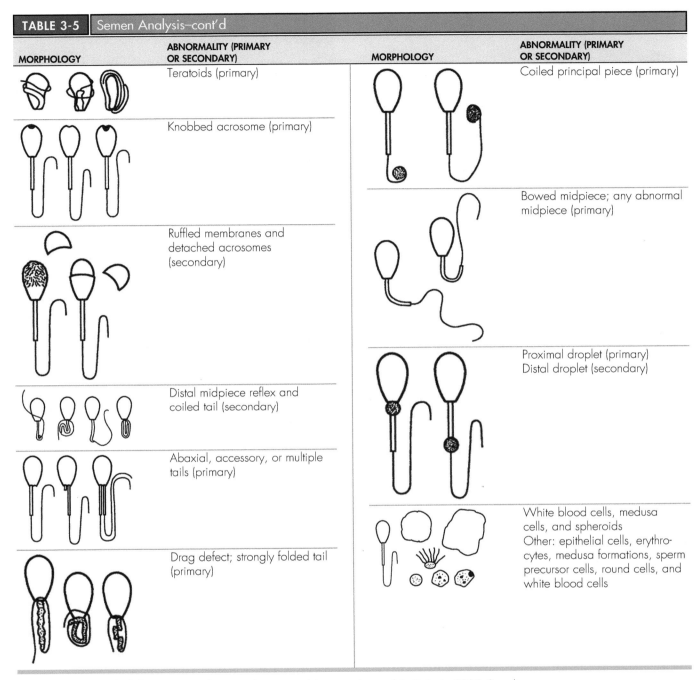

MORPHOLOGY	ABNORMALITY (PRIMARY OR SECONDARY)	MORPHOLOGY	ABNORMALITY (PRIMARY OR SECONDARY)
	Teratoids (primary)		Coiled principal piece (primary)
	Knobbed acrosome (primary)		Bowed midpiece; any abnormal midpiece (primary)
	Ruffled membranes and detached acrosomes (secondary)		Proximal droplet (primary) Distal droplet (secondary)
	Distal midpiece reflex and coiled tail (secondary)		
	Abaxial, accessory, or multiple tails (primary)		White blood cells, medusa cells, and spheroids Other: epithelial cells, erythrocytes, medusa formations, sperm precursor cells, round cells, and white blood cells
	Drag defect; strongly folded tail (primary)		

From Youngquist RS, Threlfall WR. *Current therapy in large animal theriogenology*, ed 2, St. Louis, 2007, Saunders.

BOX 3-6 | Materials Required for Electroejaculation

- Electroejaculator (box, cord, and probe)
- Collection container
- Rectal palpation sleeve

be started at the lowest level possible and the knob turned approximately 10 times before increasing the stimulate to the next level, and then the knob should be turned approximately 10 more times before jumping to another level, and so on until ejaculation occurs.

ARTIFICIAL VAGINA

AVs can be used for semen collection. Box 3-7 provides a list of materials needed for AV use. Several styles of AVs are

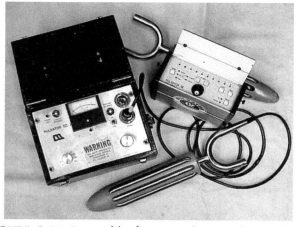

FIGURE 3-14 Two models of ruminant electroejaculators and two rectal probes. (From Bassert JM, McCurnin DM, editors: *McCurnin's clinical textbook for veterinary technicians,* ed 7, St. Louis, 2010, Saunders.)

BOX 3-7	Materials Required for Artificial Vagina Use

- Artificial vagina
- Thermometer
- Hot water
- Collection bottle
- Female in estrus, sweet steer, or phantom dummy
- Nonspermicidal jelly

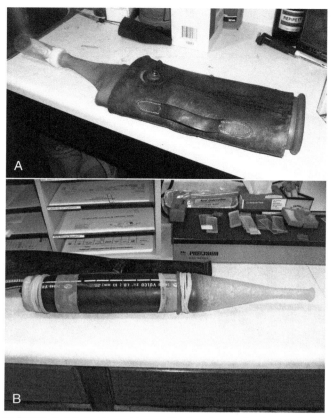

FIGURE 3-15 **A,** Missouri-type artificial vagina used on horses. **B,** Bull artificial vagina.

available, but all contain the same basic components: an outer casing, an inner lining, and a collection bottle. The outer casing provides for a secure grip on the device and protects the contents. An inner lining usually has a rubber bladder that can be filled with warm water; the male ejaculates into the inner lining. The inner lining leads to a collection bottle for containing the semen (Fig. 3-15).

The AV must be prepared for cleanliness and male comfort. The reusable rubber AV liner should be cleaned and flushed with clean hot water, soaked in isopropyl alcohol for at least 2 hours, and then air dried. Soaps and disinfectants can build up residues in the rubber that may be spermicidal and therefore are seldom used. Some rubber liners can be gas sterilized with ethylene oxide, but sterilization must be followed by 2 to 3 days of airing out; consult the manufacturer's instructions for cleaning options. Disposable AV liners are available. These liners are nontoxic to sperm, but some males do not accept the plastic liners as well as the reusable rubber liners.

Stallions are particular about the temperature of the AV. The optimal temperature inside the AV is approximately 45° C (113° F). Filling the AV with slightly warmer water allows for some heat loss before use, but the temperature of the water should not exceed 48° C (118.4° F). Some stallions need adjustments to the temperature. The liner should be checked for comfortable pressure. It should apply good contact around the penis and allow for full expansion of the penis,

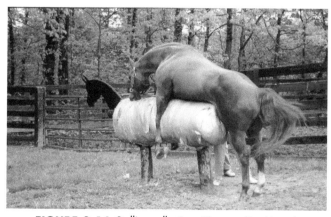

FIGURE 3-16 Stallion collection. (Courtesy Kim Myers.)

but overfilling may prevent the erect penis from entering the AV. The inner lining should be lubricated with a sterile nonspermicidal lubricant by placing the lubricant on a sterilely gloved hand and smearing the lubricant on the cranial two thirds of the liner. Finally, a gel filter is usually inserted into the AV to catch and strain out the gel fraction of the ejaculate and any impurities (Fig. 3-16).

NATURAL STIMULATION

Natural stimulation requires manual stimulation of the male. Box 3-8 contains a list of materials used for natural stimulation.

BOX 3-8	Materials Required for Natural Stimulation

- Vinyl or nitrile gloves
- Phantom dummy
- Collection container
- Filter

BOX 3-9	Materials Required for Postcoital Aspiration

- Obstetrical sleeve
- Warm water and antiseptic
- Sponge

Because of the major differences associated with semen collection in each species, specific information on semen collection can be obtained in the sections of this book on individual species. Natural stimulation is often performed for boars; a gloved hand is used. During collection of boar semen, it is important to apply constant pressure to the glans penis. Because boars have a large gel fraction of their ejaculate, a filter is used to separate it during collection.

POSTCOITAL ASPIRATION

Postcoital aspiration can be performed in camelids. Box 3-9 provides a list of materials used for postcoital aspiration. A sponge is placed into the vagina of the female just bred, and the seminal fluid is collected from the vagina for evaluation. The sponge must be sterile, and when washing the vulva before collection great care is taken to avoid allowing water to contaminate the sperm sample. Water kills sperm very quickly, so avoiding water contamination is important for proper evaluation.

SEMEN PREPARATION FOR ARTIFICIAL INSEMINATION

Frozen semen is packaged in hollow plastic French straws *(semen straws)* or in ampules. Straws have largely replaced ampules; they are easily inserted into special insemination catheters or "guns" for easy use and survive the freezing process better than ampules.

This is an overview of sperm preparation for freezing (Figs. 3-17 and 3-18). Specific details relevant to each species can be found in this book in the sections on each species. Sperm gathered for freezing is obtained using the same semen collection procedures described previously. When sperm is prepared for freezing, the sperm-rich fraction is filtered from the gel fraction of the ejaculate, evaluated, and diluted with semen extender according to the results of the semen evaluation.

Extenders are a combination of liquid and solid ingredients designed primarily to nourish the sperm and help them survive outside the male's "reproductive" tract. Extenders are also used to increase the volume of sperm if the ejaculate is to be split into two or more aliquots. Most of the many recipes for extenders contain a source of protein and simple sugars. They are buffered for pH, and sometimes antibiotics are added to reduce the incidence of bacterial venereally transmitted diseases.

ESTROUS CYCLE DETERMINATION

Planned breeding is labor intensive but allows for good record keeping and better reproductive, nutritional, and veterinary management of breeding stock. Planned breeding begins with estrous cycle determination. Knowledge of the estrous cycle and of each breeding female's stage of the reproductive cycle helps veterinary personnel and producers to be successful with breeding and even with treatment of uterine infections that can be counterproductive in the breeding process.

Most often, producers and veterinary personnel are concerned with identifying animals in estrus. Monitoring animals for estrus status is known as heat detection.

The methods available for estrous cycle staging can be performed at any time and include those described in the following paragraphs.

RECTAL PALPATION

Rectal palpation is commonly used in horses and cattle. In cattle, chute or head catch restraint is generally used (Fig. 3-19). Horses usually are restrained in stocks. Rectal palpation allows for examination of the ovaries and for the presence of follicles and their size. Follicles increase in size and become softer as the time of ovulation approaches. The follicles and corpora lutea of cattle are more superficial on the ovary than in the horse; therefore, palpation is more informative in cattle. In horses, early follicles develop inside the ovary and may be missed by palpation. Secondarily, the cervix can be examined for consistency. The cervix relaxes (dilates) and becomes *hyperemic* during estrus.

VAGINAL EXAMINATIONS

A vaginal examination is most useful in horses. It usually consists of a visual examination of the cervix through a vaginal speculum. Preparation of the *perineum* and *vulva* should be performed. A vaginal speculum (disposable or reusable) and a light source (penlight, flashlight) are required for a visual examination (Fig. 3-20).

For a manual vaginal examination, the examiner needs a sterile obstetrical sleeve and sterile, water-soluble lubricant. The cervix is observed. A relaxed, hyperemic cervix is consistent with estrogen influence (estrus), whereas a "high-dry-tight" cervix is consistent with progesterone influence (diestrus or *luteal phase*). Evaluation of the cervix is not as specific as other methods for staging the estrous cycle. It typically is used to supplement other observations (Fig. 3-21).

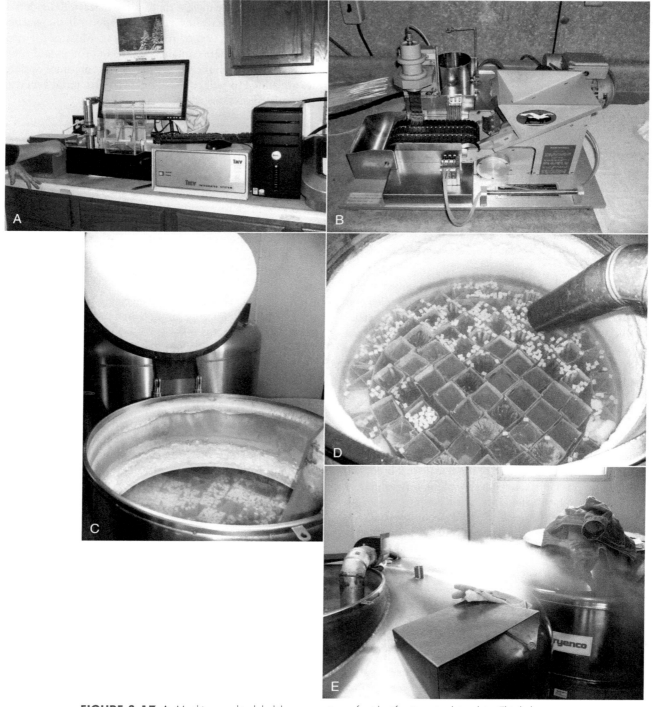

FIGURE 3-17 **A,** Machine used to label the semen straws for identification at a later date. This helps producers, technicians, and veterinarians ensure the right semen is placed in the right female. **B,** Machine used to fill semen straws before the final freeze. **C,** Tanks have very thick insulation to help keep the semen frozen with liquid nitrogen. **D,** Semen straws are often color coded to help with identification. **E,** Notice the fog produced by liquid nitrogen. When semen tanks arrive at your clinic, make sure you see some fog when you open the container because this indicates the semen has remained frozen during the shipping process.

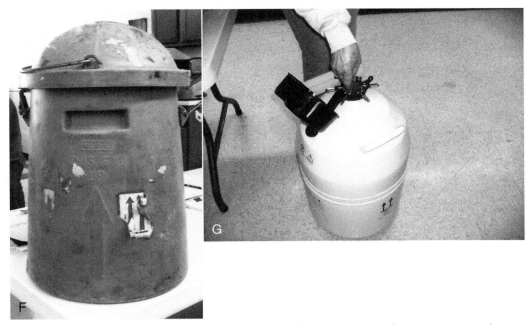

FIGURE 3-17, cont'd F, Semen is often shipped to producers or veterinary clinics in containers such as these. **G,** When semen arrives at your clinic, it is important that you transfer it to a farm tank such as this one.

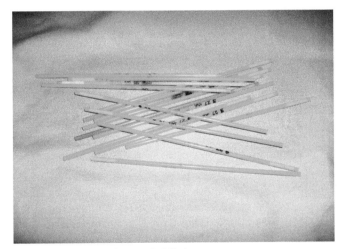

FIGURE 3-18 Semen straws.

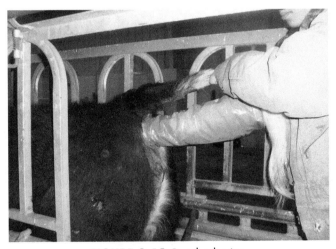

FIGURE 3-19 Rectal palpation.

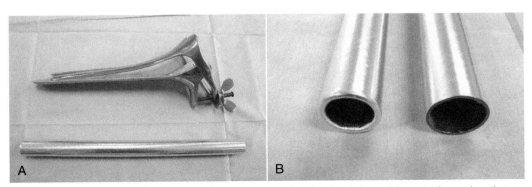

FIGURE 3-20 A, Stainless steel reusable vaginal speculum *(top)* and disposable vaginal speculum *(bottom).* **B,** The disposable vaginal speculum has a smooth rounded edge *(left)* at one end designed to be inserted into the vagina. The sharper edge *(right)* is used as a handhold.

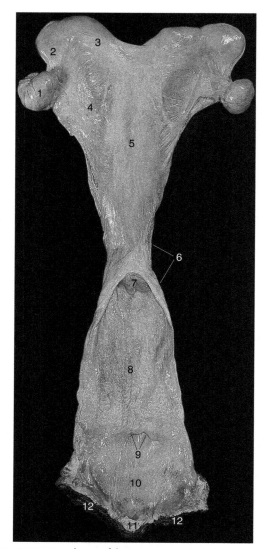

FIGURE 3-21 Dorsal view of the equine reproductive tract. The vagina and vestibule have been opened from the dorsal side. *1,* Ovary; *2,* tip of the left uterine horn; *3,* left uterine horn; *4,* broad ligament; *5,* body of the uterus; *6,* position of the cervix; *7,* external opening of the cervix; *8,* vagina; *9,* urethral opening; *10,* vestibule; *11,* clitoris; *12,* vulva. (From Flood PF, Rosenstein DS, Mandeville D: Abdominal and pelvic viscera. In Clayton HM, Flood PF: *Clinical anatomy of the horse,* Oxford, 2006, Mosby.)

> **TECHNICIAN NOTE**   Manual evaluation of the cervix is useful in horses. A hyperemic cervix is indicative of estrus. A high-dry-tight cervix is indicative of the luteal phase.

DIAGNOSTIC ULTRASOUND PER RECTUM

Diagnostic ultrasound per rectum can be used in cattle and horses. Although it is seldom necessary in cattle because of the ease of ovary palpation, it is the most accurate method for determining a *mare's* estrous cycle phase. A rectal examination is typically performed before the ultrasound study to allow palpation of the uterus and cervix. Feces from the rectum are evacuated so that the ultrasound *transducer* achieves good contact with the rectal wall. Ultrasound is superior to palpation of the ovaries in that it can visualize

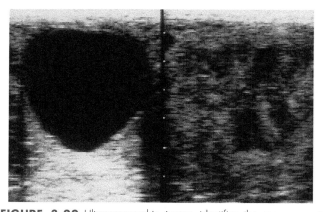

FIGURE 3-22 Ultrasonographic image identifies the *measurement* of an equine follicle for the possibility of ovulation. (From Brinsko SP, Blanchard TL, Varner DD: *Manual of equine reproduction,* ed 3, St. Louis, 2011, Mosby.)

inside the ovaries to see structures such as small follicles. It also allows precise measurement of follicle size. Follicle size is important because most mares ovulate when follicle diameter reaches 35 to 55 mm (Fig. 3-22). Individual animals usually establish a fairly consistent ovulation diameter, which can be followed from year to year to help predict the time of ovulation.

> **TECHNICIAN NOTE**   Diagnostic ultrasound per rectum is the most accurate method for estrous cycle determination in the mare.

OBSERVATION OF STANDING HEAT

Observation of *standing heat* can be useful in cattle, horses, sheep, goats, and swine. Physical signs such as a swollen vulva, vaginal discharge, increased vocalization, frequent urination, and restlessness may be seen in ruminants that are in estrus. However, the most reliable indicator of estrus is the observation of a female that allows other animals to mount her. This evaluation is often simply performed by routine visual herd checks. If animals are in groups, it is common to observe them twice a day for a minimum of 30 minutes. Animals may be observed being "ridden" or may be checked for signs of having been mounted, such as ruffled hair or hair loss in the tail-head area, or mud and dirt on top of the hindquarters. The number of the animal is recorded, and breeding is planned accordingly (Fig. 3-23). The cow that is standing for the mounting is in heat, not the animal that is mounting.

> **TECHNICIAN NOTE**   Remember that the cow that is standing for the mounting is in heat, not the animal that is mounting.

In swine, visual signs may include enlargement and reddening of the vulva, restlessness, mounting of other females, and decreased appetite. A mucoid vaginal discharge is occasionally seen. In swine, it is common for 6 to 12 gilts to be

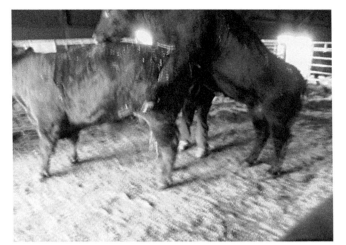

FIGURE 3-23 This cow is showing a strong mounting response. Remember the cow that is standing is the animal in heat. Cows not exposed to bulls will also ride each other and show similar responses.

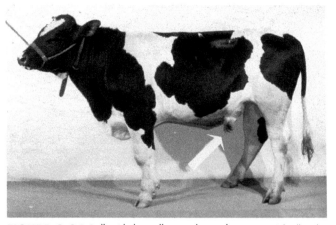

FIGURE 3-24 Bull with laterally translocated prepuce. Ideally, the newly created preputial orifice should be adjacent to the fold of the flank *(arrow)*. (From Fubini S, Ducharme N: *Farm animal surgery*, St. Louis, 2004, Saunders.)

taken to the boar for evaluation of estrus or for the boar to be walked along a line of sow stalls and the females' response documented while the boar is in front of their stalls. Females in standing heat respond to the sight, sound, and smell of a boar (intact or *vasectomized*) and seek the boar. If the boar mounts the female, the female will assume a characteristic motionless stance with the legs rigid and the ears stiff and erect ("popping the ears"). This stance is known as *lordosis*, and a female in standing heat displays this stance if pressure is placed on her back. This behavior is used to advantage by handlers; by pressing firmly down on a female's back with the hands and initiating a lordosis response, standing heat can be confirmed.

Mares are often observed for signs of estrus by teasing them with a stallion across a fence or stall door. The mare is observed for winking of the vulva, squatting, urinating, tail raising, and posturing. Some producers and veterinarians grade the response observed when teasing and assign a number that correlates with the strength of response, which should correlate with her stage of estrous.

Camelids are evaluated for cushing, which is positioning of the female in ventral recumbency.

Other methods to detect standing heat can be used that do not require direct observation of the behavior. *Heat mount detectors* or *chemical marking patches* ("rump patches") are adhesive patches with chemicals contained in a flexible, clear plastic sleeve. The patch is placed on top of the hindquarters, over the sacral spine. If an animal is mounted, the weight of the mounting animal crushes the plastic sleeve and allows the chemicals to mix, resulting in a color change. The herdsman simply checks the herd for activated rump patches, indicating standing heat.

Teaser animals, also known as *gomers* or *sidewinders* (Fig. 3-24), may also be used to mark estrus females. Teaser animals are prepared in several ways; each method has advantages and disadvantages. Intact males may be vasectomized or have the penis surgically translocated to prevent

entry into the vagina. Teaser females may be prepared by treatment with hormones, with or without spaying. Castrated males may be treated with testosterone. Once the teaser animal has been prepared, it is fitted with a marking device. The device is often a chin-ball halter or marking collar, which contains a dye reservoir. When the teaser mounts the estrus female, the riding activity applies the dye in a to-and-fro motion across the back of the estrus female. The herdsman checks the herd for the dye marks left by the teaser, thus indicating that the female is in standing heat. Females can also have temporary marking paint applied to their tail head to aid in identification of females in heat. If the paint is rubbed away, the producer knows the animal has been ridden. Electronic mounting devices can be applied to the tail head of females. When other animals ride the female wearing the device, the device sends a signal to the computer that informs the producer that the female is in heat.

VAGINAL CYTOLOGY

Vaginal cytology can be used in any large animal species. Although cyclic changes do occur in the epithelial cells lining the vagina, the changes are not as specific as in small animal species and therefore have limited practical application.

PEDOMETRY

Pedometers are devices placed on the neck or legs of cows that evaluate the number of steps the animals take. During estrus, cattle tend to take more steps, and this can be used as a mechanism to evaluate estrus.

ESTRUS SYNCHRONIZATION

Estrus synchronization is used as a management tool when breeding a large number of females. Estrus synchronization is especially useful when using AI. It may be advantageous to "synchronize" the herd so that labor and planning can be maximized for efficiency.

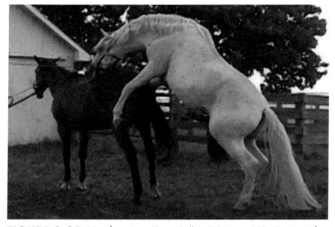

FIGURE 3-25 Hand mating. (From Sellon DC, Long MT: *Equine infectious diseases*, St. Louis, 2007, Saunders.)

Synchronization is usually accomplished by hormonal treatment with prostaglandin, progesterone, or estrogen compounds. The hormones can be used alone or in combination, depending on the desired effect. They are delivered by injection, subcutaneous implant, or intravaginal drug-releasing sponges. Some hormones can be delivered orally as a feed additive. The regimen used depends largely on the species and the management needs of the farm operation.

Subcutaneous hormone implants are used commonly in cattle and less often in small ruminants. The implants are placed on the outer (dorsal) aspect of the ear pinna, between the skin and the cartilage. Implants are injected using a special injection gun designed by the manufacturer for its individual brand of implant. The skin of the ear pinna should be cleaned before the injection.

LIVE COVER

Live cover is used in all species. Live cover refers to the physical mounting and breeding that occurs between a male and a female. The producer need not be involved in this process, other than placing the selected animals together. However, use of live cover in some production systems is rare because of the increased use of AI. Some systems used in live cover breeding include *pen mating* or harem breeding, *hand mating*, and *individual breeding*.

PEN MATING

Pen mating or harem breeding is a system in which multiple animals are placed together and allowed to mate using natural instincts. Most often, there are multiple females but only a few males.

HAND MATING

Hand mating is a system of placing one male and one female together during the female's estrus. The producer remains present during the breeding process to ensure that breeding takes place (Fig. 3-25).

INDIVIDUAL BREEDING

Individual breeding is a system of placing one male and one female together. They are left in the same pen for an extended period of time. The animals are not observed. The producer assumes that the female will eventually enter estrus and be mated during the proper time.

ARTIFICIAL INSEMINATION

Supplies include the following:
- Animal records
- Restraint
- Liquid nitrogen tank or semen cooler
- Electric thaw unit
- Thermometer
- Timer
- Semen or insemination pipettes
- Straw cutter or scissors

Other insemination equipment varies by species.

AI is commonly used in horses, cattle, and swine. AI is used more in dairy cattle than in any other farm animal. It is used in dairy goats and beef cattle and less often in sheep. AI is a procedure in which fresh or frozen semen is placed into the female's reproductive tract with the use of a pipette.

AI offers many benefits, including the following:
- Reduced potential for transmission of venereal diseases
- Ability for one sire to "breed" more females than possible with natural breeding, thus allowing fewer males to be used in the breeding program and allowing genetically superior males to exert more influence on a herd
- Ability to synchronize estrus in a herd of females and therefore have a shorter and better defined breeding season
- Reduced physical injury risk to both the male and female from natural mounting and penetration
- Facilitation of shipping and long-term storage of semen, thereby allowing wide distribution of superior genetics
- Elimination of the need to keep and care for a breeding male on the premises
- Better management of the breeding program and better planning for food, labor, and medical needs

Not all breed registries accept individuals that have been conceived by AI. Some registries allow AI, provided it is performed with the female and male on the same premises. If breed registration of offspring is desired, the animal owner should consult the breed registry for current regulations and restrictions.

An AI program can be conducted in two basic ways: (1) keep breeding males on the premises and collect fresh semen as needed for prompt use or (2) store deep-frozen *(cryopreserved)* semen from males from any geographic location and use the semen when needed. Cattle spermatozoa in particular tolerate cryopreservation extremely well, so the sperm can be kept almost indefinitely.

PREPARATION OF THE PERINEUM/VULVA FOR REPRODUCTIVE PROCEDURES

Many reproductive procedures begin with proper cleansing of the perineum and vulva, especially whenever the vagina is to be entered as part of the procedure. Cleansing is performed to prevent carrying feces and other debris inside the vagina, cervix, and uterus. Mares are often prepared for AI more intensively than other species because of their increased likelihood to contract an infection that can be detrimental to conception. In ruminants and swine, this step is often skipped when performing AI. However, similar preparation is performed in these species for other reproductive procedures.

The female should be properly restrained. The tail should be bandaged or wrapped and either held or tied to the side for the procedure. Cleansing is usually done with roll cotton soaked in warm, clean water. Mild soap should be the cleansing product of choice for AI. Povidone-iodine scrub or chlorhexidine scrub can be used if preparation for other procedures is needed. An initial cleansing of the anal area may be necessary to remove crusted feces and fecal water. Then, using scrub, the preparation is begun on the lips of the vulva and gradually extended in circular fashion to include the perineum, anus, and inner aspect of the buttocks. Water is used in the same pattern to rinse away the soap. The process is repeated as many times as necessary until no residue is seen on the cotton.

The technician should be careful to stand to the side of the hindquarters during cleansing of this area and be alert to possible kicks. Some females are sensitive to water dripping on the hocks or running down the legs. This sensitivity could cause some animals to kick. Horses in particular are sensitive to this water. Any water running down a horse's thighs and hocks should be wiped with dry cotton or a dry towel.

Once the area is prepared, the tail should not be allowed to contact the area. If defecation occurs, the entire cleaning process should be repeated. Following the veterinarian's procedures, cleansing of the area again to remove lubricant, blood, or other debris may be necessary.

HANDLING OF SEMEN FOR ARTIFICIAL INSEMINATION

Proper semen handling is critical for successful conception. Without proper handling, semen will die or become damaged, greatly decreasing the chances of successful conception.

Nitrogen tank maintenance is also important. Frozen semen should be stored in the tanks at a temperature of −196° C. It is important to keep more than 2 inches of liquid nitrogen in the tank at all times. If these requirements are met, the semen can be stored indefinitely. The tank should be kept in a clean, dry, well-ventilated environment. It is wise to store the tank elevated from the floor, if possible, to help avoid corrosion.

Before beginning the AI procedure, it is important to prepare the female as described previously. Document the female's identification, date, time, and any physical examination findings that may influence her ability to care a pregnancy to term. Next, the semen straw should be located within the nitrogen tank. Care should be taken to avoid lifting the canes out of tank to identify them. This can compromise the safety

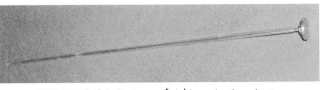

FIGURE 3-26 Bovine artificial insemination pipette.

of frozen semen. If identification can be performed without raising the canes, it should be. If it is not possible, then the canes should not be lifted out of the tank for more than 10 seconds. Identification of the appropriate straws is extremely important. Care should be taken to ensure that the proper straw is used for insemination because the cost of these straws and breedings can be thousands of dollars.

The appropriate straw should then be thawed. Only thaw one straw at a time. The straw should be thawed only once you are sure that insemination will occur immediately following the thaw. Some semen manufactures send thaw instructions with the semen; if this is done; the instructions should be followed. If instructions are not provided, then the semen should be thawed in a water bath at 35° to 37° C for 40 seconds.

Any excess water on the outside of the straw should be dried. The air bubble in the straw should be flicked to the sealed end, and the sealed end is cut. The straw is loaded into the insemination pipette or gun (varies by species) and kept warm. Keeping it warm is most often accomplished by placing it under the inseminator's clothing. Insemination should occur promptly after the thaw.

ARTIFICIAL INSEMINATION PROCEDURE

All insemination equipment must be kept clean and handled carefully to prevent contamination. Contamination can result in death of sperm and/or infection of the female's reproductive tract. Insemination should be performed with care because puncture or laceration of the reproductive tract with the equipment is possible. The AI procedure varies from species to species (Fig. 3-26). The AI procedure for each species is described in the chapters on individual species.

EMBRYO TRANSFER

Embryo transfer has become an increasingly valuable tool in reproduction. Most commercial interest in embryo transfer is for cattle, but the procedure is used by some purebred breeders of sheep, goats, and horses. The procedure is not yet widely used in swine. The process has been used mainly to obtain more progeny from genetically superior sires and dams, but more recently the potential to control certain infectious diseases has been recognized. By controlling the health status of the donor females and special handling of the embryos, pathogen-free embryos can be produced. It is safer to move pathogen-free embryos into a herd than young, potentially disease-carrying animals. Because cattle embryos can be cryopreserved in liquid nitrogen, they can be shipped to recipient cows anywhere in the world. In horses, another advantage of embryo transfer is that the donor mare can remain in competition (e.g., racing, showing) without ever becoming pregnant herself.

All stages of the embryo transfer process, from collection to microscopic evaluation to storage and finally transfer, must be conducted under conditions that are as sterile as possible. The embryos should be protected from temperature shock and evaporation of the liquid medium. Embryo transfer consists of the following basic steps:

- Superovulation: *Superovulation* is the ability to cause a single female to ovulate multiple eggs. Hormonal treatment is used to stimulate follicle development and control the timing of estrus and ovulation.
- Breeding: The donor animal is bred naturally or, more commonly, by AI.
- Embryo recovery: The donor's uterus is flushed days after ovulation to recover the embryo. The days for *flushing* are specific to each individual species. In some species a *Foley catheter* can be used to collect the embryos; in other species collection must be done with surgical methods. Modified phosphate-buffered saline (PBS) is used to collect the embryos into special collection containers that filter the embryos.
- Embryo identification: The contents of the filter cup are poured into a sterile "search dish" and examined with a stereomicroscope. Once an embryo is identified, a special pipette is used to aspirate the embryo and place it in a special culture medium. Embryos are rated for quality and classified as good, moderate, or poor. Degenerated or defective embryos are discarded.
- Embryo transfer: The embryo is transferred to a recipient female that has been hormonally synchronized to prepare her reproductive tract for pregnancy. The embryo may be transferred surgically through a standing flank procedure (preferred) or a ventral midline approach using general anesthesia, or it may be transferred nonsurgically through the vaginal-cervical route. Species-specific embryo transfer procedures are discussed further in the chapters on individual species (Figs. 3-27 to and 3-31).

PREGNANCY DETECTION

Confirming pregnancy has several important roles in a managed breeding program. It allows for planning of labor; feeding, veterinary, and space needs; and estimated budgeting for associated costs and potential profits. It also allows early identification of females with fertility problems so that diagnosis and treatment can be instituted in the hope of subsequent breeding and successful pregnancy without missing a breeding season. Failure to produce offspring each breeding season represents an economic loss to the producer.

The pregnancy detection procedure is used to identify the presence of an embryo or fetus and to estimate the gestational age of the embryo or fetus if the breeding date is unknown. It can be used to determine fetal viability by confirming the presence and vigor of the fetal heartbeat. It is also used to identify twin conceptions, which are undesirable in a horse

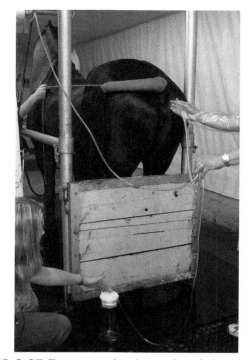

FIGURE 3-27 The mare is placed in stocks with the tail wrapped and hung in a vertical position. The technician, who is wearing a sterile sleeve, holds the sterile catheter while examining the integrity of the air cuff. The system is completed by a large-volume filter and a plastic container with flushing medium, both connected to the catheter by Silastic tubing and a V-junction. The flushing medium is collected in a graduated recipient to measure the volume recovered. (From Samper JC: *Equine breeding management and artificial insemination,* ed 2, St. Louis, 2009, Saunders.)

because the equine uterus is not designed to support and nourish more than one fetus. Competition for space and nutrition usually results in the death and abortion or *stillbirth* of both twin fetuses. Occasionally, one twin is born alive, but it typically is weak and small, and a twin foal faces a high mortality rate. Birth of living twins is rare, and survival of both is even rarer. When twin embryos or fetuses are detected, the veterinarian needs to advise the owner of options to either terminate the pregnancy or terminate one of the embryos in hope that the other may survive. Methods of twin reduction include crushing, which can be performed between 14 and 15 days and has a 95% success rate. Other methods often have an estimated 50% success rate and include crushing when there is a bicornual twin; this procedure can be performed between 16 and 60 days. Pinching can be performed between 35 and 60 days, craniocervical dislocation between 65 and 110 days, and ultrasound-guided fetal injection at 115 to 130 days. Technicians should consult their state laws concerning pregnancy diagnosis. Some states consider pregnancy diagnosis to be a diagnosis, and veterinary technicians are not allowed to perform the examination.

Various tools are available to diagnose pregnancy with greater precision. The accuracy of the many methods of pregnancy determination varies depending on the species, stage of pregnancy, and skill of the clinician. The cost of the

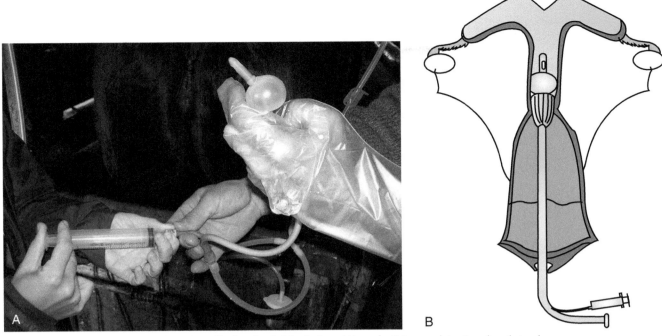

FIGURE 3-28 A, Air cuff inflated with 30 mL of air. We prefer 24-gauge latex French catheters because they are inexpensive and very soft, so minimal trauma is caused to the uterus during flushing. **B,** Correct placement of the flushing catheter, forming a tight seal at the internal cervical os after the cuff has been inflated. (From Samper JC: *Equine breeding management and artificial insemination,* ed 2, St. Louis, 2009, Saunders.)

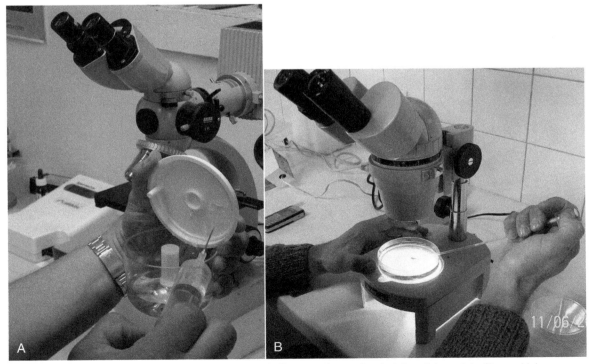

FIGURE 3-29 A, The filter content is poured off in a sterile cross-hatched Petri dish, and the filter and lid are rinsed with flushing medium to reduce the risk of embryos sticking to them. **B,** The embryos are then evaluated under a microscope. (From Samper JC: *Equine breeding management and artificial insemination,* ed 2, St. Louis, 2009, Saunders.)

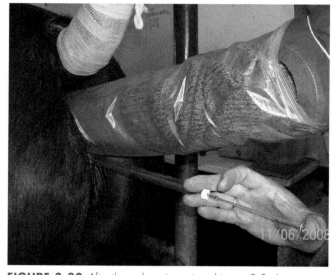

FIGURE 3-30 After the embryo is aspirated into a 0.5-mL straw, it is placed into a disposable sterile transfer gun. The embryo is transferred to the tip of a uterine horn by applying gentle pressure on the transfer gun plunger. (From Samper JC: *Equine breeding management and artificial insemination*, ed 2, St. Louis, 2009, Saunders.)

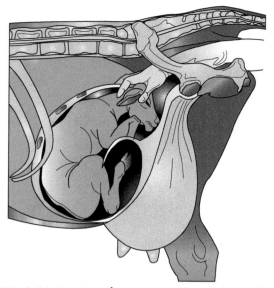

FIGURE 3-32 Detection of pregnancy in the cow by rectal palpation. Pregnancy is approaching term. (From Noakes DE, Parkinson TJ, England GCW: *Veterinary reproduction and obstetrics*, ed 9, London, 2009, Saunders.)

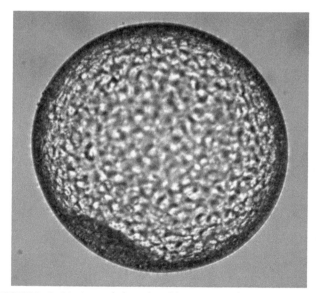

FIGURE 3-31 Expanded grade 1 blastocyst recovered 8 days after ovulation. (From Samper JC: *Equine breeding management and artificial insemination*, ed 2, St. Louis, 2009, Saunders.)

RECTAL PALPATION

In Horses

Experienced clinicians can detect the presence of a pregnancy as early as 18 to 21 days. By 28 days, pregnancy usually is easy to confirm with rectal palpation. As pregnancy proceeds, the fetus enlarges and fluid accumulates around it, thus causing the uterus gradually to "fall" over the brim of the pelvis into the abdominal cavity. This leads to a time period from approximately day 90 to day 150 when confirmation of a pregnancy may be difficult because the uterus is essentially out of reach of the palpator. After day 150, pregnancy determination is more consistent, and after approximately day 270, the fetus has enlarged to a size that can be reliably felt. Rectal palpation cannot be used to detect fetal heartbeat and can detect a living fetus only by detecting movement of the fetus in late pregnancy.

In Cattle

Rectal palpation is the most common method used in cattle. Experienced clinicians can detect pregnancies reliably as early as 25 to 30 days (Fig. 3-32).

In Sheep and Goats

A method of rectal palpation with a hollow plastic "palpation rod" *(Hulet rod)* has been described in sheep. The ewe is placed on her back (a submissive position for sheep), and the lubricated rod is inserted into the rectum and is used gently to elevate and hold the uterus against the abdominal wall, where it can be palpated with the free hand. Developed fetuses may be felt through the abdominal wall. With experience, detection of pregnant ewes may be highly accurate after 60 days of gestation. Palpation rods can be used in goats but are difficult to use because goats resent being restrained on their backs and often struggle, possibly resulting in rectal tears and abortions.

procedure is usually a necessary consideration. Accurate breeding records are helpful in selecting the best diagnostic test for a suspected pregnant animal, based on the suspected length of the pregnancy. Methods of pregnancy diagnosis include those discussed in the following paragraphs.

FAILURE TO RETURN TO ESTRUS

Many producers or owners simply use the failure to return to heat as the primary pregnancy "test." However, failure to return to heat may indicate conditions other than pregnancy, such as a pathologically *persistent corpus luteum* or *cystic ovaries.*

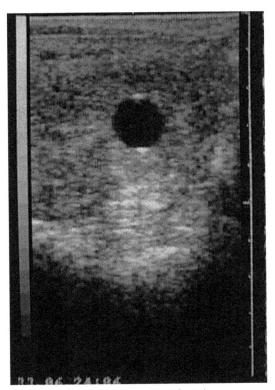

FIGURE 3-33 Ultrasound examination of 13-day pregnancy. (From Colahan PT, Merritt AM, Moore JN, Mayhew IG, editors: *Equine medicine and surgery*, vol 2, ed 5, St. Louis, 1999, Mosby.)

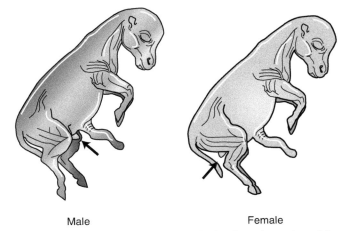

Male

Female

FIGURE 3-34 Location of the genital tubercle in the male and female fetus. (From Reef VB: *Equine diagnostic ultrasound*, St. Louis, 1998, Saunders.)

In Swine

Rectal palpation is possible in larger sows if the palpator has small arms; however, diagnosing early pregnancy is difficult.

DIAGNOSTIC ULTRASOUND PER RECTUM

In Horses

Ultrasound can reliably detect the presence of an embryo as early as 10 to 12 days (Fig. 3-33), and it is more reliable than rectal palpation for confirming twin conceptions. The fetal heartbeat can be imaged as early as 4 weeks. Another advantage of ultrasound is the ability to show the client the examination on the viewing screen and to record the examination on video or as a photograph. The hard copy can provide documentation not only for the medical record but also for the client, so it is a popular client public relations tool (the client can start a baby album). Ultrasound per rectum has the same time limitations as rectal palpation, with the time frame from day 90 to 150 being somewhat difficult to image because of the position of the uterus in the abdomen. Ultrasound per rectum can be used to determine the sex of a fetus, with the optimum time between days 60 and 75. It is accomplished by measuring the location of the developing genitals (*genital tubercle*) from the tail or umbilicus. In males, the genital tubercle is closer to the umbilicus; in females, it is closer to the tail (Fig. 3-34). This method is 99% accurate when performed by experienced clinicians. Timing of the examination is critical because the uterus begins to fall over the pelvic brim during the same time frame. Sex can also be determined by transabdominal ultrasound scanning

for specific male or female genitalia; the optimum time for this approach is 100 to 220 days. After 220 days, the size and positioning of the fetus make sex determination by any approach difficult.

In Cattle

Ultrasound can detect pregnancy as early as 12 days in cattle and 18 days in small ruminants. It is highly effective for early pregnancy diagnosis. However, confirmation of pregnancy at this stage is seldom necessary, and the added cost of the procedure is seldom justified. Ultrasound enables the clinician to perform accurate measurements and therefore may be used to estimate fetal age and determine fetal sex. Fetal sex is best determined between days 60 and 70, with high accuracy when performed by experienced clinicians. The distance between the genital tubercle and the umbilicus and tail is measured. In males, the tubercle is closer to the umbilicus, and in females, it is closer to the tail.

In Sheep and Goats

A linear array probe used in horses can be modified by taping it (and its cord) to an insemination-infusion pipette or small polyvinylchloride pipe for advancement into the rectum.

DIAGNOSTIC ULTRASOUND TRANSABDOMINAL

In Horses

Transabdominal ultrasound cannot be used while the uterus is contained within the pelvis, before approximately days 70 to 80 of pregnancy. From about day 80 until term, the method is reliable. The examination is performed through a clipped area on the ventrolateral abdomen, cranial to the mammary gland, by using a transducer that can penetrate to a depth of 20 to 30 cm (2.5 to 3.5 MHz).

In Small Ruminants

Ultrasound through the abdominal wall is commonly used in small ruminants. The procedure may be done as early as days 30 to 45, but accuracy rates greater than 95% are possible after day 60 of pregnancy. Most animals can be scanned while they are standing. Clipping a small window may be necessary for proper contact of the transducer. A 5.0-MHz transducer may be suitable for early pregnancies, but with increasing abdominal size a 3- to 5-MHz transducer is preferred. The ultrasound transducer is placed near the front of the udder, to the right side of the udder, or high in the right inguinal region, depending on the stage of pregnancy. It is aimed first toward the pelvic inlet and is slowly rotated cranially to produce a sweeping scan of the abdomen. Accurate counting of fetuses with ultrasound is difficult, but the best chance for visualization of multiple fetuses occurs between days 45 and 90. Measurement of the length of a fetus may allow estimation of fetal age. Fetal heartbeat may be seen by days 30 to 35.

DOPPLER ULTRASOUND PER RECTUM AND TRANSABDOMINAL

In Sheep and Goats

This method has been used in small ruminants after days 35 to 40 of gestation. A rectal Doppler probe is used to "hear" the fetal heart rate, which is roughly twice the maternal heart rate. After approximately 50 days, Doppler imaging may be used transabdominally and is highly accurate after 75 days. Counting fetuses with Doppler ultrasound is difficult.

In Cattle

Doppler ultrasound has been used in cattle. The fetal heart can be heard through rectal Doppler imaging by weeks 6 to 7.

In Swine

Transabdominal ultrasound is the primary method for diagnosing pregnancy in swine. Historically, *A-mode* ultrasound and Doppler ultrasound have been used most often to detect pregnancy. A-mode ultrasound is most accurate between days 30 and 90 of gestation, and Doppler is accurate from day 28 until the end of gestation. Real-time *(B-mode)* ultrasound is increasingly being used in swine. It can detect pregnancy as early as 18 days, with best accuracy after 22 days. The preferred patient position for ultrasound is standing. Ultrasound coupling gel or other coupling medium is necessary. The transducer is placed in the lower right flank, in an area approximately 5 cm caudal to the umbilicus and 5 cm lateral to the teat nipple line. The transducer is angled approximately 45 degrees dorsally and is swept slowly cranially to caudally to identify the uterus.

EXTERNAL PALPATION ("BALLOTTEMENT")

In Horses

The examiner presses both fists against the lower flank area and rapidly presses inward. Supposedly, this action rapidly displaces the pregnant uterus (if present), which then rebounds back into its original position and "bumps" the examiner's fists. This method lacks accuracy and has largely been replaced by other methods. External abdominal palpation as used in small animals is not possible in large animals.

In Cattle

This method requires a fetus of sufficient size to be "bumped" with the hands through the abdominal wall. One or both fists are placed over the right lower paralumbar fossa and are pressed rapidly inward toward the uterus. The fetus and fetal fluids are displaced momentarily by the thrust. They then rebound and give a characteristic "bump" back against the operator's hands, which are left pressed against the body wall. Sheep and goats should be beyond 100 days of gestation; cattle should be beyond 6 to 7 months of gestation. This method is not highly reliable.

ABDOMINAL RADIOGRAPHS

Although commonly used for pregnancy diagnosis in small animals, abdominal radiographs are not considered useful for this purpose in cattle, horses, and swine. Although possible in small ruminants, there is little indication for the procedure. However, it is highly reliable for pregnancy diagnosis, and it can be used to count the number of fetuses, given the high incidence of twins and triplets in small ruminants. Mineralization of the fetal skeleton, which occurs as early as days 65 to 70, is necessary for viewing the fetus on a radiograph. Best results may occur after day 90. Fasting the female may improve visualization of fetuses.

LABORATORY TESTS

Laboratory tests are typically used when rectal examination is inconclusive or impossible to perform (on small females or on wild or dangerous horses). The test results can be difficult to interpret and have limited usefulness. Many tests are not possible to perform or are not reliable until the later stages of pregnancy, well beyond the useful time frame of the normal breeding season (should rebreeding be necessary).

Progesterone Assays

In horses, progesterone assays are blood tests. Normal levels are difficult to determine because much individual variation exists. A "pregnant" level in one mare may be "nonpregnant" in another. In cattle, assays for progesterone compounds in blood, urine, and milk are available. The expense of hormonal tests is seldom justified in ruminants.

Estrogen Assays

In horses, estrogen assays are available as blood and urine tests for various analogues of estrogen but are generally not reliable until late pregnancy, after 150 days of gestation. A fecal test for estrogen is available and may be accurate after 120 days. In cattle, assays for estrogen compounds (estrone sulfate) in blood, urine, and milk are available. Tests must be carefully selected on the basis of thorough knowledge of pregnancy physiology. All tests have potential pitfalls and limited time frames during gestation when they would be useful. The expense of hormonal tests is seldom justified in ruminants.

Chorionic Gonadotropin

Chorionic gonadotropin (pregnant mare serum gonadotropin [PMSG]) is a blood test that can be used in horses. Chorionic gonadotropin is produced by the endometrial cups from days 35 to 120. Mares that abort pregnancies after the endometrial cups have formed (days 35 to 38) may continue to test positive for pregnancy until approximately 120 days after conception because the endometrial cups may continue to secrete hormones until that time.

Immunologic Tests

Immunologic tests are newer tests (enzyme-linked immunosorbent assay [ELISA], mare immunologic pregnancy test, direct latex agglutination) that are being developed for pregnancy diagnosis after 35 to 40 days. The ELISA appears to be more accurate from days 35 to 90 than the other tests; after day 90, all tests are accurate. Immunosuppressive early pregnancy factor (IEPF) testing is currently available.

Pregnancy-Specific Protein B and Pregnancy-Associated Glycoproteins

Pregnancy-specific protein B (PSPB) and pregnancy-associated glycoproteins (PAGs) have been identified in various ruminant species, including cattle, sheep, and goats. They are produced by the placenta throughout gestation and can be measured in plasma by radioimmunoassay. PSPB can be detected in blood for early pregnancy diagnosis.

ABORTION

Management of abortion should be handled carefully because of the extreme zoonotic potential. Gloves, protective clothing, masks, and boots should be worn when dealing with an abortion or handling the aborting female, fetal membranes, or fetus. The client should also be advised of this potential and instructed to follow protective measures. Females that are aborting should be separated from other animals in their herd to help prevent spread of disease if the cause is contagious. If a client calls to ask about collecting samples for submission to the hospital, advise clients to bring the placenta and the entire fetus if possible.

PARTURITION

CLINICAL SIGNS OF IMPENDING PARTURITION

After the appropriate gestation period for each species has passed, technicians and producers should prepare for *parturition*. Several clinical changes that occur before parturition can indicate the approach of parturition. For information concerning clinical signs associated with impending parturition, see the chapters on individual species.

Some of the clinical signs associated with impending parturition include swelling of the vulva, relaxation of the muscles and ligaments of the hindquarters and tail head, thick mucous discharge from the vulva, enlargement of the udder, and distention of the uterus.

In some species, specific procedures are performed before parturition. These are covered in the chapters on individual species for which these procedures are required.

LABOR

The three stages of labor are stage 1, stage 2, and stage 3.
- Stage 1 is the preparatory stage of labor, when the animal is restless and shows little interest in food. Occasional kicking at the belly and straining may occur. This is when the myometrial contractions begin. The cervix is beginning to dilate. The fetus aligns itself with the birth canal. During stage 1, the contractions force the fetus against the cervix, which further activates dilation and releases more oxytocin. Oxytocin is responsible for uterine contraction. The fetus enters the birth canal, and the chorioallantois eventually ruptures.
- Stage 2 involves expulsion of the fetus.
- Stage 3 The chorionic villi detach from the endometrial crypts, and the placenta is expelled.

Each species transitions through each stage of labor, although the time that each species or each individual spends within a given stage varies. When progress does not result within a typical time frame, the female may need assistance (Fig. 3-35). Females should be moved to an area that is large enough for the female to move around freely and house a neonate. The area should be clean and dry.

DYSTOCIA

Dystocia literally means "difficult birth." Dystocias occur more frequently in first-time (primiparous) mothers and are less likely to occur with each subsequent pregnancy. The causes of dystocia may be generally divided into fetal causes and maternal causes.

Fetal causes of dystocia are more common and include the following:
- Malformations of the fetus: "Fetal monsters" cannot conform to the shape of the birth canal and cannot pass through the birth canal on their own.
- Stillbirths: These often occur because the fetus cannot position itself for delivery.
- Large fetal size compared with the size of the birth canal: This complication commonly occurs when females are bred to males that are considerably larger or are known to sire large-birthweight offspring, as is commonly done in cattle, in hopes of increasing calf size. The larger birthweight size often exceeds the size of the dam's birth canal (especially in first-calf heifers), resulting in inability of the fetal shoulders or hips to pass without assistance.
- Abnormal fetal presentation: This is the most common cause of dystocia. It is also known as fetal malposition and is common in sheep and goats.

Maternal causes of dystocia include the following:
- Compromised birth canal, such as pelvic fracture or old injuries
- Uterine torsion
- Rupture of the supporting structures of the pelvis and abdominal wall

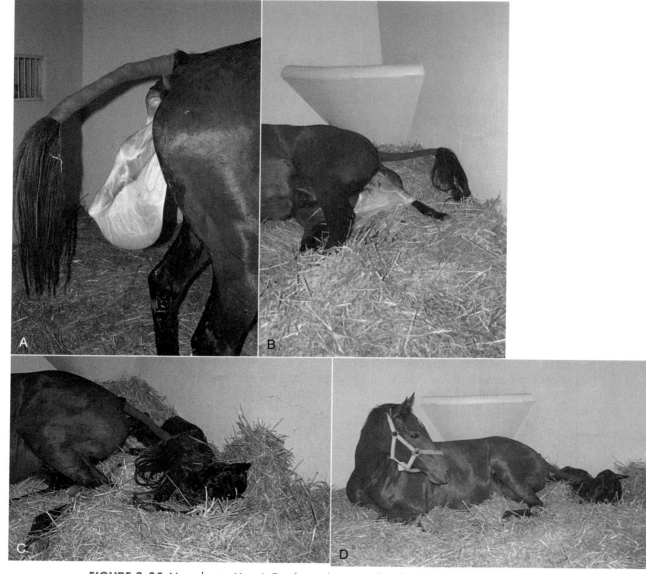

FIGURE 3-35 Normal parturition. **A,** Two feet and a nose at the vulva. One leg is always more advanced than the other to allow easy passage of the shoulders, which are the widest part of the foal. **B,** Mare is now in a recumbent position, and the foal has passed to the midcervical level. **C,** Foal with just the lower half of its hindlegs remaining in the vagina. The umbilical cord is still attached, but the amnion has been removed from the foal. **D,** Mare nickering to her foal. The mare and foal should not be disturbed at this time. (From McAuliffe SB, Slovis NM: *The color atlas of diseases and disorders of the foal,* Oxford, 2008, Saunders.)

Normally, the fetus is mobile within the uterus during the gestation period just before birth. The fetus must orient itself to the normal head-first, forelegs-extended, "head-diving" position that allows a normal delivery. Any deviation from this position likely will result in an inability of the fetus to be expelled from the uterus, especially in cattle and horses. Flexed legs, flexed neck, "belly up" posture, breech (posterior) presentation, or a fetus that is dead and cannot reposition itself all lead to delivery problems.

Signs of malposition include appearance of the nose with no hooves or just one hoof showing, hooves that are not facing toward the ground, and failure of any part of the fetus to appear at the vulva within the normal time frame for the species.

Dystocia is a true emergency situation. The technician should be familiar with the procedures and equipment used to treat dystocias to provide assistance during what is usually a tense situation for everyone involved.

> **TECHNICIAN NOTE**   Dystocia is a true emergency situation.

Signs of dystocia include a fetus that is not presenting in an appropriate amount of time for that species. (See the chapters on individual species.) Forceful straining without progress, flexed limbs or head of the fetus, and fetal hoof soles facing dorsally can all be signs of dystocia.

In any species, attending a patient with dystocia begins with restraint of the animal. The most important aspect when dealing with dystocia is keeping the clinician and assisting personnel safe. Physical restraint must be adequate for the situation because behavior is unpredictable during delivery. Females may stand or lie down with little warning. Stocks are not recommended for use with horses. The examination and treatment preferably are performed in an area where personnel can move easily to safety. Chemical restraint and/or caudal epidural may be used to minimize straining by the female (especially cattle). Examining the fetus or treating the dystocia is difficult (and dangerous) while the female is straining, often violently, to deliver the fetus.

Following establishment of proper patient restraint, the technician should begin an evaluation of the patient's general physical status. Conditions such as cardiovascular shock and hemorrhage may necessitate emergency therapy before treatment of the dystocia. Treatment of these conditions is necessary before beginning the surgical manipulations. Once the female's condition is stabilized, the veterinarian proceeds with examination of the dystocia.

A rectal examination may be performed, usually followed by a vaginal examination. The tail should be wrapped and the peritoneal area cleansed for the vaginal examination. These procedures must be performed thoroughly but promptly because time is precious. If the female is having contractions, the birth canal should be checked for possible blockage. Occasionally, a full rectum partially obstructs the female's vaginal canal, especially in smaller species. An enema may be necessary to remove fecal material. The hands should be held with the fingers and thumb together in a pointed position to enter the vulva. A slight rotating motion of the hand assists passage into the pelvic inlet. The birth canal is searched for fetuses, which may be in a sideways or breech position or may be large. In species that have multiple fetuses, two fetuses may become entangled.

> **TECHNICIAN NOTE** Preparation of the female's peritoneal area should be performed promptly but thoroughly. Time is precious!

The clinician either wears plastic sleeves or uses scrubbed hands and arms to enter the vagina, depending on personal preference. Personnel who are handling instruments or assisting with the delivery should wear disposable gloves because of the possibility of zoonotic disease transmission, which may affect the reproductive tract, the fetus, and fetal membranes. A clean area should be established for equipment, and instruments should be sterilized or disinfected. Sterile procedures are not necessary because parturition is not a sterile process, but the area and equipment should be kept as clean as possible.

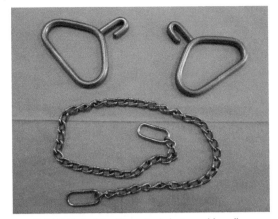

FIGURE 3-36 Obstetrical chain and handles.

Once the cause of dystocia is diagnosed and the condition of the fetus is determined, the veterinarian should advise the client of the options available and proceed rapidly to save both the mother and the neonate, if possible. The three primary methods for treating dystocias are *mutation* and delivery by *traction, fetotomy,* and *cesarean section.*

MUTATION AND DELIVERY BY TRACTION

This is the most common procedure and almost always is the first method attempted to resolve the dystocia. Basically, mutation means changing the position of the fetus so that it can be delivered. Repositioning the fetus while it is in the birth canal is extremely difficult because it often is wedged in the canal, and there simply is not enough room for maneuvering. Therefore, it usually is necessary to repel (push) the fetus back into the uterus to create enough space to reposition it. Repelling the fetus can be difficult. Sometimes the mare is placed on an incline, with her head facing downhill, to assist the fetus going back into the uterus. In extreme cases, the mare may be anesthetized or her hindquarters lifted with a hoist.

Lubrication is essential for use with tactical maneuvers, especially if the fetus is to be repositioned and/or pulled from the birth canal. It is common to use a nasogastric tube and pump to instill several liters or even gallons of lubricant into the vagina and uterus; an adequate amount should be available. The lubricant should be clean but does not have to be sterile.

> **TECHNICIAN NOTE** Always ensure that a large amount of lubricant is available if mutation and delivery by traction are the intended methods to correct dystocia.

Once the malposition is corrected (if it can be corrected), attempts are made to deliver the fetus by traction. Traction (pulling) on the fetus may be applied directly with the hands or through various instruments designed to obtain a firm hold on the fetus and/or head and neck of the fetus. These instruments should be clean and may be disinfected before and during use by placing them in a stainless steel bucket with water and disinfectant solution. The most common instruments needed are obstetrical chains and handles (Fig. 3-36).

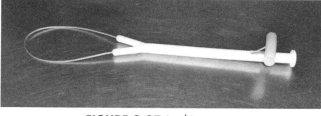

FIGURE 3-37 Lambing snare.

Obstetrical chains or straps and handles are commonly used to facilitate manual traction on the fetus. Various surgical hooks and snares also are used (Fig. 3-37).

By placing the chains (or straps) around the limbs, the clinician can bring the fetus into the proper position. The handles can be attached and passed to assistants to help the clinician apply traction. If the fetus is dead, other instruments such as *blunt eye hooks*, double-action sharp pointed cray hooks, wired surgical snares, and rope nooses may be used. Fetal extractors, commonly known as *calf jacks,* are routinely used in cattle but are not designed for use in horses because they may cause unnecessary trauma to the mare's reproductive tract. When manual traction cannot deliver the fetus in cattle, devices that create extra leverage on the fetus are commonly used. In general, the reproductive tract of cows appears to tolerate these maneuvers better than the reproductive tract of horses, with less trauma and inflammation when the maneuvers are properly performed by experienced clinicians. In general, more force may be used to extract a calf than a foal. The device most often used to increase traction and leverage on the fetus is the calf jack or calf puller. Several brands and styles of these devices are available, and all have similar components: a long central metal rod, a metal rump support, and a handle on the central rod that operates a ratchet mechanism similar to a car tire jack. These mechanical traction devices are not for use on mares or small ruminants. With these devices, mild traction can be placed on the head or limbs of the fetus to extract it. Various instruments are available to assist in applying traction; *lambing snares, pig pullers, forceps,* and *nylon cord* may be helpful. All manipulations should be done carefully to prevent damaging the mother.

> **TECHNICIAN NOTE**   Calf jacks should not be used on mares!

The traction team should work together, applying force under the direction of the clinician. Traction is always applied with gradual, smooth motions; sharp, jerking motions should be avoided. The natural pathway of delivery is not a straight line behind the female; rather, it is a curved path from the pelvis down to the ground. To simulate the natural arc of delivery, traction is applied at a 45-degree angle toward the ground, if the female is standing. If the female is recumbent, the path should be recreated as if the female were standing. Liberal amounts of lubricant should be available to assist in

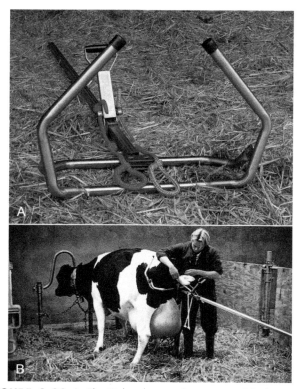

FIGURE 3-38 A, The Vink calving jack is one model of commercially available calf puller. The rump support, central supporting rod, and ratchet handle are shown. **B,** Calving jack in place on a patient with dystocia. The rump support rests on the pelvis, and the central supporting rod extends directly caudally behind the patient. The front feet and pasterns are seen extending from the vulva. The clinician has placed an obstetrical chain around each front leg of the fetus and attached the chains to the ratchet mechanism. (From Noakes DE, Parkinson TJ, England GCW: *Veterinary reproduction and obstetrics,* ed 9, London, 2009, Saunders.)

the delivery. Malposition must first be corrected; the calf jack is not a substitute for proper repositioning. After the fetus is positioned correctly, obstetrical chains or straps are strategically placed on the fetus, most commonly on the front legs. The calf jack is positioned with the rump support against the cow for stability and the central rod directed caudally behind the cow (Figs. 3-38 and 3-39). The chains are then attached to the ratchet device on the central rod. Repeated pumping action of the handle, like that used with a car jack, places increasing traction on the chains and therefore on the fetus. The central rod then can be aimed slightly up or down to alter the forces on the fetus during the extraction.

In sheep and goats, the most common cause of dystocia is abnormal presentation of the fetus. Manual mutation and traction are highly successful in treating simple malpositions in these species. Caudal epidural blocks are helpful in sheep and goats to decrease discomfort and straining. Attention to cleanliness of the patient and instruments is essential. Generous amounts of lubricant are necessary for obstetrical procedures on sheep and goats. Clipping the wool around the vulva may be necessary to cleanse the area thoroughly.

In swine, *uterine inertia* may result from exhaustion or hypocalcemia. The sow should be kept comfortably cool and

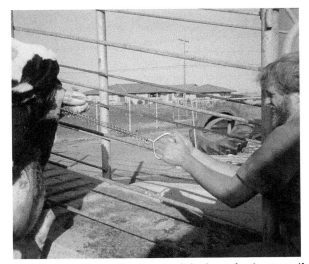

FIGURE 3-39 Chains placed around the legs of a bovine calf in a normal delivery position. (From Bassert JM, McCurnin DM, editors: *McCurnin's clinical textbook for veterinary technicians,* ed 7, St. Louis, 2010, Saunders.)

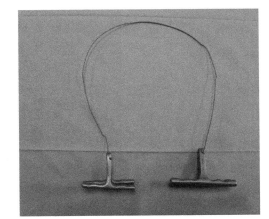

FIGURE 3-40 Wire saw and handles. The wire is supplied on a spool and cut to the desired length. The handles are then clamped to secure the ends of the wire.

may resume labor after a brief rest. Oxytocin injection may help to restore uterine contractions. If not, cesarean section may be the only option to save the female.

One common problem during parturition in swine is determining whether a sow has delivered all her fetuses. The end of parturition usually is signaled by the sow's standing and voiding a large amount of urine, followed by her lying down comfortably to allow the litter to nurse. If a question exists about possible incomplete delivery, manual examination of the uterus can be performed. However, reaching the full extent of the uterine horns is difficult. Transabdominal B-mode ultrasound can be used to detect retained fetuses.

FETOTOMY

If the fetus is dead and cannot be delivered by mutation and traction, a fetotomy may be performed. This procedure involves making one or more cuts to the fetus to amputate portions of the limbs, head, or neck and then removing the severed portions. Doing so reduces the size of the fetus and allows removal of parts that are rigid and unable to conform to the birth canal. One to three transections is generally sufficient and must be performed carefully to prevent lacerating the female's reproductive tract. The female is sedated and given a caudal epidural block for the procedure. Transections can be performed using a special guarded, handheld fetotomy knife or a Gigli wire saw (Fig. 3-40). To protect the female's reproductive tract from the sawing action, the wire is passed through a rigid metal tube (fetotome) that extends from the vulva through the cervix. The wire is placed internally and looped around the part to be removed, and the wire ends are brought to the outside the female. Handles are attached to each end, and to-and-fro motion on the handles is used to transform the wire into a cutting instrument. Once the necessary parts have been removed, traction is placed on the remaining portion to remove it. Because amputation may

create a sharp exposed piece of bone, removal must be carefully done to prevent puncturing or lacerating the reproductive tract. Liberal lubricant should be available.

Fetotomy avoids major abdominal surgical procedures and has less aftercare, quicker recovery, and fewer complications than a cesarean section. However, many clinicians are reluctant to perform the procedure because of the risk of lacerations and punctures to the female's reproductive organs. In addition, any tissue damage to the lining of the vagina and cervix can result in scar tissue and adhesions that can interfere with future attempts to conceive and carry a fetus. This risk is higher in horses than in cattle.

CESAREAN SECTION

Cesarean section is a fairly common surgical procedure in ruminants. In many cases, it is faster and safer than a fetotomy. In small ruminants, the clinician is limited by the size of the female's pelvis and reproductive tract, thus making treatment of complicated dystocias difficult. In cattle, the trauma caused by attempting vaginal delivery of a fetus may outweigh the benefits of trying to avoid the surgical procedure. Fortunately, caesarean section in cattle is a straightforward procedure with good survival rates for both the females and offspring. An additional advantage is that the procedure can usually be done using local anesthesia, with or without sedation, thereby avoiding general anesthesia. Occasionally, general anesthesia is necessary and may be safely used.

Cesarean section may be indicated in the following circumstances:
- Fetus too large for vaginal delivery
- Size of the female prohibiting vaginal manipulations by the clinician
- Failure of the cervix to dilate
- Vaginal prolapse
- Fetal emphysema (dead, partially autolyzed fetus)
- Fetus too malformed for vaginal delivery (fetal monster)
- Planned termination of pregnancy, before term, to save the life of the dam (e.g., pregnancy toxemia in sheep and goats)

POSTPARTUM COMPLICATIONS

Postpartum complications include retained placentas, uterine prolapses, ketosis, acetonemia, pregnancy toxemia, displaced abomasums, milk fever, and mastitis. These conditions should be monitored and brought to the veterinarian's attention if suspected.

NEONATAL CARE

Immediately after birth, the following should be addressed, in order:

1. Oxygenation/pulse assessment
2. Temperature regulation
3. Care of the umbilical cord and umbilicus: The umbilicus should break spontaneously at birth. It should be dipped in 0.5% chlorhexidine solution two to three times during the first 24 hours of life.
4. Nutrition (nursing): Neonates should receive colostrum, or nursing should be confirmed. The neonate should stand within 0.5 to 1 hour and be nursing within 1 to 2 hours.
5. Bonding of the female and the neonate
6. Passage of meconium: Neonates should pass this first stool in 12 hours. It is dark green to black and can cause colic if it is not passed. An enema may be necessary.
7. Adequacy of passive transfer of antibodies
8. Physical examination of the neonate

Further information about each of these requirements can be found in the chapters on each individual species.

CASE STUDY

Dr. Joyce has informed you that the mare he is examining by ultrasound is carrying twins. Should you smile from ear to ear and inform the client that the mare is pregnant with twins, saying congrats as you finish giving the good news?

CASE STUDY

Mrs. Carrier, a small cow/calf producer, calls the clinic asking about current options for pregnancy detection. She has only about five head. What options do you give her, and what are the pros and cons for each of these options?

CASE STUDY

Look at the example EPDs in Table 3-1 and select the best bull for each of the following situations.

A. Last year, rancher O had to assist calving 35% of his herd. This year he would like a lower percentage. Which bull should he choose?
B. Rancher B wants to keep the offspring from this year's matings as replacement heifers. He lives in Arizona, and feed is not plentiful. He would like to minimize feed consumption by the new replacement heifers. Which bull should he choose?
C. Rancher C wants to sell his calves at weaning. His goal is to maximize his profit. He plans to sell the calves by weight. Which bull should he choose?
D. Which bull would you want to sire the calf you are going to consume? Which bull do you think the general public wants to sire the calf they are going to consume?

SUGGESTED READING

Anderson DE, Rings DM: *Current veterinary therapy: food animal practice*, ed 5, St. Louis, 2008, Saunders.

Davis H, Riel DL, Pappagianis M, Miguel K: Diagnostic sampling and therapeutic techniques. In Bassert JM, McCurnin DM, editors: *McCurnin's clinical textbook for veterinary technicians*, ed 7, St. Louis, 2010, Saunders, pp 585-673.

Ensminger ME, Parker RO: *Swine science*, Danville, Ill, 2005, Interstate Publishers.

Fubini SL, Ducharme NG: *Farm animal surgery*, St. Louis, 2004, Saunders.

Gillespie JR, Flanders FB: *Modern livestock and poultry*, ed 8, Clifton Park, NY, 2010, Delmar Cengage Learning.

Hafez ESE: *Reproduction in farm animals*, ed 6, Philadelphia, 2000, Lea & Febiger.

Noakes DE, Parkinson RJ, England GCW: *Veterinary reproduction and obstetrics*, ed 8, London, 2009, Saunders.

Pinto CRF, Eilts BE, Paccamonti DL: Animal reproduction. In Bassert JM, McCurnin DM, editors: *McCurnin's clinical textbook for veterinary technicians*, ed 7, St. Louis, 2010, Saunders, pp 370-399.

Pugh DG: *Sheep and goat medicine*, ed 2, St. Louis, 2011, Saunders.

Smith MC, Sherman DM: *Goat medicine*, Baltimore, 1994, Williams & Wilkins.

Sonsthagen TF, Teeple TN: Nursing care of food animals, camelids, and ratites. In Sirois M, editor: *Principles and practice of veterinary technology*, ed 3, St. Louis, 2011, Mosby, pp 585-611.

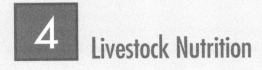

4 Livestock Nutrition

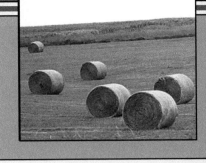

LEARNING OBJECTIVES

After reading this chapter, you will be able to

- Define the nutritional needs of livestock
- Demonstrate an understanding that poor nutrition can lead to nutrient deficiencies or toxicity
- Identify the function of each basic nutrient category
- Identify parts and functions of animal digestive systems
- Explain the differences and similarities of different types of digestive systems
- Explain various methods of determining nutrient composition of feedstuffs
- Classify common *feedstuffs* into various categories
- Identify common feedstuffs used by livestock
- Balance livestock *rations* using commonly accepted methods

KEY TERMS

Abomasum
Ash
Bile
Carbonaceous
Cardia
Cecum
Chewing cud
Chyme
Cured
Digestible energy
Dry matter
Energy feeds
Ergot
Feedstuff
Forages

Gallbladder
Gastric lipase
Glucose
Legumes
Lipase
Maintenance nutrient requirements
Modified ruminant
Net energy
Nonruminant
Nutrients
Omasum
Pancreatic amylase
Pancreatic juice
Pasture plants
Pepsin

Proteinaceous
Ration
Rennin
Reticulum
Roughages
Rumen
Ruminant
Rumination
Salivary amylase
Salivary maltase
Stocks
Tankage
Total digestible nutrients
Trypsin

ABBREVIATIONS

BCS: Body condition score
DE: Digestible energy
DNA: Deoxyribonucleic acid
ECF: Extracellular fluid
FDA: Food and Drug Administration
IV: Intravenous

MNR: Maintenance nutrient requirement
NE: Net energy
PCV: Packed cell volume
PPN: Partial parenteral nutrition
RBC: Red blood cell

RNA: Ribonucleic acid
SC: Subcutaneous
TDN: Total digestible nutrients
TPN: Total parenteral nutrition
TS: Total solids

THE IMPORTANCE OF NUTRITION

Nutrition is an extremely important aspect of the large animal industry. Without proper nutrition, disease and reproductive failure are common. Veterinarians and veterinary technicians can be major sources of nutritional information to clients. Some producers of cattle, sheep, goats, and swine consult a nutritional specialist. With these clients, the veterinarian and veterinary technician are involved with nutrition only when problems present themselves in the form of disease. For other producers, the veterinarian or veterinary technician may be the nutritional specialist. No matter what role the veterinary professional plays in nutritional decisions, an understanding of large animal nutrition is important when problems develop. As much as 90% of health-related disease in large animals can be related to improper nutrition.

> **TECHNICIAN NOTE**   As much as 90% of health-related disease in large animals can be related to improper nutrition.

TYPES OF DIGESTIVE SYSTEMS

Three types of digestive systems exist in large animal species, and these animals are classified accordingly: *nonruminants, ruminants,* and *modified ruminants.* Horses and swine are nonruminants. Cattle, sheep, and goats are ruminants. Llamas and alpaca are modified ruminants. Knowledge of these systems is important when selecting the proper feeds to be used in each species.

> **TECHNICIAN NOTE**   Horses and swine are nonruminants. Cattle, sheep, and goats are ruminants. Llamas and alpacas are modified ruminants.

In every large animal species, feed enters the mouth and travels down the esophagus to the stomach. The esophagus is connected to the stomach via the *cardia.* The stomach design is one of the major differences within large animal species. The mouth is responsible for chewing. The saliva produced within the mouth contains *salivary amylase* and *salivary maltase.* Salivary amylase is responsible for converting some starch to maltase or maltase sugar. Salivary maltase is responsible for changing maltase to *glucose.*

Ruminants do not chew their food completely before swallowing. The food goes directly to the *rumen.* Later the rumen becomes full and the animal lies down. At this time the feed is forced back into the mouth, and the feed material is chewed again. This process is known as *rumination* or *chewing cud.*

In nonruminants the stomach uses enzymes and gastric juices to digest the feed material. The gastric juice is 0.2% to 0.5% hydrochloric acid. The enzymes include *pepsin, rennin,* and *gastric lipase.* Pepsin is responsible for breaking down proteins into proteoses and peptones. Rennin is responsible for curdling milk. Gastric lipase is responsible for breaking fats into glycerol and fatty acids. Much of the fat entering the stomach is not broken down. Ruminants have four stomach compartments through which food material passes, in the following order: rumen, *reticulum, omasum,* and *abomasum.* The rumen is responsible for microbial digestion by bacteria and protozoans. The rumen and reticulum are not separate compartments but separate areas. Together they lie on the left side of the animal. The bacteria convert the low-quality protein from forages into needed amino acids. They also are responsible for producing many of the vitamins needed by the animal. The reticulum has a honeycomb appearance and is responsible for grinding the feed material. The function of the omasum is unknown, but it is thought to be responsible for grinding action and may remove water from the feed. It makes up approximately 8% of the total stomach area. The abomasum in ruminants is responsible for gastric juice digestion and is known as the true stomach because its action is similar to that of a nonruminant. It makes up approximately 7% of the total stomach.

> **TECHNICIAN NOTE**   In ruminants, the path of feedstuff through the stomachs is as follows: rumen, reticulum, omasum, and abomasum.

After feed passes through the stomach, it enters the small intestine. At this point, the feed is known as *chyme.* The chyme is mixed with *pancreatic juice, bile,* and intestinal juices. The pancreatic juices contain three enzymes: *trypsin, pancreatic amylase,* and *lipase.* Trypsin is responsible for further breakdown of proteins. Some of the peptones and proteoses are broken down into peptides. Pancreatic amylase changes starch in the feed to maltase and then to glucose. Lipase is responsible for changing fats into fatty acids and glycerol.

Bile is stored in the *gallbladder,* except in the horse because the horse does not have a gallbladder. Bile aids in digestion of fats and fatty acids. Fatty acids combine with bile to form bile salts.

> **TECHNICIAN NOTE**   Horses do not have a gallbladder.

Intestinal juices are created from the glands within the walls of the intestine and are responsible for breaking down proteins and carbohydrates to their simplest forms. After the chyme has been broken down into its simplest form, the *nutrients* can be absorbed through the intestinal wall.

Material not absorbed in the small intestine passes into the large intestine. The *cecum* connects the small intestine to the large intestine. The cecum is a small ring that has little function in most animals, except the horse. The cecum of a horse contains bacteria that allow digestion of large amounts of roughage. The large intestine is primarily responsible for water absorption and mucus production, which aid in the passage of feed through the rest of the system. Some bacterial action takes place in the large intestine. The remaining material, known as feces, passes through the large intestine into the rectum, from which it is defecated.

> **TECHNICIAN NOTE**   Horses are cecum fermenters!

NUTRIENT REQUIREMENTS

The stage of production, age, and use all contribute to the animal's nutritional requirements. An overview of nutritional requirements can be found within the sections on individual species.

CARBOHYDRATES

Carbohydrates make up a large percentage of livestock diets. Cereal grains and forages are good sources of carbohydrates. Carbohydrates are made of simple sugars. These simple sugars are held together by glycosidic bonds to create starches (complex carbohydrates). When animals consume complex carbohydrates, their bodies must break the glycosidic bonds and convert the carbohydrate to its simplest form, simple sugars. Once in simple sugar form, the sugars can be absorbed by the digestive tract. Microflora in the rumen or cecum of some nonruminants convert fiber such as cellulose into energy. However, lignin is a fiber that is considered indigestible. As plants age, the amount of lignin increases, thus making the plant less digestible. Concentrates and forages often supply carbohydrates in livestock diets.

LIPIDS

Lipids are used as a source of heat, they provide dietary energy, and they help carry fat-soluble vitamins. Fats can be classified into three groups: simple lipids, compound lipids, and derived lipids. Simple lipids are esters of fatty acids with glycerol or alcohol. Compound lipids are combined with some other chemical category, such as phospholipids, lipoproteins, or glycolipids. Derived lipids are fatty acids and sterols (e.g., linoleic acid, arachidonic acid).

PROTEINS

Amino acids are the building blocks of proteins. They can be thought of as beads in a necklace. Just as different arrangements of beads make different necklaces, different arrangements of amino acids make different proteins. There are only 23 known amino acids, and only 20 of these 23 amino acids combine to make proteins.

Proteins make up the majority of soft tissues and organs in an animal's body. Proteins are essential in young animals. They are responsible for many of the chemical reactions that take place in the body. Protein is needed for reproduction, lactation, growth, formation of enzymes and hormones, and energy production. Loss of protein can result in decreased production, anemia, weight loss, and reduced growth rates. Excesses of protein may affect reproduction.

VITAMINS

Vitamins are needed in very small amounts by animals. Vitamins are divided into two groups. Fat-soluble vitamins include vitamins A, D, E, and K; water-soluble vitamins include vitamin C and B-complex vitamins. Ruminants require water-soluble vitamins when they are ill because these animals are unable to synthesize the vitamins during illness. Rumen microbes synthesize vitamin B complex, vitamin C, and vitamin K, so these vitamins are not required by ruminants unless they are ill. Vitamin A deficiency can result in animals that are fed poor-quality forages. Vitamin A deficiency can cause night blindness, skin ailments, weak offspring, or reproductive failure.

Thiamine (Vitamin B₁)

Sources of thiamine include oats and wheat. Thiamine is required for coenzyme metabolism and nerve function, and it can help increase appetite. Deficiencies result in ataxia, blindness, heart irregularities, depression, head pressing, convulsions, brain swelling, decreased body temperatures, and even death. Toxicities are rare.

Riboflavin (Vitamin B₂)

Sources of riboflavin include alfalfa, pasture grasses, and clovers. Riboflavin is required for metabolism of other nutrients and for hemoglobin production. Deficiencies of riboflavin result in decreased growth, diarrhea, and anemia. Toxicities are rare.

Pyridoxine (Vitamin B₆)

Sources of pyridoxine include pasture grasses, corn gluten meal, and alfalfa. Pyridoxine is required for metabolism of other nutrients and nitrogen metabolism. Deficiencies result in anemia, decreased growth, anorexia, and eye discharge. Toxicities are rare.

Cobalamin (Vitamin B₁₂)

Sources of cobalamin include whey and brewer's yeast. Cobalamin is required for red blood cell (RBC) formation, deoxyribonucleic acid (DNA) synthesis, and maintenance of nerve tissue. Deficiencies result in poor reproduction and decreased coordination. Toxicities are rare.

Vitamin C

Sources of vitamin C include hay and pasture grasses. Vitamin C is required for metabolism of folic acid. It plays an important role in the strength of teeth and bones, and it also has an antioxidant effect. Deficiencies of vitamin C result in hemorrhage, enlarged joints, delayed wound healing, and ulcerated gums. Toxicities are rare in food animals.

Biotin

Sources of biotin include soybean meal and young pasture grasses. Biotin is needed for enzyme function and metabolism of other nutrients. Deficiencies result in lameness, poor reproduction, dull hair coats, poor growth, skin ulcers, eye exudate, and inflammation of the mucous membranes. Toxicities are rare.

Folic Acid

Sources of folic acid include alfalfa and wheat. Folic acid is required for choline synthesis, hemoglobin synthesis, and protein use. Deficiencies of folic acid result in anemia, diarrhea, and poor growth. Toxicities are rare.

Niacin

Sources of niacin include yeast supplements and wheat barley. Niacin is important for growth and for the release of energy from other nutritional substances. Deficiencies of niacin result in decreased growth and appetite, as well as diarrhea. Toxicities are rare.

Pantothenic Acid

Sources of pantothenic acid include wheat bran and alfalfa. Pantothenic acid is required for maintaining normal blood levels, metabolism of other nutrients, and hemoglobin production. Deficiencies result in dull hair coats, enteritis, and neurologic diseases. Toxicities are rare.

MINERALS

Minerals are inorganic materials needed in various amounts by animals for growth and for tooth and tissue formation. The total mineral content of animals and plants is called ash. Minerals are classified as either macrominerals or trace minerals.

Macrominerals
Calcium and Phosphorus

Calcium and phosphorus should be provided in a 1.4:1 to 2:1 ratio in livestock diets. Common supplements include bone meal and dicalcium phosphate.

Sodium and Chloride

Salt should be provided free choice to livestock. Deficient animals may develop muscle cramps, decreased milk production, a rough hair coat, and weight loss. Excesses of salt, although rare, can cause anorexia, salt toxicosis leading to collapse, and weight loss.

Magnesium

Magnesium works closely with calcium and phosphorus in the body. Deficiencies of magnesium can cause reduced dry matter intake or anorexia. Young animals that are magnesium deficient may develop bone and teeth malformations.

Sulfur

Deficiencies of sulfur can lead to reduced growth. Excesses of sulfur can cause clinical neurologic signs.

Potassium

Potassium maintains acid-base balance, osmotic pressure, and muscle activity. Deficiencies can lead to diarrhea, coma, and even death. Toxicity may inhibit magnesium absorption, which can lead to potassium retention.

Trace Minerals

Selenium, manganese, fluorine, iodine, zinc, chromium, copper, molybdenum, cobalt, iron, and silicon are trace minerals. Trace minerals and macrominerals both are needed to maintain healthy livestock.

Iron

Sources of iron include alfalfa and corn gluten meal. Iron is required for muscle oxygenation, enzyme activation, and hemoglobin synthesis. Deficiencies can result in anemia, pica, dull hair coats, and diarrhea. Toxicities can result in poor reproductive performance and RBC abnormalities.

Iodine

Sources of iodine include oats, wheat, molasses, and iodized salt. Iodine is required for milk production, growth, hormone synthesis, and muscle tissue development. Deficiencies can result in poor reproduction, dull hair coats, and poor growth. Toxicities can result in hyperparathyroidism and goiter.

Cobalt

Sources of cobalt include corn, wheat, and molasses. Cobalt is required for formation of vitamin B_{12}. Deficiencies can result in poor hair coats, decreased milk production, poor appetites, and poor reproductive performance. Toxicities are rare.

Zinc

Sources of zinc include corn gluten, germ meal, and wheat by-products. Zinc is required for healthy coats and skin, development of reproductive organs, and bone synthesis. Deficiencies result in irregularities in bone, poor appetite, poor growth, hair loss, delayed wound healing, and parakeratosis. Toxicities can result in poor growth, increases in appetite, stiff gait, and anemia.

Manganese

Sources of manganese include wheat, corn, and grasses. Manganese is required for proper clotting, for metabolism of other nutrients, and for bone and cartilage growth. Deficiencies can result in lameness, poor growth, and reproductive disorders. Toxicities are rare.

Chromium

Sources of chromium include wheat, corn, and vegetable oil. Chromium is required for increased insulin action, and for DNA, ribonucleic acid (RNA), and fatty acid synthesis. Deficiencies result in decreased fat metabolism, hyperglycemia, and glucosuria. Toxicities are rare.

Fluorine

Fluorine is found in almost all foods. It is required for proper bone and tooth strength. Deficiencies are rare. Toxicities result in deformation of teeth, abnormalities of bone, and the inability to use feeds properly; they and can also cause dull hair coats.

Selenium

Sources of selenium include wheat by-products and oilseed meals. Selenium is required for fatty acid oxidation, and it prevents tissue damage. Deficiencies result in muscle disease and liver necrosis. Toxicities result in paralysis, blind staggers, anemia, weight loss, and lameness.

Copper

Sources of copper include molasses, grasses, and cottonseed. Copper is required for hair pigment, skeletal structure, reproduction, absorption of iron, and hemoglobin synthesis. Deficiencies include diarrhea, lameness, anemia, and swayback. Toxicities include increased thirst, gastroenteritis, and hypersalivation.

Silicon

Sources of silicon include grains. Silicon is required for skeletal development. Deficiencies result in skeletal abnormalities. Toxicities result in calculus formation.

Molybdenum

Sources of molybdenum include grasses, alfalfa, corn, oats, and wheat. Molybdenum is required for metabolism of other nutrients, for enamel production, and for growth. Deficiencies are rare. Toxicities result in weight loss, dull hair coats, poor reproduction, and diarrhea.

WATER

Water is the most needed nutrient. It makes up 65% to 85% of an animal's body weight at birth and 45% to 60% of the body weight at maturity. Deficiencies of water reduce feed intake, which in turn reduces the animal's productivity. Water deficiency can cause increased excretion of nitrogen and electrolytes such as sodium and potassium. An animal that becomes extremely dehydrated can die.

FEEDS

Several types of feeds can be chosen to meet the nutritional requirements of large animal species. These feeds can be broken into eight categories: *roughages, pasture plants* silage, *energy feeds,* protein supplements, mineral supplements, vitamin supplements, and additives. Identification of common feed is important for client perception, but knowing what common *feedstuffs* are available to meet the animal's nutritional requirements is also important. The following discussion describes some of the more common feeds used in the large animal industry. Several very good books on livestock feeds and feeding can be used to supplement this information.

> **TECHNICIAN NOTE** Being able to identify common feedstuffs used in the large animal industry is important for client perception.

DRY ROUGHAGES AND FORAGES/PASTURE PLANTS

Roughages are also known as *forages.* Roughages are cut and *cured* so that they can be fed to livestock throughout the year. Pasture plants are roughages that have not been cut. These feeds are eaten directly from the plant in the pasture (Fig. 4-1). These products often contain 18% crude fiber. Roughages are low in energy and contain more than 18% crude fiber. Roughages are required in ruminant diets. Dry roughages and forages can be divided into two subcategories: *carbonaceous* roughages, which are low in protein; and *proteinaceous* roughages, which are high in protein. *Legumes* are proteinaceous roughages that contain nitrogen; nonlegumes do not contain nitrogen. Some of the common roughages used in large animal nutrition include the following.

Carbonaceous Roughages
Straw

Straw can be used as a feed for large animals, but more often it is used for bedding. Several types of straw available include wheat straw and oat straw (Fig. 4-2).

Stocks

Stocks can be grazed by livestock. Livestock often graze stocks during the winter months once crops have been removed from the field (Fig. 4-3).

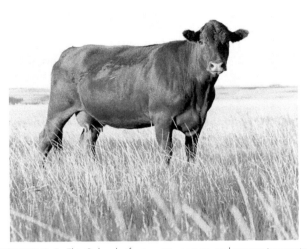

FIGURE 4-1 This Salers heifer is out to pasture and consuming pasture plants. (Courtesy American Salers Association.)

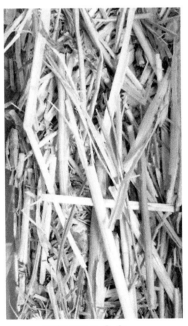

FIGURE 4-2 Straw.

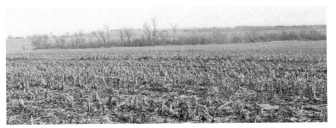

FIGURE 4-3 Corn stocks.

Proteinaceous Roughages
Clover

Several varieties of clover include alfalfa, alsike clover, red clover, white clover, sweet clover, birdsfoot trefoil, and crown vetch. In the United States, alfalfa is grown in the Midwest and the West. Alfalfa grazing by ruminants can be hazardous because alfalfa can cause bloat. Alfalfa is a good source of protein (Fig.4-4).

Hay

Hay can consist of combinations of several different species of grass, or it can be a specific type of hay. Hay in combination is often referred to as prairie hay. Some types of grasses that may be included in hay are big blue stem, Kentucky bluegrass, orchard grass, fescue, Bermuda grass, little blue stem, side oats grama, switchgrass, and smooth brome. Some could also be classified as pasture plants if they were eaten directly from the pasture (Fig. 4-5). Any of these grasses can be harvested alone and sold separately; for example, timothy hay is commonly purchased as a single grass (Fig. 4-6). Hay can be stored in several different forms: stacks, big round bales (Fig. 4-7), large square bales, and little square bales. The type of livestock system and the number of animals are considered when a producer is deciding on the type of storage form to use.

Grass hay is high in fiber but low in *total digestible nutrients (TDN)*. Sun-cured hay is the only natural food with a high vitamin D content.

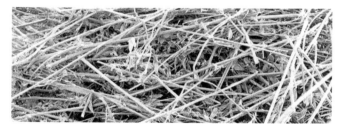

FIGURE 4-4 Alfalfa.

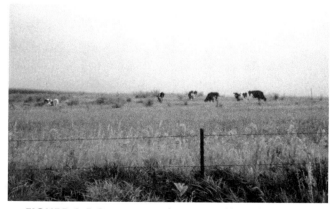

FIGURE 4-5 Pasture grasses being grazed by Holstein cows.

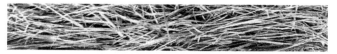

FIGURE 4-6 Timothy hay.

SILAGES

Silage is a product of fermentation of green forage crops that has been compressed and stored under anaerobic conditions in a container called a silo. Several different types of silage are available. Common forms of silage include corn, sorghum, alfalfa, and clover. Hay put up for silage is often referred to as haylage (Figs. 4-8 and 4-9). The product can be stored for long periods of time, provided the product does not come in contact with oxygen. Silage is often used

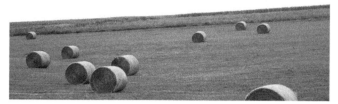

FIGURE 4-7 Big round bales.

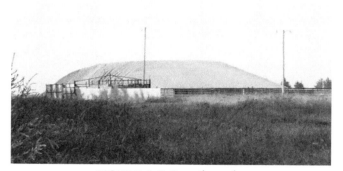

FIGURE 4-8 Corn silage pile.

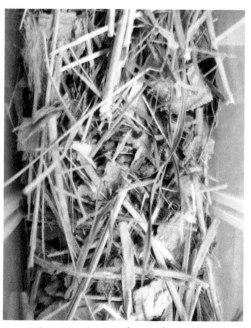

FIGURE 4-9 Grass hay and corn silage.

because the producer can use the entire plant for feed materials. When producers make silage, they chop the entire plant for feed, instead of using just the seed head as a form of feed. Silage feeds are harvested with a high moisture content, so weather can play an important role in the harvest and production of silage.

ENERGY FEEDS

Energy feeds contain less than 20% protein and less than 18% crude fiber. These products in general are high in TDN, *net energy (NE),* and *digestible energy (DE).* These feeds are low in fiber and protein. Energy grains, also known as carbonaceous concentrates, can be divided into cereal grains, sorghums, and by-product feeds.

Cereal Grains
Corn

Corn is one of the most popular feed concentrates in the Midwest. There are different types of corn. Sweet corn and popcorn are grown primarily for human consumption. Field corn is the type of corn most commonly fed to large animals. Each of the general types of corn has subtypes. The value of corn varies with its water content. Corn is graded as number 1 through 5, and moisture content is established with grade and allows for a known amount of dry matter. Corn is often further processed from the kernel that is collected at harvest to increase the digestibility of the product (Fig. 4-10).

Oats

Oats are highly palatable. This feed is great for starting young animals on feed. Oats are widely grown but are most common in the Midwest and other central states (Fig. 4-11).

Barley

Barley is commonly grown in the central and western United States (Fig. 4-12). Barley is the least palatable of the grains and can become contaminated with *ergot,* a black fungus that reduces palatability, causes abortion, and reduces blood supply to the extremities, with resulting necrosis of the lower limbs, tail, and tips of the ears. Barley tends to cause digestive disturbances if it is ground too finely, and it should make up no more than one third of the diet.

> **TECHNICIAN NOTE** Ergot can cause necrosis of the lower limbs and tips of the ears when it is ingested by livestock.

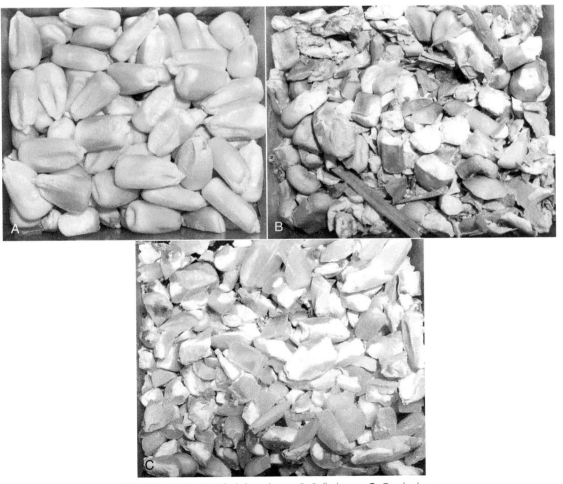

FIGURE 4-10 **A,** Whole-kernel corn. **B,** Rolled corn. **C,** Cracked corn.

Continued

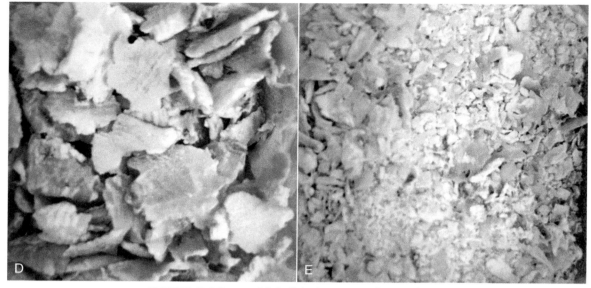

FIGURE 4-10, cont'd D, Flaked corn. E, Finely ground corn.

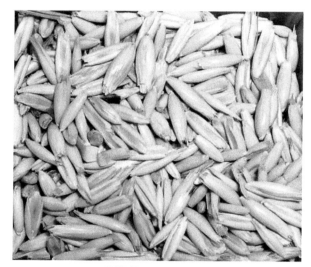

FIGURE 4-11 Oats.

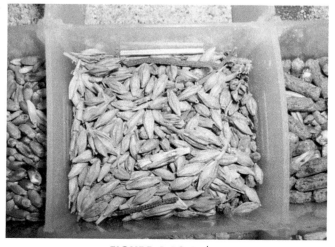

FIGURE 4-12 Barley.

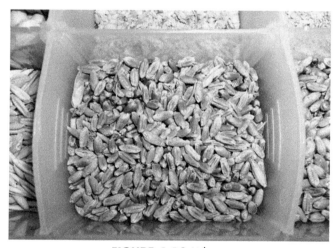

FIGURE 4-13 Wheat.

Wheat

Wheat is a good feed, having 5% of the value of corn, but it packs in the stomach. Wheat is widely grown in the United States; however, it is extremely expensive because humans compete for wheat for food consumption (Fig. 4-13).

Rye

Rye is the least palatable of the grains. It also can be contaminated with ergot, causing necrosis of the hooves, lower limbs, tail, and tips of the ears. Rye tends to cause digestive disturbances if it is ground too finely and should not make up more than one third of the diet (Fig. 4-14).

Triticale

Triticale is a hybrid between wheat and rye. It contains higher-quality protein than other grains but is limited by its low content of lysine. It is unpalatable and may contain ergot, similar to rye. Triticale should be limited to no more than 50% of the diet (Fig. 4-15).

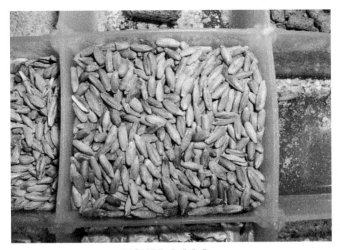

FIGURE 4-14 Rye.

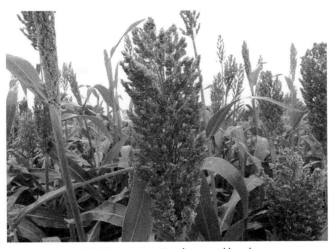

FIGURE 4-16 Sorghum seed head.

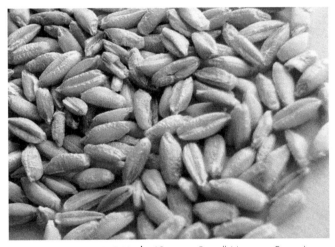

FIGURE 4-15 Triticale. (Courtesy Purcell Mountain Farms.)

Sorghum

Sorghum is quite drought resistant and is often grown and fed in areas with little rainfall. Sorghum must be processed for maximum digestibility. Several types of sorghum include kafir, milo, and several hybrids (Fig. 4-16).

By-Products
Molasses

Molasses is a by-product of the manufacturing process from sugar beets and sugar cane. It is fed in either liquid or dried form. It is a good source of energy and is quite palatable. It also can be used to help hold together loose feeds and reduce dust content.

PROTEIN SUPPLEMENTS

Protein supplements contain 20% or more of protein. These products can be broken into two categories: vegetable origin and animal origin.

Vegetable Origin

Soybean meal is the most widely used oilseed meal in the United States (Fig. 4.-17). Other oilseed meals include linseed meal, cottonseed meal (Fig. 4-18), soybean meal, and peanut meal.

Animal Origin

These types of supplements are obtained from meat or poultry packing or rendering plants, from surplus milk or milk by-products, and from marine sources. Some of these sources include *tankage* (by-product from the meat industry), blood meal, bone meal (Fig. 4-19), meat meal, and milk.

Cattle and other ruminants cannot be fed material derived from mammalian sources, such as meat, bone meal, and other animal by-products. This rule was established in August 1997 by the U.S. Food and Drug Administration (FDA) to minimize the potential of spreading transmissible spongiform encephalopathy. Tallow, blood by-products, gelatin, and milk products are excluded from regulation and are acceptable for use in ration formulation.

Nonprotein Nitrogen

Urea is not a protein supplement but a source of nitrogen that can be used by the rumen bacteria for protein synthesis (Fig. 4-20).

VITAMIN AND MINERAL SUPPLEMENTS

Several sources of mineral supplement include, but are not limited to, limestone, oyster shell, wheat germ oil, ensiled yeast, and bone meal. Minerals are often purchased in the form of a mineral block for smaller herds of livestock or for horses. Vitamins can be purchased individually and added to the ration or purchased as a mix (Fig. 4-21).

Additives

Several additives can be incorporated into a large animal diet, including hormone feed additives and anthelmintic agents. Each species and product produced from that species have specific requirements that must be followed when feed additives are used. No extralabel use of feed additives is allowed. Only FDA-approved additives are

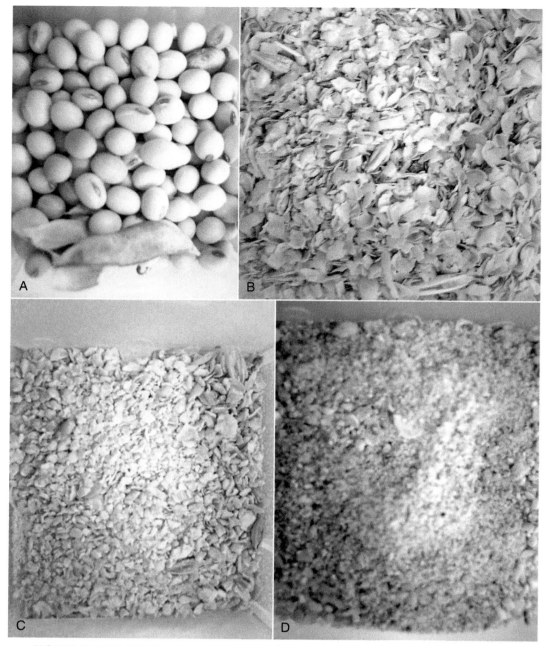

FIGURE 4-17 **A,** Whole soybeans. **B,** Soybean hulls. **C,** Crushed soybeans. **D,** Finely ground soybeans.

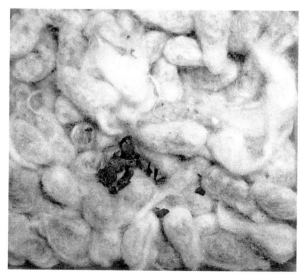

FIGURE 4-18 Cottonseed.

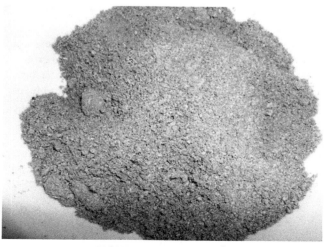

FIGURE 4-19 Bone meal.

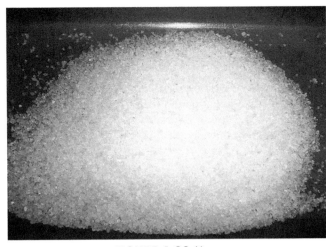

FIGURE 4-20 Urea.

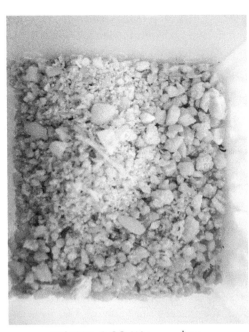

FIGURE 4-22 Wet corn gluten.

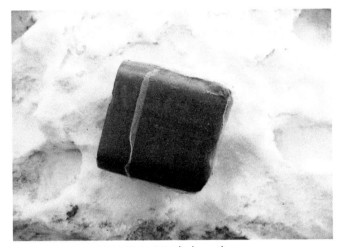

FIGURE 4-21 Block supplement.

allowed. No one, including a veterinarian, can legally prescribe the use of feed additives other than as directed on the product label.

OTHER BY-PRODUCTS
Wet Corn Gluten
Wet corn gluten is a by-product of the milling industry. The milling industry prepares starches, sugars, and corn oils for consumption by humans (Fig. 4-22).

Distillers' Grains
Distillers' grains are by-products of the ethanol industry. Wet corn gluten and distillers grains are processed using different procedures and are marketed in different product forms, depending on the company supplying the products (Fig. 4-23).

BALANCING RATIONS

Livestock diets can be purchased in bag form, and the label on the bag can be consulted for feeding amounts, but this process is too time and labor intensive when feeding extremely large

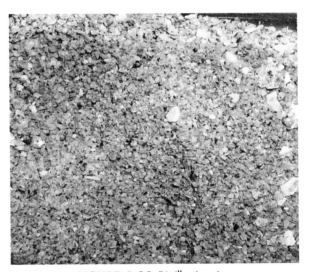

FIGURE 4-23 Distillers' grains.

herds, for two reasons: (1) the cost and (2) the amount of time and labor needed to complete the task. Therefore, owners of large animals often purchase the types of feeds described in bulk and form *rations* specific to their herd and its needs. A body condition score (BCS) may also be used by some producers before formulating a ration to identify if weight gain or loss is required. Because of the delicate balances needed to meet an animal's nutritional requirements, veterinary professionals often use the method of ration balancing. Ration balancing allows us to formulate a diet on paper and evaluate its ability to complete the animal's needs. The following steps should be used to formulate a high-quality ration for livestock. Many tools are available to help you balance rations and include online resources, computer programs, and textbooks. These resources often use the National Research

Council's information to provide information about the animal's requirements and information on what nutrients are contained in a type of food.

IDENTIFY THE ANIMAL'S NUTRITIONAL REQUIREMENTS

Tables can be used as general guidelines to determine the animal's nutritional requirements. All animals have *maintenance nutrient requirements (MNRs)*. The maintenance requirement is the amount of nutrition needed to maintain an animal in its current condition. Depending on what function is expected from the animal, nutritional requirements for growth, production, work, or reproduction can be calculated.

DETERMINE WHICH FEEDS WILL BE USED

Feeds are chosen based on the animal's digestive system, the amount of feed the animal can consume, and the best feeds available to meet the animal's nutritional requirements. The nutritional value of feeds can be found two ways: (1) tables with information about the nutritional content of feedstuffs and (2) feed testing. Feed testing is the process of collecting feed samples from 20 random spots in the bale, pile, or bin. The feed is sent to the laboratory for analysis, and the nutritional content is reported back to the owner or veterinarian. Feed testing is a more precise way of evaluating the nutritional content of potential feeds. If several types of feeds can be used to meet the animal's nutritional requirements, the choice is often made based on economics and ease of handling or storage. Consideration also should be made for palatability. If tomorrow cockle burrs were found to be high in protein, we could try to feed them to the livestock, but chances are the livestock would not eat these plants because they are unpalatable. For example, sheep dislike strong odors, a factor that should be considered when selecting feeds.

CALCULATE THE AMOUNT OF FEED TO USE IN THE RATION

Several methods can be used to determine what the animal's diet should contain to meet its nutritional requirements. Algebraic equations or Pearson square methods can be used. Computer programs are also available. Because some computer programs are extremely expensive, you should consider learning the procedure using the Pearson square method or the algebraic equation method.

CHECK THE RATION FORMULATED AGAINST THE NEEDS OF THE ANIMAL

Once the animal's diet has been calculated, it is extremely important to review the diet and ensure that all the animal's nutrient requirements will be met.

MAKE ADJUSTMENTS

If the diet does not meet all the animal's nutrient requirements, you must make adjustments, change feeds, or supplement the diet to correct the problem.

EXAMPLES
Use of Pearson Square
One limitation of using the Pearson square method is that calculations can be made using only two feedstuffs.

Identify the Animal's Nutrient Requirements
The producer has a 700-pound heifer. He wants her to gain 1.5 pounds/day. Her daily requirements according to the National Research Council tables are as follows.
- 15 pounds of dry matter intake
- 12% crude protein
- 70% TDN

Determine Which Feeds Will Be Used
The producer would like to feed the heifer what he has available. Right now the producer currently has the following:
- Barley = dry matter 88%, TDN 75%, crude protein 6%
- Sun-cured hay = dry matter 90%, TDN 89%, crude protein 26%

Calculate the Amount of Feed to Use in the Ration
To balance for TDN, proceed as follows:
1. Balance for TDN. Draw a square and place 70% in the center.
2. At the upper left corner of the square, write "barley = 75," and at the lower left corner write "sun-cured hay = 89." These numbers represent the TDN percentage in each feedstuff.
3. Subtract diagonally, from smaller from larger (75 − 70 = 5; 89 − 70 = 19), and write the numbers on the right side of the square.
4. Add the numbers on the right side of the square (19 + 5 = 24). These numbers indicate that a ration of 19 parts barley and 5 parts sun-cured hay will give a 70% TDN ration. This is a total of 24 parts.
5. Divide the barley and sun-cured hay parts by 24 to obtain the preliminary percentages of barley (19 ÷ 24 = 79.2%) and sun-cured hay (5 ÷ 24 = 20.8%) (Fig. 4-24).
6. Determine the crude protein concentration in the barley and sun-cured hay mixture. Multiply the percentage of each feedstuff in the mix by its crude protein content. Barley is 79.2% of the mix and contains 6% crude protein. Sun-cured hay is 20.8% of the mix and contains 26% crude protein. Add the results. The crude protein concentration in the mix is as follows:

Barley: $0.792 \times 6 = 4.752\%$

Sun-cured hay: $0.208 \times 26 = 5.408\%$

Check the Rations Formulated Against the Needs of the Animal
The ration was balanced for TDN, so we know it meets the animal's requirement. However, we did not balance the ration for crude protein, so we must check this percentage:

$4.752\% + 5.408\% = 10.16\%$

The heifer needs 12%; this ration does not meet the requirements needed by the heifer. The producer most likely will need to supplement with a third feed that will make up the deficiency.

Make Adjustments
Blood meal is 88.9% crude protein. If the producer supplements with crude protein, the deficiency can be corrected.

Using Algebraic Equations
Identify the Animal's Nutrient Requirements
Your client arrives at the clinic asking questions about how to feed his mature 6-year-old mare doing moderate work. The horse weighs 1100 pounds. The horse's requirements are shown in Table 4-1. This particular horse eats between 1% and 2% of its body weight in forage.

Determine Which Feeds Will Be Used
The owner would like to feed orchard grass that he has available and oats. You choose to begin the ration with the horse eating 1.75% forage (Table 4-2):

Orchard grass: 1100 pounds × 0.0175
= 19.25 pounds of orchard grass to be fed

Calculate the Amount of Feed to Use in the Ration, and Check the Ration Formulated Against the Needs of the Animal
First, calculate the total amount of each nutrient being provided by the forage (Table 4-3). Because DE is the only requirement we have not met, we can take 9.8 Mcal times the remaining nutrients to be supplied and divide by 1.35 Mcal/pound (the DE of oats) = 7.26 pounds. If you feed 7.26 pounds of oats and 19.25 pounds of orchard grass, you will have met the horse's requirements.

Make Adjustments
Because this ration meets the horse's requirements, you have completed the calculations. However, if you are concerned about the excess requirements of crude protein, calcium,

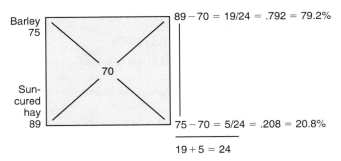

FIGURE 4-24 Pearson square method of calculating rations.

TABLE 4-1 | Dietary Requirements of Horses

REQUIREMENT	DIGESTIBLE ENERGY (Mcal)	CRUDE PROTEIN (pounds)	CALCIUM (g)	PHOSPHORUS (g)
Maintenance	16.4	1.4	20.0	14.0
Moderate work	8.2	0	0	0
Total requirements	24.6	1.4	20.0	14.0

TABLE 4-2 | Horse Ration Example: Part 1

FEED	DIGESTIBLE ENERGY (Mcal)	CRUDE PROTEIN (pounds)	CALCIUM (g)	PHOSPHORUS (g)
Orchard grass	0.77	0.1	1.5	1.04
Oats	1.35	0.11	0.36	1.54

TABLE 4-3 | Horse Ration Example: Part 2

	DIGESTIBLE ENERGY (Mcal)	CRUDE PROTEIN (pounds)	CALCIUM (g)	PHOSPHORUS (g)
Total daily requirement for the horse	24.6	1.4	20	14
Total nutrients from the forage	19.25 × 0.77 = 14.8	19.25 × 0.1 = 2	19.25 × 1.5 = 29	19.25 × 1.04 = 20
Remaining nutrients to be supplied for the concentrate	9.8	−0.6 Because you are over, consider the requirement as being met unless you are trying to be economical, then adjust	−9 Because you are over, consider the requirement as being met unless you are trying to be economical, then adjust	−6 Because you are over, consider the requirement as being met unless you are trying to be economical, then adjust

and phosphorus, you could adjust the percentage of orchard grass being fed or select another feed.

FLUID THERAPY

The animal's body consists primarily of water. The body's water is divided among three "compartments": intracellular (inside cells); extracellular (plasma water and fluid [lymph]); and transcellular (body cavities such as joints, gastrointestinal [GI] lumen, cerebrospinal fluid, thorax, abdomen). In a normal animal, the total amount of water in its body is allocated roughly as follows:

$$\text{Total body water} = 60\% \text{ intracellular fluid}$$
$$+ 30\% \text{ extracellular fluid (ECF)}$$
$$+ 10\% \text{ transcellular fluid}$$

Animals may experience diseases or conditions that cause imbalances in one or more of the compartments. Severe diarrhea, profuse sweating, and a frozen water bucket are examples of factors that can cause problems with water balance. Fortunately, during times of imbalance, water can shift between the compartments in an attempt to maintain health. However, there are limits to the amount of water that can shift without doing harm; when this limit is reached, medical intervention in the form of water supplementation is necessary to prevent complications and possibly death.

Imbalances are not limited to water. Electrolytes, pH, and nutritional substances (protein, carbohydrate, fat) may also become compromised, and medical therapy to replace or balance these items may be necessary.

In the natural state, an animal has only one body system for intake of fluids and electrolytes: the GI tract. However, it has four body systems that can lose fluids and electrolytes:

- GI tract, through loss of luminal water and electrolytes
- Respiratory tract, through water vapor in expired air and respiratory exudates
- Urinary tract (kidneys), through urine
- Integument, through sweat

An additional "route" of loss is external or internal hemorrhage. The body may recover water and electrolytes from internal hemorrhage by reabsorption, but this reabsorption is a gradual process and may not be rapid enough to prevent death in severe cases. External hemorrhage, of course, is a total loss.

Fluid therapy is basically an alternative to an animal's normal ability to drink and balance its own fluid compartments. Fluid therapy is indicated to

- Maintain fluid, electrolyte, or nutrient balance when disease prevents the animal from its normal oral intake
- Maintain fluid, electrolyte, or nutrient balance while the animal is under anesthesia
- Replace fluid or electrolytes when the animal's normal oral intake would be too slow

Calculations for replacement of water are different from calculations for replacement of substances such as electrolytes and nutrients. The calculations are considered separately here.

FLUID (WATER) CALCULATIONS

At any given moment, an animal exists in one of three states:

- Overhydrated: This condition rarely occurs naturally; it is usually the result of iatrogenic overadministration of fluids.
- Normally hydrated: The animal does not need fluids (unless necessary to maintain hydration, such as during anesthesia).
- Dehydrated: The animal needs fluid therapy (if unable to replace deficits by mouth).

The dehydrated animal is recognized by laboratory data (packed cell volume/total solids [PCV/TS] measurement) or clinical signs. Dehydration is estimated on the basis of PCV/TS and clinical signs. Guidelines for estimating the percentage of dehydration on the basis of clinical signs are available (Table 4-4).

> **TECHNICIAN NOTE**   Dehydration is estimated on the basis of packed cell volume/total solids and clinical signs.

Fluid calculations are extensively covered in other texts. Fluid calculations in large animals are basically no different from calculations in small animals; the same formulas apply. What can be difficult to appreciate is the large volume of fluids necessary in large animals compared with small animals.

TABLE 4-4	Estimating Dehydration in the Horse			
PERCENTAGE OF DEHYDRATION (%)	**HEART RATE (bpm)**	**CAPILLARY REFILL TIME (sec)**	**PCV/TS**	**COMMENTS**
<5	Normal (28-40)	Normal (<2)	Normal	Clinically silent
6-7	40-60	2	40/7	Mild dehydration; mildly delayed skin tent (2-3 sec)
8-9	61-80	3	45/7.5	Moderate dehydration; obviously delayed skin tent (3-5 sec), tacky mucous membranes
10-11	81-100	4	50/8	Approaching severe dehydration/shock; weak peripheral pulse, sunken eyes, dry mucous membranes; delayed skin tent >5 sec
12-15	>100	>4	>50/>8	Shock, collapse, death if untreated

PCV/TS, Packed cell volume/total solids.

Not only do large animals have a large amount of total body water, but also herbivores cycle a tremendous volume of water and electrolytes through their GI tracts in a 24-hour day. Literally gallons of saliva and gastric and intestinal fluids are produced and secreted into the GI tract lumen, and the animal must recover almost all these fluids to remain normally hydrated. GI diseases can be especially devastating to a large animal's hydration.

The basic formula for calculating fluid needs in any animal is as follows:

$$\text{Fluids needed} = \text{Maintenance fluids} + \text{Ongoing losses} + \text{Deficit replacement}$$

> **TECHNICIAN NOTE** Fluids needed = Maintenance fluids + Ongoing losses + Deficit replacement.

MAINTENANCE FLUIDS

The term *maintenance fluids* refers to the volume of water necessary to maintain life. This is the volume necessary to supply all the body's cells and to remove cell waste. Whether an animal drinks water normally by mouth or receives fluid therapy, the animal must have at least 2 to 4 mL/kg/hour of water. This amount may need to be slightly increased during late pregnancy and during lactation. Heavily lactating animals need approximately 1 L extra for each liter of milk produced. Fever can also increase maintenance requirements.

To emphasize the amount of fluids required in large animals, using the minimum amount of 2 mL/kg/hour, an average 500-kg horse requires at least 1 L of water per hour (24 L/day) just to sustain its life.

> **TECHNICIAN NOTE** It is often difficult for technicians to understand the large volumes of water a horse needs to sustain life.

ONGOING LOSSES

Ongoing losses are caused by the animal's primary disease or environmental conditions. Diseases may include diarrhea, gastric reflux, GI ileus, kidney disease, profuse and prolonged sweating, severe edema, hemorrhage, and loss of fluids into body cavities. Most ongoing losses cannot be strictly measured; therefore, the amount usually is an estimate. However, some losses, such as gastric reflux (via nasogastric intubation) and urine output (via indwelling urinary catheter), can be accurately measured.

> **TECHNICIAN NOTE** Conditions such as diarrhea, gastric reflux, gastrointestinal ileus, kidney disease, profuse and prolonged sweating, severe edema, hemorrhage, and loss of fluids into body cavities are causes of ongoing losses.

If the animal is healthy, this factor is zero. If the animal has a disease that causes ongoing fluid losses, medical or surgical therapy is used to try to resolve the primary disease. Once the primary disease is under control, the ongoing losses should end, and this factor will drop to zero and can be eliminated from the equation.

DEFICIT REPLACEMENT

Deficit replacement applies only to dehydrated animals. Animals that are overhydrated or normally hydrated do not have a deficit to replace. The formula for replacement of water deficit is as follows:

$$\text{Body weight (kg)} \times \% \text{ dehydration} = \text{Liters to replace}$$

Once the animal's deficit has been replaced, this factor becomes zero and can be eliminated from the equation.

> **TECHNICIAN NOTE** Deficit replacement is calculated only if the animal is dehydrated.

The speed of deficit replacement is determined by the status of the patient. Mild and moderate deficits are replaced over 12 to 24 hours. Severe dehydration, as evidenced by cardiovascular shock, is an emergency situation, and replacement often is necessary within 1 to 2 hours if the patient is to have any chance of survival.

Once the deficit has been replaced and the ongoing losses have been controlled, the animal needs only maintenance fluids to survive. If intravenous (IV) fluids are used for fluid therapy, the animal is weaned off maintenance fluids as soon as possible and is returned slowly to oral intake.

SUBSTANCE CALCULATIONS

The term *substances* refers to all nonwater items that can be measured in the laboratory, including the following:
- Electrolytes, especially sodium, potassium, and chloride
- Minerals, especially calcium and phosphorus
- Nutrients, primarily glucose and protein
- pH buffers, primarily bicarbonate

If normal values are known, the patient's values can be compared with normal levels. For any given substance, an animal is in one of three states at any given moment:
- Substance excess: The animal does not need replacement.
- Normal value: The animal does not need replacement but may need maintenance amounts to retain normal levels.
- Substance deficit: The animal may need medical therapy to replace the deficit and return the animal to normal levels (depending on the severity of the deficit and primary disease).

The formula for replacing the deficit of any measurable substance is as follows:

$$(\text{Normal value} - \text{Patient's value}) \times \text{ECF factor} \times \text{Body weight (kg)} = \text{Amount to replace}$$

The *ECF factor* refers to the percentage of an animal's total body water that is ECF. The percentage is age dependent; younger animals have a higher percentage of ECF. The following factors are used:

- 0.3 for adults
- 0.4 for older foals
- 0.5 for neonates

The mathematical units for the amount to replace depend on how the laboratory measures the substance in question. For example, if the substance is measured in milliequivalents (mEq), the answer (amount to be replaced) also will be in mEq. If the substance is measured in milligrams (mg), the answer also will be in milligrams.

Substance replacement must be done cautiously to avoid complications. The patient's blood substance levels should be monitored periodically while the patient is receiving supplementation. Bolus administration is dangerous and should be avoided. The most common substances replaced in horses are potassium, calcium, and bicarbonate.

POTASSIUM

Herbivores are highly dependent on dietary potassium to maintain normal potassium levels in the body. Horses that are off feed for longer than 24 hours typically must receive potassium supplements.

> **TECHNICIAN NOTE**   Horses that are off feed for longer than 24 hours typically must receive potassium supplements.

If a deficiency has developed, potassium replacement can be accomplished by adding potassium chloride (KCl) solution (commercially available) to the animal's IV fluids. Potassium replacement should not exceed a rate of 1 mEq/kg/hour. Excessively rapid administration can lead to life-threatening hyperkalemia, with subsequent cardiac standstill.

Once deficits have been replaced and the patient is receiving maintenance fluid levels, maintenance potassium can be given. Maintenance KCl usually can be safely added to IV fluids at 20 mEq/L for as long as the animal is off feed.

CALCIUM

Animals that are off feed, lactating, or sweating profusely may experience excessive calcium loss. If calcium is deficient, calcium can be given by the IV route. This can be accomplished in several ways. Calcium borogluconate (23%) is perhaps the most common IV supplement used. If calcium borogluconate is given too quickly, life-threatening cardiac arrhythmias may result; patients should be closely monitored during administration of any calcium supplement. Generally, the maximum rate of calcium borogluconate given by the IV route is 250 mL over 20 to 30 minutes. Unless the animal's condition is considered an emergency, calcium should be given as a gradual IV drip, with caution. Calcium-containing solutions should not be allowed to mix physically with bicarbonate solutions.

> **TECHNICIAN NOTE**   If calcium is given too quickly intravenously, life-threatening cardiac arrhythmias may result.

BICARBONATE

Most pH imbalances in herbivores result in acidosis and accompanying low levels of bicarbonate in the blood (Table 4-5). To restore normal bicarbonate levels, sodium bicarbonate solutions usually are given by the IV route. Replacement must be gradual. Typically, half of the calculated deficit is replaced over several hours, and the second half is replaced over the next 12 to 24 hours. Rapid administration can cause central nervous system dysfunction (severe depression and possible coma).

ROUTES AND METHODS OF ADMINISTRATION

The route of fluid therapy depends on the urgency for correction of the patient's deficits, as well as the patient's underlying health or disease status. If the GI tract is functional and the patient's needs are not critical, then the GI tract can be used for treatment. The treatment may be as simple as adding substances such as electrolytes, glucose, or bicarbonate to a bucket of water. Some additives are not highly palatable or may be added excessively, thus leading to poor taste, so voluntary consumption is unreliable. Whenever a water source is supplemented with additives, another source of plain fresh water should be available at all times to provide the horse with a choice. A patient's intake of both plain and supplemented water should be monitored closely.

The GI tract may also be used for replacement of fluids and other substances through nasogastric intubation. Fluids do not have to be sterile, and this saves cost. Nasogastric intubation also eliminates "patient choice" in selecting what to consume. However, the capacity of the stomach and the speed at which it can empty have limits. If these limits are exceeded, colic can result. For an average adult horse with an immediate need for replacement, a maximum volume of 8 L of fluid every 30 to 60 minutes can be given. However, this volume may be too much for some individuals, so less aggressive volumes given less frequently should be used whenever possible. Administering the fluid directly into the stomach does not mean that the fluid will be absorbed rapidly or completely. Absorption is a different process from gastric emptying.

> **TECHNICIAN NOTE**   For the average adult horse with an immediate need for fluid replacement, a maximum volume of 8 L of fluid every 30 to 60 minutes can be given.

TABLE 4-5	pH of Equine Blood
Normal pH	7.32-7.44
Acidemia	7.2-7.31
Life-threatening acidemia	<7.2

Absorption is a slower process and seldom is quick enough to treat shock or severe imbalances successfully.

Subcutaneous (SC) fluids are not used in large animals in the same fashion as in small animals. The SC route is not used to replace fluid deficits in large animals because the volumes of fluid required usually are so large that SC tissues likely would be compromised by the pressure and distention. SC fluids tend to gravitate to dependent areas of the body, where absorption is slow. In addition, few areas of loose, elastic skin are suitable for SC fluids. The lateral cervical regions and the lateral aspect of the triceps muscle mass have enough elasticity to allow administration of small volumes of fluid (<500 mL). This is occasionally done (especially in ruminants) for calcium or magnesium supplementation.

For all other situations, fluids are given by the IV route. For short-term administration, a large-diameter hypodermic needle (14- to 18-gauge) can be inserted directly into a vein and supported manually or taped to hold it in position. Fluids can be given directly through the needle into the vein through sterile rubber tubing. This method is commonly used for small volumes (<1 L) and for emergency situations when an IV catheter is not readily available. If longer-term IV fluid therapy is necessary, an IV catheter should be placed.

The tubing used for administration should be sterile and flexible. Standard IV fluid administration sets, arthroscopy tubing, "bell" IV lines, and many other choices are available (Fig. 4-25). Large-bore tubing should be used when rapid administration is necessary. If the patient is allowed freedom to wander around the stall while fluids are given, the tubing must be long enough to allow the patient to reach the borders of the stall and to lie down if it chooses. If the patient's movement is restricted, shorter tubing can be used. Special coil-style tubing for large animals is available; it stretches like a telephone cord to allow the patient to move around the stall or lie down, yet the tubing takes up slack as the patient moves. This tubing is rigid enough to provide some resistance to kinking.

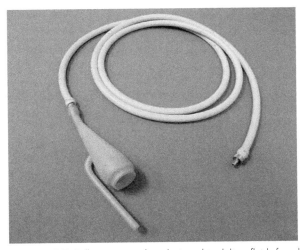

FIGURE 4-25 Bell intravenous line designed to deliver fluids from bottles by sliding the "bell" portion over the mouth of the bottle and inserting the Luer tip into a catheter or needle inserted into a vein.

One of the greatest challenges in large animal fluid administration is preventing kinking or disconnection of the administration tubing. This is most likely to occur when the patient roams around the stall or lies down and tangles the tubing around its neck or legs. Sometimes a patient must be placed in stocks or have its head tied to prevent it from wandering or lying down while fluids are being given. Regardless, large animals *must* be closely supervised when they are receiving IV fluids. Kinking can lead to blood clotting inside the catheter as a result of stagnation of fluid movement through the catheter; in this case, the catheter likely will have to be replaced. Disconnection of administration tubing from the catheter can result in either aspiration of air through the catheter into the bloodstream (air embolism) or massive external hemorrhage from the catheter, depending on the level of the catheter in relation to the heart. In either case, death can result.

Fluids can be purchased in 1-, 3-, 5-, or 6-L bags. Administration sets (especially arthroscopy tubing) can be obtained with one, two, or four heads; multiple heads allow attachment to multiple fluid bags, for convenience. For most patients, the larger-volume fluid bags (5 to 6 L) are more convenient to manage, especially if the patient requires large volumes of fluid.

Fluids can be given by gravity flow or with pressurized flow. For gravity flow, fluid bags can be hung from the ceiling on a rope and pulley system or from any point higher than the patient's catheter or needle. For pressurized administration, pressurized "squeeze" sleeves that wrap around fluid bags can be purchased. Alternatively, the fluids can be pressurized by injecting air into the fluid bag or bottle with a large syringe or hand pump. High-pressure administration is reserved for rapid, emergency situations.

Mechanized IV fluid pumps can be used for large animals but typically are used only for delivery of smaller volumes of fluids, primarily in foals and for low-volume parenteral nutrition in adults. Standard IV fluid pumps cannot exceed 999 mL/hour.

ENTERAL AND PARENTERAL NUTRITION

Various disease conditions may render an animal's GI tract incapable of intake, digestion, or absorption of food and water. For example, a mandibular fracture may prevent chewing; a pharyngeal abscess may prevent normal swallowing; and many conditions of the stomach, intestines, and colon can prevent normal digestion, absorption, or both. Non-GI diseases, such as fever, severe pain, or diseases of the central nervous system, may affect an animal's desire to eat and drink. Failure to consume adequate carbohydrates, proteins, and lipids forces the body to process its reserves and perhaps its own tissues to prevent starvation. Malnutrition has well-known deleterious effects on health and on the ability of a sick or injured animal to heal and return to health.

Patients can be partially or totally nutritionally supported. Formulas are available to calculate an animal's energy, protein, and lipid requirements; vitamins and minerals can be added if necessary. The formulas attempt to account for the patient's

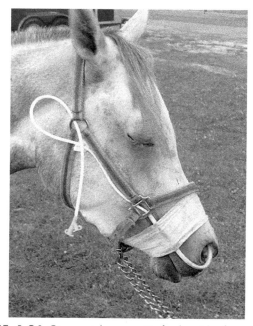

FIGURE 4-26 Commercial nasogastric feeding tube for administration of fluids or enteral feeding. (From Hardy J: Critical care. In Reed SM, Bayly WM, Sellon DC, editors: *Equine internal medicine*, ed 2, St. Louis, 2004, Saunders.)

age, body weight, and energy requirements. The patient's underlying disease may affect the calculated nutritional requirements. For example, sepsis in foals greatly increases energy needs to more than maintenance levels. Once the requirements have been calculated, the clinician can prescribe substances to meet the nutritional needs of the patient precisely.

Nutritional support can be given by enteral (GI) or parenteral routes.

Enteral Feeding

Enteral feeding is feasible only if the GI tract is capable of digestion and absorption. Liquid diets can be formulated from readily available materials and given by stomach tube. Standard nasogastric tubes can be used; however, many horses resent repeated intubation, and long-term intubation with standard nasogastric tubes often is traumatic to tissues and interferes with swallowing. To minimize the effects of repeated or long-term use of standard tubes, commercially available nasogastric feeding tubes have been developed. The tubes are narrow in diameter and made from soft plastic, resulting in less tissue trauma. The tubes are secured to the muzzle or halter and, if properly maintained, allow long-term fluid and nutritional support (Fig. 4-26). If a slurry-type diet or sticky substances have been given through any feeding tube, the tube should be flushed well after each use to prevent clogging.

Because of the interference with swallowing and the possibility of aspiration, patients with indwelling nasogastric tubes, especially large-diameter tubes, should not attempt to eat around the tube. Muzzles or stripped stalls may be necessary. A patient that is allowed access to water should be watched closely for coughing or reflux from the nostrils,

which indicates difficulty swallowing. Removal of the water source may be necessary.

Occasionally, a patient has a condition that prevents passing a nasogastric tube through the nasal cavity or pharynx. Enteral feeding still is possible by placing a feeding tube directly into the esophagus through an esophagostomy. Once the tube is removed, the esophagostomy heals by second intention with only topical care.

Parenteral Nutrition

Parenteral routes are used as an alternative to the GI tract. In large animals, the IV route is the parenteral route of choice. Nutritional support can be provided with either partial parenteral nutrition (PPN) or total parenteral nutrition (TPN). Calculations of the patient's nutritional needs are performed, and a decision is made whether to try to meet all (TPN) or part (PPN) of the patient's requirements. The decision is based on the patient's disease, physical condition, and length of time for which support will be necessary.

Sterile carbohydrate, lipid, and amino acid solutions are commercially available for IV use. The content of each solution is compared with the calculated patient's needs, and the amount required for a 24-hour period is calculated and delivered through an IV catheter.

BLOOD AND PLASMA ADMINISTRATION

Whole blood is used to treat life-threatening blood loss, RBC deficit, or platelet loss. Currently, whole blood for large animals is not commercially available because of the inability to freeze it or store it under refrigeration for more than several days. Therefore, whole blood is collected and used on an "as needed" basis.

Fresh whole blood is collected from donor horses that are confirmed negative for equine infectious anemia and are current with their vaccines. With regard to blood types, more than 30 different RBC alloantigens exist in horses, leading to more than 400,000 possible alloantigen combinations. Therefore, there is no such thing as a "universal donor." However, two alloantigens, Aa and Qa, are highly immunoreactive and are very prevalent in horses. The most desirable blood donors are negative for these alloantigens. Blood typing can be performed to identify the best potential donors (Standardbreds and Belgians have the lowest reported incidence of Qa and Aa alloantigens, followed by Quarter horses). Although negative Aa and Qa donors should reduce the risk of incompatibility, they do not totally eliminate the risk.

Major and minor cross-matching should always be done to confirm a compatible donor, even when blood types are known (Table 4-6). Unmatched transfusions, although not preferred, may be necessary in emergency situations. They can be performed with slightly increased risk; most horses can receive one or more transfusions over 3 to 4 days from a single unmatched donor. Unmatched donors preferably should be geldings; the next choice would be a female that has never been bred. A healthy adult horse can donate 15% to 20% of its total blood volume (≈5 to 10 L of blood at one

TABLE 4-6	Major and Minor Cross-Matches		
CROSS-MATCH DESIGNATION	**COMPONENTS**	**PERFORM FOR WHOLE BLOOD TRANSFUSIONS**	**PERFORM FOR PLASMA TRANSFUSIONS**
Major cross-match	Donor RBCs × recipient serum	Yes	No
Minor cross-match	Donor serum × recipient RBCs	Yes	Yes

RBCs, Red blood cells.

collection, or up to 20 mL/kg every 3 to 4 weeks). Blood volume of the adult horse is estimated as follows:

$$\text{Body weight (kg)} \times 8\% \text{ to } 10\% = \text{Total blood volume (L)}$$

Whole blood is collected using strict aseptic technique. The patient is clipped and prepared over a jugular vein. The operator should wear sterile gloves. A large-diameter needle or catheter (preferably 12 to 14 gauge) is inserted into the jugular vein (*against* the direction of blood flow to facilitate collection), sterile tubing is attached, and blood is collected by gravity or vacuum-assisted flow. Gravity collection is preferred because it causes less damage to RBCs.

Whole blood can be collected into a sterile glass or plastic container, but plastic is preferred because glass can potentially activate platelets and coagulation factors. Anticoagulant (usually citrate based) must be added to the collection container. Commercially available acid citrate dextrose (ACD) solution (2.5% to 4%) is used at a blood-to-ACD ratio of 9:1. Sodium citrate (3.2%) also can be used, in the same blood-to-citrate ratio. Commercial blood collection kits are available and convenient and provide plastic collection bags or bottles with premeasured anticoagulant and transfer tubing. Periodically during the collection procedure, the collection container should be gently swirled or rotated to assist mixing of the blood with the anticoagulant. The effects of storage on equine blood are not well known; therefore, whole blood is preferably collected and transfused promptly. Short-term refrigerated storage for several days has been reported, using citrate phosphate dextrose as the anticoagulant at 4° C (39.2° F).

The volume of blood given to the recipient depends on the underlying disease and the reason for the transfusion. Usually, whole blood is given to replace RBCs. The volume of blood to be given is related to the patient's current RBC count and not the patient's ideal normal RBC count. Several formulas have been reported and used successfully for calculating transfusion volumes. One suggested formula is as follows:

$$\begin{aligned}\text{Liters required} = &\ \text{Body weight (kg)}\\ &\times \text{Blood volume factor (mL/kg)}\\ &\times (\text{PCV desired} - \text{PCV measured})/\text{PCV of donor}\end{aligned}$$

Blood volume is factored as follows:

151 mL/kg neonate less than 4 weeks old
93 mL/kg neonate 4 to 2 weeks old
82 mL/kg foal 12 weeks to 6 months old
72 mL/kg 6 months old to adult

This formula provides only an estimate of blood to be replaced. In reality, administration of the entire calculated amount is seldom necessary.

Whole blood is given to the recipient through an IV catheter of at least 14-gauge diameter. The administration system should have an in-line filter to remove clots, and the filter should be replaced after filtering every 3 to 4 L. Even when cross-matching between donor and recipient indicates compatibility, adverse allergic reactions still may occur. Before beginning the transfusion, record the patient's heart rate, respiratory rate, and temperature. The first 50 mL of blood should be given slowly over 15 to 30 minutes, and the recipient should be closely monitored for changes in heart rate, respiratory rate, and attitude. If the patient's parameters remain stable over the introduction period, the administration rate can be increased to 15 to 20 mL/kg/hour. The patient should be closely monitored throughout the entire transfusion. The transfusion should be stopped immediately if any reactions are observed. Because bacterial contamination may be responsible for the reaction, the blood being administered should be cultured if adverse reactions are observed. Delayed reactions to transfusions may occur, so close monitoring should continue for at least 24 hours after the procedure.

Transfused equine RBCs live only 2 to 5 days on average. In rare instances when an animal is able to receive its own RBCs (autotransfusion), the life span of the cells may extend to 14 days.

Plasma transfusion is readily accomplished in the horse because of the availability of commercial plasma. Plasma may be needed to replace plasma proteins, clotting factors, or antibodies (especially in foals with failure of passive transfer). Plasma may be made "hyperimmune" to certain antigens. By exposing the plasma donor to the antigen, antibodies will be produced, with passive transfer of immunity to the recipient.

Plasma can be collected fresh or bought commercially. Fresh plasma can be collected by harvesting whole blood from donor horses and performing plasmapheresis of the whole blood. However, the equipment is expensive and usually is found only at large equine facilities. A less costly method is to collect whole blood and allow the cells to settle by gravity for several hours (at room temperature) or by centrifugation. The plasma then can be aseptically aspirated or siphoned from the settled RBCs and given to the recipient by the IV route after passing the plasma through an in-line microfilter. Plasma collected in this fashion is seldom completely free of cells and is prone to bacterial contamination.

Commercial plasma is collected from donors that are free of Aa and Qa alloantigens, and it is cell free. Controlled exposure of donor horses may produce plasma that is rich in antibodies against certain diseases. Compatibility (cross-match) testing usually is not necessary; however, if it is deemed necessary, only the minor cross-match is applicable. Commercial plasma usually is sold in 1-L plastic bags and is stored frozen. Plasma should never be thawed in a microwave oven, to avoid denaturing the plasma proteins. Rather, thawing should occur slowly in warm water. Plasma should reach at least 37° C (98.6° F) before administration. Frozen plasma generally stores safely for up to 1 year. Its expiration date should not be exceeded. If an accidental partial or complete thaw occurs, refreezing is not recommended.

The amount of plasma given to a patient varies widely, depending on the reason for the transfusion, the rate of protein breakdown and redistribution, and the quality (protein levels) of the plasma being given. No single formula exists for performing universal calculations. The veterinarian calculates replacement volumes based on patient and plasma variables. Typically, foals require 1 to 2 L to treat failure of passive transfer, and adults treated for hypoproteinemia require at least 6 L. Administration of plasma is similar to that of whole blood, given through a 16-gauge or larger IV catheter. An administration set with an in-line filter is appropriate.

Although the incidence is low, allergic reactions to plasma administration do occur. Reactions usually occur during the infusion and manifest as shivering, difficult or rapid breathing, weakness, colic, or shock. If these reactions are observed, the infusion should be stopped immediately, and a clinician should be alerted to the situation.

CASE STUDY

A prominent veterinary college has just released new data that fish oil is extremely valuable to sheep. The data suggest that fish oil can increase feed efficiency by 20%. What considerations should you make before recommending fish oil to your sheep clients?

CASE STUDY

You recently acquired a new equine client who has never owned a horse before and has oats and alfalfa available as feeds. This client would like to know how much feed should be given and whether oats and alfalfa will meet the horse's nutritional requirements. What should you do? What information will you give the client?

CASE STUDY

You are sent to a large dairy operation to sample feeds and send them to the laboratory. The dairy uses your clinic only for veterinary information and makes up a large percentage of your clinic's income. You are asked to sample the corn silage, wet distillers' grain, timothy hay, and cotton seed. You are not told where any of the feeds are located, but you know they are stored in bulk around the dairy. How will you determine which feedstuff is which, to identify the bags? Describe the procedure you will use to collect the feeds.

CASE STUDY

One of your clients currently is feeding rye. His cows' hooves are beginning to show signs of necrosis. What questions should you ask when taking the history?

SUGGESTED READING

Gillespie JR, Flanders FB: *Modern livestock and poultry*, ed 8, Clifton Park, NY, 2010, Delmar Cengage Learning.

Jurgens MH: *Animal feeding and nutrition*, ed 8, Dubuque, Iowa, 1997, Kendall/Hunt Publishing.

Topel JA: Large animal nutrition and feeding. In Tighe MM, Brown M, editors: *Mosby's comprehensive review for veterinary technicians*, ed 3, St. Louis, 2008, Mosby.

Large Animal Hospital Management

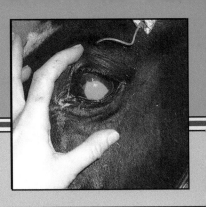

5 Daily Hospital Responsibilities

OUTLINE

LEARNING OBJECTIVES

When you finish this chapter, you will be able to

- Demonstrate a basic understanding of mobile large animal practices
- Describe the complex nature of how large animals must be transported to clinics
- Properly care for stalled patients
- Discuss the pros and cons of bedding materials
- Discuss the need for proper ventilation in a veterinary hospital
- Describe the importance of proper feeding and watering practices in the clinic as well as the importance of documentation
- Properly execute the grooming procedure
- Recognize potential complications of *recumbent* and *contagious cases* and know how to prevent such complications

KEY TERMS

Ambulatory practice
Blepharospasm
Central sulcus of the frog
Compartment syndrome
Contagious case
Decubital ulcer

Farm call
Field service
Foot bath
Hot zone
Lateral sulci of the frog
Nonambulatory

Picking
Recumbent
Skin scald
Stripping
Tuber coxae
Urine scald

HOSPITAL/CLINIC PROCEDURES

It is an unfortunate fact of life that the amount of money available for health care and veterinary medicine is often limited by the animal's production value. Most farmers provide what they can for diagnosis and treatment of their livestock, but the monetary value of the animal may fall far short of what is required for its medical or surgical treatment. It is disheartening to tell a farmer that surgery for a cow's broken leg is possible but may cost several thousand dollars while knowing that the realistic value of the cow may be only $800. In addition to maintaining the farm and the other animals on the farm, the farmer also must provide for his or her family, and at some point these economic considerations must enter the decision-making process.

The monetary value of horses usually is considerably more than that of production livestock (at least in the mind of the owner). Emotional attachment often plays a role in the owner's decision to finance a horse's treatment. In addition, many horses are accustomed to being handled and transported, and this familiarity makes transportation to a hospital more practical than with other large animals. Therefore, horses are generally more likely than livestock to be evaluated and treated at large animal clinics. However, I have met several livestock producers who feel a strong emotional attachment to their livestock and go above and beyond the economic value of the livestock.

Because of cost and practicality, not all sick large animals have the luxury of going to a hospital or clinic.

Large animals present unique circumstances and challenges for their examination and treatment. The size of these animals and herd management pose some difficulty with their transportation, so large animal work is often performed on the farm. Many large animal clinics and hospitals are available nationwide, but arrangements for transportation in trailers or livestock vans are required to reach these "haul-in" facilities. Transportation of large animals may be problematic. Not all large animal owners have a trailer or livestock van, and transportation must be arranged through a friend or professional livestock transportation company. A significant amount of time may be required to arrange for an animal's transportation, and in some parts of the country the nearest large animal hospital is several hours away. When dealing with an emergency case in which assessment and treatment are urgent, the time delay related to finding transportation, loading, and driving the animal to the hospital can have devastating consequences. Other circumstances may dictate that the animal is unable to be loaded onto a trailer, and the veterinarian must make a farm call to provide treatment.

Ambulatory practice, field service, and *farm calls* are types of large animal practices in which the veterinarian takes the necessary supplies and equipment to the farm and performs the diagnostic and treatment procedures there. Mobile veterinary units may be homemade or purchased from companies that specialize in their design. The unit may range from simple storage bins to large fiberglass units with refrigerators, running hot and cold water, and storage space for supplies and equipment. These units can be adapted to cars, vans, or trucks (Fig. 5-1).

Improvising examinations and treatments on the farm is often required and can present challenging situations, many of which can have completely successful outcomes. Accurate assessment of the facilities, personnel, and costs involved is important when planning to treat sick animals on the farm. These same factors also must be considered in the hospital environment.

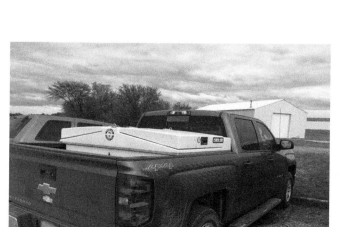

FIGURE 5-1 Typical mobile veterinary unit.

The following principles of facility care and maintenance apply to large animal hospitals and clinics, but with a little imagination and planning, most can be adapted to care for animals at their home farms.

PROPER SHIPMENT OF PARCELS

Many times in large animal practice, you will be shipping packages of samples to diagnostic laboratories for further analysis. Many of the laboratories will have their own packaging instructions. It is important to follow these instructions because improper shipping can result in the loss or damage of samples. Sometimes this damage is extensive enough that a diagnosis is unable to be made.

The goals of packaging are to protect the specimens from temperature extremes (freezing and heating) and to protect persons who may come into contact with the package from exposure to infectious agents. For this reason, it is extremely important to prevent leakage of specimens. Neither commercial carriers nor the U.S. Postal Service will deliver containers that leak.

In general, all sample containers should contain the owner's name and animal identification, written with a waterproof marker. The containers should be leakproof. Whirl-Pak (Nasco, Fort Atkinson, Wisc.) bags are a great option for samples that do not require that fluid be added. Stick-on labels often come off when condensation occurs within the packaging. It is best to send blood tubes in actual shipping boxes because the glass can be broken during shipping. Most samples require an ice pack to keep the shipping container cool. After the sample is secured, the rest of the box should be lined with a plastic bag to prevent leakage and absorbent material to soak up any spills. The exterior container should be sturdy enough to withstand trauma during shipping.

HANDLING OF VACCINES

As a veterinary technician in a large animal practice, at certain times of the year you will handle vaccines on a daily basis. Understanding the basics of vaccine handling is extremely important. You will not only use this knowledge for yourself but also will be responsible for educating producers about proper vaccine handling. Anyone who handles vaccines must fully understand the importance of proper care.

First, vaccines should always be purchased from a reputable dealer who understands the importance of proper vaccine handling. The efficacy of a vaccine is compromised if it has been mishandled even once before reaching the patient.

Vaccines should always be transported in a closed, refrigerated container (Figs. 5-2 and 5-3). Styrofoam containers are a great method of vaccine transport because an ice pack can easily be sent with the product inside the cooler (Fig. 5-4). Do not buy these ice packs. Instead, store them in a freezer after you receive shipments from your dealers. Vaccines should never be exposed to ultraviolet light. Even when processing livestock or horses, the vaccines should be kept cool. The bottles and syringes should be kept in the closed, refrigerated container when they are not being used.

When vaccines require mixing, with most modified live vaccines you should never mix up more than you can use within an hour. The efficacy of the vaccine starts to diminish once mixed, and its limit of effectiveness is 1 hour. Producers who are processing only small numbers of livestock should be sold small bottles of vaccines with fewer doses.

STOCKING AND CLEANLINESS

The mobile unit and veterinary clinic should be stocked and maintained. In a mobile unit, inventory should be taken at least daily and items restocked as necessary. Cleanliness and disinfection of the mobile unit should be routinely performed for sanitation and to maintain an acceptable appearance to clients. Dirty facilities, whether buildings or vehicles, may give the impression that the veterinarian has a disregard for sanitation or is simply too lazy to maintain his or her equipment. Technicians often are responsible for maintaining cleanliness and inventory for the mobile unit or clinic.

SHARPS HANDLING

Sharps handling requires special attention. Everyone at a veterinary practice should be trained on proper sharps handling to avoid injury. All sharps disposal containers should be labeled with a "Sharps Disposal Container" label. The label for livestock medical sharps containers must include a biohazard emblem (Fig. 5-5). Sharps containers should be kept out of reach of children and animals. The containers should be made of rigid, puncture-resistant, and leakproof material. When the container is not in use, a lid should be applied and closed tightly. Everyone should be instructed to wash their hands after handling sharps.

Disposal of sharps can be accomplished in one of two ways. You may add Portland cement or Sharp-seal (Earth-Shield, Bakersfield, Calif) to the container and then send it to an approved landfill, or you can heat the sharps until they are melted and then bury them in an identified location on the premises.

These instructions should be provided to producers so they are aware of the legal options available to them. If veterinary clinics are not using biohazard red sharps containers, the methods described earlier can be used in veterinary clinics.

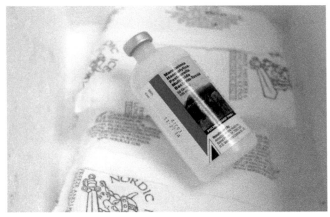

FIGURE 5-2 Vaccine bottles stored on ice for producers.

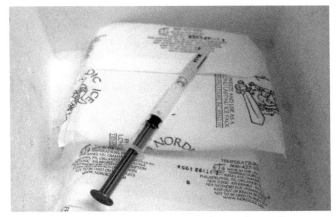

FIGURE 5-3 Vaccine syringes stored on ice for producers.

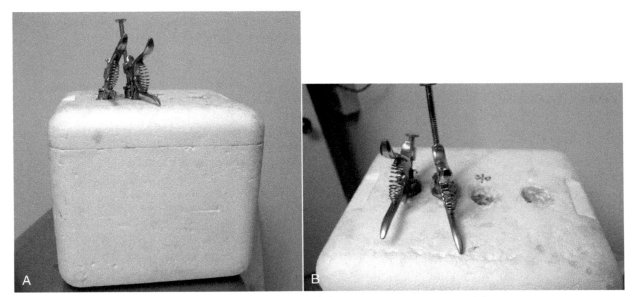

FIGURE 5-4 A and B, A Styrofoam container used for keeping vaccines in syringes cool during processing.

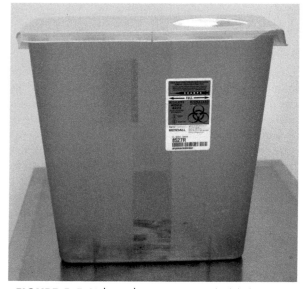

FIGURE 5-5 Biohazard container. Note the label present.

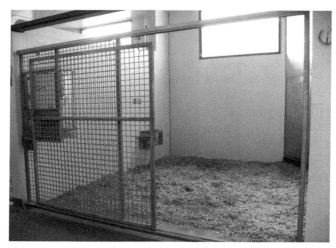

FIGURE 5-6 Typical horse stall in excellent condition and extremely clean, with great example of a cement floor.

SYRINGE CLEANING

When working with ruminants and swine, it is common to use glass barrel or plastic syringes that are reused. Proper syringe cleaning is important to avoid infection, which can lead to injection site lesions. If infections are severe enough, they can become systemic and cause death. Therefore, it is extremely important that syringes be cleaned properly.

First, the external syringe surface should be cleaned with soap, water, and a brush. Next, the inside components of the syringe should be rinsed with distilled water or deionized water that is near boiling point (hotter than 180° F). These components include the tubes and connectors. Rinsing is accomplished by drawing the water into the syringe and squirting it out. Three to five rinses should be adequate. Finally, the excess water should be squirted from the syringe and the syringe set aside to cool before it is used. Heat will kill a modified live vaccine product. Soaps and disinfectants should not be used on the internal components because they will also inactivate and kill modified live vaccines when these cleaning agents are used in these types of syringes. Periodically, at least quarterly, it is recommended to disassemble these syringes completely and clean them as previously described. After syringes have been cleaned, they should be stored in a dust-free, dry (low humidity) environment.

STALL/HOSPITAL MAINTENANCE AND CARE

In a clinical setting, livestock are commonly housed in stalls. Stalls should be cleaned daily to remove manure and wet spots (urine) (Fig. 5-6). The two basic approaches to stall cleaning are to (1) remove only the soiled bedding and try to spare as much bedding as possible *(picking)* or (2) remove all bedding, soiled or not, down to the stall floor *(stripping)*. Whether a stall is picked or stripped depends largely on the nature of the case and the habits of the animal. Some animals are very "neat," defecating and urinating in particular spots; the stalls of these patients can be successfully picked

for perhaps several days. At the other end of the spectrum are the extremely dirty animals of the world—they have no pattern to their defecations and urinations, and they may walk repeatedly through their eliminations and scatter feces and urine all over the stall. Picking for these cases is difficult. Stalls of animals with diarrhea are also difficult to pick.

For cases that lend themselves to picking, the stall should be checked at least twice daily and picked as necessary. Wet urine spots should be removed to the depth to which the urine has soaked. After removing the soiled bedding, replace as much bedding as was removed by picking. Animals that are active in their stalls may push bedding against the walls of the stall; be sure to spread this bedding back toward the center of the stall to create an even surface.

Stripping of bedding should occur at least every few days for any patient and more frequently if warranted by the nature of the case. After stripping the stall, the bedding must be completely replaced. This is obviously more expensive than picking and is more time consuming, so stripping should be done judiciously. Stripping should always be done after a patient is discharged, to allow for thorough stall cleaning and/or disinfection between patients.

When cleaning stalls, do not overlook the walls and ceiling. Cobwebs are common on stall ceilings and walls and should be removed regularly because the presence of cobwebs, dust, and other particulate matter on these surfaces reflects poorly on hospital cleanliness.

Barn aisles should be swept at least once daily. Usually, sweeping two to three times daily is required to maintain cleanliness and a neat appearance of the facility.

Stall Flooring

The two common types of stall floors are cement (concrete) and dirt/packed clay. Some older barns have wood floors, but these are not often seen in a hospital setting. Each type of flooring has advantages and disadvantages.

Cement floors (and walls) are advantageous for hospital use because they can be disinfected and steam cleaned. Portable spray-type steam-cleaning machines can be taken from stall to stall to perform thorough cleansing of stalls between patients. This is especially valuable when the previous patient had a contagious disease. If steam cleaners are not used, disinfectants can be applied directly to the surface, scrubbed, and hosed. Dirt and wooden walls and floors are difficult to disinfect adequately with these procedures. The disadvantages of cement flooring are as follows: its expense to install; decreased patient comfort, especially for animals that lie down to sleep or are recumbent as a result of their disease; and sometimes compromised drainage. Proper contouring of the floor with a central drain is vital for drainage, and patient comfort can be improved with the appropriate amount of deep bedding for the case.

Rubber mats can be placed between the cement floor and the bedding layer. Some mats are solid rubber; others have a porous waffle-type construction that improves drainage. Because liquids cannot penetrate solid mats for drainage, moisture control must be provided by absorption into the bedding material. Absorbent bedding material should be used with solid mats. Rubber mats can greatly increase patient comfort, but they are expensive and difficult to maintain and thoroughly disinfect.

Sand can be placed over the cement; however, the cement stalls cannot have drains. The major disadvantage to this type of flooring is the amount of time it takes to clean, remove, and replace the sand between patients. However, it is extremely useful for lameness cases because of the cushioning effect of sand.

Dirt floors must be constructed properly to provide acceptable drainage. Dirt floors have the obvious disadvantage of poor disinfection properties. If a contagious patient is housed on a dirt floor, the stall may have to be isolated for days or weeks following dismissal of the contagious animal before another patient can be housed safely in the stall.

Stall Bedding

Bedding material is placed on top of the stall floor to improve comfort and absorb urine and fecal liquids. The two most popular types of bedding material are wood shavings and grain straw. Other types of bedding include sawdust, peat moss, and shredded paper. Each type of bedding has pros and cons.

Wood shavings are made from softwoods or hardwoods. Softwood shavings have good absorbency, often comparable to or better than straw. Shavings are generally less dusty than straw and usually are tolerated better by horses with respiratory allergies. Shavings may provide more of a cushion effect, which may benefit patients with sore feet or legs. However, wood shavings are more likely to get under bandages and casts and are more abrasive than straw. Wood bedding products are believed to harbor more gram-negative bacteria than straw, which may be an exposure concern for neonates. Therefore, straw is preferred for pregnant animals and neonates.

Sawdust is another wood product used for bedding. However, it can be unacceptably dusty, and the particles are small enough to be inhaled. Sawdust is poor bedding for pregnant animals, neonates, and any animal with respiratory

problems. Recumbent patients and neonates may be more prone to scratching their corneas on the particles when they are lying on their sides. (Young foals do not sleep standing as many adults do.)

> **TECHNICIAN NOTE**   When sawdust is used for recumbent or young patients, the animals may be more prone to scratching their corneas on the particles when they are lying on their sides.

Wood products, whether shavings or sawdust, must be free of black walnut *(Juglans nigra)* content. Black walnut causes acute laminitis (founder) in horses, although the exact route of toxin entry into the horse is not yet understood. When purchasing wood product bedding, ask the distributor to identify the types of wood in the product. Black walnut produces shavings and sawdust that are dark; however, other safe types of wood can produce similar dark colors. If dark shavings/sawdust particles are visible, avoid using the product unless the contents are known to be free of black walnut. Many distributors are not aware of black walnut's toxicity to horses.

> **TECHNICIAN NOTE**   Do not use black walnut shavings around horses!

Straw is usually oat or wheat. Oat straw is more absorbent than other straw types, although straw in general is not highly absorbent compared with other types of bedding. Straw is naturally dusty, and dustiness increases if the straw blades are chopped short. Straw is generally poor bedding for respiratory cases and gastrointestinal (GI) cases. Some animals eat straw bedding; straw has little nutritional value but may increase the likelihood of digestive problems in the horse if it is eaten in large quantities.

> **TECHNICIAN NOTE**   Straw eaten in large quantities may increase the likelihood of digestive problems in horses.

Peat moss is highly absorbent, and horses will not eat it. Peat moss is unlikely to harbor fungi and is not considered likely to contribute to respiratory conditions. Peat moss is cushiony when applied deeply and, combined with its absorbency, may be excellent bedding for recumbent ("downer") cases. Peat moss should be stored in well-ventilated areas only.

Shredded paper products are highly absorbent bedding materials with little dust. Paper products usually are good for patients with respiratory allergies and other respiratory cases. However, newsprint can leave stains on the patient.

> **TECHNICIAN NOTE**   Newsprint used as bedding can leave stains on the patient.

Stall/Stable Ventilation

Ventilation must be adequate not only in the barn aisles but also in individual stalls. Barn aisles usually are easy to ventilate by opening barn doors. Stalls usually are difficult to ventilate unless they have windows. Poorly ventilated stalls may benefit from stall fans, which may be easily provided by using inexpensive floor fans hung outside the stall and above ground level on ropes or attached with duct tape. Key issues with ventilation are preventing drafts and keeping dust levels to a minimum. In addition, ammonia vapor is generated by urine in the stall. Ammonia is a respiratory irritant and may exacerbate respiratory diseases, especially in foals. Proper ventilation and stall cleaning to remove wet spots minimize ammonia vapor.

DAILY PATIENT CARE

Feeding Patients

Depending on the patient's disease, special feeding may be required. If the animal has difficulty chewing or swallowing, the food may need to be moistened or even made into gruel. The clinician will prescribe any special diet necessary for the patient. Sick horses are seldom fed concentrates because of increased concerns for developing GI problems. Sometimes patients cannot be fed any food, and occasionally even water must be withheld for successful management of a particular disease. This is especially true of GI diseases. If these patients are depressed, they may not have an interest in food or water. Horses that are being withheld food and water sometimes eat or chew anything they can—bedding, wooden doors/walls, buckets, and so forth. Managing these horses may require placing a muzzle on them. Muzzles are not always effective because some horses can find inventive ways to eat around them, and other horses can remove muzzles. If it is vital that the horse take nothing by mouth (nil per os [NPO]), it is better to remove all bedding and use rubber mats or inedible bedding such as peat moss.

> **TECHNICIAN NOTE**   Horses housed in veterinary clinics are rarely fed concentrates.

Although eating from the ground occurs on farms, this procedure should not be allowed in a hospital setting and should be discouraged on the farm. Manure and urine can contaminate the feed. Hay can be suspended in a hay net or placed in a hay rack. Hay nets and slat-type hay racks should be higher than shoulder level to prevent hooves from becoming entangled in them if the animal paws with the front legs.

> **TECHNICIAN NOTE**   Do not feed horses on the ground!

Animals should have access to supplemental salt and/or trace minerals, which can be provided in the form of loose salt or the more traditional block form (salt/mineral brick or "lick"). Giving each patient a full block is unnecessary; the blocks can be divided with a hammer or small saw for short-stay patients. Discard salt licks between patients as part of thorough stall cleaning.

> **TECHNICIAN NOTE**   A hammer can be used to break up salt blocks into smaller pieces for short-stay patients.

Record the types and amount of feed offered to the animal, as well as what the animal actually eats. Some animals may eat their hay but refuse their grain, or vice versa. Some may eat fresh grass if it is available but refuse hay. Some may eat only a portion of what is put in the stall. What the animal eats *and* does not eat can be important information for the clinician.

Watering Patients

Water provision is a vital part of animal care. Fresh water provided daily is an absolute necessity. Water can be provided in the stall by using either manual or automatic methods. Manual watering involves filling a water container, usually a bucket, with a water hose. Automatic waterers are convenient for human caretakers but are not always helpful in a hospital setting. Most animals do not have access to these devices on their home farm and therefore do not know how to use them. The waterers make a noise when they refill that repels many horses. Automatic systems are difficult to disassemble for thorough disinfection. Perhaps the greatest drawback in a hospital setting is the inability to track a patient's water intake accurately. With an automatic system, no convenient way exists to monitor the amount of water entering the bowl under normal circumstances.

> **TECHNICIAN NOTE**   Fresh water provided daily is an absolute necessity. Water may have to be refilled multiple times per day.

Manual watering is preferable in the large animal hospital. Standard water buckets hold 5 gallons, so some animals may require two 5-gallon buckets in their stalls. Water containers should be checked more than once per day and filled as necessary. The amount of water consumed by an animal is important information and should be recorded at each "bucket check." Animals may not drink adequate amounts of water in the hospital setting because of stress, illness, or water that tastes different from what they are accustomed to on their home farm. Water consumption is particularly important to monitor in GI patients.

Because opinions vary on what a "full bucket" means, it is useful to standardize a full bucket by marking the fill level with tape or a nontoxic paint mark. This marking provides consistency by having all caretakers fill the bucket to the same level. When estimating the amount of water consumed by the animal at each bucket check, do not assume that the amount of water missing from the bucket has actually been consumed by the horse. Some animals play with their water buckets (with their mouths or by pawing with the forelimbs) and spill large quantities of water on the floor. Animals may place their noses in their buckets and splash their water without actually drinking. Therefore, you should check the stall floor in the area of the bucket to see whether most of the water has been spilled or whether it has, in fact, been consumed by the horse. Record the approximate amount of water consumed, and refill the bucket to the fill line.

Some animals benefit from electrolyte water solutions. Electrolyte water is generally made by adding a commercially prepared electrolyte powder to a standard volume of water. Potassium chloride can be made with 6 to 10 g of electrolyte salt per liter of water. Many animals drink electrolyte water during hot weather to replace losses through sweat evaporation (horses primarily), and some simply seem to enjoy the alternative to plain water. Horses with diarrhea may selectively drink electrolyte and bicarbonate solutions; bicarbonate water is made by adding 10 g of baking soda per liter of water. Electrolyte water should never be used as the sole water source. Instead, it should be provided as a supplement to plain, fresh water.

Water buckets should generally be placed at or above shoulder level so that the animal's legs will not get caught in them. Rubber buckets are easy to disinfect and last longer than metal buckets, which have a tendency to become crushed and may rust. In cold weather, water sources may freeze, and either the ice must be physically broken and removed or ice formation must be prevented with commercially available electric water warming coils.

> **TECHNICIAN NOTE** Electrolyte water should never be used as the sole water source.

Grooming

The importance of daily grooming in horses should not be overlooked. Grooming not only is essential for patient cleanliness but also provides an opportunity to find developing or previously undetected problems. Swellings, lacerations, discharges, skin infections, and changes in attitude all can be observed during grooming. Livestock should be kept clean (standard condition), but daily grooming is not essential.

Grooming should consist of the standard steps of curry combing, brushing, and hoof cleaning. The curry comb is the first step of grooming (Fig. 5-7). The curry comb is used on the fleshy (muscular) parts of the body only (i.e., not on the face or below the knee and hock). It is used in a circular motion, firmly, to loosen deep-seated dirt and bring it to the surface, where it can be brushed off the horse.

> **TECHNICIAN NOTE** Never use curry combs on a horse's face or below the knee or hock.

Brushes come in many varieties of bristle stiffness and bristle materials (Fig. 5-8). In general, stiff bristles should be used only on the fleshy parts of the body. Soft bristles can be used anywhere on the body, with special care on the face. Brushing should be done with short strokes, by flicking the brush up and away from the coat at the end of the stroke. Flicking the brush kicks dirt particles off the horse, and this is the purpose of brushing. Brushing is always done in the direction of the lay of the hair.

> **TECHNICIAN NOTE** When brushing, always brush with the grain of the hair.

A towel can be used after brushing to remove any leftover surface debris. Moist towels can be used to clean eye and nose discharges and the perineal region. The forelock, mane,

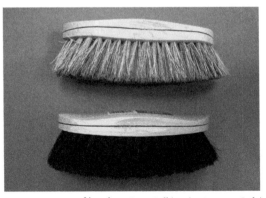

FIGURE 5-8 Types of brushes. **Top,** Stiff bristle. **Bottom,** Soft bristle.

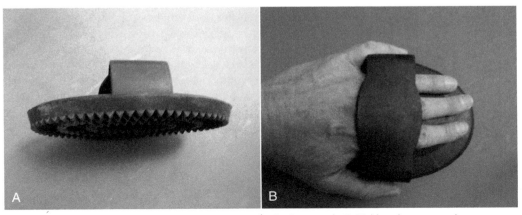

FIGURE 5-7 Grooming using a curry comb. **A,** Curry comb. **B,** Holding the curry comb.

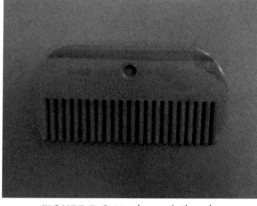

FIGURE 5-9 Metal mane/tail comb.

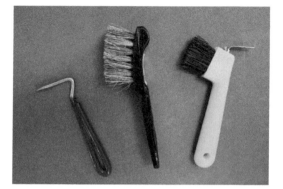

FIGURE 5-10 Plain hoof pick, hoof brush, and combination hoof pick/brush.

and tail hairs are combed with a plastic or metal mane/tail comb (Fig. 5-9). Do not try to pass the comb through large amounts of hair at once; separate the hairs into small sections and comb each section individually.

Hoof cleaning is done with a hoof pick and brush. Several designs of picks and combs are available (Fig. 5-10). The hoof must be elevated to clean the bottom of the hoof, which is a critical surface to clean. The most common deficiency of hoof cleaning is failure to clean the recesses of the bottom of the hoof completely. The *lateral sulci of the frog* and the *central sulcus of the frog* are recesses of the hoof that should be thoroughly picked to help prevent bacterial and fungal infections (Fig. 5-11). Most people do not realize that the horse does not feel routine hoof picking unless trauma or infection has exposed sensitive tissue. Therefore, their tendency is to pick so lightly that the cleaning is not effective. Unless sensitive tissue is exposed, use firm pressure on the hoof pick and brush.

> *TECHNICIAN NOTE* Unless sensitive tissue is exposed on the hoof, firm pressure with the hoof pick and brush is necessary to ensure proper cleaning.

Patient cleanliness may affect the animal's sense of well-being. Many horses are accustomed to grooming and enjoy it. Patient cleanliness also has a tremendous impression on the client. When clients visit their horse and when they pick up

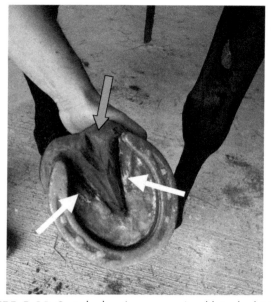

FIGURE 5-11 Central sulcus *(green arrow)* and lateral sulci *(white arrows)* of the frog.

their horse at the end of hospitalization, the patient should be "spotless." The reputations of the veterinarians and of the hospital rely on keeping patients and their surroundings clean.

> *TECHNICIAN NOTE* When clients visit or when the patients are discharged, clients expect their animals to be clean. Doing so gives the hospital a good reputation.

SPECIAL CASES

Two types of cases require special considerations: contagious cases and recumbent ("downer") patients.

Isolation of Contagious Cases

Respiratory diseases usually are spread by direct contact with respiratory secretions. The secretions may be spread directly by coughing, sneezing, or nose-to-nose contact or indirectly by carrying secretions from infected animals to uninfected animals on clothing, equipment, hands, and so on. The animals themselves can rapidly spread infection throughout a barn. It has been estimated that a coughing horse can propel respiratory droplets as far as 30 yards.

Infectious GI diseases typically cause diarrhea. Animals with diarrhea can produce gallons of fecal water in a 24-hour period, and the excrement commonly contains an astounding number of infectious organisms. Like the infectious agents of respiratory diseases, GI infectious organisms may spread by direct or indirect contact. In most equine hospitals, diarrhea is so potentially contagious that any horse with loose or diarrheic stool is treated as contagious until proven otherwise.

> *TECHNICIAN NOTE* It is common practice to consider horses with diarrhea as contagious until proven differently.

Adding to the dilemma of contagious disease is that horses may begin to shed the infectious organisms before they become overtly ill, and sometimes shedding occurs in the complete absence of clinical signs ("carrier" animals). This is especially true of GI infections with *Salmonella* species.

The ramifications of an infectious disease outbreak in a hospital setting cannot be overemphasized. When otherwise healthy animals that are hospitalized for routine procedures become sick with a contagious disease while under the care of the hospital (or shortly after their discharge from the hospital), the result can be a public relations disaster. *Salmonella* in particular is associated with a negative connotation among equine owners. *Salmonella* infection is difficult to eliminate from a barn, the bacterium has many strains that are highly resistant to current antibiotic therapy, and it has a well-known carrier state in horses. Owners are aware of these facts, and word will spread throughout a horse community if a hospital fails to contain a case of *Salmonella* infection successfully. Therefore, it is best to overreact to a potentially contagious disease rather than underestimate the potential for spread of the disease to other horses in the hospital. Confirmed and potentially *contagious cases* should be isolated from the general hospital population.

> **TECHNICIAN NOTE**   Confirmed and potentially contagious cases should be isolated from the general hospital population.

Many hospitals have stalls that are reserved for use only by patients with contagious cases. Larger facilities may even have barns dedicated to this purpose. In facilities with no dedicated isolation area, isolation can be accomplished with a little improvisation. If no separate building is available for isolation, the animal ideally should be placed in an area of the barn with minimal "traffic flow." This area usually is a stall in an outer corner of the facility, as opposed to a centrally located stall. Isolation stalls should have flooring and walls that can be reliably disinfected; dirt floors and wooden walls are not the best choices for isolation areas.

Once a stall is identified as housing an isolation case, it should be clearly marked "Isolation," and an isolation protocol should be instituted. When setting aside a stall for isolation, it is advisable not to post specific disease diagnostics where they can be viewed by the public. The patient's diagnosis or suspected diagnosis is privileged, private information and is potentially damaging to the hospital and to the sick animal's owner and home farm if the information is made public.

> **TECHNICIAN NOTE**   Isolation stalls should be clearly marked with "Isolation" signs.

The ideal isolation stall has an entrance that is open to the outside perimeter of the barn rather than the main barn aisle. With this setup, the animal can enter and exit the stall without

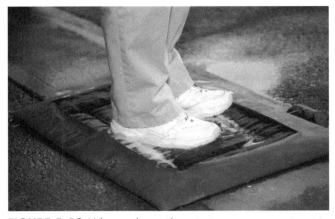

FIGURE 5-12 When working with contagious cases, separate equipment, including brushes, lead ropes, towels, and plastic booties, is used for each patient, to prevent cross-contamination to other horses. (From Sellon DC, Long MT: *Equine infectious disease*, St. Louis, 2007, Saunders.)

walking down the main aisle; it also allows the staff to clean the stall without carrying bedding and excrement through the main areas of the barn, where contamination could occur. Ideally, an isolation stall also has a clearly defined *"hot zone"*. around it. The hot zone is an area that no one should enter without permission or without proper personal protective gear. The hot zone can be defined with tape or paint on the barn floor or even hay bales stacked to restrict traffic around the stall. The stall can be further isolated by hanging sheets or blankets on all stall walls if the walls are not solid.

> **TECHNICIAN NOTE**   Hot zones are areas that no one should enter without permission or without proper personal protective gear.

An isolation protocol should be established in every hospital. This protocol should clearly identify all aspects of handling a contagious or potentially contagious case. The protocol should identify criteria for what constitutes an isolation case, how the case will be isolated, and how the case will be handled after it is isolated. The isolation protocol should be specific and strictly enforced.

Because many diseases can be transferred indirectly on fomites, the stall cleaning implements and grooming tools used for a patient in isolation should be dedicated solely to that patient (Fig. 5-12). These items should be kept in the hot zone and should not travel to any area of the hospital where uninfected animals are housed or walked. In addition, examination tools such as stethoscopes, thermometers, syringes, adhesive tape, and other equipment should be either dedicated to the isolation case or disinfected before they are used on another patient. The cardinal rule is that *anything that enters the isolation hot zone does not leave the hot zone until it is disinfected.*

> **TECHNICIAN NOTE**   Anything that enters the isolation hot zone does not leave the hot zone until it is disinfected.

Many facilities find it helpful to put a treatment cart or shelving in the hot zone that contains the commonly used items for the case. Items may include grooming tools, syringes and needles, rectal sleeves, medications, thermometer, stethoscope, latex gloves, alcohol, povidone-iodine (Betadine) solutions, halters, and lead ropes. These items are disinfected or discarded after conclusion of the isolation case.

In addition to dedicated supplies for the patient, an established protocol for personal protective apparel must be in place for any staff handling the case. Some cases may be so potentially contagious that only certain staff members will be designated each day to work with the case. For example, staff members who work with foals or immunocompromised patients would be prevented from entering any isolation hot zones because the threat of transmitting microbes to neonates or immunocompromised patients is an unnecessary risk. Another consideration is that some infectious diseases are zoonotic, placing staff at risk for contracting the disease. Personal protection cannot be overemphasized.

Contagious microbes are present on the stall floor. Therefore, special attention should be paid to footwear and preventing the spread of microbes through the hospital on shoes or boots. Several approaches may be taken to footwear protection in the hot zone. Anyone entering the hot zone may remove his or her shoes and wear rubber boots (or slip them on over the shoes) on entering the hot zone and then step in a disinfecting solution designed for dipping or scrubbing the boots upon entering *and* exiting the area *(foot bath)*. Another approach is to provide disposable foot covers to pull over the shoes or boots. Disposable foot covers are made of plastic or surgical drape-type material and are readily available through medical supply companies.

Employees' hands should be protected with disposable examination gloves or rectal sleeves. If clothing needs to be protected, disposable or reusable surgical gowns can be placed in the hot zone for staff use. Some diseases may warrant donning protective caps and surgical masks. The isolation protocol should specifically identify the personal protective measures to be taken. Regardless of the protective clothing worn, hands should always be washed immediately after any contact with isolation equipment or patients; this is for protection of other patients *and* the technician. Handwashing between patients is good practice even when working with noncontagious animals in any hospital or clinic setting.

> **TECHNICIAN NOTE** Wash your hands after handling any patient, and wash your hands between patients.

Patients should not leave the isolation area until they are discharged to go home or until the conditions that required isolation are resolved. Occasionally, the patient's disease requires surgical treatment or radiology or other diagnostics that can be provided only in certain areas of the hospital. If the patient must be taken to these areas, walking the animal through main barn aisles should be avoided. The patient should be brushed thoroughly to remove loose debris, and the

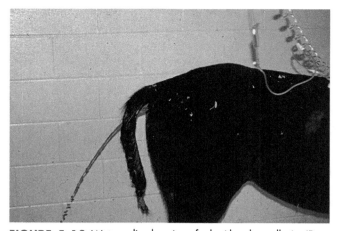

FIGURE 5-13 Watery diarrhea in a foal with salmonellosis. (From McAuliffe SB, Slovis NM: *The color atlas of diseases and disorders of the foal,* St. Louis, 2009, Saunders.)

feet should be picked out. Just outside the stall, the animal's hooves should be scrubbed thoroughly with a dilute bleach solution (1:64; 2 oz of bleach per 1 gallon of water). After the diagnostic or surgical procedure is completed, disinfect all equipment and floors contacted by the isolated animal.

> **TECHNICIAN NOTE** Before taking a contagious animal beyond its hot zone, its hooves should be scrubbed thoroughly with dilute bleach solution.

Often overlooked when planning for an isolation case is trash disposal. Large garbage bags should be available in the hot zone, and a protocol should be established for disposal of the bag once it is full. Bags should be tied shut before they are transported out of the isolation area. The trash should always be treated as potentially contagious material.

Traffic in and out of hot zones should be limited. These areas should be entered only when necessary. The patient's medical treatments should be combined as best as possible with feeding, watering, and stall cleaning schedules. Limit not only the number of people handling the case but also the number of times they handle the case. Similarly, the patient should be restricted from entering areas where healthy patients are kept. If the horse will be hand walked for exercise, use the back stall door or put the horse in a corner stall where it does not have to travel down barn aisles.

An animal with diarrhea should not be fed off the ground because it risks continual reinfection of the patient (most diarrheal diseases are transmitted by the fecal-oral route) (Fig. 5-13). Hay nets, hay racks, and feed buckets suspended above ground level are alternatives. Attention should be paid to limiting contamination of the patient and the stall. This requires frequent cleaning, which usually is necessary more than once per day. The patient's hindquarters should be kept clean to minimize contamination and prevent scalding of the perineal area from diarrhea. Thorough cleansing of soiled tails is important. However, tail bathing is time consuming and places staff at risk for personal contamination. A better approach is to prevent tail soiling by placing a tail bag on the patient. As soon as diarrhea is observed, wash the tail with warm water and mild detergent. A tail bag is easily constructed from a rectal sleeve to keep the tail free of diarrheic stool, and this bag should be changed every 24 to 48 hours.

> **TECHNICIAN NOTE**   In horses with diarrhea, a tail bag should be placed to reduce the amount of time a technician has to spend cleaning the tail.

Diarrhea scalds the skin of the perineum and hindlimbs. These areas should be cleansed as necessary with warm water and mild soap. Vigorous scrubbing should be avoided. Desitin (vitamin-enriched petrolatum) ointment is helpful in preventing and treating *skin scald* in these areas.

After conclusion of a contagious case (dismissal or euthanasia), all equipment, the stall, and the hot zone must be disinfected. Laundry (e.g., towels, blankets, gowns) should be shaken free of bedding while still in the stall and placed in a plastic bag that is tied or taped shut before it is taken to the laundry room. Hot zone laundry should be washed separately using detergent and 1 cup of bleach. All other porous materials, such as tape rolls, unopened syringes, needles, examination gloves, cotton swabs, and gauze, should be discarded because no effective way exists to clean and disinfect these items. Thermometers should be stripped of any string or tape and wiped down with dilute bleach mixture (1 cup of bleach per 5 gallons of water). Items that will be reused, such as stomach tubes or pumps and stethoscopes, should be cleaned initially inside the hot zone, a dilute bleach mixture applied, and then sealed in plastic bags for transport to other areas of the hospital, where these items can be further disinfected or sterilized in gas or steam autoclaves.

Ideally, the stall should be steam cleaned if the equipment is available. Otherwise, the stall can be scrubbed with an appropriate disinfectant; dilute household bleach is suitable for most contagious cases (2½ cups of bleach per 5 gallons of water). Apply the dilute bleach and allow it to air dry; do not rinse it. The stall ceiling, walls, doors, and floor should be cleaned; do not forget the outside surfaces of the stall walls and doors. Stall-cleaning implements, grooming tools, buckets, treatment cart, and other similar material should be soaked in the bleach mixture for at least 10 minutes and allowed to air dry; these items do not leave the hot zone until disinfection procedures are completed. Some facilities go through the entire disinfection procedure twice and may even culture the stall and implements before removing their hot zone status. Dilute bleach may not be appropriate for use after certain diseases; appropriate disinfectants for specific diseases usually can be identified by consulting reference texts or appropriate disease experts (Fig. 5-14).

Recumbent Cases

Recumbent cases or *nonambulatory* animals refer to animals that preferentially spend most of their time lying on the ground or are physically unable to stand because of their disease.

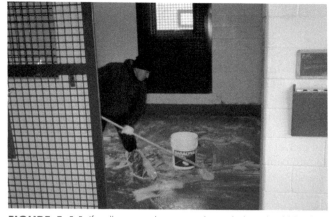

FIGURE 5-14 If stalls cannot be steam cleaned, they should be thoroughly scrubbed with the appropriate disinfectant. (From Sellon DC, Long MT: *Equine infectious diseases*, St. Louis, 2007, Saunders.)

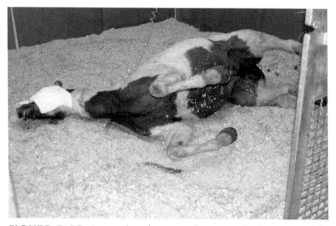

FIGURE 5-15 A recumbent horse can be extremely dangerous while it is having spasms or is attempting to stand. (From Sellon DC, Long MT: *Equine infectious diseases*, St. Louis, 2007, Saunders.)

The typical diseases responsible for recumbency usually produce severe musculoskeletal pain, profound weakness, or neurologic dysfunction. Recumbent large animals present significant and sometimes unique problems. Many of the same problems are seen in recumbent small animals, but the size of large animals increases both the risk of problems and the difficulty in preventing and treating complications when they occur.

Another factor to keep in mind when working with recumbent large animals is the animal's nature to stand. Domestic large animals are species of prey, and survival instinct drives them to try to stand on their own legs. This instinct may lead to violent and persistent attempts to stand, although they may not succeed. These animals may do great damage to themselves and their surroundings during their struggle to stand, and personnel working with such patients must be alert and cautious when working around them (Fig. 5-15).

> **TECHNICIAN NOTE**   Recumbent large animals often attempt to stand. It is important to be aware of your surroundings and protect yourself and the animal from danger.

Recumbent cases require intensive care, typically around-the-clock devotion to the patient. When deciding whether to pursue care for the recumbent case, the facilities and staff available must be considered and realistically evaluated. The owner must be informed about the time requirements, labor requirements, and costs related to providing around-the-clock care.

When managing a recumbent animal, the complications described in the following paragraphs must be anticipated and measures instituted in an attempt to prevent them. Realize that complications still may occur even in well-managed cases despite every attempt made to prevent complications. Simply too many variables are involved for any preventive measure to be 100% effective.

Problems associated with recumbency include *decubital ulcers, compartment syndrome,* eye trauma, limb trauma, respiratory disease, bladder dysfunction, and GI dysfunction.

Decubital ulcers are commonly known as pressure sores. When animals lie in one position for extended periods of time, circulation is compromised. Compromise to both arterial and venous blood supply may occur if the body weight of the animal exceeds the pressure inside these vessels. If the pressure outside the vessel (body weight) exceeds the pressure inside these vessels (blood pressure), the vessel will collapse. Areas particularly prone to developing decubital ulcers are those with bony prominences; these areas lack fleshy muscle and skin, which cushion other areas and help prevent this complication. The areas most prone to developing decubital ulcers are the *tuber coxae* (point of the hip), lateral prominences of the shoulder and hock, and orbital/zygomatic arch area of the head.

> **TECHNICIAN NOTE**   The most common locations for decubital ulcers are the tuber coxae, lateral prominences of the shoulder and hock, and orbital/zygomatic arch area of the head.

Prevention of decubital ulcers is attempted through proper bedding and patient repositioning. Bedding for recumbent cases should be deep but not rigid enough to compromise the blood circulation. Deep layers of straw or shavings, thick foam pads, waterbed mattresses, and peat moss all can provide resilient bedding that applies fairly even pressure against the patient's body.

Repositioning typically means rolling the patient from one lateral recumbent position to the opposite recumbency (i.e., left lateral to right lateral recumbency, and vice versa). Rolling ideally is performed every 2 hours. Rolling large animals usually requires two to three people and may be dangerous unless the patient is completely paralyzed or unconscious. Patients with some ability to move their limbs may resist rolling by violent limb movements; personnel must use extreme care during the rolling procedure to prevent injury to themselves and the patient. Occasionally, to make the procedure safe for staff and patient, heavy sedation or anesthesia is necessary in these patients.

> **TECHNICIAN NOTE**   Repositioning a recumbent patient is ideally done every 2 hours.

Repositioning is best accomplished using a three-point system. Ropes are placed around the forelimb pasterns, the hindlimb pasterns, and the head/halter or neck. The ropes should be placed carefully, especially around the pasterns. A slip knot can be placed in the rope, which can be swung over the hoof and pastern from a safe distance. The person placing the rope should stand out of reach of the leg's range of motion to avoid being struck by the leg or hoof if the animal struggles. Once the rope is in place, a staff member should walk the rope around the animal's body and assume a position on the dorsal side of the patient. When the limb ropes have been secured, the head/neck rope can be secured. The head/neck rope should be long enough so that the staff member is not within striking distance of the front hooves; grasping the halter with the hands is not advisable as a substitute for a head rope unless the animal is completely immobile. All personnel should be out of striking range of the legs (unless the animal is completely immobile) before the actual rolling procedure begins. All the ropes are drawn taut, and, on verbal cue, the animal is rolled over into the opposite recumbency. Bedding and padding should be rearranged as necessary to cushion the animal in its new position.

Compartment syndrome is not uncommon in recumbent large animals, regardless of the cause of recumbency. Recumbent animals of all species are susceptible to compartment syndrome, but the heavy body weight of large animals exacerbates the problem. Muscle compartments are areas where some muscles in the body are encased in dense connective tissue called fascia, which has little elasticity. Compartment syndrome is caused by the collapse of vessels inside a muscle compartment when the heavy body weight of the animal presses down on the compartment's blood and lymphatic vessels. Collapse of vessels eventually compromises nutrition and waste elimination for the muscle and nerve cells inside the compartment and results in various degrees of muscle and nerve dysfunction. In recumbent animals, rolling and proper bedding are the primary methods of attempted prevention. Compartment syndrome is a significant problem in anesthetized animals.

> **TECHNICIAN NOTE**   Rolling and proper bedding are the primary methods of preventing compartment syndrome.

Eye trauma is a consideration in recumbent large animals because of the position of their eyes. The eyes are wide set in large animals, an anatomic feature typical in animals of prey. Wide-set eyes allow a larger, wider field of vision that may let the animal see predators more readily. However, when the eyes are located laterally on the head, they are exposed to trauma more than eyes placed in a more median position. When large animals lie in lateral recumbency, the head basically rests on the orbit and eye. Therefore, the eye rests on

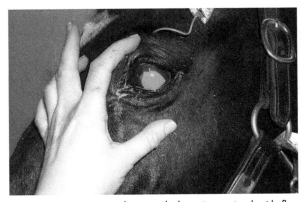

FIGURE 5-16 Patient with corneal ulceration stained with fluorescein. (From Bassert JM, Thomas J: *McCurnin's clinical textbook for veterinary technicians*, ed 8, St. Louis, 2014, Saunders.)

the bedding material and is susceptible to trauma unless protective measures are applied. The most common eye trauma is corneal ulceration caused by abrasions from the bedding. Corneal ulcers are recognized by the classic signs of tearing and *blepharospasm* (squinting), and they are confirmed by fluorescein staining of the cornea (Fig. 5-16). Prevention is attempted through the use of nonabrasive materials in the head area, such as smooth pads or a cloth to cover abrasive surfaces and possibly protective headgear such as eye cups or helmets. A small inflated 12-inch tire inner tube can be placed underneath the eye area to lift it off the ground surface.

> **TECHNICIAN NOTE** Corneal ulceration resulting from abrasions from bedding material can occur in recumbent patients.

Leg trauma may occur if the recumbent animal is not completely paralyzed and is capable of leg motion. These animals may try repeatedly and unsuccessfully to rise because their natural instinct is to try to stand. These unsuccessful attempts can lead to significant musculoskeletal trauma, especially from thrashing of the legs. Recumbent animals should have leg protection provided by leg bandages, which generally should be applied to all four limbs. In a recumbent horse, horseshoes should be removed to minimize trauma if the horse strikes itself (or personnel) with its hooves.

> **TECHNICIAN NOTE** Horseshoes should be removed in recumbent patients, and all four legs should be bandaged.

Recumbent patients are at increased risk for developing respiratory problems. The risk often relates to the patient's primary disease and probably is increased by gravity-induced congestion of the "down" (lower) lung. Regular rolling of the patient is helpful in reducing the risk of pleuritis and pneumonia associated with recumbency.

Bladder and rectum evacuation may be issues in recumbent patients, especially in neurologic cases in which the bladder and rectum may not be capable of normal emptying. Abnormal emptying usually relates to the muscular sphincters that control emptying of the bladder and/or rectum and falls into one of two categories: (1) sphincters that are too tight and therefore prevent normal emptying and (2) sphincters that are too relaxed and cannot retain the contents of the storage organs. Some animals will not void while lying down even if neurologic and sphincter functions are normal. These animals may void only if they are assisted to stand or are elevated in a body sling to a standing position.

To aid fecal voiding, the diet (if the patient can eat) should be highly digestible and as moist as possible. Warm mashes and fresh grass are good choices for most patients. Fecal output should be monitored. If output is insufficient, regular rectal evacuation (at least twice daily) will be required using a gloved hand and liberal lubrication. If the anal sphincter is lax or the patient has diarrhea, fecal material will flow freely from the anus. Fecal water and urine can cause skin scald, which is a condition characterized by irritation and inflammation of the skin. The perineal area of recumbent patients should be cleansed often, and the perineum and inner thigh regions may benefit from application of ointments such as Desitin. Bedding in the hindquarter area should be checked often and changed as necessary.

Bladder management of recumbent patients is critical to prevent pressure damage to the urinary tract and urinary tract infections. Unlike in small animals, in large animals manual expression of the bladder is not possible externally and may be accomplished only occasionally internally through rectal palpation. However, bladder expression through the rectum risks perforating the rectal wall; generally avoid it except in select cases.

When the bladder sphincter cannot contract fully, urine may dribble out of the bladder, sometimes almost continuously. Although the obvious external problems in this situation are *urine scald* and wet bedding, remember that internally the bladder is distended with stagnant urine and is susceptible to infection (bacterial cystitis). When the bladder sphincter cannot relax, urine accumulates and distends the bladder, thus leading to multiple problems including rupture of the bladder or ureters from the high internal pressures. In these cases, the clinician must provide an exit for the urine, and in large animals this means bladder catheterization. Catheters may be either indwelling (Foley) or intermittently inserted (mare or stallion urinary catheter) several times per day. Catheterization of any type greatly increases the risk of bladder infection, and catheterized animals often receive prophylactic antibiotics while they are being treated. Great attention to sterile technique should be followed during bladder catheterization.

Some patients may be capable of standing with the assistance of ropes or slings (Fig. 5-17). Slings are useful only for patients who have some limb control; they are intended to assist, not substitute for, the ability to stand. When completely immobile patients are placed in a sling, they simply

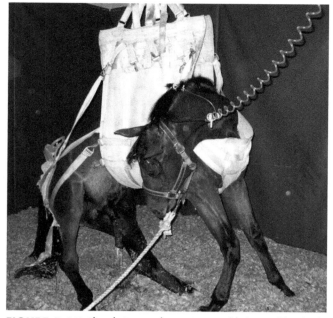

FIGURE 5-17 Sling being used on a 2-year-old Thoroughbred colt. (From Sellon DC, Long MT: *Equine infectious diseases*, St. Louis, 2007, Saunders.)

slump and have difficulty breathing; they even may slide out of some slings. Assisted standing should be performed as often as is reasonable given the patient's disease and staff or equipment available. Many patients will eat, defecate, and urinate only when standing. Cleaning and grooming, physical examination, and some treatments are easier to perform when the patient is standing.

> **TECHNICIAN NOTE** Slings are useful only for patients who have some limb control.

Food or fresh water, or both, can be offered to a patient that is capable of oral intake. The patient's disease dictates whether this is possible or even advisable. When oral intake is offered, the patient should be in sternal recumbency to minimize the risk of aspiration of material into the lungs. Hay bales or supporting pads can be used to hold the patient in sternal recumbency because many recumbent animals cannot hold themselves in this position. If food or water will be given through a nasogastric tube, the animal should be kept in sternal recumbency, if possible, for the intubation procedure.

DISINFECTION AFTER PATIENT DISMISSAL

Following a patient's release, either after successful treatment or because of loss of the patient through death, the patient's stall, grooming tools, and medical equipment and supplies should be cleaned and disinfected before they are used on another patient. The stall should be stripped of food and bedding, and the stall walls, ceiling, and floor should be cleaned thoroughly. The level of disinfection depends on whether the case had a

contagious disease and the nature of the contagious disease, if present. In most cases, dilute bleach (1 cup of household bleach per 5 gallons of water) is an economical and effective disinfectant. Some disease organisms may require stronger bleach solutions (1 part bleach to 10 parts water) or special commercially prepared disinfectants, such as quaternary ammonium compounds, phenolic compounds, or iodophors.

Isopropyl alcohol may be adequate for some pieces of medical equipment, such as stethoscopes, when the patient had no known contagious condition.

Before any disinfectant is applied, all organic matter (e.g., blood, discharges, excrement, bedding) should be removed. Quaternary ammoniums and bleach are ineffective in the presence of organic matter. Phenols and iodophors are considered to have some activity in the presence of organic matter, but activity becomes less reliable with increasing amounts of debris. Organic matter can be removed by scrubbing with brushes and brooms or by using a portable steam cleaner if available. Brushes, mops, and brooms can be used to apply the disinfectant solution to the stall surfaces. Dilute bleach can be allowed to air dry on the treated surfaces.

Stall-cleaning tools and grooming tools ideally should be disinfected after use on any patient. Avoid transporting these items through uncontaminated areas of the hospital until the items have been disinfected.

Water and feed buckets and pans should always be cleaned and disinfected between patients, regardless of case history. Buckets and pans should be scrubbed with brushes and soaked for at least 10 minutes in diluted bleach. Buckets should be rinsed thoroughly with water before they are used for the next patient. Hay nets can be disinfected by soaking them in dilute bleach.

Well-managed hospitals have an established protocol for disinfection that covers both noninfectious and infectious case situations. When in doubt about the diagnosis, it is best to assume that the case is contagious and disinfect accordingly. Some facilities perform microbial cultures on the stall after disinfection procedures and do not let another animal into the stall until culture results are negative for infectious organisms.

> **TECHNICIAN NOTE** Proper disinfection for contagious and noncontagious cases is essential for quality veterinary care.

CASE STUDY

A case of *Streptococcus equi* "strangles" has just been confirmed in one Dr. Jones' patients. The horse is going to be staying in clinic with you. Your practice is new and does not have a current contagious case protocol. You have been assigned the task of writing the new protocol. You have several veterinary assistants and doctors who will be using the protocol. Write a contagious case protocol for this busy practice.

CASE STUDY

Mr. Cook has a 1200-pound stud has just been diagnosed with West Nile virus. The stud is extremely valuable, and the owner is willing to pay for its treatment. The stud is recumbent and will need around-the-clock care. You have been assigned the task of creating the animal's care schedule. What considerations will you make? Write a care plan specific to this case. Consider all aspects of a contagious case.

SUGGESTED READING

Bassert JM, McCurnin DM, editors: *Clinical textbook for veterinary technicians*, ed 7, St. Louis, 2010, Saunders.

Sirois M: *Principles and practice of veterinary technology*, ed 3, St. Louis, 2011, Mosby.

Speirs VC: *Clinical examination of horses*, St. Louis, 1997, Saunders.

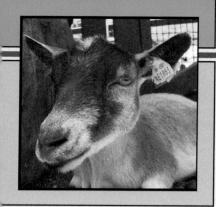

Admissions, Medical Records, and Physical Examinations

OUTLINE

LEARNING OBJECTIVES

When you have completed this chapter, you will be able to

- Explain the importance of identification in a veterinary practice
- Effectively document identification for each species
- Explain the importance of identifying the caretaker of the animal responsible for decisions
- Explain the procedure for loading and unloading livestock and horses from trailers
- Identify common medical records
- Explain the importance of medical records
- Perform a *physical examination* on any large animal species
- Assist in a *neurologic examination*
- Prepare and assist for a colic examination

KEY TERMS

Ankle band
Auscultation
Ballottement
Bishoping
Borborygmi
Capillary refill time
Chestnut
Cyanosis
Ear notching
Ecchymotic hemorrhage
Electronic identification tag
Eructation
Extralabel drug use
Flank
Food Animal Residue Avoidance and Depletion Program
Freeze branding

Hot branding
Ileus
Insurance examination
Lameness
Loss of use insurance
Marking
Mortality insurance
National Animal Identification System
National Farm Identification and Records System
Neurologic examination
Panel tag
Petechial hemorrhage
Physical examination
Points
Poll

Premises registration
Prepurchase examination
Pulse deficit
Purpuric hemorrhage
Ramp trailer
Skin pinch test
Skin turgor
Slant-load trailer
Step-up trailer
Stock Trailer
Surgical insurance
Temporary marking paint
Toxic line
Two-horse trailer
Withdrawal times

KEY ABBREVIATIONS

A-V: Atrioventricular
CN: Cranial nerve
CRT: Capillary refill time

EID: Electronic identification
FARAD: Food Animal Residue Avoidance and Depletion Program

ID: Identification
NGT: Nasogastric tube

ADMISSIONS

Although all large animals have the potential to be kept at a veterinary clinic for treatment, horses and young animals are kept most often. The following admissions and medical records can be used in any location, and blanks can be provided to producers, thus allowing them to maintain a thorough record of the animal's treatments and health on the farm.

Animals usually arrive at the clinic accompanied by their owners, although sometimes employees or family members of the owner, horse trainers, or agents arrive with the animal. In the case of professional transportation companies—used primarily with horses—the owner/agent rarely travels with the horse, and the van driver may be the only person arriving with the animal. Therefore, determining who is in charge of the decision-making processes for the animal is important. Depending on the circumstance, the owner, trainer, employee, family member, or agent of the animal may be responsible for the decisions. Determine who this person is and obtain his or her contact information (e.g., telephone numbers). Treatment is often delayed until permission can be obtained from the owner or agent, so accurate information is essential, especially for emergency cases.

Horses are often transported with protective gear such as leg wraps, head bumpers, or blankets. Much of this gear is not necessary during the hospital stay and should be sent home with the owner/transporter. If this is not possible, place these items in a plastic bag or storage bin and mark it clearly with the horse's name so that the items can be returned when the horse is discharged. Although these items usually are not expensive, their loss could make the hospital seem disorganized and result in poor client public relations.

> **TECHNICIAN NOTE**   Quality public relations should be practiced at all times, on the phone, in person, and by your actions. Professionalism, Professionalism, Professionalism!

LOADING AND UNLOADING LIVESTOCK AND HORSES

One of the potentially most dangerous situations for a technician is loading or unloading livestock or horses from trailers. Working as a veterinary technician, at some point in your career you will be loading and unloading livestock or horses.

Most horses are trained to load and unload from trailers. Most likely, you will not be involved in the loading or unloading of these animals because the owners will be present and take on the responsibility themselves. However, in some cases the person dropping off the animals does not have much experience with horses, and you may be enlisted to help in the loading or unloading process. In addition, the veterinary professional may be asked to assist with the loading or unloading of animals that are not trained to load or unload. The most important factor when loading or unloading horses is patience.

In the ideal situation, the horse loads or unloads uneventfully and calmly. Some horses jump into or out of trailers and may possibly land on the handler. This is a dangerous situation, and technicians should be aware of this possible behavior whenever handling horses around trailers.

The two most common trailer designs into which horses are loaded are ramp trailers and step-up trailers (Fig. 6-1). *Ramp trailers* often have back doors that lower to the ground and double as a ramp. The horse is walked up the ramp into the trailer. *Step-up trailers* require the animal to step up into the trailer to load. With these types of trailers, horses are more likely to jump in or out of the trailer when loading or unloading.

When loading a horse onto a trailer, you should remain calm (horses often sense fear in their handlers, and this is most likely to cause a more dangerous situation) and walk at the level of the *poll* (Fig. 6-2). Do not pause or hesitate when you reach the point at which the horse will have to step up or onto the ramp. Pausing or hesitating gives the horse a split

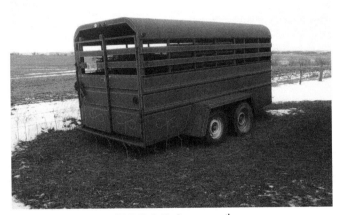

FIGURE 6-1 Step-up trailer.

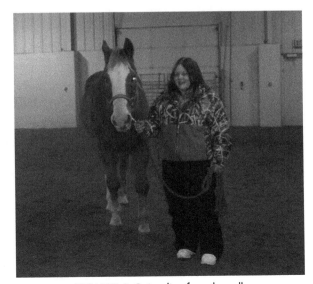

FIGURE 6-2 Leading from the poll.

second to think about what it is being asked to do. If you hesitate, continued attempts may be much more difficult. If the situation calls for redirection, never stop moving; keep forward movement and circle the horse back around to try again. If the horse is not going to load smoothly, the horse most likely will pull back on the lead rope once it is asked to step onto the ramp or into the trailer. Young horses or horses with a lack of training may pull back when they approach the trailer or even when they are inside the trailer. A horse that pulls back inside the trailer can cause a very dangerous situation because it may rear or lunge forward on top of the handler. To avoid this situation, never place yourself in front of the horse. You should always lead from the poll.

> **TECHNICIAN NOTE**   Never pause or hesitate when you reach the point at which the horse will have to step up or onto the ramp. If you have to redirect the horse, always keep forward motion and circle away from the trailer.

Trailer layouts include *two-horse trailers* (Fig. 6-3), *stock trailers,* and *slant-load trailers.* A two-horse trailer does not allow you to enter the trailer with the horse. In this type of trailer, the animals have to enter themselves. You will need to lead the horse to the trailer with forward motion and then give slack in the lead rope to allow for entrance. Some horses are used to having the lead rope draped over the neck as they load onto the trailer. Once the animal is loaded, the gate on the back of the trailer should be calmly but quickly closed to prevent the horse from backing off the trailer.

In a stock trailer, the horse will have a lot of room to move laterally inside the trailer. The horse is secured to a side wall once it is inside. In this type of trailer, the technician steps inside the trailer with the horse while loading and confidently

leads it to the location where it will be tied and secured with trailer straps. Lead ropes are often used to secure horses inside trailers, although cross ties are the safest method for doing so. If a lead rope is used to secure the horse inside a trailer, it is important to tie it with a quick-release knot. When you are securing the horse inside a trailer, remember to leave no more than a foot and a half of slack in the rope. If the horse were to pull back after the rope is secured, the rope could trap the handler inside the trailer between the wall of the trailer and the rope, thereby causing a dangerous situation. Horses should always be secured in a trailer with trailer ties or lead ropes if possible. The safety of the technician, owner, and veterinarian is the most important aspect of loading, and safety should always be considered first. If tying a horse in the trailer is determined to be too dangerous, you may have to leave the horse untied and free to move around throughout part of the trailer. Most of these types of trailers have partitions that separate the trailer into halves or thirds (Fig. 6-4); if used, the partition should be calmly but quickly closed to prevent escape of the horse.

> **TECHNICIAN NOTE**   If using a lead rope to secure a horse inside a trailer, always use a quick-release knot.

In a slant-load trailer (Fig. 6-5), the horse may be asked to load through a narrow area at the back of the trailer and then stand at an angle within the trailer. Once the horse is in the proper position, a partition is closed to allow another horse to be loaded beside it or to secure the animal from lateral movement during the ride. Extreme care should be taken when closing partitions in slant-load trailers because the handler often is in the proximity of the animal's hindlimbs.

Figure 6-6 shows the correct procedure for loading a horse onto a trailer. When unloading a horse from any of these trailers, the safest way to ask the horse to exit the trailer is to back it out of the trailer. Extreme care should be taken when doing so because a horse often reacts by lunging forward when stepping off or onto the ramp. Always keep your eyes open and your attention on the horse. Horses that are

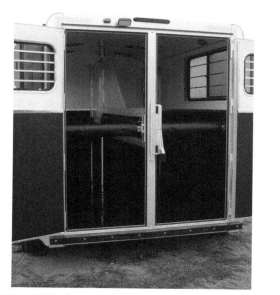

FIGURE 6-3 Two-horse trailer. (Courtesy Stidham Trailers, Chickasha, OK .)

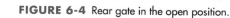

FIGURE 6-4 Rear gate in the open position.

allowed to walk off a trailer in a forward motion may often jump off trailers, with the potential for causing severe injury if they were to jump on the handler.

> *TECHNICIAN NOTE* When loading or unloading horses, always keep your eyes open and your attention on the horse.

When problems arise while attempting to load or unload a horse from a trailer, the best approach is preparation. People have thousands of ideas and tips for getting a horse to load on a trailer. In your preparation, have a conversation with the veterinarian in advance of any of these situations to determine the veterinarian's wishes and ideas about loading techniques before any incidents occur.

When livestock are loaded onto trailers, there is still an element of danger associated with the procedure. However, gates and alleyways tend to make the job easier. The most important aspect to remember when loading livestock is their point of balance; if you are behind the animal, the animal will move forward. By providing a narrow alleyway and encouraging the animal to move forward from behind, the animal will most likely load uneventfully. The animal may hesitate when loading onto the trailer, but noise or a light tap with a paddle will usually encourage the animal to load. The most common problem that occurs when loading livestock onto trailers is trying to load an animal through an alleyway that is too wide. If the animal has the ability to turn around in the alleyway, it will most likely choose this route instead of the trailer. Adjustable alleyways set to the proper width can make loading a smoother process (Figs. 6-7 and 6-8). Remember that stress decreases production, so loading and unloading livestock should always be done calmly.

> *TECHNICIAN NOTE* Stress decreases production! Loading and unloading livestock should always be done calmly.

MEDICAL RECORDS

The medical record should be started immediately when the animal arrives. Time can be saved by filling out basic information over the telephone when the owner/agent or

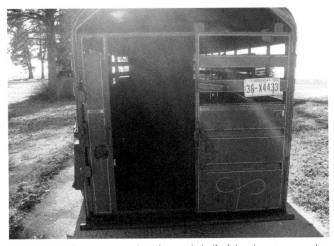

FIGURE 6-7 In some stock trailers, only half of the door is opened to allow easier loading from alleyways.

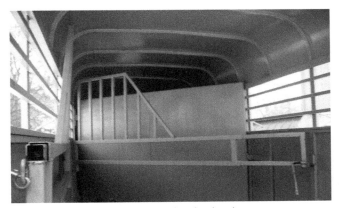

FIGURE 6-5 Slant-load trailer.

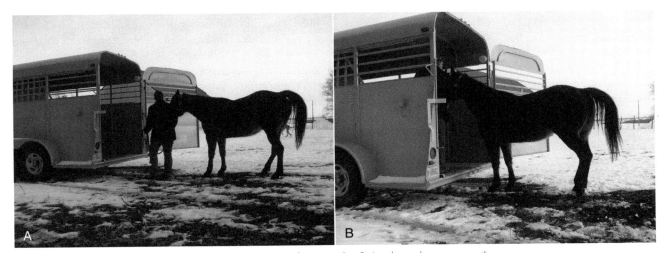

FIGURE 6-6 A, Approaching a trailer. **B**, Loading a horse on a trailer.

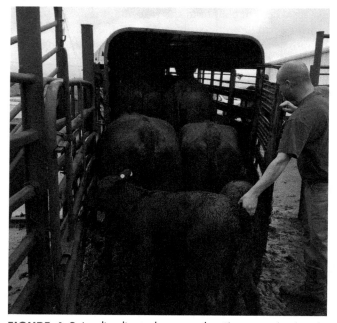

FIGURE 6-8 Loading livestock on a trailer. The person loading the livestock is seen from the camera's point of view. Notice the gates on either side of the cattle that form an alleyway. (Courtesy E-Z Mobile Livestock Weigh Systems.)

BOX 6-1	Abbreviations Commonly Used in Medical Charting of Physical Exams

AD: Right ear
ADR: Are not doing right
AS: Left ear
AU: Both ears
BAR: Bright, alert, and responsive
BCS: Body condition score
DD or Ddx: Differential diagnosis
DDN: Dull, depressed, and nonresponsive
Dx: Diagnosis
ECG: Electrocardiogram
HR: Heart rate
Hx: History
IM: Intramuscular
IOP: Intraocular pressure
LA: Large animal
LOC: Level of consciousness
MLV: Modified live vaccine
MM: Mucous membrane
OD: Right eye
OS: Left eye
OU: Both eyes
R/O: Rule out
SOAP: Subjective, objective, assessment, plan
Stat: Immediately
TPR: Temperature, pulse, and respiration
TV: Tidal volume
Tx: Treatment
WNL: Within normal limits
Wt: Weight

referring veterinarian makes the animal's appointment. The basic information should include patient signalment and billing information. A treatment authorization form is advisable because it is a cost estimate form. Cost estimates can help prevent misunderstandings with the owner/agent, especially when an animal with a complicated medical or surgical case is to be treated. The cost of diagnosis and treatment of large animals usually far exceeds the cost of comparable procedures in small animals, primarily because of the large body weight and number of staff required to care for large animals. For example, pharmacy charges for use of the same drug in a horse versus a large dog may be 10 to 25 times higher for *each* dose of the drug in the horse because of body weight alone. Many hospitals also include a charge sheet in the medical record so that each procedure performed and related supplies can be tracked for billing purposes. A list of abbreviations often used in medical record forms can be found in Box 6-1

One aspect unique to the horse industry is the widespread use of insurance. Although small animal insurance is becoming more common, equine insurance has existed for many years. Equine insurance has three common types. *Mortality insurance* covers the value of the horse in case of death. The insurance company pays the owner the estimated worth of the horse if it dies, although there may be exclusions for certain causes of death. Because of the potential for fraud, it is sometimes necessary to obtain permission from the insurance company before treatment and/or euthanasia is performed. *Surgical insurance* covers specific costs of surgery and hospitalization, with some limitations, similar to human health insurance policies. Permission from the insurance company must often be obtained before elective and

some emergency surgical procedures are performed. *Loss of use insurance* states specifically the intended use of the horse, and if the horse cannot perform its intended use because of illness or injury, the owner may be reimbursed. Insurance companies must often be included in the decision-making processes for the patient; therefore, it is important to obtain this information as part of the medical record.

A basic physical examination form or patient flow sheet should be included for all animals for recording temperature, pulse, respiration, bowel movement/urination, and food/water consumption information. Monitoring these parameters is vital even in healthy animals. When animals are moved to a clinic/hospital environment, they typically are stressed by the transportation and by their placement in an unfamiliar environment. The water and food sources likely are different from those at their home farm, and their intake may change and lead to gastrointestinal (GI) problems. Equally important to the animal's "intake" is its "output"; defecations and urinations are important to note. A history of temperature, respiration, and heart rate while the animal is at the clinic is important diagnostic information.

> **TECHNICIAN NOTE**   Several commonly used medical forms can be viewed on the Evolve website.

A treatment form is useful for recording and planning diagnostics and treatments and should provide a place for the technician/clinician to initial each procedure as it is performed. Other parts of the medical record depend on the nature of the case and may include radiology, ultrasound, endoscopy and laboratory reports, surgical procedures, and other pertinent information. Treatment records should accurately identify each animal treated, the type of medication, the dose and route that the medication was given, and the withholding time (if any) that was recommended to the owner. Recording the drug lot numbers is also advisable.

Medicating any food production animal is often complicated by the production of meat and milk products destined for human consumption. To prevent certain drugs and other chemicals (e.g., pesticides) from entering the human food chain, withdrawal intervals *(withdrawal times)* have been established for many of the substances used in food-producing animals. The withdrawal interval is the time between administration of a known dose of a drug or chemical to an animal and the time that the animal's meat, milk, and eggs are presumably safe for human consumption. The U.S. Food and Drug Administration (FDA) is the agency responsible for drug approval and for establishing withdrawal intervals for drugs approved for use in food animals, based on scientific evidence. Withdrawal intervals are printed on the labels of approved substances. Residue-contaminated meat or milk has significant economic and legal consequences for the farmer, and sometimes the farmer may see the veterinarian (and veterinary staff) as being responsible for contamination by failing to follow proper procedures or giving inaccurate advice.

> *TECHNICIAN NOTE* Withdrawal times help to keep the nation's food supply safe, and producers should always be informed of withdrawal times.

Many drugs are not approved for use in food animals but may be desirable or necessary to use in certain situations. This is referred to as *extralabel drug use.* Withdrawal intervals are not printed on the labels of such drugs. To guide veterinarians on the extralabel use of drugs in food animal species, the *Food Animal Residue Avoidance and Depletion Program (FARAD)* is a convenient source of information. FARAD is the primary resource for recommendations for withdrawal times after extralabel drug use in food animals. It is a computer-based decision support system that provides current label information on withdrawal times of approved drugs, a database of scientific articles with data on drug residues and pharmacokinetics of nonapproved drugs, and official tolerances of drug and pesticide residues in meat, milk, and eggs. (FARAD may be contacted at www.farad.org or by phone at 1-888-USFARAD. FARAD is sponsored through the U.S. Department of Agriculture [USDA]). An iPhone application from FARAD is also available and is very useful during field calls.

> *TECHNICIAN NOTE* Extralabel drug use is the use of drugs in situations not approved for the drug.

A form for recording client communications is important for documentation. All client communications should be summarized; the time, date, and method of communication should be recorded; and the form should be signed.

If euthanasia is to be performed, a euthanasia consent form should be included. If the owner/agent is not available to sign the euthanasia form, permission can be verbally obtained over the telephone. Facsimile communication is another means for obtaining necessary signatures. Sometimes the need for euthanasia is not immediately known, but euthanasia becomes necessary later, with little notice. For example, the animal in an emergency situation may suddenly "crash and burn" and require immediate euthanasia to prevent suffering; the time delay involved in trying to contact the owner/agent may result in unnecessary suffering. In these cases, having the owner/agent sign a euthanasia consent form when the animal first arrives at the hospital allows the clinician to euthanize the animal humanely in a truly crisis situation and then contact the owner after dealing with the crisis.

The medical record can be kept on a clipboard or in a binder and placed on the patient's stall door or kept in a central nursing station of the hospital. Patient confidentiality should be considered when choosing a location for the patient's medical record. Procedures, medications, and diagnostic test results are not intended to be public information. If the hospital allows visitors, and most do, the reputation of a farm, ranch, horse, trainer, or stable may be jeopardized if this private information becomes public. The medical record should be in a form that allows it to travel around the hospital with the animal for its various procedures but be accessed only by hospital personnel.

> *TECHNICIAN NOTE* Confidentiality is extremely important! Medical records are not public information, and the wrong information could jeopardize a farm, ranch, trainer, or stable. Failure to comply with this confidentiality could result in the loss of business or in lawsuits.

PATIENT IDENTIFICATION

No matter what document you are filling out, each document should have a patient identification (ID) area on the form. Patient ID should be performed during the admissions process.

Proper patient ID is essential; surgery and even euthanasia have been performed on the wrong animal because of inadequate or inaccurate ID. It is important not only to record an animal's *markings* in the medical record but to have some method of identifying the animal itself and the animal's housing (e.g., stall, crate, or pen). It is common practice to place a card on the housing door or gate as a form of patient ID. The patient's signalment is usually recorded on the card; again, be sensitive to issues of confidentiality when displaying this information. To identify a patient, patient ID tags can be made. (Small animal plastic ID collars are well suited for this use.) Form the ID tag or band into a circle, and tape or braid it to the animal's mane, forelock, tail, pastern, or halter.

> **TECHNICIAN NOTE**   Proper patient identification is essential to ensure the proper treatment on the right animal.

Patients are described by sex, breed, age, permanent or temporary ID, coat color, and markings. Descriptions in the patient signalment of color and natural markings may not be enough to distinguish an individual animal; for example, a description of a black Angus cow on a purebred Angus ranch would not be very informative, considering that almost all the animals on this operation are black cows. Therefore, an effort must be made to identify each animal as specifically as possible.

Technicians should be familiar with the proper terms for the species being housed. A table of common terminology for each species can be found at the beginning of each species section. Slight variations in these terms may exist among different breeds, geographic locations, and common jargon.

Markings may be natural or artificial (humanmade). Artificial ID can be temporary or permanent. Temporary artificial forms of ID include *panel tags, electronic identification (EID)* tags, metal clips, collars, *ankle bands, temporary marking paint,* brisket tags, and tail tags. Common forms of permanent artificial ID include lip tattoos, freeze brands, hot brands, *ear notching,* and microchips. Natural markings include hair color, color patterns, scars, hair whorls, muscle indentations, and *chestnuts.* Natural markings should be defined for all large animals, but they are often defined more extensively in horses. Colors are kept fairly simple for other livestock, considering that most animals of the same breed look almost exactly the same.

PANEL TAGS

Panel tags are commonly used as a form of ID in cattle, swine, sheep, and goats. The tags can be placed in the middle third of the ear and worn like an earring (Fig. 6-9). Individual producers use a variety of tag colors, sizes, and number/letter systems to identify each individual animal. No set numbering or lettering system is used in any species of livestock, so technicians should not assume that the way one producer uses a tag is the same way every other producer uses the tags. These tags can easily be removed if the animal is sold, and the animal can be retagged with a tag relevant to the new producer's system (Fig. 6-10). A panel tag can easily be ripped out or removed, making it a temporary form of ID.

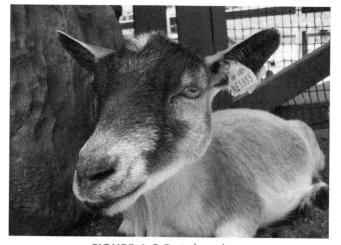

FIGURE 6-9 Typical panel tag.

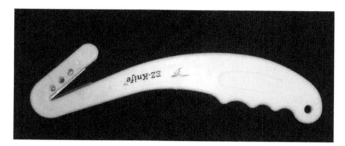

FIGURE 6-10 Tag remover.

ELECTRONIC IDENTIFICATION TAGS

EID tags are becoming more popular. The USDA is implementing the *National Animal Identification System.* This system will help animal health officials more effectively track animals during a disease outbreak and quickly find other animals that may be infected. The system will be put into place in three phases. The first phase is *premises registration.* The USDA is asking producers to register their farms and ranches as locations where livestock are raised. The second phase is animal identification. The EID tags are placed in all livestock and stay with the animal until death (Fig. 6-11). The third stage of the system is an animal tracking database where information about the livestock will be stored. The system is in the beginning of implementation and is not fully under way.

Dairy producers have in place a system known as the *National Farm Identification and Records System.* It is a voluntary system for maintaining records within the dairy industry. Some producers are using it as a means of gathering better information about their herds.

> **TECHNICIAN NOTE**   Ask producers about the meaning of their panel tags before using them as a form of identification. Not all producers use panel tags in the same way.

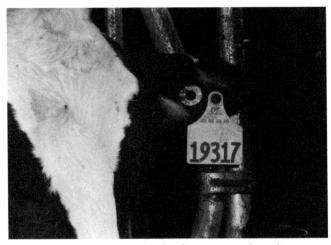

FIGURE 6-11 Electrical identification tag and panel gag.

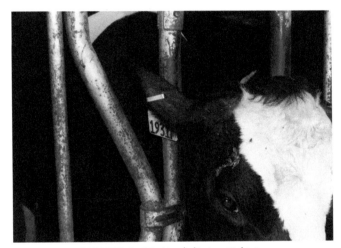

FIGURE 6-12 Metal clip in a Holstein.

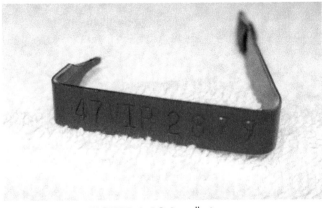

FIGURE 6-13 Brucellosis tag.

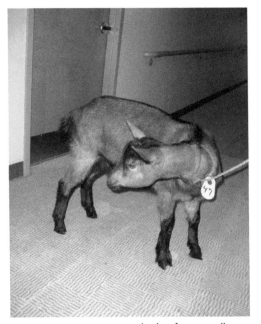

FIGURE 6-14 Goat with identification collar.

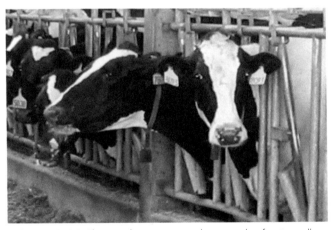

FIGURE 6-15 These cattle are wearing electronic identification collars.

Orange metal clips are also placed in heifers that have been vaccinated for brucellosis (Fig. 6-13). These orange metal tags are always placed in the right ear along with a tattoo that helps to signify that those heifers have undergone brucellosis vaccination. Other livestock such as sheep and goats may also be identified using metal clips.

COLLARS

Collars are commonly used in goats and dairy cattle (Fig. 6-14). Some collars carry an electronic device that allows automated equipment to identify the individual animal, record milking yields, or control the animal's diet (Fig. 6-15).

ANKLE BANDS

Ankle bands are commonly used in dairy cattle (Fig. 6-16). They can be numbered, but most often a color is used to signify a group or a problem with the animal.

METAL CLIPS

Metal clips are commonly used in cattle as a more secure form of ID. These clips are less likely to be ripped out than panel tags but are not as easy to read from a distance (Fig. 6-12). To read metal clips, the cattle must be restrained.

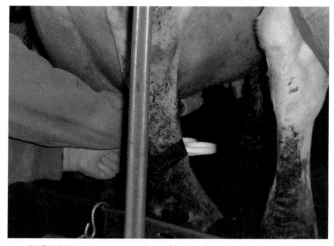

FIGURE 6-16 Notice the ankle band on the back right leg.

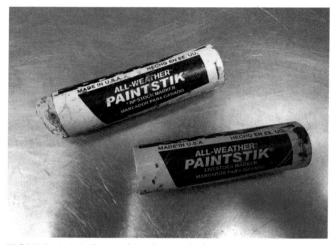

FIGURE 6-17 The producer has marked the animal with temporary marking paint.

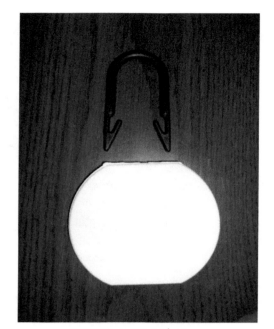

FIGURE 6-18 Brisket tags.

TEMPORARY MARKING PAINT

Temporary marking paint is used in all large animal species. It is a waterproof paint similar to car paint that can be applied to the animal. This temporary form of ID rubs off after time but is useful for heat detection, pregnancy checking, or identifying an individual or group of individuals for a short period of time (Fig. 6-17).

BRISKET TAGS

Brisket tags can be used in cattle as another form of identification. They work in much the same way as panel tags (Fig. 6-18).

EAR NOTCHING

Ear notching is a permanent form of ID that is commonly used in goats, horses, and pigs. Ear notching is done in cattle but not as a form of ID. Ear notching in cattle is used for collection of tissue in the testing for bovine viral diarrhea. The universal ear notching system is not the only system of ear notching used by producers. Technicians should obtain clarification about the type of system being used (Fig. 6-19).

> **TECHNICIAN NOTE** Always talk with producers about the meaning of their ear notching system.

TATTOOS

Heifers are commonly tattooed as part of the brucellosis vaccination procedure. Other species that are commonly tattooed as a form of ID include goats and swine. Racehorses commonly have tattoos placed on the labial mucosa (inner lining) of the upper lip (Fig. 6-20). The tattoo is usually a combination of numbers and letters that identify the year of birth and the horse's registration number. Lip tattoos are usually applied to racehorses when they enter race training, most often as 2 year olds.

HOT BRANDS AND FREEZE BRANDS

Brands may be required by certain breed registries. Some producers have their own brands for ID of animals that belong to their farm or ranch. Often registries mandate the type, configuration, and location of the brand. However, any owner can brand an animal with a symbol of his or her choice wherever he or she prefers. Brands are usually placed on the side of the neck, over the triceps muscle on the forelimb, or on the hip/thigh area of the hindlimb. The two types of branding are freeze branding and *hot branding* (Fig. 6-21). *Freeze branding* destroys the hair pigment, which is derived from cells called melanocytes. Freeze branding uses branding irons dipped in liquid nitrogen. The iron is applied for a predetermined time necessary to kill the melanocytes but spares the follicle cells that grow the hair (Fig. 6-22). The hair eventually grows back white

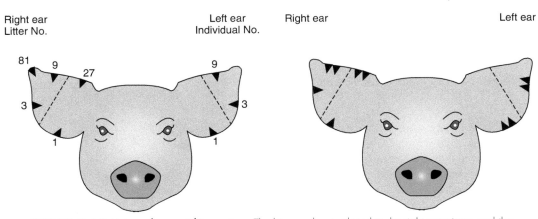

FIGURE 6-19 Universal ear notching system. The litter number is placed in the right ear pinna, and the individual pig number is placed in the left ear pinna. The pig on the *right* shows litter number 76, individual pig number 8.

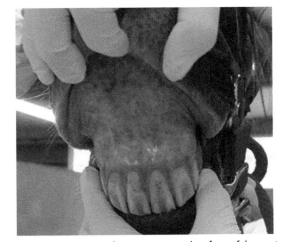

FIGURE 6-20 Tattoo on the upper mucosal surface of the equine lip. (From Sellon DC, Long MT: *Equine infectious diseases*, ed 2, St. Louis, 2014, Saunders.)

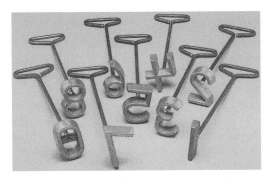

FIGURE 6-22 Freeze branding irons. (From Sonsthagen T: *Veterinary instruments and equipment: a pocket guide*, ed 3, St. Louis, 2014, Mosby.)

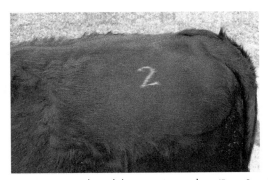

FIGURE 6-23 Freeze brand showing pigment loss. (From Sonsthagen T: *Veterinary instruments and equipment: a pocket guide*, ed 3, St. Louis, 2014, Mosby.)

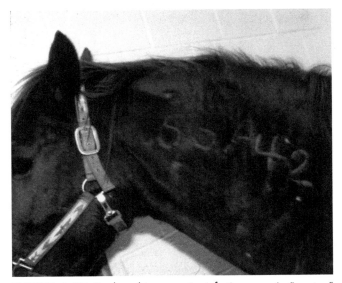

FIGURE 6-21 Hot brand in an equine infectious anemia "reactor." (From Sellon DC: Equine infectious anemia. In Sellon DC, Long MT, editors: *Equine infectious diseases*, ed 2, St. Louis, 2014, Saunders.)

(no pigment) in several months (Fig. 6-23). Gray horses can be freeze branded, but the iron is applied longer to kill not only melanocytes but also the hair follicles so that hair does not regrow. The result is a bald brand. In horses, freeze brands can be placed high along the crest of the neck and may be obscured by the mane. Be sure to look beneath the mane for freeze brands and other markings. Hot branding is considered by some to be more painful than freeze branding, which numbs the nerves within seconds of application of the freeze branding iron.

However, many people who have performed hot brand procedures maintain that the discomfort of the animal is minimal during the procedure and is comparable to that produced by freeze branding. The goal of hot branding is to kill the hair follicles, thus producing a hairless scar.

MICROCHIPS

Microchips can be placed in any large animal, but because of the cost associated with microchipping, the only species in which they are commonly used is the horse. Microchips can be inserted subcutaneously in horses and are usually placed in the neck area (Fig. 6-24). Microchips are encoded for the individual horse and require a special sensor to scan the horse and read the ID code. This form of ID is gaining popularity in the horse world. In ruminants, you may see use of rumen boluses that contain a microchip as a form of ID.

MARKINGS

Markings should be recorded for all livestock; however, markings are most useful in the horse. The six "markings" on domestic animals are the four legs, the head, and the tail. Markings are usually white and are described as such. In particular, white markings are the most distinguishing (Fig. 6-25). Leg and face markings are often described subjectively; for example, what one person calls a "full sock" is a "low stocking" to another, and this may be problematic. No standard level has been established at which a sock becomes a stocking, a coronet becomes a pastern, and so on. Similar confusion exists with facial markings (i.e., no standard landmarks for strictly defining strips, stripes, and blazes). To minimize confusion, it is preferable either to use a diagram to draw and label the markings (Fig. 6-26) or to use a camera to photograph the animal for definitive ID. Drawings should be as accurate as possible; for example, stars are not always in a perfect diamond shape, although they are often drawn that way. Stars are usually irregular in shape; in addition, they may be located above, at, or below eye level. These details are important. Facial markings are often continuous; for example, a star may be continuous with a strip or stripe. When describing continuous facial markings, use a dash between the markings (e.g., star–strip, star–strip–snip). Photographs are especially useful for breeds with complicated coat patterns, such as Paint Horses, Appaloosas, and Pintos, which are difficult to draw accurately. A lack of markings on a leg or face is also recorded for accuracy and to prevent fraudulent altering of medical records. Clearly indicate which body part lacks the markings and write "none" (e.g., left forelimb—none). Within a clinic it can be beneficial to communicate a standard description for each marking. Box 6-2 lists standard marking descriptions.

COAT COLOR

Coat color should be identified as a form of ID for every animal. In most livestock species the colors are relatively simple, for example, red or black. However, with horses

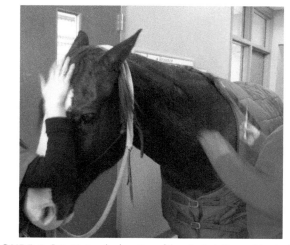

FIGURE 6-24 Notice the location of the alcohol. This will be the location of chip placement.

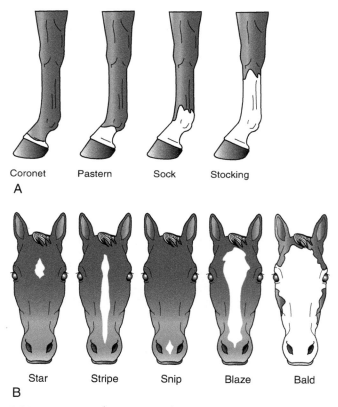

FIGURE 6-25 White point markings. **A,** Common leg markings. **B,** Common face markings.

the color may not be straightforward. With more than 400 breeds of horses, no standard universal definition for coat color is available.

Coat color should always be recorded, although it is not a highly individual feature (Fig. 6-27). Coat colors are not often distinguishing, especially among several breeds with little variation in coat color (e.g., most Standardbreds are bay). Each horse breed registry defines its own acceptable and unacceptable coat colors and patterns, and these

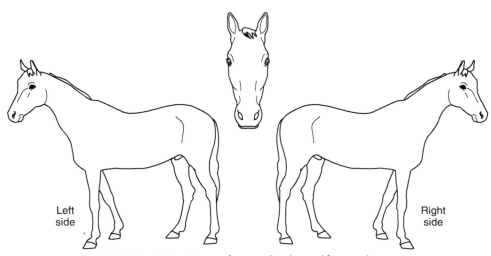

FIGURE 6-26 Diagram for recording leg and face markings.

BOX 6-2	Standard Marking Descriptions

Bald: Wide white marking that goes behind at least one eye
Blaze: Thick white line outside the bridges of the nasal bones
Coronet: White marking that forms a thin white line around the coronet band
Pastern: White marking below the level of the pastern that does not cross the pastern at any point
Snip: Small marking between the nostrils anywhere on the dorsal aspect of the face, on the bottom third of the head
Sock: White marking that crosses the pastern at any point and does not cross the knee or hock at any point
Star: Small marking between the eyes located anywhere from the poll to the bottom third of the forehead
Stocking: White marking that crosses the knee or hock at any point
Stripe: Thin white line within the bridges of the nasal bones

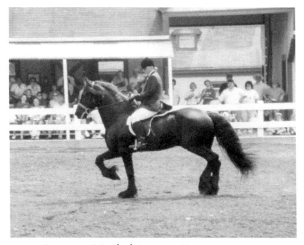

FIGURE 6-28 Black Friesian. (Courtesy Kim Myers.)

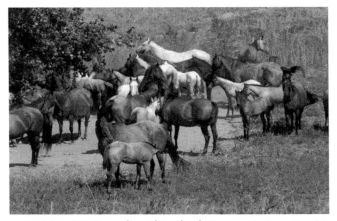

FIGURE 6-27 Coat color within a herd. (Courtesy the Pitzer Ranch.)

definitions may not be in agreement with those of other breeds. Foals present another challenge because a foal's coat color may be different from that of its eventual adult coat. The best example of this is the gray coat color; these horses usually are born black and lighten to gray with age, eventually progressing to what appears to be pure white. For purposes of patient ID, record the coat color at the time of admission, not the anticipated adult color.

The following is a generalized overview of coat color. It may not work for every breed association and is not a complete list of colors.

Black
Black is a truly black horse; it cannot have brown areas anywhere. The color cannot fade at all during the year. The horse can, however, have *points* (Fig. 6-28).

Brown
A black horse that becomes brown anywhere on the body during the year, usually on the muzzle and flank, is considered brown. Brown therefore can be any shade of black down to a lighter brown but cannot have any red hue (Fig. 6-29).

Chestnut
A brown horse with a red hue is called a chestnut (Fig. 6-30).

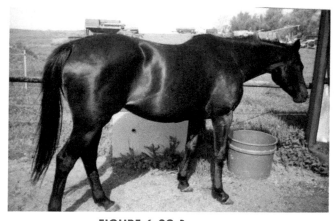

FIGURE 6-29 Brown mare.

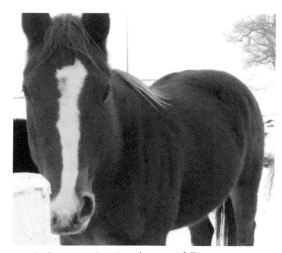

FIGURE 6-31 Sorrel mare in full winter coat.

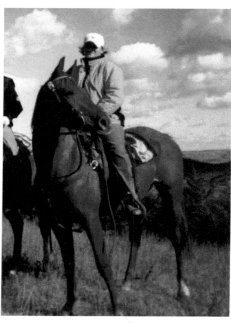

FIGURE 6-30 Chestnut mare.

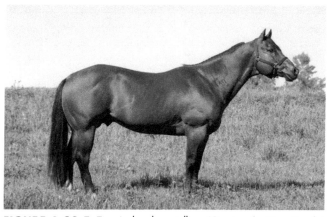

FIGURE 6-32 Ty Two Jack, a bay stallion. (Courtesy the Pitzer Ranch.)

Sorrel

A brown horse with a dull red hue is called a sorrel. The only breed that recognizes this color is the American Quarter Horse Association (AQHA). Within the AQHA you must distinguish between a sorrel and a chestnut; the distinction is made on the brightness of the red coat. All other breeds of horses do not differentiate this color and just call the horse a chestnut (Fig. 6-31).

Bay

A brown, chestnut, or sorrel horse with black lower legs, mane, and tail is a bay (Fig. 6-32).

Dun

A dun has yellow tan as the main body color and the same black lower legs, mane, and tail as a bay. The dun has a dorsal stripe: a dark line down the middle of the horse's back (Fig. 6-33).

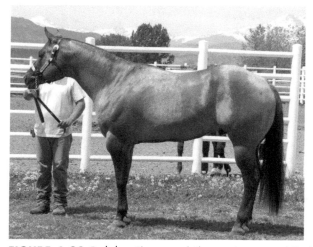

FIGURE 6-33 Red dun. Phenomenal Play, an International Buckskin Horse Association (IBHA)/American Quarter Horse Association (AQHA) stallion by Phenomenal Creation out of Ima Cool Playgirl Act, owned by Wild Basin Ranch, Longmont, Colo. (Courtesy Wild Basin Ranch, Longmont, Colo.)

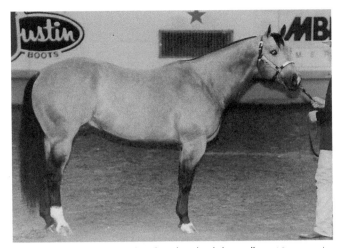

FIGURE 6-34 Two Eyed Red Buck, a buckskin stallion. (Courtesy the Pitzer Ranch.)

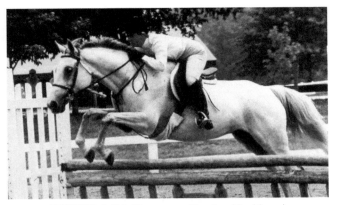

FIGURE 6-36 Gray mare. (Courtesy Kim Myers.)

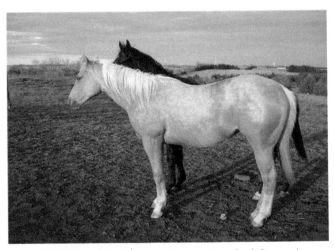

FIGURE 6-35 Palomino. (Courtesy Fran Smith Roemer.)

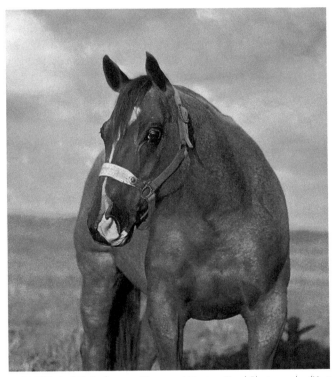

FIGURE 6-37 Red roan. (Courtesy Western Pearl Photography/Kori Simmons.)

Buckskin

A buckskin is the same color as a dun but does not have a dorsal stripe (Fig. 6-34).

Palomino

A palomino is the same allover color as the dun and buckskin, with a white or blonde mane and tail (Fig. 6-35).

Gray

A horse can look white to a layperson but is referred to as gray by equine professionals because the skin of most of these horses is black (Fig.6-36). (If the skin is pink, then the horse is referred to as white, but this is rare.)

Roan

A roan's coat color is salt and pepper. One strand is white and the next strand is colored. They are often red or blue and sometimes referred to as strawberry roan, red roan, or blue roan for the appropriate color. The head of the horse is solid in color and does not have the roan pattern (Fig. 6-37).

HAIR WHORLS

Hair whorls are often used as a form of ID in horses. All horses have hair whorls (also known as swirls or cowlicks), which can be used for ID purposes (Fig. 6-38). Certain whorl locations are common to all horses, so whorls at these locations are not considered distinguishing features of an individual. Whorls on the flanks and over the trachea are common to all horses and seldom are helpful in definitive ID. However, some whorls occur at locations that are useful for ID. All horses have at least one whorl on the forehead between the eyes, but the whorl may be located above, below, or at the level of the eyes. The whorl may be right or left of the midline, and some horses may have two or even three whorls in this area. When properly recorded, the forehead whorls are useful. The other areas to check for distinguishing whorls are along the crest of the neck and along

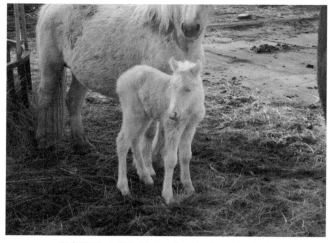

FIGURE 6-38 Notice the whorls on this foal.

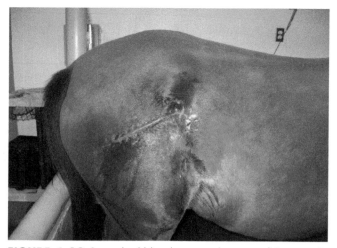

FIGURE 6-39 Scars should be documented as part of the animal's identification.

the jugular grooves. Do not assume that if there is a whorl on one side of the horse there will be a corresponding whorl on the other side. The standard written symbol for whorls is a simple "X" recorded on the horse's diagram or photograph.

MUSCLE IDENTIFICATION

Muscle indentations above the jugular groove on the side of the neck are uncommon. These indentations are readily seen and felt and usually are unilateral. They are generally assumed to result from trauma, although the animal may not have a history of known trauma to the area. Owners may simply fail to observe the trauma if the skin is not broken. Horsemen and horsewomen refer to these indentations as *wizard's thumbprints* or *warlock's thumbprints*. Because they are unusual, muscle indentations should be recorded as part of the patient ID.

SCARS

Scars occur in two visible forms, those with hair and those without. Usually, if a scar has hair, the hair is white. Scars should be described by location, length, shape, and the presence or absence of hair (Fig. 6-39).

CHESTNUTS

Chestnuts occur on the medial aspect of all limbs (Fig. 6-40). Chestnuts are the evolutionary remnants of the digital pad of the first digit. They are small (1 to 3 cm), ovoid, raised areas of cornified tissue proximal to the carpus on the forelimbs and at the level of the tarsus on the hindlimbs. They are seldom useful for ID purposes.

AGE

Age is another component of the signalment and should be included with the animal's ID, for example, a 6-year-old, sorrel mare with white star and left hind stocking. Age is best confirmed with registration papers if the animal is registered with a breed association, although many animals, even horses, do not have breed registries, and their owners are relied on for information on the animals' age. Examination of the teeth is a well-accepted method of aging animals, but it requires experience to be accurate. Teeth can be intentionally

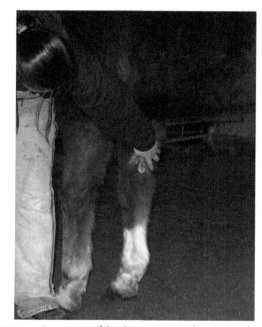

FIGURE 6-40 Location of the chestnuts on the front limbs of the horse.

altered for deceptive purposes to make them appear younger, a practice known as *bishoping* in horses. Aging by teeth is further explained in each species section.

HISTORY AND BASIC PHYSICAL EXAMINATION OF HORSES

The history and physical examination are the most important parts of the animal's record and serve as the starting point for identifying the patient's problems. "Problems" are any conditions that require medical or surgical treatment *or* that compromise the animal's quality of life. Most clinicians use a problem-oriented approach to diagnosis and treatment; this provides a logical method to work through any medical or surgical case. A thorough history and a complete physical examination are essential for successful problem solving.

HISTORY

The physical examination process always begins with taking the history and inspecting the animal's environment. Because large animals are usually kept in herd situations, conditions affecting one animal may have consequences for the others on the farm. The history should focus not only on the individual but also on the management of the entire group. Food and water sources, pasture management, herd health programs, introduction of new animals, feeding practices, toxin exposure, and environmental stresses are among the factors that should be explored. Many owners attempt treatment of animals before they call the veterinarian, and owners should be asked about any treatments and/or medications that the patient was given. This is fairly common in large animal practice, especially with production animals; economic factors often dictate whether the owner calls the veterinarian immediately or attempts to solve the problem independently. Owners may be reluctant to admit this information and may need to be asked specifically whether they have treated the animal and what they may have attempted for treatment.

> **TECHNICIAN NOTE** Histories should focus not only on the individual but also on the management of the entire herd.

It is essential that you not appear to pass judgment on the farmer's/owner's practices during the history taking and inspection of the facilities. Simply record the facts and allow the veterinarian to make any suggestions or assessments of management practices.

> **TECHNICIAN NOTE** Do not pass judgment during the history-taking process. Your job is to gather the facts!

Several approaches are available for taking a patient's history. If owners are allowed to give the history without any guidance, they typically provide a rambling discourse that leaves out essential information, fails to follow a time line, and includes unnecessary information. Some experienced owners provide an excellent history with little coaching, but most owners do not know how to give a concise, useful summary of their animal's condition. Approaches to history taking range from letting an owner talk without any guidance to the "inquisition" approach where the person taking the history asks specific questions. Some clients may need these extremes, but most respond best to the middle-of-the-road approach of "coaching." In the coaching approach, the person taking the history lets the owner tell his or her story but asks specific questions along the way to guide the owner and ensure details are not missed. Most owners do not know what information is significant and what is not, so the person taking the history must attempt to obtain the relevant information and prevent the owner from going off on a useless tangent. Owners also seldom appreciate the value of a time line and tend to wander through the time sequence. The questioner must try to keep the information in a sequential format.

Once the history is obtained, it must be evaluated for accuracy. Some information may be difficult to evaluate, and some may be misleading. Some owners give false information to spare embarrassment; they do not want to appear ignorant or admit they may have made a mistake.

History taking should be tailored to the patient's problems. For example, if a contagious disease is suspected, the patient's vaccination history, possible exposure to other infected animals, and health management practices of the farm should be investigated. If the animal is going to be admitted to the hospital, it can be valuable to know whether an animal has a tendency to eat its bedding or has a known sensitivity or allergy to certain types of bedding. This information seems to be more relevant when dealing with the equine patient. When the animal is admitted to the hospital, its at-home diet should be recorded. This information should include the type and amount of roughage (hay or grazing), concentrates (grains), and any supplements, as well as the normal feeding schedule. The at-home diet should be simulated as closely as possible in the hospital because radical changes in types and volumes of feed can cause GI problems, especially in horses.

PURPOSE OF THE PHYSICAL EXAMINATION

Physical examinations may be performed for several reasons. Any time an animal is being evaluated for a problem, a physical examination should be performed. The physical examination can set the baseline for repeat examinations and can be used to gather essential information in making a diagnosis. After completing a physical examination of a patient, the technician may be in doubt about whether certain findings are significant or of sufficient concern to warrant alerting the clinician in charge of the case. It is helpful to establish "when to call" guidelines as part of the patient's treatment orders. The clinician should establish ranges for examination parameters that need urgent attention, such as "if temperature >102.5° F, call Dr." or "if heart rate > 60 bpm, call Dr." Other reasons for performing physical examinations include insurance examination and prepurchase examinations.

An *insurance examination* is required by the insurance company before a horse can receive insurance coverage. It may range from a basic examination to a thorough, in-depth examination. The type of insurance and the animal's value dictate the depth of examination required by the insurance company. The *prepurchase examination,* conducted before completing the sale of an animal, is a common procedure in equine practice. A seller and a buyer are identified, and the veterinarian performing the examination is presumed to be working in the buyer's best interest (the veterinarian is paid by the buyer). Like the insurance examination, the prepurchase examination is dictated by the intended use of the horse and its estimated value. It may be a simple physical examination or an in-depth examination including biopsies, blood samples, endoscopy, electrocardiogram/echocardiogram, and diagnostic imaging. Prepurchase examinations are often a source of lawsuits against the veterinarian, usually because of a misunderstanding of the purpose of the examination. Owners often believe that the examination is a guarantee for the future of the horse, yet the veterinarian has no crystal ball. Most veterinarians are keenly aware of this fact and go to great lengths to document the findings of prepurchase examinations and not overstate their findings as predictions of future performance. The technician should understand the potentially sensitive nature of the insurance and prepurchase examination and help ensure accuracy and privacy of the results.

> **TECHNICIAN NOTE** Prepurchase examinations are paid for by the buyer. Prepurchase examinations are not a guarantee of the animal's future performance.

BASIC PHYSICAL EXAMINATION

The basic physical examination typically includes temperature/pulse/respiration (TPR), heart/lung *auscultation,* abdominal auscultation, hydration status, examination of mucous membranes, and height/weight measurement. More in-depth evaluations are covered under specific body systems.

Visual Observation

The physical examination of any animal should begin with an initial visual observation of the animal from a distance and should include watching their gate and mental awareness. The animal's posture, behavior, body condition, and alertness are easily observed. More specific signs, such as breathing pattern and respiratory noises, body swellings, skin wounds, and muscle atrophy, may also be noted.

Fecal and Urine Observation

The character of feces and urine is available for observation and should be evaluated. Fecal character varies among animals and their types of diet. Cattle defecate 12 to 18 times per day, and their feces have a semisolid "cow-plop" consistency, without a distinct form. Goats produce formed feces in the shape of small, solid pellets. Sheep feces also are pelleted. Horses have an apple look to their fecal material. Swine fecal material is in a soft tubular form. Llamas and alpaca feces are pelleted, and these animals often use communal feces piles. The color of the feces depends on the diet, ranging from green to dark brown. In ruminants, the presence of undigested roughage fibers is not normal and may indicate dysfunction of the rumen/reticulum.

> **TECHNICIAN NOTE** Undigested roughage fibers in ruminant feces may indicate dysfunction of the rumen/reticulum.

If an animal urinates, a mental note of this should be taken because it can be extremely important to the veterinarian's diagnosis. It is always a good idea to catch urine at this time if possible because most animals urinate shortly after being restrained, and if you are not watching for it,

you will miss your opportunity. Techniques for urine collection are discussed in later chapters, but for many species we have no reliable way of collecting urine other than the wait and see approach.

Respiratory Rate

The number of respirations per minute can be counted several ways: (1) using a stethoscope to listen to air movement in the trachea or chest; (2) using a hand to feel movement of air in and out of a nostril; and (3) most commonly, simply counting chest excursions (rise and fall of the thoracic wall) per minute.

The respiratory rate is best taken by counting chest excursions from a distance, before herding or handling. The excitement and fear of herding or being restrained can cause dramatic increases in respiratory rate, especially in hot environmental temperatures, that do not reflect the true respiratory rate of the animal at rest.

Respirations should be characterized by their effort and depth. Respiration may be described as shallow, deep, labored, gasping, and other nonspecific terms. Horses normally use a combination of thoracic and abdominal muscles to breathe; this is called costoabdominal breathing. Some painful conditions of the chest may lead to increased use of the abdominal muscles to breathe, referred to as an "increased abdominal component to the respiratory pattern." Normal horses cannot breathe through the mouth. If mouth breathing is observed, it should be noted and brought to the attention of the clinician. Ruminants are capable of open-mouth breathing, though it is usually considered to be a sign of distress or heat stress (usually when environmental temperature exceeds 85° F). An abdominal breathing pattern is normal.

> **TECHNICIAN NOTE** Open-mouth breathing in ruminants is often a sign of distress or heat stress.

Respiratory noises are not uncommon in horses and may be significant. Noises may be characterized as wheezing, whistling, honking, snoring, or fluttering. Noises may be heard only at rest or perhaps only during exercise. It is important to note the horse's activity at the time the noise is heard. Equally important to note is whether the noise occurs during inspiration, expiration, or both. When one is standing next to a ruminant or auscultating the thorax or trachea, occasional low-pitched fluttering sounds are heard; this is *eructation* (burping), which is normal in ruminants. Eructation rates are approximately 18 per hour in cattle and 10 per hour in sheep and goats.

Respiration rate may increase during hot weather or following physical activity. Foals have a high respiratory rate at birth because of the residual fluid in the lower airways. Newborn foals may have a respiratory rate of 80 to 90 breaths per minute; this slows to 60 to 80 in the first 5 to 10 minutes after birth and gradually decreases to 20 to 40 for the first week or 2 weeks of life.

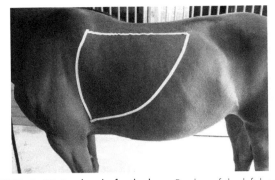

FIGURE 6-41 Landmarks for the lung. Borders of the left lung field for auscultation.

Lung Auscultation

Despite the large size of these species' lungs, breath sounds may be difficult to hear. A quiet environment is important for an accurate evaluation.

The borders of the lung fields in each species are the same for the right and left sides of the chest (Fig. 6-41). The lung field basically consists of a cranioventral area and a caudodorsal area; part of the cranioventral field is obscured by the shoulder musculature and cannot be heard. The stethoscope is placed in several locations within the lung field to listen to several breaths at each location (Fig. 6-42). The lungs are best auscultated between ribs 6 and 11 in swine. The borders for lung auscultation in the ruminant are between rib number 5 cranially and rib number 11 caudally. If necessary to induce deep breathing for lung auscultation, the nostrils and mouth (because ruminants can mouth breathe) can be held closed for about a minute to stimulate deeper breathing and a higher respiratory rate. Normally, air movement in and out of the airways should be heard and should not be accompanied by wheezing or gurgling or by moist sounds. The clinician should be alerted if abnormal noises are heard. Equally significant may be the absence of breath sounds, as occurs in some respiratory diseases; the clinician should be alerted that no breath sounds are detected.

Lung auscultation should always be performed on both sides of the chest. Respiratory diseases and other abnormalities do not necessarily affect both lungs and pleural cavities equally, and results of auscultation may be different over the right and left lungs.

Lung Percussion

Lung percussion can be performed by using a spoon or a solid snap of the finger moving from the dorsal aspect of the lung field ventrally while listening to the sounds through your stethoscope. If a change in sound can be identified and heard at the same level across the chest, concern for fluid accumulation in the chest is warranted.

Pulse Rate

The pulse rate is taken by palpation of arteries. Veins do not have palpable pulses because of the low blood pressures inside veins.

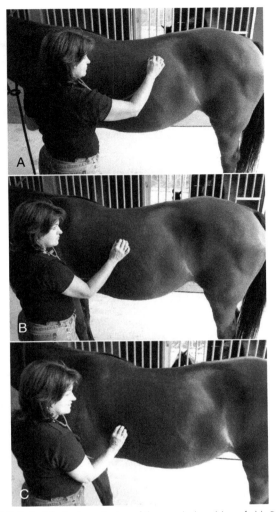

FIGURE 6-42 A, Auscultation of the caudodorsal lung field. **B,** Auscultation of the midthorax. **C,** Auscultation of the cranioventral lung field.

Strictly speaking, heart rate and pulse rate are not the same; heart rate refers to the number of heartbeats per minute (bpm); pulse rate refers to the number of palpable arterial pulse waves per minute. In normal animals, heart rate and pulse rate are equal.

Auscultation of the heart is used properly for taking heart rate, not pulse rate. This is because some heart abnormalities may produce audible heart sounds that are not necessarily accompanied by an arterial pulse. For accuracy, if the heart is auscultated, the arterial pulse should be simultaneously palpated to ensure that each audible heartbeat is accompanied by a palpable pulse wave. If each audible heartbeat is not accompanied by a pulse wave (a condition called a *pulse deficit*), the clinician should be notified.

Arterial pulses in horses may be palpated at several locations. The most convenient location is over the facial artery where it courses over the ventral aspect of the mandible, rostral to the origin of the masseter muscle (Fig. 6-43, *A*). Two or more fingers are lightly rolled back and forth across the mandible to identify the facial artery/facial vein bundle. Once identified, the bundle is firmly pressed against the

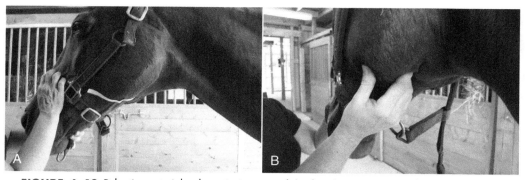

FIGURE 6-43 Palpating arterial pulses. **A,** Location of the facial artery. **B,** Press the vascular bundle against the medial aspect of the mandible.

mandible to feel the arterial pulse (Fig. 6-43, *B*). If the bundle is pressed too tightly, the artery may be occluded, and the pulse may not be easily felt. A common mistake is not being patient when palpating large animal pulses; heart rates are much lower in large animals than in small animals.

Other arteries are available for taking the pulse in the horse. The transverse facial artery is located in a horizontal depression about 1 inch caudal to the lateral canthus of the eye and just below the zygomatic arch (Fig. 6-44). The coccygeal artery supplies the tail and is located along the ventral midline of the tail (Fig. 6-44, *C*). The dorsal metatarsal artery is located between metatarsals 3 and 4 (cannon bone and lateral splint bone) on the hindlimbs (Fig. 6-44, *D* to *F*). The lateral and medial digital arteries also can be palpated where they course over the abaxial aspect of the proximal sesamoid bones of each leg or just proximal to the collateral cartilages of each hoof (Fig. 6-44, *G*). The carotid artery, like all arteries, has a pulse wave but is difficult to palpate accurately in large animals because of its deep position and is seldom useful for palpation.

In swine, common pulse points are the auricular (ear) artery along the ear pinna and the coccygeal artery of the tail; the femoral artery may be available in recumbent animals. In small pigs, the heart rate may be felt directly over the heart by placing the hand against the chest wall just behind the left elbow.

In cattle, the pulse can be palpated readily at the facial artery, but the coccygeal, median (forelimb), and great metatarsal (hindlimb) arteries are also available. The femoral artery is most convenient in sheep and goats.

The features of the pulse to note are its rate and rhythm. The rate is recorded as number per minute. Pulse rhythm is recorded as regular or irregular. Irregular rhythm likely indicates an arrhythmia of the heart. The most common irregularity of the pulse in horses is caused by a heart arrhythmia called second-degree atrioventricular (A-V) block. This arrhythmia is caused by failure of the electrical current generated by the atria to reach the ventricles, that is, an intermittent "blockage" of current occurs at the A-V node, which normally acts as an electrical gate between the atria and ventricles. This "blockage" results in dropped beats, but usually in a *regular pattern.* Typically, the dropped beat occurs every third or fourth heartbeat

and is readily identified by palpating the pulse. The regular rhythm is interrupted by a single "lost" (dropped) beat, with the "lost" beats occurring at regular intervals (e.g., beat–beat–beat–silence–beat–beat–beat–silence). Even though second-degree A-V block is usually a normal finding in horses, it should be noted in the medical record. Horses with this arrhythmia may have very low resting heart rates, less than 28 bpm. This arrhythmia is more common in fit horses and should disappear in any horse when the horse is exercised. It is thought to be caused by increased tone from the vagal nerve, which is part of the parasympathetic nervous system.

Pulse quality is often described as strong, bounding, weak, thready, or other nonspecific terms. Pulse quality is subjective; its usefulness depends on the experience of the person assessing the pulse and should not be overinterpreted.

Heart Auscultation

Auscultation of the heart should be performed on left and right side of the chest, although most of the heart valves and sounds are heard best from the left side. The right side should not be overlooked; some murmurs are audible only on the right side and will be missed if the animal is auscultated only from the left. Auscultation should be done in a quiet environment, so the animal may have to be taken to another area of the barn or hospital for ideal evaluation.

> **TECHNICIAN NOTE**   Most heart sounds are heard best from the left side. However, the technician should listen to both left and right sides when performing a physical examination.

The landmarks for basic auscultation of the heart are the same on either side of the chest and are the same for both horses and cattle. The landmarks for dorsoventral position of the heart are the level of the shoulder joint for the heart base and the point of the elbow (olecranon) for the heart apex (Fig. 6-45). The craniocaudal position is defined by the caudal border of the triceps muscle, which roughly divides the heart into cranial and caudal halves. Using these landmarks, the position of the heart can be estimated and generally corresponds to the fourth or fifth intercostal space.

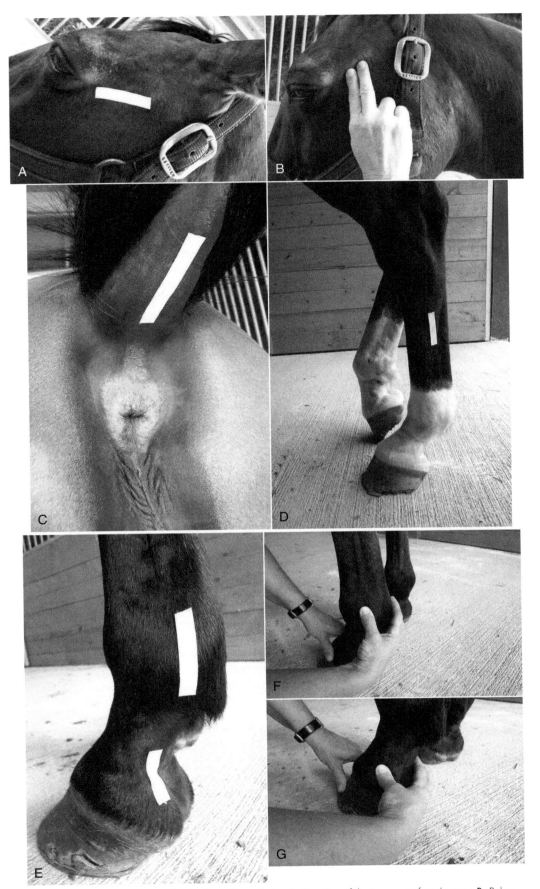

FIGURE 6-44 Locating and palpating other arteries. **A,** Location of the transverse facial artery. **B,** Palpation of the transverse facial artery. **C,** Location of the coccygeal artery. **D,** Location of the dorsal metatarsal artery. **E,** Location of the lateral digital artery over the lateral proximal sesamoid bone and proximal to the lateral collateral cartilage. **F,** Palpation of the digital arteries over the proximal sesamoid bones. **G,** Palpation of the digital arteries proximal to the collateral cartilages.

Usually, the heart is best heard cranially to the caudal border of the triceps muscle. However, the triceps muscle is too thick to allow the heart sounds to be heard through it. Therefore, it is essential to place the head of the stethoscope directly against the chest wall but stay deep to the triceps muscle. This is easily accomplished by gently using a hand to lift the muscle slightly away from the chest wall before the stethoscope is positioned (Fig. 6-46). Another approach is to move the forelimb to a more forward position, as if the animal were taking a step forward, which moves the triceps cranially. However, many animals are reluctant to hold this position for any length of time, and this position is nearly impossible to achieve in cattle.

Cardiac sounds are normally only S1 and S2 in cattle (unlike the horse, in which any combination of S3 and S4 may accompany S1 and S2). The heart rate is counted as beats per minute. The cardiac sounds S1 (lub) and S2 (dub) are components of one heartbeat. A common error, especially made by those accustomed to small animal auscultation, is to count S1 and S2 as separate beats, essentially doubling the actual heart rate. The heart rate in large animals is slow, and the heart sounds usually are loud and distinct, thus leading to the possible confusion.

> **TECHNICIAN NOTE**   The cardiac sounds of S1 (lub) and S2 (dub) are components of one heartbeat.

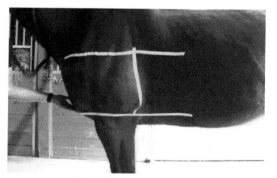

FIGURE 6-45 Landmarks for the heart. The *horizontal marks* indicate the level of the shoulder and elbow joints. The *vertical mark* indicates the caudal border of the triceps muscle.

Auscultation is also used to detect abnormal heart sounds or murmurs. Murmurs are not uncommon in horses. Most murmurs are physiologic, normal heart sounds and are simply the result of large volumes of blood moving at high speeds through the heart valves. Because of the large heart size, these sounds are readily heard and are referred to as ejection murmurs. Ejection murmurs are commonly heard in horses and should disappear when the horse is exercised. True cardiac disease is unusual in horses but is usually accompanied by murmurs or other abnormal sounds. The clinician should be alerted whenever abnormal sounds are heard because the sounds may need to be characterized and investigated further. Murmurs are assessed for loudness and for the time of their occurrence in the cardiac cycle (systolic or diastolic). The horse may be exercised to see whether the abnormal sound disappears, stays the same, or becomes louder with exercise. Using these criteria, the clinician decides whether further diagnostic tests are warranted.

Body Temperature

Temperature is almost always taken rectally, by using a standard mercury thermometer or a digital thermometer. Rarely, vaginal temperature is used. Although any thermometer may be used on large animals, special large animal thermometers are commonly available. Large animal thermometers are typically 5 inches long and have a thicker glass casing than regular thermometers. In addition, they often include a ring top, which allows the user to attach a string (Fig. 6-47). Strings are helpful for two reasons: (1) aspiration of the thermometer into the rectum and (2) pushing the thermometer out of the rectum. Some animals pull the anus inward when the thermometer is in place (particularly horses), which occasionally results in aspiration of the thermometer into the rectum. This is potentially serious if the thermometer breaks inside the rectum or the animal strains to defecate; perforation of the rectum may occur and can be life-threatening. The presence of the thermometer in the anus may also stimulate defecation; if this occurs, the thermometer passes out of the rectum and falls to the ground, often breaking. Broken thermometer glass can puncture hooves or skin or may be eaten as the animal browses for food. Because of these complications, it is common either to maintain a firm grip on the

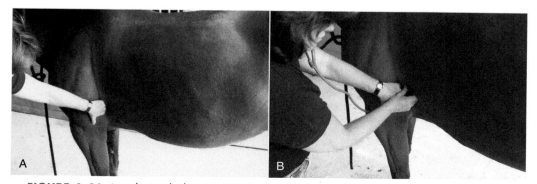

FIGURE 6-46 Auscultating the heart. **A,** Gently lift the triceps muscle away from the chest wall. **B,** Place stethoscope against the chest wall, deep to the triceps muscle.

thermometer for the entire procedure or to tie a string to the ring top and secure the string to the animal's tail hairs or hair coat (never the skin!) with a clothespin or alligator clamp. If the horse aspirates the thermometer, the string can be used to retrieve it gently or to follow the string manually into the rectum to retrieve the thermometer. If the horse pushes the thermometer out of the rectum, the secured string should prevent it from falling on the ground. Do not attach a piece of string longer than 12 inches because longer strings allow the thermometer to dangle on the legs, and this causes some animals, especially horses, to kick.

> **TECHNICIAN NOTE** Always clip thermometers to the hair or physically hold the thermometer until you obtain a reading.

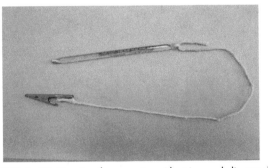

FIGURE 6-47 Ring-top thermometer with string and clip attached.

Placing the rectal thermometer requires some tact. The thermometer should be lubricated with petroleum jelly, mineral oil, water, "poor man's lube" (which is defecated fecal material—useful in animals that have normally loose stools), the time-honored method of spitting a small amount of saliva on the thermometer tip, or dipping the thermometer in the animal's water bucket. The practice of using fecal material, spitting on the thermometer, or dipping the thermometer in the water bucket gives the impression of disregard for sanitary procedure. Even if the thermometer has been properly disinfected, owners view it as a piece of equipment that has been in other animals' rectums and has no place in their animal's water bucket.

To insert the thermometer, stand next to the animal's hindquarters and face caudally (Fig. 6-48, *A*). Do not stand directly behind the animal unless it is restrained in a squeeze chute. If the animal resists by kicking, the technician can stand behind a stall door or a stack of hay bales for protection. Grasp the tail near the base and elevate it or push it to the opposite side of the animal. It is not necessary to "crank" the tail to an extreme position—this only meets with resistance by the animal. Another trick is to apply gentle pressure to the inside of skin beside the anus, and a horse that is clinching its tail down onto its anus will sometimes lift its tail. Move the tail only enough to gain clear entrance to the anus (Fig. 6-48, *B*). Some animals respond best to gentle rubbing of the perianal area before touching the anus with the thermometer. It is often good practice to let the animal know what is coming rather than jamming the thermometer in the anus with no warning. The anal opening is identified either by look or by

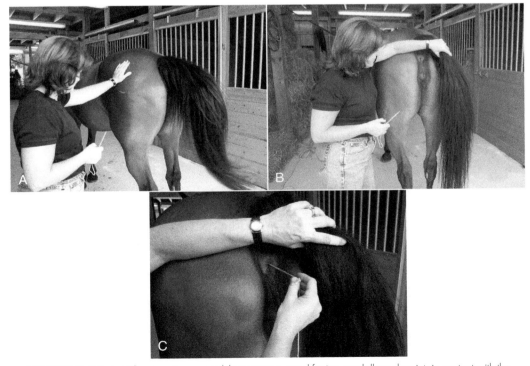

FIGURE 6-48 **A,** When inserting a rectal thermometer, stand facing caudally and maintain contact with the horse. **B,** Grasp the tail at the base and move it gently to the side. **C,** Insert the thermometer.

feel, and the thermometer is gently inserted with a twisting motion (Fig. 6-48, *C*). When taking the rectal temperature of the goat, a dark brown, waxy material may be seen near the anus; this secretion is normal and is produced by sebaceous glands under the tail head. Never force the thermometer if it does not easily advance because the rectal wall can be perforated with very little force. If the animal strains in resistance, try distracting it by offering feed or, in the case of the horse, having someone tap on its forehead. The thermometer usually passes horizontally, but some horses require tipping the thermometer slightly upward (dorsally).

The thermometer should be advanced several inches into the rectum, then either held by hand or clipped to the tail hairs (Fig. 6-49, *A*) or coat hairs (Fig. 6-49, *B*). It should be left in place for at least 60 seconds (mercury type) or until the audible/visual signal is heard or seen (digital type). Placement of a digital rectal thermometer in a steer is shown in Figure 6-50.

Normal temperature varies by age, breed, and environment of the animal. Body temperature is typically lowest in the morning. Temperatures outside of the normal range for animals may be normal for some individuals or could be altered by exercise or hot weather, so these situations should always be considered. Other circumstances may influence temperature. Draft horses tend to have low rectal temperatures. Neonatal foals may lack some ability to generate body heat and often have low body temperatures immediately after birth. Temperature of older foals may average approximately 1° F higher than in adults for the first few days to weeks after birth. Rectal procedures such as rectal examination may allow air to enter the rectum, leading to a balloon effect in which the rectum fills with air. This will falsely lower rectal temperature; therefore, temperature should be taken before any rectal procedure. If the rectum contains feces, the thermometer tip may be inadvertently inserted into a fecal ball. This is the most common cause of unexpectedly low readings. If this occurs, the procedure should be repeated.

> **TECHNICIAN NOTE**   Consider all environmental factors when taking rectal temperatures.

Abdominal Auscultation

A stethoscope is used to listen to abdominal sounds, which are created by movements of the intestines. This is commonly

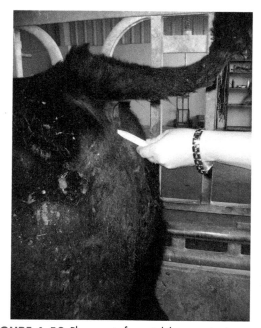

FIGURE 6-50 Placement of a rectal thermometer in a steer.

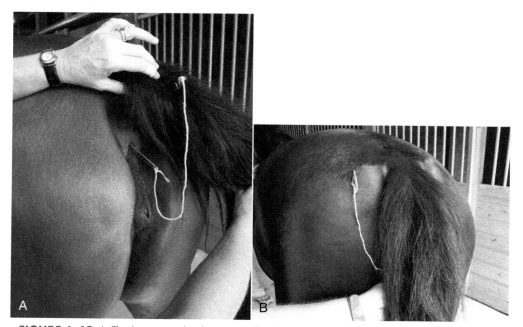

FIGURE 6-49 **A,** The thermometer has been inserted and secured with the clip to the tail hairs. **B,** Thermometer secured to hair coat with the clip.

referred to as GI motility. This term is somewhat of a misnomer because some sounds are generated by passive movement of gas and liquids in the intestines without any actual propelling motion by the intestinal musculature. Therefore, it is not completely accurate to assume that all intestinal sounds are caused by functional intestines. This becomes important in the patient with GI disease. Sick portions of intestine may have little or no purposeful motility, yet passive fluid and gas sounds may be heard. Experience is required to distinguish active from passive sounds.

Abdominal auscultation in the horse should be performed on both sides of the animal. The common site for auscultation is the *flank*, the area between the pelvis and the caudal margin of the rib cage. The flank is normally slightly depressed. The point of the hip is the dorsal extent of the flank area (Fig. 6-51). The flank is only part of the total abdominal wall, and auscultation can be performed at any location on the abdominal wall. Horses may be sensitive in the flank and abdominal area, so these areas should be approached slowly and gently. A good method is to place the hand with the stethoscope on the horse's back and slowly slide it to the flank or lower abdominal area.

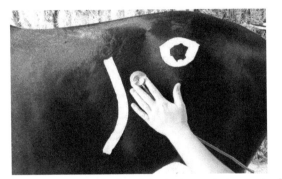

FIGURE 6-51 Landmarks for abdominal auscultation in the flank area are the point of the hip (tuber coxae) and the last rib.

> **TECHNICIAN NOTE** When performing abdominal auscultation in the horse, place your hand with the stethoscope on the horse's back and slowly and gently slide it to the flank or lower abdominal area.

A standard four-point auscultation usually is sufficient for most patients. The stethoscope is used to auscultate the upper flank and the lower flank on both sides of the abdomen. The four points are referred to as the upper left, upper right, lower left, and lower right quadrants (Fig. 6-52 and Box 6-3). Results of the auscultation at each location are recorded as follows:

0 = No motility heard
+1 = Hypomotility
+2 = Normal motility
+3 = Hypermotility

Intestinal motility sounds, also called *borborygmi*, have been described as sounding like thunder rumbling or an approaching freight train. These sounds are usually associated with coordinated, normal patterns of large intestinal motility. The number of borborygmi per minute is counted in each abdominal quadrant; the stethoscope should be left in place *at least 1 minute* at *each* of the four points to obtain an accurate count. "Normal" motility is considered to be one to three

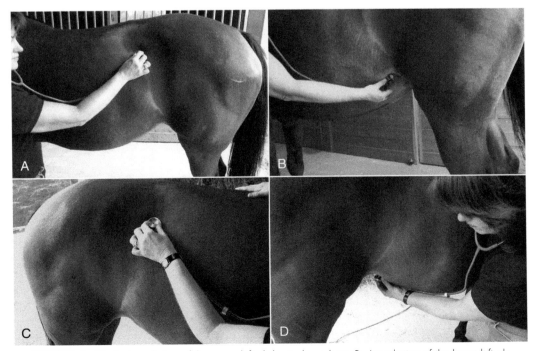

FIGURE 6-52 A, Auscultation of the upper left abdominal quadrant. **B,** Auscultation of the lower left abdominal quadrant. **C,** Auscultation of the upper right upper abdominal quadrant. **D,** Auscultation of the lower right abdominal quadrant.

borborygmi per minute in each abdominal quadrant. More than this rate is considered to be hypermotility, and less than this rate is considered to be hypomotility. Complete absence of borborygmus is equated with intestinal standstill, properly termed *ileus*. Ileus typically indicates serious intestinal disease and is often associated with increased morbidity and mortality. Remember, however, that gas and fluid "tinkling" sounds may still be heard in the patient with ileus. These are passive sounds and should *not* be confused with functional intestine.

> **TECHNICIAN NOTE** When performing abdominal auscultation, the technician should listen to all four quadrants on both the left and right sides. The technician should listen to each quadrant for at least 1 minute.

Evaluation of the ruminant abdomen includes assessment of rumen contractions. The rumen occupies most of the left side of the abdominal cavity. The number of rumen contractions per minute may be counted by auscultation directly over the caudolateral rib cage or paralumbar fossa on the left side. Contractions sound like a deep rumbling or thunderstorm noise that becomes gradually louder as the contraction approaches the stethoscope. Rumen contractions can also be counted by *ballottement* (palpation) by pressing both fists firmly into the left paralumbar fossa (use one fist in the sheep and goat). The fists are allowed to remain against the body wall for 1 minute. Each rumen contraction is felt as a wave passing under the hands that pushes the hands slightly outward (Fig. 6-53). The normal animal has one to two contractions per minute. Hypomotility and absence of motility (ileus) are abnormal findings; hypermotility of the rumen also is unusual. Auscultation of the right side of the abdomen usually reveals few sounds; this is normal in ruminants.

The shape of the abdomen is observed by standing behind the animal and facing the head. The overall shape of the

> **BOX 6-3 | Four-Point Abdominal Auscultation**
>
> The four-point auscultation is recorded using a grid that identifies each abdominal quadrant as follows:
>
> | Upper left quadrant | Upper right quadrant |
> |---|---|
> | Lower left quadrant | Lower right quadrant |
>
> Results of the auscultation at each location are recorded as follows:
> 0 = No motility heard
> +1 = Hypomotility
> +2 = Normal motility
> +3 = Hypermotility
> For example, a horse with hypomotility in the lower right quadrant and a normal number of borborygmi in all other quadrants would be recorded as follows:
>
> $$\frac{+2|+2}{+2|+3}$$

right and left abdominal "silhouettes" should be similar, and the overall outline of the cow should resemble a pear (i.e., wider at the lower flanks than at the paralumbar fossae). The paralumbar fossae normally should be flat or slightly sunken. Accumulation of gas within certain portions of the GI tract (tympany or "bloat") can produce asymmetry and enlargement of the abdominal wall. Severe abdominal gas accumulation causes enlargement of the paralumbar fossa on both sides of the animal, changing the shape from a pear to an apple. The most common location for bloat, the rumen, appears as an enlargement of the left paralumbar fossa; this has been referred to as a "papple" shape, in which the left side resembles an apple and the right side a pear (Figs. 6-54 and 6-55).

> **TECHNICIAN NOTE** Bloat in ruminants is identified by enlargement of the left paralumbar fossa.

Gas accumulations can also be detected by percussion and auscultation with the stethoscope. The stethoscope is held in place with one hand while the other hand is used to snap a finger against the abdominal wall at several locations around the stethoscope head. In order to elicit the distinctive ping noise, you must almost snap your finger hard enough to cause minimal pain in your fingertips. Gas accumulations make a resonant "ping" sound, like a high-pitched drum. Pings generally indicate abnormal position or contents of

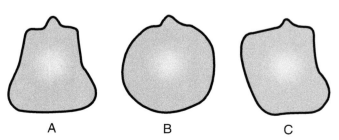

FIGURE 6-53 Ballottement of the rumen contractions.

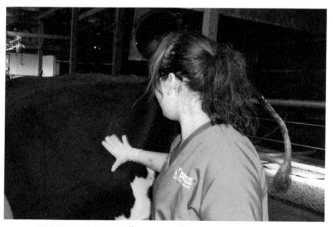

A   B   C

FIGURE 6-54 Shapes of the ruminant abdomen, observed from behind. **A,** Normal pear shape. **B,** Abnormal apple shape. **C,** Abnormal "papple" shape.

one or more GI tract organs. Solid organs and non-GI organs cannot accumulate gas and therefore do not ping (except the uterus, which is extremely rare). Pinging should be performed on both sides of the abdomen and may detect abnormalities before they are visible as external enlargement of the abdomen (Figs. 6-56 to 6-58).

During a colic examination, it is important to listen to the lower abdomen around the midline to evaluate for sounds of the ocean; this can be important in identifying sand colic (e.g., colic induced by consuming sandy soil).

Mucous Membranes

Mucous membranes are tissues that have the ability to make and secrete mucus. The color of mucous membranes is helpful for disease diagnosis. Several mucous membranes are readily visible to the examiner: the gums (gingiva) (Fig. 6-59, *A*), conjunctiva of the eye (Fig. 6-59, *B*), lining of the nostrils (Fig. 6-59, *C*), the prepuce, and the inner surfaces of the vulva in females (Fig. 6-59, *D*). The inner surface of the ear pinna does not secrete mucus and therefore is not a mucous membrane, although it may be useful for detecting icterus and evidence of clotting disorders.

If full opening of the mouth is necessary for examination, placing the fingers into the interdental space and pressing on the hard palate encourages the mouth to open. The tongue can be quickly grasped and brought to the side at the commissure of the lips, where it encourages the animal to keep the mouth open. Alternatively, use of a mouth speculum may be indicated. The tongue of cattle is strong and has a single deep transverse groove across its dorsal surface; this groove is often mistaken for a laceration. The molars of ruminants

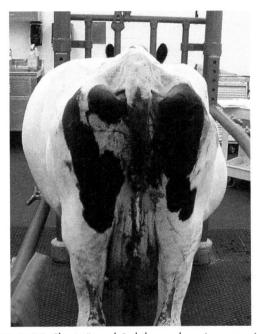

FIGURE 6-55 Classic "papple" abdomen shape in a cow with ruminal bloat. (From Fubini SL, Ducharme NG: *Farm animal surgery*, St. Louis, 2004, Saunders.)

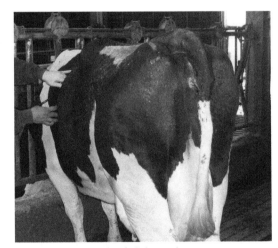

FIGURE 6-57 Example of abdominal percussion or "pinging."

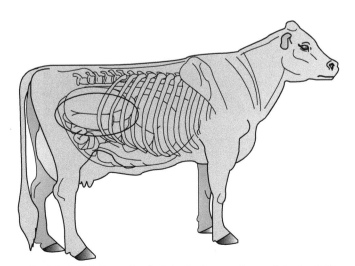

FIGURE 6-56 Example of abdominal percussion or "pinging." The *shaded area* indicates the location of resonance (ping) associated with accumulation of air in the cecum resulting from cecal volvulus. (From Fubini SL, Ducharme NG: *Farm animal surgery*, St. Louis, 2004, Saunders.)

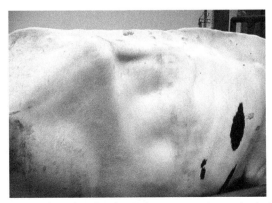

FIGURE 6-58 Right side of a Holstein cow with cecal volvulus (rib cage visible to the *right*, tuber coxae and pelvis to the *left*). Observe distention in the right paralumbar fossa, corresponding to the area of abdominal "ping." (From Fubini SL, Ducharme NG: *Farm animal surgery*, St. Louis, 2004, Saunders.)

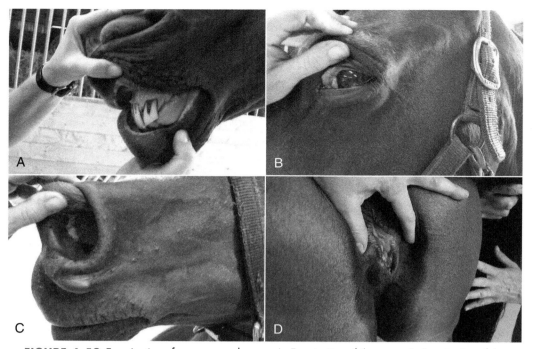

A

B

C

D

FIGURE 6-59 Examination of mucous membranes. **A,** Examination of the gums. **B,** Examination of the conjunctiva. **C,** Examination of the mucosa of the nares. **D,** Examination of the vulva in the female.

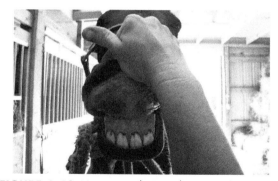

FIGURE 6-60 Mucous membrane color. Normal gum color.

may be sharp and jagged, and caution must be used whenever the hands are placed into an animal's mouth. When examining the mouth and head, and especially with cattle, be aware of the possibility of being struck by the animal's head if it is not properly restrained.

The mucous membrane color usually is light to dark pink (Fig. 6-60). The color may change with abnormalities of blood perfusion and oxygen content of the blood and other diseases. *Cyanosis* is a bluish tint that usually indicates extremely low oxygen content in the tissue. Brickred coloration indicates bacterial septicemia, septic shock, or both (Fig. 6-61). Endotoxic shock in the horse has the unique characteristic of producing a purple gum line along the margins of the teeth, referred to as the *toxic line*. Yellowish coloring of the gums indicates icterus, which usually is related to hepatic dysfunction or abnormal hemolysis of red blood cells. Pale mucous membranes may indicate anemia or poor perfusion; however, the gums of

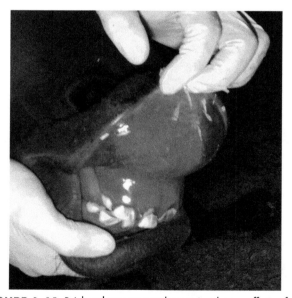

FIGURE 6-61 Brick-red mucous membranes in a horse suffering from severe diarrhea, colic, and endotoxemia. (From Bassert JM, McCurnin DM: *McCurnin's clinical textbook for veterinary technicians,* ed 7, St. Louis, 2010, Saunders.)

some horses normally are pale pink and do not indicate disease in these animals.

> **TECHNICIAN NOTE**   Endotoxic shock in the horse has a unique characteristic of producing a purple gum line along the margins of the teeth; this is referred to as the toxic line.

Clotting disorders may create reddish spotting of the mucous membranes. Small pinpoint hemorrhages less than 1 mm in diameter are called *petechial hemorrhages*. Hemorrhages 1 mm to 1 cm in diameter are called *ecchymotic hemorrhages*. Larger hemorrhages are referred to as *purpuric hemorrhages*.

Mucous membranes are also assessed for moisture and are commonly described as moist, dry, tacky, or other subjective terms. This information is less useful than the color of the membranes.

Hydration Status

The hydration status of an animal is important information. It can be measured with laboratory tests or estimated from the physical examination. Two main methods of assessing hydration of the animal on physical examination are the skin turgor test and the *capillary refill time* (CRT).

The *skin turgor* test is also known as the *skin pinch test*. The loose skin over the point of the shoulder is briefly and firmly pinched with the fingers and allowed to retract to its original position. In normally hydrated animals, the skin snaps back to its original position in approximately 1 second or less. In dehydrated animals (>5% dehydration), the response is prolonged to more than 1 second. In severely dehydrated animals, the skin may take 8 seconds or longer to retract. Skin turgor is less reliable in obese animals; fat in the cervical area may falsely improve the skin snap.

The CRT is assessed by pressing briefly but firmly on the gums with a fingertip to produce a "blanched" white spot (Fig. 6-62). The time for the original color to return to the blanched spot is counted in seconds. "Cranking" a horse's lips widely apart to access the gums is not necessary; the lips need to be elevated only enough to see the gum line. Original color should return in less than 2 seconds. Dehydration and shock prolong the CRT. Severe dehydration and severe shock may greatly prolong the CRT to 5 to 8 seconds.

> **TECHNICIAN NOTE** Prolonged capillary refill time (CRT) may be indicative of severe dehydration or severe shock.

Height and Weight Measurement

Height and weight measurement may serve different purposes. Height measurement in horses may be required as part of the insurance and prepurchase examinations, for breed registration, and for entry into certain horse show classes. Hip height in cattle can also be an important measurement, and you may be asked to perform this measurement as well. Weight measurement is generally used for calculating the proper dose of drugs and therapeutic substances and for formulating the animal's diet.

Height measurement may seem like a benign procedure to the novice horseman or horsewoman, but it can be a major

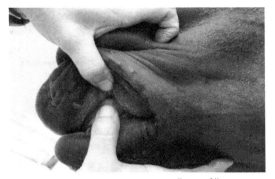

FIGURE 6-62 Assessing capillary refill time.

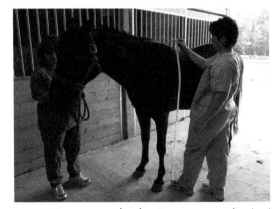

FIGURE 6-63 Measuring height. Proper position for the height/weight tape for measuring height.

issue for many horse owners. Registration of an individual into a particular breed may depend on the height of the adult animal; unregistered animals have little reproductive value.

Height in horses may be estimated roughly or measured precisely. Ponies are less than 14.2 hands high.

Rough estimates can be made with a height/weight tape. This instrument is essentially a tape measure, marked in hands (1 hand = 4 inches). Height is ideally measured with the horse on a firm surface. The horse's head should not be elevated or lowered but should be in a horizontal position, paralleling the ground. The tape is secured on the ground with a foot just behind a forelimb (Fig. 6-63, *A*). The tape is then stretched vertically to the withers, and the height is read at the level of the most caudal mane hair or the highest point of the withers. Although this is the standard procedure, I have seen variations in the locations where the measurements should be started and stopped. Therefore, if the measurement is being performed for a show or association, it is to your benefit to confirm how the measurements should be taken (Fig. 6-63, *B*). The tape gives an approximation of the animal's height.

For precise determination of height, commercially made rigid measuring rulers are available. These rulers are made of metal and include carpenter's bubble levels to ensure that the ruler is not tilted when the measurement is taken. Again, the animal should be on firm ground, with the head and neck held level with the ground, and the measurement should be

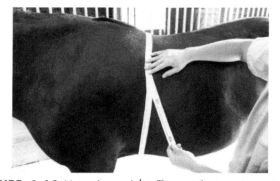

FIGURE 6-64 Measuring weight. The weight tape is positioned around the thorax at the girth.

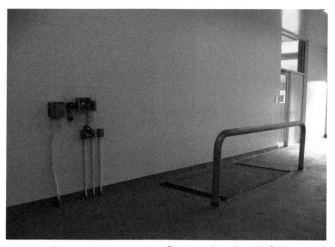

FIGURE 6-65 Equine walkover scale within the floor.

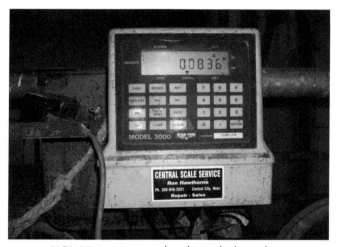

FIGURE 6-66 Livestock scale attached to a chute.

taken at the last mane hair or highest point of the withers, depending on the registry or rules of competition.

Weight can be roughly estimated with the height/weight tape or taken specifically with a livestock scale. The height/weight tape has one side calibrated for weight measurement. The weight tick marks are based on measurements at the girth of the horse. The tape is applied to encircle the horse at its girth, the area behind the withers just behind the forelimb (Fig. 6-64). The weight tape is formulated from logarithms of normal animals and may be inaccurate for extremely thin or obese animals. The build of an animal may also affect the results. Height/weight tapes for cattle are not accurate for horses. Another calculation for weight in horses is as follows:

$$\frac{\text{Heart girth} \times \text{Heart girth} \times \text{Body length}}{330} = \text{Weight (pounds)}$$

This calculation tends to be more accurate than other methods when a scale is not available.

Precise weights for large animals can be obtained with standard livestock scales or digital livestock scales. Walkover-style digital scales are popular at many hospitals and clinics (Figs. 6-65 and 6-66). When taking multiple cattle weights as the animals follow each other through the chute, it is important to remember to zero the scale or tare the scale every 5 to 10 head. This helps to keep the weight measurements accurate because added fecal material in the chute will alter the weights with time. In addition, most of these chutes are suspended, and just the movement of the cattle through the chute can alter the actual weight being displayed.

NEUROLOGIC EXAMINATION

The purpose of the "neuro examination" is threefold:
1. Confirm that neurologic disease is present, or not.
2. Localize where disease is occurring in the nervous system (Box 6-4).
3. Arrive at a diagnosis or formulate a list of possible diagnoses (rule-out list). Further diagnostic tests are usually required to confirm the specific neurologic disease from a list of rule-outs.

The technician may assist in the performance of neurologic examinations. Truly neurologically affected animals must be handled cautiously. Certain diseases can produce ataxia and other deficits that predispose the animal to stumbling and

---

BOX 6-4 | Basic Localization of Neurologic Lesions

Central Nervous System
- Cerebrum
- Cerebellum
- Brainstem (medulla)
- Spinal cord

Peripheral Nervous System
- Peripheral nerves
- Neuromuscular junctions

---

perhaps falling, possibly injuring the handler. Even recumbent animals with "neuro" cases (unless they are completely paralyzed) must be respected for the potential damage that can be caused by thrashing legs and struggling efforts to stand.

The neurologic examination is similar to that performed in small animals, with a few modifications. If the patient is presented in recumbency, additional modifications may be necessary. Minimal equipment is needed for a basic examination; however, referral to a well-equipped hospital may be required if further diagnostics are necessary.

BOX 6-5	Cranial Nerves

- CN 1: Olfactory nerve
- CN 2: Optic nerve
- CN 3: Oculomotor nerve
- CN 4: Trochlear nerve
- CN 5: Trigeminal nerve
- CN 6: Abducens nerve
- CN 7: Facial nerve
- CN 8: Vestibulocochlear (auditory) nerve
- CN 9: Glossopharyngeal nerve
- CN 10: Vagus nerve
- CN 11: Spinal accessory nerve
- CN 12: Hypoglossal nerve

The basic neurologic examination consists of the following steps:

1. History and general physical examination
2. Observation
   a. Behavior
   b. Mental status (level of awareness or consciousness)
   c. Posture and coordination: Head, body, and limbs are observed for abnormalities such as head tilt, weakness, ataxia, and involuntary movements such as tremors, muscle asymmetry, tetany, and myoclonus
3. Cranial nerve (CN) examination (Box 6-5)
   a. Smell: CN 1: Smell is difficult to assess but is usually evaluated by noting reactions to isopropyl alcohol, food, feces, and so forth, held close to the nostrils. Problems with olfaction are rare in horses.
   b. Menace reflex: CN 2/CN 7: Vision is assessed by the menace reflex, which is performed by making a gesture toward the eye and watching for closure of the eyelid and/or withdrawal of the head. The test also assesses CN 7, which is necessary to close the eyelid. The test is best performed with several fingers spread apart to avoid creating and pushing a current of air against the cornea. The cornea can feel air currents and initiates closure of the eyelid, even in a blind animal. The menace reflex is not fully developed in neonatal foals until approximately 2 weeks of age.
      Vision may also be assessed by walking the horse through an obstacle course. To prevent "cheating," you may need to blindfold one of the horse's eyes to assess vision accurately in the opposite eye.
   c. Pupillary light reflex: CN 2/CN 3: When a light is directed into one eye, the pupils of both eyes should constrict in response. The "direct response" is the constriction of the pupil on the same side as the light, and the "consensual response" is constriction of the opposite eye. Proper function of both CN 2 and CN 3 is necessary for a normal pupillary light reflex but is not a test of vision; blind horses may have normal pupillary light responses.
   d. Pupil symmetry: CN 2/CN 3: The pupils are assessed for miosis (constriction), mydriasis (dilation), and anisocoria (pupils of different size).

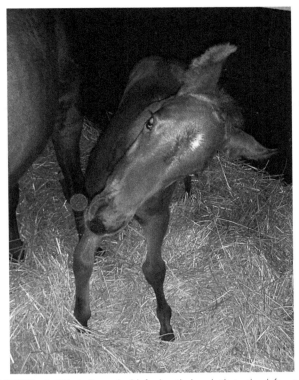

FIGURE 6-67 A 2-month-old foal with head tilt to the left, ptosis (drooping) of the left eyelid, drooping left ear pinna, and deviation of the muzzle to the right. (From McAuliffe SB, Slovis NM: *Color atlas of diseases and disorders of the foal,* St. Louis, 2008, Saunders.)

   e. Eye position: CN 3/CN 4/CN 6/CN 8: The position of the eye within the orbit is assessed at rest and while the head is rotated slowly from side to side. Abnormal position at rest (strabismus) and abnormal eye movement (nystagmus) may occur. When the horse's head is elevated, the normal response is for the eyes to try to remain horizontal, thus causing a natural ventral rotation; this is sometimes referred to as the doll's eye effect.
   f. Facial sensation: CN 5/CN 7: A blunt object is used to touch or lightly pinch the areas of the face, ears, and mouth. The horse should respond with movement of muscles in the area or withdrawal of the head. It is important to touch both the medial canthus and the lateral canthus of each eye because of separate innervation of each location.
   g. Facial symmetry: CN 5/CN 7: The muscles of the head are observed for atrophy and loss of muscle tone. Drooping of the ear, lips, and/or eyelids is abnormal. Deviation of the muzzle to one side is also abnormal (Fig. 6-67).
   h. Hearing: CN 8: Hearing is difficult to evaluate, and assessment is usually done by clapping or producing a loud noise and watching for a response. Deafness in horses is rare.
   i. Tongue pull: CN 12: The tongue is pulled out of the mouth to one side, and the horse should retract it back into the mouth within several seconds. The test is repeated to the opposite side (Fig. 6-68). The tongue

should also be inspected for atrophy of one or both sides, which occasionally occurs.

j. Swallowing: CN 9/CN 10: Abnormal swallowing may cause water, feed, or saliva to dribble from the mouth or nostrils.

4. Gait assessment

a. Observation of the horse at the walk and trot performed on a straight line and in circles.

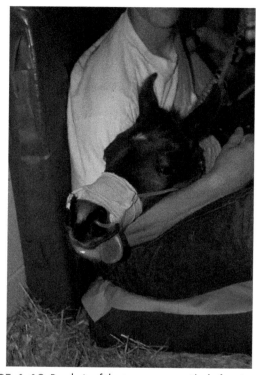

FIGURE 6-68 Paralysis of the tongue seen with dysfunction of cranial nerve 12. (From McAuliffe SB, Slovis NM: *Color atlas of diseases and disorders of the foal*, St. Louis, 2008, Saunders.)

b. Circling: Sometimes called "spinning," the horse is turned in very tight circles, and the coordination of the limbs is observed. The handler should turn the horse's head sharply to one side so that the hindquarters respond by moving away from the handler. This is maintained until the horse has turned 360 degrees several times. The procedure is repeated on both sides of the horse. Falling, stepping on itself, failing to lift the legs, or wide circumduction of the outside limb may be abnormal behavior (Fig. 6-69).

c. Backing: Limb coordination of the horse is observed. Dragging the legs or stepping on itself may be abnormal.

d. Incline walking: The horse is walked up and down an incline while limb coordination is observed.

e. Elevated head walking: The handler holds the lead rope in one hand and uses the other hand to elevate the horse's head (beneath the chin) so that the nostrils are level with the poll. The horse is then walked in a straight line. Elevating the head may accentuate proprioceptive deficits. This test may also be performed on an incline; the handler must be extremely careful not to position himself or herself directly in front of the horse in case the horse stumbles and falls.

5. Postural reactions

a. Sway reaction: This test is performed either by pushing sideways on the horse's forequarters or hindquarters or by pulling the horse sideways by the tail ("tail pull" or "tail sway" test). Normal horses should make an effort to resist the push or pull. The tail pull must be performed cautiously so that the handler is not kicked; it is safest to grasp the tail near its end, to create some space between the handler and the horse. The handler should stay laterally even with the hindquarters, not lagging behind the hindquarters, where a kick is possible. The test is repeated on both sides

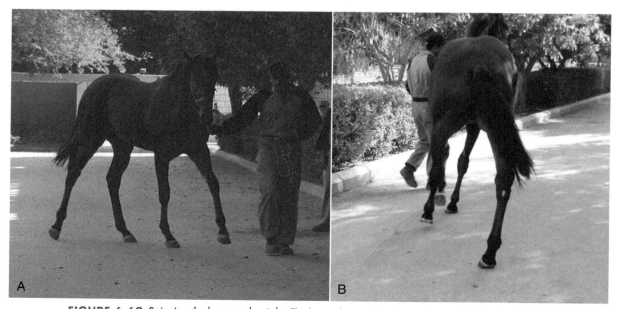

FIGURE 6-69 Spinning the horse to the right. The horse shows wide circumduction of the hindlimbs, truncal sway at the turn (**A**), and the hypermetric movement of the left forelimb (**B**). (From McAuliffe SB, Slovis NM: *Color atlas of diseases and disorders of the foal*, St. Louis, WB Saunders, 2008.)

and may also be performed while the horse is walked in a straight line.

b. Placing responses: A leg is lifted and set down in an abnormal position, such as a base-wide stance or a cross-legged position (Fig. 6-70). The normal response is for the horse to reposition the leg directly beneath itself within several seconds. This test is variable in individuals and may be difficult to evaluate.

c. Hopping: This test is difficult to perform in large animals. One person handles the head and one performs the maneuver. One of the horse's legs is elevated while lateral pressure is applied to the shoulder (for a forelimb) or hip (for a hindlimb) area to encourage the horse to hop sideways on three legs (Fig. 6-71).

6. Spinal reflexes
   a. Anal/perineal reflex: The anus and perineal area are gently prodded with a blunt instrument. The anus should contract in response. The handler must take care to stand to the side of the horse (similar position to taking rectal temperature) to avoid being kicked (Fig. 6-72).
   b. Patellar reflex/triceps reflex: The patellar tendon or triceps tendon is struck with a soft rubber mallet. This test is difficult to perform accurately in nonrecumbent animals and may elicit a kick from some individuals.
   c. Withdrawal reflexes: A hemostat or blunt probe is used to press or pinch the skin of the limbs. The normal animal will withdraw (flex) the limb in response. The evaluator should avoid the path of the flexed limb because flexure may be forceful and rapid, producing injury.

7. Tail tone: Most horses resist elevation of the tail. A limp or weak tail may be abnormal.

8. Cutaneous sensation
   a. Panniculus response: A blunt instrument is used to stimulate (by pinching or pricking) the skin across the neck and body lightly. Twitching of the cutaneous muscles in response is normal and should be brisk (Fig. 6-73).
   b. Limbs: The skin over the limbs is similarly stimulated, to look for areas of decreased or absent sensation.

Following the basic neurologic examination, the clinician makes an initial assessment of the animal's condition and recommends treatment or further diagnostic tests. Box 6-6 and Figure 6-74 cover special diagnostics.

COLIC EXAMINATION

Colic is a nonspecific term that means "abdominal pain." Although most cases of colic in horses are caused by diseases of the GI system, other organ systems such as the urinary and reproductive tracts are also located in the abdomen and can cause colic when they are diseased. Some musculoskeletal conditions can also effectively mimic colic.

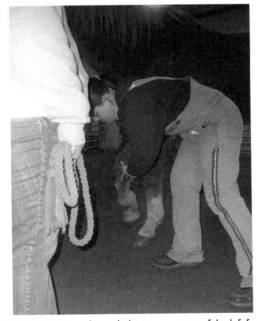

FIGURE 6-70 Cross-legged placing response of the left forelimb.

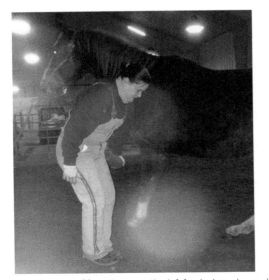

FIGURE 6-71 Lateral hopping test. The left forelimb is elevated while pressure is applied to the shoulder to encourage hopping to the right.

> **TECHNICIAN NOTE** Colic means abdominal pain.

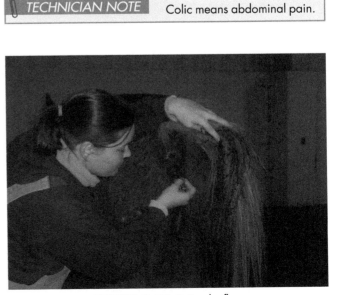

FIGURE 6-72 Perineal reflex.

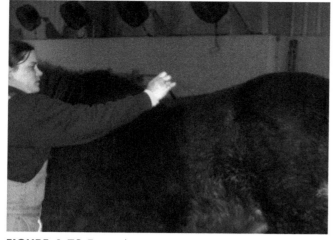

FIGURE 6-73 Testing the cutaneous sensation of the trunk by gently pressing with a blunt instrument, such as a ballpoint pen.

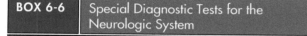

BOX 6-6	Special Diagnostic Tests for the Neurologic System

Diagnostic Imaging
- Plain film radiographs: The head and cervical regions can be radiographed. Sedation or general anesthesia may be necessary. The thoracolumbar spine and sacral spine are difficult to image, except perhaps in small individuals.
- Contrast radiography (myelogram): In large animals, this procedure is used for cervical spinal cord evaluation. General anesthesia is required. The procedure is performed with the animal in lateral recumbency. Injection of contrast medium is performed at the atlantooccipital space. The head is elevated during and for approximately 5 minutes after injection of contrast medium to encourage caudal flow of contrast material away from the brain. Owners should be warned of the risk of seizures and other possible reactions. Recovery from general anesthesia in neurologically affected animals presents additional patient risk (see Fig. 6-74).
- Computed tomography/magnetic resonance imaging: Currently available equipment limits imaging to the head and cranial cervical regions.
- Nuclear scintigraphy: This technology can be used to image the vertebral column.

Electrodiagnostics
The following are possible in large animals:
- Electroencephalogram
- Electromyogram
- Auditory brainstem response testing
- Nerve conduction studies

Horses with colic usually display easily observed signs of pain and discomfort. However, mild colic may be missed by inexperienced horse owners, and stoic horses may not show the full extent of their discomfort. Signs of colic pain may include one or more of the following:
- Sweating
- Pawing with the front feet, which may become so persistent that horses wear away areas of the hoof wall

- Frequent posturing to urinate but expelling little or no urine
- Looking back at the flanks
- Crouching as if preparing to lie down
- Lying down for prolonged periods of time
- Rolling on the ground
- Grinding the teeth (bruxism)
- Quivering upper lip
- Signs of self-trauma that may accompany severely painful conditions, often seen best on the head and face (especially the periorbital region) as a result of repeated thrashing of the head against the ground
- Increased respiratory and pulse rates
- Kicking at the abdomen with the hind feet
- Groaning
- Standing with the back arched ("hunched up")
- Playing with water but not drinking
- Lying on the back
- Dog-sitting (uncommon)

In addition to signs of pain, various other clinical signs may occur depending on the underlying disease and severity of the underlying disease:
- Dehydration
- Cardiovascular shock
- Abdominal distention
- Abnormal mucous membrane color
- Abnormal feces or absence of feces
- Abnormal rectal temperature

Colic should be considered an emergency situation, and a veterinarian should be consulted immediately. If you are talking to a client about colic over the telephone it is best to advise the client not to give any pain medications until the veterinarian has had a chance to examine the animal. Many horse owners have pain medication at the farm and will try to use it because they believe that it can make the animal feel comfortable; however, this often hides the extent of pain the horse is having once the veterinarian is able to examine the animal. Veterinarians often use the severity of colic to determine their diagnosis and treatment protocol, so the administration of pain medication by the client can compromise the recovery of the horse. Therefore, advise clients not to treat the animal unless a veterinarian has told them to do so.

> **TECHNICIAN NOTE**   You should always advise clients not to give pain medications to a horse experiencing colic unless a veterinarian has instructed them to do so. The veterinarian will evaluate the situation, determine the urgency for a colic examination, and advise the client on how to manage the horse until it can be examined.

> **TECHNICIAN NOTE**   Colic is an emergency situation!

The goals of the colic examination are to diagnose the cause of the colic and then provide appropriate medical and/or surgical treatment to resolve the condition. Unfortunately,

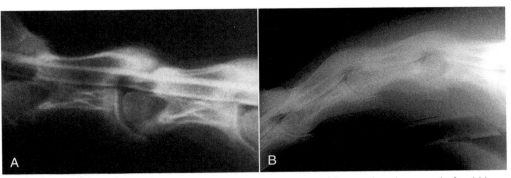

FIGURE 6-74 **A** and **B,** This myelogram is showing the narrowing of the spinal cord as a result of wobbler syndrome. (**A,** From Speirs VC: *Clinical examination of horses,* St. Louis, 1997, Saunders; **B,** from Auer JA: *Equine surgery,* ed 3, St. Louis, 2006 Saunders.)

BOX 6-7	Classification of Types of Colic*

1. Tympanic (gas) colic
2. Simple intestinal obstruction
3. Strangulating intestinal obstruction
4. Nonstrangulating intestinal infarction
5. Peritonitis
6. Enteritis/colitis
7. Gastrointestinal ulceration
8. Nongastrointestinal pain (urinary, reproductive, musculoskeletal)

*Some cases may involve a combination of two or more types of colic.

BOX 6-8	Setup Checklist for Basic Colic Examination

Nose twitch
Thermometer
Stethoscope
Rectal sleeve
Lubricant (nonsterile)
Nasogastric tube (assorted sizes)
Stomach pump
Dose syringe
Stainless steel bucket and warm water
Adhesive tape, 1-inch width
Ethylenediamine tetraacetic acid (EDTA) and serum
   Vacutainer blood tubes
Vacutainer sleeve and 20-gauge Vacutainer needles (18-, 19-, 20-gauge × 1½-inch needles; 3-, 6-, 12-mL syringes)
Clippers
Disposable razor
Latex examination gloves
Sterile latex gloves
Skin preparation materials (scrub, alcohol, gauze 4 × 4s)
IV catheters/materials for IV catheterization
Local anesthetic
Sedative/analgesic drugs

IV, Intravenous.

arriving at a specific diagnosis for the cause of colic is not often possible because of the limitations of the tools used for the examination, relative to the size and anatomy of the equine abdomen. A large portion of the abdomen cannot be palpated rectally or visualized with radiographs, ultrasound, or even laparoscopy. Even exploratory abdominal surgery is limited in visualization and ability to exteriorize certain parts of the abdomen. Despite the infrequency of a specific diagnosis, successful treatment of colic is often achieved. The reason for this success is, in part, the commonly used strategy of categorizing colic based on clinical signs and laboratory tests; once colic is categorized, rational treatment can be instituted (Box 6-7).

The technician performs a valuable role in assisting the veterinarian in the colic examination and should be familiar with the basic elements of the examination (Box 6-8). The veterinarian does not perform every component of the examination in each case and may alter the sequence of the examination based on the situation at hand. For instance, if shock is identified, treatment of shock may be instituted before the rest of the examination is completed. The components of the colic examination include the following:
- Observation
  - Pain: The horse is observed for signs and severity of colic. Pain assessment can be the single most important piece of information obtained during a colic examination. In patients with severe pain, the rest of the examination may not be possible until pain is controlled.
  - Attitude
  - Environmental surroundings
- History taking (Box 6-9)
  - General husbandry and management practices
  - History of the current colic episode
- Basic physical examination
  - Temperature
  - Pulse rate and rhythm
  - Respiratory rate and character
  - Physical condition/evidence of self-trauma
  - Mucous membrane color
  - CRT
  - Abdominal auscultation and percussion

BOX 6-9	History Taking of Patients With Colic

General Husbandry and Management
Environment/habitat
Feed types and sources
Feeding schedule
Water sources
Use of horse/daily routine
Routine/preventive health care program
Parasite control program
Medical/surgical history of patient

History Related to Current Colic Episode
Duration of colic (when first observed)
Progression of colic (pain increasing, decreasing, or static)
Recent feed consumption (what and when)
Recent water consumption
Recent medical problems/trauma
Recent medications
Possibility of exposure to foreign bodies or toxins
Pregnancy status
Previous colic episodes (diagnosis, treatments given, response)
Last defecation (character, volume, and time)
Response to treatment (if given)

- Nasogastric intubation
- Rectal examination
- Diagnostic sampling
  - Abdominocentesis
  - Blood work
  - Fecal specimen
    - Parasite evaluation
    - Presence of sand
    - Fecal culture
- Diagnostic imaging (only in selected cases)
  - Abdominal radiographs
  - Diagnostic ultrasound
  - Gastroscopy
  - Thermography
  - Laparoscopy

Nasogastric intubation is used as a diagnostic tool during the colic examination and as a treatment tool. Because horses cannot vomit, the stomach can become so distended with gas and ingesta that the stomach ruptures internally. Gastric rupture is a fatal condition, with or without surgical intervention. Therefore, intubation can be a lifesaving maneuver by providing an exit for accumulated gas and liquid. The stomach contents that are voided through the nasogastric tube (NGT) are referred to as *reflux*. Reflux may be gas, liquid, or a combination of both. Gas reflux cannot be accurately measured, but liquid reflux can be collected in a bucket and measured (Fig. 6-75). As diagnostic tools, the type and amount of reflux provide important information.

In some cases, the NGT is used to administer medications directly into the stomach. This can be safely done only in horses that are not having gastric reflux. Small volumes are given through a dose syringe, and larger volumes are pumped directly

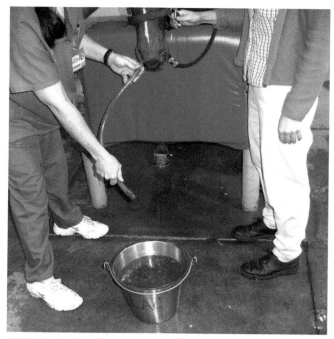

FIGURE 6-75 Collecting gastric reflux into a bucket. Note that one hand is used to stabilize the tube near the nostril. (From Sellon DC, Long MT: *Equine infectious diseases,* St. Louis, 2007, Saunders.)

from a bucket with a stomach pump. In colic cases, water is the most common treatment given by intubation. The water should be lukewarm. Substances such as electrolytes, bicarbonate, Epsom salts, activated charcoal, and mineral oil may be added to the water. Some of these substances are in powder form and should be dissolved well to prevent clogging the stomach pump. Mineral oil can be given with or without water (note that mineral oil stains clothing). After treatment, the NGT should be flushed thoroughly with warm or hot water and disinfectant; the outside of the tube should also be cleaned. Air can be flushed to clear the tube, or the tube can be hung vertically to dry. The stomach pump should also be flushed with warm water and disinfectant. The pump should be regularly disassembled to allow cleaning and lubrication of the inside of the barrel. A small rubber gasket ring inside the barrel of the pump around the plunger wears out with use and should be checked for cracking and stretching. It is easily replaced.

The rectal examination is commonly performed for the diagnosis of colic. The procedure is potentially hazardous to both the clinician and the patient. The clinician is placed in a vulnerable position at the rear of the horse, and the equine rectum is easily torn. Rectal tears can be life-threatening. Effective restraint, either physical or chemical, is imperative to control the patient. Equipment for the clinician is simple: a nonsterile, arm-length plastic sleeve and nonsterile lubricant are all that are required. Some clinicians wear a latex examination glove over the plastic rectal sleeve. In addition, clinicians usually have a preference for performing the examination with the right or left hand.

Clients often view the rectal examination as a crystal ball, and sometimes it can be just that. However, although important information is usually obtained from the "rectal," its limitations must be understood. Some animals are simply too small or too uncooperative to be examined safely. The human arm can reach only about one third of the total area of the abdomen, so many abdominal problems may be beyond the reach of the clinician. The procedure is a blind one, and determining precise anatomy when dealing with 100 feet of movable intestines in an abnormal animal can be difficult. Still, it is one of the most valuable diagnostic tools of the colic examination.

The rectal examination usually provides an opportunity to collect fresh feces. With feces grasped in the hand, the rectal sleeve is turned inside-out. The hand is removed, and the sleeve is tied shut to form a temporary container for the feces for transport to the clinic. It is standard to perform a gross fecal examination for consistency, color, odor, blood, mucous strands, and parasites. If sand-related colic is suspected, feces can be mixed with a generous amount of water, mixed well, and allowed to settle in the rectal sleeve. Sometimes direct observation of the sand is possible. The fingers are then used to check for a gritty feel of the settled material.

Abdominal radiographs are highly useful in foals. The small size and lack of solid intestinal contents of these animals increases the possibility of diagnostic-quality films. Portable radiograph machines may be used, and lateral and dorsoventral projections are possible with sedation or general anesthesia. Radiography in adult horses is limited to lateral projections of the dorsal abdomen only, and portable machines do not have sufficient strength for this use. Few diseases can be diagnosed in adults through abdominal radiographs.

Abdominal ultrasound is useful in equines of all sizes but has limited ability to penetrate deeply into the abdomen. It is best used for diagnosing problems located close to the abdominal wall (outer circumference of the abdominal cavity). Sometimes sand can be identified in the lower abdomen by ultrasound.

After gathering information from the colic examination, the clinician formulates a treatment plan. Referral to a hospital setting may be recommended for surgery, intensive care, or further diagnostics not available in the field. Treatment plans vary considerably depending on the diagnosis, individual horse variables, available staff and facilities, and economic considerations. Severe pain is often an indication for surgical exploration of the abdomen or at least referral for further diagnostic evaluation, although there are exceptions. Common treatments for mild to moderate cases include restricted oral intake of food and water, fluid therapy, analgesic drugs for control of pain, hand walking, and nonsteroidal antiinflammatory drugs. Patients are usually put on "colic watch" for frequent monitoring of pain and vital signs. Careful records should be kept to track the horse's progress and treatments, whether on the farm or in a hospital/clinic.

OPHTHALMIC EXAMINATION

Because of their pronounced lateral location on the skull, the eyes of the horse are predisposed to trauma; injuries to the orbit, eyelids, and globe are fairly common in horses. Lacerations of the eyelids, conjunctivitis, and corneal ulceration are some of the more common traumatic diseases of the equine eye. Intraocular diseases such as recurrent anterior uveitis ("moon blindness") and cataracts also occur. Abnormal growths such as sarcoids, melanomas, and squamous cell carcinoma may affect the periorbital tissues. Blockage of the nasolacrimal ducts occurs with some frequency.

TECHNICIAN NOTE Because of the location of equine eyes, horses commonly experience eye trauma.

Eye problems are notorious for going unreported until it becomes obvious to the owner that the problems are not getting better on their own. Unfortunately, this delay allows the disease to progress, sometimes to a severe state. Owners do not realize the significance of certain clinical signs. For example, the combination of tearing (excessive lacrimation) and squinting (blepharospasm) can be especially significant and represents an urgent need for veterinary evaluation; these signs often indicate corneal ulceration or recurrent uveitis. Both conditions require urgent medical attention. Owners also tend to use scissors to snip off tags of tissue when eyelid margins have been lacerated, resulting in permanent defects and chronic corneal ulceration. Some owners try to treat eye problems with leftover eye ointments from other horses and do not realize that use of certain ointments can be disastrous for some diseases. Veterinarians should be consulted promptly for all suspected eye problems, even when clinical signs may not be very impressive to the owners. Eye lacerations can be sutured if it has been less than 6 to 8 hours from the time of injury. However, without further resection of tissue, which is not always possible, lacerations more than 6 to 8 hours old should be healed by second intention. Therefore, if you are taking a phone call or consulting on an eye injury, the time since the injury should be considered.

Most ocular problems are irritating or painful, and horses may try to rub the affected eye in response. It is imperative that this action be prevented because rubbing can cause even more trauma to the eye. Protective hoods and eye cups can be used to cover the affected eye (Fig. 6-76). In severe cases, cross-tying the horse may be necessary.

Examination and medication of the eyes are important in equine practice. Although referral to board-certified ophthalmologists is an option, most eye problems are diagnosed and treated in the field. The ophthalmic examination is usually performed in a dark environment. A penlight and ophthalmoscope are necessary for the basic examination; most field practitioners prefer a handheld direct ophthalmoscope (Fig. 6-77). The examination requires good restraint of the patient's head. Use of a nose twitch and sedatives may be necessary.

Depending on the extent of the examination, topical anesthesia of the cornea and conjunctiva may be required. Topical anesthesia is achieved with ophthalmic anesthetic solutions (0.5% proparacaine HCl or 0.5% tetracaine HCl). Dilation of the pupil may also be required for examination of the retina (1% tropicamide ophthalmic solution). Instilling topical medications into the eye must be done carefully; if the horse throws its head, the medication container can be jabbed into the eye, thereby creating possibly severe trauma. To minimize this risk, the hand holding the medication

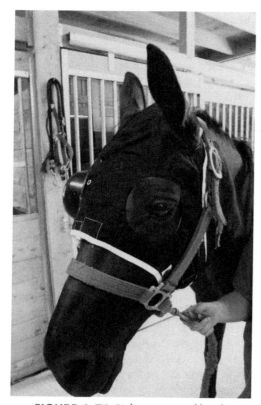

FIGURE 6-76 Right eye cup and hood.

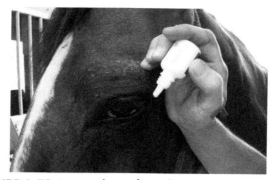

FIGURE 6-78 Proper technique for medicating the eye. Note that the hand is stabilized against the horse's head.

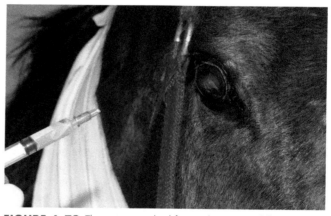

FIGURE 6-79 The easiest method for applying topical fluorescein to horses is to place a sterile fluorescein strip in a 3-mL syringe, fill the syringe with sterile eyewash and replace the plunger, and then squirt the solution through the hub of a 25-gauge needle in which the actual needle has been manually broken off. (From Gilger B: *Equine ophthalmology*, ed 2, St. Louis, 2011, Saunders.)

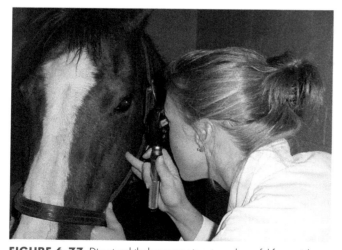

FIGURE 6-77 Direct ophthalmoscopy is extremely useful for rapid ocular examination in horses and can be used to identify most lesions of the equine ocular fundus. The working distance to the horse's head is short. (From Gilger B: *Equine ophthalmology*, ed 2, St. Louis, 2011, Saunders.)

should always be rested against the horse's head so that if the head moves, the hand will move with the head (Fig. 6-78). Horses typically resist having the eyelids forced wide open, but this is seldom necessary to place a topical solution effectively. Simply everting only the lower eyelid and placing the solution or ointment into the lower conjunctival sac are successful and tolerated well by most patients.

Because blinking and squinting can interfere with the examination, blocking sensation and motor control of the eyelids may be necessary. Various nerve blocks in the periorbital region are available to desensitize and paralyze the eyelids to facilitate the examination. Whenever a skin preparation of the eye area is necessary, surgical scrub soaps and alcohol must be used carefully or not at all. Soaps can be highly irritating if they run into the eye and may cause permanent damage. Rather, diluted surgical antiseptic solution (povidone-iodine solution diluted 50% with sterile saline) can be used in the same manner as scrub soap. Alcohol, which is also highly irritating, can be replaced with sterile saline solution for rinsing.

Because corneal lesions are prevalent in horses, staining the cornea often is necessary. Fluorescein stain strips can be placed directly against the eye, although many horses resist this method. An alternative method of staining is to aspirate 2 to 3 mL of sterile saline (or sterile eyewash solution) into a 3-mL syringe, remove the plunger, and dip the dye strip to color the saline. The plunger is replaced, and the stained saline is given (with the needle removed!) by lifting the upper eyelid and gently irrigating the cornea. No more than 1 to 2 mL is necessary to stain the cornea effectively (Fig. 6-79). After applying the stain, 2 to 3 mL of plain saline is used to flush excess dye off the cornea. A penlight or ultraviolet light

(Wood lamp) is used to highlight and search for any areas of retained dye. Areas of staining indicate that the superficial layer of the cornea has been damaged.

LAMENESS EXAMINATION

The musculoskeletal system consists of the skeleton and the associated structures that allow it to move. Bone, articular cartilage, ligaments, tendons, synovial structures, and muscles are the primary components. Injuries and disease of these structures are prevalent in horses. The musculoskeletal system is perhaps the most common body system evaluated and treated by the equine practitioner.

Swelling, discharge, and muscle atrophy are among the possible manifestations of musculoskeletal disease, but the most common clinical sign is an abnormal stance or gait, referred to as *lameness*. The three reasons for lameness are as follows:

- Pain (inflammation), the most common reason
- Mechanical interference, without pain, such as scar tissue restriction of a full range of motion
- Neurologic lameness caused by disease of the neurologic system

Detecting the source of lameness can be a daunting task for the clinician. Many problems have no obvious external signs. Often, lame horses have more than one problem. The horse usually has one primary problem, but secondary problems often result from the horse's response to the primary problem. This creates a "chain reaction" situation that can be difficult to unravel. The temperament, size, and strength of the patient create additional challenges.

The goals of the lameness examination are as follows:
1. Identify the location of the problem or problems.
2. Determine a specific diagnosis for each problem.
3. Plan therapy.

The lameness examination consists of five basic steps. The veterinarian tailors the basic examination to accommodate patient variables, client considerations, and other variables such as facilities and weather. The technician may assist by taking the history, providing restraint, and assisting in diagnostic techniques such as local anesthesia, sampling, and diagnostic imaging. The basic examination consists of the following:

History

Unless you are dealing with an experienced horse owner/trainer, it is best to guide the client through the history rather than letting him or her ramble. Questions should include the following:

- Signalment: What is the horse's age, breed, sex, and use/sport? Some diseases affect only animals of certain ages or have increased incidence in particular breeds. Each equine sport has commonly associated lameness problems that help to direct the clinician to specific areas of the horse.
- Has the horse had previous health or lameness problems?
- How long has the horse been lame?
- Was the onset sudden or gradual?

- Does the lameness get better or worse with exercise?
- Is there any known trauma or reason for the horse to be lame?
- Has the owner given any treatment or medication?
- Does the lameness show any pattern? Is the lameness associated with certain surfaces, gaits, or activities?

Observation

The horse is observed at rest (standing) and in motion.

At Rest

The horse is first observed from a distance for obvious problems such as swelling and muscle atrophy. The conformation of the horse—how the horse is put together anatomically—is also noted. Conformational faults (abnormal conformation) can predispose the horse to certain lameness problems. How the horse stands may also have significance; some painful problems cause the horse to "point" a leg. As a generality, a foreleg that is held in front of vertical position (as viewed from the side) indicates lower leg pain. A foreleg that is held behind vertical position may indicate upper leg pain. Holding a hindleg in front of vertical position may indicate upper leg pain.

In Motion

The horse is observed at various gaits. The usual method is to observe the horse moving directly away from and directly toward the clinician, and then from the side as the horse moves in both directions. The ground surface can affect the lameness; horses are usually more comfortable on soft surfaces and are less likely to show lameness. Harder surfaces such as asphalt may be necessary to show the problem to the observer, especially in horses with low-grade pain. The sounds heard when the hooves strike a hard surface can be revealing. Rough surfaces such as stone or gravel can make sound horses appear lame and should be avoided.

Horseshoes may protect the affected leg from fully displaying pain, especially if the problem is in the hoof. Removal of the shoes may be necessary to evaluate the lameness fully.

The horse is an athletic animal that uses its head and neck as a "balancing arm" when it is in motion. The way the horse uses its head and neck tends to change when the horse is in pain, and the clinician will need to observe the carriage of the head and neck. The handler should hold the head loosely so that abnormal head and neck movements can be seen.

Walk
- Walk in straight line
- Walk up and down an incline
- Backing up

Trot
- Trot in straight line
- Trot in circle (both directions)
- Flexion tests

The trot is usually the most informative gait. The trot has weight borne on two legs at a time, which is more than the other gaits. The increased weight bearing helps to accentuate most forms of lameness. The handler should encourage

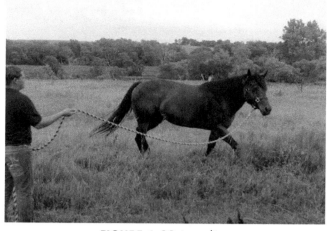

FIGURE 6-80 Lunge line.

BOX 6-10	Gait Faults

Gait faults refer to abnormal leg actions that occur while the horse is in motion. They are usually related to abnormal conformation or the method of shoeing. Gait faults are not necessarily associated with lameness, but they can predispose horses to certain lameness problems. Examples of gait faults include the following:
- Paddling: Hoof is thrown laterally after it leaves the ground.
- Winging: Hoof is thrown medially after it leaves the ground.
- Interfering: One limb hits the other.
- Plaiting: One hoof is placed directly in front of the other.
- Forging: Sole of a front hoof is hit by the toe of the back hoof of the same side.
- Overreaching: Heel of a front hoof is stepped on by the back hoof of the same side.
- Scalping: Front of a back hoof is struck with the front hoof of the same side.

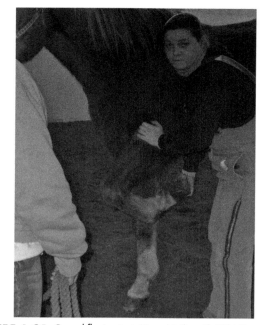

FIGURE 6-81 Carpal flexion test. (From McIlwraith CW, Trotter GW: *Joint disease in the horse,* St. Louis, 1996, Saunders.)

a slow trot (jog) from the horse rather than a fast trot; fast trotting obscures many lameness conditions.

Trotting in circles may be done on a lead line or a lunge line (Fig. 6-80). The lead line requires that the handler run in a circle with the horse. Alternatively, the horse can be placed on a lunge line (long lead line) if the horse is accustomed to it. The lunge line allows the handler to stand still while the horse circles around the handler; the length of the line controls the diameter of the circle. Circles accentuate the stresses on the inside aspects of the legs; for instance, circling the horse to the right (clockwise) increases the stress on the lateral aspect of the right legs and the medial aspect of the left legs. The smaller the circle is, the greater the force.

If circling is done on a hard surface, the horse may slip if the diameter of the circle is too tight. Larger circles are preferred on these surfaces.

The horse is observed for gait faults and lameness (Box 6-10). Especially significant are head nodding and hip hiking. Holding the head up distributes more weight to the hindlegs, and the horse takes advantage of this when in pain.

When a front leg is painful, the horse can transfer weight to the hind end by elevating the head when the painful front leg hits the ground. The opposite effect occurs with hindleg pain. When the painful hindleg hits the ground, the horse lowers its head to shift more weight to the front leg. This head action is referred to as a *head nod* or *head bob* and is a valuable tool for the clinician.

Hip hiking refers to the croup rising on one side when the hindlimb on the same side is painful, similar to a human's hip carriage when a leg is painful. It is a protective "splinting" type of motion that prevents full weight bearing on the painful limb.

Flexion tests are done to evaluate joint pain. Sensory nerve endings for synovial joints are located in the joint capsule. For the test, one or more joints are manually flexed ("cramped") with moderate force to stretch the joint capsule (Fig. 6-81). The clinician maintains the flex for a time (which varies according to the size of the joint; <1 minute for small joints, 1 to 2 minutes for larger joints) and then asks for the horse to be immediately jogged away in a straight line. It is normal for the horse to take three to four "off" strides, but it should quickly return to soundness—a negative test result. If the horse does not quickly return to a normal trot, the test result is positive, and the joints tested by the flexion warrant further investigation.

1. Canter/gallop: This is not usually necessary.
2. Specific exercise: It may be necessary to see the horse exercise with a rider on its back, pulling a cart, jumping, and so forth, to observe the lameness problem.

After the horse is observed in motion, the clinician grades the lameness. Different grading systems are available, but most clinicians use a five-grade system to describe the lameness (Box 6-11).

BOX 6-11	Lameness Severity Grading Scale

Grade 0 = Normal
Grade 1 = Difficult to see under any condition; obscure
Grade 2 = Difficult to see, except under certain conditions
Grade 3 = Consistently seen at the trot
Grade 4 = Obvious lameness at all gaits
Grade 5 = Non–weight bearing

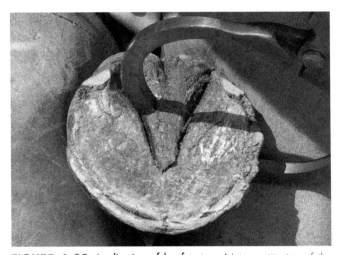

FIGURE 6-82 Application of hoof testers. Note positioning of the arms of the testers at midfrog and midheel wall. (From Floyd A: *Equine podiatry*, St. Louis, 2007, Saunders.)

Palpation

The horse is palpated, to look for areas of pain, heat, and swelling. The legs are palpated in a weight-bearing stance, and then the leg is elevated and the palpation is repeated. Knowledge of normal anatomy is essential. If the horse has shoes, the wear pattern on the shoes can be revealing; the shoe type and fit should also be noted. If the horse is barefoot, the wear pattern on the hoof wall can similarly provide information about weight bearing. Hoof testers are used to find sources of pain within the hoof wall because structures inside the hoof cannot be palpated (Fig. 6-82). Thorough palpation includes the neck, back, and hips. Although primary problems in these areas are unusual, secondary pain is often created in these areas from abnormal weight bearing in the legs (Figs. 6-83 to 6-88).

Local Anesthesia

"Nerve blocks" and "joint blocks" are often, but not always, necessary. They are used for the following reasons:
- To confirm the location of a suspected problem
- To assess the significance of a problem when more than one problem is found
- To try to localize the problem to a smaller region of a leg when the initial examination fails to find a problem

The goal of the procedure is to block pain perception. Local anesthetics can be deposited directly over nerves or directly into joints and other synovial structures to desensitize them.

By understanding which anatomical structures are supplied by individual nerves, the clinician can find the source or sources of pain in a leg through a process of elimination. In other words, if an area is blocked and the horse still feels pain, then the problem must reside in another area. The clinician then chooses another area to desensitize, and so on, until the painful structure or area is located.

The clinician may block a specific structure, if it is suspicious, or start low on the leg and work proximally to find the anatomical level where the problem is located. Basically, a block is placed, and then the clinician watches the horse while it is in motion to see whether the lameness has changed or disappeared. If the lameness is still present, then the source of pain has not been found, and another block is necessary to find the source. However, if the lameness is improved or disappears altogether, the clinician knows to look in the blocked area for the problem. "Looking" usually involves diagnostic imaging to obtain a specific diagnosis.

The procedure begins with cleaning the leg of dirt and debris. Skin preparation is different for nerve blocks and joint blocks. Synovial structures such as joints, bursae, and tendon sheaths must have a sterile skin preparation. Clipping for synovial structure blocks is preferable but not always possible, depending on the horse's circumstances. The owner should be consulted before any clipping is performed.

TECHNICIAN NOTE Anytime an animal must be clipped for a procedure, it is best to ask the owner for permission.

Some of these animals are show animals, or their hair is valuable, so owners are willing to take the risks of not clipping to perform the procedure. I recommend that after the skin has been prepared, povidone-iodine solution (not scrub) be dabbed to saturate the skin and the skin allowed to air dry before the clinician performs the block. A clean preparation technique using a standard scrub/alcohol preparation is suitable for most peripheral nerve blocks unless the nerve is located in an area where there is a risk of entering a synovial structure. A standard sterile preparation is used in these situations.

Veterinarians have preferences for where to perform the preparation and block, the needle size/length, amount of anesthetic, and whether the block is performed with the leg weight bearing or elevated. Most veterinarians prefer a fresh, previously unopened container of anesthetic for synovial structures to avoid the risk of possible contamination in previously opened bottles.

TECHNICIAN NOTE Most veterinarians prefer a fresh, previously unopened container of anesthetic for synovial structures to avoid the risk of possible contamination in previously opened bottles.

Restraint is extremely important because patient movement can cause injury to the patient or clinician. Rarely

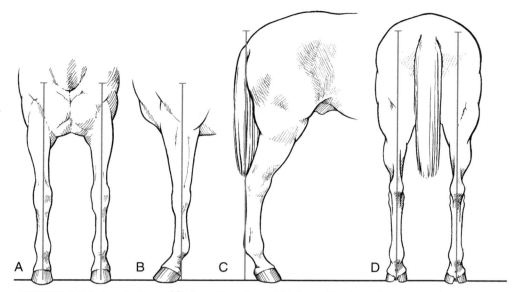

FIGURE 6-83 A to D, Normal findings. (From Ross MW, Dyson SJ, editors: *Diagnosis and management of lameness in the horse,* ed 2, St. Louis, 2012, Saunders.)

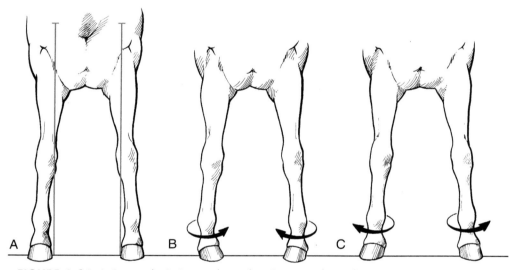

FIGURE 6-84 A, Base wide. **B,** Base wide, toed in. **C,** Base wide, toed out. (From Ross MW, Dyson SJ, editors: *Diagnosis and management of lameness in the horse,* ed 2, St. Louis, 2012, Saunders.)

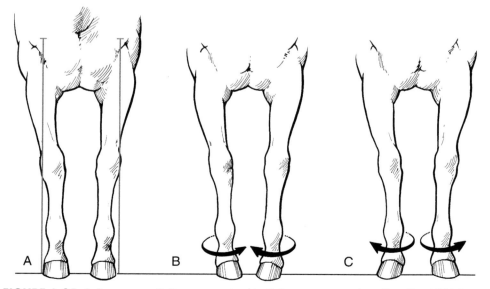

FIGURE 6-85 A, Base narrow. **B,** Base narrow, toed in. **C,** Base narrow, toed out. (From Ross MW, Dyson SJ, editors: *Diagnosis and management of lameness in the horse,* ed 2, St. Louis, 2012, Saunders.)

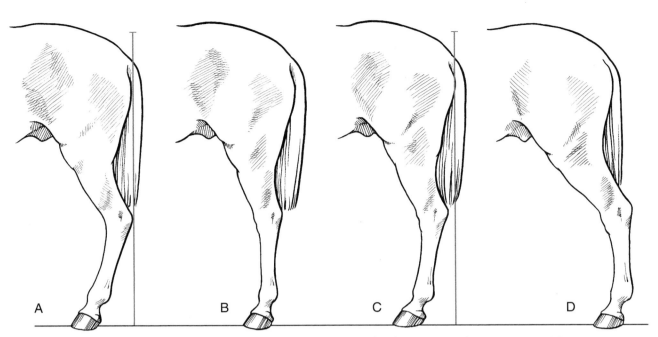

FIGURE 6-86 A, Sickle hocks. **B,** Post legged. **C,** Camped under. **D,** Camped out. (From Ross MW, Dyson SJ, editors: *Diagnosis and management of lameness in the horse,* ed 2, St. Louis, 2012, Saunders.)

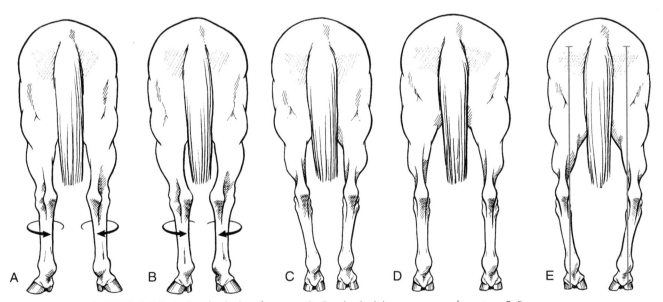

FIGURE 6-87 A, Cow-hocked conformation. **B,** Cow-hocked, base-narrow conformation. **C,** Base-narrow conformation. **D,** Base-wide conformation. **E,** Bowlegged conformation. (From Ross MW, Dyson SJ, editors: *Diagnosis and management of lameness in the horse,* ed 2, St. Louis, 2012, Saunders.)

can blocks be performed without some form of physical restraint, such as a twitch. Insertion of the needle is painful, and the clinician should alert the restrainer when the needle is about to be placed. At that time, the strength of restraint is increased (e.g., tighten the twitch, grasp an elevated leg more firmly) until needle insertion is complete. The veterinarian may direct the technician to either maintain or loosen the restraint, depending on the patient's responses.

After the injection is completed, the block needs time to take effect. This time may range from 5 minutes for superficial nerves to 30 minutes for some joints. The horse may need to be walked during this time to help distribute the local anesthetic. The horse is then evaluated after the block has been given sufficient time to take effect. The gaits and circumstances that showed the lameness best before the block are repeated after the block to assess the results most effectively.

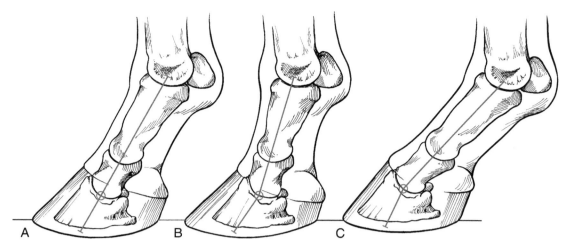

FIGURE 6-88 **A,** Ideal. **B,** Strait pasterns. **C,** Back at the pastern. (From Ross MW, Dyson SJ, editors: *Diagnosis and management of lameness in the horse,* ed 2, St. Louis, 2012, Saunders.)

Special Diagnostics

Special diagnostics may include the following:

- Radiographs (plain films with and without contrast techniques)
- Xeroradiographs
- Diagnostic ultrasound
- Thermography
- Nuclear scintigraphy
- Magnetic resonance imaging
- Computed tomography
- Arthrocentesis
- Rectal examination (for fractured pelvis or sublumbar pain)
- Biopsy (muscle, bone, synovial membrane)
- Force-plate gait analysis
- High-speed cinematographic (video) gait analysis

CASE STUDY

Dr. Overton asked you to go on a farm call to a local horse breeding farm. When you arrive at the farm, the client asks you to go to the pasture and bring the Buckskin, Palomino, and Bay horses back to the barn. How do you know which horses to collect from the pasture? Please describe your answer in depth.

CASE STUDY

You have been traveling with Dr. Hille all day, and it is 4:30 PM. You have just received a call to Mr. Kuhl's place. The veterinarian performs a physical examination and notes in the chart findings of blood coming from the eyes, nostrils, and anus of the deceased cow. You are only a few minutes from the clinic, and the veterinarian decides to run you back to the clinic so that you can continue the plans you have to go out with friends this evening. On the way back to the clinic, the veterinarian tells you that one of his differential diagnoses is anthrax. Your plans for the evening are with some of Mr. Kuhl's neighbors. Should you tell them about the differential diagnosis?

CASE STUDY

A new technician has just started her externship at your clinic. Dr. Fritz has asked her to perform a physical examination on the mare in the stocks while he helps a client in the front lobby. The technician proceeds with the examination and spends about 4 minutes performing the abdominal auscultation. This was the final step of her examination, and she tells you that she is finished. What mistake did she probably make doing the abdominal auscultation?

SUGGESTED READING

Bassert JM, McCurnin DM, editors: *McCurnin's clinical textbook for veterinary technicians,* ed 7, St. Louis, 2010, Saunders.

Bentz AI, Gill MS: Large animal medical nursing. In Bassert JM, McCurnin DM, editors: *McCurnin's clinical textbook for veterinary technicians,* ed 7, St. Louis, 2010, Saunders, pp 713–768.

Fubini SL, Ducharme NG: *Farm animal surgery,* St. Louis, 2004, Saunders.

Pugh DG: *Sheep and goat medicine,* St. Louis, 2002, Saunders.

Sheldon CC, Sonsthagen T, Topel JA: *Animal restraint for veterinary professionals,* St. Louis, 2006, Mosby.

Sirois M: *Principles and practice of veterinary technology,* ed 3, St. Louis, 2011, Mosby.

Smith MC, Sherman DM: *Goat medicine,* Baltimore, 1994, Williams & Wilkins.

Sonsthagen TF: Physical restraint. In Sirois M, editor: *Principles and practice of veterinary medicine,* ed 3, St. Louis, 2011, Mosby, pp 323–344.

Speirs VC: *Clinical examination of horses,* St. Louis, 1997, Saunders.

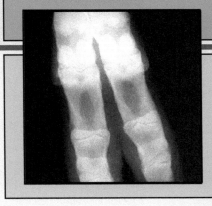

7 Diagnostic Imaging for Large Animals

LEARNING OBJECTIVES

When you finish this chapter, you will be able to

- List and explain the functions of livestock
- Demonstrate a basic understanding large animal radiographic techniques
- Produce large animal radiographs safely
- Demonstrate a basic understanding of large animal radiographic equipment
- Describe the different types of radiographic imaging
- Demonstrate a basic understanding of common problems that arise during large animal radiographic procedures
- Be able to prepare the patient for radiographic procedures properly
- Be able to perform basic standard radiographic views
- Demonstrate a basic understanding of nuclear scintigraphy
- Demonstrate a basic understanding of computed tomography
- Demonstrate a basic understanding of magnetic resonance imaging
- Demonstrate a basic understanding of thermography
- Demonstrate a basic understanding of diagnostic ultrasound
- Be able to prepare a patient for diagnostic ultrasound
- Understand the importance of proper ultrasound equipment care
- Demonstrate a basic understanding of endoscopy
- Understand the importance of proper endoscope care

KEY TERMS

Caudal
Collimator
Cranial
Distal
Dorsal
Dosimetry
Dosimeter
Electromagnetic radiation
Genetic damage

Fixed radiograph machine
Lateral
Medial
Mobile radiograph machine
Palmar
Plantar
Proximal
Portable radiograph machine
Primary beam

Radiation
Radiograph
Rostral
Scatter radiation
Somatic damage
Ventral
X-ray radiation

ALARA: As low as reasonably achievable
CC: Caudal to cranial
CdCr: Caudocranial
CR: Computed radiology
CrCd: Craniocaudal
DLPMO: Dorsolateral-palmar/dorsolateral-plantar medial oblique

DMPLO: Dorsomedial to palmar/dorsomedial to plantar lateral oblique
DP: Dorsal-palmar/dorsal-plantar
DR: Digital radiology
kVp: Kilovolt peak
LM: Lateromedial
mA: Milliamperage
mAs: Milliamperage per second
ML: Mediolateral

MPD: Maximum permissible dose
NCRP: National Committee on Radiation Protection and Measurements
OFD: Object film distance
SV: Sievert
SID: Source image distance (also known as FFD or film focal distance)

DIAGNOSTIC IMAGING: OVERVIEW

Diagnostic imaging of large animals is similar to imaging of small animals. All the imaging modalities used for small animals are also possible in large animals, although they may be limited in usefulness and availability because of the larger size of the animal. The limitations are usually related to an inability of the equipment to accommodate the size of the large animal patient or to penetrate the patient to a sufficient depth. Another restriction is that large animal imaging often takes place on the farm and therefore requires use of portable equipment; portable equipment frequently lacks the output power of stationary equipment, thus limiting the ability to obtain diagnostic-quality images of thick body parts.

I would consider this chapter to contain clinical procedures for each of the individual animals outlined in this textbook. However, because many veterinary technician programs teach large animal imaging in their diagnostic imaging classes, I chose this chapter to remain separate. This allows instructors and students to find this information in the textbook very quickly while teaching or learning these techniques because imaging may not be covered in primary large animal nursing classes. The principles of radiology are kept mostly to the equine species. However, all these views apply equally to the ruminant species and swine. Radiographs are taken in these species when valuable livestock display the need.

Many excellent texts are available to the technician that detail the principles of diagnostic imaging. The actual principles of imaging are basically the same for small and large animals; they need only to be adapted for the patient's location, size, and available equipment. This chapter emphasizes practical concerns and adaptations for large animals. The reader is encouraged to refer to other texts for in-depth discussion of imaging physics.

DIAGNOSTIC RADIOLOGY

The principles of taking a high-quality, diagnostic radiograph are the same for large and small animals. However, large animal radiology is unique because of the conformation of the patient and because most *radiographs* are obtained in a standing, awake patient. The temperament of the animal often further limits the ability to position the patient for ideal film studies.

SAFETY

The physical safety of the people handling these large animals and the safety of the animals themselves must always be the first concerns.

> **TECHNICIAN NOTE** The physical safety of the people handling large animals and the safety of the animals are always your first concerns.

One must also take into consideration the financial investment needed to perform these studies, and protecting the equipment should be considered as well. A standard portable x-ray tube that is not digital costs approximately $10,000 new. Digital units can cost more than $100,000. Large animals tend to be apprehensive about radiographs. Most radiograph machines make strange noises, generate bright light for collimation, and generally must be positioned within 40 inches of the patient. Ideally, the film cassette should be placed to contact the patient's skin, and this may alarm the animal, causing it to move away or perhaps kick. The patient is often in pain from an injury or condition, hence the need for a radiograph to be taken, which adds to the "fear factor." Personnel and equipment are therefore in vulnerable positions, with a patient that is often suspicious of the situation. Physical or chemical restraints, or both, must be selected carefully, and personnel should not be placed in dangerous, compromising positions. Common sense handling—including moving slowly and speaking calmly—is necessary. It also helps to let the animals know what is coming (i.e., rather than slapping a cassette against the leg with no warning, it helps to rub the area gently a few times to accustom the animal to touch at that location, and then place the cassette against the animal's skin).

> **TECHNICIAN NOTE** Always touch the patient in the area where the cassette will be placed before placing the cassette against the animal's skin.

If the machine produces noise, the rotor can be activated once or twice to reproduce the noise before positioning the patient for the actual film. This noise should be initiated at a distance from the patient in case the noise does create some anxiety for the patient.

Radiation safety is the next concern, once physical safety has been addressed. Small, *portable radiograph machines* present no less danger than the larger, fixed machines in hospitals and clinics; radiation is dangerous, regardless of the source. Radiation is the propagation of energy through space and matter. *Electromagnetic radiation* is the type of radiation created when performing radiographic procedures. Electromagnetic radiation varies depending on the wavelength it produces. Sources of radiation to which veterinary technicians can be exposed in the veterinary hospital include radiography, computed tomography (CT), fluoroscopy, and nuclear studies. All living cells are susceptible to radiation damage; affected cells may be damaged or killed. The cells that are most likely to be damaged are those that are rapidly dividing. People who are growing are particularly sensitive. Gonadal, neoplastic, and metabolically active cells also fall into this category. These types of cells include bone, lymphatic, dermis, blood forming, and epithelial tissues.

The two types of radiation damage are somatic and genetic. *Somatic damage* is damage that can happen immediately or can manifest in the body of the recipient for a lifetime. Somatic damage is more extensive when the body is exposed to a single massive dose of radiation rather than to smaller cumulative doses of radiation. Death is possible if a person is exposed to an extremely high level of radiation at one time. Types of somatic damage include cancer, cataracts, aplastic anemia, and sterility. *Genetic damage* results in injury to the genes of reproductive cells. This type of damage does not present itself until the damaged individual reproduces and the mutated genes create a child.

Because of the serious nature of radiation exposure, several steps to protecting yourself are necessary. To help monitor radiation exposure, veterinary professionals should wear *dosimetry* badges known as *dosimeters*.

> **TECHNICIAN NOTE**   Dosimetry badges should be worn at all times during radiographic exposure.

These badges should be worn by personnel at all times during the radiographic procedure. By monitoring the level of radiation you are exposed to, you can help limit your lifetime exposure through management. For example, if only one person ever takes radiographs, that person's exposure will be extremely high, so it is important to rotate staff taking the radiographs to help limit and spread the exposure to everyone. Small exposures are less dangerous than massive doses of exposure. Dosimetry badges can be set up to be worn several different ways, and you should check with your federally approved dosimetry badge reading company to ensure proper location of the badge during the procedure. No special activation of these badges is required; all you have to

do is wear the badge. When the badge is not in use, it should be kept in a separate location away from where any procedures that create radiation exposure will be performed and kept with the control badge sent with each batch of badges. The badges are sent in on a regular basis, and the amount of radiation received during the time period in which the badge was worn is reported. Each individual should monitor this dose and compare it with the maximum permissible dose (MPD). The MPD is the amount of radiation a person can be exposed to within a given period of time, and it guides individuals on what level of radiation exposure is safe. This MPD is set by the National Committee of Radiation Protection and Measurements (NCRP). The MPD for occupationally exposed individuals who are more than 18 years old is 0.05 Sievert (SV)/year; another unit of measurement you may hear quoted is rem. The occupational exposure for rem is 5 rem/year, and this is because 1 SV = 100 rem.

> **TECHNICIAN NOTE**   The MPD for occupationally exposed individuals older than 18 years is 0.05 SV/year or 5 rem/year.

Any person less than 18 years old is not allowed to enter the area where radiographs are being performed unless that person is ordered by a human medical physician. This is because young persons are highly susceptible to radiation damage, given that they are still growing.

> **TECHNICIAN NOTE**   Any person less than 18 years old is not allowed to enter an area where radiographs are being taken.

Personnel exposure can result from exposure to the *primary beam* radiation, x-ray tube housing leakage, and scatter radiation. Exposure to the primary beam is the result of technical error and can be avoided by *not* placing any part of your body, whether covered by protective equipment or not, within the *collimator* beam. The collimator beam is the light on the machine used to highlight the area of the patient you will be imaging. This light has the highest level of radiation, and protective equipment is not designed to prevent that type of exposure. In addition, collimation of the area you are imaging not only provides a safer environment for you, but also produces a higher-quality image.

X-ray tube housing leakage can also be prevented by ensuring that the radiographic machine you are using is evaluated yearly by a radiographic equipment expert for leakage.

However, scatter radiation cannot be prevented, so personal protection must be implemented. Scatter radiation is also known as secondary radiation. Scatter radiation is produced when the primary beam interacts with objects in its path. The amount of scatter generated depends on the intensity of the beam, the composition of structure being radiographed, the kilovolt peak (kVp) level, and the thickness of the patient. Because most large animal radiographs involve higher levels of radiation, for all these reasons it is extremely important that protective equipment be used when dealing with these patients. Personal protective equipment includes lead aprons, thyroid collars, lead gloves, protective goggles, and radiation badges. Everyone involved in the procedure should be wearing this protective equipment, even if a mechanical cassette holder with an extension arm is used or these staff members are behind the machine (Fig. 7-1).

Proper care of this equipment is important to help ensure that it is always providing the maximum amount of protection. Aprons should be hung vertically, gloves should be hung vertically, cracked apparel should be replaced, and apparel should be inspected quarterly for damage.

Other rules that should be implemented within the hospital to keep personnel safe include removing all unnecessary personnel from the radiographic suite; only the operator and necessary restrainers should be present when exposures are being made. Persons less than 18 years old or pregnant women should not be allowed in the radiographic suite while it is in use unless written documentation from their human physician is supplied. The personnel within the hospital should be rotated through the duty of radiographic imaging to minimize

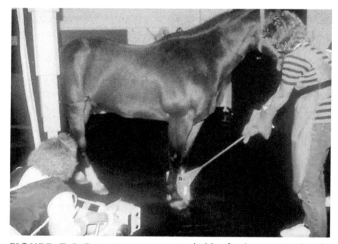

FIGURE 7-1 Extension arm cassette holder for large animal radiography. Note that the technician is wearing lead gloves, even though the cassette holder is in use. (From Partington BP: Diagnostic imaging. In Bassert J, Thomas J, editors: *McCurnin's clinical textbook for veterinary technicians,* ed 8, St. Louis, 2014, Saunders.)

exposure. Mechanical restraints should be used on patients whenever possible, and chemical restraint should be used when needed. The distance between the primary beam and the personnel taking the image should always be maximized if possible. This will help decrease the amount of scatter generated. In general, taking a radiograph requires three people: one to tend the horse's head, one to operate the radiograph machine, and one to position the film cassette. Cassette holders can be purchased or homemade, to provide distance from the primary beam. Hay bales and buckets can also serve to prop up film cassettes for cooperative patients. These devices should be used whenever the situation allows (Fig. 7-2).

Avoiding the need for retaking radiographs also decreases personnel exposure. To help prevent having to retake radiographs, situations plan your radiographic procedure carefully before beginning. Excellent communication skills with your teammates helps avoid these situations. Use of a technique chart helps prevent retakes as well. A technique chart is a chart that tells you what kVp, time, and milliamperage (mA) are required for each type of radiograph you are going to perform, as well as its thickness. This chart is made specifically for your machine and will help ensure a high-quality image each time you take a radiograph. This will help you to ensure you are following the ALARA rule. ALARA stands for as low as reasonable achievable. This means that when selecting your mA, kVp, and time, use the lowest setting possible to achieve the best image.

If using film, maintain your darkroom chemicals in good operating condition and have your x-ray machine calibrated annually by a qualified expert. Ensure that you know emergency procedures associated with your machine, and perform quality control tests annually. An exposure log that identifies the patient and type of study should also be kept.

The safety of the equipment must also enter the safety equation; radiograph machines and film cassettes are expensive, and they can also injure the patient. Because of the close distance of these items to the patient, the equipment is vulnerable and must be protected while the radiograph is taken. After the film is taken, the equipment should be removed from the immediate vicinity of the patient. Exposed and unexposed cassettes should be kept out of the area of the procedure for protection; they should also be kept in distinctly separate stacks to prevent accidental double exposure. Having

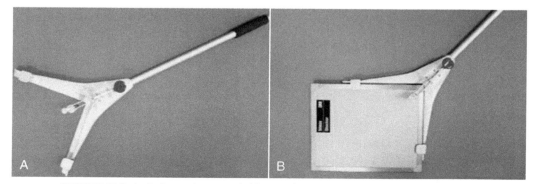

FIGURE 7-2 **A,** Radiograph cassette holder. **B,** Film cassette inserted in the cassette holder.

a marking system to identify exposed cassettes provides an additional safeguard against double exposure. Double exposure will require you to expose yourself to radiation again, and this increases your risk for radiation injury over time.

EQUIPMENT

Radiograph machines are mobile, fixed, or portable.

Mobile machines are the least frequently used; these large machines, designed for human hospitals, are rolled from room to room. In large animal practice, they are found only in hospital settings and are somewhat cumbersome to move and position. However, they are powerful and useful for thick body parts that smaller machines cannot penetrate (Fig. 7-3).

Fixed machines are mounted to either floor or ceiling tracks, to allow limited mobility within the radiograph procedure room. These machines have the highest output capabilities of any of the radiograph machine types; even so, they may not be able to penetrate thick body parts, such as the pelvis on large individuals. Collimation and illumination tend to be superior; however, the noise generated by the rotors tends to be louder than that of the other machines (Fig. 7-4).

Most large animal radiographs are made with portable machines; these "farm call" units are small enough to be taken almost anywhere there is an electrical power source (Fig. 7-5). They have limited output capability in terms of kVp (average, 90 kVp maximum) and mA (average, 20 mA maximum); therefore, longer exposure times (S) must be used to compensate. The collimators on some portable machines may not be lighted, thus creating an inability to aim the primary beam and control the exposure field reliably. Portable machines are usually used on the farm, in barns or paddocks where the quality of electricity—the "line voltage"—may be low or erratic.

Portable machines have a minimum line voltage required to produce high-quality radiographs; a line voltage indicator on the machine measures the strength of the incoming electricity. If the line voltage is low, turning off radios, electrical fences, barn lights, heaters, and other devices often increases the voltage to an acceptable range.

Because of the limited power of portable machines, their ability to penetrate thick body parts is restricted. Assuming an average 1000-pound horse, the quality of radiographs of the following areas is usually compromised when a portable machine is used:

- *Caudal* areas of the skull
- Caudal cervical vertebrae
- Shoulder joint
- Craniocaudal view of the elbow joint
- Cranioventral thorax

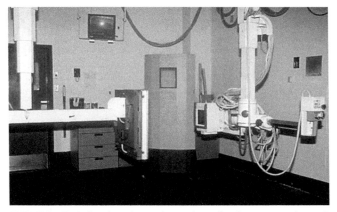

FIGURE 7-4 Fixed radiograph machine for large animals, with ceiling-mounted x-ray tube and film cassette holder. (From Partington BP: Diagnostic imaging. In Bassert J, Thomas J, editors: *McCurnin's clinical textbook for veterinary technicians*, ed 8, St. Louis, 2014, Saunders.)

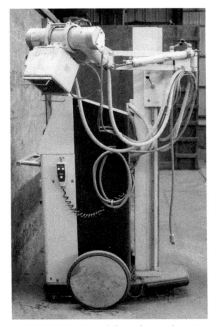

FIGURE 7-3 Mobile radiograph unit.

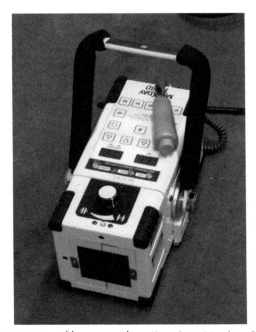

FIGURE 7-5 Portable x-ray machine. (From Sirois M, editor: *Principles and practice of veterinary technology*, ed 3, St. Louis, 2011, Mosby.)

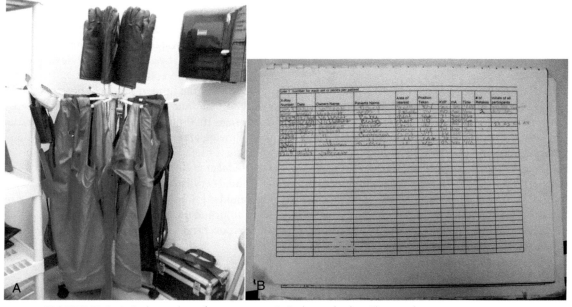

FIGURE 7-6 A, Radiographic safety equipment. B, Radiographic log. The x-ray log is just as important as your safety equipment and should be kept for legal purposes and for helping to solve safety issues if they arise.

- Pelvis
- Caudocranial view of the stifle joint
- Abdomen

When studies of these areas are necessary, the patient usually must be referred to a facility with a more powerful radiograph machine, such as a fixed type.

A cassette holder is often used to increase the space between the film and the holder, to make these procedures safer for the veterinary technician. An example of this equipment is shown in Figure 7-2.

Pictures of safety equipment are shown in Figure 7-6 and include gown, gloves, thyroid shield, goggles, and dosimeter.

Hoof positioners are also available and can help not only to position the patient but also to improve the quality of image obtained, as shown in Figure 7-7.

GENERAL CONCEPTS AND SETTINGS

In general, it requires three people to take large animal radiographs. One person is required for restraint. Another person holds the machine, and a third holds and positions the cassette.

When radiographs are generated from the machine, the energy in the form of an x-ray beam is directed at a film that captures the image. Therefore, when taking radiographic images, the machine and film must be in perfect alignment with each other (Fig. 7-8). Once the image is captured on the film, it is then processed to make the image visible. Processing of the film varies depending on the type of radiographic unit used and is discussed in the next section (on other types of radiography).

Five basic properties of *x-ray radiation* are constant, and they can help you to understand the concepts involved in generating a high-quality image.

1. Radiation can be generated by exciting an electron with heat

The inside of an x-ray machine has two sides, and they are located on opposite ends. They are known as the cathode and the anode. The cathode side consists of a filament and a focusing cup. The anode side consists of a target area and focal spot that is positively charged. When the tungsten cathode filament is heated, it excites the electrons of the tungsten, and they fly off the filament toward the anode because it is positively charged and the electrons are negatively charged. It is similar to the old saying, "opposites attract." When the electrons collide with the anode, the energy in the electron is released from the electron in the form of x-ray radiation and is directed at the patient. Of the energy produced at this location, 99% is in the form of heat, and only 1% actually becomes radiation. This is one reason that portable machines are limited in their ability to produce images of thick anatomy. The heat ruins the machine. Fixed machines have a rotating anode that dissipates the heat, so more energy can be produced without melting the target area. Portable machines have a stationary anode. The hotter the filament, the more electrons are released. This is directly proportional; therefore, more heat leads to the more electrons, and this means more radiation. The more electrons released, the more radiation is produced. The more radiation produced, the better the chance is that it will reach the film and turn it dark. The heat is controlled by milliamperage (mA). The amount of milliamperage available is controlled by the electricity available. This is another reason that portable x-ray units are limited in their ability to produce images of patients' anatomy that is extremely thick. If you increase the mA, you will make the film darker because

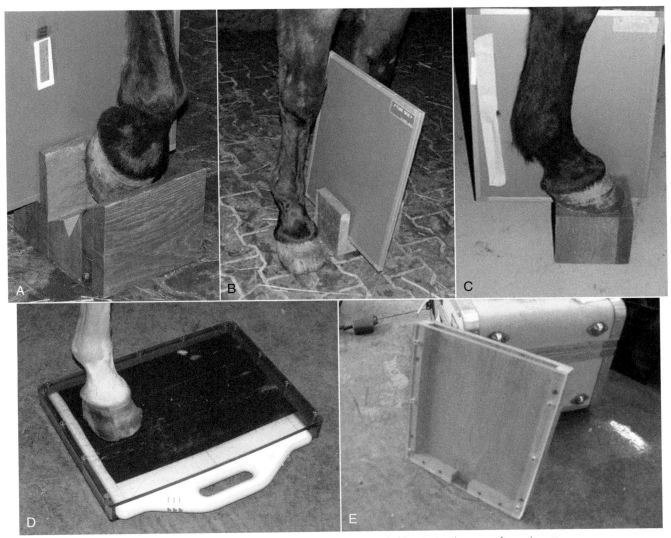

FIGURE 7-7 Hoof positioner and its use. **A,** Wood cassette holder. **B,** Another type of wood positioner. **C,** Wood block for elevation of the hoof. **D,** Cassette insert being used. **E,** Cassette holder without a cassette inserted. (From Brown M, Brown L: *Lavin's radiography for veterinary technicians,* ed 5, St. Louis, 2013, Saunders.)

you are producing more energy, which in turn can reach the film. Think of it this way: If you throw 1 ball, what is the chance of hitting your classmates? If you throw 100 balls at your classmates, what are the chances that you are going to hit someone? Better, and that is why the film becomes darker (Fig. 7-9).

2. Time is important

Time settings can be adjusted when taking radiographs. Time settings on your x-ray machine control how long the filament will be heated. The following example is theoretical and has no clinical basis, but it will help you understand the concept: If you heat the filament for 1 minute and it produces 5 electrons, how many electrons will be produced in 2 minutes? The answer is 10 electrons. So if you increase the time, you increase the amount of radiation produced. This means that you will make the film darker. If you decrease the time, you will make the film lighter. This is why you have a setting

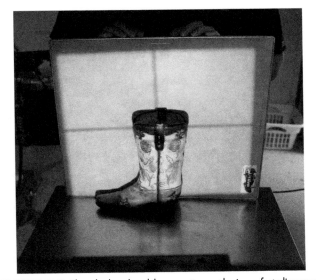

FIGURE 7-8 The tube head and the cassette must be in perfect alignment.

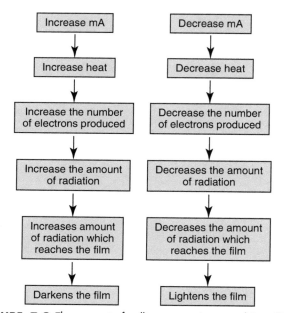

FIGURE 7-9 The concept of milliamperage (expressed in milliamperes [mA]) and milliamperage per second (mAs) as it applies to radiograph exposure.

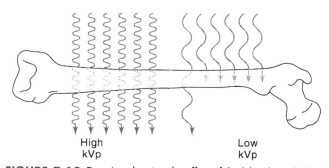

FIGURE 7-10 Drawing showing the effect of the kilovolt peak (kVp) level on x-ray beam penetration. High-kVp settings produce a more-penetrating x-ray beam, with a higher percentage of x-rays reaching the film. (From Lavin LM: *Radiography in veterinary technology*, St. Louis, ed 4, 2006.)

known as mAs (see Fig. 7-9). It is milliamperage multiplied by time (milliamperage per second). Because they both control the amount or quantity of radiation, they can be used together to control the machine.

3. Wavelength is variable

The x-ray machine generates energy that travels in the form of waves. Shorter wavelengths produce more energy, which produces more penetrating power. Longer wavelengths have less energy and have less penetrating power (Fig. 7-10). The length of the wave is measured using frequency; shorter wavelengths have higher frequencies. Frequency is defined as the number of cycles that pass a stationary point in 1 second and is measured in cycles per second. Hence thicker patients require higher frequencies to pass through the patient and create an image on the other side where the cassette is located. The wavelength is controlled by kVp. The higher the kVp, the shorter the wavelength will be, the more penetrating power will be available, and the darker the film will be. In general, the kVp controls the quality of the x-ray study. When a technique chart is not available and you have to estimate the kVp needed, Sante's rule can be used to identify a starting point for kVp. Sante's rule is defined as follows:

$$2 \,(\text{Thickness}) + \text{SID} + \text{GF} = \text{kVp}$$

The source image distance (SID) is the distance from the x-ray machine to the patient. In large animals, we can change this distance dramatically because we have more freedom to move the x-ray machine. SID is measured in inches. GF is the abbreviation for grid factor. In small animal practice, the table on which the patient is positioned has a grid, so a factor of 10 is often used for this number. However, because our patients are not positioned on tables in large animal medicine, this factor is set to zero. When you are measuring the thickness of your patient, you should measure from the bottom of the movable metal elbow and not from the top, and you should always measure this in centimeters (Figs. 7-11 and 7-12).

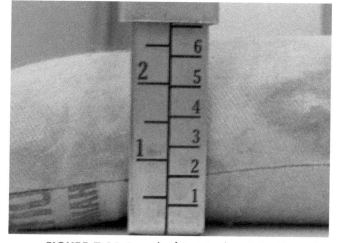

7 cm
The thickness the x-ray beam must penetrate
2 (Thickness in cm) + SID + GF = kVp setting
(2 × 7) + 40 + 0 = 54

FIGURE 7-11 Example of Sante's rule. *GF,* Grid factor; *kVp,* kilovolts peak; *SID,* source image distance.

4. X-rays travel in a straight line, so distance is important

That x-rays travel in a straight line is important for you to remember because you must keep the machine and the cassette directly opposite from each other. It is also important because scatter radiation, our major concern for safety, also travels in straight lines. This principle is also a factor in determining what will happen if you vary your SID. Standard SID is 40 inches. In small animal radiology, this number cannot be changed because a table with a grid is being used, and movement of the SID will result in improper focus of the grid unless you are taking tabletop radiographs. In large animals, however, no table is used, and that means no grid that has to be focused. This allows us to change SID to accommodate our patients' needs (Fig. 7-13). For example, if you had a horse that was extremely anxious about the noise generated by the machine, you could increase your SID and accommodate accordingly by increasing the mAs or kVp. kVp can be compensated for by adjustments using Sante's rule.

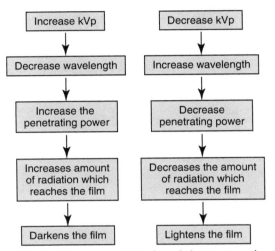

FIGURE 7-12 The concept of kilovolt peak (kVp) as it applies to radiographic exposure.

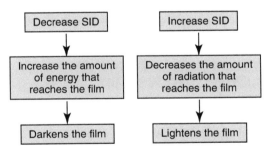

FIGURE 7-13 The concept of source image distance (SID) as it applies to radiographic exposure.

5. The amount of absorption depends on the atomic number, the physical density of the object, and the energy of the x-rays

When the x-ray radiation passes through the patient, some of the radiation is stopped by the patient. The amount stopped by the patient depends on the composition of the area. This is a great time to explain that when x-rays come in contact with the film, they turn the film black. If radiation does not contact the film, it will be clear when the image is processed. Therefore, in the case of bone, which has a high atomic number and high physical density, not that many photons (units of energy) actually reach the film, so bone looks white when it is visualized on the film. In contrast, lung, which is filled with air, has a very low atomic number and low physical density, so fewer photons are stopped as they pass through the patient. This means that many photons pass through the patient and reach the film, thus causing the film to be black after processing (Fig. 7-14).

VIEWING RADIOGRAPHS

Radiographs should be viewed on an evenly lit view box in a semidark room. When placing images on the view box, all laterally positioned anatomical features should read from left to right, so the *dorsal* aspect of the leg should be on the left and the caudal aspect of the leg on the right if you are standing looking at the view box. The *proximal* aspect of the limb should be toward the top and the *distal* aspect of the

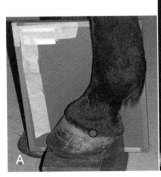

FIGURE 7-14 A and **B,** Radiographic density as exemplified by a hoof. The densities present as a result of bone, cartilage, fat, and so forth stop the radiation from reaching the film. The higher the subject density, the more radiation it stops, as evidenced by the radiograph. Where the radiation reaches the film, it turns black after processing. That is why lungs are black. Where the radiation is blocked from reaching the film (e.g., bone), it is white after processing. All shades of gray, representing varying degrees of density, may be seen in radiographs. When no exposure to radiation is present, the film is clear. (From Brown M, Brown L: *Lavin's radiography for veterinary technicians,* ed 5, St. Louis, 2013, Saunders.)

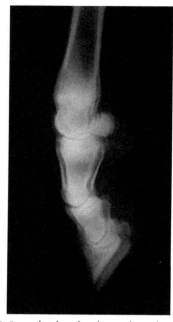

FIGURE 7-15 Properly placed radiograph on the view box when a lateral projection is being viewed.

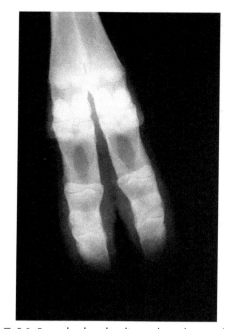

FIGURE 7-16 Properly placed radiograph on the view box when a nonlateral projection is being viewed.

limb toward the bottom of the view box (Fig. 7-15). All other views should be placed as though the horse was standing looking at you (Fig. 7-16).

MAKING ADJUSTMENTS

You can do everything right and get a bad radiograph. You can do everything wrong and get a good radiograph. Therefore, it is inevitable that you will have to retake an image at some point. Figure 7-17 is a flow chart that can be used to help make adjustments when needed. When using the flow chart, you must always answer the first question, "Is the film too light or too dark?" Let us say it is too light. You know you are going to have to increase either kVp or mAs. So now you must ask yourself the second question, to identify which one needs to be changed. Let us say that the film contained detail. Then you would need to increase mAs to correct this film. If mAs is to be adjusted, it is best to adjust it by 30% to 50%; if kVp is to be adjusted, it is best to adjust it by 10%. As you obtain more practice, you will become more familiar with what type of adjustment needs to be made to correct the image.

Another adjustment I have found useful was not designed for this purpose but works just as effectively. The air gap technique was designed to help reduce scatter radiation when taking images of large animals because a grid is not used. However, I have found it effective for horses that are uncooperative and nervous about the equipment or move when touched with the cassette. The SID is increased to 6 feet, to allow the noise from the machine to be farther away. The object film distance (OFD) is increased to 6 inches. The OFD is usually zero; it is the distance between the patient and the cassette. The purpose is to decrease scatter, but I have found it successful for horses that shy away when the cassette is applied to the leg. By adjusting both the OFD and the SID,

you decrease the magnification that would normally occur when there is an increased OFD (Fig. 7-18).

MAKING A TECHNIQUE CHART

When making a technique chart, it is important to have your x-ray machine services ensure that everything is working properly. Then if you are using standard film, clean your processor and change the chemicals to ensure that it is working properly. Ninety percent of all errors in radiography occur in the darkroom. Make sure that all the screens in your cassettes are of the same age, speed, and manufacturer. This removes any variability from cassette to cassette within the hospital. Then choose a horse of average size, weight, and bone structure. Select an mAs that will allow a low time setting. Most often in veterinary medicine, because we cannot tell our patients to stand still, we use the lowest time setting with the highest kVp. Then select your kVp based on Sante's rule. Using the adjustment flow chart shown in Figure 7-17, take a new radiograph each time until you acquire the perfect radiograph for that location. Using the mA, time, SID, and kVp from that image, you should follow these rules to create the chart:

- Caudal areas of the skull
  - Subtract 2 kVp from the original kVp for each centimeter decrease from the original measurement.
  - Add 2 kVp from the original kVp for each centimeter increase from the original measurement up to 80 kVp.
  - Add 3 kVp for each centimeter increase that places the kVp at more than 80 up to 100.
  - Add 4 kVp for each centimeter increase that places the kVp higher than 100.

Another method of making a technique chart involves keeping your radiology log at work. When you record in

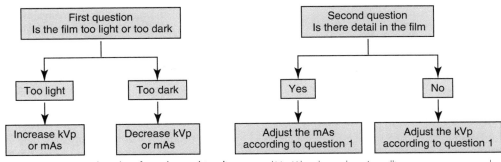

FIGURE 7-17 Flow chart for radiographic adjustments. *kVp*, Kilovolts peak; *mAs*, milliamperage per second.

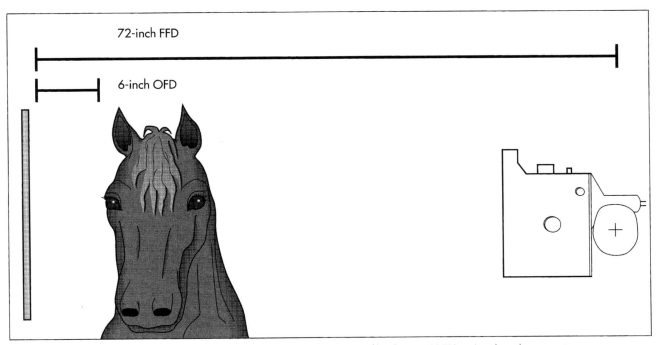

FIGURE 7-18 Air gap technique. By increasing the object film distance (OFD) to 6 inches, the scatter is allowed to pass by the cassette without affecting the film. Next, increasing the focal-film distance to 72 inches decreases the magnification and penumbra that occurred from increasing the OFD. (From Han C, Hurd C: *Practical diagnostic imaging for the veterinary technician*, ed 3, St. Louis, 2004, Mosby.)

your log, always record the mA, kVp, time, and SID, and then make notes about the quality of the radiograph you achieved at those settings. With time, you will be able to review the log, obtain an idea of the perfect settings, and make your technique chart using the previously mentioned guidelines.

OTHER TYPES OF RADIOGRAPHY

Most radiographs are made using standard radiograph machines and radiographic film and cassettes. Xeroradiographs ("blue pictures") are also made with standard radiography machines, but they use electrostatically charged plates to form latent images, which are then exposed to a charged powder (toner) to form a heat-transferred image to plastic-coated paper. Xeroradiographs provide excellent bone detail and better soft tissue visualization than conventional radiographs, but they require much higher exposures to form an image (as much as seven times higher); this creates

additional safety risks to personnel. In addition, the equipment is expensive and not economical for most practices. "Xeros" are useful when routine radiographs do not provide sufficient detail for a diagnosis.

Digital radiology, also known as computed radiography (CR) is another form of radiographic imaging. The plate is placed in a laser reader, where it is scanned with a laser beam and digitized for viewing on a computer monitor. The images can be enhanced and manipulated by the computer and printed out as hard copy. Storage of images as computer files saves office space, and images can be transferred electronically to other veterinarians and veterinary radiologists.

Digital radiology, also known as digital radiography (DR) is a second type of digital imaging often used in small animal practices. Sensors are placed in the table or on a portable cassette. The sensors capture the image, which is transferred directly to a computer. DR is available in both mobile and stationary forms.

COMMON PROBLEMS
Motion

The most common error in large animal radiography that prevents the acquisition of diagnostic-quality radiographs is motion, which produces a blurred image ("moving picture") (Fig. 7-19). Long exposure times are frequently necessary in large animal radiography, especially with portable machines. Longer exposure times mean more time for motion to occur as the image is being made.

Motion has three possible sources:
1. Radiograph machine: This problem is associated with portable machines, which are often handheld during film taking. This motion source can be alleviated by using tripods or other stands that can be purchased for the machines or by improvising support with hay bales, buckets, or boxes when possible.
2. Patient: This is difficult to control with an awake patient. Even swaying from leg to leg can be enough to ruin the quality of an image. Effective restraint is essential. Chemical restraint must be used judiciously; oversedation can make a patient wobbly and unable to stand still.
3. Film cassette: Because cassettes are usually handheld directly or with a mechanical extension arm, the person holding the cassette must hold it as still as possible. This is a difficult task, given the weight of the cassette and lead-lined gloves. Whenever possible, resting the cassette on the ground or a solid object may help to steady the cassette. In addition, only high-speed film/screen combinations should be used for general large animal radiography.

Movement of any one of the foregoing during an exposure will be captured on the radiograph film. Before each radiograph is taken, all three sources should be evaluated as part of a mental checklist, with the goal of making each one as stationary as possible.

Height of Primary Beam

The object of most large animal radiographs is the distal limb, especially the foot. Radiographic principles require that the anatomical part of interest be positioned in the center of the x-ray beam; this minimizes distortion. When the hoof is on the ground, the center of the hoof will be 1 to 2 inches above the ground. Unfortunately, no radiograph machine can center a beam at that level. Even small portable machines generate a beam that is centered at a minimum of 3 to 4 inches above ground. Therefore, for foot films, because the beam cannot be lowered to foot level, the foot must be raised to the level of the center of the beam (Fig. 7-20, A). This can be accomplished by using positioning blocks or foot stands (Fig. 7-20, B). These can be commercially obtained or made of wood (wood blocks that are 4 × 4 inches and 2 × 4 inches are popular), Plexiglass, or other sturdy material that can support the horse's weight (Fig. 7-21). The device should be wide enough to prevent it from tipping over while the horse is standing on it; it must at least the width of the horse's hoof. The horse's foot is placed on the positioning device only while the film is taken. Once the film is made, the device should be removed and set safely aside; the horse should not be allowed to stand on the support unattended.

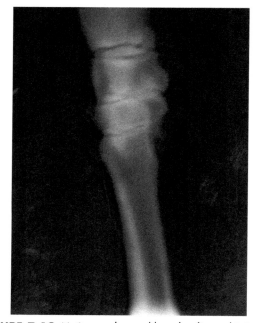

FIGURE 7-19 Motion produces a blurred radiographic image.

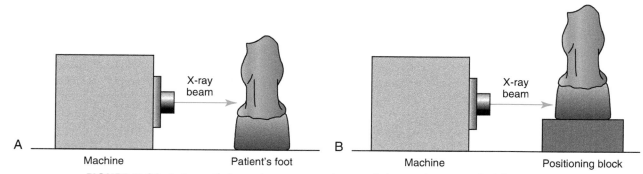

A | Machine | Patient's foot

B | Machine | Positioning block

FIGURE 7-20 A, Even with the machine resting on the ground, the x-ray beam is too high for structures in the foot. **B,** Elevation of the foot to the level of the x-ray beam, using a positioning block.

LABELING SYSTEM

Understanding that the distal limb of one leg is indistinguishable radiographically below the knee or carpus and stifle from the distal limb of any other leg is essential in both the equine and ruminant species. The reason for this resemblance is the similar bone structure of all limbs distal to the carpus and tarsus (Fig. 7-22).

Without proper identification, the clinician cannot tell a right distal limb from a left one or a front distal limb from a rear limb. Horses have had surgical procedures performed on the wrong leg because of errors in film identification. Lower leg films must always be accurately identified with some type of marker as either "right" or "left," and either "front" or "hind." The location of the marker is important for conventional marking systems for all images other than *lateral* projections. The marker is placed lateral to the sagittal plane of the joint. When taking lateral projections, the marker is placed *cranial* or dorsal to the joint (Fig. 7-23). Radiographic views

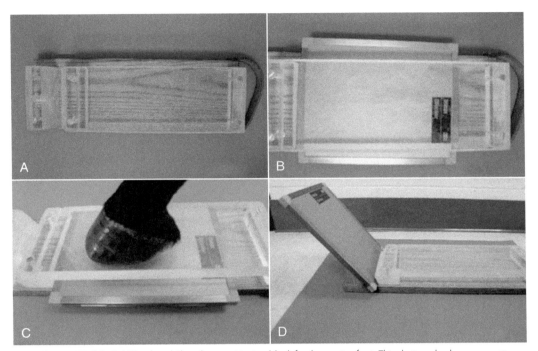

FIGURE 7-21 A, Wood and Plexiglass positioning block for the equine foot. This design also has a cassette tunnel that protects the cassette for stand-on views. **B,** Position of the cassette for stand-on radiographic views. **C,** Position of foot and cassette for stand-on views of the foot. **D,** Slots provide additional support for film cassettes.

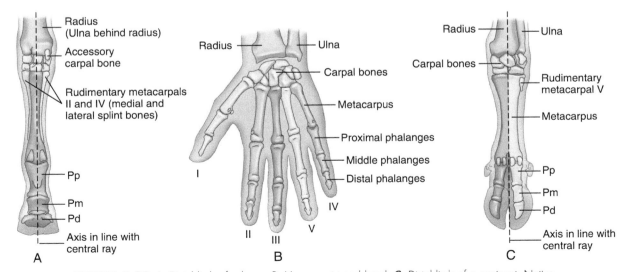

FIGURE 7-22 A, Distal limb of a horse. **B,** Human wrist and hand. **C,** Distal limb of a ruminant. Notice the anatomical similarities among the species. Also note that a horse's four limbs do not differ radiographically below the carpus and tarsus. *Pd,* Distal phalanx; *Pm,* middle phalanx; *Pp,* proximal phalanx. (From Brown M, Brown L: *Lavin's radiography for veterinary technicians,* ed 5, St. Louis, 2013, Saunders.)

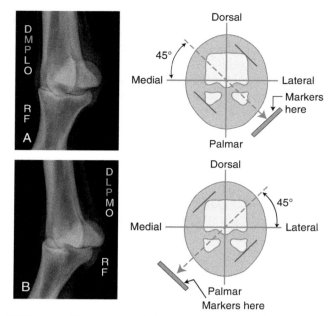

FIGURE 7-23 Description of the terminology of the oblique views on a fetlock radiograph. The *dotted lines* are the direction of the beam, and the *red lines* are the surfaces of the limbs being imaged. **A,** Lateral oblique or dorsoproximal 45-degree medial-palmarodistolateral oblique (DPr45M-PaDiLO). Following the rule and taking the middle two and outer two letters, you are looking at the dorsolateral and palmaromedial surfaces of the limb/medial sesamoid. **B,** Medial oblique or dorsoproximal 45-degree lateral-palmarodistomedial oblique (DPr45L-PaDiMO). Following the rule and taking the middle two and outer two letters, you are looking at the dorsomedial and palmarolateral surfaces of the limb/lateral sesamoid. *DMPLO,* Dorsomedial-palmarolateral oblique; *DLPMO,* dorsolateral-palmaromedial oblique; *RF,* right forelimb. (From Brown M, Brown L: *Lavin's radiography for veterinary technicians,* ed 5, St. Louis, 2013, Saunders.)

are named by the direction of the x-ray beam, from the radiograph machine to the film cassette. The first word (or initial) of the view identifies the location of the radiograph machine, and the second word (or initial) indicates the location of the film cassette. For example, if the machine is on the lateral aspect of the limb, and the film cassette is placed on the *medial* aspect of the leg, a lateromedial (LM) radiograph is produced. If the positions of the machine and cassette are reversed, a mediolateral (ML) view results (Fig. 7-24). The standard radiographic views used for the lower legs are, as in small animals, the LM view and the *dorsal-palmar/dorsal-plantar* view.

To obtain additional information to the two standard 90-degree views, it is common in large animals also to obtain oblique (angled) views of the lower legs. The four common oblique radiographic views are named by the direction of the radiographic beam (from radiograph machine to film cassette). The oblique views are made at 45-degree angles to the standard 90-degree views (Fig. 7-25). Oblique views of the distal limbs must be accurately marked because they are also indistinguishable from one another below the carpus or tarsus.

When labeling views, each label has three standard parts. The first part of the label should be left or right. Is this a left or right forelimb or hindlimb? Second is the description of the beam, for example, dorsolateral-palmaromedial oblique. Third is a description of the area, for example, cannon bone. If you are going to label one radiograph, it would be, for example, right forelimb dorsolateral-palmaromedial oblique of the cannon bone. These terms are often abbreviated RF DLPMO cannon bone.

Patient Preparation

The surface of the patient should be cleaned before taking radiographs. Shavings, dried mud, and other debris can create subtle images that interfere with interpretation of the film. Some topical medications contain iodine, and because iodine is radiopaque, it should be washed thoroughly from the area.

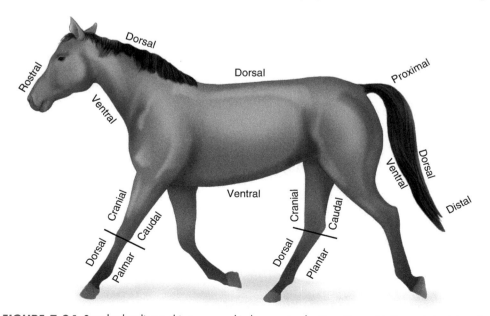

FIGURE 7-24 Standard radiographic terms used in large animals. (From Brown M, Brown L: *Lavin's radiography for veterinary technicians,* ed 5, St. Louis, 2013, Saunders.)

Bandages should be removed if possible. Although radiographs can penetrate bandages and even casts, these materials may obscure subtle anatomical lesions. If it is not safe or feasible to remove a bandage or cast, slightly longer exposure time or higher kVp can be used to help compensate for the added thickness.

Foot Radiographs

Preparation of the foot is important for high-quality films. The hoof should always be cleaned to remove dirt, gravel, and bedding. If necessary, a brush and water with mild soap can be used to clean the hoof wall, sole, and recesses of the frog.

Horseshoes should be removed whenever possible. Metallic horseshoes and nails obscure clear vision of the anatomical

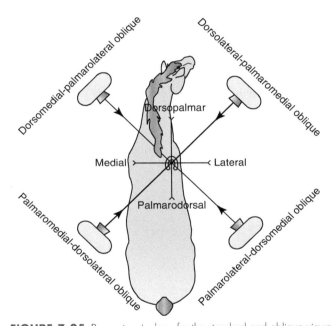

FIGURE 7-25 Proper terminology for the standard and oblique views of the right forelimb of a horse, according to the position of the radiograph machine. (Adapted from Lavin LM: *Radiography in veterinary technology*, ed 3, St. Louis, 2003, Saunders.)

structures within the hoof (Fig. 7-26). However, owners are understandably reluctant to have the shoes removed; there is additional expense and time involved in having the farrier replace the shoe. Rarely, the veterinarian may be able to see hoof lesions without removing shoes, but in most cases, the owner should be advised that the shoes should be removed to have the best chance of obtaining diagnostic-quality radiographs. The client's consent should always be obtained before pulling the horse's shoes. Because many horses tend to chip and crack their hooves if left unprotected, a temporary duct tape "hoof bootie" or commercial rubber boot can be used to protect the hoof until the farrier can return to replace the horseshoe.

The deep grooves of the sole (central sulcus of the frog and lateral sulci of the frog) are naturally occupied by air. The air creates artifacts—dark gas lines—on dorsopalmar/plantar (straight and oblique) hoof radiographs. These gas lines mimic fracture lines and may obscure true lesions. The gas lines can be eliminated by filling the grooves with something other than gas; semisolid radiolucent materials such as Play-Doh or putty are commonly used to pack the grooves and eliminate the air pockets (Fig. 7-27). The packing material should be pressed firmly into the grooves to fill them deeply and completely; however, overfilling should be avoided. Filling beyond the margins of the grooves is unnecessary, and overfilling may actually create more artifacts that obscure accurate interpretation of the film.

After packing the hoof grooves, the packing material should be covered before the horse is allowed to set the foot down on the ground. Covering the material is necessary to prevent gravel, bedding, and other debris from sticking to the material and causing artifacts. A paper towel or piece of brown paper pressed over the packing is all that is necessary to cover and protect the area (Fig. 7-28).

Head and Throat Radiographs

Metallic buckles and billets are radiopaque. Halters with metal should be removed and replaced with halters without metal.

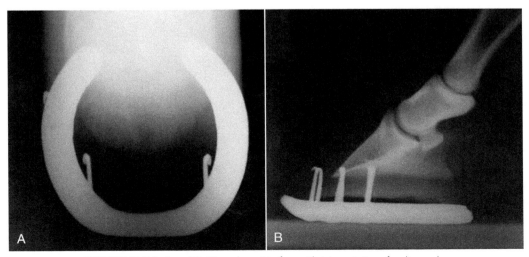

FIGURE 7-26 A and B, Horseshoes interfere with interpretation of radiographs.

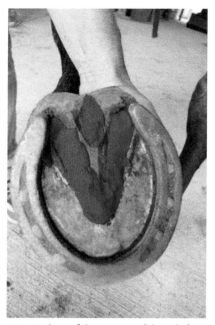

FIGURE 7-27 Packing of the grooves of the sole for radiographs.

Because of the machine lights and noise, as well as the need to press film cassettes against the head, most horses do not stand quietly for radiographs of the head area. Sedation is almost always required to obtain diagnostic films of this highly detailed region.

Pelvic Radiographs

Because of the extreme thickness and anatomical structure of the pelvic region, lateral views of the pelvis are possible only on small equids. The ventrodorsal view is available for larger animals but requires a frog-leg position in dorsal recumbency, obtainable only with the patient under general anesthesia. Patient preparation for general anesthesia is therefore required for this procedure.

STANDARD RADIOGRAPHIC VIEWS

Although the number of radiographic views of an anatomical part is limited only by the imagination, standardized views for each part have emerged to provide consistency in interpretation of radiographic films. Table 7-1 lists the standard radiographic views for the limbs, as well as common supplemental views.

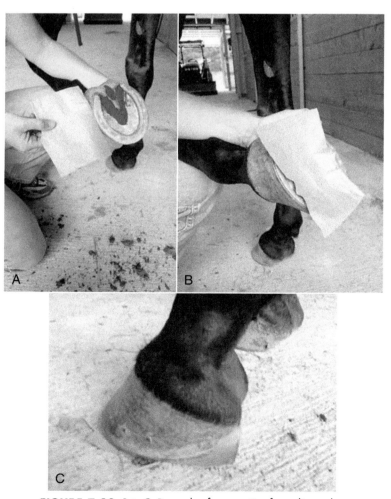

FIGURE 7-28 A to **C,** Proper hoof preparation for radiographs.

TABLE 7-1	Radiographic Views of the Equine Limbs	
ANATOMICAL PART	**STANDARD RADIOGRAPHIC VIEWS**	**SUPPLEMENTAL VIEWS**
P3/hoof	Straight DP 60-degree DP (stand-on) Lateromedial	60-degree DP oblique (stand-on)
Navicular bone	Lateromedial 60-degree DP (stand-on) 45-degree flexor tangential (stand-on)	30-degree DP (stand-on) 45-degree DP (stand-on) 60-degree DP oblique (stand-on)
Pastern	Lateromedial Straight DP Oblique (MLO, LMO)	30-degree DP
Fetlock	Lateromedial Flexed lateromedial Straight DP Oblique (MLO, LMO)	Hanging DP Flexor skyline Proximodistal oblique (MLO, LMO)
Metacarpus/metatarsus	Lateromedial DP Oblique (MLO, LMO)	
Carpus	Lateromedial Flexed lateromedial DP Oblique (MLO, LMO)	Flexed skyline (distal radius) Flexed skyline (proximal row carpal bones) Flexed skyline (distal row carpal bones)
Radius	Lateromedial Craniocaudal (AP)	Oblique (MLO, LMO)
Elbow	Mediolateral Craniocaudal (AP)	
Shoulder	Mediolateral	
Tarsus	Lateromedial DP Oblique (MLO, LMO)	Flexed skyline Flexed lateromedial
Tibia	Lateromedial Craniocaudal (AP)	Oblique (MLO, LMO)
Stifle	Lateromedial Craniocaudal (AP)	Flexed lateromedial Flexed skyline Oblique (MLO, LMO)
Pelvis	Ventrodorsal	Ventrodorsal oblique

AP, Anteroposterior; *DP,* dorsopalmar/dorsoplantar; *LMO,* lateromedial oblique; *MLO,* mediolateral oblique; *PA,* posteroanterior.

Foot

Distal Limb Anatomy
Lateromedial
- Abbreviation: LM
- Oblique in degrees: 0
- Elevation from floor in degrees: 0
- Beam center: at the sole of the foot
- Positioning: weight bearing, up on a wood block, and perpendicular to the ground

Dorsopalmar
- Abbreviation: DP
- Oblique in degrees: 0
- Elevation from floor in degrees: 0
- Beam center: middle of the hoof wall between the coronary band and sole

- Positioning: weight bearing, up on a wood block, and perpendicular to the ground

Dorsopalmar or Dorsoplantar 65 Degrees
- Abbreviation: DP 65
- Oblique in degrees: 65
- Elevation from floor in degrees: 0
- Beam center: coronary band
- Positioning: positioning device required

Dorsolateral-Palmaromedial or Dorsolateral-Plantarolateral Oblique
- Abbreviation: DLPMO
- Oblique in degrees: 45
- Elevation from floor in degrees: 0
- Beam center: coronary band
- Positioning: positioning device required

Dorsomedial-Palmarolateral or Dorsomedial-Plantarolateral Oblique
- Abbreviation: DMPLO
- Oblique in degrees: 45
- Elevation from the floor in degrees: 0
- Beam center: coronary band
- Positioning: positioning device required

Skyline of the Navicular Bone
- Abbreviation: skyline navicular
- Oblique in degrees: 0
- Elevation from the floor in degrees: 65
- Beam center: through the heal bulbs
- Positioning: cassette within a tunnel; horse standing on the tunnel

Fetlock
Lateromedial
- Abbreviation: LM
- Oblique in degrees: 0
- Elevation from the floor in degrees: 0
- Beam center: fetlock joint
- Positioning: weight bearing and perpendicular to the ground

Dorsopalmar or Dorsoplantar
- Abbreviation: DP
- Oblique in degrees: 0
- Elevation from the floor in degrees: 0
- Beam center: fetlock joint
- Positioning: weight bearing and perpendicular to the ground

Dorsolateral-Palmaromedial or Dorsolateral-Plantaromedial Oblique
- Abbreviation: DLPMO
- Oblique in degrees: 45
- Elevation from the floor in degrees: 0
- Beam center: fetlock joint
- Positioning: weight bearing and perpendicular to the ground

Dorsomedial-Palmarolateral or Dorsomedial-Plantarolateral Oblique
- Abbreviation: DMPLO
- Oblique in degrees: 45
- Elevation from the floor in degrees: 0
- Beam center: fetlock joint
- Positioning: weight bearing and perpendicular to the ground

Metacarpus/Metatarsus
Dorsopalmar or Dorsoplantar
- Abbreviation: DP
- Oblique in degrees: 0
- Elevation from the floor in degrees: 0
- Beam center: center of diaphysis
- Positioning: weight bearing and perpendicular to the ground

Lateromedial
- Abbreviation: LM
- Oblique in degrees: 0
- Elevation from the floor in degrees: 0
- Beam center: center of diaphysis
- Positioning: weight bearing and perpendicular to the ground

Dorsolateral-Palmaromedial Oblique or Dorsolateral-Plantaromedial Oblique
- Abbreviation: DLPMO
- Oblique in degrees: 45
- Elevation from the floor in degrees: 0
- Beam center: center of diaphysis
- Positioning: weight bearing and perpendicular to the ground

Dorsomedial-Palmarolateral or Dorsomedial-Plantarolateral Oblique
- Abbreviation: DMPLO
- Oblique in degrees: 45
- Elevation from the floor in degrees: 0
- Beam center: center of diaphysis
- Positioning: weight bearing and perpendicular to the ground

Carpus
Lateromedial
- Abbreviation: LM
- Oblique in degrees: 0
- Elevation from the floor in degrees: 0
- Beam center: carpal joint
- Positioning: weight bearing and perpendicular to the ground

Dorsopalmar
- Abbreviation: DP
- Oblique in degrees: 0
- Elevation from the floor in degrees: 0
- Beam center: carpal joint
- Positioning: weight bearing and perpendicular to the ground

Dorsolateral-Palmaromedial
- Abbreviation: DLPMO
- Oblique in degrees: 45
- Elevation from the floor in degrees: 0
- Beam center: fetlock joint
- Positioning: weight bearing and perpendicular to the ground

Dorsomedial-Palmarolateral
- Abbreviation: DMPLO
- Oblique in degrees: 45
- Elevation from the floor in degrees: 0
- Beam center: carpal joint
- Positioning: weight bearing and perpendicular to the ground

Flexed Lateromedial

- Abbreviation: flexed LM
- Oblique in degrees: 0
- Elevation from the floor in degrees: 0
- Beam center: carpal joint
- Positioning: leg held with the carpus in flexion but directly below the proximal forelimb; carpus not completely flexed; some space left between the forearm and cannon bone

Skyline of Third Carpal Bone

- Abbreviation: skyline of third carpal
- Oblique in degrees: 0
- Elevation from the floor in degrees:45
- Beam center: carpal joint
- Positioning: leg held with the carpus in flexion and the cannon bone parallel to the ground

Tarsus
Lateromedial

- Abbreviation: LM
- Oblique in degrees: 0
- Elevation from the floor in degrees: 0
- Beam center: tarsal joint
- Positioning: weight bearing and perpendicular to the ground

Dorsoplantar

- Abbreviation: DP
- Oblique in degrees: 0
- Elevation from the floor in degrees: 0
- Beam center: tarsal joint
- Positioning: weight bearing and perpendicular to the ground

Dorsolateral-Plantaromedial Oblique

- Abbreviation: DLPMO
- Oblique in degrees: 45
- Elevation from the floor in degrees: 0
- Beam center: tarsal joint
- Positioning: weight bearing and perpendicular to the ground

Dorsomedial-Plantarolateral Oblique

- Abbreviation: DMPLO
- Oblique in degrees: 45
- Elevation from the floor in degrees: 0
- Beam center: tarsal joint
- Positioning: weight bearing and perpendicular to the ground

Radius and Elbow
Mediolateral

- Abbreviation: LM
- Oblique in degrees: 0
- Elevation from the floor in degrees: 0
- Beam center: center of diaphysis

- Positioning: weight bearing and perpendicular to the ground

Craniocaudal

- Abbreviation: CrCd
- Oblique in degrees: 0
- Elevation from the floor in degrees: 0
- Beam Center: center of diaphysis
- Positioning: weight bearing and perpendicular to the ground

Craniolateral-Caudomedial Oblique

- Abbreviation: CrLCdMO
- Oblique in degrees: 45
- Elevation from the floor in degrees: 0
- Beam center: center of diaphysis
- Positioning: weight bearing and perpendicular to the ground

Craniomedial-Caudolateral oblique

- Abbreviation: CrMCdLO
- Oblique in degrees: 45
- Elevation from the floor in degrees: 0
- Beam center: center of diaphysis
- Positioning: weight bearing and perpendicular to the ground

Tibia
Lateromedial

- Abbreviation: LM
- Oblique in degrees: 0
- Elevation from the floor in degrees: 0
- Beam center: center of diaphysis
- Positioning: weight bearing and perpendicular to the ground

Caudocranial

- Abbreviation: CdCr
- Oblique in degrees: 0
- Elevation from the floor in degrees: 0
- Beam center: center of diaphysis
- Positioning: weight bearing and perpendicular to the ground

Craniolateral-Caudomedial Oblique

- Abbreviation: CrLCdMO
- Oblique in degrees: 45
- Elevation from the floor in degrees: 0
- Beam center: center of diaphysis
- Positioning: weight bearing and perpendicular to the ground

Craniomedial-Caudolateral Oblique

- Abbreviation: CrMCdLO
- Oblique in degrees: 45
- Elevation from the floor in degrees: 0
- Beam center: center of diaphysis
- Positioning: weight bearing and perpendicular to the ground

Stifle
Lateromedial
- Abbreviation: LM
- Oblique in degrees: 0
- Elevation from the floor in degrees: 0
- Beam center: center of stifle joint
- Positioning: weight bearing and perpendicular to the ground

Caudocranial
- Abbreviation: DP
- Oblique in degrees: 0
- Elevation from the floor in degrees: 0
- Beam center: center of stifle joint
- Positioning: weight bearing and perpendicular to the ground

Caudolateral-Craniomedial Oblique
- Abbreviation: CLCMO
- Oblique in degrees: 45
- Elevation from the floor in degrees: 0
- Beam center: center of stifle joint
- Positioning: weight bearing and perpendicular to the ground

Skull
Lateral
- Abbreviation: LAT
- Oblique in degrees: 0
- Elevation from the floor in degrees: 0
- Beam center: suspected lesion
- Positioning: no rotation

Dorsoventral
- Abbreviation: LAT
- Oblique in degrees: 0
- Elevation from the floor in degrees: 0
- Beam center: suspected lesion
- Positioning: no rotation

Oblique of Maxillary Teeth
- Abbreviation: maxillary oblique
- Oblique in degrees: 90
- Elevation from the floor in degrees: 30
- Beam center: suspected lesion
- Positioning: no rotation

Oblique of Mandibular Teeth
- Abbreviation: mandibular oblique
- Oblique in degrees: 90
- Elevation from the floor in degrees: 45
- Beam center: suspected lesion
- Positioning: no rotation

Cervical Spine
Lateral
- Abbreviation: LAT
- Oblique in degrees: 0
- Elevation from the floor in degrees: 0
- Beam center: can be cranial, middle, or caudal cervical spine, over suspected lesion
- Positioning: weight bearing and perpendicular to the ground

Thorax
Lateral
- Abbreviation: LAT
- Oblique in degrees: 0
- Elevation from the floor in degrees: 0
- Beam center: center in one of four quadrants—caudodorsal, caudoventral, craniodorsal, cranioventral
- Positioning: weight bearing and perpendicular to the ground

Pelvis
Ventrodorsal
- Abbreviation: VD
- Oblique in degrees: 0
- Elevation from the floor in degrees: 0
- Beam center: linea alba
- Positioning: weight bearing and perpendicular to the ground

NUCLEAR SCINTIGRAPHY

Scintigraphy is a method of imaging that emphasizes physiology rather than anatomy. Whereas a radiograph or ultrasound scan takes an image of a patient's anatomy, scintigraphy takes an image of a patient's physiologic processes. This is accomplished by administering a radioactive compound, allowing the compound to accumulate within the patient, and then measuring the amount of radioactivity emitted from the patient. A gamma camera is used to measure the radioactivity.

The properties of the radioactive compound determine where in the body the compound is likely to accumulate, according to the body organs that process the compound; this is the physiologic part of the image process. The radioactive compound, or radiopharmaceutical, is made by attaching a radioisotope to another compound that has an affinity for certain body organs, such as iodine for the thyroid or phosphonates for bone. Technetium-99m is the most common radioisotope used for the radiolabel.

Most large animal scintigraphy is performed to evaluate the musculoskeletal system; skeletal scintigraphy is also known as a "bone scan." The patient is sedated for the procedure. Technetium-labeled diphosphonate is given intravenously to the patient, and the diphosphonates are incorporated into the patient's bone, taking the radioactive technetium "tags" with them. The radioactivity over the bone is then measured, and high emission of radiation is assumed to reflect areas of increased blood flow in the bone or uptake by osteoblasts—an indication of inflammation or new bone formation. These areas of increased radioactivity are commonly called "hot spots."

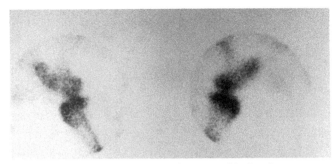

FIGURE 7-29 Nuclear scintigraphic scan of both stifle joints in a lame horse. Note the increased radioactivity (blackness) of the right stifle as compared with the left stifle joint. The horse had degenerative joint disease (chronic arthritis) in the right stifle. (From Lavin LM: *Radiography in veterinary technology*, ed 3, St. Louis, 2003, Saunders.)

Scintigraphy is helpful in detecting lesions when radiography and ultrasonography have not confirmed a diagnosis or cannot penetrate deeply enough, especially in the regions of the upper limbs, shoulders, and pelvis. Scintigraphy can also screen large areas of the patient (Fig. 7-29).

Only clinics or hospitals that are licensed to handle and dispose of radioactive materials and waste can perform this procedure. The patient must usually be isolated for several days until the radioactive material is cleared from the body; excrement requires special handling. Each state has regulations for licensing and operating these facilities.

COMPUTED TOMOGRAPHY

CT (or "CAT scan," as it was once known) is restricted to examination of the head, cranial cervical spine, and distal limbs in the adult horse. The spinal cord, thorax, and abdomen can be imaged in miniature horses and small foals, depending on the diameter of the equipment. CT equipment is expensive; therefore, it is found only in specialized facilities. Another consideration is that the patient must be under general anesthesia to prevent motion during the scan. The cost of a CT scan is high—reflecting both the cost of the equipment and the cost of general anesthesia. CT is used only when other diagnostic methods have failed to provide a diagnosis.

CT is essentially a series of thin, cross-sectional radiographs. When viewing the images, it helps me to think of the anatomical location being sliced very thinly, such as with an egg slicer, and I can then view each slice individually. The part to be imaged is placed inside a donut-shaped ring called a gantry. The gantry contains a small x-ray tube and multiple radiation detectors to receive the radiograph beam from different angles. The gantry rotates around the patient and takes multiple radiographic images. The images are collected and assimilated by a computer, resulting in a gray-scale cross-sectional image of the part. The computer can be used to enhance different types of tissue digitally.

As technology progresses, larger gantries may allow CT scans of larger body parts in adult horses. CT is generally superior to magnetic resonance imaging (MRI) for bone lesions.

MAGNETIC RESONANCE IMAGING

MRI is now possible for large animals. The physics of MRI is complex but basically involves placing the body part to be studied in a powerful magnetic field. The magnetic field causes alignment of all the hydrogen nuclei (protons) in the body part; then, radiofrequency pulses are sent through the part. This temporarily excites the magnetized protons, which emit radiofrequency signals when they return to the original magnetized state. These signals are detected and transformed into images by a computer. Ionizing radiation is not used in the procedure.

The usefulness of MRI in large animals is currently restricted by the physical capacity of the equipment. The head, cervical spinal cord, and lower legs can be imaged in an adult horse. The cost of the equipment is high, and therefore MRI is not widely available at this time. Similar to CT, general anesthesia is required, and the cost of the procedure is high as a result of the expensive equipment and the cost of general anesthesia. MRI tends to be superior to CT for soft tissue imaging.

THERMOGRAPHY

Diagnostic thermography uses a "heat camera" to scan the body surface temperature of the patient. This technique is popular because it is noninvasive, and the equipment has become more affordable and portable. Thermography can be used to examine specific body parts or used for whole body screens as part of regular "wellness" examinations of the legs. The primary use of thermography is to locate "hot spots," which may indicate inflammation (Fig. 7-30). Heat is one of the cardinal signs of inflammation. Thermography is best used to locate inflammation near the body surface. Areas of inflammation deep within the thorax or abdomen cannot be seen with thermography.

False-positive (increased heat) readings are likely with thermography unless the conditions of the examination are closely controlled. The patient should be shielded from environmental heat sources such as the sun. Bandages, tack, and blankets can all cause a local increase in heat; patients should have these removed 2 hours before the examination. Topical medications should also be removed. The area of the examination should be less than 86° F to prevent sweating; 70° F is ideal. The area should be free of drafts.

The patient should be placed in the examination area and allowed approximately 20 to 30 minutes to acclimate to the room's temperature.

Artifacts are easily produced on a thermogram, and any hot spots should be closely inspected for possible insignificant sources of heat or cold. Insects and insect bites can produce artifact hot spots on a thermogram. Injection procedures such as diagnostic nerve and joint blocks produce inflammation and cause artifact hot spots on the scan; it may be necessary to wait up to a week before performing thermography on patients that have had injections in the area of interest. In addition, areas where the hair has been clipped

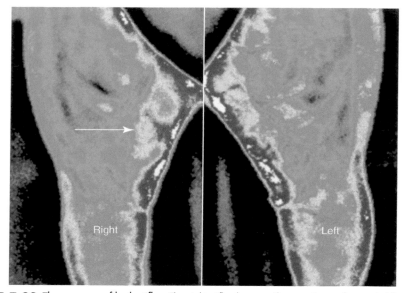

FIGURE 7-30 Thermogram of both stifles. The right stifle shows a "hot spot" over the medial femorotibial joint. (From Turner TA: Diagnostic thermography, *Vet Clin North Am Equine Pract* 17:95–113, 2001.)

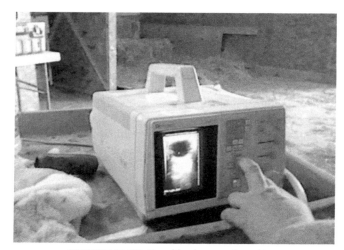

FIGURE 7-31 Portable ultrasound machine.

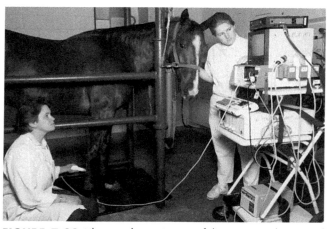

FIGURE 7-32 Ultrasound examination of the metacarpal region of the horse. (From Lavin LM: *Radiography in veterinary technology*, ed 3, St. Louis, 2003, Saunders.)

alter the surface temperature of the skin and may create artifacts. Generally, if possible, the thermogram should be performed before the horse is clipped or injected.

Thermography is useful to locate the general area of an injury, but it lacks the detail necessary for a specific diagnosis in most cases. Typically, once a hot spot is identified with thermography, radiography or ultrasound must be used to define the problem accurately.

DIAGNOSTIC ULTRASOUND

Ultrasound employs high-frequency sound waves that are beyond the range of human hearing. Depending on the frequency, ultrasound waves can be used either for diagnostic imaging (diagnostic ultrasound or "sonogram") or for therapeutic treatment of soft tissue injuries (therapeutic ultrasound). Because diagnostic ultrasound and therapeutic ultrasound serve different purposes, they require

different equipment, and the equipment is not interchangeable (Fig. 7-31).

Ultrasound is generally superior to standard radiographs for visualizing soft tissues. Radiographs are generally superior for imaging bony structures (Fig. 7-32).

Diagnostic ultrasound commonly uses sound waves in the frequency range of 2 to 10 megahertz (MHz). The waves are generated by a transducer, which is a handheld attachment to the ultrasound machine. The sound waves penetrate the patient's tissues and are reflected by tissue interfaces (i.e., the junctions between different tissue types and tissue contents) (Fig. 7-33). The transducer receives these reflected waves or "echoes" and relays them to the ultrasound machine. The ultrasound machine processes the waves into a visual image that displays on a video screen. The image is generated as a series of dots; the brightness of each dot corresponds to the amplitude of the reflected sound wave. Very bright areas are called hyperechoic

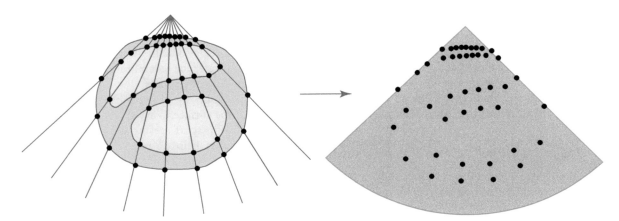

FIGURE 7-33 Ultrasound waves are reflected by tissue interfaces *(left)*. The images are converted into a series of dots to form a B-mode sonogram. (Adapted from Powis RL: Ultrasound science for the veterinarian, *Vet Clin North Am Equine Pract* 2:3–27, 1986.)

TABLE 7-2	Ultrasound Transducer Probes and Common Applications	
FREQUENCY (MHZ)	**COMMON APPLICATIONS**
10.0	Superficial tendons, ligaments, bone surfaces, eyes, jugular vein, umbilicus
7.5	Superficial tendons, ligaments, bone surfaces, eyes, jugular vein, umbilicus, male reproductive organs
5.0	Female reproductive system (per rectum), abdominal viscera (per rectum), muscles
2.5–3.0	Heart, pleural cavity, superficial aspects of lungs, kidneys, liver, spleen, abdomen (outer 10–18 inches), cranial mediastinum, deep muscle, and bone surfaces

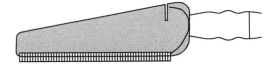

FIGURE 7-34 A standard linear array transducer. (Adapted from Reef VB: *Equine diagnostic ultrasound*, St. Louis, 1998, Saunders.)

and generally indicate a more solid tissue; black areas are called anechoic and generally indicate liquid. If an area generates less brightness than expected, the area is called hypoechoic.

The frequency of the ultrasound waves greatly influences the quality of the ultrasound examination. The higher the frequency, the shorter the wavelength; this leads to better resolution (definition) of the image, but the tradeoff is low penetration (depth) of the scan. Conversely, low-frequency waves penetrate more deeply into the patient but with less resolution. Transducers are usually limited to the production of a single frequency; therefore, several transducers must be purchased to give the practitioner the ability to scan a variety of anatomical structures (Table 7-2).

Two basic types of transducers are used. Linear array transducers have ultrasound crystals, which emit the ultrasound waves, arranged in a row (Fig. 7-34). This system emits ultrasound from multiple points along the transducer and produces a rectangular image (Fig. 7-35). Sector scanner transducers have one or more ultrasound crystals that rotate or oscillate to produce a pie-shaped image (Fig. 7-36). Variations of sector scanners, such as the annular array and phased array, are also available for some machines; these are

more expensive machines used mostly for cardiac studies such as color-flow Doppler echocardiography.

Two common types of display modes are used for ultrasound examinations. B (brightness) mode is the most commonly used; the brightness of the dots corresponds to the strength of the returning echoes. The examination is conducted in real time, but the real-time image can be frozen at any time on the screen for closer study or for recording onto camera or video film. The other type of display is M (motion) mode, which is used primarily for echocardiography (Fig. 7-37). M mode is essentially "B mode in motion" across the viewing screen. The image is a "trace" over time of the movements of the heart structures that allows measurement of wall thickness, valve motions, and chamber capacities.

The maximum depth of penetration for most ultrasound machines is 30 to 40 cm. This depth does not allow complete examination of the entire thoracic or abdominal cavity from the exterior of the patient. The abdomen has the additional option of internal ultrasound examination through the rectum; however, rectal examinations are limited by the length of the examiner's arm, and some regions of the abdomen cannot be completely evaluated. Despite these limitations, ultrasound is an invaluable tool in the examination of these body cavities.

PATIENT PREPARATION

Air reflects sound waves and produces an essentially meaningless image. For this reason, no air can be present between the patient and the transducer during the examination.

The patient's hair coat traps air and creates numerous little air pockets. The best-quality images are obtained if the hair is clipped; if the hair is coarse, shaving may also be necessary (Fig. 7-38). The owner's permission should be obtained before clipping the patient; occasionally an owner may object

to this procedure. The owner must understand that failure to remove hair can compromise the scan, especially when trying to find subtle lesions. In these cases, thoroughly soaking the area with water for several minutes before the examination may improve the results.

After clipping, the clipped hairs must be thoroughly wiped from the surface to avoid creating artifact reflections. In addition, skin scurf creates artifacts; softening the scurf with warm water helps to remove it. Dirt, topical medications, and any other debris should also be removed.

A coupling medium is used to provide a continuous path, free of air, for the ultrasound waves between the transducer and the patient. Usually, commercial ultrasound coupling gel is used. Coupling gel can be bought in bulk and portioned into individual containers for more convenient use. Other gels such as OB lubricant and KY Jelly can be used. The use of mineral oil is discouraged for use on the skin; it causes scurf in many horses, is difficult to remove, and can damage

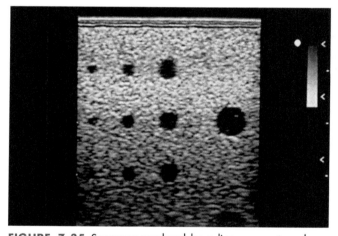

FIGURE 7-35 Sonogram produced by a linear array transducer. (From Reef VB: *Equine diagnostic ultrasound*, St. Louis, 1998, Saunders.)

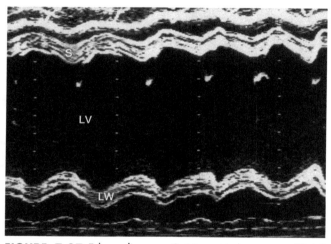

FIGURE 7-37 Echocardiogram. *S,* Interventricular septum; *LV,* left ventricle; *LW,* left ventricular wall. (From Lavin LM: *Radiography in veterinary technology*, ed 3, St. Louis, 2003, Saunders.)

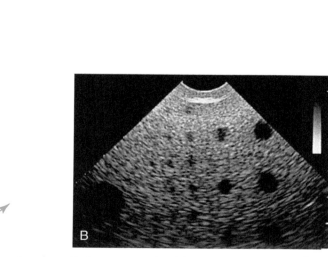

A

B

FIGURE 7-36 **A,** Sector scanner transducer. **B,** Sonogram produced by a sector scanner transducer. (Adapted from Reef VB: *Equine diagnostic ultrasound*, St. Louis, 1998, Saunders.)

the transducer head. Coupling gels should be thoroughly removed from the skin after the examination because they may be irritating to the skin if allowed to dry. The ultrasound waves emitted from the transducer have a focal zone, similar to a camera or radiograph machine (Fig. 7-39). Objects that are closer to the transducer than the focal zone, or beyond the focal zone, will not be in focus. This commonly occurs when trying to examine structures that are superficial (near the skin) and is referred to as a near-field artifact. To compensate, "standoffs"—jellylike synthetic pads—are used to back the transducer away from the skin, thus allowing the skin and structures just beneath the skin to fall within the transducer's focal zone. Standoffs may be built into some transducer heads, whereas others are handheld. Standoffs are easily damaged by excessive pressure and sharp objects, and they should be handled carefully. The handheld pads are usually stored in a refrigerator and should be allowed to warm to room temperature for best results.

REPRODUCTIVE ULTRASOUND

Reproductive ultrasound examinations are commonly used in large animal practice to image the ovaries and uterus. These examinations are performed to diagnose pregnancy (as early as 10 days), detect twin pregnancies, determine the sex of a fetus, identify disorders of the uterus and ovaries, and confirm the stage of the female's estrous cycle (Fig. 7- 40). These examinations are performed through the rectum, except in the case of late gestation, when the fetus is best

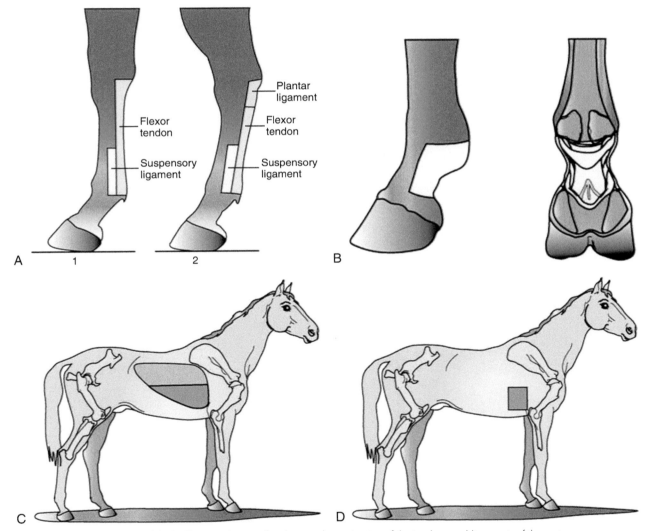

FIGURE 7-38 A, Clipping diagram for ultrasound examination of the tendons and ligaments of the metacarpus (1) and metatarsus (2). The areas marked "Suspensory ligament" are clipped if the suspensory branches are to be evaluated. **B,** Clipping diagram for ultrasound examination of the tendons and ligaments of the pastern. **C,** Clipping diagram for noncardiac ultrasound examination of the right thorax *(dark gray)*. The *lighter gray area* is added if abnormal lung sounds are auscultated in the dorsal lung field. **D,** Clipping diagram for cardiac ultrasound examination from the right side. The window is centered over the right fourth intercostal space and covers the area from the point of the elbow to the point of the shoulder. For examination from the left, the window is centered over the third to fifth intercostal spaces. Note that the forelimb is positioned cranially to open up the window.

Continued

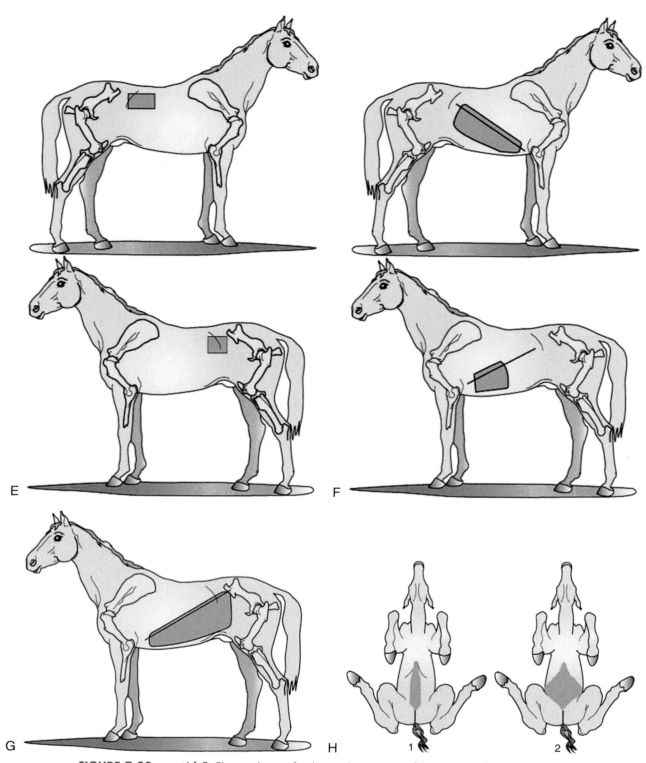

FIGURE 7-38, cont'd E, Clipping diagram for ultrasound examination of the right and left kidneys. F, Clipping diagram for ultrasound examination of the liver from both sides of the horse. G, Clipping diagram for ultrasound examination of the spleen. H, Clipping diagram for umbilical or bladder examination (1) and general abdominal examination (2) in the foal. (Adapted from Reef VB: *Equine diagnostic ultrasound*, St. Louis, 1998, Saunders.)

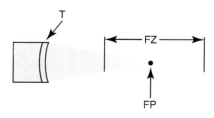

FIGURE 7-39 The transducer (T) operates in a focal zone (FZ) with a focal point (FP). (From Powis RL: Ultrasound science for the veterinarian, *Vet Clin North Am Equine Pract* 2:3–27, 1986.)

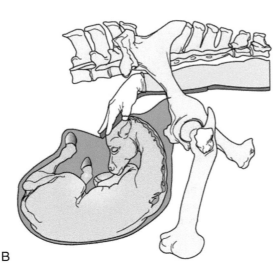

FIGURE 7-40 A, A 16-day pregnancy, visualized rectally with a 5-mHz probe. **B,** Rectal ultrasound examination of a fetus. (**A,** From Torbeck RL: Diagnostic ultrasound in equine reproduction, *Vet Clin North Am Equine Pract* 2:227–252, 1986; **B,** adapted from Reef VB: *Equine diagnostic ultrasound*, St. Louis, 1998, Saunders.)

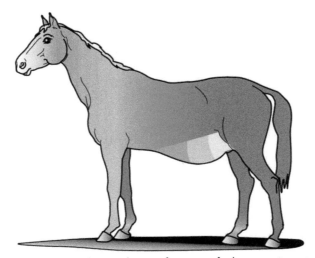

FIGURE 7-41 Clipping diagram for a mare for late gestation external ultrasound. (Adapted from Reef VB: *Equine diagnostic ultrasound*, St. Louis, 1998, Saunders.)

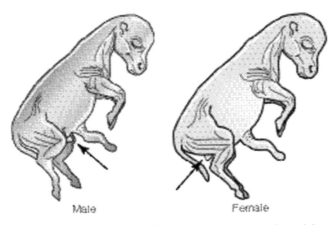

Male   Female

FIGURE 7-42 The genital tubercle is located closer to the umbilicus in the male and closer to the tail in the female. (Adapted from Reef VB: *Equine diagnostic ultrasound*, St. Louis, 1998, Saunders.)

imaged from the exterior (Fig. 7-41). Some patients resent rectal examination; care must be taken to protect the operator and the equipment from kicks and patient movement. Stocks, hay bales, stall doors, and doorways can be used as barriers against kicking and excessive movement.

Fetal sex determination ("sexing") is best performed between days 60 and 75 of gestation. Sexing requires locating the genital tubercle. In males the genital tubercle is located near the umbilicus, and in females the genital tubercle is closer to the tail (Fig. 7-42). Before day 60, the genital tubercle is located between the hindlimbs and has not yet migrated sufficiently to enable the operation to predict sex easily. After day 75, the fetus has grown to a size and location that often prevents visualization of the genital tubercle.

CARE OF ULTRASOUND EQUIPMENT

Transducers are expensive and are the most easily damaged part of an ultrasound machine. Hard impacts can damage the ultrasound crystals. The surface is susceptible to scratching from abrasive materials. Built-in standoffs are susceptible to punctures and cuts. The transducer cable should never be folded; rather, it should be loosely coiled to prevent breaking the cable wires.

The manufacturer specifies which cleaning agents are safe to use on the transducer. These instructions should be followed to prevent damage to the surface of the transducer. Abrasive cleaning agents and pads should never be used to clean transducer heads.

Cold weather can affect ultrasound examinations by altering the properties of coupling gels and standoff pads. If possible, examinations should not be performed in extreme cold. When performing examinations in a cold environment, the coupling gel should be applied and allowed to warm to the patient's skin temperature before the examination is conducted. Standoff pads also benefit from warming before use; placing the pad against the body for several minutes can warm the pad in a cold environment if another heat source is not available.

Ultrasound machines should be kept covered when not in use. If the machine is to be used for ambulatory work, a hard case is desirable to protect the unit while it is being transported.

ENDOSCOPY

Endoscopes come in two basic varieties: rigid and flexible. Rigid endoscopes are used for arthroscopy, laparoscopy, thoracoscopy, and rhinoscopy (especially evaluation of the sinuses). An external light source provides illumination for the procedure. The insertion tube is made of metal and should not be bent or flexed. The operator can observe directly through the eyepiece, but more commonly, a light from an external, stationary light source is transmitted to the tip of the endoscope, and the other bundle returns a visual image from the tip back to the operator's eyepiece. The tube also contains a system of wires and interlocking rings that allow the tip to be moved or deflected in different planes; this allows the endoscope to be directed around curves and corners and provide views in multiple directions. Most endoscopes have additional internal channels for passing instruments (e.g., biopsy or grasping forceps) and channels for air, water, and/or suction systems (Fig. 7- 43).

The flexible endoscope consists of three main parts: The control handpiece contains the eyepiece, deflection knobs, air, suction and water controls, and entrances to instrument channels. The insertion tubing is the long tube that is inserted into the patient; it is usually marked with gradations for length at 10-cm intervals. The light guide cable connects the control handpiece to the external light source and transmits light to the light fiber bundle (Fig. 7-44).

The operator controls the endoscope with the control handpiece by observing through the eyepiece and manipulating the tip with the deflection knobs. A video camera and screen are used for viewing. Rigid endoscopes are relatively short (most are <18 inches) compared with flexible endoscopes, which are up to 3 m (9 feet) long.

The flexible fiberoptic endoscope is basically a flexible, nonmetallic tube that houses two bundles of fibers. Because endoscopy is usually performed on standing, awake horses, additional staff may be required to restrain the patient.

Only the operator can view the conveyed images through the eyepiece. Video endoscope systems that project images onto a larger video viewing screen are available; this is made possible by attaching an external video camera to the endoscope eyepiece. The video screen allows bystanders to view the examination. Video image endoscopes that use a microchip and electric charges instead of fiberoptic bundles to carry images back to a viewing screen are also available. Permanent records of an endoscopic examination can be made with still photographs and video recordings, either by using a video recording system or by attaching still cameras to the eyepiece with an adapter ring.

The most common use of endoscopy in equine practice is for examination of the upper respiratory tract. These examinations are usually performed with the horse at rest, but with the

advent of the treadmill, a dynamic examination can now be performed to visualize problems that may not be apparent at rest (Fig. 7-45). Upper respiratory examinations are conducted by introducing the endoscope through a nostril and passing it through the nasal cavity; most horses resent this procedure and must be physically and/or chemically restrained. The procedure is similar to nasogastric intubation, and the same safety precautions used for nasogastric intubation should be followed whenever the endoscope is introduced through the nares.

Gastroscopy, the next most common use of endoscopy, was developed primarily to assess gastric ulceration in horses. Standard endoscopes (<110 cm) are not long enough to reach the stomach except perhaps in miniature horses and young foals; for adults, a scope 3 meters long is recommended. Endoscopes for gastroscopy are therefore more expensive

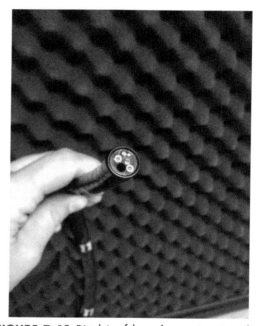

FIGURE 7-43 Distal tip of the endoscope insertion tube.

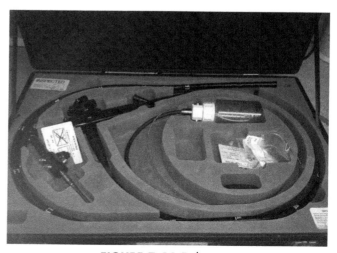

FIGURE 7-44 Endoscope.

than standard scopes. The endoscope is passed through a nostril to the pharynx and then down the esophagus to the stomach, similar to the path used for nasogastric intubation. Once the endoscope tip is in the stomach, the stomach is inflated with air to facilitate visualization; this may produce some discomfort to the patient. Gastroscopy requires fasting of the patient before the examination and sedation of the patient during the examination for best results.

Urinary tract endoscopy is also possible in both sexes. By passing the endoscope through the urethral orifice, the urethra and bladder of both males and females can be visualized. Sedation of the male is necessary to relax and extend the penis for passage of the endoscope through the urethra; females have wider and shorter urethras and may be more tolerant of the procedure (Fig. 7-46). To reduce the risk of

introducing bacteria into the urinary bladder, the endoscope should be cold sterilized and the patient properly cleansed, similar to preparation for passing a urinary catheter. (Clean the glans penis in the male and the vulva in the female.)

In the female, the endoscope can be used to evaluate the vagina, cervix, and uterus. The tail should be wrapped and held or tied to keep it away from the perineum during preparation and examination. The perineal area is thoroughly cleansed with water and mild soap, centering on the vulvar lips and progressing outwardly 4 to 6 inches, similar to preparation for vaginal and uterine reproductive procedures. The person passing the endoscope should wear sterile gloves. Sterile lubricating jelly is applied to the outer surface of the endoscope, except over the optic surface of the tip. Depositing lubricant over the endoscope tip should be avoided because the lubricant can obscure the lenses and instrument channels. Alternatively, sterile water can be used to lubricate the tip and does not obscure vision through the lenses. The uterus must be inflated with air to balloon the walls of the uterus; this is necessary for visualization within the organ. Sedation is usually required because the procedure causes some discomfort when the uterus is inflated with air.

Surgical procedures can be performed through the endoscope. Most of the procedures are performed on the upper respiratory tract in standing, sedated horses and are well tolerated. Electrosurgery can be performed by passing coagulation electrodes or snares through the instrument channel of the endoscope and applying extreme heat to a lesion. More recently, laser surgery has been performed in horses, with the surgeon using the endoscope for visualization and guidance of the laser. Laser light energy can be carried through special flexible fiber bundles, which are small enough to pass through the instrument channel of the endoscope. The surgeon can visualize lesions through the endoscope and can advance the laser fiber tip to deliver the laser energy to the affected area.

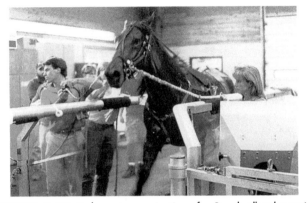

FIGURE 7-45 Endoscopic examination of a Standardbred exercising on a treadmill. The endoscopist is observing the examination on a video monitor (not included in the photograph). The equipment to the horse's left is the treadmill control panel. (From Traub-Dargatz JL, Brown CM: *Equine endoscopy*, ed 2, St. Louis, 1997, Mosby.)

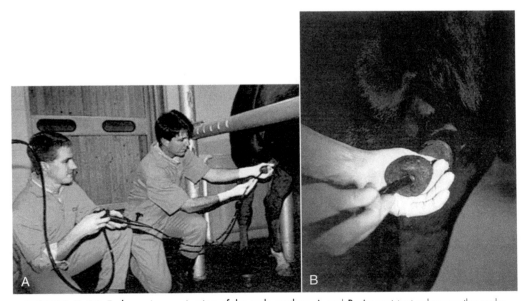

FIGURE 7-46 Endoscopic examination of the male urethra. **A** and **B**, An assistant advances the endoscope through the urethral opening at the tip of the glans penis, under guidance of the endoscopist. (From Traub-Dargatz JL, Brown CM: *Equine endoscopy*, ed 2, St. Louis, 1997, Mosby.)

CARE OF THE ENDOSCOPE

The endoscope should be inspected before each use for cracks in the external surface of the insertion tubing and debris on the tip. Damage to the fiber bundles is assessed by looking through the eyepiece; if the image is blurred or dim, and cleaning the lenses and adjusting the eyepiece focus do not improve the image, it is likely that fiber damage has occurred. The endoscope should not be used if it is damaged; repairs are necessary.

Mobility of the tip should be checked by turning the deflection knobs and watching the response of the tip; do not manually bend the tip to check its mobility. Deflection cables can stretch or even break; if the scope does not bend appropriately, the deflection cables may need to be replaced.

All connections of the endoscope to the light source, including air, water, and suction systems, should be checked before use. The water source should be filled before the examination; distilled water is preferred to tap water. In some cases, sterile fluids may be indicated.

Perhaps the most important rules for handling an endoscope are never to bend any part of the tubing at an acute angle and never twist or crush the insertion tubing. Sharp bending or twisting can break fibers. Similarly, compression can break fibers. Broken fibers cause small black dots (pixels) to appear on the image, and if the image is compromised by the black dots, expensive repairs will be necessary to replace the fiber bundles. Cold conditions increase the likelihood of fiber breakage.

Immediately after an endoscopic examination, the equipment should be cleaned thoroughly. Secretions, lubricants, and medications can dry and crust on the outer surface and tip of the insertion tube and clog the tube's internal channels. The manufacturer's specific cleaning instructions should be followed. The external surface of the endoscope tubing can be cleaned with water and mild surgical soap, by using a soft cloth or soft brush. Cotton swabs can be used to clean the tip of the scope, especially the lenses and channel openings.

The internal channels of the scope are cleaned by immersing the tip of the endoscope in a solution of water and mild soap or mild surgical soap and then applying suction. If suction cannot be applied, cleaning solutions can be flushed through the channels with large syringes. A channel cleaning brush (provided with the scope) is used to clean the instrument channels of debris more completely. All soap should be thoroughly rinsed before storing the scope or using it on another patient. Clean water or distilled water is then used for a final rinse of the channels. Residual water should be flushed from the channels with an air flush or air suction.

Endoscope control handpieces are either fully immersible or nonimmersible. Immersible scopes can be placed in disinfecting solutions or water after protective caps are placed on the handpiece. The control handpiece on nonimmersible scopes should not become wet and must be cleaned with a damp cloth.

The outside of the instrument should be dried with a soft towel, and the endoscope should be hung to dry. The drying rack should support the control handpiece and allow the insertion tubing to hang vertically for gravity drainage.

If disinfection is necessary, the manufacturer's recommendations for acceptable disinfectant solutions should be followed. A tray, plastic basin, or clean sink can serve as a reservoir for the disinfectant solution, by allowing the endoscope tubing to be loosely coiled and immersed in the disinfectant for the appropriate contact time. Disinfecting solutions cannot substitute for proper physical cleaning of the instrument.

Sterilization may be required, especially after use on suspected infectious cases. Cold sterilization by immersing the control handpiece and insertion tube in liquid sterilizing solutions is the most common way to sterilize an endoscope. Special sterilizing basins are available for immersion of the scope. Gas sterilization with ethylene oxide may sometimes be used to sterilize an endoscope. Steam autoclaving is not a sterilizing option for the endoscope, but it may be possible for some of the endoscope accessories. The manufacturer's recommendations for sterilization procedures should be consulted.

CASE STUDY

You are challenged with training a new assistant on how to assist you with taking large animal radiographs. Write down how you would explain the terminology so she understands what you want her to do when you give her the view you will be taking. Make sure it does not take more than 10 minutes.

CASE STUDY

Your practice just acquired a new endoscope and you are in charge of its care. What do you need to make sure everyone knows about cleaning it?

SUGGESTED READING

Brown M, Brown L: *Lavin's radiography for veterinary technicians*, ed 5, St. Louis, 2013, Saunders.

Clayton HM, Flood PF, Rosenstein DS: *Clinical anatomy of the horse*, St. Louis, 2005, Mosby.

Farrow CS: *Veterinary diagnostic imaging: the horse*, St. Louis, 2006, Mosby.

Han C, Hurd C: *Practical diagnostic imaging for the veterinary technician*, ed 3, St. Louis, 2004, Mosby.

Han C, Hurd C, Bretz C: Diagnostic imaging. In Sirois M, editor: *Principles and practice of veterinary technology*, ed 2, St. Louis, 2004, Mosby.

Kraft SL, Roberts GD: Modern diagnostic imaging, *Vet Clin North Am Equine Pract* 17:1–189, 2001.

Lavin LM: *Radiography in veterinary technology*, ed 3, St. Louis, 2003, Saunders.

McCurnin DM, Bassert JM, editors: *Clinical textbook for veterinary technicians*, ed 6, St. Louis, 2006, Saunders.

Rantanen NW: Diagnostic ultrasound, *Vet Clin North Am Equine Pract* 2:1–261, 1986.

Reef VB: *Equine diagnostic ultrasound*, St. Louis, 1998, Saunders.

Thrall DE: *Textbook of veterinary diagnostic radiology*, ed 6, St. Louis, 2012, Saunders.

Traub-Dargatz JL, Brown CM: *Equine endoscopy*, ed 2, St. Louis, 1997, Mosby.

Horses in Veterinary Practice

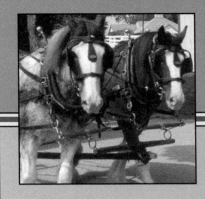

Equine Husbandry

OUTLINE

LEARNING OBJECTIVES

When you have completed this chapter, you will be able to

- Describe the zoologic classification of the species
- Proficiently use terminology associated with this species
- List normal physiologic data for the species and be able to identify abnormal data
- Identify and know the uses of common instruments relevant to the species
- Describe prominent anatomical or physiologic properties of the species
- Identify and describe characteristics of common breeds
- Describe normal living environments and husbandry needs of the species
- Describe specific reproductive practices of the species
- Describe specific nutritional requirements of the species

KEY TERMS

Ab libitum
Blepharospasm
Caslick operation
Colostrum
Draft horse
Dry matter
Feathering
Founder
Lameness

Light horse
Lochia
Meconium
Miniature horse
Nonsurgical transvaginal recovery
Omphalophlebitis
Overo
Patent ductus arteriosus
Phantom

Pony
Retained placenta
Tobiano
Tovero
Valgus
Varus
White muscle disease
Windswept

ZOOLOGIC CLASSIFICATION

The following is the zoologic classification of horses:

Kingdom	Animal
Phylum	Chordata
Class	Mammalia
Order	Perissodactyla
Family	Equidae
Genus	*Equus*
Species	*Caballus*

TERMINOLOGY AND PHYSIOLOGIC DATA

Box 8-1 lists common terminology used to describe the age and breeding status of horses. Box 8-2 lists normal physiologic data for horses.

COMMON EQUINE INSTRUMENTS

The accompanying Evolve website contains pictures and descriptions of common equine instruments.

BOX 8-1	Terminology

Mare	Female after third birthday
Broodmare	Female being used for breeding
Stallion	Intact male between 2 and 3 years of age
Gelding	Castrated male of any age
Foal	Young horse, from birth to weaning (usually 4–7 months old)
Weanling	Young horse, from weaning to first birthday
Yearling	Horse 1–1½ years old
Long yearling	Horse 1½–2 years old
Colt	Intact male between 2 and 3 years of age
Filly	Female between 2 and 3 years of age

BOX 8-2	Normal Physiologic Data

Temperature
99° F–101.5° F
102° F may be normal in warm weather or for an individual

Pulse Rate
Adults: 28–44 beats/min
Athletic horses: <28 beats/min is common
Foals at birth: 60–80 beats/min
Foals first 2 weeks of life: 70–100 beats/min

Respiratory Rate
6–12 breaths/min

Adult Weight
Varies by breed

ANATOMICAL TERMS

Figures 8-1 and 8-2 will help you review the terms for body parts and areas of horses, as well as the names of bones and joints.

BREEDS OF HORSES

COMMON DRAFT HORSE BREEDS
Brabant

Height: 16.2 to 17 hh
Weight: Approximately 2000 pounds
Color: Many
Breed association: Belgian Draft Horse Corporation of America
Website: http://www.belgiancorp.com/

The Brabant is also known as the Belgian Heavy Draft horse. Its principal breeding area began around Brabant, Belgium. The Brabant is a massive, powerful horse approximately 16.2 to 17 hh (hands high). It is short backed and compact. It has very strong, short, sturdily built legs, with ample *feathering*. The head is small in proportion, square and plain, but the expression is intelligent. The breed is notable for its kind temperament (Fig. 8-3).

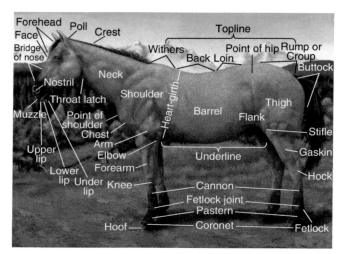

FIGURE 8-1 Parts of the horse.

Clydesdale

Height: 16.2 to 18 hh
Weight: 1600 to 2400 pounds
Color: Bay, brown, black, sorrel, roan
Breed association: Clydesdale Breeders of the United States
Website: http://www.clydesusa.com/

The Clydesdale originated in the Clyde Valley, Scotland. The breed typically stands around 16.2 hh, although some are larger and can weigh more than a ton. The legs often appear long and have abundant silky feathering. The joints should be big, the hocks broad and clean, knees flat, and neck long. Cow hocks are a breed characteristic and are not viewed as a fault. Colors are usually bay or brown, but grays, roans, and blacks are also found. Leg and facial markings are common in this breed (Fig. 8-4).

Percheron

Height: 16.2 to 17.3 hh
Weight: 1600 to 2600 pounds
Color: Usually black or gray, but many other colors also
Breed association: Percheron Horse Association of America
Website: http://www.percheronhorse.org/

The Percheron originated in the Perche region of Normandy in France. The horse on average stands 16.2 hh. The body is broad and deep chested. The head is pleasing, with a broad square forehead, straight profile, and large mobile ears. The neck is long and arched in the top line. The withers are more prominent than in most heavy breeds and allow for considerable slope in the shoulders, which is reflected in their free-moving action. The legs are short and powerful. The hooves are hard, blue horn, with little feathering on the lower limbs. The usual colors are dappled gray or black, but occasional bay, chestnut, and roan are also accepted (Fig. 8-5).

Shire

Height: 16.2 to 19 hh
Weight: 1800 to 2200 pounds

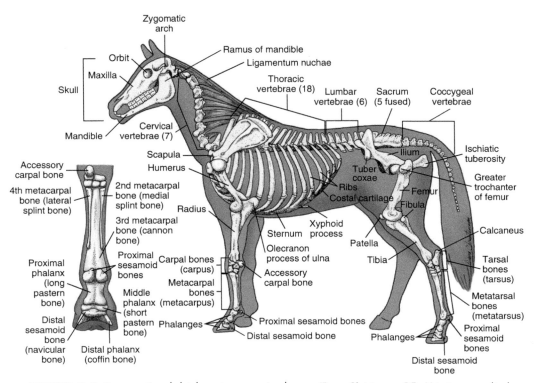

FIGURE 8-2 Comparative skeletal anatomy: equine bones. (From Christenson DE: *Veterinary medical terminology*, ed 2, St. Louis, 2008, Saunders.)

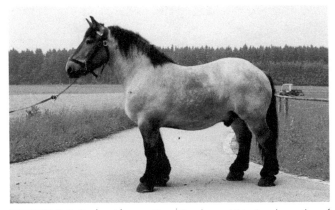

FIGURE 8-3 Brabant horse. (From Sambraus HH: *A colour atlas of livestock breeds*, London, 1992, Mosby-Wolfe.)

FIGURE 8-4 Clydesdale horses. (Courtesy Kim Myers.)

Color: Bay, brown, black, gray, chestnut/sorrel (rare)
Breed association: American Shire Horse Association
Website: http://www.shirehorse.org/

The traditional centers of breeding for the Shire horse are the English counties of Leicestershire, Staffordshire, and Derbyshire, as well as the Fen country of Lincolnshire. The Shire typically stands more than 17 hh tall. It is one of the biggest horses in the world and weighs more than a ton. The neck is relatively long for a draft horse, and it runs into deep oblique shoulders, which are wide enough to carry a collar. The legs are clean, hard, and muscular. The hocks should be broad and flat and set at the correct angle for optimum leverage. The hooves should be open; they should be wide across the coronet and

have plenty of length in the pasterns. The lower legs carry heavy but straight and silky feathering. Black with white feathering is still the most popular coat color, but numerous gray teams are seen, and bay and brown are also acceptable (Fig. 8-6).

Suffolk Punch

Height: 16.1 to 16.3 hh
Weight: 1980 to 2200 pounds
Color: Chestnut
Breed association: American Suffolk Horse Association
Website: http://www.suffolkpunch.com/

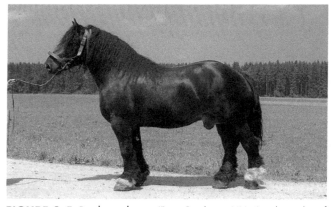

FIGURE 8-5 Percheron horse. (From Sambraus HH: *A colour atlas of livestock breeds*, London, 1992, Mosby-Wolfe.)

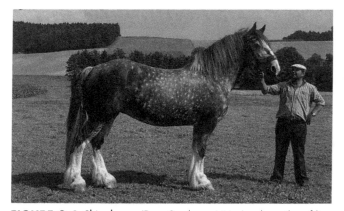

FIGURE 8-6 Shire horse. (From Sambraus HH: *A colour atlas of live-stock breeds*, London, 1992, Mosby-Wolfe.)

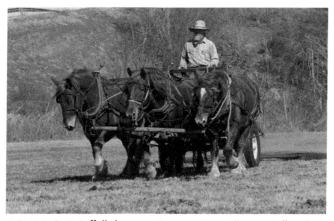

FIGURE 8-7 Suffolk horses. (Courtesy Toni Albers, Maffei-Albers Photography.)

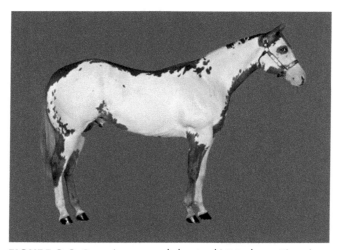

FIGURE 8-8 Overo (pronounced oh vair′ oh) Paint horse. These horses usually are white, and the white does not cross the back of the horse between its withers and its tail. Generally, at least one and often all four legs are dark. Generally, the white is irregular and is rather scattered or splashy. Head markings are distinctive, often bald faced, apron faced, or bonnet faced. An overo may be either predominantly dark or white. The tail usually is one color. (Courtesy American Paint Horse Association.)

The Suffolk Punch developed in the English county of East Anglia. Every Suffolk can trace its descent to a single stallion, Thomas Crisp's Horse of Ufford. The average height for a Suffolk is 16 to 16.3 hh. Its gaits are distinctive. The hindlegs must be close together, and cow hocks are rarely found. The quarters are huge, rounded, and powerfully muscled. The breed has a strongly crested neck, and the forearms are very muscular with good bone and minimal feathers. All Suffolks are "chestnut." The Suffolk Horse Society, formed in 1877, recognizes seven shades, ranging from a pale, almost oatmeal color to a dark, almost brown shade. The most usual is a bright, reddish color (Fig. 8-7).

COMMON LIGHT HORSE BREEDS
American Paint

Height: 15 to 16 hh
Weight: Approximately 1100 pounds
Color: Combination of white and any color of the equine spectrum
Breed association: American Paint Horse Association
Website: http://www.apha.com/

Each Paint horse has a particular combination of white and any color of the equine spectrum: black, bay, brown, chestnut, dun, grullo, sorrel, palomino, buckskin, gray, or roan. Markings can be any shape or size and located virtually anywhere on the Paint's body. Although Paints come in a variety of colors with different markings, they have only three specific coat patterns: *overo*, *tobiano*, and *tovero*. Horses of this breed can be registered in the American Paint Horse Association (APHA). The APHA is the second largest breed association in the United States (Figs. 8-8 to 8-10).

> **TECHNICIAN NOTE**　The three specific coat patterns within the American Paint breed are overo, tobiano, and tovero.

Andalusian

Height: Approximately 15.2 hh
Weight: Approximately 1130 pounds
Color: Many

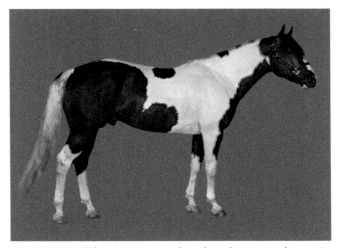

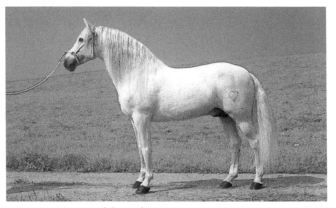

FIGURE 8-11 Andalusian horse. (From Sambraus HH: *A colour atlas of livestock breeds,* London, 1992, Mosby-Wolfe.)

FIGURE 8-9 Tobiano (pronounced tow be yah′ no) Paint horse. The dark color usually covers one or both flanks. Generally, all four legs are white, at least below the hocks and knees. Generally, the spots are regular and distinct as ovals or round patterns that extend down over the neck and chest, giving the appearance of a shield. Head markings are like those of a solid-colored horse: solid or with a blaze, strip, star, or snip. A tobiano may be either predominantly dark or white. The tail is often two colors. (Courtesy American Paint Horse Association.)

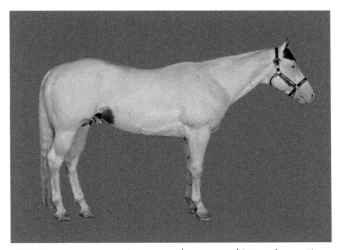

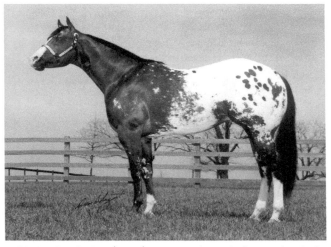

FIGURE 8-12 Appaloosa horse. Appaloosa Stallion Rocket Finder MMR. (Courtesy Don Shugart, Appaloosa Horse Club.)

FIGURE 8-10 Tovero (pronounced tow vair′ oh) Paint horse. These horses have dark pigmentation around the ears that may expand to cover the forehead or eyes. The color of one or both eyes is blue. Dark pigmentation around the mouth may extend up the sides of the face and form spots. Chest spots are seen in varying sizes. These may also extend up the neck. Flank spots range in size. These are often accompanied by smaller spots that extend forward across the barrel and up over the loin. Spots, varying in size, are present at the base of the tail. (Courtesy of the American Paint Horse Association.)

Breed association: International Andalusian and Lusitano Horse Association
Website: http://www.ialha.org/

Andalusian horse breeding is still centered in the province of Andalusia in southern Spain. The average height for an Andalusian is 15.2 hh. The horse has a commanding presence with lofty and spectacular paces. The facial profile is convex, and the eyes are almond shaped. It has a natural balance and a rather sloped croup (Fig. 8-11).

Appaloosa

Height: Approximately 16.0 hh
Weight: Approximately 1250 pounds
Color: Many colors, blanket or leopard pattern
Breed association: Appaloosa Horse Club
Website: http://www.appaloosa.com/

The name Appaloosa comes from the breed's point of origin in the Palouse region covering parts of Washington and Idaho. Appaloosas are known for their distinctive color, intelligence, and even temperament. Four identifiable characteristics are coat pattern, mottled skin, white sclera, and striped hooves. To receive regular registration, a horse must have a recognizable coat pattern or mottled skin and one other characteristic. The seven basic coat patterns are blanket, blanket with spots, roan, roan blanket, roan blanket with spots, spots, and solid. Appaloosas that meet these requirements can be registered with the Appaloosa Horse Club (ApHC) (Fig. 8-12).

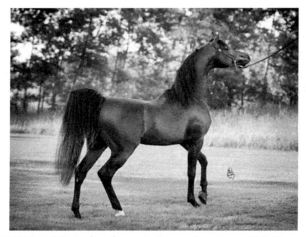

FIGURE 8-13 Arabian horse. Arabian stallion Maasai PVF. (Courtesy Stuart Vesty.)

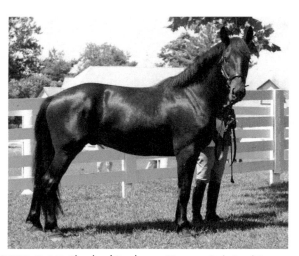

FIGURE 8-14 Cleveland Bay horse. (Courtesy Right Lead Equestrian.)

> **TECHNICIAN NOTE**   The seven basic coat patterns within the Appaloosa breed are blanket, blanket with spots, roan, roan blanket, roan blanket with spots, spots, and solid.

Arabian

Height: 14.1 to 15.1 hh
Weight: 800 to 1100 pounds
Color: Many colors, blanket or leopard pattern
Breed association: Arabian Horse Association
Website: www.arabianhorses.org/
The origin of the Arabian is unclear, but evidence suggests that it existed on the Arabian Peninsula around 2500 BC and was maintained there in its pure form. The body is compact, the back is short and slightly concave, and the croup is long and level. The legs are long, slender, hard, and clean, and the tendons are clearly defined. The head tapers to a very small muzzle with large flared nostrils. The mane and tail hair are fine and silky. During movement the tail is carried arched and high. A dished forehead is common in the breed (Fig. 8-13).

> **TECHNICIAN NOTE**   It is common to see a dished forehead on horses of Arabian descent.

Cleveland Bay

Height: 16 to 16.2 hh
Weight: 850 to 1200 pounds
Color: Bay
Breed association: Cleveland Bay Horse Society of North America
Website: http://www.clevelandbay.org/

The Cleveland Bay (CB) horse is one of the oldest native breeds of England, originating in the northern regions. Cleveland Bays are classified as a light draft breed, not "warm blood," although it is thought that purebreds have no draft blood. They are primarily known for their solid bay color, large ears, blue/black

hooves, clean legs, and calm, kind personality. The Cleveland Bay Horse Society (CBHS) in the United Kingdom maintains a closed stud book for purebreds. An upgrading program exists, but entries are rare. Until 2005, purebreds in the main studbook were limited to a solid bay color, but a very small star was allowed. Current rules accept purebreds with "excessive" white, slight roaning, and chestnuts (which remain very rare), but they are listed as mismarked on registration papers. Fewer than 1000 purebreds exist worldwide, with approximately 180 in North America. Cleveland Bay crosses, often referred to as "partbreds" or "sport horses," are sometimes misidentified as purebreds. This is an indication of the strong influence the breed has on other breeds when crossed. Separate registries for crosses are maintained by the CBHS and CBHS Australasia (Fig. 8-14).

Missouri Fox Trotter

Height: 14 to 16 hh
Weight: 900 to 1200 pounds
Color: Many
Breed association: Missouri Fox Trotting Horse Breed Association
Website: http://www.mfthba.com/

The Missouri Fox Trotter originated with the settlers from Kentucky, Tennessee, and Virginia who made their home in the Ozark Hills of Missouri. The body is well muscled, fairly deep, and noticeably wide. Although usually sufficiently compact, it may have some length in the back. The chest is wide and deep. The shoulders are strong, and the breed has rounded withers. The breed stands on average between 14 and 16 hh tall. The predominant coloration is chestnut in all shades, usually with white markings, although any color is accepted (Fig. 8-15).

Morgan

Height: 14.1 to 15.2 hh
Weight: Approximately 1000 pounds
Color: Many
Breed association: American Morgan Horse Association
Website: http://www.morganhorse.com/

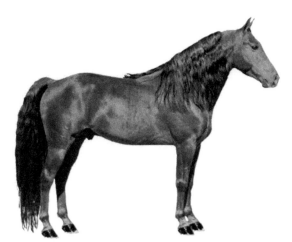

FIGURE 8-15 Missouri Fox Trotter. Missouri Fox Trotter Grand Central. (Courtesy Dawn Lindsay.)

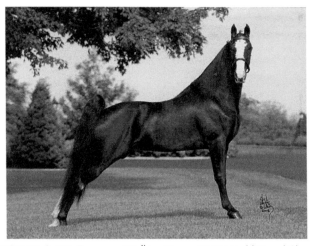

FIGURE 8-17 Tennessee Walking Horse. 2002 World Grand Champion Tennessee Walking Horse Out On Parole. (Courtesy Tennessee Walking Horse Breeders' and Exhibitors' Association, Lewisburg, Tenn.)

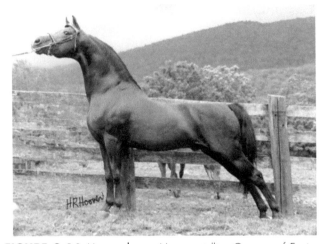

FIGURE 8-16 Morgan horse. Morgan stallion Courage of Equinox (Chasley Superman × Katy Bennfield). (Courtesy Hal Hoover, American Morgan Horse Association.)

The Morgan horse gained its name from one phenomenal stallion named Figure, who later became known as Justin Morgan, after a former owner. The breed is regarded as the first American Breed, with Figure's birthplace believed to be Springfield, Massachusetts. The present-day Morgan stands between 14.1 and 15.2 hh. The Morgan is easily recognized by a proud carriage, upright graceful neck, and distinctive head with expressive eyes. Deep bodied and compact, the Morgan has strongly muscled quarters. The intelligence, willingness, zest for life, and good sense of the Morgan are blended with soundness of limb, athleticism, and stamina. Morgans can be registered with the American Morgan Horse Association (AMHA) (Fig. 8-16).

Tennessee Walking

Height: 15 to 16 hh
Weight: 900 to 1200 pounds
Color: Many
Breed association: Tennessee Walking Horse Breeders' and Exhibitors' Association
Website: http://www.twhbea.com/

The Tennessee Walking horse evolved in the state of Tennessee in the midnineteenth century. The breed is deep bodied and short-coupled, with a head that tends to be rather plain. It carries its head much lower than a Saddlebred, and the horse moves with far less elevated action. The breed stands between 15 and 16 hh. Predominant colors are black and all shades of chestnut, sometimes with prominent white markings (Fig. 8-17).

American Saddlebred

Height: 15 to 16 hh
Weight: 1000 to 1200 pounds
Color: Many
Breed association: American Saddlebred Horse Association
Website: http://www.saddlebred.com/

The American Saddlebred originated in the southern United States and was initially called the Kentucky Saddler. The principal breeding area is still the Kentucky Bluegrass Country around Lexington. The horse typically stands approximately 16 hh. The quarters are smoothly muscled with a near-level croup and a high-set tail. The hindlegs, despite length in the shanks, are well formed, with long musculature, clean hocks, and flat, hard fetlock joints. The neck is long and elegant; its juncture with the withers ensures a distinctively high carriage in movement. The head is neat and fine with no fleshiness through the jowl (Fig. 8-18).

American Standardbred

Height: 15 to 17 hh
Weight: 800 to 1200 pounds
Color: Bay predominates, but other colors seen
Breed association: United States Trotting Association
Website: http://www.ustrotting.com/

The American Standardbred was first established in the eastern United States. Its body is long and low but is still

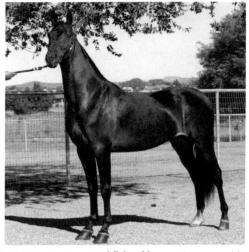

FIGURE 8-18 American Saddlebred horse. Three-year-old American Saddlebred mare Heirizona Rose. (Courtesy Norman Freeman.)

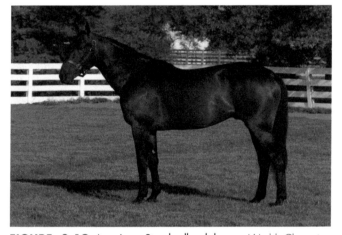

FIGURE 8-19 American Standardbred horse. World Champion trotter Donato Hanover, now standing stallion service at Hanover Shoe Farms. (Monica Thors, Courtesy Hanover Shoe Farms.)

powerful and deep through the girth. The overall build is powerful. The croup usually is higher than the withers, to give enormous propulsive thrust to the quarters. It has strong forearms. The head is plain but not unattractive, although it is heavier and less refined than that of the Thoroughbred (Fig. 8-19).

Thoroughbred

Height: 15 to 17 hh
Weight: Approximately 1000 pounds
Color: Many
Breed association: The Jockey Club
Website: http://www.jockeyclub.com/

The Thoroughbred first evolved in England during the seventeenth and eighteenth centuries. The body is typically long in its proportions. The quarters and the loins are strong. The hindlegs are long. The forearms are fine, long, and muscular. The head is refined and alert with no hint of fleshiness

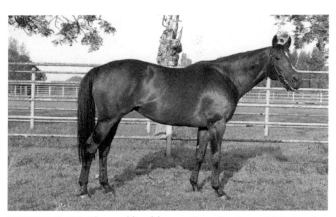

FIGURE 8-20 Thoroughbred horse. (From Sambraus HH: *A colour atlas of livestock breeds*, London, 1992, Mosby-Wolfe.)

in the jowl. The head blends into a long, gracefully arched neck that in turn joins symmetrically with the shoulders. The shoulders are long and very well sloped with prominent withers (Fig. 8-20).

Quarter Horse

HEIGHT: 14.3 to 16 hh
WEIGHT: Approximately 1000 pounds
COLOR: Many
BREED ASSOCIATION: American Quarter Horse Association
WEBSITE: http://www.aqha.com/

The Quarter horse originated in the United States during the colonial era and was developed for racing the quarter mile. The breed has a refined head with a straight profile that is distinctively shorter and wider than that of the Thoroughbred. These horses usually stand between 14.3 and 16 hh. They are compact and well muscled. The underline is longer than the back. The quarters are muscular. Horses of the breed can be registered with the American Quarter Horse Association (AQHA). The Quarter horse is one of the most popular breeds in the United States and has the largest breed registry in the world (Fig. 8-21).

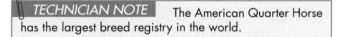

TECHNICIAN NOTE The American Quarter Horse has the largest breed registry in the world.

COLOR ASSOCIATIONS

Registries have opened that accept horses (and sometimes ponies and mules) of almost any breed or type, with color being the only requirement for registration or at least the primary criterion. These are called "color breeds." Unlike in "true" horse breeds, few if any unique physical characteristics are required, nor is the stud book limited to certain breeds or offspring of previously registered horses. As a general rule, the color also does not always breed on (in some cases, because of genetic improbability), and offspring without the stated color are usually not eligible for recording with the

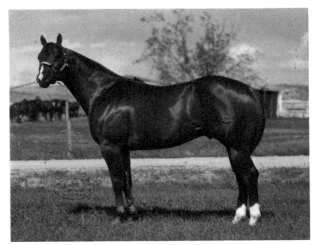

FIGURE 8-21 American Quarter horse. Watch Joe Jack, an American Quarter Horse Association legend. (Courtesy Pitzer Ranch.)

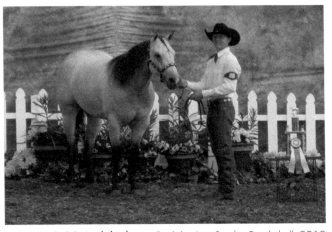

FIGURE 8-22 Buckskin horse. Buckskin Ima Smokin Bombshell, 2012 buckskin filly by Smokeys Shiney Jack and out of HS Prissys Harlan. (Courtesy Jessica Shefferd.)

color breed registry. Several horses can be double registered; this means that a horse can be registered with two different associations. This most commonly occurs when a horse is a specific color and can be registered with its breed association, as well as a color association. The following are a few of the more common color associations.

Buckskin

Height: Variable
Weight: Variable
Color: Buckskin
Breed associations: American Buckskin Registry Association, Inc.; International Buckskin Horse Association
Websites: http://www.americanbuckskin.org/; www.ibha.net/

The American Buckskin Registry Association, Inc. has been dedicated to the preservation and promotion of buckskin, dun, red dun, and grulla horses since 1963. The modern Buckskin (dun), technically a color breed, is actually a descendant from ancient time, the color being an indication of a strong heritage. In the West, horses of the buckskin, dun, red dun, and grulla hues trace to the Mustang—Spanish Barb descendants that originated in Spain as the Sorraia. Other Buckskins brought to this country can be traced to the Norwegian Dun, descendants of the nearly extinct Tarpan horses. The flourishing numbers of Buckskin horses found today are the strongest living descendants of the ancestral breeds. Along with a mixture of other bloods, Buckskins can be found in all breed types (Fig. 8-22).

Palomino

Height: Variable
Weight: Variable
Color: Palomino
Breed associations: Palomino Horse Breeders of America; Palomino Horse Association
Websites: http://www.palominohba.com/;
http://www.palominohorseassoc.com/

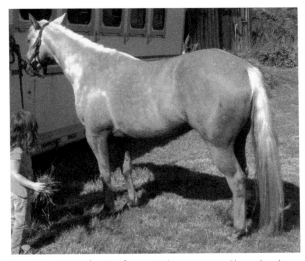

FIGURE 8-23 Palomino horse. Palomino mare Shezadazzlinggoldpine, call name Chloe, owned and trained by Joy and Jason Dorn and shown by Tashayla Dorn. (Courtesy Joy and Jason Dorn.)

The Palomino cannot be granted true breed status because of the variations in size and appearance. Therefore, it is classified more as a color than a breed; however, horses can be registered in the Palomino Horse Breeders of America (PHBA) (Fig. 8-23). Palomino horses registered with the associations of the American Quarter Horses, American Paints, American Holsteiners,, Pintos,, Appaloosas, Thoroughbreds, American Saddle Horses, Arabians, Half Arabians, Morgans, Tennessee Walking Horses, Mountain Pleasure Horses, Morabs, Quarabs, Missouri Fox Trotters, and Rocky Mountain Horses are eligible for registration with the PHBA, provided the horses meet the color and white rules.

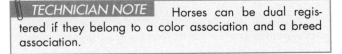

TECHNICIAN NOTE Horses can be dual registered if they belong to a color association and a breed association.

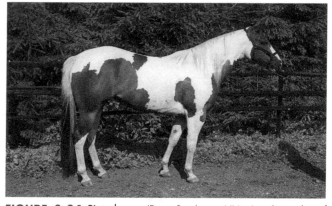

FIGURE 8-24 Pinto horse. (From Sambraus HH: *A colour atlas of livestock breeds,* London, 1992, Mosby-Wolfe.)

Pinto

Height: Variable
Weight: Variable
Color: Pinto
Breed associations: Pinto Horse Association of America, Inc.; National Pinto Horse Registry
Websites: http://www.pinto.org/;
   http://www.pintohorseregistry.com/

The name Pinto comes from the Spanish *pintado* ("painted"). The primary difference between a Paint and a Pinto is this: All Paints are Pintos, but not all Pintos are Paints. This is a good guideline, because the Paint registry's primary criteria are those of bloodlines rather than color, whereas the Pinto association's criteria are primarily concerned with color and not bloodlines. The Pinto Horse Association of America was formed to encourage the promotion of quality horses, ponies, and miniatures with color and to establish a registry for maintaining their show records and pedigrees.

Although there is a Pinto association, the Pinto cannot be granted true breed status because of the variations in size and appearance (Fig. 8-24).

> **TECHNICIAN NOTE**   All Paints are Pintos, but not all Pintos are Paints.

COMMON PONY BREEDS
Pony of America

Height: 11.2 to 13.2 hh
Weight: 500 to 800 pounds
Color: Many
Breed association: Pony of Americas Club, Inc.
Website: http://www.poac.org/

The breed originated from the efforts of one man, Leslie Boomhower of Mason City, Iowa. The breed standard calls for a pony that had the appearance of a miniature Quarter Horse/Arabian cross, with Appaloosa coloring and some of that breed's features. These ponies usually are between 11.2

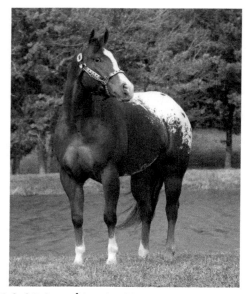

FIGURE 8-25 Pony of America. (Courtesy Joyse Banister, Pony of the Americas Club.)

and 13.2 hh tall. All the ponies are inspected before full registration is issued to ensure that they meet the breed specification. Emphasis is given to substance, refinement, and a stylish straight, balanced action marked by notable engagement of the hocks under the body (Fig. 8-25).

American Shetland Pony

Height: 11.2 to 13.2 hh
Weight: 500 to 800 pounds
Color: Many
Breed association: Pony of Americas Club, Inc.
Website: http://www.poac.org/

The breeding of the American Shetland pony was originally centered in the state of Indiana, following the large importations of ponies from the Scottish Shetland Islands that began in 1885. The pony typically stands up to 11.2 hh. The withers are unusually prominent for a pony and contribute to the slope of the shoulder. The girth is a good depth, and the legs are longer than in other ponies (Fig. 8-26).

Welsh Pony

Height: 12 to 15 hh
Weight: 500 to 750 pounds
Color: Many
Breed association: Welsh Pony & Cob Society
Website: http://www.welshpony.org/

Welsh ponies belong firmly to the Principality of Wales. For centuries they have been bred on the Welsh hills and uplands. The Welsh pony can be classified into four sections—A, B, C, and D—with A being the smallest and D being the tallest. Ponies across all four sections can vary in height from 12 to 15 hh. The Welsh Pony stud book is located with the Cob stud book. The pony has a flowing outline that is symmetrical and balanced in its proportions. It is full of quality

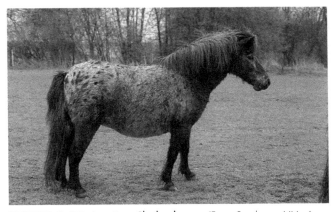

FIGURE 8-26 American Shetland pony. (From Sambraus HH: *A colour atlas of livestock breeds*, London, 1992, Mosby-Wolfe.)

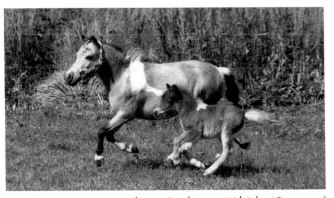

FIGURE 8-28 Miniature horse, Sunshine at Midnight. (Courtesy of American Miniature Horse Association.)

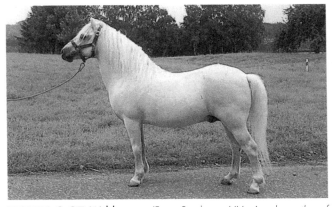

FIGURE 8-27 Welsh pony. (From Sambraus HH: *A colour atlas of livestock breeds*, London, 1992, Mosby-Wolfe.)

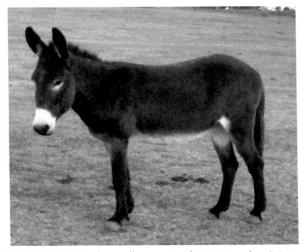

FIGURE 8-29 Donkey, call name Angel. (Courtesy of Leah Patton.)

and pony character. The forelimbs are long and well muscled. The head shows Arabian influence (Fig. 8-27).

MINIATURE HORSES
Miniature Horse

Height: Less than 34 inches
Weight: 150 to 250 pounds
Color: Many
Breed association: American Miniature Horse Association
Website: http://www.amha.org/

Many of the miniature horses have several breed influences, but the Falabella, founded in South America, is one of the main influences. The miniature horse cannot exceed 34 inches in height measured from the last hairs of the mane. The breed should be small, sound, and well balanced and should have correct conformation. Refinement and femininity should be seen in the mare. Boldness and masculinity should be seen in the stallion; the general impression should be one of symmetry, strength, agility, and alertness. Horses of this breed can be registered with the American Miniature Horse Association (AMHA) (Fig. 8-28).

> TECHNICIAN NOTE Miniature horses cannot exceed 34 inches in height.

DONKEYS AND MULES

The donkey or ass is a domesticated member of the Equidae family. A male donkey is called a jack. A female donkey is called a jenny (Fig. 8-29).

A mule is a cross between a male donkey and a female horse. A hinny is a cross between a female donkey and a male horse. Almost all mules and hinnies are infertile and unable to reproduce. A female mule that has an estrous cycle is called a molly. A molly can occur naturally or can be accomplished through hormone manipulation. Mollies have short thick heads with long ears and come in a variety of colors (Fig. 8-30).

REPRODUCTION

The normal reproductive course for any large animal species is discussed in Chapter 3. Table 8-1 lists specific equine breeding information. Figure 8-31 illustrates the equine estrous cycle.

Owners frequently have additional concerns about breeding mares early during the breeding season. Mares are seasonally polyestrous. They have estrous cycles from early spring to fall and are anestrous during the late fall and winter months.

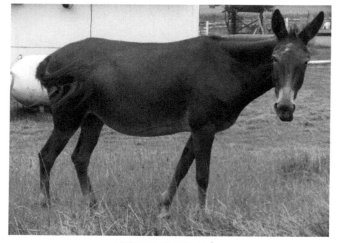

FIGURE 8-30 Mule.

TABLE 8-1	Equine Breeding Information

Male Reproductive Parameters

Length of spermatogenesis	57 days
Length of copulation	20–60 sec
Site of semen deposition	External cervical os
Ejaculate volume (mL)	60–100 mL
Total sperm ($\times 10^{-9}$)	5–19
Total normal motile sperm ($\times 10^{-9}$)	1.1

Stallion Total Scrotal Width

Any age	8 cm

Female Reproductive Parameters

Type of estrous cycle	Seasonally polyestrous (long day breeder)
Duration of estrus	2–12 days (average, 5–7)
Time of ovulation	Last 48 hr of estrus
Optimal time of breeding	Every 24–48 hr while the mare is in heat
Maternal recognition of pregnancy in days	12–14 as a result of embryo mobility
Source of progesterone per gestation day	0–150: corpus luteum >150: placenta
Type of placenta	Diffuse
Gestation period for light breeds	305–365 days
Birth weight	Varies by breed
Litter size	1 (twins are rare and undesirable)
Weaning age	4–7 mo

Pregnancy Diagnosis in Days After Ovulation

Ultrasound	>11 days
Transrectal palpation	>35 days
Progesterone	18–20 days
Estrone sulfate	>150 days
Equine chorionic gonadotropin	40–110 days

This means that, under natural conditions, horses usually breed and conceive in the spring and summer and are delivered approximately 11 months later—in spring or early summer. In certain horse breeds, all horses born in a calendar year are considered to be the same age and must compete against each other, regardless of the month they are born. It is advantageous to have foals born early in the year so that they will be bigger and stronger than foals born in late spring or summer of the same year. This is especially important in the racing breeds. Larger body size and muscle mass may also be considerations in horse show halter conformation classes in some breeds that value heavier muscling (e.g., Quarter Horses, Paint Horses, Appaloosas). If a mare fails to breed successfully or has an early embryonic loss, the mare will not cycle again for approximately 3 weeks. If she is bred again, an embryo can be detected by ultrasound only after almost 2 weeks. If several unsuccessful attempts are made to breed and conceive or if time is taken to treat a uterine infection or other disease, the month will now be May or June, and the resulting foal (if successful conception does occur) will be born "too late" the following year to be competitive.

> **TECHNICIAN NOTE**
> - All horses' birthdays are January 1 for competition purposes.
> - Mares are seasonally polyestrous. They have estrous cycles from early spring to fall and are anestrous during the late fall and winter months.

One approach to compensate for the naturally short breeding season is the use of artificial lighting. Artificial lighting during the winter months can "fool" the mare's system by increasing the photoperiod to which she is exposed, thus resulting in winter estrous cycles. This is done to create a longer breeding season, usually so that foals can be born as early the following year as possible. A longer breeding season also allows more time for repeated attempts to breed and conceive in case something goes "wrong." Artificial lighting is provided beginning in December in gradually increasing increments until 16 total hours of light exposure per day are achieved. Most mares respond with estrous cycles beginning in January or February.

SEMEN COLLECTION IN THE STALLION

Artificial vaginas (AVs) are most commonly used to collect semen from stallions. Most collections are made into a handheld AV while the stallion mounts a mare in estrus ("jump" mare); however, some stallions can be trained to mount and ejaculate into an inanimate mounting dummy mare ("*phantom*"). Phantoms can be adjusted to a comfortable height for the stallion and reduce the risk of injury to the stallion from unwilling mares. The AV can be built into the phantom.

The technician wears gloves and prepares the stallion by washing the penis with warm water. The stallion is usually encouraged to have an erection by exposing him to a mare in heat, and the penis is cleaned while the erection is maintained.

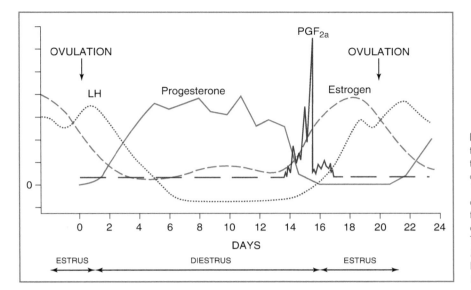

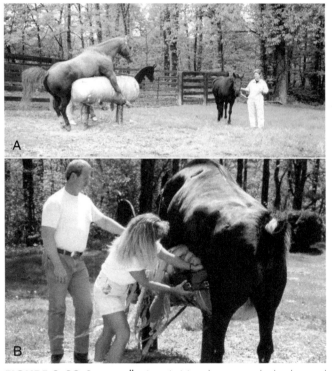

FIGURE 8-31 Equine estrous cycle. Estrus is 4 to 7 days long, and luteinizing hormone peaks after ovulation. Diestrus begins around 2 days after ovulation. Progesterone is high throughout a 14- to 15-day diestrus. If a pregnancy signal is not secreted by the early embryo by days 14 to 16, prostaglandin is released from the uterus, goes to the corpus luteum, and causes luteolysis (luteal death). The cycle then starts over. *LH*, Luteinizing hormone; *PGF*, prostaglandin F. (From Bassert JM, McCurnin DM: *McCurnin's clinical textbook for veterinary technicians*, ed 7, St. Louis, 2010, Saunders.)

If a jump mare is being used, she also needs to be prepared. The tail should be wrapped or bandaged, and the perineal area should be washed with antiseptic scrub and clean water. Usually, the mare needs to be restrained to prevent injury to the stallion and personnel. A twitch is commonly used, and sometimes hobbles are placed around the hindlimbs to prevent kicking.

The actual collection procedure is potentially dangerous. Breeding behavior in horses is usually aggressive and sometimes violent, and personnel are in vulnerable positions. Many facilities require personnel to wear helmets. The procedure requires a minimum of one person to handle the mare, one to handle the stallion, and one person to perform the collection into the AV. The usual method is to restrain the mare and then lead the stallion to approach the mare from her left side. The stallion is allowed to mount the mare, and the semen collector quickly moves in to grasp and divert the penis into the AV before it can enter the mare. The hands are then used to stabilize the AV alongside the mare while the stallion ejaculates. The AV is aimed slightly downward so that the ejaculate flows into the collection bottle (Fig. 8-32).

Following the collection procedure, the mare and stallion are quickly separated. The mare's perineal area is again cleansed, and the mare is examined for trauma to the legs and body. The stallion's penis is also cleansed, and he is examined for any evidence of genital or bodily trauma.

SEMEN STORAGE

The semen should be protected from exposure to air, sunlight, and extreme heat or cold. Fresh semen is used immediately. Cooled semen is usually kept in plastic bags housed in a special insulated container (the Hamilton Equitainer [Hamilton Research, Ipswich, Mass.] is most popular). Cooled semen should be left in the container until it is ready to be used, and it should be used within 24 hours. It is not necessary to warm cooled semen; the warmth of the mare's reproductive tract is sufficient. After the mare is prepared, the plastic bags containing the semen are opened. The semen

FIGURE 8-32 Semen collection. **A,** Note the mare in the background is used to tease up the stallion. **B,** Deviation of the penis into the artificial vagina. (Courtesy Kim Myers.)

is aspirated into 35- or 60-mL syringes. At least 1 to 2 mL of semen should be left for semen analysis (to be performed immediately before or after the insemination procedure). Nonspermicidal syringes that do not have a rubber plunger are commercially available.

Frozen semen is stored in 0.5- to 5.0-mL straws in liquid nitrogen; the straws require brief thawing in a warm water bath just before use (Fig. 8-33). Some of the straws are designed for insertion into special insemination guns rather than aspiration of the semen into a syringe.

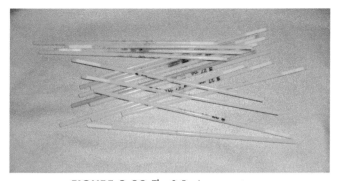

FIGURE 8-33 The 0.5-mL semen straws.

> **TECHNICIAN NOTE**   The 0.5-mL semen straws are most commonly used for storage of frozen semen.

The standard insemination dose for equines is 500 million progressively motile sperm per insemination if the sperm is cooled or fresh. If the sperm is frozen, a dose of 240 to 300 million progressively motile sperm per insemination is often used. Using the results of the semen analysis, a single ejaculate from a stallion can be split into several insemination doses for use on one or more mares. "Extenders" are commonly added to the semen. Extenders are a combination of liquid and solid ingredients designed primarily to nourish the sperm and help them survive outside the stallion's reproductive tract. Extenders are also used to increase volume if the ejaculate is to be split into two or more aliquots. Most of the many recipes for extenders contain a source of protein and simple sugars. They are buffered for pH, and antibiotics are added to reduce the incidence of venereally transmitted bacterial disease. The benefits of extended semen are well documented.

ARTIFICIAL INSEMINATION

For best success with mare insemination, the ovaries should be monitored with transrectal ultrasound during estrus. Using this system allows clinicians to observe a follicle greater than 35 mm in diameter. At that time, the mare would be inseminated and a dose of human chorionic gonadotropin or deslorelin given to induce ovulation, which will occur within 48 hours. When using frozen semen, a smaller window of opportunity exists, and mares are often examined by ultrasound every 6 hours and inseminated when ovulation is detected. In mares, the site of semen deposition during artificial insemination is intrauterine and transcervical. Insemination should be performed within 48 hours before ovulation if the sperm is fresh or cooled. It is more important that timing of insemination be closer if frozen semen is being used because of viability and longevity concerns. For that reason, if frozen semen is being used, the insemination should be performed from 12 hours before ovulation to 6 hours after ovulation. The mare is restrained in stocks. Preparation of the perineum is performed as described in Chapter 3. The veterinarian or technician, wearing a sterile plastic sleeve, manually places an 18- to 20-inch sterile insemination pipette through the cervix into the uterus; a vaginal speculum can also be used for assistance. A finger is introduced through the cervix, and the pipette is guided through the cervical canal into the uterus. The syringe containing the semen is attached to the pipette, and the semen is slowly administered. At recommended sperm concentrations for the mare, the volume to be infused is often 10 to 100 mL. At this time, some clinicians or producers massage the clitoris or cervix for a few minutes to stimulate uterine contractions. The pipette and hand are slowly removed from the vagina. To discourage straining and expulsion of the semen, it is common to walk the mare for several minutes after the procedure.

Performing multiple inseminations, every 24 to 48 hours, is common while the mare is in heat. Ultrasound examinations are commonly used to follow development of the follicle and confirm ovulation so that inseminations can be optimally timed. This is especially useful when the volume of semen available is limited.

> **TECHNICIAN NOTE**   Ultrasound is commonly used to monitor development of the follicle and confirm ovulation in the mare.

EMBRYO TRANSFER

The donor mare is monitored closely (through palpation or ultrasound examination) for time of ovulation or is hormonally manipulated to induce ovulation. The donor mare is bred by natural or, more commonly, artificial insemination. The donor's uterus is flushed 7 to 9 days after ovulation to recover an embryo (or possibly two embryos, if twin conception occurs); this is called *nonsurgical transvaginal recovery.* A two-way Foley catheter is positioned through the cervix and secured by inflating the cuff. Several liters of specially prepared saline solution are infused (1 L at a time) and then drained by gravity flow into a special collection container that contains a filter cup to trap the embryo (Fig. 8-34).

The contents of the filter cup are poured into a sterile "search dish" and are examined with a stereomicroscope (15×). Once the embryo is identified, a special pipette is used to aspirate the embryo and place it in a special culture medium. The embryo is kept at room temperature until transfer, which should occur within 2 hours after recovery. Embryos may also be placed in a special embryo transport medium and stored (or shipped) for transfer within 12 to 24 hours.

The embryo is transferred to a recipient mare that has been hormonally synchronized to prepare her reproductive tract for pregnancy. The embryo can be transferred surgically through a standing flank procedure (preferred) or a ventral midline approach using general anesthesia, or it can be transferred nonsurgically through the vaginal-cervical route. The recipient carries the pregnancy and is delivered of and raises the foal. Parturition and lactation are the same as in naturally conceived pregnancies.

Potentially, an embryo may be recovered from each estrous cycle; therefore, a single mare may provide an average

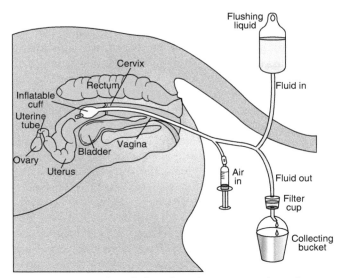

FIGURE 8-34 Embryo flushing through a two-way Foley catheter.

of six to eight embryos per breeding season. Some breed registries do not allow embryo transfer or limit the number of foals per year that can be registered to a single dam. Superovulation, which uses hormonal manipulation to induce ovulation of multiple eggs during a single estrous cycle, has been successful in cattle but has not been perfected in horses.

> *TECHNICIAN NOTE* Some breed registries do not allow embryo transfer or limit the number of foals per year that can be registered to a single dam.

CLINICAL SIGNS AND PREPARATION FOR IMPENDING PARTURITION

Gestation in horses averages 330 to 345 days, although up to 360 days is not uncommon. Mares commonly have a longer gestation with their first foal, with subsequent pregnancies lasting approximately 5 days less. Statistically, most foalings (80%) occur at night.

> *TECHNICIAN NOTE* Most foalings occur at night.

The time of parturition is indicated by clinical signs, although they are not sufficiently reliable to predict the exact time with certainty. Edema of the legs and a plaque of edema on the ventral abdomen are commonly seen in late pregnancy, but these signs are not helpful in predicting the time of foaling. The udder enlarges about 2 to 4 weeks before foaling, although enlargement may be minimal in maiden mares. The teats may "wax," which refers to the leakage and subsequent drying of a small quantity of *colostrum* from each teat that produces a waxlike cap on the end of each teat. Parturition often follows 24 to 48 hours after waxing is observed; however, this is not always reliable, and some mares do not wax. Other possible signs

are mild swelling of the vulva, discharge from the vulva, and relaxation of the pelvic ligaments (detected by palpating the muscles around the tail head for a soft "jiggling like Jell-O" effect).

Rectal temperature may be helpful in some mares. Normally, body temperature is slightly higher at night than in the morning. If the nighttime temperature is not higher than the morning temperature, the mare may foal within 36 hours. This method is not highly accurate.

To improve the ability to predict parturition, tests for the calcium level in mammary secretions have been developed. Calcium concentration rises sharply as the time of foaling approaches. The test is actually more accurate for predicting when foaling is not likely to occur than for predicting when it will occur. Calcium levels less than 400 ppm (10 mM/L) usually mean that foaling is unlikely. At levels greater than 400 ppm, most mares foal within 48 hours, and the remainder within another 48 hours. Samples can be run in a laboratory or evaluated with commercially available test kits. Water hardness test kits can also be used. Distilled water should be used for diluting the milk samples because the calcium in tap water alters the results.

PARTURITION
Stage 1

As the mare actually begins stage 1 of labor (preparatory stage), restlessness, pacing, sweating, and disinterest in food are common. Many mares lie down and get up repeatedly and may posture to urinate frequently. Stage 1 may last from 2 to 4 hours on average. The mare should be separated from other horses. The tail should be wrapped, and the perineal area should be washed with mild soap. If a *Caslick operation* has been performed but the sutures are not yet removed, they should be opened with sharp, disinfected surgical scissors. No anesthetic is necessary because the scar tissue bridge lacks innervation. The mare should be observed closely for the second stage of labor.

> *TECHNICIAN NOTE* Stage 1 may last from 2 to 4 hours on average.

Stage 2

Delivery of the fetus in horses is rapid compared with other species. Survival of the species requires that the foal be delivered rapidly, be able to stand quickly, and be capable of keeping up with the moving herd. Some mares even remain standing during the birth procedure. Supervising or "attending" a foaling is desirable to ensure the well-being of both mare and newborn foal. The delivery can be observed and emergency assistance provided if dystocia is identified. It is best not to interfere with the birth process and remain at a distance unless difficulty is suspected or observed.

Stage 2 of labor begins with the release of several gallons (8 to 20 L) of chorioallantoic fluid ("water breaking"); delivery of the fetus is usually complete within 20 to 30 minutes. The normal presentation is head and front limbs first, in a "head-dive" position; the soles of the hooves should face the ground. The feet rupture the white amnion, which is the membrane immediately surrounding the fetus; a small volume of additional fluid may be expelled. Because the equine placenta separates rapidly from the uterine wall, the foal loses its "oxygen line" and cannot survive being retained in the uterus or pelvic canal for long periods of time (unlike other species, in which the placenta separates gradually from the uterine wall). If no part of the fetus is seen from the vulva within 20 minutes of the water breaking, the likelihood of dystocia is high. If the foal is not fully delivered and breathing on its own within 30 to 45 minutes, dystocia should be assumed, and emergency assistance should be obtained. Dystocia is always a true emergency.

> **TECHNICIAN NOTE** Stage 2 of labor is usually completed within 20 to 30 minutes. If the foal is not delivered in 30 to 45 minutes, consider dystocia, which is an emergency.

Stage 3

Stage 3 of labor, passage of the placenta and fetal membranes, should occur within 2 to 4 hours. If passage does not occur within 4 to 6 hours, the placenta is considered to be retained, and a veterinarian should be consulted. Equines are susceptible to developing uterine infection, with possible septicemia and endotoxemia, as complications of a *retained placenta*. Clients should never be encouraged to pull on the retained membranes or tie weights to the placenta. Rather, the mare should be confined and the tail wrapped. The exposed membranes can be tied to themselves (with twine) to keep them from dragging on the ground or being kicked by the mare until the veterinarian arrives.

> **TECHNICIAN NOTE** If the placenta is not passed within 4 to 6 hours, it is considered to be retained.

DYSTOCIA

The incidence of dystocia in mares is low compared with other large animal domestic species; however, when dystocia does occur in a horse, the consequences may be disastrous, and recovery of a live foal is not often achieved.

The most common cause of dystocia in horses is fetal malposition. Normally, the fetus is mobile within the uterus during gestation. Just before birth, the fetus must orient itself to the normal head-first, forelegs extended, "head-diving" position that allows a normal delivery (Fig. 8-35).

Any deviation from this position will likely result in an inability to be expelled from the uterus (i.e., dystocia). Flexed legs, a flexed neck, "belly up" posture, breech (posterior) presentation, or a fetus that is dead and cannot reposition itself all lead to delivery problems.

Signs of malposition include appearance of the nose with no hooves or just one hoof showing, hooves that are not facing the ground, and failure of any part of the fetus to appear at the vulva within 20 to 30 minutes after rupture of the chorioallantoic sac ("water breaking"). Another sign of dystocia is the presence of strenuous contractions with no progress for 10 minutes. Other signs of dystocia include hoof soles facing dorsally, a foal in a dorsopubic position, or a foal with a posterior presentation and flexion of the head, neck, or limbs. Finally, if a red bag appears during delivery, this is an emergency. This is a red chorioallantois that will appear unruptured at the vulva. If this occurs, it is important to break the bag immediately and begin assisting in parturition.

Physical restraint must be adequate for the situation. Behavior is unpredictable during delivery (stage 2 of labor), and mares may stand or lie down with little warning. Stocks are not recommended. It is preferable to perform the examination and treatment in an area where personnel can easily move to safety. Chemical restraint or caudal epidural anesthesia, or both, may be used to minimize straining by the mare. Examining the fetus or treating the dystocia while the mare is straining, often violently, to deliver the fetus is difficult (and dangerous).

> **TECHNICIAN NOTE** Stocks are not recommended as a form of restraint during parturition.

Once the mare is restrained, a rectal examination can be performed, usually followed by a vaginal examination. The tail should be wrapped and the perineal area cleansed for the vaginal examination. These procedures must be performed thoroughly but promptly because time is precious. The clinician either wears plastic sleeves or uses scrubbed hands and arms to enter the vagina, depending on personal preference. Sterile procedures are not necessary; parturition is not a sterile process, but nonetheless it should be kept as clean as possible.

Once the cause of the dystocia is diagnosed and the condition of the fetus is determined, the veterinarian advises the client of the options available and must proceed rapidly to save both mare and foal, if possible. Options include mutation and delivery by traction, which are the first methods attempted during equine dystocia, fetotomy, and cesarean section.

> **TECHNICIAN NOTE** Mutation and delivery by traction are often the first methods attempted to correct dystocia in the mare.

Cesarean Section

Because of the complication rate associated with the procedure, cesarean section is generally the last resort for removal of a fetus. Unlike in cattle, which tolerate cesarean section as a standing surgical procedure through the flank, the procedure in horses is usually performed through a ventral midline incision with the horse under general anesthesia and in

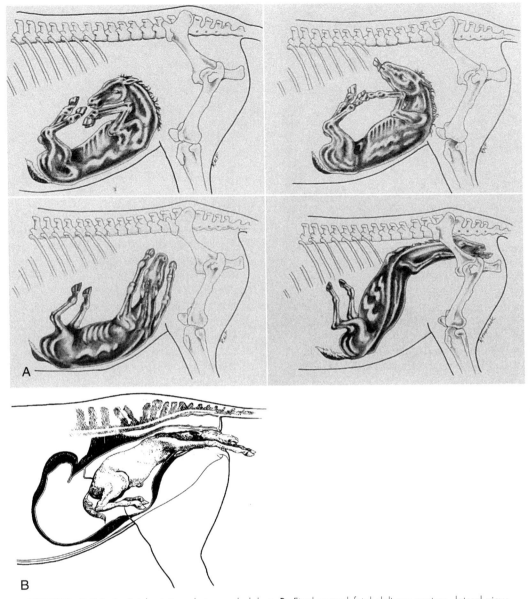

FIGURE 8-35 **A,** Fetal rotation during early labor. **B,** Final normal fetal delivery posture, lateral view. (From Colahan PT, Merritt AM, Moore JN, Mayhew IG, editors: *Equine medicine and surgery,* vol 2, ed 5, St. Louis, 1999, Mosby.)

dorsal recumbency. Infection (especially peritonitis), septicemia, laminitis, hemorrhage, and retained placenta are not uncommon following cesarean section. Recovery of a live foal from the procedure is unusual, primarily because of the time delay between the onset of dystocia and the surgical treatment by cesarean section. However, a team of assistants should be prepared to receive and care for the foal if it is alive. If alive, the foal is usually depressed from the effects of the general anesthetic drugs, and resuscitation drugs and equipment should be available.

> **TECHNICIAN NOTE** Cesarean section in horses is often performed as a last resort.

NEW MARE AND FOAL CHECK

After an uncomplicated delivery, it is common practice for the veterinarian to examine both mare and foal within the first 24 hours after birth (Fig. 8-36). The client should be instructed to save the placenta for examination by placing it in a plastic garbage bag (wear gloves) and refrigerating it (if possible) until the veterinarian arrives. The placenta should be kept out of reach of dogs and cats because they often try to eat it or carry it away.

The veterinarian will give the mare a thorough physical examination, followed by a rectal, vaginal, and perineal examination to check for trauma from parturition. The uterus is commonly lavaged to dilute and expel *lochia*

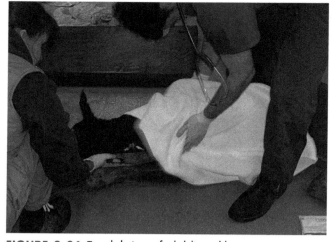

FIGURE 8-36 Towel drying a foal delivered by cesarean section in a sternal position to stimulate respiration. (From McAuliffe SB, Slovis NM: *Color atlas of diseases and disorders of the foal*, St. Louis, 2008, Saunders.)

(postpartum accumulation of fetal fluids and blood in the uterus). The veterinarian will examine the placenta to ensure that it has been completely expelled and will check for thickening and discoloration, which could indicate placentitis or other abnormalities.

The foal will receive a thorough physical examination, as described in the following section on routine care of the neonatal foal. Blood is drawn for passive transfer (antibody) testing, and often a complete blood count (CBC) is obtained. Further examination and blood work depend on any abnormalities that are detected during the course of the evaluation.

ROUTINE CARE OF THE NEONATAL FOAL

The neonatal period is the period following birth, which most clinicians consider to be the first 4 to 5 days of life. This period is one of susceptibility to many diseases and conditions that can be threatening to the immediate and long-term health of the foal; indeed, many of the diseases are life-threatening. An estimated 2% of all foals born alive die before they are 48 hours old. Long-term consequences of neonatal diseases may alter the animal to the point of preventing it from achieving its intended use or athletic potential.

> *TECHNICIAN NOTE* An estimated 2% of all foals born alive die before they are 48 hours old.

The outward appearance of a foal can be deceptive. Some foal diseases are obvious to the observer through external clinical signs; unfortunately, however, many foal diseases begin with only vague clinical signs that untrained personnel fail to recognize (Table 8-2). Failure to recognize these early signs leads to delays in diagnosis and treatment and, combined with the tendency of foals to deteriorate rapidly, results

TABLE 8-2	Neonatal Timeline
TIME AFTER BIRTH	**NORMAL CLINICAL FINDINGS**
30–60 sec	Spontaneous breathing begins
5 min	Heart rate ≥60, respiratory rate ≥60
30–60 min	Foal stands
60–180 min	Foal nurses
<10 hr	First urination
<24 hr	First defecation (meconium)

in many foals being presented to the clinician in emergency conditions and too late for successful treatment.

Good neonatal care is a combination of sound management practices and recognition of normal and abnormal conditions. Once delivery is complete, the following needs of the newborn must be addressed:
1. Oxygenation and pulse assessment
2. Temperature regulation
3. Care of the umbilical cord and umbilicus
4. Nutrition (nursing)
5. Bonding of mare and foal
6. Passage of meconium
7. Adequacy of passive transfer of antibodies
8. Physical examination of the foal

OXYGENATION AND PULSE ASSESSMENT

The first priority immediately after delivery is to ensure a clear airway. Any amnion (whitish fetal membrane) remaining over the nostrils should be removed. The force of passing through the birth canal squeezes most of the fluid from the upper airways; even so, the nostrils should be cleared with the fingers and wiped with a clean towel (see Fig. 8-36). A large bulb syringe can be used to aspirate fluid from each nostril. The foal is placed in a sternal position with the head and neck extended, and the body is rubbed vigorously with dry towels to stimulate breathing. If breathing does not occur within 1 minute, resuscitation should be given. First, the foal's neck should be extended. The mouth and one nostril should be held shut and the open nostril used to blow air into the lungs (confirmed by observing the chest rising). Both nostrils should be open for exhaling. The process is repeated several times and, if unsuccessful, continued at a respiratory rate of 20 to 30 per minute until the foal makes its own efforts to breathe. Alternatively, a nasotracheal tube (8- to 10-mm internal diameter, 45- to 55-cm length) can be inserted through one nostril, the cuff inflated, and the foal manually resuscitated as described earlier or mechanically ventilated with an Ambu-bag or mechanical ventilator at a rate of 20 to 30 per minute (Figs. 8-37 and 8-38).

> *TECHNICIAN NOTE* If a foal is not breathing on its own, resuscitation is done at a rate of 20 to 30 breaths per minute until the foal attempts to breathe on its own.

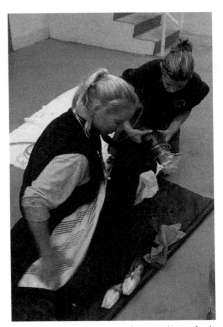

FIGURE 8-37 Ambu-bag being used to ventilate a foal with room air being delivered by terminal cesarean section. This foal required Ambu-bag ventilation for 40 minutes before spontaneous respiration occurred. Thereafter, the foal made an uneventful recovery and went home 3 days later. (From McAuliffe SB, Slovis NM: *Color atlas of diseases and disorders of the foal*, St. Louis, 2008, Saunders.)

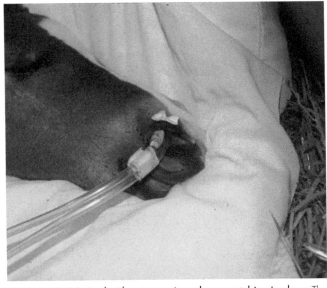

FIGURE 8-38 Foal with nasogastric and oxygen tubing in place. The nasogastric tube is sutured to the muzzle, and the oxygen tubing is taped to the nasogastric tube. If oxygen tubing alone is being used, it should be sutured directly to the muzzle. (From McAuliffe SB, Slovis NM: *Color atlas of diseases and disorders of the foal*. St. Louis, 2008, Saunders.)

The respiratory rate can be quite variable immediately after birth, but it should be at least 60 breaths per minute at 5 minutes after birth. This rate will stabilize at 60 to 80 breaths per minute over the first hour after birth and then decline over the next few hours to 30 to 40 breaths per minute. This rate will persist for the first few weeks of life.

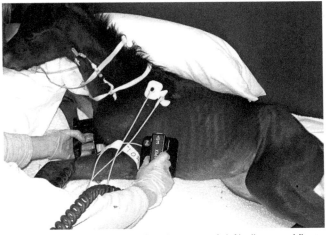

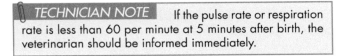

FIGURE 8-39 Correct sites for placement of defibrillator paddles in the foal. (From McAuliffe SB, Slovis NM: *Color atlas of diseases and disorders of the foal*, St. Louis, 2008, Saunders.)

The pulse should be evaluated for rate and strength. The pulse should be at least 60 beats per minute at 5 minutes after birth. The pulse rate usually elevates to more than 100 over the first hour and then declines to 75 to 100 for the first week of life.

The respiratory rate and pulse rate are highly useful indicators of well-being in the newborn foal. If either remains less than 60 at 5 minutes after birth, a veterinarian should be consulted promptly (Fig. 8-39).

> **TECHNICIAN NOTE** If the pulse rate or respiration rate is less than 60 per minute at 5 minutes after birth, the veterinarian should be informed immediately.

TEMPERATURE REGULATION

Neonatal foals are highly sensitive to hypothermia. Drying the foal with towels removes amniotic fluids from the hair coat and is the first step to warming the body. If the environmental temperature is cold, heat lamps can be used. Heat lamps should be kept at least 4 feet away from the foal to prevent overheating and burns, which occur at approximately 103° F (39.4° C). Deep bedding helps to keep foals warm; straw is generally the preferred bedding for foals. Drafts should be prevented.

> **TECHNICIAN NOTE** When heat lamps are being used to warm a foal, they should be no closer than 4 feet from the foal to prevent overheating and burns.

Rectal temperature of the neonate ranges from 99° F to 101.5° F (37.2° C to 38.6° C). Efforts to warm a foal should begin at a rectal temperature of 100° F (37.8° C). Heat lamps, warm water pads or bottles, and blankets can be used. Electric heating blankets and heating pads should not be placed directly against the skin because of the possibility of causing thermal burns.

CARE OF THE UMBILICAL CORD AND UMBILICUS

The umbilical cord should not be cut unless necessary to prevent strangulation of the foal or entanglement around the mare's legs; these are rare occurrences. If the cord must be cut, hemostats should be placed over the stump to prevent hemorrhage (Fig. 8-40). Once the strangulation or entanglement is relieved, the stump should be shortened to within several inches of the foal's abdomen and the hemostats kept in place for 4 to 6 hours to prevent hemorrhage.

Whenever possible, nature should be allowed to take its course. Usually, the mare and foal lie quietly for several minutes, and then the umbilical cord breaks naturally when the mare stands. The umbilical cord has a natural breakpoint about 1 to 2 inches from the foal's abdomen. The process of natural rupture causes spasm of the blood vessel walls, helping to control hemorrhage. If the cord continues to bleed actively and manual pressure for several minutes fails to stop the bleeding, a hemostat can be placed across the stump for several hours. The smallest size hemostat possible that will control the hemorrhage should be used; large hemostats tend to dislodge easily when a foal tries to stand and move around.

Traction should never be put on the umbilical cord such that the tension pulls directly on the foal's abdominal wall. If manual rupture of the umbilical cord is necessary, press one hand flat against the umbilicus for support of the abdominal wall and use the other hand to grasp the cord several inches from the abdomen and apply traction to take advantage of the natural breakpoint.

The umbilical stump should be dipped in an antiseptic solution to cauterize the stump and minimize the bacterial population. Dilute povidone-iodine solution (3%) and dilute chlorhexidine solution (1:4 dilution) have been successfully used; tincture of iodine may cause unnecessary tissue damage. The stump is dipped two to three times daily for the first week of life; a large, clean syringe case (20- or 35-mL size) makes a convenient container for the antiseptic and helps minimize splashing. Fill the container with antiseptic, center the opening over the umbilical stump, and press the container upward against the abdominal wall to "dunk" the umbilical stump effectively several times. Antiseptic should never be forced up or poured into the umbilical stump. The urachus, which is included in the stump, is short and communicates directly with the bladder, thus providing a potential pathway for the irritating antiseptic to enter the bladder and cause chemical cystitis. Special care is necessary to avoid this complication if the procedure is done on a recumbent foal; this complication is less likely to occur if it is performed on a standing foal.

The umbilicus should be checked at least twice daily for *omphalophlebitis* and possible formation of abscesses. Moisture, redness, swelling, pain, and exudation indicate the need for veterinary evaluation. Other common complications include persistent patent urachus and umbilical hernia (for more information, see Chapter 11).

NUTRITION (NURSING)

The suckling reflex is assessed by placing one or two fingers in the foal's mouth. This action should stimulate a vigorous suckling effort in response (Fig. 8-41). The suckling reflex is not present at birth; it develops rapidly after birth, beginning at about 5 minutes, and it should be vigorous by 20 minutes.

The foal must stand to nurse. On average, a foal should make efforts to stand by 30 to 60 minutes after birth and should be nursing by 60 to 180 minutes (average, 120 minutes) (Fig. 8-42). Just observing the foal's head in the vicinity of the mare's udder is not an indication that the foal is actually nursing. The foal should be observed actually taking the teat into the mouth and swallowing. Milk should be seen on and around the lips. A foal may need assistance finding the teat and getting it into the mouth the first few times it tries to nurse.

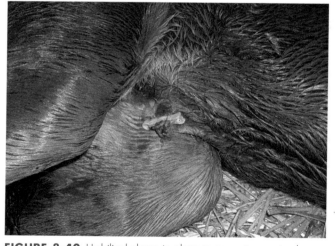

FIGURE 8-40 Umbilical clamp in place to prevent excessive hemorrhage, which may be caused by manual tearing or cutting of the umbilical cord. (From McAuliffe SB, Slovis NM: *Color atlas of diseases and disorders of the foal*, St. Louis, 2008, Saunders.)

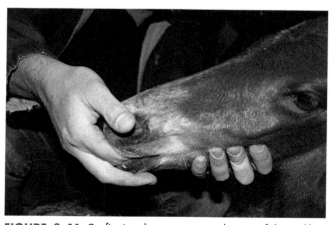

FIGURE 8-41 Confirming the presence or absence of the suckling reflex. (From McAuliffe SB, Slovis NM: *Color atlas of diseases and disorders of the foal*, St. Louis, 2008, Saunders.)

> **TECHNICIAN NOTE** Foals should make efforts to stand approximately 30 to 60 minutes after birth.

Some mares resent the foal's attempts to nurse and may even try to kick the foal. These horses are usually maiden mares or mares with painful udders. The mare may need to be twitched or sedated to allow the foal to nurse. The problem usually improves over several days; warm compresses may help lessen udder swelling and pain.

Foals are totally dependent on milk as a source of energy because they are not born with large stores of carbohydrate or fat. Hypoglycemia develops rapidly in foals that do not nurse or that nurse poorly, and the condition is potentially life-threatening. Foals should naturally nurse every 1 to 2 hours. One possible clue to decreased nursing by the foal may be the mare's development of a distended udder with excess milk. Milk may be observed streaming from the teats. Failure to nurse or infrequent attempts to nurse will usually signal a more significant problem, and complete physical examination of the foal is warranted. Hypoglycemia is confirmed by analysis of blood glucose levels; supplementation should begin when blood glucose falls to less than 90 mg/dL. Blood glucose of 60 mg/dL requires emergency treatment, and death may occur at 40 mg/dL.

> **TECHNICIAN NOTE** Death may occur in foals with a blood glucose level less than 40 mg/dL.

Several options are available for feeding orphan or rejected foals. Pan or bucket feeding and bottle feeding are most commonly used (Box 8-3). If bottle feeding is used, nature

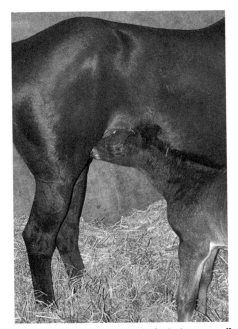

FIGURE 8-42 Normal behavior with foal showing affinity for its dam. (From McAuliffe SB, Slovis NM: *Color atlas of diseases and disorders of the foal*, St. Louis, 2008, Saunders.)

should be simulated as best as possible (Fig. 8-43). Rubber ewe nipples for lambs are preferred to cow nipples. Human infant nipples can be used for neonates but sometimes require slight enlargement of the nipple hole. The foal's head and neck should be extended during the feeding but not elevated above the level of the withers; elevating the head and neck increases the chance of aspiration of milk into the lungs.

BOX 8-3	Guidelines for Feeding Orphan and Rejected Foals

Options for Feeding
- Mare's milk: This is the best choice.
- Cow's milk: Use 2% milkfat. Add 80 g of dextrose or glucose per 1 gallon of milk or 4 tsp of jelly pectin per 1 quart of milk (20 g/L). Do not add table sugar (sucrose), corn syrup, or honey. Do not use long term.
- Goat's milk: Feed unaltered. If gastrointestinal (GI) disturbances occur, modify as recommended for cow's milk. Do not use long term.
- Commercial mare's milk replacers: These are sold as powders and are reconstituted with warm water. Foals may find these unpalatable. Soft stools are common and are not of concern. GI problems, especially diarrhea, tend to occur with milk replacers, especially when foals are not gradually introduced to the product or when the product is not changed regularly. Discard any unused, unrefrigerated, reconstituted product at each feeding or at least two to three times daily. Keep feeding containers clean.

Feeding Schedule

0–1 weeks of age	Feed at least every 2–3 hours.
1–2 weeks of age	Feed every 3–6 hours. Sick foals may need more frequent (every 2 hours) feedings.
2–4 weeks of age	Give 3–6 feedings per day. Begin offering solid food (creep feed or grain) and small quantities of hay or fresh pasture grass. A salt/mineral block should be provided, and fresh water should be available at all times.
4–6 weeks of age	Feed two to three times daily. Increase solid food intake.
>6 weeks of age	Stop feeding milk/milk substitute if solid food intake is adequate.

Amount to Feed
Divide daily total into the number of feedings:

Days 0–2	10%–15% body weight (kg) daily in milk or milk substitute
Days 3–4	Increase to 20%–25% body weight daily in milk or milk substitute; continue until 5 weeks of age
>5 weeks	17%–20% body weight daily in milk or milk replacer

Formulas to calculate precise energy needs are available. Healthy foals need a minimum of 100 kcal/kg/day. Sick foals need a minimum of 180 kcal/kg/day. In general, healthy average-sized foals should gain an average 0.5–1.5 kg/day of body weight.

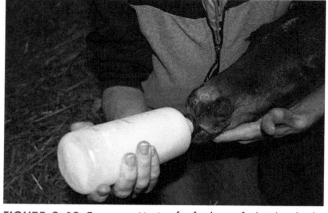

FIGURE 8-43 Correct positioning for feeding a foal with a bottle. (From McAuliffe SB, Slovis NM: *Color atlas of diseases and disorders of the foal*, St. Louis, 2008, Saunders.)

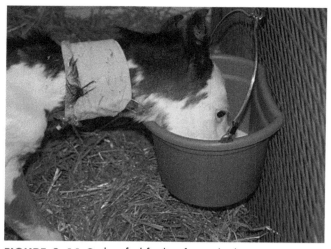

FIGURE 8-44 Orphan foal feeding from a bucket. (From McAuliffe SB, Slovis NM: *Color atlas of diseases and disorders of the foal*, St. Louis, 2008, Saunders.)

Some veterinarians recommend offering the bottle under the handler's armpit to simulate natural bumping and udder-seeking behavior. Foals should be encouraged to use a pan or bucket as soon as possible to minimize human imprinting. Buckets and pans should be shallow and wide (Figs. 8-44 and 8-45). The container should contain enough liquid so that the foal does not bump its nose on the bottom of the container, which may startle the foal and make it reluctant to "trust" the container. The foal may need to be introduced to drinking from the container by taking advantage of the suckling reflex. The handler should moisten his or her fingers with the milk substance, place the fingers in the foal's mouth, and slowly guide its mouth to the liquid by submerging the fingers.

Nurse (foster) mares provide another alternative but are seldom available in most parts of the country. A nurse mare is a mare that has lost her foal or had her foal intentionally removed. The lactating mare is then leased to the client in hopes that she will accept the client's motherless foal and nurse it as her own. Draft horse breeds and draft cross breeds are popular for nurse mares because of their temperament and their milk production. However, draft mares may actually produce volumes of milk that are excessive for smaller light horse breed foals, resulting in excessively rapid weight gain and growth and related developmental orthopedic diseases. Lactating goats have occasionally been successfully used as "nurse goats."

BONDING OF MARE AND FOAL

The mare and foal should be subject to as little interference as possible so that natural bonding can occur. On rare occasions, a mare rejects her foal. Usually, the rejection is related to the immediate environment of the mare; too much human interference, loud noises, dogs, or other horses that can be seen or heard by the new mother all have been associated with rejection of foals. Mares and newborns that are housed indoors are best kept in fairly isolated stalls in low-traffic areas.

> **TECHNICIAN NOTE**   Mares and newborn foals should be kept in a fairly isolated stall with low noise levels and low traffic.

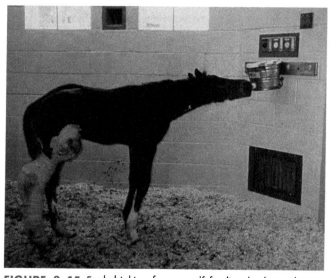

FIGURE 8-45 Foal drinking from a calf feeding bucket with teat. (From McAuliffe SB, Slovis NM: *Color atlas of diseases and disorders of the foal*, St. Louis, 2008, Saunders.)

Mares tend to be very protective of their foals. Some mares may even show aggression toward humans. One person should be responsible for handling the mare when work on or around the foal is necessary. The mare should be restrained first before an attempt is made to approach or restrain the foal. The handler should not try to prevent the mare from seeing or being close to the foal; this will upset even a "good" mare. Let the mare be as close to the "action" as possible, and keep procedures organized and brief.

PASSAGE OF MECONIUM

Meconium is the term for fetal feces. The fetus naturally swallows amniotic fluid, which is processed by the gastrointestinal (GI) tract to a waste material that accumulates in the colon and rectum. The material is usually hard, dark, and in the form of clumped pellets. Meconium should be defecated after birth; however, it is often difficult and painful to pass.

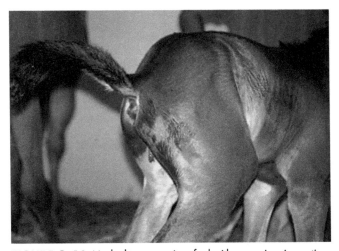

FIGURE 8-46 Marked tenesmus in a foal with meconium impaction. (From McAuliffe SB, Slovis NM: *Color atlas of diseases and disorders of the foal*, St. Louis, 2008, Saunders.)

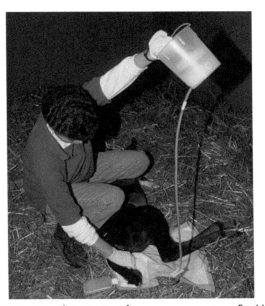

FIGURE 8-47 Administration of a soapy enema using a flexible tube inserted into the anus. (From McAuliffe SB, Slovis NM: *Color atlas of diseases and disorders of the foal*, St. Louis, 2008, Saunders.)

Foals typically strain to pass the material and may need several attempts to expel the clumped mass (Fig. 8-46). For this reason, it is routine to give newborn foals an enema. A standard human pediatric sodium phosphate enema (Fleet enema) is commonly used; no more than 1 pint total volume should be instilled at a time. An alternative is a warm mild soap and water enema given through soft rubber tubing with gravity flow. The enema must never be forced; if resistance is encountered, the enema should be stopped and a veterinarian consulted.

> **TECHNICIAN NOTE** It is common to administer an enema to newborn foals to aid in the passage of meconium.

Enemas may be repeated every 4 to 6 hours until the meconium passes (Figs. 8-47 and 8-48). If the meconium is not passed in 24 hours or if colic is observed at any time, a veterinarian should be consulted. More aggressive therapy may be necessary. Owners should never be advised to try to remove the meconium themselves. Meconium impactions are the leading cause of colic in neonatal foals and may be severe enough to require surgical correction. Signs of meconium impaction are frequent posturing and straining to defecate without producing feces, frequent swishing of the tail as if the foal were agitated, restlessness, decreased nursing, rolling, and possible abdominal distention.

> **TECHNICIAN NOTE** Meconium impactions are the leading cause of colic in neonatal foals.

ADEQUACY OF PASSIVE TRANSFER OF ANTIBODIES

Colostrum (first milk) is essential for passive transfer of immunity to foals. Equids are unique in that passive transfer of antibodies across the placenta does not occur; therefore, the foal is completely dependent on colostrum for passive

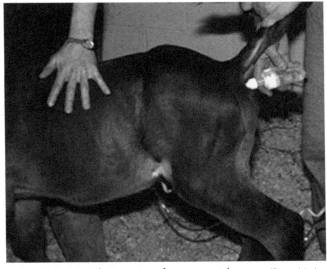

FIGURE 8-48 Administration of a commercial enema. (From McAuliffe SB, Slovis NM: *Color atlas of diseases and disorders of the foal*, St. Louis, 2008, Saunders.)

antibody transfer until its own immune system matures. The foal's immune system is not fully capable of producing protective antibody levels until close to 8 weeks of age.

> **TECHNICIAN NOTE** Passive transfer of antibodies across the placenta does not occur in horses. Foals depend on colostrum for passive transfer until close to 8 weeks of age, when their own immune system matures.

Neonatal bacterial septicemia is the leading cause of sickness and death in foals from 0 to 7 days of age; mortality is approximately 75%. (For more information on neonatal bacterial septicemia, see Chapter 11.) The leading risk factor for developing septicemia is failure to obtain adequate antibody levels from colostrum. For a foal to receive this natural protection, several processes must be successful:

- The mare must produce colostrum, and the colostrum must be available in the udder.
- The colostrum must have sufficient levels of antibody.
- The foal must ingest sufficient quantities of colostrum in the first 18 hours of life before the intestine loses its ability to absorb large proteins (absorption is best in the first 6 hours).

> *TECHNICIAN NOTE*   The leading cause of sickness and death in foals from 0 to 7 days of age is neonatal septicemia.

Rather than guessing whether colostrum intake and absorption have been adequate, it is common practice to obtain a blood sample from the foal and confirm the foal's antibody (immunoglobulin G [IgG]) levels. The radial immunodiffusion test provides the most specific quantitative measurement, but it usually requires that the sample be sent to a referral laboratory and takes 24 hours to run. This delay in obtaining results may delay treatment. Newer "foal-side" field test kits based on latex agglutination or enzyme-linked immunosorbent assay are fast and convenient; they can be run on serum, plasma, or whole blood. Most test kits are semiquantitative (i.e., the results are given as a range, rather than a specific number), which is quite adequate for clinical use. The optimum time to test the foal's blood is debated; however, blood is usually drawn within the first 18 to 24 hours of life.

> *TECHNICIAN NOTE*   It is common practice to test immunoglobulin G levels of foals.

Antibody levels have been correlated with the level of protection in the foal, and the foal is placed into one of four categories on the basis of test results (Table 8-3).

Antibody levels alone do not determine whether a foal becomes sick. High antibody levels do not guarantee health; foals with high antibody levels can still become septicemic.

TABLE 8-3	Antibody Levels	
ANTIBODY LEVEL (mg/dl)	CATEGORY OF PROTECTION	RISK FOR DEVELOPMENT OF NEONATAL SEPTICEMIA
>1200	Excellent	Minimal
400–800	Adequate	Low
200–400	Partial failure of passive transfer	Increased
<200	Total failure of passive transfer	High

Foals with low antibody levels can remain healthy with good management practices, such as stall sanitation, cleanliness, warmth, good nutrition, minimizing contact with other animals, and frequent monitoring of temperature, pulse, and respiration (TPR) and of physical condition for early detection of problems. Usually, however, it is prudent to supplement low antibody levels when they are identified. The veterinarian will discuss treatment options and risks with the client.

> *TECHNICIAN NOTE*   Antibody levels alone do not determine whether a foal becomes sick.

Problems with colostrum production and consumption should be identified and addressed as soon as possible. Potential problems include the following:

- Some mares may leak colostrum just before or immediately following parturition. Colostrum is recognized by its straw color and sticky texture.
- Rarely, mares may fail to produce colostrum. Grazing on fescue grass during pregnancy is the most common cause. Mares should be removed from fescue before the last trimester of pregnancy. If a mare is agalactic, an alternative source of colostrum will be needed.
- Mares may produce colostrum that is deficient in antibody levels. Colostral antibody levels can be readily assessed using a colostrometer. If a colostrometer is not available, a commercial test kit can be used in making an estimate. Poor-quality colostrum may need to be supplemented.
- Orphan foals, rejected foals, and foals too weak to nurse may need colostrum from alternative sources.

Alternative sources of colostrum may or may not be readily available. Many breeding farms maintain a supply of frozen colostrum for emergency use; colostrum "banks" exist in some parts of the country. Colostrum can be collected from healthy mares; mares with foals can spare 250 mL of colostrum and still have plenty for their own foal. After the mare gives birth, the foal is allowed to nurse. Then, the udder is cleaned with mild soap and water and a soft cloth, and colostrum is milked into a clean glass jar or zipper lock bag, sealed, and marked with the mare's name and date of collection. The colostrum can be used immediately or stored frozen for up to 1 year. Frozen colostrum should not be thawed in a microwave oven to avoid denaturing proteins (antibodies are proteins) and destroying normal bacterial flora (which are needed by the foal's intestinal tract). Instead, colostrum can be thawed gradually in a warm water bath. The colostrum then can be given to a foal in need by bottle or nasogastric intubation. Administration must occur during the first 18 hours after birth to be effective.

The amount of colostrum necessary to protect a foal depends on the amount ingested and the amount of antibody in the colostrum. The amount of antibody in colostrum can be measured by sending a sample to a laboratory for protein analysis, but this may incur needless delay. For field measurements, a colostrometer is easy and quick to use. Commercial kits for assessing colostrum are also available.

The colostrometer measures the specific gravity of colostrum, which correlates with the IgG level. Readings should be made with the colostrum at room temperature (i.e., at the same temperature as the instrument). Adequate colostrum has more than 3000 mg/dL IgG, which corresponds to a specific gravity greater than 1.060 on the colostrometer. Once the IgG content has been determined, the specific volume of colostrum necessary to provide 70 g or more of total of IgG can be calculated and given to the foal. As a rule of thumb, 2 pints of colostrum (with adequate antibody level) provide the minimum goal for most foals. To prevent overdistending the stomach, up to 1 pint can usually be given per feeding, and at least 1 hour should be allowed between feedings.

If colostrum is not available, commercial plasma can be given by nasogastric tube. This reduces the complications of placing an intravenous (IV) catheter and minimizes the risk of adverse reactions. Nonplasma high-level antibody products have become available for nasogastric intubation. Bovine colostrum is tolerated and absorbed by the foal's GI system but is likely to afford only partial and short-lived protection for the foal. Mild diarrhea has been observed following administration of bovine colostrum to foals.

> **TECHNICIAN NOTE** Colostrum can be stored frozen for 1 year. Do not thaw colostrum in the microwave.

Foals more than 18 hours old and those with GI diseases cannot be supplemented through the GI tract. The only option available for these foals is IV plasma or immune serum transfusion. Plasma transfusion in foals is performed similarly to adults, except that it is preferable to sedate the foal and restrain it in lateral recumbency for the IV catheterization and transfusion procedures. As a rule of thumb, 1 L of "regular" (not hyperimmune) commercial plasma will elevate the IgG level of a normal foal by 200 mg/dL.

Regardless of the route of therapy, the foal should be retested after treatment to ensure that adequate protection has been achieved. Serum IgG levels should be rechecked 8 to 12 hours after treatment.

PHYSICAL EXAMINATION OF THE FOAL

Box 8-4 lists guidelines for evaluating the neonatal foal.

Heart Auscultation

A continuous "machinery murmur" over the left heart base indicates a *patent ductus arteriosus*. In horses this is normal and should gradually disappear by 4 days of age.

> **TECHNICIAN NOTE** Patent ductus arteriosus is normal before 4 days of age in the foal.

Lung Auscultation

Lung sounds are moist for the first hours after birth because of the presence of fetal fluids. Even after fetal fluids have cleared, foal lungs continue to sound harsh. Auscultation is not a reliable indicator of lung disease in foals. Foals can have normal lung sounds yet have severe lung disease. The reason is the prevalence of interstitial pneumonia in foals, which does not affect the alveoli and airways. If alveoli and airways are not affected, the classic signs of cough, nasal discharge, and abnormal lung sounds will not be present. Therefore, lung disease in foals is best detected by external signs, such

---

BOX 8-4	Basic Evaluation of the Neonatal Foal

Temperature
99° F–101.5° F
>102° F is febrile

Pulse Rate
≥60 at 5 minutes
75–100 for first week of life

Respiratory Rate
≥60 at 5 minutes, 60–80 for first 1–2 hours, decreases to 30–40 for first month

Mucous Membrane
Dark pink to pink to pale pink
Mild icterus is not uncommon; usually a normal finding but may indicate disease

Capillary Refill Time
1–2 sec

Ear Pinnae
Examine for icterus and petechiae, which may indicate septicemia

NUTRITIONAL REQUIREMENTS FOR THE HORSE

AGE	CRUDE PROTEIN (%)	CALCIUM (%)	PHOSPHORUS (%)	DIGESTIBLE ENERGY (DE) (Mcal/kg)	EST TOTAL FEED CONSUMED (% BODY WEIGHT/DAY)
Nursing foal (2–4 months)	16.0	0.9	0.6	3.3–3.8	0.5–0.75
Weanling (4–6 months)	14.5	0.7–0.8	0.4–0.5	2.9	2.5–3.5
Yearling (12–18 months)	12.0–12.5	0.4–0.5	0.25–0.3	2.65–2.8	2–3
2 years old	11	0.35	0.2	2.5	2–2.5
Mature (ranges depend on exercise level)	8–11.5	0.25–0.35	0.2–0.25	2–2.85	1.5–3.5
Stallion during breeding season	10	0.3	0.25	2.4	1.5–2.5
Pregnant mare	8–11	0.25–0.5	0.2–0.35	2–2.45	1.5–2.0
Nursing mare	11–13	0.35–0.5	0.25–0.35	2.45–2.6	2–3

as increased respiratory rate, increased respiratory effort ("pumping"), abdominal breathing, and flared nostrils.

Gastrointestinal Tract

Reflux of milk from the nostrils may indicate a cleft palate. Foals should be watched for abdominal distention. GI motility sounds, which are primarily fluid and gas sounds in the neonate, should occur every 10 to 20 seconds.

After the foal passes meconium, normal "milk feces" should be seen. Milk feces have a soft or pasty consistency and are yellowish to tan.

Mild diarrhea normally occurs around days 5 to 10, corresponding with the mare's first heat cycle after parturition ("foal heat"); this is referred to as "foal heat diarrhea." It is seldom severe, is not normally accompanied by fever, and rarely requires any treatment; it is self-limiting within several days of onset. The cause is unknown.

> **TECHNICIAN NOTE**   Foal heat diarrhea occurs between 5 and 10 days of age.

A veterinarian should be consulted for any diarrhea that is accompanied by fever, dehydration, or loss of appetite or that persists more than 2 to 3 days.

Urination

The first urination should occur by 10 hours of age. Normal urine volume in a foal is 148 mL/kg/day (Fig. 8-49). Urine specific gravity is low compared with that in adults, with a range from 1.001 to 1.012. Foals should be observed for stranguria, or difficulty urinating, during the first few days of life (Fig. 8-50).

Ocular Examination

Scleral and conjunctival hemorrhage is commonly observed after birth and usually affects both eyes. Increased pressure during passage through the pelvic canal is believed to cause the hemorrhage. It resolves without treatment over several days.

The corneas and lenses should be clear and transparent; however, congenital cataracts sometimes are seen. The menace reflex, which is used to evaluate cranial nerves II (optic) and VII (facial), is not fully developed until 2 weeks of age. The pupillary light response may also be slow (but present) during this time.

Foals must be watched carefully for entropion of the lower eyelid. Dehydrated foals quickly develop entropion, which results in hairs rubbing on the cornea and subsequent development of corneal ulcers. Corneal ulcers can form rapidly and quickly progress to infection, rupture, or both, of the globe. Treatment of entropion is an urgent situation. Entropion is treated by everting the affected lid with a subcutaneously injected "bleb" of procaine penicillin G or by temporary suturing of the lid in the correct position (Fig. 8-51).

Blepharospasm (squinting) and tearing are the hallmarks of corneal ulcers and are the earliest clinical signs. Cloudiness of the cornea and "milk spots" may not be present initially; therefore, they cannot be relied on as the only telltale signs of an ulcer. When any of these signs are observed, a veterinarian should be consulted immediately. The eye will need thorough evaluation, and topical and systemic medication may be necessary. Patients with severe cases may require surgical treatment.

Musculoskeletal System

The hooves of the neonate are covered by fetal hoof pads, which appear as irregular, yellowish, soft material covering the sole of each hoof. The hoof pads fall off or wear away quickly as the foal bears weight. No special treatment is required.

Fractured ribs, which are caused by the high pressures on the foal as it passes through the pelvic canal of the mare, are not uncommon. When rib fractures occur, multiple adjacent ribs commonly are involved. Swelling may or may not

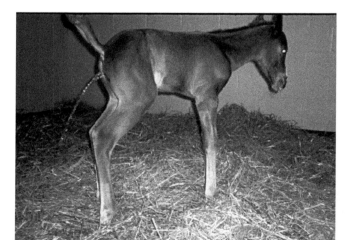

FIGURE 8-49 Filly urinating normally. Note no ventroflexion of the back. (From McAuliffe SB, Slovis NM: *Color atlas of diseases and disorders of the foal*, St. Louis, 2008, Saunders.)

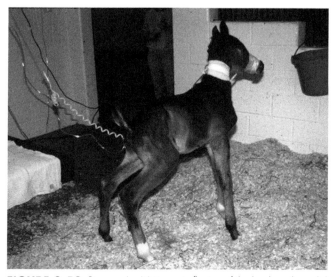

FIGURE 8-50 Stranguria. Note ventroflexion of the back and caudal position of hindlegs. (From McAuliffe SB, Slovis NM: *Color atlas of diseases and disorders of the foal*, St. Louis, 2008, Saunders.)

be seen initially but typically develops and is mild. Palpation may reveal the fractured ends if they are displaced. Auscultation over the fracture may reveal a clicking sound with each inspiration. Ultrasound can be used to identify questionable fractures. Fractured ribs almost always heal without special treatment, but occasionally bleeding into the pleural cavity and punctured heart or lungs may occur. The foal should be restricted to a stall for approximately 3 weeks to allow the fracture to stabilize. Pressure in the area of fractured ribs should be avoided.

> **TECHNICIAN NOTE** Fractured ribs may be seen in newborn foals as a result of the pressure as the foal passes through the birth canal.

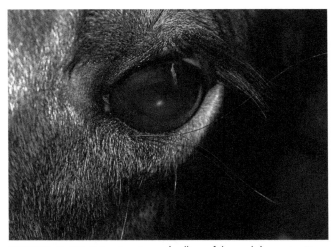

FIGURE 8-51 Entropion, inward rolling of the eyelid margin. (From McAuliffe SB, Slovis NM: *Color atlas of diseases and disorders of the foal,* St. Louis, 2008, Saunders.)

Joints should be watched for effusion (swelling), heat, and pain. Any joint swelling, with or without *lameness,* should be considered suggestive of a septic process (bacterial infection), and a veterinarian should be consulted.

The gait of the neonate can be difficult to assess. Exaggerated leg movements are normal, and spinal reflexes may be increased (hyperreflexive). Foals may naturally stand with a base-wide stance.

Legs should be evaluated for limb deformities. The two primary types of limb deformities are flexural and angular.

- Flexural deformity: Flexural deformity is assessed by viewing the legs from the lateral (side) position. Before birth, the musculoskeletal soft tissues (muscles, tendons, and ligaments) of the limbs have not supported weight. When the foal first stands and bears weight, these unused soft tissues are seldom accustomed to the tension, and flexural deformities commonly occur. One or more legs may be affected. The two varieties of flexural deformity are (1) soft tissues that are too "loose" and (2) soft tissues that are too "tight." When the soft tissues are too loose, the fetlock is hyperextended and appears as a "dropped ankle." As the foal begins to move around, the soft tissues adapt to weight bearing, and the condition usually corrects spontaneously within several days. In more advanced cases, the hoof may not sit flat on the ground; the toe is elevated off the ground, and the weight is rocked back on the heels (Fig. 8-52). Veterinary evaluation should be sought for these cases. These foals are at risk for damaging the lower leg joints and tendons and severely bruising (often abscessing) the heels. They should be confined to a stall or small pen to prevent running and excessive exercise until the tissues strengthen and the hoof rests normally on the ground. A common practice is to place heel extensions (using special shoes

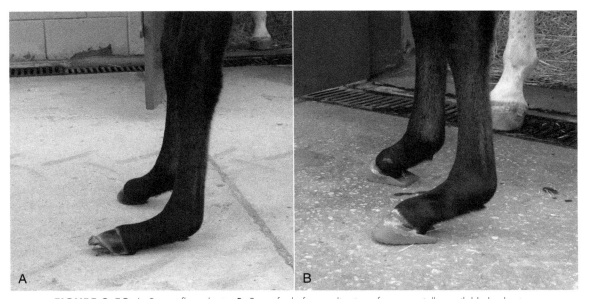

FIGURE 8-52 A, Severe flexor laxity. **B,** Same foal after application of commercially available heel extensions. Note improvement in the pastern angle. However, a longer heel extension would be more suitable. (From McAuliffe SB, Slovis NM: *Color atlas of diseases and disorders of the foal,* St. Louis, 2008, Saunders.)

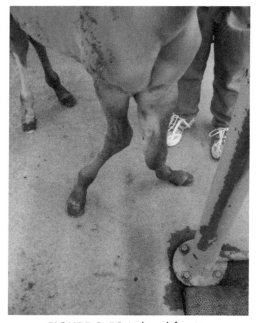

FIGURE 8-53 Valgus deformity.

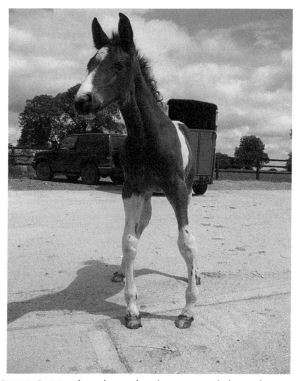

FIGURE 8-54 Bilateral carpal and metacarpophalangeal varus angular deformity. (From McAuliffe SB, Slovis NM: *Color atlas of diseases and disorders of the foal,* St. Louis, 2008, Saunders.)

or thin plywood blocks) on the affected hooves. The heel extensions force the hoof to sit flat on the ground by preventing the ability to rock back on the heels. These heel extensions are worn until the legs have strengthened. When the tissues are too tight, commonly referred to as "contracted tendons," the appearance of the leg depends on which tendons and ligaments are involved. The forelimbs are more commonly affected than are the hindlimbs. The normal fetlock angle may diminish, giving an upright, straight, "post-legged" appearance. Knuckling over at the fetlock may occur in severe cases. Other foals may have a clubfoot appearance, and the heel may not rest flat on the ground. Veterinary evaluation is necessary to identify which structures are too tight and to select the appropriate therapy. Radiographs may be necessary to assess the health of bones and joints. Therapy may include dietary management, IV administration of tetracycline, application of extended toe shoes, use of splints or casts, and even surgical treatment in some cases. Patients with severe cases may not respond to any combination of medical or surgical therapy.

- Angular deformity: Angular deformity is assessed by viewing the legs from a craniocaudal (front-back) position. The leg appears crooked or deviated from the midline, usually in the vicinity of the carpus or tarsus, although less commonly the fetlock area is affected. The two varieties of angular deformities are (1) *valgus,* when the deviation is away from the body's median plane (Fig. 8-53); and (2) *varus,* when the deviation is toward the median plane (Fig. 8-54). Occasionally, a foal is born with a varus deformity of one limb and a matching valgus deformity of the opposite limb. This occurs more commonly in the hindlimbs and is believed to be caused by malpositioning in the uterus during late

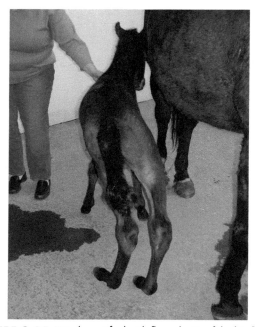

FIGURE 8-55 Windswept foal with flexor laxity of the hindlimbs.

gestation. Foals with this appearance are referred to as windswept foals (Fig. 8-55). Depending on the severity, treatment may or may not be required. Radiographs are recommended to determine the cause of the deformity so that therapy can be prescribed. Mild angulations may respond to corrective trimming or shoeing.

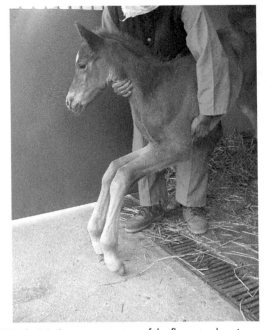

FIGURE 8-56 Severe contracture of the flexor tendons in a newborn foal. (From McAuliffe SB, Slovis NM: *Color atlas of diseases and disorders of the foal*, St. Louis, 2008, Saunders.)

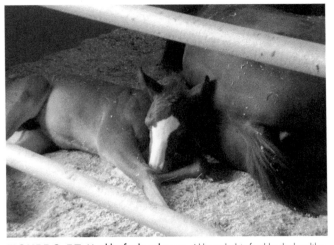

FIGURE 8-57 Healthy foal and mare. Although this foal looks healthy, it is important to perform a postpartum examination.

More severe angulations may require splints or even surgical treatment to correct the deformity. If bone damage is involved, complete straightening of the leg may not be possible, even with surgical intervention (Fig. 8-56).

IDENTIFICATION AND CARE OF THE SICK NEONATAL FOAL

A foal is not simply a miniature version of an adult. The function of organ systems, nutritional needs, and distribution of body water are quite different in neonates (Fig. 8-57). Some neonatal problems are obvious—crooked legs, hernias, and lameness can be readily seen by most observers. However, many serious neonatal diseases begin with vague clinical signs that untrained personnel may fail to detect. One of the most important characteristics of sick neonates is their tendency to "crash and burn," often within a matter of hours. Adopting a "wait and see" attitude frequently leads to disaster, requiring heroic measures to save the foal—often without success.

Certain conditions may predispose a foal to developing illness. When any of the following conditions are observed, the foal is considered to be a "high-risk" foal:
- Mare with fever, systemic disease, or vaginal discharge during pregnancy
- Abnormal placenta
- Prolonged delivery or dystocia
- Mare with agalactia or colostrum leakage before parturition
- Premature or dysmature foal
- Twin foal
- Orphaned or rejected foal

- Failure to ingest colostrum
- Delivery by cesarean section

High-risk foals should be watched very closely for development of abnormalities. Frequent monitoring of TPR and frequent physical examinations should be performed. Passive antibody transfer status should be determined with a blood test for IgG and treatment instituted as necessary. Attention to stall sanitation and a warm, dry environment are essential. The umbilicus should be treated three to four times daily and watched closely for signs of infection. If any abnormalities are detected in these foals, early evaluation and treatment offer the best chance of a successful outcome.

Sick foals seldom have only one problem, although often only one problem is readily apparent. Astute clinicians carefully evaluate all body systems for problems and provide treatment as necessary. In addition, because the immune system does not respond well until several weeks after birth, careful attention must be paid to sanitation and sterile technique when treating and examining foals, to avoid creating additional problems from iatrogenic contamination.

> **TECHNICIAN NOTE** Sanitation is very important when dealing with foals.

Injections, diagnostic sampling, and IV catheter and feeding tube maintenance require strict attention to cleanliness. Stall sanitation is a must; urine and feces should be removed frequently. Hand washing before and after contact with the foal is important. Many procedures on the foal are performed by restraining the foal on the ground in lateral recumbency, and working at ground level requires extra care to prevent contamination of equipment and supplies. The ground under the foal should be covered with a clean sheet, towel, or drape to form a barrier against bedding and excrement.

The level of care required for a sick foal may range from a heat lamp and blanket to complete 24-hour care in a neonatal intensive care unit. Some recumbent foals may struggle

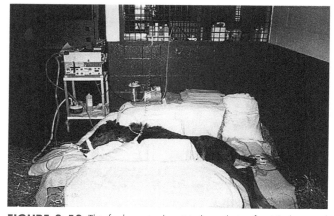

FIGURE 8-58 This foal required assisted ventilation for 10 days and then was gradually weaned off the ventilator. Such foals often require extensive physical therapy and assistance in rising for a number of weeks after removal from the ventilator. (From McAuliffe SB, Slovis NM: *Color atlas of diseases and disorders of the foal,* St. Louis, 2008, Saunders.)

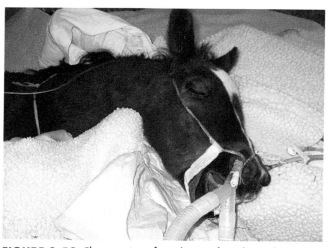

FIGURE 8-59 Close-up view of attachment of ventilator tubing to endotracheal tube. Intensive nursing care is required for foals on ventilators. (From McAuliffe SB, Slovis NM: *Color atlas of diseases and disorders of the foal,* St. Louis, 2008, Saunders.)

frequently, thus risking tangling fluid and oxygen lines, and require at least one person literally to sit with them at all times (Fig. 8-58). Once a sick foal has been evaluated and its needs determined, client communication is important to determine what treatment options are available and reasonable to pursue. Care for many foal diseases is labor intensive and expensive.

The following patient needs may need to be addressed:

- Nursing care: This includes warmth, cleanliness, and care of complications of recumbency (pressure sores, constipation, urine scalding).
- Nutritional care: This care includes pan or bottle feeding, indwelling nasogastric tube, or IV feeding (partial or total parenteral nutrition); hypoglycemia develops rapidly in neonates that are not nursing normally, so blood glucose levels may need to be monitored three to four times daily.
- Immune status: Treatment is given if antibody levels are low.
- Respiratory support: Supplemental nasal oxygen may be needed, as well as a mechanical ventilator for severe cases (Fig. 8-59).
- Fluid therapy: IV fluids may be indicated to maintain normal hydration, electrolyte, and acid-base balance.
- GI ulceration: The incidence of gastric (and duodenal) ulceration is very high in sick equine neonates; many receive oral or IV antiulcer medications for prophylaxis or treatment.
- Disease-specific medication and treatment: Antibiotics, antiinflammatory drugs, or joint lavage may be indicated, depending on the foal's specific medical or surgical problems.
- Neonatal diseases: For more information on neonatal diseases, see Chapter 11.

Depending on the facilities, the severity of the foal's disease, and other factors, the mare may or may not be able to stay with the foal during its medical treatment. This decision is not always easy. If the mare is to remain with the foal, she should be allowed as close to the foal as possible. If a partition is needed to keep the mare physically apart from the foal, as is often necessary to prevent entanglement

in fluid or oxygen lines, the partition should allow the mare to be as close to the foal as possible and maintain visual contact. If the foal is unable to nurse, the mare should be milked every 2 to 4 hours to encourage continued lactation while the foal recovers. Occasionally, it is in the best interests of the mare, foal, and staff to remove the mare from the foal, which is essentially early weaning. Separation must be complete, removing sight, smell, and sound of the foal. Sedation of the mare may be required. To end lactation, hand milking is stopped, and carbohydrates in the mare's diet are reduced.

> **TECHNICIAN NOTE**   When foals are unable to nurse, the mare should be milked every 2 to 4 hours to encourage continued lactation.

Restraint of the foal in lateral recumbency is often necessary. One person should be responsible for restraining the head and neck, with care taken to protect the downward (lower) eye. Care should be taken to avoid interfering with breathing by accidentally compressing the trachea or throat or occluding the nostrils. If the foal is capable of leg motion, usually one person has to restrain the forelimbs and another person has to restrain the hindlimbs. Limbs should never be restrained by grasping only the distal parts of the limbs, such as the pasterns. The primary restraining force should be applied just proximal to the carpus or tarsus, with lighter force applied to the distal limbs if necessary.

DIGESTIVE SYSTEM AND NUTRITION

Table 8-4 lists dental formulas and a dental eruption table (Fig. 8-60).

Equine teeth can be used to estimate age. Eruption of teeth can provide an estimate of age in younger animals. As horses age, wear patterns are used to estimate age. Other indications

TABLE 8-4	Equine Dental Formulas and Dental Eruption Table

Deciduous: dental formula: 2(I3/3 C0/0 PM3/3) = 24 total

Permanent: dental formula: 2(I3/3 C0–1/0–1* PM3–4/3–4† M3/3) = 36, 38, 40, or 42 total

Eruption	I1	Birth–1 wk
	I2	4–6 wk
	I3	6–9 mo
	C	—
	PM1	Birth–2 wk
	PM2	Birth–2 wk
	PM3	Birth–2 wk
Eruption	I1	2½ yr
	I2	3½ yr
	I3	4½ yr
	C*	4–5 yr
	PM1†	5–6 mo
	PM2 (first cheek tooth)	2½ yr
	PM3 (second cheek tooth)	3 yr (upper), 2½–3 yr (lower)
	PM4 (third cheek tooth)	4 yr (upper), 3½–4 yr (lower)
	M1 (fourth cheek tooth)	9–12 mo
	M2 (fifth cheek tooth)	2 yr
	M3 (sixth cheek tooth)	3½–4 yr

*Canines in the female are usually absent or very small and seldom erupt.
†Premolar 1 (wolf teeth) are frequently absent or fail to erupt. Lower PM1 is unusual. Gender does not affect the presence of wolf teeth.

of age include the occlusal angle, the infundibulum, the Galvayne groove, and the 7-year hook.

The occlusal angle is the angle of the caudal incisors (Fig. 8-61). This angle is close to 180 degrees in newly erupted teeth and declines to approximately 90 degrees around the age of 20 years.

The infundibulum is also known as the "cup." These cups are the grooves in the occlusal surface. In young horses, the grooves in the occlusal surface are deep, but the grooves wear and eventually go away as horses age. As the cups disappear, an enamel spot or mark is left behind, and the pulp cavity is exposed, causing a yellow mark in the dentin that is known as the dental star (Figs. 8-62 to 8-66; see Fig. 8-61).

The Galvayne groove is a depression that runs down the labial surface of the upper third incisor (Fig. 8-67). It is thought to appear at age 10 years. It runs halfway down the tooth at 15 years, runs the entire length of the tooth at 20 years, disappears from the top half of the tooth at 25 years, and disappears completely at 30 years of age.

The 7-year hook is a hook created when the maxillary teeth are longer than the mandibular teeth, thus causing a hook to form. This hook is most obvious at age 7 years and gradually disappears and then recurs at approximately 13 years. The hook is not considered an accurate age estimator.

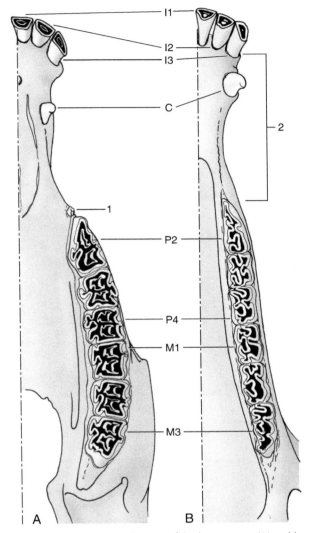

FIGURE 8-60 Permanent dentition of the horse, upper (A) and lower (B) jaws. *1,* Wolf tooth (P1); *2,* diastema. (From Dyce KM, Sack WO, Wensing CJ: *Textbook of veterinary anatomy,* ed 4, St. Louis, 2010, Saunders.)

DIGESTION

The horse is classified as a hindgut fermenter. Horses are grazers; they eat frequently but only small amounts because their stomachs have relatively little capacity. The stomach of a horse holds only 2 to 4 gallons at any given time. The horse's esophagus is between 50 and 60 inches long and can contract in only one direction. Horses cannot regurgitate or throw up. The horse's stomach and small intestine undergo enzymatic digestion. Stomach ulcers can become a problem in some equine patients. The small intestine of the horse is approximately 50 to 70 feet long, making up 30% of the entire GI tract. Roughages move through the small intestine much more slowly than do concentrates. On average, grains take 2 hours to pass through the small intestine of a horse, and roughages require 8 hours. The hindgut of the horse uses microbial fermentation, which takes place in the large intestine and cecum. The cecum of the horse is approximately 4 feet long and holds approximately 7 to 9 gallons. The large colon

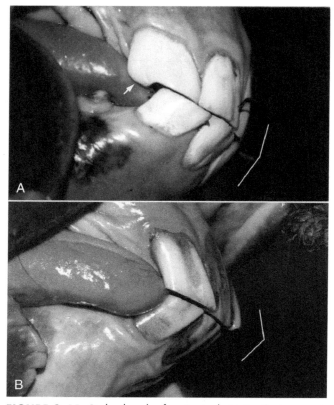

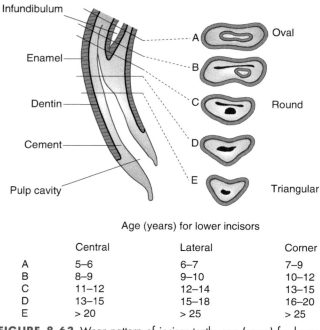

FIGURE 8-63 Wear pattern of incisor teeth: age (years) for lower incisors. (From Knottenbelt DC: *Saunders equine formulary*, ed 2, Oxford, 2006, Saunders.)

Age (years) for lower incisors			
	Central	Lateral	Corner
A	5–6	6–7	7–9
B	8–9	9–10	10–12
C	11–12	12–14	13–15
D	13–15	15–18	16–20
E	> 20	> 25	> 25

FIGURE 8-61 Occlusal angle of equine teeth. Notice the increase in angle between **A** and **B**. **A** also shows a 7-year hook. (From Baker G: *Equine dentistry*, ed 2, Oxford, 2005, Saunders.)

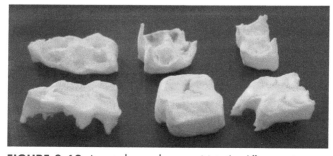

FIGURE 8-62 Assorted premolar caps. Note the differences in cups. (From Allen T: *Manual of equine dentistry*, St. Louis, 2003, Mosby.)

of the horse is approximately 12 feet long and holds approximately 14 to 18.5 gallons. The small colon of the horse is approximately 12 feet long and holds approximately 5 gallons. Food takes 36 to 72 hours to pass completely through the equine GI tract. Another unique characteristic of the horse is that it does not have a gallbladder; bile is excreted continuously. The horse is not the only animal that does not have a gallbladder, but it is the only large animal discussed in this book that does not have a gallbladder.

> **TECHNICIAN NOTE**
> - Horses are hindgut fermenters.
> - Horses cannot regurgitate or throw up.
> - Horses do not have a gallbladder.

When rations are formulated for horses, roughages are commonly used. Carbohydrates supply 80% to 90% of a horse's diet. Roughages are traditionally cheaper than concentrates, and horses can easily meet their nutritional requirements with a larger amount of roughage and a smaller amount of supplemented concentrate, although the concentrate is not always necessary. Any type of roughage should be clean, dry, and free of mold or toxins. Any type of diet change should be made gradually over 7 to 10 days. Water should be supplied *ab libitum*. Horses consume 5 to 12 gallons of water per day.

> **TECHNICIAN NOTE**
> - Equine diets should be changed only gradually over 7 to 10 days.
> - Horses drink 5 to 12 gallons of water per day.

ROUGHAGES

Even though roughages are commonly consumed by horses, a few types of roughages should be avoided in horses. Feeding straw or corn stalks to horses is not recommended because of the low nutritional value of these substances and the increased potential for compaction within the GI tract. In addition, meeting a horse's nutritional requirement would be difficult using these types of feedstuffs. Silages are also not recommended for use in equine diets. Silages can often have mold and mycotoxins present in the feed. Horses are more sensitive than other species to mold and mycotoxins, which can cause GI problems if they are consumed by a horse. Sweet clover poisoning can occur in horses fed sweet clover and can cause multisystem hemorrhages. Fescue grass is contaminated with the endophyte *Acremonium coenophialum*.

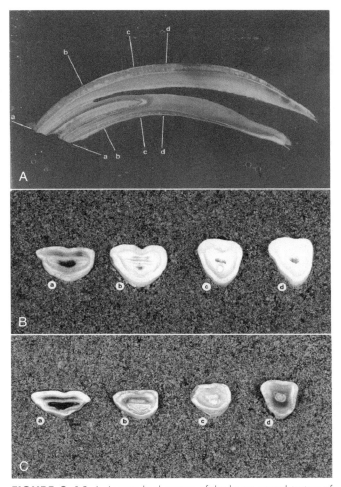

FIGURE 8-64 **A,** Longitudinal section of the lower central incisor of a Standardbred horse (4 years old). **B,** Lower central incisor of a 5-year-old Standardbred horse. Cross-sections at various levels as indicated in **A.** In sections *c* and *d,* the pulpal cavity is open. **C,** Occlusal tables of the lower central incisor of Standardbreds at 5 years *(a),* 8 years *(b),* 14 years *(c),* and 20 years *(d)* of age. In occlusal tables *c* and *d,* the pulpal cavity is occluded by secondary dentin. (From Baker G: *Equine dentistry,* ed 2, Oxford, 2005 Saunders.)

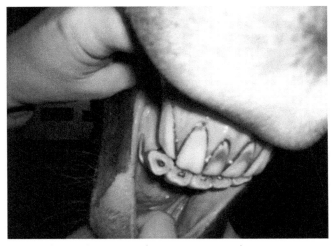

FIGURE 8-65 Note the wear patterns on these incisors.

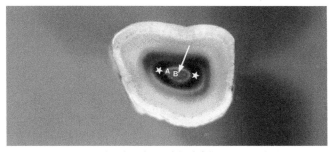

FIGURE 8-66 Occlusal surface of the left lower central incisor (401) of a 15-year-old draft horse. The dental star consists of a dark peripheral rim *(asterisk)* and a central white spot *(arrow).* The white spot is composed of secondary dentin (*A*) and a core of tertiary dentin (*B*). (From Baker G: *Equine dentistry,* ed 2, Oxford, 2005, Saunders.)

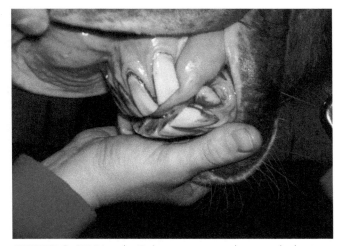

FIGURE 8-67 Note the Galvayne groove on the upper third incisor.

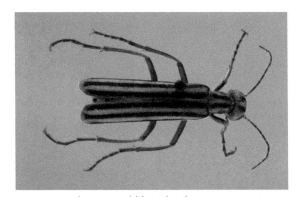

FIGURE 8-68 **Three-striped blister beetle** (From Orsini JA, Divers TJ, editors: *Equine emergencies: treatment and procedures,* ed 4, St. Louis, 2014, Saunders.)

The fungus produces a toxin that can cause lameness, agalactia, poor weight gain, and increased TPR. No treatment is available for fescue toxicity, so fescue grasses should not be fed to horses. Another problem can arise when horses are fed alfalfa contaminated with blister beetles, which are toxic. A striped blister beetle contains approximately 5 mg of the toxin cantharidin, which, when consumed, can cause ulcers in the mouth or throat, colic, and diarrhea (Fig. 8-68).

TECHNICIAN NOTE
- Horses are not commonly fed silages because horses have higher sensitivity to mold and mycotoxins.
- Fescue grass can be contaminated with the endophyte *Acremonium*, which produces a toxin that causes reproductive problems in mares if it is consumed.

CONCENTRATES

Oats, corn, wheat, and barley are common grains fed to horses. As horses increase the amount of exercise they perform, their energy requirements increase as well. Depending on the stage of pregnancy, the energy requirements of horses may increase 20% to 30%. Energy is often supplied to these horses in the form of concentrates. Higher protein levels are needed in young growing horses. Sometimes concentrates are supplemented with protein, often in the form of soybean meal or linseed meal. Excess amounts of protein can cause strong ammonia odors that can cause respiratory irritation if stalls are not cleaned regularly. Other supplements that may be used include fat supplements and fermentable fiber. Beet pulp, rice, and wheat bran all are types of fermentable fiber that can be used in conjunction with psyllium to increase the fiber content in the diet to help prevent sand colic in horses.

FEEDING CONSIDERATIONS BY AGE

Gestating mares can be maintained on a maintenance ration for the first 90 days of gestation. As pregnancy progresses, the mare's energy requirements increase. The mare will need 20% more energy, and the horse should be transitioned to concentrate containing 11% crude protein. During the last 3 weeks of gestation, the energy requirement of the mare increases again, and adequate amounts of calcium and phosphorus should be supplied. A good guideline is that the mare should gain 10% of her body weight during pregnancy. During lactation, mares should be fed a diet similar to that of yearlings.

TECHNICIAN NOTE   During gestation, a mare should gain 10% of her body weight.

At approximately 1 to 2 weeks of age, foals should begin receiving small amounts of creep feed, which should contain 16% crude protein. Young foals that are not gaining weight can have their creep feed top dressed with milk replacer to encourage growth. Starting at 2 to 3 months of age, foals can be fed 1 pound of concentrate per day. This amount is increased by an additional 1 pound of concentrate for every month of age through weaning; however, this amount should never exceed 7 to 9 pounds of grain. At weaning, foals should then be offered 1 pound of roughage for every 100 pounds of body weight along with their concentrate ration. This should be continued until 12 months of age.

TECHNICIAN NOTE   At 2 to 3 months of age, foals can be fed 1 pound of concentrate per day, and this amount can be increased by an additional 1 pound for every month of age through weaning.

Yearlings and 2-year-old horses should be provided roughage free choice. These horses can also be supplemented with a concentrate containing 13% crude protein. When mature horses are being fed, their *dry matter* intake should be approximately 1.75% of their body weight. Concentrates can be offered in small amounts to nonactive horses, and amounts can increase as the amount of work being performed increases. Stallions can be fed as mature horses with supplemental grain during the breeding season.

When considering the feeding of horses that are being exercised or worked, the horses can be classified into one of three categories: light work, moderate work, or heavy work. Horses classified as doing light work are being exercised or worked for less than 1 hour per day. Most horses being ridden are classified as horses performing light work. Horses classified as performing moderate work are involved in active competition and are sweating daily on a regular basis. Horses classified as performing heavy work are horses involves in endurance activities such as endurance racing, polo, cross-country competition, or horse racing.

TECHNICIAN NOTE   Lightly working horses are horses that perform 1 hour or less of work per day.

Lightly working horses require a crude protein level between 8.5% and 10% (this level can increase up to 13% if horses are being supplemented with fat or if low-quality roughage is being fed). They should be provided 1% to 2% of their body weight in roughages and 0.5% to 1% of their body weight in concentrate. Moderately and heavily working horses need 8.5% to 14% crude protein in their diets. Moderately working horses need 1% to 2% of their body weight in roughages and 0.75 to 1.5% in grain. Heavily working horses need 1% to 1.5% of their body weight in roughage and 1% to 2% of their body weight in grain (Fig. 8-69).

When horses are being worked, it is important to remember to cool them down before allowing them to drink water. Horses allowed to drink immediately after exercise, while they are still hot, are more likely to *founder* or have digestive disturbances.

MINERALS

Roughages supplied in the equine diet are often rich enough in potassium to meet the horse's requirements. The calcium-to-phosphorus ratio for horses should be approximately 2:1. Excessive amounts of calcium can impair the function of trace minerals and compromise the absorption of phosphorus. Extreme amounts of calcium can also be responsible for secondary nutritional hyperparathyroidism. Deficiencies in the calcium-to-phosphorus ratio can cause abnormal bone growth or contribute to weak bones, which can manifest as lameness.

0—Emaciated	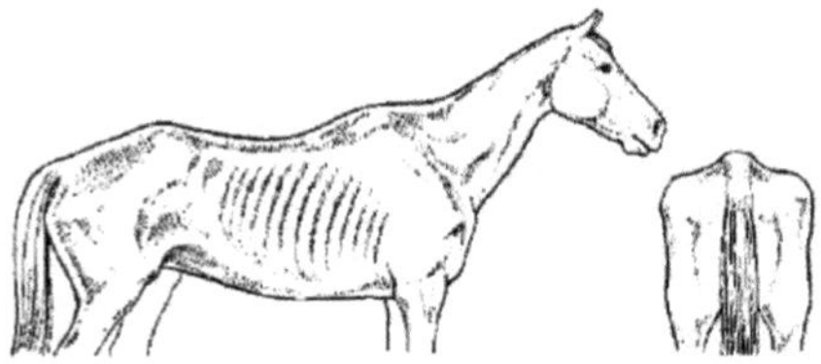	• No fatty tissue can be felt—skin tight over bones • Shape of individual bones visible • Marked ewe-neck • Very prominent backbone and pelvis • Very sunken rump • Deep cavity under tail • Large gap between thighs
1—Very thin	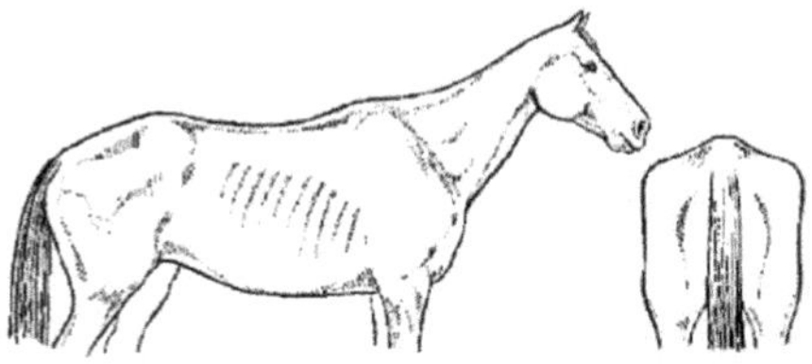	• Barely any fatty tissue—skin more supple • Shape of bones visible • Narrow ewe-neck • Ribs easily visible • Prominent backbone, croup, and tail head • Sunken rump; cavity under tail • Gap betweent thighs
2—Very lean	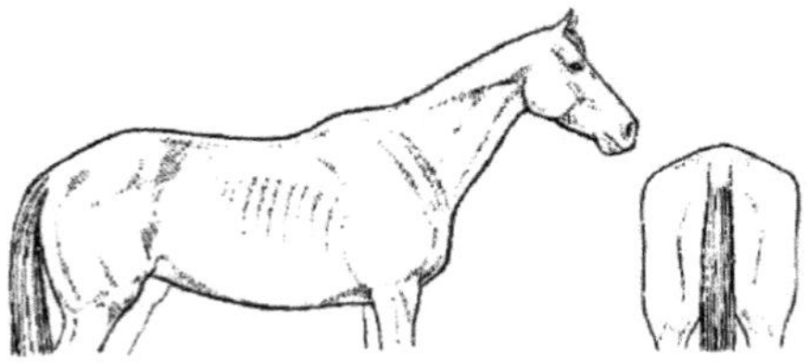	• A very thin layer of fat under the skin • Narrow neck; muscles sharply defined • Backbone covered with a very thin layer of fat but still protruding • Withers, shoulders, and neck accentuated • Ribs just visible, a small amount of fat building between them • Hip bones easily visible but rounded • Rump usually sloping flat from backbone to point of hips, may be rounded if horse is fit • May be a small gap between thighs
3—Healthy weight	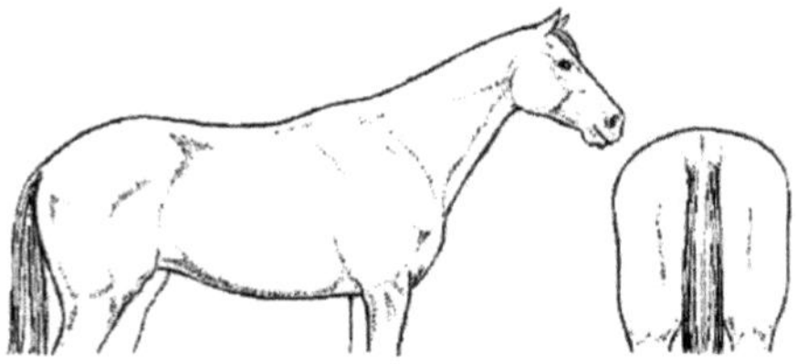	• A thin layer of fat under the skin • Muscles on neck less defined • Shoulders and neck blend smoothly into body • Withers appear rounded over tips of bones • Back is flat or forms only a slight ridge • Ribs not visible but easily felt • A thin layer of fat building around tail head • Rump beginning to appear rounded • Hip bones just visible
4—Fat	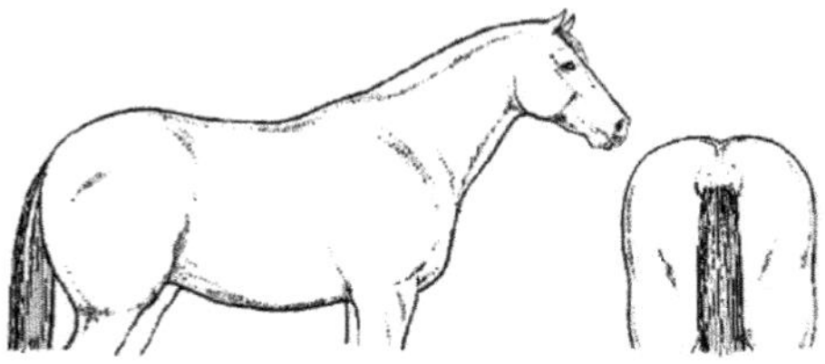	• Muscles hard to determine beneath fat layer • Spongy fat developing on crest • Fat deposits along withers, behind shoulders, and along neck • Ribs covered by spongy fat • Spongy fat around tail head • Gutter along back • Rump well rounded • From behind rump looks apple shaped • Hip bones difficult to feel
5—Obese	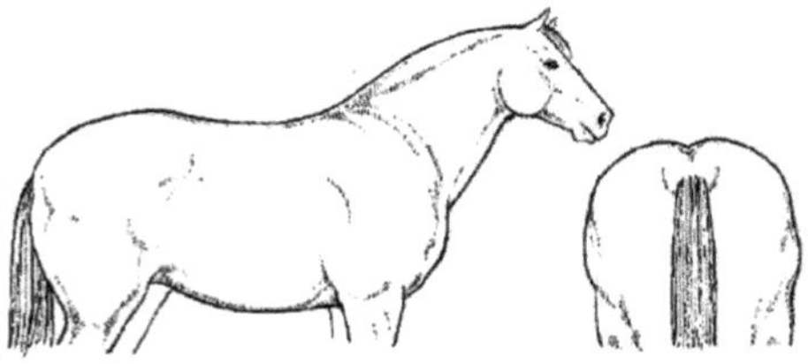	• Horse takes on a bloated or blocky appearance • Muscles not visible—covered by a layer of fat • Pronounced crest with hard fat • Pads of fat along withers, behind shoulders, along neck, and on ribs; ribs cannot be felt • Extremely obvious gutter along back and rump • Flank filled in flush • Lumps of fat around tail head • Very bulging apple-shaped rump, bony points buried • Inner thighs pressing together

FIGURE 8-69 Body condition score.

> *TECHNICIAN NOTE*
> * Excess amounts of calcium can cause secondary nutritional hyperparathyroidism.
> * The calcium-to-phosphorus ratio for horses should be approximately 2:1.

Although uncommon, magnesium deficiency can cause nervous conditions in the horse that manifest as staggering and convulsions. Sodium chloride is often supplied in the equine diet with the use of salt blocks. A salt block should always be made available for ab libitum consumption by horses. Horses that are being worked often perspire during exercise and should be supplemented with loose salt in their concentrate ration. Horses lose 30 grains of salt in every pound of perspiration.

Iodine is extremely important in pregnant mares. Deficiencies in iodine can be responsible for fetal abnormalities, weak foals, and foals with enlarged thyroid glands. Mares deficient in iodine may experience goiter, are at increased risk for a retained placenta, and can have a longer gestation period. Excesses in iodine can cause the same abnormalities seen with deficiencies in iodine. Copper is needed for proper iron use and is important for cartilage, pigment, and bone formation. Anemia can be seen in horses with deficiencies of copper. Zinc deficiencies can cause poor wound healing and hair loss. *White muscle disease* can be seen with deficiencies of selenium and vitamin E. Mares with deficiencies of selenium and vitamin E may have reduced fertility and are at greater risk for retained placenta. Excess amounts of selenium can cause dyspnea or sudden excitability. If excesses are continued for long periods, lameness and hoof deformity can occur.

CASE STUDY

Mrs. Rockwell calls regarding a miniature foal born yesterday. The foal is depressed and refuses to eat. You ask her please to bring the foal in for a physical examination. The doctor orders a chemistry panel. On the panel, the foal is found to have a blood glucose reading of 90 mg/dL. What will the doctor ask you to do next? What could possibly happen if the foal's blood glucose drops to 40 mg/dL?

CASE STUDY

Mrs. White raises Clydesdales. Her champion halter mare gave birth to a foal 5 days ago. Mrs. White has noticed that the umbilical cord has continually remained damp since birth. The foal seems to drip fluid from its umbilicus randomly. The doctor is called to Mrs. White's farm to examine the foal. The doctor confirms it is a patent urachus. What is the typical treatment protocol?

SUGGESTED READING

American Miniature Horse Association: <www. amha.org/> (Accessed 06.04.15.)

American Morgan Horse Association: <www. morganhorse.com/> (Accessed 06.04.15.)

American Paint Horse Association: <www.apha.com/> (Accessed 06.04.15.)

Appaloosa Horse Club: <www.appaloosa.com/> (Accessed 06.04.15.)

Beech J: Neonatal equine disease, *Vet Clin North Am Equine Pract* 1:1–263, 1985.

Bentz AI, Gill MS: Small animal medical nursing. In Bassert JM, McCurnin DM, editors: *McCurnin's clinical textbook for veterinary technicians*, ed 7, St. Louis, 2010, Saunders, pp 674–712.

Edwards EH: *The encyclopedia of the horse*, New York, 2001, Dorling Kindersley.

Lewis LD: *Feeding and care of the horse*, ed 2, Baltimore, 1996, Williams & Wilkins.

Mitchell CF, Moore RM, Gill MS: Large animal surgical nursing. In Bassert JM, McCurnin DM, editors: *McCurnin's clinical textbook for veterinary technicians*, ed 7, St. Louis, 2010, Saunders, pp 1056–1092.

Pinto CF, Eilts BE, Paccamonti DL: Animal reproduction. In Bassert JM, McCurnin DM, editors: *McCurnin's clinical textbook for veterinary technicians*, ed 7, St. Louis, 2010, Saunders, pp 370–399.

Teeple TN: Nursing care of horses. In Sirois M, editor: *Principles and practice of veterinary technology*, ed 3, St. Louis, 2011, Mosby, pp 569–584.

Vaala WE: Perinatology, *Vet Clin North Am Equine Pract* 10:1–271, 1994.

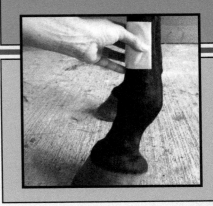

9 Equine Clinical Procedures

LEARNING OBJECTIVES

After reviewing this chapter, you will be able to

- Set up and prepare the patient for each procedure, perform the procedure (when appropriate), or assist the clinician in performing diagnostic sampling and medication procedures
- Properly insert and maintain an intravenous catheter and monitor the catheter for complications
- Explain the rationale and indications for each of the clinical procedures described
- Set up materials and equipment, and prepare the patient as needed for the procedure
- Provide assistance to the veterinarian when performing the procedure, or perform the procedure when it may be appropriate for a veterinary technician to do so
- Perform or assist with necropsy and sample collection procedures, and maintain a safe environment during these procedures

KEY TERMS

Atlantooccipital space
American Association of Equine
  Practitioners (AAEP)
Anaphylactic shock
Balling gun
Caps
Centesis
Clinching
Cutdown
Ependymal

Epistaxis
Farrier
Feed additives
Floating
Hematoma
Lumbosacral space
Nasogastric intubation
Pneumothorax
Poultices
Pruritus

Sinocentesis
Smegma
Subarachnoid space
Subcutaneous emphysema
Sweats
Thrombophlebitis
Trephining
Turbinates

KEY ABBREVIATIONS

BTT: Blue top tube
CSF: Cerebrospinal fluid
GRNTT: Green top tube
GTT: Gray top tube

IM: Intramuscular
IV: Intravenous
LTT: Lavender top tube

RTT: Red top tube
SC: Subcutaneous
SST: Serum separator tube

DIAGNOSTIC SAMPLING

Diagnostic sampling refers to obtaining samples of body fluids or tissues for the purpose of analysis. The results of the analysis are then used to aid the clinician in making a diagnosis and in planning and monitoring treatment.

Body fluids that can be collected include venous and arterial blood, abdominal fluid, pleural fluid, airway fluid, joint fluid, cerebrospinal fluid (CSF), feces, and urine. The technician should be familiar with where the procedure is performed, proper preparation (prep) for the procedure, which tests will be performed on the fluid, and the rationale behind the procedure. Details on processing and performing laboratory tests are beyond the scope of this text and are covered in detail in many excellent references.

In general, "normal" body fluids (other than blood) have the following characteristics:

- Their clarity is transparent (not cloudy).
- They are nonodorous.
- They have low white blood cell (WBC) counts.
- They have no or few red blood cells (RBCs); the procedure itself (i.e., obtaining the sample) can cause some bleeding into the fluid.
- They have no bacteria (if obtained from closed body cavities).
- They have low protein levels.

Tissue samples include skin and mucosal scrapings or swabs, fine needle aspirates, and biopsy tissue sections. These procedures are performed similarly in all species, and the reader is referred to other sources for in-depth coverage of these topics.

Restraint for each of these procedures varies depending on the behavior of the horse. Most procedures can be performed with the use of a halter and stocks. However, sometimes sedation is required.

VENOUS BLOOD SAMPLING

Equipment box for venous blood sampling:
- Alcohol
- 20-gauge × 1½-inch needle or Vacutainer needle
- Syringe or Vacutainer

Blood samples may be collected from arteries or veins. Preference for arterial or venous blood is dictated by the type of analysis to be performed. Almost all blood samples are venous. Veins are more accessible (located more superficially) and are less prone to *hematoma* formation than are arteries.

Sites for venous blood sampling include the jugular vein (Fig. 9-1), cephalic vein, lateral thoracic vein, saphenous vein, and coccygeal vein. Any vein that can be identified, occluded, and accessed safely may be used. The technician should use an approach and preparation similar to that for an intravenous (IV) injection, described in the section on parenteral injection techniques.

Sites for arterial blood sampling are more difficult to access, especially in unsedated patients. The transverse facial artery and the dorsal metatarsal artery are most

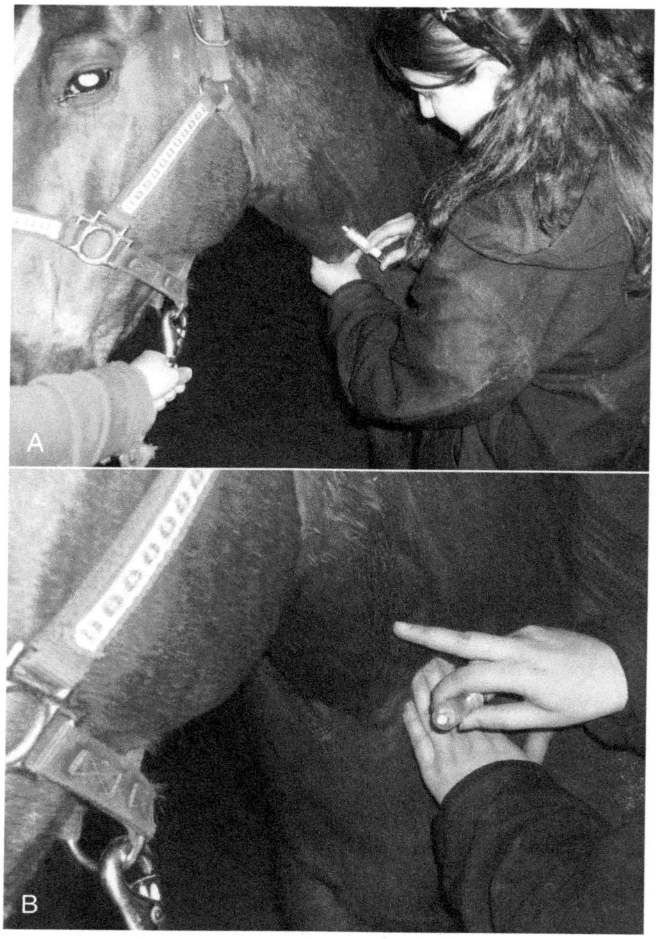

FIGURE 9-1 **A,** Location of the jugular vein. **B,** Use of a Vacutainer for blood collection from the jugular vein.

commonly used, especially in anesthetized patients. Arteries are prone to development of hematomas after needle withdrawal, so firm pressure should be applied directly to the puncture site (minimum of 1 to 2 minutes) to minimize this risk.

Blood can be collected by aspiration into a syringe or Vacutainer (Becton, Dickinson, and Company, Franklin Lakes, NJ) tube. When patients are needle shy, it may be advisable to use a 20-gauge (ga) needle and Luer syringe to aspirate the blood and then transfer it to a vacuum tube. For direct blood draws into Vacutainer tubes, 1½-inch-long Vacutainer needles are available for large animal use.

Processing and analysis of blood samples are discussed in detail in other texts. Table 9-1 lists normal complete blood count values. Table 9-2 lists normal blood chemistry values for horses.

Handling and storage of samples are important. When drawing blood, it is important to try to collect enough blood to run three of each tests required; this will allow enough blood if an error occurs. Lipemic and hemolyzed samples can alter values. If multiple tubes must be filled, it is best always to fill the anticoagulant tube first, to decrease the risk of sample clotting. Never shake anticoagulant tubes;

TABLE 9-1	Normal Complete Blood Count Values	
Packed cell volume (%)	Increased with polycythemia, dehydration, stress, in neonates, and high globulin levels; decreased with anemia, bleeding, overhydration, and in weanlings	32–52 (42)
Hemoglobin (g/dL)	Increased with polycythemia; decreased with anemia	11–19 (15)
Red blood cells ($\times 10^6$ μL)	Increased with polycythemia and dehydration; decreased with anemia and overhydration	6.5–12.5 (9.5)
Total protein (g/dL)	Increased in dehydration and in lipemic samples; decreased with overhydration	6.0–8.0
White blood cells ($\times 10^3$/μL)	Increased with acute local inflammation, toxicity, and bacterial infections; decreased with marrow diseases, radiation, drug therapy, and certain viruses	5.5–12.5 (9)
Platelets ($\times 10^5$/μL)	Decreased with marrow hypoplasia, equine infectious anemia, septicemia, epistaxis, immune-mediated hemolytic anemia, disseminated intravascular coagulation, ehrlichiosis	1–6 (3.3)
Mean corpuscular volume (MCV) (fL)	Increased with B_{12} and folic acid deficiency; decreased with iron deficiency	34–58 (46)
Mean corpuscular hemoglobin (MCH) (pg)	Increased with hemolysis; decreased with iron deficiency	15.2–18.6
Mean corpuscular hemoglobin concentration (MCHC) (g/dL)	Increased with hemolysis, lipemia, and Heinz bodies	31–37 (35)
Bone marrow myeloid-to-erythrocyte (M:E) ratio		0.94–3.76:1 (1.64:1)
DIFFERENTIAL, ABSOLUTE		
Segmented neutrophils (segs)		30%–65% 2700–6700 (4700)
Bands		0%–2% 0–100 (2)
Lymphocytes		25%–70% 1500–7500 (3500)
Monocytes		0.5%–7% 0–800 (400)
Eosinophils		0%–11% 0–925 (375)
Basophils		0%–3% 0–170 (50)

instead, rock them. Samples should be processed within 4 to 6 hours, or the plasma and serum should be removed and placed in the refrigerator. If glucose is in question, the sample should be run immediately. Always label your tubes with the patient's full name and date. Other items to consider writing on the tubes include zoonotic disease suspects, chemotherapy patients, and time-specific samples. Tubes should always be stored upright (Table 9-3).

BLOOD GAS SAMPLES

Equipment for blood gas samples:
- Alcohol
- 25-ga needle
- 3-mL syringe
- Rubber stopper
- Heparin
- Ice
- Thermometer

Blood gas analysis is used most often in assessing patients with respiratory disease and for monitoring patients under general anesthesia. The analysis determines the oxygen content, carbon dioxide content, and pH of the blood sample. Arterial blood is usually preferred to venous blood for blood gas analysis because it more accurately reflects the ventilation status of the animal. Blood gas analysis as an anesthetic monitoring tool is more common in large animals than small animals.

> **TECHNICIAN NOTE**   Arterial blood is often preferred to venous blood for blood gas samples because it more accurately reflects the ventilation status of the animal.

Samples for blood gas analysis must not clot and must not be contaminated by atmospheric air. Typically, a 25-ga needle and a 3-mL syringe are used to obtain the sample.

TABLE 9-2	Normal Blood Chemistry Values	
Blood urea nitrogen (mg/dL)	Increased with kidney disease, azotemia, and uremia	10.4–24.7
Creatinine (mg/dL)	Increased with kidney disease	0.9–2.0
Glucose (mg/dL)	Decreased in fatty liver disease; increases with diabetes and stress	62.2–114
Albumin (g/dL)	Increased with dehydration; decreased with brucellosis, chronic liver disease, glomerular disease, hyperglobulinemia, hypertension, malnutrition, and malabsorption	2.5–3.8
Total bilirubin (mg/dL)	Increased in animals with liver disease, bile duct obstruction, jaundice, or hemolytic anemia; can be normal if horse is fasted for more than 24 hours	0.3–3
Aspartate aminotransferase (AST) (µg/L)	Increased in liver disease or with muscle damage; can be increased after exercise	115.7–287
γ–Glutamyltransferase (GGT) (µg/L)	Increased with hepatocellular and cholestatic liver disease, hepatocyte necrosis, and cholestasis	2.7–22.4
Creatine kinase (µg/L)	Increased with muscle disease	34–165.6
Alkaline phosphatase (µg/L)	Increased with liver disease and cholestasis, steroids, and growth	70.1–226.8
Lactate dehydrogenase (DH) (µg/L)	Increased with hepatocyte damage, muscle damage, and hemolysis	102.3–340.6
Sodium (mEq/L)	When increased can cause neurologic disorders and hypertension; decreases can be due to *Escherichia coli* infection, polyuria or polydipsia, weight loss, and anorexia	133.3–147.3
Potassium (mEq/L)	Increases can result from severe metabolic acidosis; decreases can be caused by anorexia, increased renal excretion, abomasal stasis, intestinal obstruction, enteritis, and weight loss.	2.8–4.7
Chloride (mEq/L)		97.2–110.1
Calcium (mg/dL)	Increased with kidney stones, renal failure, and some cancers; Decreased in renal disease and bone disease	10.4–13.4
Phosphorus (mg/dL)	Increased in renal failure; decreased with osteomalacia, rickets, and tetany	2.3–5.4
Magnesium (mg/dL)	Decreased with fever and hypersalivation	1.8–2.7

TABLE 9-3	Shows Techniques for Completing a Complete Blood Count
COMPONENT	**TECHNIQUE**
PVC	Fill a capillary tube ¾ of the way full, and seal the end with clay. Repeat. Now you have two blood-filled capillary tubes. Place them in the centrifuge and spin for 3–5 minutes. Record the color and transparency of the plasma. Then using a PCV card, record the percentage
Total protein	After completing the PCV, break the capillary tube just above the buffy coat (a white line separating the plasma and RBCs) Place a drop of plasma on the refractometer lens and look through the refractometer. Record the value
WBC estimate	Under 40×, count 10 fields, counting each WBC seen; then divide that number by 10 and multiply by 2000
WBC differential	Under 1000×, identify and classify 100 WBCs. Each classification then becomes a percentage
nRBC correction	While performing your differential, keep tract of any nRBC seen. Then take the observed TWBC × 100 / 100 + nRBC
Platelet estimate	Under 100× in the monolayer, count platelets in 10 different fields; divide by 10. Then multiply by 15,000–18,000
MCV	PCV (%) × 10 / RBC count × 10^6/µL
MCH	PCV (%) × 10 / RBC count × 10^6/µL
MCHC	HGB (g/dL) × 100 / PCV (%)

HGB, Hemoglobin; *MCH*, mean corpuscular hemoglobin; *MCHC*, mean corpuscular hemoglobin concentration; *MCV*, mean corpuscular volume; *nRBC*, nucleated red blood cells; *PCV*, packed cell volume; *RBC*, red blood cell; *TWBC*, total white blood count; *WBC*, white blood cell.

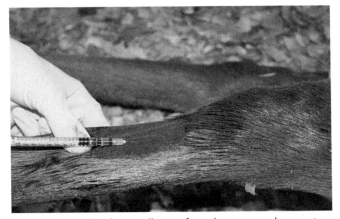

FIGURE 9-2 Blood gas collection from the metatarsal artery in a neonate. A small diaper dampened with water and placed in the microwave for 20 seconds was placed over the artery for 30 seconds before collection. The warm compress allowed for dilation and easy visualization of the artery. Topical application of a local anesthetic cream may decrease movement before collection. (From McAuliffe SB, Slovis NM: *Color atlas of diseases and disorders of the foal*, St. Louis, 2008, Saunders.)

To prevent coagulation of blood, just enough heparin is aspirated to fill the needle and appear in the needle hub. No air or air bubbles should be in the syringe. At least 1 mL of blood is drawn from an artery or vein, and the needle is immediately capped with a rubber stopper to keep air from contacting the sample (rubber stoppers from blood tubes work well). The syringe-needle-cap combination is placed on ice and is promptly analyzed. The sample should be run within 10 minutes but may yield accurate results for approximately 1½ hours if the sample is maintained on ice and kept airtight. The patient's temperature should be taken at the time of collection, and the analysis must be corrected for body temperature (Fig. 9-2).

TECHNICIAN NOTE Samples used for blood gas analysis cannot be exposed to atmospheric air or allowed to clot.

URINE COLLECTION

Equipment for urine collection:
- Voided
  - Collection container
  - Possibly furosemide (syringe and needle)
  - Examination gloves
- Catheterization
  - Tranquilizer (syringe and needle)
  - Antimicrobial soap
  - Water
  - Stallion catheter for males
  - Mare catheter or metal Chambers catheter for females
  - 60-mL syringe (catheter or Luer tip depending on the catheter used)

- Sterile gloves
- Sterile lubricating jelly
- Sterile collection container

The purpose of urine collection is to obtain a sample of urine for laboratory analysis. Indications for urine collection include urinary tract disease, various systemic diseases, and toxicologic or pharmacologic analysis. Cystocentesis is not feasible in large animals; therefore, sampling is limited to voided urine collection and bladder catheterization. Cystocentesis is not used in adults because of the inability to stabilize the bladder and the possibility of perforating the intestines during the procedure. Cystocentesis has been successfully performed in foals and small ponies and miniature horses, but it is a risky procedure and is not often attempted.

TECHNICIAN NOTE Because of the size of animals and possible complications, cystocentesis is not often performed in large animals.

Voided urine is not sterile and therefore is not suitable for culture and sensitivity testing. Urine is collected into a clean container when the horse urinates. When catching a sample of voided urine, it is best to avoid the initial urine stream and collect a midstream sample. The initial urine stream tends to contain more mucus and cell debris and may not be representative of the content of the urine. Urination is sometimes facilitated with diuretic drugs such as furosemide to reduce the time spent waiting for a voided sample. When analyzing diuretic-induced urine samples, the effects of the drug on parameters such as urine specific gravity must be considered. To prepare for a voided collection, you will need a clean container, examination gloves, and possibly diuretic drugs. Some racehorses are trained to urinate on command. Each horse is trained with a different command, so it is a good idea to ask the client about the horse's training. To begin, the horse should be restrained. If diuretics are to be administered, they should be given now. Once the horse begins to urinate, allow the initial portion of the urine stream to pass, and then catch the midstream urine in a clean container; finally, cap the container.

TECHNICIAN NOTE
- If a diuretic is used before collecting a urine sample, the effects of the diuretic on urine specific gravity should be considered.
- When catching voided urine, it is best to collect a midstream sample.

Catheterization of the bladder risks contamination of the urine with bacteria that accumulate on the catheter as it passes through the urethra. Therefore, culture results of catheterized samples must be interpreted with caution. Because cystocentesis is not feasible in large animals, catheterized

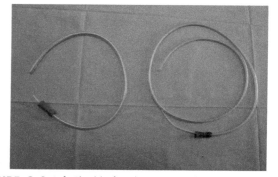

FIGURE 9-3 *Left,* Flexible female urinary catheter and stylet. *Right,* Flexible male urinary catheter and stylet.

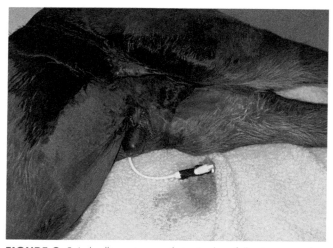

FIGURE 9-4 Indwelling urinary catheter in place following surgical repair of a bladder wall defect. The condom fitted at the end of the catheter acts as a one-way valve that allows urine to flow out but prevents air from entering and inflating the bladder. (From McAuliffe SB, Slovis NM: *Color atlas of diseases and disorders of the foal,* St. Louis, 2008, Saunders.)

urine samples are the accepted compromise for microbial testing. Urine collection using catheterization is a sterile procedure, so you should prepare the following equipment before the procedure: a urinary catheter (stallion catheter for males; mare catheter or metal Chambers catheter for females [Fig. 9-3]), a 60-mL syringe (catheter or Luer tip depending on the catheter used), sterile gloves, sterile lubricating jelly, and a sterile collection container (plastic or glass).

> **TECHNICIAN NOTE**   Culture results from catheterized samples must be interpreted with caution because bacteria can accumulate on the catheter as it passes through the urethra.

To begin, the horse should be restrained standing, but the procedure can be performed with the animal in lateral recumbency.

Males

Tranquilization is usually required to cause relaxation and extension of the penis. The catheterization procedure induces discomfort; therefore, personnel should position themselves cranially to avoid being kicked with the hindlegs. Additional physical restraint may be necessary. Catheterization of the bladder is performed through the urethra. In males, the urethral entrance is on the end of the glans penis. Following extension of the penis, the tip of the glans penis is prepared with at least three applications of antimicrobial soap and water rinses. The tip of the catheter should be well lubricated with a sterile lubricant. The urethral opening is identified, and the lubricated catheter is passed into the urethra and is slowly advanced into the bladder. If the catheter has a stylet, it must be withdrawn to allow urine flow through the catheter. Urine sometimes flows freely from the catheter and may be collected in a sterile container. If urine does not flow freely, a sterile 60-mL syringe is used to aspirate urine from the bladder (Fig. 9-4).

> **TECHNICIAN NOTE**   The penis should be prepped with at least three applications of antimicrobial soap and water rinses.

Females

The tail is tied or held to the side, and the perineum is prepared with at least three applications of antimicrobial soap and water rinses. The clinician's gloves should be well lubricated with a sterile lubricant. Physical restraint may be necessary; sedation is occasionally necessary. In females, the urethral entrance is located in the floor of the vestibule-vagina junction (Fig. 9-5). The procedure from this point is carried out similar to that of male catheterization.

After the procedure has been performed, all soap residues should be removed to prevent scalding of the skin and mucosal surfaces. Catheterization may cause temporary irritation of the urethra, thus leading to increased frequency of urination for 1 to 2 days.

> **TECHNICIAN NOTE**   It is important to inform clients that urinary catheterization may lead to increased frequency of urination for 1 to 2 days.

> **TECHNICIAN NOTE**   Calcium carbonate crystals are normal and common in horse urine.

Evaluation of the Urine Sample

Common urine analysis procedures include the following:
- Gross evaluation: Normal horse urine is clear to cloudy and yellow. The cloudiness reflects a relatively large amount of mucus, which is normal in the horse.
- Urine specific gravity.
- Chemical analysis: Values are determined using reagent test strips ("dipsticks") or machine analysis, or both.
- Urine sediment evaluation: Calcium carbonate crystals are normal and common in horse urine.
- Microbial culture and sensitivity: These tests are performed if infectious disease is suspected or confirmed.

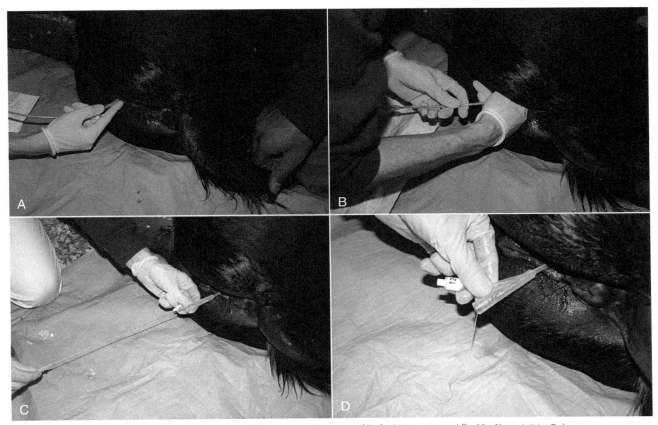

FIGURE 9-5 A to **D,** Placement of a urinary catheter in a filly foal. (From McAuliffe SB, Slovis NM: *Color atlas of diseases and disorders of the foal,* St. Louis, 2008, Saunders.)

FECAL COLLECTION

Equipment for fecal collection:

- Collection container
- Glove
- Sleeve

Fecal collection is performed for parasitic evaluation or microbial culture, or both. Indications for fecal collection include suspected intestinal parasite infestation or suspected intestinal bacterial, viral, or protozoal infection.

Feces can be collected from the ground by using a glove or clean container or from the rectum by using a glove or rectal sleeve. A hand is inserted into the glove or sleeve and is used to grasp the feces. Then, while maintaining a grasp on the feces with the hand, the glove or sleeve is simply turned inside out. This maneuver keeps the feces inside the glove or sleeve, and physical contact with the fecal material is avoided. The glove or sleeve is tied in a knot above the feces and is transported to the laboratory. Sample sizes for large and small animals are similar; large animals do not require voluminous fecal samples.

> **TECHNICIAN NOTE**   The same amount of fecal material is needed for a large animal fecal analysis as is needed in small animals.

Evaluation of Fecal Samples
Common Features Evaluated on Fecal Samples

The following observations should be made when performing a fecal laboratory analysis:

- Gross evaluation: Normal equine feces are mostly solid, in formed fecal balls. Color is light to dark green. Mucous coating may indicate that the feces have been retained longer than normal.
- Parasitic evaluation: Testing includes fecal flotation without or without quantitative techniques and with or without larval culture.
- Fecal culture and sensitivity: These tests are especially important when *Salmonella* is suspected. *Salmonella* testing usually requires daily samples for 3 to 5 days; at least 10 g of feces should be submitted for each sample.

ABDOMINOCENTESIS (ABDOMINAL TAP)

Equipment for abdominocentesis:

- Clippers
- Surgical scrub and alcohol
- Sterile gloves
- Ethylenediamine tetraacetic acid (EDTA)
- Serum (plain) blood tubes/red top tube
- Adult:18 or 19-ga × 1½-inch needle
- Obese adult: 20-ga × 3-inch spinal needle

- Foal: 20-ga × 1-inch needle
- Blunt trocar or cannula for severely bloated patients
- No. 15 scalpel blade
- Local anesthetic: syringe /25-ga × ⅝-inch needle
- Sterile 4 × 4 gauze
- Clean cloth or towel
- Skin suture or staple (may be placed)
- Antibiotic ointment

The purpose of an abdominocentesis is to obtain a sample of abdominal (peritoneal) fluid for analysis. The fluid is produced by the cells of the peritoneum, which line the abdominal wall and the outer surfaces of the abdominal organs. Abnormalities of abdominal organs may change the character of the abdominal fluid and provide clues for the diagnosis of abdominal disease.

The procedure can be readily performed in the clinic or in the field. Indications for abdominocentesis include abdominal disease, gastrointestinal (GI) or non-GI in origin, and chronic weight loss.

> **TECHNICIAN NOTE**   Some indications for abdominocentesis are abdominal disease, gastrointestinal (GI) or non-GI in origin, and chronic weight loss.

It is important that all the appropriate equipment be prepared before beginning the procedure. You will need sterile gloves, EDTA and serum (plain) blood tubes, a needle (18- or 19-ga × 1½-inch needle for most adults, 18-ga × 3-inch spinal needle for large or obese horses, 20-ga × 1-inch needle for foals), a blunt trocar or cannula for severely bloated patients, a no. 15 scalpel blade if using a trocar or cannula, local anesthetic and syringe, with a 25-ga × ⅝-inch needle for anesthesia of the skin (for foals or if using a trocar or cannula), sterile 4 × 4 gauze if using a trocar or cannula, and a clean ground cloth or towel for foals.

Adults are restrained in a standing position for the procedure; foals are restrained in lateral recumbency. The procedure is usually performed at the most dependent (lowest) point of the abdomen, on the ventral midline or slightly to the right of the ventral midline (Fig. 9-6).

The hair should be clipped, and sterile skin preparation should be performed (Fig. 9-7). Performing the procedure without clipping the hair is possible, but special care must be taken to prepare the area properly, and the client should be warned about the slightly increased risk for introducing infection.

Local anesthesia is seldom necessary in most patients when hypodermic or spinal needles are used. However, local anesthesia of the skin is routinely performed for foals or whenever a trocar or cannula is used. A final skin preparation is performed after the anesthetic is injected subcutaneously.

Patient restraint is sometimes necessary, although the procedure is well tolerated, and many horses require minimal, if any, restraint. The patient should be prevented from walking during the procedure.

Personnel should stand as far cranially as possible to avoid being kicked during the procedure. Patients typically flinch when the needle is passed through the skin but rarely kick.

A small stab incision through the skin is performed if the trocar or cannula method is being used; syringe needles do not require a skin incision. The clinician advances the needle, trocar, or cannula until fluid is obtained. Fluid is collected by gravity flow into the sample collection tubes. The EDTA tube sample should be collected first because most of the laboratory analysis will use this sample. At least 1 mL of fluid should be obtained to prevent false laboratory results, which can occur if the ratio of EDTA to abdominal fluid is too high.

> **TECHNICIAN NOTE**   At least 1 mL of fluid should be obtained to prevent false laboratory results, which can occur if the ratio of EDTA to abdominal fluid is too high. If bacterial disease is suspected; as little as one drop of fluid is sufficient for this use.

The serum (plain) tube is used to collect samples for culture if bacterial disease is suspected; as little as one drop of fluid is sufficient for this use. Abdominal fluid may be difficult to obtain, sometimes requiring several attempts.

Bleeding is common after the needle is removed. This bleeding is caused by incidental perforation of skin vessels, which are difficult to avoid because they can rarely be seen. Manual pressure over the site stops the bleeding. If a stab incision was made, the clinician may elect to place a simple skin suture or skin staple to close the incision.

The area should be cleaned gently, and antibiotic ointment should be applied daily for 2 to 3 days. Complications such as infection or abscessation of the site are uncommon.

Evaluation of Abdominal Fluid

Common evaluations performed on an abdominocentesis sample include the following:

- Gross visual examination: Normal abdominal fluid is pale yellow, clear, and odorless. Its consistency is similar to water.
- Total protein level.
- RBC and WBC counts.
- Packed cell volume.
- Microscopic evaluation.
  - Cytology: Direct smear, air dried, stained.
  - Gram stain if bacteria are observed.
- Microbial culture and sensitivity: These tests are performed if infection is suspected or confirmed.
  - Ancillary tests: These may include pH, enzyme, and other chemistry studies; seldom necessary.

ARTHROCENTESIS (JOINT TAP)

Equipment for abdominocentesis:

- Clippers
- Surgical scrub and alcohol
- Povidone-iodine
- Sterile gloves
- EDTA

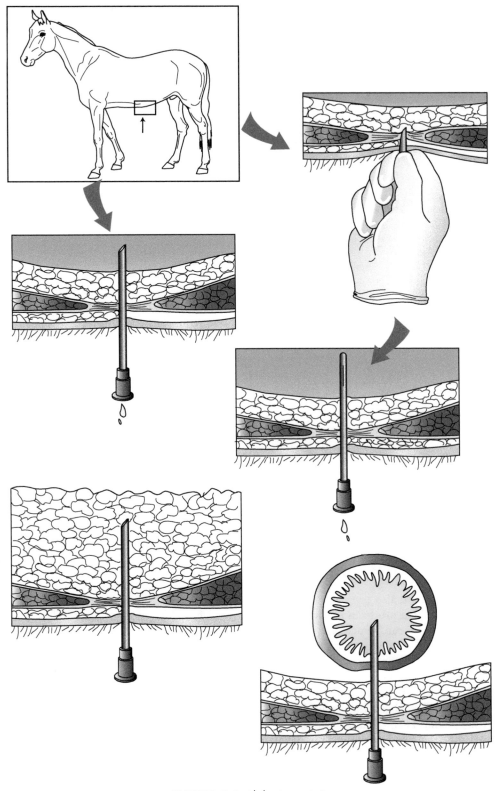

FIGURE 9-6 Abdominocentesis.

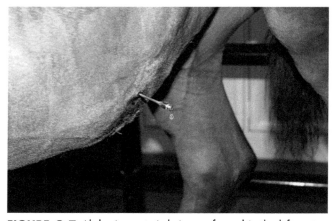

FIGURE 9-7 Abdominocentesis being performed in the left ventro-lateral abdomen. This site was chosen in this foal based on ultrasound findings of localized peritonitis. (From McAuliffe SB, Slovis NM: *Color atlas of diseases and disorders of the foal*, St. Louis, 2008, Saunders.)

- Serum (plain) blood tubes/red top tubes
- Needle (size varies)
- Sterile 6- or 12-mL syringe
- Local anesthetic, syringe, and needle
- Medication that will be injected (if being performed)
- Antibiotic ointment
- Bandaging material

Arthrocentesis is performed to obtain synovial fluid from a synovial joint for analysis. All synovial joints contain synovial fluid, which is produced by the cells of the synovial membrane. Disease of the joint often changes the characteristics of the fluid, and the sample can be used to aid in the diagnosis of various joint diseases and of tendon sheath and bursal disease.

> **TECHNICIAN NOTE**   Arthrocentesis can be used to aid in the diagnosis of various joint diseases and of tendon sheath and bursal disease.

Tendon sheaths and bursae are also synovial structures lined by a synovial membrane that produces synovial fluid. Many tendon sheaths and bursae can be accessed for fluid collection in the same manner as the joints. Analysis of these samples is similar to that of joint fluid.

Arthrocentesis and centesis of other synovial structures can be performed in the clinic or in the field. It is common practice to use the procedure to medicate the synovial structure. After the fluid sample has been obtained, the selected medication is injected into the structure before the needle is removed.

> **TECHNICIAN NOTE**   It is common practice to use arthrocentesis to medicate the synovial structure. The medication is injected before the needle is removed.

Before beginning the procedure, it is important to collect all the following supplies, to perform the procedure: sterile gloves; EDTA and serum (plain) blood tubes; a needle

(depends on many factors, especially location and depth of the joint, size of the patient, temperament of the patient, and the clinician's preference); sterile 6- or 12-mL syringe; local anesthetic, a syringe, and a needle (if skin block is necessary, e.g., foals, deep synovial structures, and patients that resist the procedure); and the medication to be injected, if applicable.

> **TECHNICIAN NOTE**   Local anesthesia can be needed for arthrocentesis in foals, deep synovial structures, or patients that resist the procedure.

Patient restraint depends on many factors, including the anatomical location of the synovial structure, the restraint method, and the clinician's preference. Restraint is required for most cases and ranges from minimal restraint to more severe physical restraint. In some cases, chemical sedation or even general anesthesia is necessary. Most arthrocentesis is performed with the horse standing and weight bearing, although some structures are accessed with the leg elevated. Some synovial structures are accessible from more than one location (Fig. 9-8). The patient must be motionless while the needle is in the joint because motion can bend or break the needle, and the cartilage and synovial membrane surfaces of the joint can be severely lacerated or punctured.

The hair should be clipped and the skin sterilely prepared. It is possible to perform the procedure without clipping the hair, but special care must be taken to prepare the area properly, and the client should be warned about the slightly increased risk for introducing infection. In either case, after the final alcohol scrub, I recommend applying povidone-iodine solution to the area and allowing it to air dry. The solution remains on the patient until the procedure is completed.

Local anesthesia is usually necessary for the skin and subcutaneous (SC) tissue if a large needle is to be used, such as for the hip and shoulder joints. Local anesthesia is sometimes required for horses that resist the procedure. It can be provided as a small anesthetic bleb at the skin puncture site or by regional anesthesia of peripheral nerves on the limbs. Most horses do not require local anesthesia for lower leg arthrocentesis.

> **TECHNICIAN NOTE**   Local anesthesia is usually necessary for the skin and subcutaneous tissue if a large needle is used for arthrocentesis of the hip and shoulder joints.

Once the needle enters the synovial structure, fluid may flow freely or not at all. Occasionally, the clinician uses a sterile syringe to aspirate the synovial fluid. The sample for the EDTA tube should be collected first because most of the laboratory analysis will use this sample. At least 1 mL of fluid should be obtained to prevent false-negative and false-positive laboratory results, which can occur if the ratio of EDTA to fluid is too high. The serum (plain) tube is used to collect samples for culture if bacterial disease is suspected; as little as one drop of fluid is sufficient for this use.

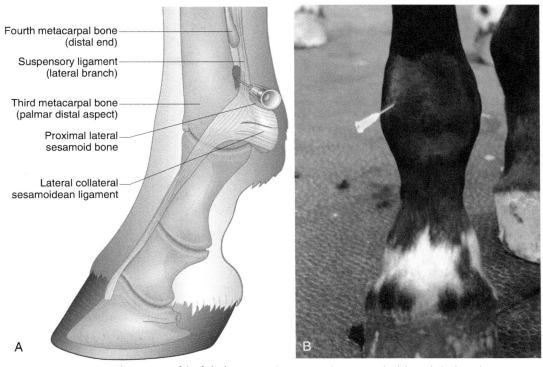

Fourth metacarpal bone
(distal end)

Suspensory ligament
(lateral branch)

Third metacarpal bone
(palmar distal aspect)

Proximal lateral
sesamoid bone

Lateral collateral
sesamoidean ligament

A

B

FIGURE 9-8 Arthrocentesis of the fetlock joint. **A,** The joint can be approached through the lateral aspect of the palmar or plantar pouch. **B,** The fetlock joint also can be entered cranially on either side of the extensor tendon. The fetlock is readily entered at this site when there is marked effusion of the joint. The advantage of this site is that inadvertent penetration of the metacarpal or metatarsal blood vessels is less likely. (From McAuliffe SB, Slovis NM: *Color atlas of diseases and disorders of the foal,* St. Louis, 2008, Saunders.)

> **TECHNICIAN NOTE** At least 1 mL of fluid should be obtained during arthrocentesis if the sample is to be added to EDTA to prevent false laboratory results.

After the fluid samples are collected, medication can be injected through the needle into the synovial space.

Bleeding from the skin is not unusual after needle withdrawal and is controlled with direct pressure. If bleeding occurs, the blood is cleaned from the skin, and antibiotic ointment is placed over the injection site. Bandaging depends on several factors. Often the joint disease itself requires some form of bandaging. Otherwise, many clinicians prefer to cover the injection site for 24 hours to minimize the risk of infection. This practice becomes more essential with structures closer to the ground (i.e., the distal limbs).

> **TECHNICIAN NOTE** Many clinicians prefer to bandage the injection site for 24 hours after arthrocentesis to help minimize the risk of infection.

Exercise is also dictated by the nature of the joint disease, the horse's occupation, and the type of medication injected into the joint (if this was performed).

Evaluation of Synovial Fluid

Common procedures include the following evaluations and measurements:
- Gross visual examination: Normal synovial fluid is yellow, clear, and odorless. The fluid should have viscosity (i.e., be "stringy"); watery consistency is abnormal.
- Total protein level.
- RBC and WBC counts.
- Packed cell volume.
- Microscopic evaluation.
  - Cytology: Direct smear, air dried, stained.
  - Gram stain if bacteria are observed.
- Microbial culture and sensitivity: These tests are performed if infection is suspected or confirmed.
  - Ancillary tests: These may include pH, enzymes, chemical mediators of inflammation, and other chemistry studies; cartilage fragment analysis and mucin clot tests are no longer routinely performed.

CEREBROSPINAL FLUID COLLECTION

Equipment for cerebrospinal fluid collection:
- General anesthetic agent for atlantooccipital space
- Sedative for lumbosacral
- Clippers
- Surgical scrub and alcohol
- Rope
- Sterile gloves

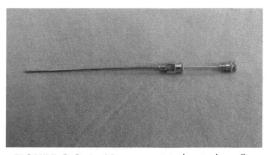

FIGURE 9-9 An 18-gauge × 3-inch spinal needle.

- Sterile 12- or 20-mL syringe
- EDTA
- Serum (plain) tubes/red top tubes
- 18-ga × 3-inch spinal needle
- 8-inch spinal needle
- Local anesthetic, 12-mL syringe, and 20-ga × 1½-inch needle
- Antibiotic ointment

CSF is collected from the *subarachnoid space* for analysis. CSF is produced by *ependymal* cells in the ventricles of the brain and flows in the subarachnoid space around the brain and spinal cord. CSF also flows through the ventricles of the brain and the central canal of the spinal cord but cannot be safely accessed in these locations. Collection of CSF is used to diagnose brain and spinal cord disease and to differentiate peripheral nervous system disease.

> **TECHNICIAN NOTE** CSF collection is used to diagnose brain and spinal cord disease and to differentiate peripheral nervous system disease.

Diseases of the central nervous system may produce changes in the character and composition of CSF; therefore, CSF is used as a diagnostic aid in neurologic disease.

CSF in the subarachnoid space can be readily accessed for sampling at two locations: the atlantooccipital space (also referred to as the cisterna magna) and the lumbosacral space. These procedures are significantly different in technique, but the CSF obtained from either location is essentially the same, as are the laboratory analysis procedures.

Before beginning the procedure, collect the following equipment: sterile gloves; sterile 12- or 20-mL syringe; EDTA and serum (plain) tubes; a needle (18-ga × 3-inch spinal needle for atlantooccipital tap [Fig. 9-9], 8-inch spinal needle for lumbosacral tap); local anesthetic, a 12-mL syringe, and a 20-ga × 1½-inch needle for lumbosacral tap; or general anesthetic (injectable or inhalation) for atlantooccipital tap.

Atlantooccipital Space Collection

The *atlantooccipital space* can be safely accessed only with the patient under general anesthesia. Although the procedure carries the risks of general anesthesia, it is a brief procedure, and injectable anesthesia can be used. CSF is technically easy to obtain at this location. If the patient is ataxic, as many neurologic patients are, the risk of self-injury during

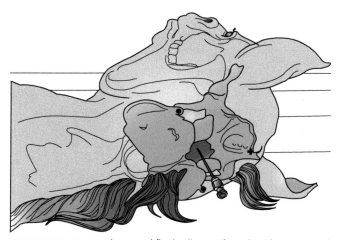

FIGURE 9-10 Cerebrospinal fluid collection from the atlantooccipital space.

the anesthetic recovery period is increased and may be unacceptable. The atlantooccipital space is located just caudal to the poll, on the dorsal midline, at the level of the wings of the atlas (Figs. 9-10 and 9-11). This procedure must be performed with the horse under general anesthesia; therefore, proper preparation for anesthesia is required. The patient is placed in lateral recumbency. A rope is usually placed around the nose and is pulled caudally to ventroflex the head and neck; this opens up the atlantooccipital space and facilitates needle placement. The patient is clipped and sterilely prepared for the procedure. The needle is advanced by the clinician, paying careful attention to anatomical landmarks, until the bevel is confirmed to be in the subarachnoid space. With atlantooccipital taps, fluid usually flows freely from the needle and can be collected from the needle hub. Fluid may flow freely from the lumbosacral space but usually needs to be collected by gentle aspiration with a sterile syringe because it cannot be easily collected by gravity flow with the needle in its vertical position. Fluid is usually collected into both EDTA and serum tubes; more than 1 mL should be placed in the EDTA tube.

> **TECHNICIAN NOTE**
> - CSF collection from the atlantooccipital space requires general anesthetic risk.
> - The atlantooccipital space is located just caudal to the poll, on the dorsal midline, at the level of the wings of the atlas.

Lumbosacral Space Collection

The *lumbosacral space* is usually accessed in the awake, standing patient; this avoids the risk of recovery from general anesthesia. However, the lumbosacral space is technically more difficult to enter, and patients may display violent reactions to pain from the procedure. The lumbosacral space is located on the dorsal midline, at the level of the wings of the ilium (Fig. 9-12). The procedure is performed in the standing patient, usually with sedation. Care must be taken not to oversedate the horse, which may cause excessive body swaying.

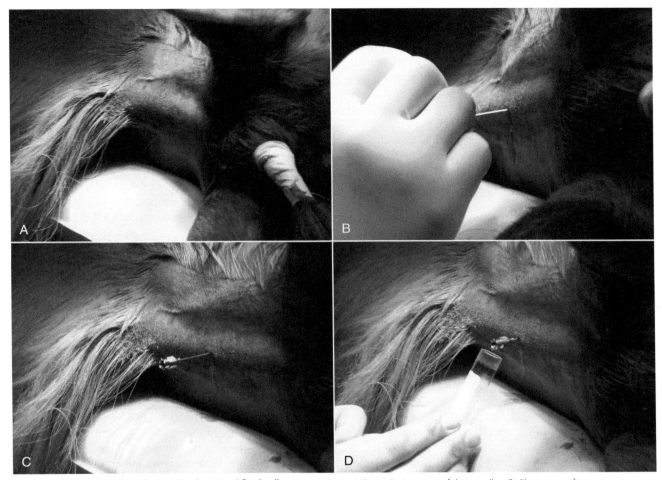

FIGURE 9-11 Cerebrospinal fluid collection. **A,** Prepared site. **B,** Insertion of the needle. **C,** Placement of the needle. **D,** Collection of the fluid. Note the drop at the hub of the needle. (Courtesy Nebraska Equine.)

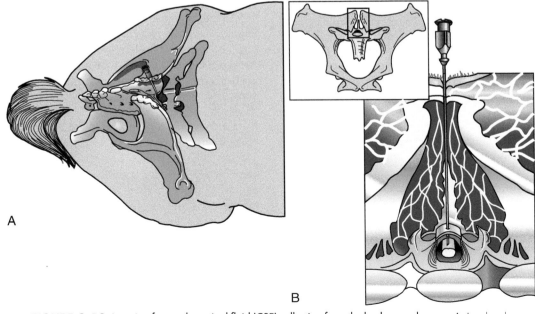

FIGURE 9-12 Location for cerebrospinal fluid (CSF) collection from the lumbosacral space. **A,** Landmarks for CSF collection from the lumbosacral space. **B,** Collection of CSF from the lumbosacral space. (From Speirs VC: *Clinical examination of horses,* St. Louis, 1997, Saunders.)

Because the patient must stand still during the procedure, stocks are highly desirable to restrict movement. The horse must also stand squarely with weight distributed evenly on all legs because leaning makes the procedure difficult to perform. The patient is clipped and sterilely prepared for the procedure, and local anesthesia of the skin, SC tissues, and deeper tissues is performed. A final preparation is performed after the local anesthetic is injected. The procedure is then performed as if you were collecting fluid from the atlantooccipital space.

After the procedure, blood is cleaned from the site, and antibiotic ointment is placed over the area. Minimal local swelling is expected. Infection and abscessation at the site are uncommon.

> **TECHNICIAN NOTE**   After collection of CSF, minimal local swelling is expected. Infection and abcessation at the site are uncommon.

Evaluation of Cerebrospinal Fluid

CSF fluid should be analyzed as soon as possible because of rapid deterioration of cells.

Common procedures include the following evaluations and measurements:
- Gross visual examination: Normal CSF is clear, colorless, and odorless. It has the consistency of water.
- Total protein level.
- RBC and WBC counts: A hemocytometer is often required for accurate counts.
- Microscopic evaluation
  - Cytology: This uses direct smear, which is air dried and stained.
  - Gram stain is performed if bacteria are suspected or confirmed.
- Microbial culture and sensitivity: These tests are performed if an infectious cause is suspected or confirmed.
- Serology: Antibody titers for some neurologic diseases are commonly performed on CSF.
- Ancillary procedures: Glucose, pH, electrolyte, and enzyme levels are occasionally measured.

THORACOCENTESIS (CHEST TAP)

Equipment for thoracocentesis:
- Ultrasound is not required but is extremely helpful
- Aspiration machine if necessary
- Clippers
- Surgical scrub and alcohol
- Sedation
- Sterile gloves
  EDTA
  Serum (plain) tubes/red top tube
  Large-gauge syringe needle at least 3 inches long
  Catheter (14 or 16 ga) × 3 inches long
  Trocar or cannula at least 3 inches long
  Anesthetic, a 6-mL syringe, and a 20- or 22 ga ×
  Inch needle
  Scalpel blade

- Sterile 35- or 60-mL Luer-tip syringe
- Three-way stopcock
- Antibiotic ointment

Thoracocentesis is performed to obtain a sample of pleural fluid for analysis. Collection of pleural fluid can be useful for any disease that produces pleural effusion, including diseases of the pleural cavity (pleuritis, pleuropneumonia), diseases of the lungs (pneumonia, pleuropneumonia), some cardiac diseases, and some neoplastic diseases.

Pleural fluid is produced by the cells of the pleura, which line the pleural cavities and surface of the lungs. This fluid surrounds the lungs and is entirely different from samples of fluid and cells collected from the airways of the lungs (transtracheal wash or aspirate, bronchoalveolar lavage [BAL]). The pleural cavities normally are closed body cavities, whereas the respiratory airways openly communicate with the outside world.

Normally, there is little accumulation of pleural fluid in the pleural cavities, and access to the fluid is often difficult in normal horses. However, diseases of the pleural cavity and external surfaces of the lungs may change the character and quantity of the pleural fluid, by increasing volume and thereby making access easier.

In most horses, the right and left pleural cavities communicate through a small "hole" in the caudal mediastinum. Disease of a pleural cavity may "plug" this communication with fibrin and other exudates. Therefore, pleural effusion or abnormal pleural fluid in only one pleural cavity is possible, whereas the other cavity may be essentially normal.

Diagnostic ultrasound examination is extremely valuable in detecting pleural fluid. Ultrasound can identify accumulation of pleural fluid and guide the clinician in selecting the specific location for performing thoracocentesis. The procedure is sometimes performed on both right and left pleural cavities.

Before beginning the procedure, collect the following materials: sterile gloves; EDTA and serum (plain) tubes; a needle (clinician's preference for large-gauge syringe needle at least 3 inches long); an IV catheter (14 or 16-ga) at least 3 inches long; a sharp trocar or cannula (at least 3 inches long); local anesthetic, a 6-mL syringe, and a 20- or 22-ga × 1- or 1½-inch needle; a no. 15 scalpel blade; a sterile 35- or 60-mL Luer-tip syringe; and a three-way stopcock.

The patient is restrained in a standing position. The sample is taken from the right or left lateral thoracic wall, through an intercostal space. The specific location is usually determined following ultrasound examination, usually toward the ventral aspect of the lateral thoracic wall (Fig. 9-13).

The procedure is usually performed with the horse under sedation, although physical restraint alone may be sufficient for some horses. The patient must stand still for the procedure. The patient is clipped and sterilely prepared. The preparation is performed after the intercostal site is determined by ultrasound or physical examination. Local anesthesia of the skin, SC tissue, and deeper tissues is performed, and a final scrub of the area is performed after the local anesthetic is deposited.

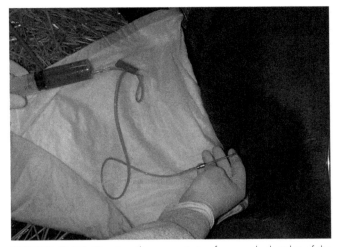

FIGURE 9-13 One-time thoracocentesis of one or both sides of the thoracic cavity can be achieved using a teat cannula. This has the advantage of requiring a smaller incision and is particularly useful in neonates. Here the teat cannula has been attached to the syringe via an extension set to prevent air entering the thoracic cavity. Ideally, a three-way stop cock should also be in place. (From McAuliffe SB, Slovis NM: *Color atlas of diseases and disorders of the foal*, St. Louis, 2008, Saunders.)

The needle is advanced through the intercostal space into the pleural cavity. Care is taken to avoid iatrogenic pneumothorax, which occurs if the needle allows free passage of air from the atmosphere into an open space in the pleural cavity. For this reason, it is common to control the entrance of the needle hub with a three-way stopcock or other valve.

> *TECHNICIAN NOTE* Care must be taken to prevent iatrogenic pneumothorax. This is usually accomplished using a three-way stopcock or other valve.

Once the needle bevel enters an area of fluid accumulation, the fluid often flows freely from the needle and can be collected directly into the sample tubes. Sometimes the pleural fluid contains fibrin or other exudates that can occlude the bevel and limit fluid flow through the needle. Gentle aspiration with a sterile syringe may facilitate sample collection. Samples are collected into both EDTA and serum (plain) tubes.

After the diagnostic samples are collected, the needle is in often left in place, and as much pleural fluid as possible is drained from the pleural cavity. Sometimes drainage must be assisted by manual or machine aspiration.

After the procedure, bleeding is controlled with manual pressure over the puncture site. The area should be cleaned, and topical antibiotic ointment should be applied. The patient should be observed for signs of pneumothorax, which include elevated respiratory rate, dyspnea, cyanosis, and possibly collapse.

> *TECHNICIAN NOTE* Signs of *pneumothorax* include elevated respiratory rate, dyspnea, cyanosis, and possibly collapse.

Evaluation of Pleural Fluid

Common procedures include the following evaluations and measurements:

- Gross visual examination: Normal pleural fluid is transparent, clear to light yellow in color, and odorless. It has the consistency of water.
- Total protein level.
- RBC and WBC counts.
- Microscopic evaluation
  - Cytology: This uses direct smear, which is air dried and stained.
  - Gram stain is performed if bacteria are suspected or confirmed.
- Microbial culture and sensitivity: These tests are performed if infectious cause is suspected or confirmed.

Ancillary procedures: Other chemistry studies are occasionally performed.

TRANSTRACHEAL ASPIRATION (TRANSTRACHEAL WASH)

Transtracheal aspiration is used to obtain a representative sample of material from the lower respiratory tract airways by "washing" the material from the tracheal lumen. It is assumed that the material in the trachea accurately reflects the condition of the lower airways—bronchi, bronchioles, and alveoli. The procedure is useful for diagnosis of lower respiratory tract disease.

> *TECHNICIAN NOTE* Transtracheal aspiration is useful for diagnosis of lower respiratory tract disease.

The respiratory airways are internal epithelial surfaces that communicate with the environment through the nose and mouth. Because this is not a closed body cavity, microorganisms are normally present on the airway surfaces and are commonly recovered in the diagnostic samples. This may make diagnosis of infectious disease and interpretation of culture results difficult. Two methods can be used to obtain samples: endoscopic and percutaneous.

Endoscopic approach

Equipment needed for endoscopic transtracheal aspiration:

- Sedative, a needle, and a syringe
- Fiberoptic endoscope
- Sterile, long narrow-gauge polyethylene tubing
- 100 to 200 mL of sterile saline
- Two to three sterile 60-mL syringes
- EDTA tubes
- Serum (plain) tubes/red top tubes

For endoscopic collection, a fiberoptic endoscope is placed through the nasal cavity to enter the tracheal lumen. Special tubing is placed through the biopsy channel of the endoscope to perform the wash. The advantages of this method are that it is noninvasive and it allows visual examination of the upper airways and trachea. The disadvantages are patient resistance to the presence of the endoscope and

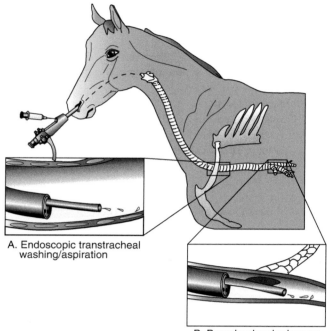

A. Endoscopic transtracheal washing/aspiration

B. Bronchoalveolar lavage

FIGURE 9-14 Endoscopic technique for transtracheal wash and bronchoalveolar lavage.

the questionable accuracy of microbial samples recovered with this technique. Because the endoscope must travel through the nasal cavity, pharynx, and larynx before it enters the trachea, the tip of the endoscope may acquire contaminants.

The following equipment should be prepared before using the endoscopic method: fiberoptic endoscope; long, narrow-gauge polyethylene tubing (sterile); sterile saline (100 to 200 mL); two to three sterile 60-mL syringes; and EDTA and serum (plain) tubes.

Most horses resist placement of the endoscope, so restraint of the head is essential and is usually accomplished with a nose twitch. The patient is restrained in a standing position as the endoscope enters through a nostril (Fig. 9-14). The endoscope is passed through the nasal cavity into the trachea. The tubing is passed through the biopsy channel of the endoscope until it enters the trachea. Sterile saline in a 60-mL syringe is rapidly injected through the tubing, and the syringe is used to aspirate as much fluid as possible back into the tubing and syringe. Recovery of only a few milliliters of the injected saline is common. Up to 300 mL of saline can safely be used to perform the wash; any saline that reaches the alveoli will be absorbed by the body. The majority of saline will not be recovered into the syringes. No special aftercare is necessary.

> **TECHNICIAN NOTE**   As much as 300 mL of saline can be safely used to perform a transtracheal wash. Any saline that reaches the alveoli will be absorbed by the body.

Percutaneous approach

Equipment needed for percutaneous transtracheal aspiration:

- Sedative, a needle, and a syringe
- Clippers
- Surgical scrub and alcohol
- Sterile gloves
- Local anesthetic and a 25-ga needle
- No. 15 scalpel blade
- 14-ga teat cannula or IV catheter or syringe needle
- Sterile polyethylene or red rubber catheter
- 100 to 200 mL of sterile saline
- Two to three sterile 60-mL syringes
- Sterile 4 × 4 gauze squares
- Elastic adhesive tape
- EDTA tubes
- Serum (plain) tubes/red top tubes
- Antibiotic ointment

In percutaneous collection, the sample is taken directly from the trachea through the skin. This method is perceived to be a sterile procedure that yields more accurate microbial samples than the endoscopic method. The disadvantage is that it is an invasive procedure with possible complications; however, complications are uncommon.

> **TECHNICIAN NOTE**   Percutaneous collection is perceived to be a sterile procedure that yields more accurate microbial samples; however, it is an invasive procedure.

The following equipment should be prepared for percutaneous collection: sterile gloves; local anesthetic, a 3-mL syringe, and a 25-ga needle; a no. 15 scalpel blade; a 14-ga teat cannula or IV catheter or syringe needle; sterile polyethylene or red rubber catheter (small enough to pass through the needle, at least 12 inches long); sterile saline (100 to 200 mL); two to three sterile 60-mL syringes; sterile 4 × 4 gauze squares; elastic adhesive tape; and EDTA and serum (plain) tubes.

The horse should be restrained in a standing position because the collection takes place on the ventral midline of the neck, over the middle third of the cervical trachea. The tracheal rings are easily palpated on ventral midline; the needle is placed between tracheal rings (Figs. 9-15 to 9-20). The skin over the ventral trachea is clipped and sterilely prepared. Local anesthetic is deposited by the SC route, and a final preparation is performed.

The patient should be discouraged from elevating its head during the actual wash procedure; holding the head and neck level with the ground is ideal.

> **TECHNICIAN NOTE**   The head and neck should be held level with the ground during percutaneous transtracheal aspiration.

Note that chemical sedation may be necessary for some patients. However, certain sedatives may interfere with the cough reflex, which is desired during this procedure to help bring up material from the lower airways.

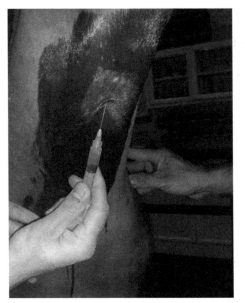

FIGURE 9-15 An area measuring 3 cm × 3 cm over the proximal third of the trachea is clipped and surgically prepared. Approximately 1 mL of lidocaine is infused subcutaneously. (From McAuliffe SB, Slovis NM: *Color atlas of diseases and disorders of the foal*, St. Louis, 2008, Saunders.)

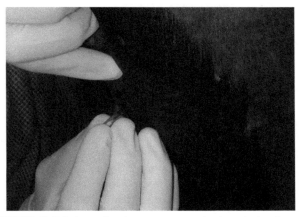

FIGURE 9-16 A small stab incision is made through the skin and subcutaneous tissue using a no. 15 scalpel blade. (From McAuliffe SB, Slovis NM: *Color atlas of diseases and disorders of the foal*, St. Louis, 2008, Saunders.)

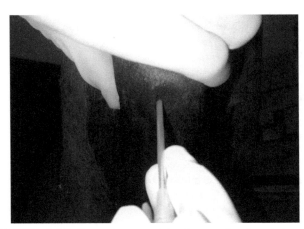

FIGURE 9-17 The trachea is stabilized in one hand, and the cannula is punctured through the trachea between two cartilage rings. (From McAuliffe SB, Slovis NM: *Color atlas of diseases and disorders of the foal*, St. Louis, 2008, Saunders.)

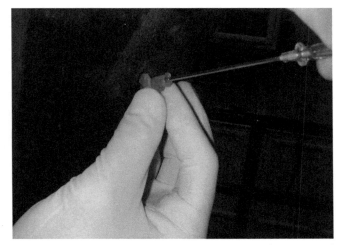

FIGURE 9-18 The stylet is removed, and the urinary catheter is passed down into the tracheal lumen to the level of the thoracic inlet. (From McAuliffe SB, Slovis NM: *Color atlas of diseases and disorders of the foal*, St. Louis, 2008, Saunders.)

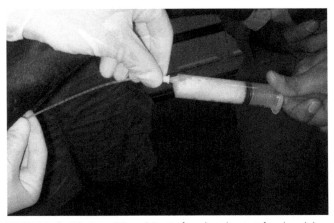

FIGURE 9-19 From 30 to 35 mL of sterile saline is infused and then aspirated. No changes in relative cell counts occur in samples stored for 24 hours at 4° C in a capped syringe. If delays longer than 24 hours are expected, contact your local laboratory to identify a proper fixative solution before sending the sample for analysis. (From McAuliffe SB, Slovis NM: *Color atlas of diseases and disorders of the foal*, St. Louis, 2008, Saunders.)

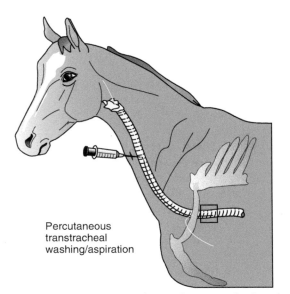

Percutaneous transtracheal washing/aspiration

FIGURE 9-20 Percutaneous technique for transtracheal wash and bronchoalveolar lavage.

TECHNICIAN NOTE   The cough reflex is desirable
during the percutaneous transtracheal aspiration procedure.

Personnel should not stand directly in front of the horse,
to avoid being struck with the forelimbs. A stab incision is
made through the skin only. The needle of choice is passed
through the incision and enters the trachea between tracheal
rings. Once the needle is confirmed to be in the trachea,
the sterile tubing is placed through the needle to enter the
trachea. The wash procedure is identical to that in the endoscopic
technique. Once fluid has been collected into the
syringes, it is injected into the EDTA and serum tubes and
other diagnostic media as desired.

After the procedure, bleeding is controlled with manual
pressure. The incision site should be cleaned and covered
with antibiotic ointment. A light pressure wrap is applied,
and sterile 4×4 gauze squares are placed over the site
and are secured by encircling the neck several times with
4-inch–diameter elastic adhesive tape, with care taken not
to occlude blood flow or breathing. The wrap is removed in
24 hours.

TECHNICIAN NOTE   A light pressure wrap is
applied to the collection site after the procedure. The wrap
should stay in place for 24 hours.

Complications may include infection or abscessation of
the puncture site and SC emphysema. *Subcutaneous emphysema*
is common but seldom causes any clinical problem; the
air is eventually reabsorbed. Covering the incision with a
pressure wrap reduces the amount of air accumulation.

TECHNICIAN NOTE   Complications of the percutaneous
transtracheal aspiration procedure include subcutaneous
emphysema and infection or abcessation of the
puncture site.

Evaluation of Transtracheal Fluid

Common procedures include the following evaluations and
measurements:
- Gross visual examination: Normal samples are odorless
  and slightly cloudy because of the presence of mucus,
  cells, microorganisms, and debris.
- Microscopic evaluation
  - Cytology: Direct smear, air dried, stained. Mucus is
    normally seen. Bacteria also are normally seen and
    may represent normal bacterial flora. In herbivores,
    plant material, pollen, and fungal hyphae may be seen
    and are not necessarily associated with disease; however,
    their presence should be noted.
- Gram stain is performed if bacterial disease is suspected
  or confirmed.
- Microbial culture and sensitivity: These tests are performed
  if an infectious cause is suspected or confirmed.

BRONCHOALVEOLAR LAVAGE

Equipment needed for BAL:
- Endoscope
- Sterile tubing
- BAL catheter
- Local anesthetic
- 100 to 200 mL of sterile saline
- Two to three sterile 60-mL syringes
- EDTA tubes
- Serum (plain) tubes/red top tubes

BAL is another method for collecting lower airway fluid
samples and is similar to the transtracheal wash procedures.
Usually, an endoscope is passed as far as possible into the
trachea or bronchi, and sterile tubing is passed through the
endoscope as far as possible into the lower airways, presumably
coming to rest in a bronchus or bronchiole (see Fig.
9-14). It is possible to pass tubing directly from the nares
through the trachea without using an endoscope. The lavage
is performed similarly to transtracheal aspiration, by injecting
large aliquots of sterile saline and attempting to recover
as much of the fluid as possible by aspirating with a syringe
after each saline injection. Catheters for BAL procedures are
commercially available. Local anesthetic is often infused into
the bronchi to decrease the cough reflex; coughing does not
enhance this procedure and is not desirable.

TECHNICIAN NOTE   Coughing is not desirable
and does not enhance the bronchoalveolar lavage
procedure.

BAL samples are believed to reflect the condition of the
lower airways more accurately than transtracheal samples because
they are obtained farther down the respiratory tract. The
potential disadvantage is that the region of lung sampled with
BAL may or may not be abnormal; there is no way to ensure
that the tubing lodges in a diseased area of the lung. Evaluation
of the fluid is similar to that for transtracheal wash samples.

MEDICATION TECHNIQUES

ORAL MEDICATION

Many medications are delivered by the oral route. These
medications may be supplied in powder, tablet, or liquid
form. Different strategies are available to deliver each of
these drug forms.

Feed Additives

Feed additives and equipment:
- Mortar and pestle or baggie and hammer
- Applesauce, molasses, sweet feed

Oral medications may be given as *feed additives,* added to
the horse's dry feed, usually grain. The advantages of this approach
are primarily convenience; powders and liquids can
be added to the feed directly. There is no need to catch and
restrain the horse with this method.

Placing whole tablets into the feed is seldom successful; therefore, crushing the tablets into a powder is preferred. Tablets can be crushed by using a mortar and pestle or by the time-honored method of placing the tablets in a plastic bag and hitting them with a hammer against a hard surface. Large volumes of tablets can be ground with a standard food blender. Many large hospitals grind high volumes of tablets and store them in plastic containers for use over several days.

> **TECHNICIAN NOTE**
> * Large pills can be crushed by placing the pills in a plastic bag and hitting them with a hammer. Pills also can be ground using a standard food blender.
> * Adding crushed pills to molasses, applesauce, pudding, or peanut butter and then pouring the pills onto feed can help ensure equine consumption. These methods are not foolproof.

The disadvantages of this method are many. Medications often have an objectionable taste, causing horses to reject their food. Taste can be disguised with substances such as molasses, syrup, applesauce, pudding, and peanut butter, but some horses still reject the medicated feed. Attempts to hide the medicine in an apple or carrot also have mixed results. Another pitfall of powdered feed additives is their tendency to "fall through" or "sift" through the grain to the bottom of the feed tub as the horse eats. This results in underdosing because much of the dose settles to the bottom of the feed tub and is not consumed. Using sweet feed (which has molasses) or other sticky substances can improve delivery of the powder by preventing it from sifting through the feed. Another problem is that many horses spill grain from their mouths when they eat, and this causes medication to land on the ground. Delivering medications by adding them to the feed can be a highly unreliable method of dosing horses and other large animals.

Dose Syringes
Equipment needed for dose syringe delivery:
* Dose syringe
* Medication

Dose syringes can be used to deliver medications directly into the mouth. To use this method, the medication must be in a liquid or paste form. Powders can be mixed with a liquid medium such as molasses or applesauce to form a paste but must not be made into thick pastes, which are difficult to push through the opening of the syringe. Contrarily, the liquid medium should not be too watery, which may result in spillage from the mouth. A thick syrup consistency is ideal.

> **TECHNICIAN NOTE** When pastes are made to be given orally, they should not be too thick or too thin.

Dose syringes bought commercially usually are capable of delivering up to 500 mL of liquid. This large volume is seldom necessary to deliver most common medications. A 60-mL catheter-tip syringe is useful for smaller volumes. The opening of Luer-tip syringes is too small to make delivery of medication into the mouth feasible. This situation can be corrected by carefully cutting the Luer tip off any syringe and enlarging the opening to dime size or slightly smaller. The 20-, 35-, and 60-mL Luer-tip syringes that have been modified in this way are ideal for delivery of most oral medications.

When using any type of dose syringe, the fingers should be used to open the horse's lips before introducing the syringe (Fig. 9-21, A). Jamming the syringe into the mouth without warning may alarm and possibly injure the horse. The syringe should be introduced near the commissure of the lips. The lips should be slightly parted with the fingers or thumb, and the tip of the syringe should be carefully introduced toward the interdental space (Fig. 9-21, B). Once in the mouth, the syringe should be directed caudally between the cheek and the cheek teeth (Fig. 9-21, C). Avoid introducing the syringe over the incisors because the horse can bite and break the syringe (Fig. 9-22, A). Also avoid aiming the syringe over the base of the tongue, which increases the horse's ability to spit out the medication and also increases the possibility of squirting the liquid into the trachea (Fig. 9-22, B). Most horses try to spit medication out of the mouth. This reaction can be discouraged by elevating the chin after dispensing the medication and waiting for the horse to swallow. "Jiggling" the throat while the chin is elevated is an old trick to encourage swallowing. Regardless of the method used, the technician should always observe the horse after delivering oral medication to be sure the dose is consumed and not spat out on the ground.

> **TECHNICIAN NOTE** Always observe the horse following administration of oral medication to ensure that the horse does not spit out the medication.

The *balling gun* is an instrument designed to administer large tablets to large animals. It is a poor choice for medicating horses. The balling gun must be placed deep into the mouth, over the base of the tongue, and horses typically resist it by throwing their heads. Unfortunately, this may lead to lacerations and puncture wounds of the larynx and pharynx.

> **TECHNICIAN NOTE** A balling gun is a poor choice for oral medication of horses.

Nasogastric Intubation
Equipment for nasogastric intubation:
* Lubrication
* Nasogastric tube
* Syringe pump
* Tape
* Cap
* Umbilical tape or string

Nasogastric intubation is a variation of oral dosing. It involves placing a long, plastic "hose" from the nostril to the pharynx, where it enters the esophagus and is advanced into the stomach. The advantages of nasogastric intubation include reliable delivery of the entire dose to the patient and the ability to use the nasogastric tube as a diagnostic tool in addition to a medication tool. Disadvantages include trauma to the horse's turbinates, larynx, and pharynx, which can result in nosebleeds, abscesses, and inflammation and swelling. The turbinates are fragile, and nosebleeds occasionally occur, even with the most skilled technician. Nosebleeds are especially likely if the horse throws its head during the procedure.

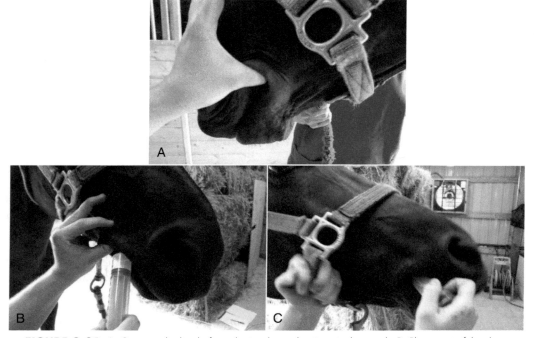

FIGURE 9-21 **A,** Opening the lips before placing the oral syringe in the mouth. **B,** Placement of the dose syringe near the commissure of the lips. **C,** Proper positioning of the oral syringe.

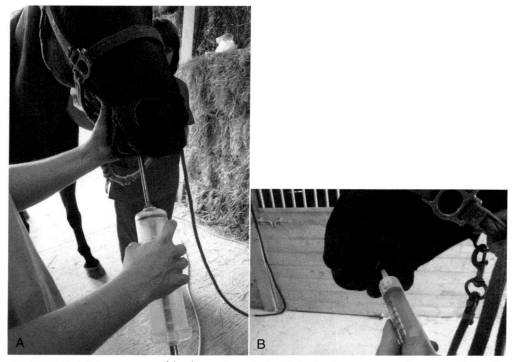

FIGURE 9-22 Improper use of the dose syringe. **A,** Avoid placing the syringe over the incisors. **B,** Avoid delivering medication across the interdental space.

If a nosebleed (epistaxis) occurs, the volume of the resulting hemorrhage may be impressive to the layperson, but remember that the quantity is usually small in terms of the total blood volume of a horse. Elevating the horse's head and possibly applying cold water or cold compresses over the nose may help. Unless the horse has a bleeding disorder, the hemorrhage is rarely life-threatening and stops on its own. Horses with nosebleeds typically snort frequently, spraying blood droplets in every direction. Be prepared for this response.

> **TECHNICIAN NOTE** Epistaxis commonly occurs during nasogastric intubation. Elevating the head and possibly applying cold water or cold compresses over the nose may help.

Another disadvantage of nasogastric intubation is the possibility of "tubing the lungs," which occurs when the tube enters the trachea rather than the esophagus. Placing the tube in the trachea usually elicits coughing but is not a problem if the tube is withdrawn promptly. Problems occur when the tube is left in the trachea and liquids are delivered through the tube. The liquids run down the trachea and bronchi into the lungs, resulting in life-threatening pneumonia. Every precaution must be taken to prevent delivering medications into the trachea.

Another difficulty with nasogastric intubation is that horses resent this procedure. Restraint is necessary with almost all horses, unless they are moribund. Physical restraint may be insufficient, and chemical restraint often is necessary. Because the tube is being placed through a nostril, personnel involved in the procedure should stand to the side of the head and forequarters, out of reach of a possible strike with the front hooves.

Once a nasogastric tube is placed into the stomach, it should not be allowed to slide in and out, which could lead to accidental entry into the trachea. The person handling the head of the horse is often responsible for stabilizing the tube's position. The tube should be held firmly, and resting the hand against the horse's muzzle or halter helps keep the tube in the desired position if the horse moves its head.

Delivery of medication through the tube can be accomplished in several ways. A funnel can be placed into the opening of the tube, held above the level of the stomach, and the fluid poured into the funnel. This method is slow and somewhat cumbersome. Alternatively, a dose syringe containing the medication can be attached to the tube opening and the plunger pushed to deliver the medication. The most common method is to place the medication or liquids to be delivered into a bucket or plastic jug and use a stomach pump to deliver the contents (Fig. 9-23). Whatever the method of delivery, liquids should never be forced against back pressure. The capacity of an average (1000-pound) horse's stomach is 4 to 5 gallons, and approaching or exceeding this volume is risky. Typically, 1 gallon of fluid is the maximum given at one dosing, although this may be repeated at 30-minute or 1-hour intervals in urgent situations.

Most commercial nasogastric tubes are made of clear plastic materials. Nasogastric tubes come in several diameters, from foal size through large horse size (Fig. 9-24, A). Nasogastric tubes can be purchased with two options of openings at the stomach end of the tube (Fig. 9-24, B). A single opening at the stomach end is available; however, this type of tube tends to plug with debris (undigested material) once it enters the stomach. Tubes are also available with side ports, which are small holes in the sidewall of the tube, near the end of the tube, in addition to the large main opening at the end of the tube. The addition of side ports makes blockage less likely. Side ports can be added to

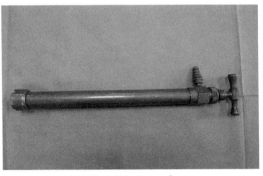

FIGURE 9-23 Stomach pump.

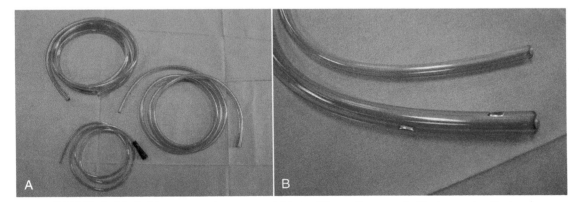

FIGURE 9-24 A, Nasogastric tubes are available in different diameters. **B,** Single opening *(top)* and multiple side ports *(bottom)*.

tubes using a piece of heated metal (e.g., a nail) to melt several penetrating holes into the tube. All nasogastric tubes should have smooth edges on the main end hole and all side ports; sharp edges tend to grab and tear nasal tissue, with resulting nosebleed.

Nasogastric tubes are never placed without lubrication on the outside of the tube. Water is the most common lubricant, but petroleum jellies such as obstetrical lubricants (OB lubes) also can be used. The lubricants need not be sterile. Mineral oil is a readily available alternative. However, it is irritating to the mucous membranes of the nose and droplets may be inhaled into the lungs, so its use for this purpose is discouraged.

> **TECHNICIAN NOTE**   Nasogastric tubes should never be placed without lubrication on the outside of the tube.

An idiosyncrasy of the tubes is their sensitivity to temperature; they stiffen in cold temperatures. Excessively stiff tubes tend to cause nosebleeds. Soaking tubes in warm water before use softens them.

One advantage of using a nasogastric tube is that it can be left in place for 24 to 48 hours, thus allowing staff to medicate the horse or monitor stomach contents without having to replace a tube every few hours. If the tube is to be left in place, it should be secured to the halter (Fig. 9-25). Adhesive tape is usually used to secure the tube to the halter, although clinicians have preferences regarding how and where to secure the tube. Regardless of the method, the tube should not be secured with large loops through which a horse could place a hoof. This is important because horses with indwelling tubes are often being treated for abdominal pain (colic), which is often accompanied by lowering the head and pawing with the front feet. If the feet are put through the tube loops, the tube can be ripped from its position in the stomach. It is helpful to mark the position of an indwelling tube with a simple ring of adhesive tape at the level of the nostril so that the staff can easily see whether the horse has dislodged the tube from its original position (Fig. 9-26).

> **TECHNICIAN NOTE**
> • A nasogastric tube can be left in place for 24 to 48 hours.
> • Mark the position of an indwelling tube with a simple ring of adhesive tape at the level of the nostril so that the staff can easily see whether the horse has dislodged the tube from its original position.

Some clinicians believe that the nasogastric tube provides a possible route for air to enter the stomach and lead to bloat. These clinicians usually cap the external opening of the tube with a syringe plunger or syringe case to prevent aspiration of air. Other clinicians do not believe that aspiration of air is a problem and leave the tube open. This is based on the clinician's preference because data have not shown that either approach is problematic.

> **TECHNICIAN NOTE**   Some clinicians believe that the external opening of the tube should be capped to prevent bloat.

Removal of the nasogastric tube requires some skill to avoid causing nosebleeds. Removal should not become a "taffy pull," where the operator grabs the tube in one place and pulls it completely out of the nose. Most horses have the tendency to throw their head upward, especially when the last 12 to 24 inches of the tube is removed, effectively turning

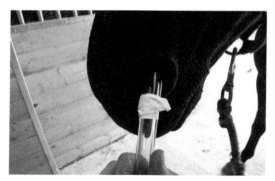

FIGURE 9-26 Proper position of the tube is marked with adhesive tape at the level of the nostril.

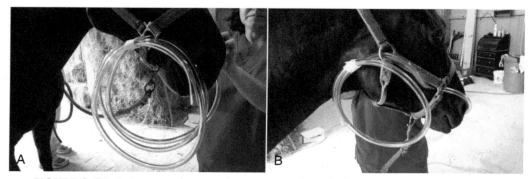

FIGURE 9-25 **A,** One way of securing the nasogastric tube to the halter. **B,** Another way of securing.

the tube into an "intranasal whip" and causing a nosebleed. The operator should keep the hands close to the nostril, retrieve a 12-inch section with one hand, then regrasp with the other hand and withdraw another 12 inches, and so on. In this manner, the handler removes the tube in short segments and maintains control of the tube at all times.

> **TECHNICIAN NOTE** Nasogastric tubes should be pulled out hand over hand, by grasping the tube at 12-inch intervals to prevent a whiplike action as the tube is removed.

When a tube is removed, liquid material often is located inside the tube. If this material is not controlled, it can dribble out of the tube as it is withdrawn and be inhaled into the lungs as the tube is withdrawn. Covering the external opening of the tube during its removal is important because it prevents liquids from flowing out of the tube. Either cover the external opening with a thumb or finger or crimp the tube by folding it over double during removal.

> **TECHNICIAN NOTE** The nasogastric tube should be capped or crimped to prevent the tube's contents from being aspirated into the lungs while the tube is being removed.

ENEMAS

Equipment needed for enema:
- Enema tube
- Enema solution
- Syringe pump

This once popular route is rarely used today for medication of large animals. It is still used for its ability to stimulate bowel movements in some cases of GI disease, although its usefulness is debated. Enemas are commonly given to newborn foals to encourage passage of meconium (fetal feces). Human pediatric enema solutions can be used for equine neonates and require no special equipment.

Older animals require delivery of larger volumes of fluid. Fluids should be warm and nonirritating. Delivery is accomplished through a tube or hose that has been adapted for this purpose. Enema tubes can be made from any flexible rubber or plastic tubing with smooth siding. Side ports should be removed to prevent accidental catching of the rectal mucosa in the ports. A single opening at the end of the tube should be made and the edges smoothed and rounded. Old nasogastric tubes are commonly used for enema tubing.

> **TECHNICIAN NOTE** Enema fluids should be warm and nonirritating.

Insertion begins with restraint of the patient. This procedure is not painful but does produce some discomfort. The operator should stand to the side of the horse during the entire procedure. The tip of the hose is lubricated and is gently inserted several inches into the rectum. The hose should not be inserted more than 12 inches and should never be forced if resistance is encountered. Once the hose is inserted, the desired enema solution is administered by gravity flow (safest) or the use of a large-dose syringe or pump. Fluids should never be forced against resistance because of the risk of rupturing the rectum. Generally, 1 to 3 gallons of liquid can be given to an average (1000-pound) adult horse. When fluids begin to flow out of the anus or resistance is encountered, the administration is stopped.

> **TECHNICIAN NOTE** The tip of the enema tube should be lubricated, and it should never be forced if resistance is encountered during placement.

The horse's urge to void the rectum usually is rapid, and the enema fluids are expelled in projectile fashion. The operator is encouraged to stand well to the side of the horse's rear end and be prepared for rapid voiding of most of the enema volume.

PARENTERAL INJECTION TECHNIQUES

Equipment needed for parenteral injections:
- Alcohol
- 4 × 4 gauze
- Syringe
- Needle
- Injection material

Syringes and needles can be used to deliver injections by many routes. The route selected depends on many factors, including the U.S. Food and Drug Administration–approved routes of injection (listed on the label of all medications), tractability of the patient, capability of the person performing the injection, toxicities of the medication, and temperament of the patient. The most common routes of injection are intramuscular (IM), IV, SC (also called SQ), and intradermal (ID).

Before any parenteral injection, the skin should be cleaned appropriately. Some procedures, such as IV catheterization and joint injections, require sterile preparation of the skin. However, for most routine injections, cleaning of the skin and hair with isopropyl alcohol is sufficient. The alcohol can be placed on a cotton swab or gauze 4 × 4 square and then used to wipe the intended injection site vigorously. Wipe repeatedly until the cotton or gauze is essentially clean. A common mistake is to wipe only over the hair; the alcohol should thoroughly soak the skin. Even if the skin over the site appears to be clean, alcohol should be used, even though it does not thoroughly disinfect the skin. Scrubbing with alcohol removes some debris and makes a positive impression on the client.

> **TECHNICIAN NOTE** Preparation for joint injections and intravenous catheterization requires sterile skin preparation. Other injection methods can be performed after a thorough scrubbing of alcohol.

If the horse is being medicated with injectable drugs, multiple injections are often required over several days. This tends to make the horse sore, especially if large volumes of drug are given at each injection. It is helpful to have a rotation plan for the injections, where the location of the shot is rotated to prevent overuse of a single site. For instance, the jugular veins can be alternated at each injection for IV injections. For IM injections, the left side of the neck can be used first, then the left hindquarter, then the right side of the neck, then the right hindquarter, and so forth.

> **TECHNICIAN NOTE**   It is important to rotate injection sites if medication is to be administered in large volumes or for several days.

Intramuscular Injections

Strictly speaking, any skeletal muscle that can be accessed safely can be used for an IM injection. However, several muscles that are more readily accessible than others include the brachiocephalicus, pectoral, gluteal, semitendinosus, and triceps brachii.

Muscles do not have unlimited capacity for injection. It is recommended that the maximum volume of injection be limited to 15 mL in any single location. In smaller muscle bellies, such as the pectoral and semitendinosus, 5 to 10 mL is the maximum volume. In large draft horses, these volumes can be increased by an additional 5 mL. Some common medications, such as procaine penicillin G, require volumes of approximately 30 mL at each treatment in an average horse; this dose must be split into two sites of 15 mL each. Two separate injection sites can be used, or the needle can be placed for administration of half the dose, then the bevel partially withdrawn to the level of the subcutaneous tissue, redirected at a 45-degree angle to the first injection angle, and reinserted along this new line. The second half of the dose can then be administered.

> **TECHNICIAN NOTE**   Injection volume for intramuscular use in most muscles is 15 mL. In smaller muscles the volume is 5 to 10 mL, and in draft horses the volume can be increased by 5 mL.

Some drugs are toxic or injurious if they are accidentally injected by the IV route. Therefore, all IM injections should be "screened" before the drug is delivered to ensure that the bevel of the needle is not in the lumen of a blood vessel. This is accomplished by stabilizing and aspirating the syringe—pulling gently backward on the plunger—before injecting. If blood is seen in the needle hub or syringe, the needle should be withdrawn and discarded, and a new needle should be inserted and aspirated again before injecting.

> **TECHNICIAN NOTE**   If blood is visualized on aspiration of the syringe, the needle should be withdrawn and discarded, and a new needle should be inserted and aspirated again before injecting.

Selecting a diameter and length of syringe needle depends on the size of the muscle to be injected, the volume to be delivered, and the consistency of the medication. Thicker medications require larger diameters. In general, most IM injections are done with a range of 18- to 22-ga needles; the length is usually 1 to 1½ inches. Foals and ponies require the shorter length; smaller muscles such as the pectoral also need the 1-inch length. Thin horses with little muscle mass are also candidates for shorter needles.

> **TECHNICIAN NOTE**   Most intramuscular injections are done with a range of 18- to 22-ga needles, and the length is usually 1 to 1½ inches. Foals, smaller muscles, and thin horses require shorter needles (e.g., 1 inch).

Following IM injections, bleeding from the injection site is common. This blood is usually from skin vessels that were punctured during insertion of the needle and does not imply that the needle bevel was in a blood vessel at the time of injection. The bleeding can be controlled with hand pressure over the site. Bleeding leaves red stains on the hair coat, which is unsightly in light-colored horses. Cleaning this blood from the horse, by using peroxide or alcohol, rather than leaving a large blood stain gives a better impression to the client.

Injection abscesses are a potential complication of IM injections. They are more likely to occur when injections are given through dirty skin and seem to occur more often after administration of biologic products, such as vaccines, than other products. As with any abscess, part of the treatment is providing drainage. Drainage occurs best when it is ventral, allowing gravity to assist the process constantly. Of the commonly used injection sites, the pectoral and semitendinosus muscles provide the best access for ventral drainage. Conversely, the brachiocephalicus and gluteal muscles provide poor drainage access.

Several methods have been described for giving IM injections to horses, and each has its advantages and disadvantages. To my knowledge it has never been proven that one method is superior to another. Some clinicians believe that the needle should be inserted into the muscle first and the syringe attached next. The benefit of using this type of method is that if the horse jumps, the weight of the syringe is not hanging on the needle, thus causing the needle to bounce up and down in the skin and leading to tissue trauma. However, the argument is that the hub of the needle is exposed to the environment again, even though it is a brief time. Some people like to pinch the skin before inserting the needle. The skin over the neck is somewhat loose, and some prefer a technique where the skin is first pinched with one hand before the injection (Fig. 9-27, *A*). While this skin pinch is maintained, the needle is inserted approximately 1 to 2 inches directly caudal to the skin pinch (Fig. 9-27, *B*). Pinching the skin accomplishes two things: (1) it distracts from the pain of the needle; and (2) when the skin is released, it slides caudally to cover the IM needle track, providing a physiologic "bandage." Other people prefer to use the back of the hand to tap on the horse's neck lightly as if they were patting them. Then without hesitation they turn their hand over in rhythm with their patting and insert the needle. The advantage is that the horse does not even know it is coming, and many horses do not even notice it. It also decreases the chance that a horse will become trained to it because most horses are patted on the neck by owners as a reward. Once the needle is removed, the horse is patted again as a reward, which allows another form of reward, as well as a check for bleeding. Each clinician and technician will have a favorite method. However,

it is nice to ask clients whether they have a preference to the method used.

Intramuscular Injection Sites

Lateral cervical. The most common site for IM injection is the lateral aspect of the neck, in the brachiocephalicus or serratus ventralis muscle. This area is easy to access, and personnel can stand to the side of the forequarters, where a strike or kick is less likely. The landmarks for safe injection are (1) a hand's width ventral to the crest of the neck (Fig. 9-28, *A*), (2) a hand's width dorsal to the jugular groove (Fig. 9-28, *B*), and (3) a hand's width cranial to the cranial border of the scapula (Fig. 9-28, *C*). These landmarks outline a large triangle (Fig. 9-28, *D*), and the injection can be safely administered anywhere in this area. After the skin is cleansed, the needle is inserted at an angle perpendicular to the skin and is inserted to its full depth. The needle should be stabilized

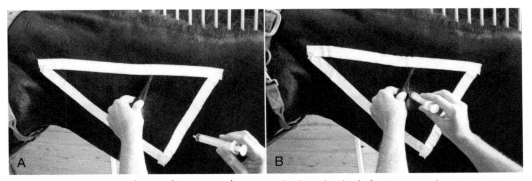

FIGURE 9-27 Lateral cervical injection technique. **A,** Pinching the skin before intramuscular injection into the neck. **B,** Inserting the needle caudal to the skin pinch.

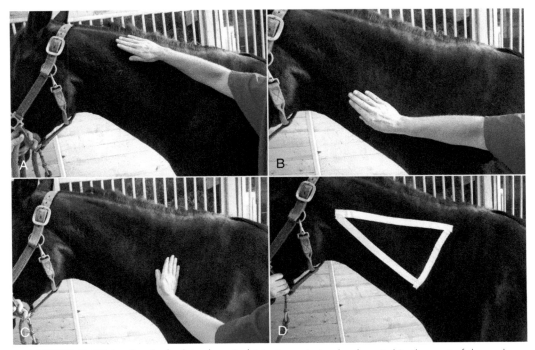

FIGURE 9-28 Landmarks for lateral cervical injections. **A,** Landmark ventral to the crest of the neck. **B,** Landmark dorsal to the jugular groove. **C,** Landmark cranial to the scapula. **D,** Borders for intramuscular injections into the lateral cervical area.

while its position is checked by gentle aspiration, and then the medication is delivered.

The lateral cervical area is contraindicated for IM injection in nursing foals. Soreness usually follows IM injection, and foals with sore necks tend to avoid nursing. Other sites such as the semitendinosus are better choices in nursing foals.

Pectoral Muscle. The pectoral muscles are suitable for smaller volumes of injection, less than 5 mL in most cases, although larger horses can receive up to 10 mL per injection. In general, a 1-inch needle is used. This muscle is somewhat movable in the standing horse, and one hand should be used to stabilize the muscle belly while the other hand inserts the needle at a 90-degree angle to the skin (Fig. 9-29). Be sure to stand to the side of the forequarters, out of range of a potential forelimb strike.

The pectoral muscles have good ventral drainage compared with other IM sites, which is an advantage if an injection abscess develops.

Triceps Muscle. The triceps muscle is generally used when all other common sites have been exhausted. It is not suitable for large injection volumes and should be avoided in any performance animal unless absolutely necessary out of fear of causing soreness or scarring the triceps, which is the main muscle that propels the forelimb. Soreness and scarring could produce lameness and poor performance.

Gluteal Muscles. The gluteal muscle actually consists of several muscle bellies in the rump area. The skin overlying this area is thick and fairly tight, and more force is required to penetrate it with a needle than in other locations. For this reason, small-diameter needles should be used cautiously; 18- to 20-ga syringe needles are recommended for most medications.

The landmarks for safe injection are (1) a hand's width lateral to the spine (dorsal midline) (Fig. 9-30, *A*), (2) a hand's width caudal to the tuber coxae (Fig. 9-30, *B*), and (3) a hand's width dorsal to the greater trochanter of the

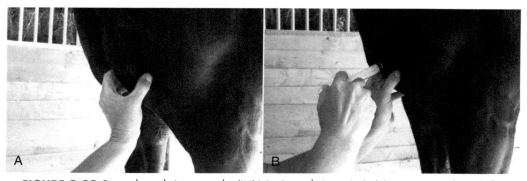

FIGURE 9-29 Pectoral muscle intramuscular (IM) injection technique. **A,** Stabilizing a pectoral muscle for IM injection. **B,** Inserting the needle at a 90-degree angle to the skin.

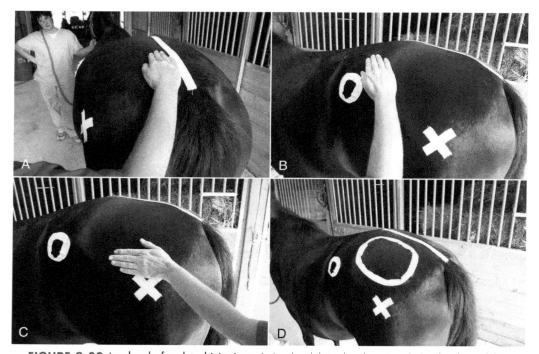

FIGURE 9-30 Landmarks for gluteal injections. **A,** Landmark lateral to the spine. **B,** Landmark caudal to the tuber coxae (point of the hip). **C,** Landmark dorsal to the greater trochanter of the femur. **D,** Boundaries for safe intramuscular injection into the gluteal muscle.

femur (Fig. 9-30, *C*). These landmarks define a circular area, and injections can be safely given within these boundaries (Fig. 9-30, *D*).

The technician should stand beside the flank or area of the point of the hip and face caudally during the injection. In general, the farther cranially the technician stands, the more likely he or she will avoid a kick from a hindleg.

Horses do not like to be surprised with needles. If the needle is thrust into the animal with no warning, a kick is a common response. This area does not have a lot of loose skin, so using the tapping method is useful. Use the base of the hand to thump the skin firmly three or four times just before inserting the needle. This action serves as notice that something is about to happen (alternatively, if the horse's attitude makes thumping unwise, at least try to rub the area firmly). The area is thumped, and then the needle is immediately inserted perpendicular to the skin, to its full depth. It is recommended not to leave the syringe attached to the needle during insertion because horses may kick or "dance around" after the needle is inserted. If a horse moves around and the technician cannot hold on to the syringe, the weight of the syringe essentially will turn the needle into an IM blade, lacerating muscle fibers and blood vessels as the syringe wobbles above the skin (Fig. 9-31, *A* and *B*).

> **TECHNICIAN NOTE**   It is recommended not to leave the syringe attached to the needle during insertion. However, I must say that in some situations attaching a syringe after the needle has been inserted is not possible in some young horses or older horses that are needle shy, and having the needle attached, with prompt injection of the fluid, is necessary.

Once the needle is inserted and the horse is still, one hand should stay committed to holding the needle hub for the rest of the procedure (Fig. 9-31, *C*). Attach the syringe, aspirate to check position, and then deliver the medication. The syringe and needle are withdrawn as a unit when the injection is complete.

The gluteal muscles should be avoided in racehorses and other performance horses that "drive off the hind end," to avoid causing possible muscle soreness or scarring.

Semitendinosus Muscle. The semitendinosus muscle is well suited to smaller injection volumes, less than 10 mL. As with injection in the gluteals, the handler must care to prevent being kicked. The proper site for injection is at the most prominent area of the buttocks as viewed from a lateral position (Fig. 9-32, *A*). The needle is inserted in a caudal-to-cranial direction, perpendicular to the skin (Fig. 9-32, *B* and *C*). The needle must avoid the sciatic nerve, which lies in the easily visible groove on the caudolateral aspect of the thigh (Fig. 9-32, *D*). Another reason to avoid the groove is that the substance may not be injected "intra" muscularly if the needle is put into the groove. The needle should be inserted before the syringe is attached, in case the horse moves or kicks. An alternative approach that provides additional safety from kicks is to stand on the opposite side of the horse (i.e., stand beside the left hindquarters and insert the needle into the right semitendinosus muscle) and reach across the buttocks to insert the needle.

Intravenous Injections

Injections can be given into any vein that is visible or palpable and safely accessed. By far, most IV medications are given into the jugular vein.

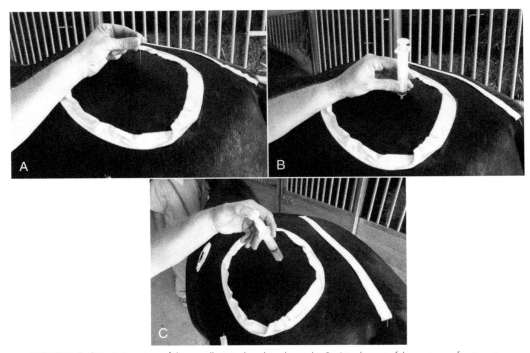

FIGURE 9-31 A, Insertion of the needle into the gluteal muscle. **B,** Attachment of the syringe after insertion of the needle. **C,** Avoid giving the injection without stabilizing the syringe hub.

Needles for IV injections range from 14 to 22 ga in diameter and 1 to 1½ inches in length, depending on the viscosity of medication to be injected and the size of the vein.

The 14-ga needle is used for rapid fluid infusions and administration of euthanasia solutions, which must be injected rapidly. I prefer a 19-ga × 1½-inch length for most equine IV injections and a 20-ga × 1-inch length for foals. It is highly recommended to place the needle first, confirm its position, and then stabilize the needle hub while attaching the syringe and while injecting.

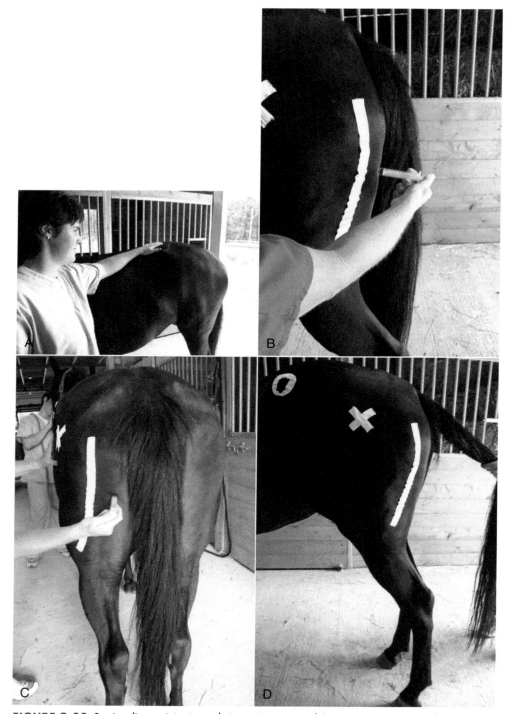

FIGURE 9-32 Semitendinosus injection technique. **A,** Location of the most prominent area of the buttocks. **B,** Insertion of the needle from cranial to caudal into the semitendinosus muscle. **C,** Proper technique for intramuscular semitendinosus injection. **D,** Location of the sciatic groove.

> **TECHNICIAN NOTE** It is highly recommended to place the needle first during an IV injection, confirm entrance into the vein, stabilize the needle hub, and then attach the syringe and inject.

Some controversy exists regarding the direction of IV injections. Some clinicians prefer to inject with the flow of blood in the vein; others inject against the blood flow. Injecting against the direction of blood flow creates turbulence, which some fear may cause clotting of the blood. Although this argument makes some intuitive sense, to my knowledge the superiority of one method over the other has never been proved. Personal preference dictates the technique used.

IV injections should always begin by distending the vein and then visualizing or palpating the vein to identify its course. Best results are obtained when the needle mimics (parallels) the course of the vein. Trying to hit a vein from an angled or skewed approach is more difficult to accomplish. Once the needle is aligned over the distended vein, the needle is tilted to a 45-degree angle to the skin and is advanced through the skin in a single smooth motion and into the vein. Unlike IM injections, the needle should not enter perpendicularly to the skin.

The speed of injection depends on the intent of the drug and possible side effects. Euthanasia solutions and some anesthetics are intentionally given as bolus. Other medications have serious complications if they are given too rapidly by the IV route. Most substances are best delivered by a slow injection technique, which allows them to mix and dilute with the blood.

> **TECHNICIAN NOTE** Consult the veterinarian regarding to the rate of injection when performing an intravenous injection.

Intravenous Injection Sites

Jugular Vein. The jugular vein is used for most IV procedures in large animals. It is readily accessible, and personnel can position themselves away from strikes and kicks from the hooves. It is also the largest-diameter peripheral vein, which makes identification and puncture easier than in other veins.

The jugular vein lies just below the skin in the jugular groove. The anatomy of this area is important; the carotid artery and vagosympathetic nerve trunk lie deep to the jugular vein and parallel to it. It is possible to insert a syringe needle such that it goes completely through or around the jugular, thus penetrating the carotid artery and, rarely, the vagosympathetic trunk.

> **TECHNICIAN NOTE** It is possible to insert a syringe needle such that it goes completely through or around the jugular, thus penetrating the carotid artery and, rarely, the vagosympathetic trunk during a jugular vein injection.

A "carotid stick" Has several possible consequences. Large hematomas can result, and although they seldom are life-threatening, they can take days to weeks to resolve and pose a risk for infection. The blemish they produce can keep a horse from the sale ring, show ring, or race, thus leading to unhappy clients. Blood in the carotid artery travels rapidly to the brain. When the brain receives a bolus of certain drugs injected into the carotid artery, horses may collapse, have seizures, display dementia, and even die of cardiac or respiratory arrest. Horses may recover from these effects but may be left with permanent neurologic defects. Injecting any compound into the carotid artery must be avoided.

> **TECHNICIAN NOTE** Carotid stick can cause large hematomas that can keep horses from the sale ring, show ring, or race, thus leading to unhappy clients, and some medications can lead to death if they are given in the artery.

The risk of accidental carotid injection can be minimized in several ways. Whenever possible, the cranial half of the jugular groove should be used for vein access (Fig. 9-33). In the cranial half of the jugular groove, the omohyoideus muscle is interposed between the jugular vein and the carotid artery, thereby affording some protection to the artery (Fig. 9-34). However, this muscle is not thick enough to prevent a carotid stick, and other precautions should still be taken.

It is recommended to insert the needle first, without the syringe, so that the needle's position can be confirmed. When the needle is placed in the jugular vein and the vein is distended by manual pressure, blood should flow freely from the hub of the needle. However, this blood is not under high pressure as it exits the hub, and, because it is venous blood, it does not display a pulse effect. In contrast, carotid arterial blood is under high pressure and may squirt up to several feet out of the needle hub; in addition, the blood often displays a pulsing effect. The color of the blood exiting the hub has been used as a criterion for needle location, with dark blood assumed to be jugular venous blood and bright red blood assumed to be arterial. However, this method is highly unreliable and is not recommended.

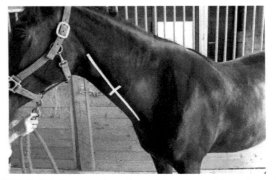

FIGURE 9-33 Demarcation of cranial and caudal portions of the jugular groove.

Once the needle has been inserted and its position in the jugular vein has been confirmed, one hand should be committed to stabilizing the needle hub while the syringe is attached and the medication delivered. Maintaining the position of the needle prevents accidental advancement into the carotid artery, as well as accidental injection into the perivascular tissues. Some medications are highly irritating when they are injected outside the vein and can lead to large areas of inflammation, skin slough, and permanent scarring. The technician should be certain that the needle bevel rests inside the lumen of the jugular vein to avoid these complications.

> **TECHNICIAN NOTE**   Some medications if injected outside of the vein can cause inflammation, skin sloughing, and permanent scarring.

After the injection, the needle is removed, and finger pressure is applied to the venipuncture site to prevent bleeding. Sedated horses or horses that hold the head lower than the heart can experience blood loss into the SC tissues around the venipuncture site that leads to hematomas. Elevating the head and applying manual pressure can prevent hematoma formation. Similar precautions should be taken with accidental puncture of the carotid artery; elevate the head and apply firm pressure to the area for at least 5 minutes.

> **TECHNICIAN NOTE**   After administering an injection into the jugular vein, the technician should apply manual pressure and elevate the animal's head to prevent hematoma formation. If the carotid artery is entered, pressure should be applied to the site for at least 5 minutes.

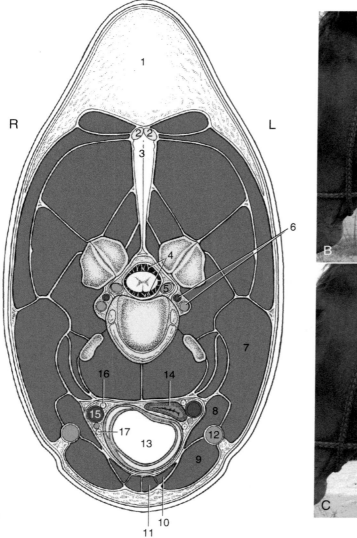

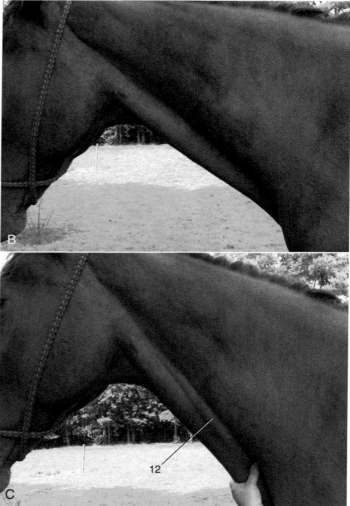

FIGURE 9-34 A, Cross-section of the cranial portion of the neck. **B,** The external jugular vein is not visible, but it is raised (**C**) when occluded in the jugular groove. *1,* Crest; *2, 3,* funicular and laminar parts of nuchal ligament; *4,* subarachnoid space; *5,* internal vertebral venous plexus; *6,* vertebral artery and vein; *7,* brachiocephalicus; *8,* omohyoideus; *9,* sternocephalicus; *10,* sternothyroideus; *11,* sternohyoideus; *12,* external jugular vein; *13,* trachea; *14,* esophagus; *15,* common carotid artery; *16,* vagosympathetic trunk; *17,* recurrent laryngeal nerve. (From Dyce KM, Sack WO, Wensing CJG: *Textbook of veterinary anatomy,* ed 4, St. Louis, 2010, Saunders.)

Lateral Thoracic Vein, Cephalic Vein, Saphenous Vein, and Coccygeal Vein. These veins can be accessed when the jugular vein is not an alternative for IV injection. They are considerably smaller than the jugular vein, and injections of large volumes are slower and technically more difficult. For most purposes, a 1-inch syringe needle is adequate.

The lateral thoracic vein runs along the ventrolateral aspect of the thorax (Fig. 9-35). Clipping the hair can facilitate visualizing this vein if the hair coat is long. Blood in the vein flows cranially toward the brachial vein.

The cephalic vein (forelimb) and saphenous vein (hindlimb) are leg veins that are difficult to access in standing horses (Fig. 9-36). They are more useful for sedated patients or horses or foals in lateral recumbency that are under anesthesia or sedation. The handler should take precautions to prevent being kicked while accessing these veins. Motion of the legs can easily dislodge the needle during injection.

The coccygeal vein lies on the ventral midline of the tail, adjacent to the coccygeal artery. It is best accessed near the base of the tail (Fig. 9-37). Use of this vein should be restricted to only small volumes of nonirritating substances. Any swelling or perivascular scarring in this area may occlude the coccygeal artery, which is the main (and only) arterial supply to the tail. The entire tail may slough if occlusion occurs. This site should be avoided if possible.

Subcutaneous Injections

SC injections are easiest to perform in fleshy areas where the skin is loose and elastic, which allows the technician to lift the skin and slide the needle between the tented skin and the underlying muscle tissue. The most common place for SC injections in large animals is under the skin of the lateral aspect of the neck.

The skin is tented (Fig. 9-38, *A*), and the needle is advanced into the "tent" at an angle nearly paralleling the surface of the neck (Fig. 9-38, *B*). Once the needle bevel is completely in the SC space, the skin is released and the injection made. Releasing the skin allows the technician to

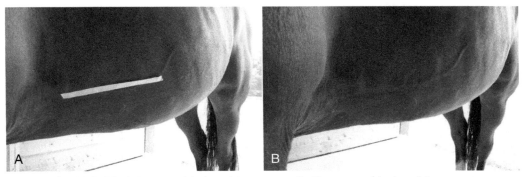

FIGURE 9-35 **A,** Location of the lateral thoracic vein. **B,** Closer view of the lateral thoracic vein.

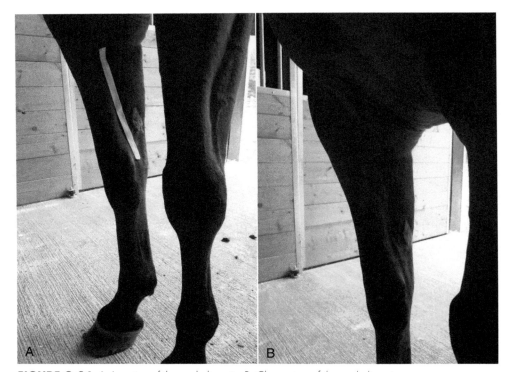

FIGURE 9-36 **A,** Location of the cephalic vein. **B,** Closer view of the cephalic vein.

observe the "skin bleb," which usually confirms correct delivery of the injection. When the needle is properly placed, the animal has little resistance to injection.

SC injections are not suitable for large volumes of fluid in large animals; therefore, the SC route is not used for fluid therapy as it is in small animals. Syringe needles from 20- to 25-ga × 1-inch length are used.

Intradermal Injections

ID injection is rarely used to administer medications. It is used mainly for diagnostic testing in large animals for tuberculosis (cattle) and skin testing for allergies.

Only volumes less than 1 mL can be injected into the skin at a single site. A 25-ga needle is the largest size used for ID injections. After the skin is cleansed, the needle is laid nearly parallel to the skin, with the bevel up, and is advanced into the skin. This is a shallow injection, and care must be taken

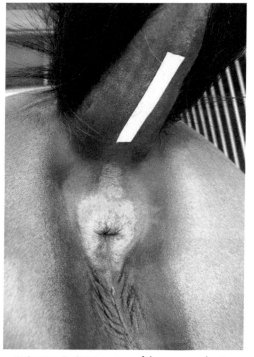

FIGURE 9-37 Location of the coccygeal vein.

not to enter the SC tissue. The syringe plunger is gently withdrawn to ensure that the bevel is not within a blood vessel; if no blood is aspirated, the injection is completed. A visible bleb should appear in the skin (Fig. 9-39).

Adverse Reactions

Adverse reactions may occur following administration of any medication. Some reactions are allergic (hypersensitivity or immune mediated), and the manifestations may be local or generalized (anaphylaxis). *Anaphylactic shock* may be life-threatening, leading to respiratory distress, collapse, and death. Most local allergic reactions (skin wheals, hives, or facial edema) are not life-threatening, but they can be uncomfortable for the horse *(pruritus)*. If facial edema is severe, breathing may be compromised. A veterinarian should be consulted when any allergic reaction is suspected.

> **TECHNICIAN NOTE**   A veterinarian should be consulted when any allergic reaction is suspected.

Adverse vaccine reactions are uncommon. They may produce anaphylactic reactions, but these are rare. Most vaccine reactions are mild and localized, consisting of muscle soreness at the injection site (especially stiff neck), swelling at the injection site, mildly elevated temperature (<101.5° F), and 24 to 48 hours of depression and loss of appetite. Abscesses may develop. Cold compresses at the injection site and administration of a nonsteroidal antiinflammatory drug such as phenylbutazone may be helpful in the acute phase of a local reaction. If a firm swelling develops over the next several days, an abscess may be organizing; hot packs may be warranted. If body temperature is greater than 101.5° F at any time or if depression and loss of appetite continue for more than 48 hours, the veterinarian should be consulted.

> **TECHNICIAN NOTE**   Clients should be informed that if the body temperature is greater than 101.5° F at any time or if depression and loss of appetite continue for more than 48 hours following injections, the veterinarian should be consulted.

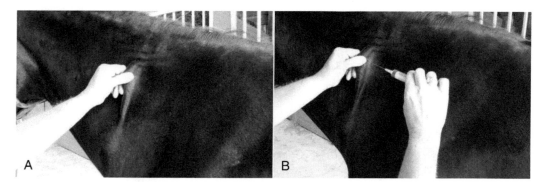

FIGURE 9-38 **A,** Elevating the skin for subcutaneous injection. **B,** Injection technique for subcutaneous injection.

Reactions may be related to the rate of administration, which is usually a problem with IV medications. Bolus administration of some drugs, especially those with potassium or calcium, may have adverse effects on the cardiovascular system.

Reactions may occur with inadvertent IV injection of drugs that are not intended for IV use or accidental injection into the carotid artery of drugs that are intended for other routes. Possible effects include dementia, collapse, and death.

> **TECHNICIAN NOTE**   Possible side effects from accidental injection into the carotid artery include dementia, collapse, and death.

Chemical damage to tissue may occur with improper injection techniques. This is most common with perivascular injection of drugs intended for IV use. Phenylbutazone and barbiturates are the most common examples of this complication. If these drugs are injected outside a vein, severe tissue inflammation and necrosis may occur.

> **TECHNICIAN NOTE**   If phenylbutazone or barbiturates are injected outside a vein, severe tissue inflammation and necrosis may occur.

> **TECHNICIAN NOTE**   Procaine penicillin G should be given only by intramuscular injection.

Procaine penicillin G, a commonly used antibiotic in horses, is approved only for IM injection. Two types of adverse reactions are associated with use of this drug. True penicillin allergy occurs rarely and usually manifests as skin wheals or hives. Horses with true penicillin allergy should not receive penicillin drugs after the allergic reaction is observed. More common than allergy, however, is poor injection technique, which results in accidental injection into the bloodstream. When the drug then reaches the brain, dementia, hyperesthesia, and collapse may occur. This type of reaction is related to the procaine portion of the drug and is not an allergic reaction. Most horses recover from a procaine reaction. These animals may safely receive doses of the drug in the future, provided the doses are not again injected directly into the bloodstream. These two types of reactions are often confused by clients, who report that their horse had an allergic reaction to penicillin, when in fact the horse most likely had a reaction to a bloodstream injection. Careful questioning of the client usually distinguishes the type of reaction the horse actually experienced.

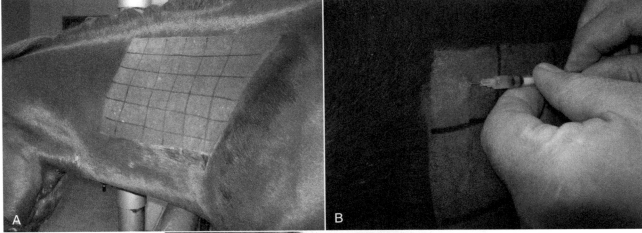

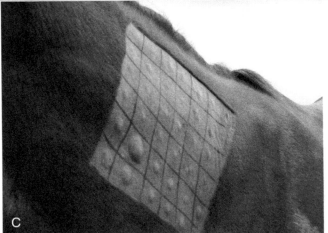

FIGURE 9-39 A, Preparation for allergy testing. B, Intradermal injection. C, Results of allergy testing plot. (Courtesy Nebraska Equine.)

Adverse systemic reactions warrant immediate treatment. If the medication is still being administered, it should be stopped immediately, and the patient should be evaluated. Treatment may range from simply keeping the animal warm, to treatment with corticosteroids, epinephrine, or IV fluids, to emergency establishment of a patent airway with nasotracheal intubation or even tracheostomy. The clinician should be alerted whenever an adverse reaction is suspected. An emergency "crash kit" containing emergency drugs and tracheostomy equipment is essential in any practice (Box 9-1), and it should be readily available.

INTRAVENOUS CATHETERIZATION

IV catheterization has become a readily available, commonplace procedure in equine medicine. Catheters may be placed for short-term use, as for induction and maintenance of anesthesia, emergency fluid administration, and euthanasia. Long-term use is also possible for patients requiring long-term fluid therapy or IV medication. If properly placed and maintained, catheters are safe to use and save the pain and discomfort of multiple IV perforations.

Catheter Selection

Catheters are available in different lengths, diameters, and materials. Selection of catheters should not be a "one-size-fits-all" proposition but should be adapted to the patient and the patient's needs. To minimize the risk of *thrombophlebitis,* the shortest-length, smallest-diameter, least-reactive catheter that will accomplish the treatment goals should be chosen.

The length of the catheter must be carefully considered. Catheters are either long (5 to 6 inches) or short (2 to 3 inches). Short catheters, which are stiff, can be used successfully in foals and small ponies but must be used carefully in larger patients. If a horse has turned its head to the side, the catheter tip may perforate the vein when the horse returns the head to a forward-facing position. Short catheters are not suitable for long-term use. However, the risk for thrombophlebitis increases with increasing catheter length.

> **TECHNICIAN NOTE**   Catheters are either long (5 to 6 inches) or short (2 to 3 inches).

Catheter diameter is another factor that must be considered. The primary factor in choosing diameter is the "need for speed" (i.e., how rapidly the medication or fluid must be delivered). The most commonly used diameters are 10, 14, and 16 ga. The 10-ga catheters are recommended for emergency administration of large fluid volumes. The 16-ga catheters are useful for repeated IV medication, with or without small IV fluid volumes. For most general purposes, a 14-ga catheter is the most commonly used, especially when administration of large volumes of maintenance fluids is necessary. Because the risk of thrombophlebitis rises as catheter diameter increases, the smallest diameter that can accomplish the treatment goals should be chosen.

BOX 9-1   Equine Emergency Crash Kit

Drugs*
Atropine 1% injection
Calcium gluconate 23%
Diazepam 5 mg/mL injection
Dopamine 200 mg/20 mL injection
Doxapram 20 mg/mL injection
Epinephrine 1:1000 injection
Glycopyrrolate injection
Lidocaine 2% injection
Prednisolone sodium succinate injection
Sodium chloride 0.9%
Xylazine 100 mg/mL injection

Syringes and Needles†
60 mL (1)
20 ga × 1 inch (5)
30 mL (2)
20 ga × 1½ inches (10)
20 mL (3)
18 ga × 1½ inches (10)
12 mL (5)
18 ga × 3½ inches (2)
6 mL (5)
18 ga × 6 inches (2)
3 mL (5)
14 ga × 3 inches (2)

Catheters†
10 to 12 ga × 5½ inches (5)
16 ga × 5½ inches (3)
Extension set (2)
Administration set (2)

Airway Supplies†
Endotracheal tube 14 mm (1)
Endotracheal tube 9 mm (1)
Oral speculum/bite block (1)
Air syringe 60 mL (1)
KY (sterile lubricating) jelly (1)
Tracheostomy tube, self-retaining
Disposable scalpel handle (1)
Disposable no. 10 blade (3)
Forceps, Kelly (2)

Miscellaneous
Adhesive tape, 1-inch diameter
Heparin flush
Surgical skin stapler

---

*Be sure an emergency drug dose/dilution chart is readily available.
†Number in parentheses indicates quantity of that item.

> **TECHNICIAN NOTE**   The primary factor in choosing the diameter of a catheter is the "need for speed."

Catheters are constructed from different materials. These materials vary in tissue reactivity (i.e., the tendency to cause inflammation or initiate the clotting cascade). The materials also affect mechanical properties, such as the tendency to kink and ease of insertion. In addition, tissue reactivity affects the tendency to cause thrombophlebitis, and this tendency is related primarily to the softness of the material. Stiff materials are associated with a higher risk of thrombophlebitis. Some of the more commonly available catheter materials are polypropylene, Teflon, polyurethane, and silicone. Polypropylene is the stiffest and most reactive of the materials. Polypropylene catheters are usually large in diameter, which makes them desirable for emergency IV fluid administration. However, because of their reactivity, they should not be used for more than 24 hours and should be replaced if IV therapy is still necessary after that time. Teflon and polyurethane have moderate stiffness/reactivity and can be used safely for 7 days on average if properly maintained. These IV catheters are the most popular currently in use. Silicone is the most pliable and least reactive material. With sterile placement and careful maintenance, silicone catheters have been safely left in place for 4 weeks. However, silicone catheters are available only in smaller diameters, and this restricts their use for fluid therapy to small volumes only. The low reactivity makes silicone a popular choice for neonates.

> **TECHNICIAN NOTE**
> - Polypropylene catheters have the largest diameter, but they should not be used for more than 24 hours because of their reactivity.
> - Silicone catheters can be safely left in place for 4 weeks.
> - Teflon and polyurethane can safely stay in place for 7 days.

Catheter Sites

Almost all IV catheters in large animals are placed in the jugular vein. Although the esophagus usually lies on the left side of the trachea, penetration of the esophagus by the catheter is unlikely, and either jugular vein can be used safely. If the jugular veins are not usable, the next choice is usually the lateral thoracic vein (Fig. 9-40). The median, cephalic, and saphenous veins of the legs are available but are difficult to enter because of the tendency of these veins to collapse once the catheter is introduced, thus making advancing the catheter to its proper depth difficult. In addition, even if the catheter is successfully placed, motion of the legs makes it difficult to prevent kinking and dislodgement. Leg veins are easier to access when the patient is lateral recumbency than when standing.

Intravenous Catheter Placement Technique

Equipment needed for intravenous catheter placement:
- Clippers
- Surgical scrub and alcohol
- Local anesthetic, syringe, and needle
- Catheter

- Cap, a three-way stopcock, and an extension set
- Heparin flush
- 2-0 nonabsorbable suture
- Suture needle or 20-ga syringe needle
- Adhesive tape or Superglue
- Iodine ointment
- Cotton ball
- Antimicrobial ointment
- 4 × 4 gauze
- Elastic adhesive tape

In general, the location for perforation of the vein should be as far "upstream" (with regard to the direction of blood flow) as possible. If the first attempt at insertion is unsuccessful, further attempts can be made "downstream." This minimizes irritation to endothelium that is trying to heal from unsuccessful punctures.

> **TECHNICIAN NOTE** When a catheter is placed, perforation of the vein should be as far "upstream" (with regard to the direction of blood flow) as possible to allow room for a second attempt if the first is unsuccessful.

Aseptic technique should be followed. The hair is clipped, and a surgical scrub should be performed. Occasionally, owners request that the hair not be clipped. In that case, catheters can be inserted safely if aseptic technique is followed, but owners should be warned of an increased risk of infection.

After clipping, the skin should be surgically prepared with an appropriate scrub solution, followed by isopropyl alcohol wipes. A minimum of three scrub and alcohol applications should be performed. Examination gloves should be worn when preparing the skin.

> **TECHNICIAN NOTE** Occasionally, owners request the hair not be clipped for intravenous catheter placement. It is important to convey to them the increased risk of infection associated with not clipping.

Local anesthesia of the skin over the vein is hardly ever necessary. However, it should always be performed in foals and in individuals that are needle shy. If local anesthesia is used, no more than 1 mL of anesthetic should be given. Placing large blebs of anesthetic makes visualization and palpation of the vein difficult and is no more effective than the smaller volume. Local anesthetic is delivered with a 25-ga needle into the SC tissue.

Cutdowns are sometimes performed in other species to facilitate IV access. This procedure involves local anesthesia of the skin, followed by a small skin incision. The catheter is then introduced directly into the vein. Cutdowns are hardly ever necessary in horses unless the desired site of insertion is obscured for some reason.

Insertion technique is similar to the technique for venipuncture. The insertion angle should mimic the course of

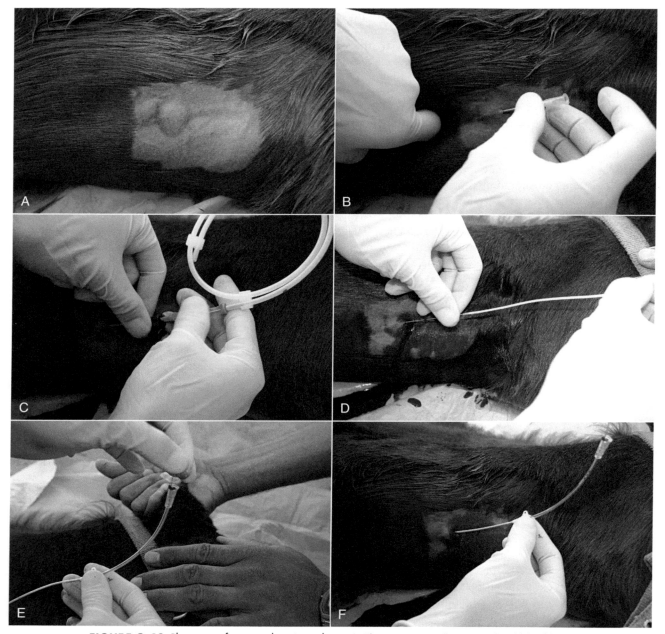

FIGURE 9-40 Placement of an over-the-wire catheter. **A,** The site is surgically prepared. A bleb of local anesthetic is then placed at the site. **B,** A 14-gauge needle is inserted into the vein. **C,** The J-wire is advanced through the needle. **D,** The needle is removed over the wire. **E,** The catheter is advanced over the tip of the wire. The wire is fed up through the catheter until it can be grasped at the plastic hub of the catheter. **F,** The catheter is passed through the skin and advanced down the vein. It is of utmost importance not to let go of the J-wire at any stage. (From McAuliffe SB, Slovis NM: *Color atlas of diseases and disorders of the foal,* St. Louis, 2008, Saunders.)

the vein, and the catheter should enter at a 45-degree angle to the skin (Fig. 9-41, *A* and *B*). Once the tip of the catheter is in the vein, blood should flow freely from the hub. At this point, the catheter stylet should be withdrawn only 1 to 2 inches; this gives the catheter some rigidity as it is advanced fully into the vein (Fig. 9-41, *C*). Full removal of the stylet before the catheter is advanced invites kinking of the catheter. With the stylet slightly withdrawn, the catheter

and stylet are carefully advanced, as a unit, fully into the vein (Fig. 9-41, *D*). Once the catheter hub is touching the skin and blood flows freely from the catheter, the stylet can be withdrawn and discarded.

One of the most common errors in catheter insertion is allowing the vein to collapse during advancement of the catheter. Distention of the vein greatly enhances the chances for success. The technician should develop a

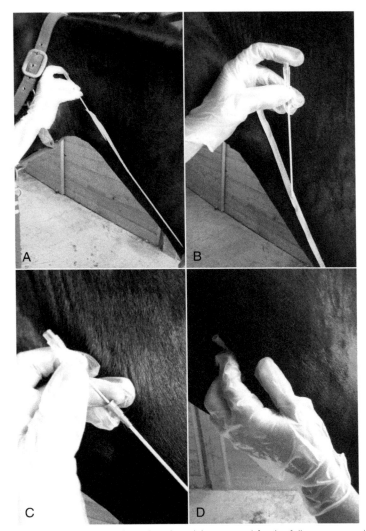

FIGURE 9-41 The skin should be clipped and sterilely prepared for the following procedure. **A,** Proper insertion angle for an intravenous (IV) catheter. **B,** Improper approach for insertion of an IV catheter. **C,** Partial withdrawal of the stylet. **D,** The catheter is advanced until the hub reaches the skin.

technique that allows advancement of the catheter with one hand while the other hand maintains occlusion of the vein.

> **TECHNICIAN NOTE** One of the most common errors in catheter insertion is allowing the vein to collapse during advancement of the catheter. To avoid this problem, remember to maintain good occlusion during placement.

Immediately after insertion and confirmation of proper location in the vein, the catheter should be capped with an injection cap, three-way stopcock (Fig. 9-42), or extension set. The type of cap depends on the medications and/or fluids to be delivered. After the catheter is capped, it should be promptly flushed with heparin flush solution to prevent clotting of the catheter.

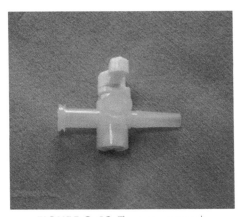

FIGURE 9-42 Three-way stopcock.

The next step is to secure the catheter hub to the skin. Catheter stabilization is extremely important. In humans, catheter motion is the number one factor leading to the development of phlebitis. Several methods are used for securing catheters. The most secure attachment is made by suturing the hub directly to the skin. Nonabsorbable suture material (2-0 diameter) is ideal for this use. A standard suture needle (cutting or reverse cutting) or a 20-ga syringe needle can be used to place the suture through the skin. It is then tied to incorporate the catheter hub and bind it tightly to the skin. Placement of one or two skin sutures usually is sufficient. Another stabilization method is the traditional "butterfly" made from adhesive tape and placed around the hub. The butterfly is secured to the skin with sutures or skin staples. Butterflies tend to allow more motion of the catheter than direct suturing and therefore are not suitable for long-term catheters. Using Superglue to bond the hub directly to the skin is another method. Superglue should not be the only method of stabilization because it is the least reliable method available. However, it is a useful addition to the other methods.

> **TECHNICIAN NOTE**   After the catheter is capped, it should be promptly flushed with heparin flush solution to prevent clotting of the catheter.

Once the catheter is placed and secured, the skin around the insertion site should be lightly coated with an antibacterial or povidone-iodine ointment. Further dressing of the catheter site depends on the patient's circumstances. All long-term catheters and catheters in foals should be covered with sterile 4 × 4 gauze squares and secured with an elastic adhesive tape around the neck, with care taken not to constrict blood flow in the vein (Fig. 9-43). A cotton ball with antibiotic ointment works well. Catheters in recumbent patients should be protected to prevent contamination from the bedding and ground.

Catheter Maintenance

The principles of IV catheter maintenance are similar in all species. Maintaining cleanliness, minimizing motion, flushing regularly to prevent clotting, and observing closely for evidence of problems are essential.

The area around the catheter must be kept clean. If protective dressings are used, they should be changed as needed. Injection caps and three-way stopcocks should be replaced every 24 to 48 hours. Alcohol should be used to clean injection caps, which should be allowed to air dry before any injection is made through the cap. Hands should be clean or covered with gloves whenever the catheter is handled. Whenever the catheter must be manipulated, it should be stabilized to prevent motion, which increases the risk of complications.

> **TECHNICIAN NOTE**   Injection caps and three-way stopcocks should be replaced every 24 to 48 hours when used with an intravenous catheter.

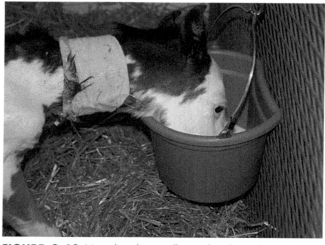

FIGURE 9-43 Note the plastic adhesive bandage placed to help hold the catheter in place. (From McAuliffe SB, Slovis NM: *Color atlas of diseases and disorders of the foal*, St. Louis, 2008, Saunders.)

Heparin flush can be made by diluting heparin in normal saline (10 international units heparin per milliliter of normal saline). Approximately 10 mL of heparin flush is used to clear the catheter thoroughly. The catheter should be flushed after administration of every medication. Medications should never be allowed to mix in the catheter because they may react chemically to form crystals and precipitates that can be harmful to the patient or clog the catheter. Catheters should be flushed a minimum of four times daily, even if they are not being used for medication. Flushing should be easy to perform and meet a minimum of resistance. Resistance usually indicates clotting inside the catheter or kinking of the catheter; in either case, the catheter usually will have to be replaced.

> **TECHNICIAN NOTE**   Medications should never be allowed to mix in the catheter.

Catheters must be closely watched for problems. The catheter itself should be checked for mechanical failure; typically, catheters fail at the junction of the hub and the barrel. Liquid may be seen dripping from this area while it is being injected. If the patient is receiving IV fluids, the skin and hair near the insertion site may be wet from leakage. Mechanical failure is an indication for removal of the catheter.

> **TECHNICIAN NOTE**   Typically, catheters fail at the junction of the hub and the barrel. Catheters should be monitored for leaks or wet spots in the dressings.

The insertion site should be watched closely for thickening, swelling, pain, and purulent exudate. The vein should be gently palpated beyond the length of the catheter for cordlike swelling, which could indicate thrombus formation. These routine "catheter checks" should be performed several times per day, and the clinician should be alerted if problems are detected. Most commonly, skin swelling around the insertion site is caused by local SC infection or inflammation and less commonly indicates true thrombophlebitis. However, distinguishing SC inflammation from IV inflammation can be difficult. The catheter should not be removed without first consulting the clinician.

Thrombophlebitis is inflammation of a vein with concurrent thrombus formation. Thrombus formation may begin on the catheter itself or on damaged areas of the vein walls created by insertion or use of the catheter. Once thrombus formation begins, the thrombus may grow to a size large enough to obstruct blood flow completely. The thrombus may be complicated by bacterial colonization (septic thrombophlebitis). Bacteria may come from the patient's own bloodstream (septicemia) or may travel down the catheter from the catheter hub or insertion site (ascending infection). Poor insertion technique, lack of cleanliness, and excessive motion of the catheter all are associated with increased risk of thrombophlebitis.

If one jugular vein thromboses, the other jugular vein usually can provide adequate drainage of the head. However, if both jugular veins thrombose, severe swelling of the head typically results.

> **TECHNICIAN NOTE** If one jugular vein thromboses, the other jugular vein usually can provide adequate drainage of the head. However, if both jugular veins thrombose, severe swelling of the head typically results.

Other veins drain the head, but they are smaller in diameter and cannot provide sufficient drainage to prevent edema formation. Swelling of the head may be life-threatening if breathing is compromised. Forced elevation of the head by tying it above the level of the heart will discourage further fluid accumulation. Feed should be offered well above ground level.

If thrombophlebitis is confirmed, the catheter must be removed. The tip of the catheter should be cultured for bacteria by cutting off the tip with sterile scissors and placing the tip into a sterile container for submission to the laboratory. Hot packs should be applied to the inflamed area several times per day. Once the skin has dried, topical dimethyl sulfoxide (DMSO) gel or liquid can be applied to help reduce swelling. DMSO should not be applied to broken or wet skin. The insertion site should be kept free of exudates and covered with an antibacterial ointment.

Once a vein is affected with any degree of thrombophlebitis, all use of the vein must stop (Fig. 9-44). All staff should be alerted to the location of the affected vein, and other veins must be used instead.

Thrombosis is not always permanent. The body has mechanisms to break down clots and may partially or completely resolve the thrombi. However, the lining of the vein is usually left with irregularities that can initiate more thrombi, and other veins should be preferentially used if catheterization is ever necessary in the future.

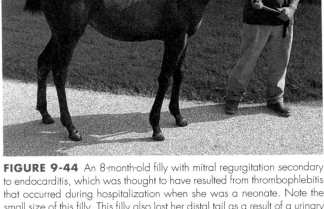

FIGURE 9-44 An 8-month-old filly with mitral regurgitation secondary to endocarditis, which was thought to have resulted from thrombophlebitis that occurred during hospitalization when she was a neonate. Note the small size of this filly. This filly also lost her distal tail as a result of a urinary catheter that was taped too tightly to the tail. (From McAuliffe SB, Slovis NM: *Color atlas of diseases and disorders of the foal*, St. Louis, 2008, Saunders.)

> **TECHNICIAN NOTE** The insertion site of the catheter should be watched closely for thickening, swelling, pain, thrombus formation, and purulent exudate.

Use of IV catheters to obtain blood samples is strongly discouraged. This practice increases the risk of clotting in the catheter, and blood samples may be tainted with drug residues inside the catheter.

> **TECHNICIAN NOTE** The use of intravenous catheters to obtain blood samples is strongly discouraged.

Catheter Removal

After a catheter is removed, care must be taken not to allow hematoma formation at the insertion site. Firm pressure should be applied directly over the insertion site for at least 1 minute. Do not occlude the vein downstream from the insertion site because this can cause blood to back up and exit through the puncture site. Elevating the head after removing a jugular catheter minimizes the risk of hematoma formation.

Once bleeding has stopped, the insertion site should be cleaned, and an antibacterial ointment should be placed directly into and around the location. Bandaging the area is optional in most cases.

SHOE REMOVAL

Horses are shod for several purposes. Preventive shoeing is most common and is used to support and protect the hooves. Modifications can be made to the trimming and shoeing to influence the way the hoof supports weight and how it behaves in motion, to improve traction on slick surfaces such as ice, or to improve performance for a particular sport. Therapeutic or prescription shoeing is used to treat specific problems and can be used on one or more hooves as necessary. Therapeutic shoes often are temporary until the primary problem has healed (Fig. 9-45).

> **TECHNICIAN NOTE** Hooves grow an average of one fourth of an inch per month. Every 5 to 8 weeks, the shoes must be removed and the hooves trimmed to prevent overgrowth.

Horseshoes do not stop the hoof from growing. Hooves grow an average of one fourth of an inch per month, although individual variation is noted. Every 5 to 8 weeks, the shoes must be removed, and the hooves must be trimmed to prevent overgrowth. The horse may be reshod after trimming. In some cases, the old shoes can be reused (reset), but shoes eventually wear out and must be replaced. Bent shoes need to be replaced. Trimming and shoeing must be performed by knowledgeable professionals. Farriers usually perform the trimming and shoeing for most horses. Trimming and shoeing are a regular expense for most horse owners and may be significant, especially when special shoeing is required. Many shoes must be handmade or carefully adjusted by the farrier, and the time required for the farm call and farrier's time and materials must be compensated. The owner must also schedule a time to be present for the shoeing, which is another potential inconvenience.

> **TECHNICIAN NOTE** Farriers usually perform the trimming and shoeing for most horses.

When shoes must be removed for veterinary purposes, several points should be kept in mind. First, unless it is an emergency, the owner should be consulted before removing shoes. When shoes are removed for a veterinary reason, the veterinarian is actually creating another bill (the farrier's) in addition to the veterinary bill because the *farrier* must be called to replace the shoe. A little client education about the reason that the shoes must be removed is wise. Sometimes the expense of replacing the shoes is prohibitive, or the horse may be difficult to shoe, and the owner may request that the clinician try to "work around" the shoes. However, the owner must understand the possible limitations that this places on the examination. Shoes should be removed carefully so that they can possibly be used for a reset, which saves money. For this reason, removed shoes should never be discarded. In a clinic setting, removed shoes should be identified with marking tape and returned to the owner when the horse is discharged.

> **TECHNICIAN NOTE** The owner should be consulted before a shoe is removed. If the shoe is removed, it should be returned to the owner.

Horseshoes are removed for various reasons. Overgrown hooves, injured hooves, lameness examination, hoof radiographs, preparation for surgical procedures, and recovery from general anesthesia are some indications for shoe removal. Additionally, horses may step or twist on their shoes and partially dislodge them. When shoes are loose or twisted, the potential for further damage to the foot and leg is high, and the shoes should be removed immediately.

> **TECHNICIAN NOTE** Dislodged shoes and shoes that are loose or twisted can cause further damage to the foot and leg and should be removed immediately.

The horse should be adequately restrained. All steps of shoe removal are done with the leg elevated. Shoe removal is a fairly straightforward procedure. To remove a shoe, you must understand how the shoe is held to the hoof. Shoes are usually attached with nails, although "glue-ons" have become popular for situations where nails cannot be easily used, such as for foals. If extra stability must be added to the shoe, side clips or rims can be added to the shoe and positioned against the hoof wall (Fig. 9-46). Clips and rims supplement the lateral stability of the shoe but do not replace nails for holding the shoe on the hoof.

Horseshoe nails are shaped such that they follow a slightly curved path when driven with the hammer. Nails are driven from the bottom of the hoof wall, through the insensitive portion of the wall until they exit through the side of the hoof wall approximately ¾ to 1 inch from their point of entry (Fig. 9-47, *A* and *B*). Once the nail exits, the sharp point of the nail is removed, and the remaining protruding portion is folded over 180 degrees and is pressed flat against the hoof; this is referred to as *clinching* the nail. This folded portion (the clinch) secures the nail and prevents it from backing out of the hoof. It is also this bent portion that must be removed

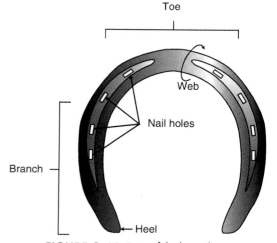

FIGURE 9-45 Parts of the horseshoe.

or straightened to remove the nail and therefore the shoe (Fig. 9-47, *C*). Shoe removal involves three steps.

CLINCH REMOVAL

Counting the number of nail heads confirms the number of clinches to be removed. Two main methods are used for clinch removal. The first method is to file off the clinches

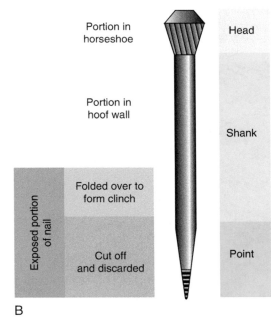

with a metal file or hoof rasp (Fig. 9-48). This must be done carefully to avoid removing large areas of periople (outer surface of the hoof). If the clinches are "buried" in the hoof wall, filing them off may be difficult without creating much surface damage to the hoof wall. Rasping may be more comfortable for sensitive hooves. The second method is to cut (or straighten) the clinches with a clinch cutter and hammer (Fig. 9-49). The clinch cutter has two blades, wide and narrow, each with a flattened top that can be struck with a hammer. The clinch cutter is positioned so that the selected blade is under the clinch and facing proximally along the hoof wall. The blade should be held as flat as possible against the hoof to engage the clinch but avoid gouging the hoof wall. The hammer is struck until the clinch is cut off or straightened enough to remove the nail safely (Fig. 9-50).

> **TECHNICIAN NOTE** Counting the number of nail heads confirms the number of clinches to be removed.

NAIL REMOVAL

Nail removal is done by pulling the nail out from the head. Crease nail pullers are designed to grasp the nail by the head and pull it from the shoe (Fig. 9-51). Pull-offs can be used to grasp nails with protruding heads. Individual nail removal is

FIGURE 9-46 Horseshoe with side clip. (Courtesy Nebraska Equine.)

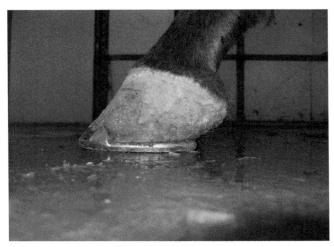

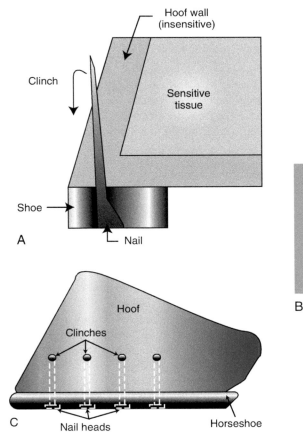

FIGURE 9-47 **A,** Diagram of horseshoe nail driven properly through the hoof wall. **B,** Parts of the horseshoe nail. **C,** Diagram of horseshoe, nails, and clinches.

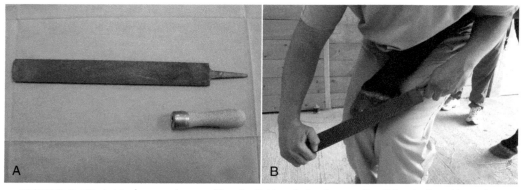

FIGURE 9-48 **A,** Hoof rasp and optional handle. **B,** Use of a hoof rasp to file off the clinches of horseshoe nails.

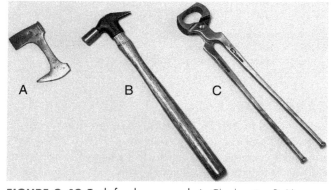

FIGURE 9-49 Tools for shoe removal. **A,** Clinch cutter. **B,** Hammer. **C,** Shoe pull-offs. Note the knobs on the handles of the pull-offs. (From Colahan PT, Merritt AM, Moore JN, Mayhew IG, editors: *Equine medicine and surgery*, vol 2, ed 5, St. Louis, 1999, Mosby.)

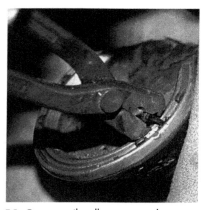

FIGURE 9-51 Crease nail pullers are used to remove each nail. (From Colahan PT, Merritt AM, Moore JN, Mayhew IG, editors: *Equine medicine and surgery*, vol 2, ed 5, St. Louis, 1999, Mosby.)

not always necessary. Often when the clinches have been removed, the act of pulling off the shoe pulls the nails out with the shoe, but this must be done carefully. All nails should be retrieved from the area so that none are left on the ground to injure other horses or people (Fig. 9-52).

> **TECHNICIAN NOTE**   All nails should be retrieved from the area so that none are left on the ground to injure other horses or people.

SHOE REMOVAL

Shoe removal is done with shoe pullers ("pull-offs"). Shoe pullers look very similar to hoof trimmers ("nippers"), but pull-offs have small knobs on the ends of the handles. Nippers should never be used to pull nails or remove shoes because this will dull the cutting edges. Removal begins with elevation of the branches (heels) of the shoe and proceeds toward the toe (Fig. 9-53). The jaws of the pull-off are placed between one shoe branch and the hoof, and the handles are closed to push the jaws together. The handles are then rolled toward the midline of the toe, thus prying the shoe off the hoof (the toe should be well supported before any leverage is applied to the pull-offs). This is repeated on the other branch of the shoe and is then repeated as needed,

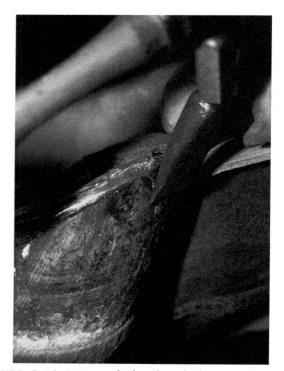

FIGURE 9-50 Cutting a clinch with a clinch cutter. The clinician elevates the hoof and positions the clinch cutter blade beneath the clinch. A hammer is used to strike the clinch cutter and remove the clinch. (From Colahan PT, Merritt AM, Moore JN, Mayhew IG, editors: *Equine medicine and surgery*, vol 2, ed 5, St. Louis, 1999, Mosby.)

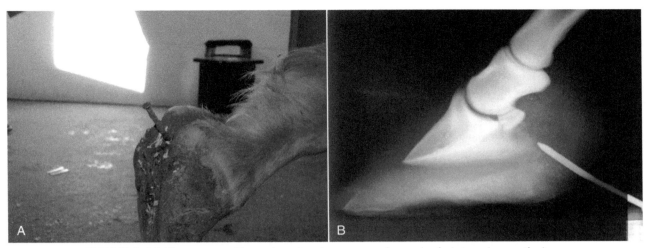

FIGURE 9-52 This is not a nail from a horseshoe, but it is a good example of what can happen if a horse were to impale itself with a nail. **A,** A nail embedded in a hoof. **B,** A radiograph that identifies the nail's location.

progressing toward the toe and alternating sides until the shoe is free. The pull-off handles should not be rolled toward the outside edge of the hoof wall; this tends to tear off pieces of the hoof wall.

> *TECHNICIAN NOTE* The pull-off handles should not be rolled toward the outside edge of the hoof wall; this tends to tear off pieces of the hoof wall.

Removal must be performed carefully to prevent damaging the hoof wall. Failure to remove clinches completely or to be aware of side clips can result in large chips and cracks, which likely will be problematic. Some methods of clinch removal (especially rasping) can scuff the outer layers of the hoof and damage the periople layer; damage to this layer can bother some clients. It is desirable not to bend shoes during removal in case they can be reset, but aluminum shoes are somewhat soft and commonly bend during removal. Most owners are aware of this.

After the shoe is removed, the unshod hoof is prone to chipping and cracking, especially if the horse is on hard surfaces. Chipping and cracking are unsightly and may interfere with the ability to replace a shoe (which makes farriers and owners quite unhappy). Hoof cracks can also extend into sensitive tissue and become a source of lameness. To minimize this risk, a hoof rasp can be lightly used to round off any sharp edges on the bottom of the hoof wall where it meets the ground. Covering the hoof wall and sole with duct tape after shoe removal can also reduce the risk of chipping.

> *TECHNICIAN NOTE* Chipping or cracking the hoof wall during shoe removal can interfere with the ability to replace the shoe. All attempts should be made to prevent this.

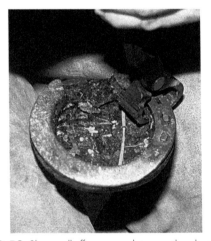

FIGURE 9-53 Shoe pull-offs are used to pry the shoe away from the hoof, beginning at the heels and progressing toward the toe. (From Colahan PT, Merritt AM, Moore JN, Mayhew IG, editors: *Equine medicine and surgery*, vol 2, ed 5, St. Louis, 1999, Mosby.)

EXTERNAL COAPTATION

External coaptation refers to the use of bandages, splints, and casts. It should not be confused with external fixation, which is a method of fracture fixation using metal pins that are placed through bone, exit the skin, and are secured to an external frame.

Indications for external coaptation include the following:

- Reduce (compress) dead space to prevent formation of hematomas/seromas during treatment of surgical or traumatic wounds.
- Reduce skin motion around a surgical or traumatic wound.
- Minimize wound contamination by protecting the wound from environmental exposure or from absorbing drainage and discharge.
- Hold medications against a surgical or traumatic wound.
- Prevent further injury to tissues after an initial injury.
- Compress open wounds to retard development of exuberant granulation tissue ("proud flesh").

- Prevent self-mutilation of a wound.
- Immobilize a limb or joint.
- Provide supplemental support to a joint or limb.
- Protect limbs during transportation.
- Protect limbs during work or performance.
- Apply pressure to control hemorrhage.

The basis of a good bandage is padding. This becomes especially important on the lower legs (distal to the carpus/tarsus), where there is no muscle tissue to provide protection for the tendons, ligaments, and neurovascular structures.

> **TECHNICIAN NOTE**   Failure to apply adequate padding can have disastrous consequences, including pressure sores, pressure necrosis, and inflammation of tendons and ligaments, all resulting from compromise or complete strangulation of blood supply.

Failure to apply adequate padding can have disastrous consequences, including pressure sores, pressure necrosis, and inflammation of tendons and ligaments, all resulting from compromise or complete strangulation of blood supply. Tendinitis of the superficial or deep digital flexor tendons may result from lack of padding ("bandage bow"). Pressure sores and necrosis of the skin and SC tissues ("cording") may also occur, with permanent scarring or regrowth of white hairs in the damaged area, or both. Complete strangulation of the blood supply to the area may cause gangrene and sloughing of a part. If this occurs in a lower leg area that has little collateral circulation, the results may threaten the horse's career or even the horse's life. Usually, it is better to use too much padding than too little. However, too much padding can prevent a good fit and can result in slipping and bunching up of the bandage, which also may lead to compromised blood flow. Proper bandage fit is as much an art as it is a science. The goal should be a snug, firm fit—not too tight or too loose—and padding is the most important key to achieving proper fit.

> **TECHNICIAN NOTE**   Padding is the most important aspect of external coaptation.

Bandages should be applied evenly to prevent problems: The pressure applied by a bandage should be even throughout the length of the bandage. A bandage should not be applied tightly in one region and loosely in another. All layers of a bandage should be applied in the same direction, and each layer of the bandage should be applied under a constant tension that is appropriate for that layer. Each layer of a bandage has a different function and therefore is applied under a different tension from the other layers.

> **TECHNICIAN NOTE**   The pressure applied by a bandage should be even throughout the length of the bandage.

Bandages can cause pressure sores, especially over bony prominences of the legs. The accessory carpal bone, calcaneus (point of the hock), proximal sesamoid bones, and heel bulbs are prone to developing pressure sores and should be well padded in an effort to prevent this complication. Another approach to prevention is the use of relief incisions—small incisions through constrictive layers of the bandage made directly over the pressure point—to effectively remove constriction and rubbing by the bandage at that spot.

> **TECHNICIAN NOTE**   Bony prominences should be well padded, or the constrictive layers of the bandage should be cut over the area to help prevent pressure sores.

Bandages should be monitored at least once daily. Depending on the type of bandage and temperament of the patient, bandage checks may needed several times per day. Bandage checks should include examination for dislodgment, tightness (too tight or too loose), soiling, strikethrough (absorbed wound exudate appearing on the surface of the bandage), swelling around the margins of the bandage, and unraveling of material. If any of these problems are seen during the bandage check, the clinician should be alerted. One of the most important parameters to check in patients with leg bandages is increased lameness, not only in the bandaged leg but also in the other legs. Bandages should not increase lameness in any leg. When lameness is observed, the clinician should closely evaluate the bandage. A bandage change is usually required in this circumstance.

> **TECHNICIAN NOTE**   Bandages should be checked at least once daily.

Bandages should also be watched for "patient tampering." This is not common in large animals, but it does occur. Patients' chewing on their bandages is the most common form of tampering and can be difficult to control. One approach is to try to limit physical access to the bandage by tying or cross-tying the patient. Neck cradles are available, which are the large animal version of the Elizabethan collar. Neck cradles are usually constructed from smooth wooden slats, bound together with leather or string (Fig. 9-54). Another strategy is to place unpleasant-tasting liquids or pastes on the outer surface of the bandage. However, many of these substances are irritating to skin, so care must be taken not to apply them to the skin adjacent to the bandage. Caustic chemicals should not be used to discourage bandage chewing because of possible damage to the tissues of the mouth and eyes if the horse rubs its head or chews on the bandage.

> **TECHNICIAN NOTE**   If unpleasant-tasting liquids are used to prevent bandage tampering, it is important that the chemical used not cause irritation to the skin, eyes, or gastrointestinal system if ingested.

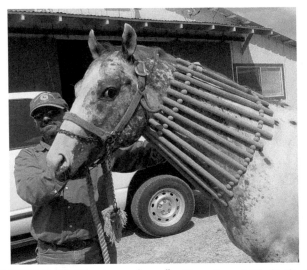

FIGURE 9-54 Wooden neck cradle. (From Bassert JM, McCurnin DM, editors: *McCurnin's clinical textbook for veterinary technicians*, ed 7, St. Louis, 2010, Saunders.)

Even if complications are not seen, bandages still must be routinely changed for sanitation and to inspect the healing of the injured area. The purpose of the bandage and the patient's demeanor dictate how frequently routine bandage changes are necessary.

Many types of bandages are available. Choosing the type of bandage for a patient depends on several factors:

- Anatomical location of the bandage
- Available materials
- Patient factors (confinement, temperament, and training)
- Experience of the personnel applying the bandage
- Purpose of the bandage

Always ask "What am I trying to accomplish with this bandage?" and then select the most appropriate bandage for the situation. The best bandage may not be the same for every patient or every situation.

LEG BANDAGES AND SPLINTS

Many types of leg bandages and splints are available. This discussion emphasizes bandages and splints with primarily medical uses.

Exercise Bandages and Wraps

These bandages are designed to provide additional support or protection, or both, for the legs during exercise. The need for exercise bandages is determined by the horse's "profession" and by the horse's tendency to strike its own legs (interfering) accidentally. The bandages are usually worn only during exercise or turnout and are removed afterward. Indications include the following:

- Protection of lower legs during turnout or exercise: This may be accomplished by wrapping only the metacarpus or metatarsus (cannon area) or the entire distal limb down to the coronary band. Commercial "boots" are available to protect specific areas, such as the splint bones or the fetlocks. These boots usually have padding incorporated

into them and are secured with hook-and-loop or buckle straps. They are constructed of leather or Neoprene rubber (Fig. 9-55).
- Protection of the hoof and heel bulbs: If a horse has a tendency to step on the heels of its front feet with its back feet, commercial rubber "bell boots" can be placed around the pasterns of the forelimbs to cover the heels. Bell boots can be combined with lower limb wraps to provide complete coverage of the lower leg, heels, and coronary band (Fig. 9-56).
- Support of lower legs during turnout or exercise: It is commonly believed that bandages can provide significant support to the tendons and ligaments of the lower legs. However, when the body weight and biomechanical force of a horse moving at speed are compared with the strength of bandaging materials, support wraps probably do not provide more than 5% to 10% additional support to the lower leg. Nevertheless, support wraps are commonly used.

Shipping Bandages

When horses are transported, they are subject to sudden vehicle stops, starts, and turns. Horses that are thrown off balance may slip, fall, or step on themselves, thereby causing serious injury. Some horses kick while they are in the transportation stall, and this can produce injury. Some individuals strongly resist loading into the trailer or van and can injure themselves in the struggle. Protecting the legs of the horse for transportation is essential.

Proper protection includes, at the minimum, complete lower leg coverage from below the carpus or tarsus to the hoof, including the coronary band. This can be provided by bandaging the cannon and pastern, in addition to covering the coronary band with the bandage or a bell boot.

Commercially available shipping wraps that cover the entire lower leg, including the coronary band, are available. They offer some padding for protection and are washable. Shipping boots come in lower leg and full leg lengths (Fig. 9-57).

Hoof Bandages

This family of bandages is generally used to cover open surgical or traumatic hoof wounds. Hoof bandages also can be used to protect the hoof from external damage, such as preventing chipping of the hoof wall after removal of horseshoes (especially useful for lameness examinations on hard surfaces). Hoof bandages, wraps, and covers can be made from standard bandaging materials, applied as prescription horseshoes by farriers, or purchased commercially.

Before a hoof bandage is placed, any open wounds should be cleaned, and appropriate topical medications should be applied. The rest of the hoof should be clean and dry. The treatments and bandaging should be performed on a clean surface, which can be provided by spreading paper or cloth towels under the horse. If the horse accidentally sets a foot down during treatment, the clean towel will prevent contamination of open wounds. Once open wounds have been treated, a bandage or other covering must be placed for protection.

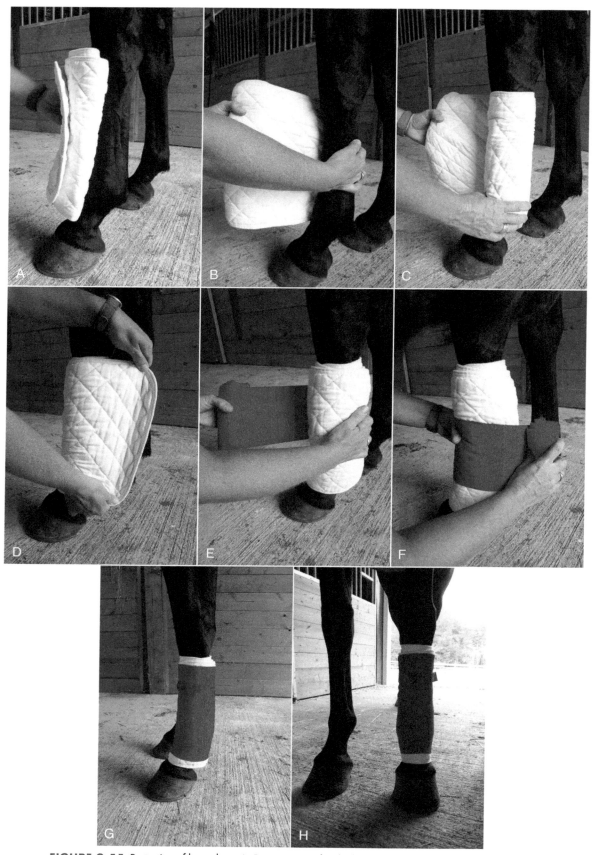

FIGURE 9-55 Protection of lower legs. **A,** Proper sizing of quilted cotton to cover the metacarpus or metatarsus. **B,** The bandage is started by placing the edge of the roll on the medial aspect of the limb and unrolling it in a cranial direction. **C,** The padding is unrolled evenly, avoiding wrinkles. **D,** Completed padding layer. **E,** The securing layer is started at the middle of the padding, again beginning on the medial aspect and unrolling in a cranial direction. **F,** Note use of the free hand to stabilize the bandage to prevent "spinout." **G,** Side view of finished bandage. Note that 1 inch of padding is exposed at the top and bottom of the bandage. **H,** Front view of finished bandage.

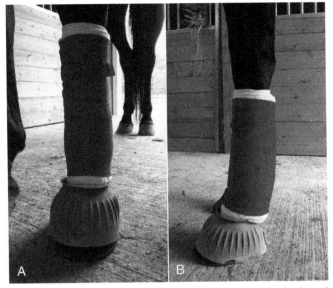

FIGURE 9-56 A, Addition of a bell boot to protect the heels and coronary band. **B,** Side view of bell boot.

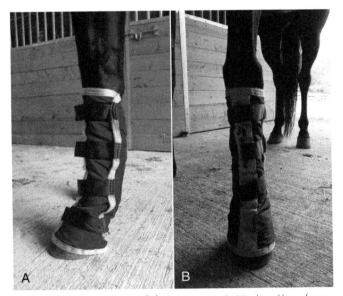

FIGURE 9-57 Commercial shipping wrap. **A,** Hook-and-loop fasteners are positioned on the lateral aspect of the leg to prevent catching. **B,** Note coverage of the heels and coronary band.

> **TECHNICIAN NOTE**   Apply hoof bandages in a clean, dry area, or provide a towel in case the horse steps down onto the foot during treatment.

One way to cover the entire hoof is with a commercial hoof boot. Commercial hoof boots (e.g., EZ Boots, EasyCare, Tucson, Ariz.) are made of rubber and are available to fit all sizes of hooves. These boots have metal bindings that secure them in position. Boots must fit snugly or they will be easily dislodged, especially in wet or muddy conditions. This can have disastrous consequences if an open wound is exposed by loss of a boot.

Hooves can also be protected by bandaging. In general, the material for hoof bandages should be waterproof and durable. Elastic and nonelastic bandaging tape can be used for wrapping the foot, but duct tape is more durable, more waterproof, and less expensive.

Several rules apply to using tape "booties." Because of the risk of constricting blood flow to the hoof, nonelastic tapes should not be applied on or above the coronary band, and elastic tapes should be used cautiously above the coronary band. As long as tape is confined to the hoof wall only, it can be applied tightly to produce a snug fit. Too much tape on the sole can cause discomfort; therefore, use only enough to provide a reasonably thick covering that will stay in place.

> **TECHNICIAN NOTE**   Nonelastic tapes should not be applied on or above the coronary band, and elastic tapes should be used cautiously above the coronary band.

Horseshoes can be designed to protect and cover healing hoof wounds. Hoof pads can be applied to cover an injured area and are appropriate when the injury does not require direct topical care. Treatment plates (i.e., "boiler plates") are metal plates that are fixed to a horseshoe with three to four screws. The metal plate completely covers the sole but can be removed with a screwdriver to allow full access to the sole (Fig. 9-58). Treatment plate shoes are useful for protecting open sole wounds between topical treatments, such as soaking and application of topical medications. Owners can be easily instructed on maintaining and removing treatment plates and frequently find these shoes more convenient and less expensive than the alternative of daily bandage changes. Depending on the construction of the shoe (i.e., whether the screw heads are exposed or recessed into the shoe), the horse may or may not be able to have limited turnout exercise.

Distal Limb Bandages
The distal limb bandage is the most common bandage used for medical purposes. It is used almost exclusively for inflammatory conditions of the lower leg, but it can also be applied for protection and support.

Inflammatory conditions are accompanied by swelling, and one of the main purposes of this type of bandage is to limit or reduce swelling by applying firm compression. The distal limb bandage is applied from the top of the metacarpus or metatarsus to just below the coronary band. It should not be placed to cover only the cannon area. Because the bandage is designed to apply compression, lymphatic and venous drainage of parts of the leg distal to the compression may be compromised (this is true of any bandage). Swelling of the pastern often results if compression is applied only to the cannon area; therefore, the entire pastern down to and including the coronary band should be included in the bandage. Compression is not an issue below the coronary band.

Before the bandage is applied, topical medications are applied if indicated. If wounds are present, they are cleaned, and

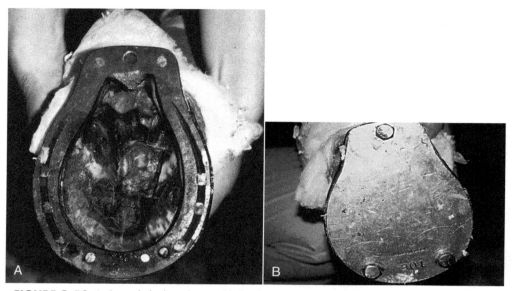

FIGURE 9-58 A, Screw holes have been added to this treatment plate shoe. **B,** The treatment plate in position to cover the sole. (From Wildenstein MJ: Horseshoeing. In Colahan PT, Merritt AM, Moore JN, Mayhew IG, editors: *Equine medicine and surgery,* vol 2, ed 5, St. Louis, 1999, Mosby.)

an appropriate topical wound medication is applied (if indicated; some wounds may be left dry). If no wound is present, topical medications are seldom necessary, although occasionally topical treatments such as sweats or poultices are applied.

Restraint of the patient is critical to successful application of the bandage; it is not possible to bandage a moving target properly. If the horse moves its leg during application, the layers already applied often have to be removed and the whole bandaging process started again from the beginning. Most horses are easily bandaged with no restraint, but some may require mild or moderate restraint. Ideally, the horse should bear weight on the leg during bandage application, although sometimes pain from an inflammatory condition makes weight bearing difficult or impossible.

Having all bandaging materials assembled beforehand, unwrapped and ready for use, and within easy reach of the person applying the bandage is important.

The five standard layers of the distal limb bandage can be modified slightly to accommodate the underlying condition of the leg. Layers 1 and 2 are necessary only if wounds are present; otherwise, they can be omitted. The standard layers, from innermost to outermost, are the wound dressing, the layer to hold the wound dressing, the padding, the securing layer, and the finishing layer, as described in the following subsections.

> **TECHNICIAN NOTE**   Layers 1 and 2 of a leg bandage can be omitted if a wound is not present.

Wound Dressing

If an open or sutured wound is present, a wound covering is usually placed directly against the wound (Fig. 9-59). The nature of the wound determines the type of covering. The thickness of the covering is dictated by the amount of compression to be applied to the wound by the bandage and the

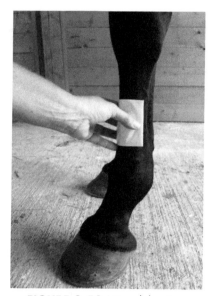

FIGURE 9-59 Wound dressing.

anticipated amount of exudate absorption needed. Common choices include the following:

- Dry 4 × 4 gauze squares are useful to absorb fluid if wound exudation or bleeding is expected. The gauze may be sterile or nonsterile, according to the needs of the wound.
- Nonstick pads (e.g., Telfa) are useful to minimize trauma to the new epithelial cells during the epithelialization phase of wound healing.
- Saline-soaked gauze is sometimes useful to encourage wound granulation.
- Petrolatum-impregnated wound coverings are useful to cover clean, sutured incisions and lacerations. The petrolatum prevents the pad from sticking to the sutures and incision line.

- Gauze rolls can lie passively over suture lines to increase the amount of pressure applied by the securing layer of the bandage.

Layer to Hold Wound Dressing

If a wound dressing is used, it must be held in place against the wound. This layer must not be used to apply compression; the goal is to keep the wound dressing passively in position over the wound. Elastic materials are generally preferred to minimize the risk of strangulation. Common choices for this layer include the following:

- Roll gauze, brown or white. For large animals, the gauze rolls should not be less than 3 inches wide; 4 or 6 inches is preferable. The gauze may need to be sterile, depending on the nature of the wound. Roll gauze is rather inelastic and can cause constriction of blood flow if it is applied too tightly. Kling roll gauze has more elasticity than standard roll gauze.
- Elastic foam rubber: This material is self-adherent and very flexible. It tears easily under tension, which makes the possibility of strangulation extremely low. It is easy to apply without any special instruments and readily conforms to the leg (Fig. 9-60).
- Elastic adhesive tape.

Padding

Whenever compression is applied, adequate padding must be used to prevent strangulation of the blood supply. In general, the more compression to be applied, the thicker the padding required. The padding layer is applied passively, without pressure. Quilted cloth pads, towels, and even disposable diapers can be used for the padding layer. However, sheet cotton is the preferred material.

> *TECHNICIAN NOTE* The more compression to be applied, the thicker the padding required.

Sheet cotton is available by the dozen or in large quantities by the bale (200 sheets). If indicated, sheet cotton can be wrapped and sterilized in an autoclave. The sheets are rectangular and must be folded over to reduce their size to fit the lower leg. The length of the horse's lower leg dictates the pattern used to fold the sheets. Regardless of the folding pattern, the cardinal rule for adequate padding is to use a minimum of three sheets in a distal limb bandage (when folded over, this produces six layers of cotton). Occasionally, the sheets are so thin that four sheets are required to produce sufficient padding.

> *TECHNICIAN NOTE* The cardinal rule for adequate padding is to use a minimum of three sheets when applying a distal limb bandage.

When sheet cotton is used, the securing layer may have difficulty "biting" into the sheets because the material has a fairly smooth surface. Nonsterile, 6-inch-wide, brown roll

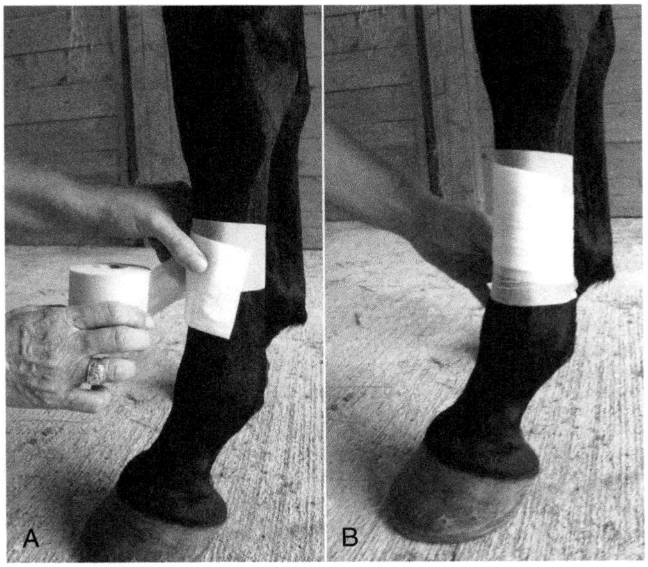

FIGURE 9-60 **A,** Use of Foam-air over wound dressing. **B,** Completed layer to hold wound dressing in position.

gauze can be applied circumferentially over the sheet cotton to provide a better "bite" for the securing layer. The gauze also helps to conform the padding more closely to the leg (Fig. 9-61).

Roll cotton can be used for padding, but it is difficult to work with and often leads to uneven thickness and bunching of the layer. However, roll cotton is useful for adding bulk over a distal limb bandage, as is done in the application of splints.

Securing Layer

The securing layer is the only layer that is used to apply compression. Compression is applied from distal to proximal, as evenly as possible over the entire length of the wrap. The layer is applied by spiraling the bandage material around the leg; compression is applied by placing the layer under tension as it is unrolled. The amount of tension controls the amount of compression. For more compression, pull the layer into more tension as it is applied. Common securing materials are the following:

- Cloth bandages: These are usually supplied as rolls of cloth material referred to as derby wraps or flannel wraps. Ace (3M, St. Paul, Minn.) elastic self-adhering bandages can also be used. Cloth bandages are washable but tend to lose their elasticity over time. Because they stretch markedly and unevenly, they are difficult to use to apply evenly distributed compression. Because they are usually secured with hook-and-loop straps, tape, or large safety pins, reliable compression is difficult to maintain. In addition, cloth bandages typically are too short to cover the full length of the bandage adequately.
- Elastic self-adhesive tape (Table 9-4): For large animals, the minimum width is 3 inches, but 4- to 6-inch tape is preferable. The self-adhesive properties of the tape help to provide consistent compression throughout the length

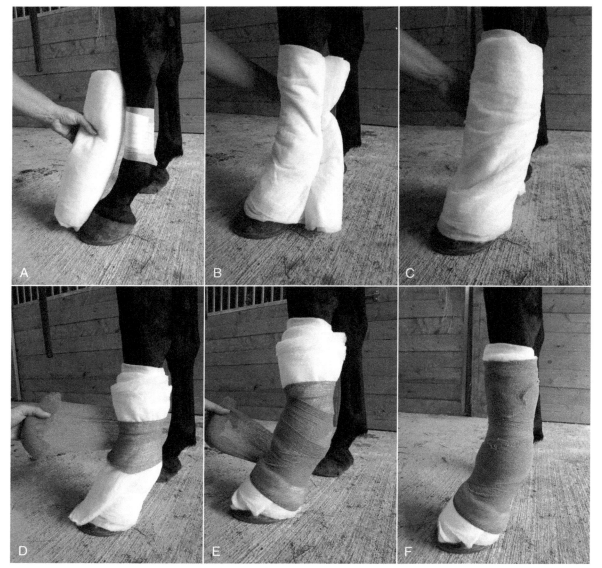

FIGURE 9-61 A, Proper length of padding for a distal limb wrap. **B**, Sheet cotton is unrolled evenly around the leg. **C**, Finished padding layer. Note the smoothness of the material. **D**, Brown gauze is used to further conform the padding, beginning at the middle of the bandage. **E**, The gauze is continued distally before spiraling proximally. **F**, Finished gauze layer.

TABLE 9-4	Bandaging Tapes	
TYPE	**PROPERTIES**	**TRADE AND COMMON NAMES**
Elastic, self-adhesive	Adheres to itself but not to other surfaces	Vetrap (3M, St. Paul, Minn.), Co-Flex (Andover Healthcare, Salisbury, Mass.)
Elastic, adhesive	Has adhesive coating that allows it to adhere to itself and other surfaces	Elastikon (Johnson & Johnson, New Brunswick, NJ), Conform (Kendall/Covidien, Minneapolis, Minn.)
Nonelastic, adhesive	Has adhesive coating that allows it to adhere to itself and other surfaces	Adhesive tape, duct tape

of the bandage. This is the most popular choice for the securing layer.

- Elastic adhesive tape: The minimum width for large animal use is 3 inches, but 4 inches is preferable. The expense of these types of tapes often precludes their use for this layer. They are most often used for the finishing layer.
- Nonelastic adhesive tape: The lack of elasticity increases the chance of strangulation; therefore, this tape is not often used for the securing layer. However, this material is suitable for holding splints in place over a padded distal limb wrap.

> **TECHNICIAN NOTE**   The securing layer is the only layer that is used to apply compression.

Finishing Layer

This layer is optional, depending on the underlying condition and the clinician's preference. Finishing is provided by covering the top or bottom, or both, of the bandage with elastic adhesive tape. The purpose is to prevent bedding and other debris from entering the bandage. It also can help prevent slipping of the bandage, although it should not be relied on as 100% effective for this purpose.

Typically, the tape is wrapped two to three times around the top or bottom, or both, of the bandage, overlapping the bandage and the adjacent skin or hoof wall. The tape should not apply compression; it should be applied to stick to the skin or hoof passively (Fig. 9-62).

To apply the bandage, first gather bandaging supplies and have them ready for use. If necessary, restrain the patient and try to keep the leg in a fully weight-bearing position. The principles of bandage application are as follows:

1. Apply any topical medications or treatments, and clean and dress wounds. Clean and dry the leg before applying the padding.
2. When unrolling bandage materials, it is standard practice to begin on the medial aspect of the leg and unroll cranially to establish the direction of the "bandage spiral" (Fig. 9-63, A). Once a direction has been established, all layers of the bandage should follow the same direction. When unrolling materials, the material should unroll around the leg like a carpet unrolling on a floor (think of the leg as the floor) (Fig. 9-63, B and C).
3. If the padding material has been folded (to achieve proper length), the open (free) edges of the material should be placed distally.
4. The length of the padding layer should cover the coronary band distally and extend proximally to the top of the metacarpus or metatarsus. Always leave at least 1 inch of padding exposed at the proximal and distal ends of the bandage.
5. The securing layer must usually be "seated" before it can be pulled tautly to apply compression. Seating the material involves circling the padding layer several times, starting near the middle of the bandage and proceeding distally with minimal tension. When the securing material is within 1 inch of the distal margin of the padding layer, the seating is complete, and compression can now be applied in a proximal direction. Once the material is seated, it is easier to apply compression, and the padding is less likely to "spin out" (i.e., spin around the leg while the bandage is being applied) (Fig. 9-64).
6. After the material is seated, the securing layer is applied tautly to apply compression. The layer is applied by spiraling around the leg from distal to proximal, overlapping each previous spiral by half the width of the material. The tension on the tape should be even with every pass, over the entire length of the bandage (Fig. 9-65, A). The purpose of the bandage determines the amount of tension; some conditions require more compression than others. Most elastic tapes have a waffle or ribbed appearance on the roll. Pulling the tape tautly until the waffle or rib pattern disappears is the minimum amount of tension to apply (Fig. 9-65, B and C). The bandage should be stabilized with the free hand (the hand not holding the tape roll) to prevent spinout during application of the tape.
7. Be sure that the padding layer does not bunch up as the securing layer is placed because bunched-up areas tend to rub and cause pressure sores. Bunching tends to occur at the pastern-fetlock area, where the change in angulation and diameter of the leg makes a good form fit difficult to achieve. Using 6-inch brown roll gauze over the padding helps conform the padding to the leg, thus making application of the securing tape easier.

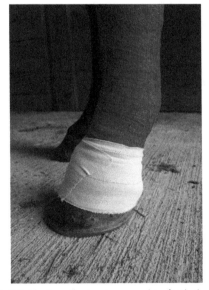

FIGURE 9-62 Elastic adhesive tape used to finish the bottom of a distal limb bandage.

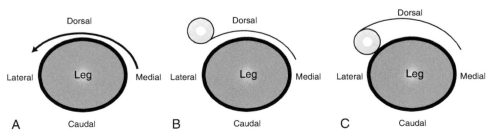

FIGURE 9-63 **A,** Proper direction to unroll bandage material. **B,** Proper way to unroll bandage materials. **C,** Improper way to unroll bandage material.

8. Check the bandage for proper fit before finishing the bandage. One finger should be able to fit snugly between the bandage and the skin at the proximal and distal ends of the bandage. If two or more fingers can be inserted, the bandage may be too loose. The midsection of the bandage can be checked by thumping the wrap with a finger; proper compression usually results in a "watermelon thump"

sound. Be sure that 1 inch of padding is exposed at the top and bottom of the wrap (Fig. 9-66).

Full Limb Bandages

For conditions of the carpus or upper limb (antebrachium) of the forelimb, or both, and the tarsus or upper

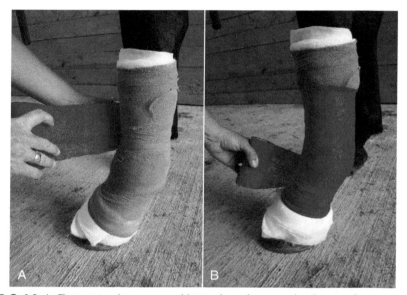

FIGURE 9-64 **A,** The securing layer is seated by applying the material with minimal tension around the middle of the bandage. **B,** The tape is then applied distally.

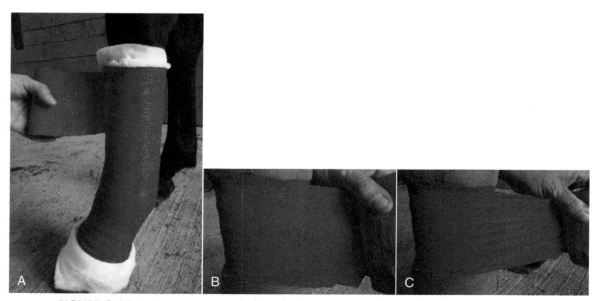

FIGURE 9-65 **A,** Compression is applied in a distal-to-proximal direction by pulling the tape to the desired tension as it is unrolled. **B,** The waffle pattern of the tape is visible when the tape is under insufficient tension. **C,** The waffle pattern disappears when the proper tension is applied to the tape.

limb (gaskin) of the hindlimb, or both, a full limb bandage should be used. A common error is trying to bandage these areas with a wrap that encircles only the upper leg. This practice should be avoided for two reasons. First, applying compression to only the upper leg can lead to edema of the lower leg. Second, even with use of adhesive tapes, these bandages are usually doomed to slip down the leg. Therefore, they must be "buttressed" against a supporting structure to prevent slipping. For these reasons, the full limb bandage is applied in two parts (commonly referred to as a double-decker bandage).

> *TECHNICIAN NOTE* Even with use of adhesive tapes, full limb bandages are usually doomed to slip down the leg.

A standard distal limb bandage (padding and securing layer) is applied to the lower leg first. This bandage supports the upper leg bandage and applies compression to the lower leg. The upper bandage is applied next and is essentially a repeat of the distal limb bandage, with wound dressings used as necessary. The upper bandage is applied so that it overlaps the lower bandage by 2 to 3 inches (Fig. 9-67).

Pressure sores are likely to form over the point of the accessory carpal bone and the point of the calcaneus (point of the hock). Use of extra padding over these bony prominences may decrease this complication, but relief incisions may achieve the same result. A relief incision is a small, vertical incision made through the securing and padding layers, directly over the bony prominence. The incision provides spot relief of compression and rubbing. Relief incisions must be made carefully to prevent accidental laceration of the skin (Fig. 9-68).

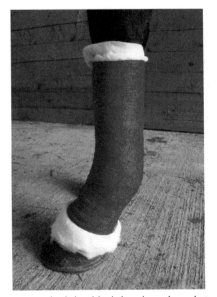

FIGURE 9-66 Finished distal limb bandage, lateral view. Note that padding is exposed at both ends of the bandage, no bunches or wrinkles are seen, and no "waffling" pattern to the tape is visible.

Additional concerns exist for strangulation and pressure sores over the gastrocnemius tendon (Achilles tendon) in the hindlimb. This area should be liberally padded if any compression is to be applied. The bandage should be monitored closely for complications.

Full limb bandages can be finished with elastic adhesive tape to prevent debris from collecting under the bandage. The double-decker method can allow bandage changes of the upper wrap only, provided the lower wrap is in good condition.

Limb Splints
Splints are applied to try to immobilize a joint, bone, or soft tissues following severe, destabilizing injuries. They can be used temporarily to transport an injured patient or used long term to support healing of tissues during conservative treatment or following surgery.

> *TECHNICIAN NOTE* Splints can be used temporarily to move an injured patient or long term to support healing tissues during conservative treatment or following surgery.

The simplest type of splint is the Robert Jones splint bandage (Fig. 9-69). This is basically a distal limb or full limb bandage with a large amount of padding. The most common method is to apply a standard distal limb or full limb bandage first and then add a thick layer of padding over the outside of the standard bandage. Roll cotton is ideal for the additional padding. It is bulky but conforms well if roll gauze is used to seat it. The padding is conformed and seated with roll gauze, and a securing layer is applied to finish the bandage.

The outermost securing layer for splints should be a nonelastic adhesive tape. Because the goal of splints is immobilization, nonelastic tape is more likely than elastic tape to restrict movement. Standard adhesive tape (3- to 4-inch width) or duct tape is ideal for this use.

> *TECHNICIAN NOTE* Duct tape is ideal for use as the securing layer of a splint.

Splints are usually made with supporting struts incorporated into them for additional support and immobilization. Struts can be made from wooden poles, broomsticks, metal rods, and casting tape (molded to the patient's leg). Polyvinylchloride pipe is extremely strong and can be cut using a hacksaw and metal file to fit the patient (Fig. 9-70). Struts should be cut to fit the entire length of the splint bandage, with care taken to remove, contour, or pad any sharp edges that could injure the patient.

> *TECHNICIAN NOTE* Struts can be made from wooden poles, broomsticks, metal rods, polyvinylchloride pipe, and casting tape.

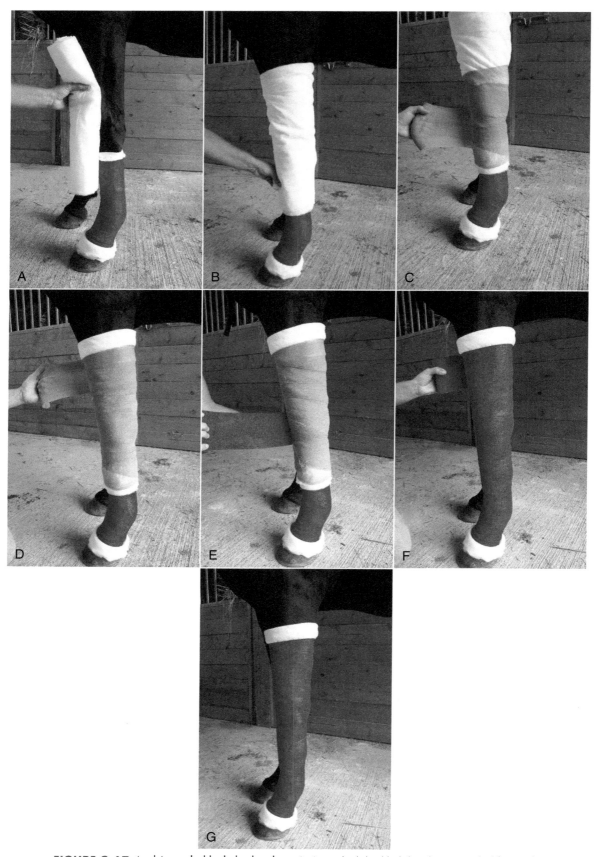

FIGURE 9-67 Applying a double-decker bandage. **A,** A standard distal limb bandage is applied first, and then the "double deck" is positioned. **B,** Completed padding layer. **C,** The gauze is seated similarly to a distal limb bandage. **D,** Completed gauze layer. **E,** The securing layer is seated at the middle of the padding layer, similar to a distal limb bandage. **F,** Compression is applied in a distal-to-proximal direction. **G,** Finished securing layer.

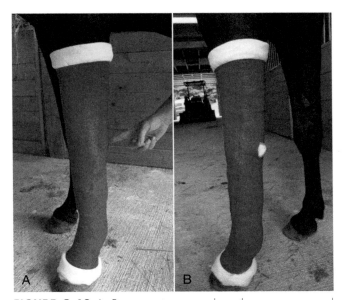

FIGURE 9-68 A, Bony prominences such as the accessory carpal bone are prone to pressure sores. **B,** A small relief incision is made through the securing layer directly over the bony prominence to prevent a pressure sore.

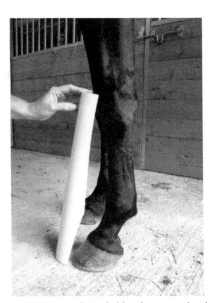

FIGURE 9-70 Sizing a polyvinyl chloride strut to the desired length. This strut is suitable for a distal limb splint.

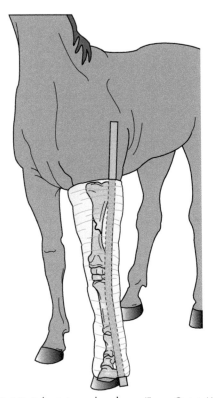

FIGURE 9-69 Robert Jones bandage. (From Orsini JA, Divers TJ, editors: *Equine emergencies: treatment and procedures,* ed 4, St. Louis, 2013, Saunders.)

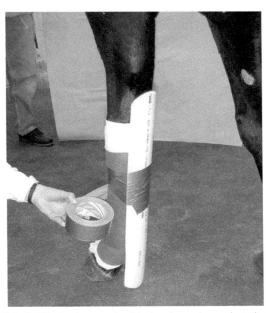

FIGURE 9-71 Applying a distal limb splint with a polyvinyl chloride supporting strut. (From Bassert JM, McCurnin DM, editors: *McCurnin's clinical textbook for veterinary technicians,* ed 7, St. Louis, 2010, Saunders.)

A standard distal limb or full limb wrap is applied to the leg first. More padding can be added over the standard wrap to increase the bulk of the padding layer. Enough padding should be added to reduce mobility of the leg and protect the leg from rubbing by the struts. One or more struts are then positioned and secured firmly with nonelastic adhesive tape or duct tape (Fig. 9-71).

The anatomy of the leg dictates the proper location of struts. All joints of the forelimb (below the shoulder) and hindlimb (below the hip) can normally move only in a craniocaudal direction. Therefore, to prevent craniocaudal motion, struts should be placed on the cranial or caudal aspects of the limb, or both. If the struts are placed medially or laterally, no solid material will prevent motion in the craniocaudal plane. The patient's injury dictates whether one or two struts are necessary.

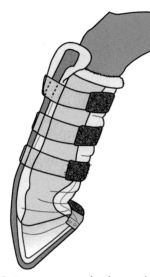

FIGURE 9-72 Emergency metal splint applied over a distal limb bandage.

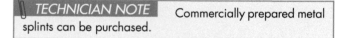
> **TECHNICIAN NOTE**   The struts must be placed cranially and caudally to prevent motion.

Immobilization of a joint usually requires immobilization of the joint above and the joint below the injured joint. The shoulder and hip are located too proximally to be supported by a bandage or splint. Similarly, the elbow and stifle cannot be completely immobilized by splints because of the inability to immobilize the joints above them (i.e., the shoulder and hip joints). Modified Thomas splints have been adapted for large animal patients; they restrict, but do not completely immobilize, the elbow and stifle joints.

Commercially prepared metal splints have been developed (e.g., Kimzey splint, Kimzey, Woodland, Calif.) and can be purchased in different lengths and sizes (Fig. 9-72). These splints are used mostly for emergency immobilization of a part, usually for transportation and protection until the wound can be evaluated at a hospital or clinic. The splint is secured with hook-and-loop straps. A standard distal limb bandage or full limb bandage can be applied under the splint for additional protection of soft tissues.

> **TECHNICIAN NOTE**   Commercially prepared metal splints can be purchased.

Splints can provide good immobilization if they are properly applied; however, complete immobilization is not possible because splints use bandaging materials that are not rigid. If complete immobilization is required from external coaptation, a cast must be used.

Limb Casts

Casts are superior to splints for providing immobilization of the limbs. However, they are subject to the same mechanical

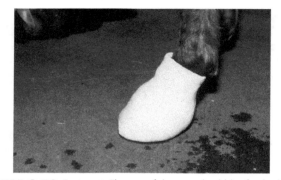

FIGURE 9-73 Foot cast. The top of the cast should be finished with elastic adhesive tape. (From Auer JA, Stick JA: *Equine surgery,* ed 2, St. Louis, 1999, Saunders.)

limitations as splints for treating the upper joints of the forelimbs and hindlimbs.

Casting material is usually a combination of fiberglass with resins. For large animal use, 3- to 4-inch width is preferred. Fiberglass is lighter and stronger than older plaster materials and cures faster. Fiberglass is difficult to conform to the leg, but this difficulty is easily overcome with experience. Fiberglass is also relatively radiolucent, which allows some ability to monitor healing of bone with radiographs without having to remove the cast. Large animal casts are of several types.

1. A foot cast incorporates the entire hoof and extends proximally to a level between the coronary band and the fetlock, depending on the underlying condition. This cast is used for conditions of the hoof and some pastern conditions (Fig. 9-73).
2. A lower limb cast incorporates the entire hoof and extends proximally to the top of the metacarpus or metatarsus.
3. A full limb cast incorporates the entire hoof and extends to just below the level of the elbow on the forelimb or just below the stifle on the hindlimb.
4. A tube cast (sleeve cast) is the only type of cast that does not enclose the hoof. The cast extends from the fetlock to just below the elbow or stifle. This cast is used mostly for foals with angular limb deformities or flexural deformities of the lower leg. Use of the foot and pastern is maintained with this type of cast.

Cast application is almost always done with the patient under general anesthesia because the patient must be motionless during application and initial curing of the cast material. In addition, awake patients may be in too much pain to allow manipulation of the leg into the proper position for a cast. The risks of general anesthesia and especially recovery from anesthesia must be weighed against the risks of an improperly applied cast.

> **TECHNICIAN NOTE**   The consequences of a poorly fitting cast are potentially disastrous.

The consequences of a poorly fitting cast are potentially disastrous. Strangulation, ulceration, fractures, dislocations, and refusal to bear weight on the cast are real concerns with any cast, and poor fit greatly increases the likelihood of these complications. The exception is the foot cast, which can be placed on awake, standing, cooperative patients under ideal circumstances. In some emergency situations when anesthesia is impossible or impractical, temporary limb casts have been placed without general anesthesia, to allow transportation of the patient to a treatment facility.

Clinicians have individual preferences about how to clean the leg and prepare it for the cast, whether or not to use orthopedic felt padding, and what type of additional padding or covering to use underneath the cast. Talcum powder, powdered boric acid, or corn starch is sometimes rubbed into the skin to help absorb moisture. The underlying condition of the leg determines the need for topical medications and additional wound dressings. Bulkiness of materials should be minimized. In general, the less bulk beneath the cast, the better the fit that can be obtained.

> **TECHNICIAN NOTE**   Cast applications are almost always done with the patient under general anesthesia.

The bottom (weight-bearing) surface of the cast in large animals requires an additional protective layer to prevent wearing away of the cast. Clinicians may prefer to add a metal walking bar, a piece of rubber tread, a piece of plywood, or an acrylic such as methylmethacrylate that can be spread over the bottom of the cast (Fig. 9-74). All casting materials to be used should be identified and assembled before anesthesia is induced.

Because the hoof is included in almost all casts, it should be cleaned as thoroughly as possible. It is not wise to enclose a dirty hoof in a high-moisture, poorly aerated environment such as a cast because fungal or bacterial infections ("thrush") of the hoof can easily result. Trimming or paring of the frog, sole, and hoof wall helps remove the outer layer of debris and contaminants. Any infected areas should also be removed by trimming. A scrub brush is used to clean off all surfaces of the hoof completely, with a povidone-iodine scrub or solution. The hoof should then be rinsed and dried. The sulci of the sole and frog can be packed with cotton or gauze soaked in povidone–iodine solution if thrush is a concern.

> **TECHNICIAN NOTE**   The hoof should be thoroughly cleaned and dried before a cast is applied.

Casting tape is available in rolls; 3- to 4-inch width is appropriate for large animals. The rolls are activated by immersing them in warm water. The application of the casting tapes on the patient typically requires at least three people (in addition to the anesthetist): one person to unwrap and moisten the tape rolls, one to two people to hold the leg in proper position, and one to two people to actually apply and mold the casting material. The step-by-step casting process is

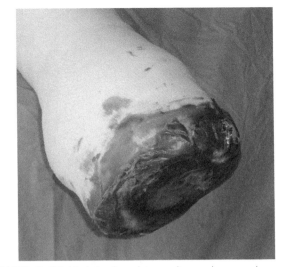

FIGURE 9-74 Methylmethacrylate acrylic can be spread across the bottom of the cast for protection. (From Bassert JM, Thomas J, editors: *McCurnin's clinical textbook for veterinary technicians*, ed 8, St. Louis, 2014, Saunders.)

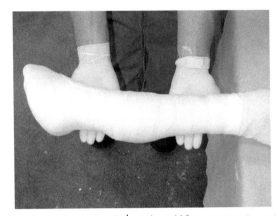

FIGURE 9-75 **Preventing indentations.** When assisting in cast application, keep the hands open and hold the fingers together to avoid leaving indentations. (From Bassert JM, Thomas J, editors: *McCurnin's clinical textbook for veterinary technicians*, ed 8, St. Louis, 2014, Saunders.)

similar to casting in small animals. When molding the material to the limb, it is important not to make indentations in the casting tape. Keeping the hands open and holding the fingers together help prevent making indentations, which can lead to pressure sores (Fig. 9-75).

Some anesthetic time must be devoted to the curing process. The cast should be hard before the patient is allowed to recover. Finishing the proximal end of a cast with an elastic adhesive tape is common to prevent bedding, feces, and other debris from collecting inside the cast and causing pressure sores and irritation (Fig. 9-76).

Strict stall rest is mandatory for casted patients. The most common cause of cast complications is excessive motion of the leg in the cast. Horses should not be forced to move unless absolutely necessary. Contrary to popular belief, excessively deep stall bedding can cause the patient to stumble and should be avoided.

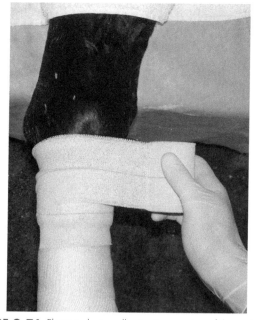

FIGURE 9-76 Placing elastic adhesive tape on top of the cast to form a seal prevents debris from getting down inside the cast. (From Bassert JM, Thomas J, editors: *McCurnin's clinical textbook for veterinary technicians,* ed 8, St. Louis, 2014, Saunders.)

> **TECHNICIAN NOTE**　Horses in casts should not be forced to move unless absolutely necessary.

Patients with casts are high priority with regard to monitoring and case care. Many things can go wrong in a hurry in patients with a cast, with grave consequences. The patient and cast should be checked for fit, cracking, heat, drainage, smell, swelling, redness, inflammation, irritation, discomfort, and pain. A clinic or hospital setting is highly preferred for these cases so that trained personnel can monitor the patients. Complete patient and cast monitoring should be done at least twice per day. Box 9-2 details the components of cast monitoring.

Suspected complications warrant immediate evaluation. Life-threatening consequences are possible, and a "let's look at it in the morning" attitude is not prudent. When casts are confirmed or suspected of causing a problem, a cast change is often necessary. A decision is made whether or not to recast the leg. General anesthesia will be necessary if another cast is contemplated.

Client education on casts should include warnings about cast (pressure) sores. Cast sores are expected in most patients, especially when the cast is left in place for longer than 1 week. Cast sores may be superficial, requiring minimal care. However, cast sores also can lead to deep, full-thickness wounds that may require significant care, including the possibility of skin grafts, to heal. These sores may lead to permanent scarring, including regrowth of white hair. The consequences of skin damage must be weighed against the consequences of trying to heal the leg's injury without a cast.

BOX 9-2　Monitoring of the Casted Patient

The "cast check," which should be done at least twice a day, should include evaluation of the following:

1. Temperature, pulse, and respiration (TPR): Elevation in temperature, pulse, or respiration may indicate inflammation or infection. Even mild increases in pulse or respiration may be early indicators of pain associated with inflammation. Close evaluation of the casted limb and the contralateral limb (especially the hoof for laminitis) should be performed.
2. Hot spots: Feel the cast for hot spots (areas of heat), which often indicate underlying inflammation such as a pressure sore. Some heat directly over wounds is expected. Pressure sores also generate heat and commonly develop over the heel bulbs, proximal sesamoid bones, accessory carpal bone, and the calcaneus. Distal limb casts tend to create sores at the top of the cast, over the dorsal aspect of the cannon bone. This area should be watched carefully for cast pressure sores.
3. Odor.
4. Exudate: The porous nature of fiberglass may allow exudates to appear on the surface of the cast. Depending on the nature of the underlying condition, exudation may or may not be expected. The clinician should be alerted if exudate is seen.
5. Swelling: Check the areas around the margins of the cast for swelling.
6. Wear: The bottom of the cast over the sole of the foot must be closely examined for excessive wear. If the leg shifts distally in the cast because of excessive wear, pressure sores and even strangulation of the leg may occur.
7. Cast integrity: Check the integrity of the cast (cracks, separation of layers).
8. Inflammation: Check the opposite limb for inflammation, especially over the digital tendons and the hoof. All hooves should be closely monitored for laminitis (heat, increased rate and strength of pulse, constantly shifting weight, reluctance to bear weight).
9. Weight bearing: The most important assessment is how the horse uses the cast, including willingness to bear weight. This should be observed several times a day. Any change in use, such as going from willingness to bear weight to refusal to bear weight on the cast, frequently indicates an underlying problem that must be carefully and immediately investigated.

> **TECHNICIAN NOTE**　It is important to inform clients about the possibility of cast sores.

Clients should always be warned about complications developing in the other legs. One of the most common complications of casts is laminitis in the other legs, especially in the contralateral limb. This complication is related to pain in the casted leg (from the cast, the underlying condition, or both), which forces the horse to spend increased time supporting its weight on the opposite, uncasted leg. The increase in weight bearing may also cause significant inflammation of tendons and ligaments in the opposite leg. When laminitis develops

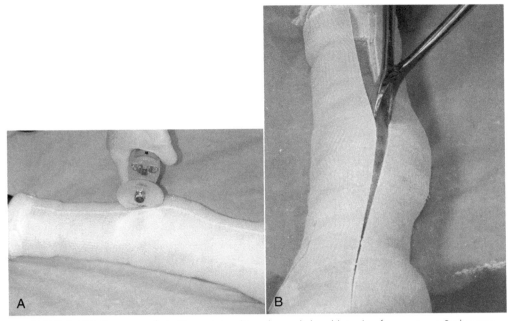

FIGURE 9-77 Cast removal. **A,** The cast is split on the medial and lateral surfaces using a Stryker saw, and the cut is continued under the foot. **B,** Once the cast is completely cut, the two halves are separated with cast spreaders. (From Bassert JM, Thomas J, editors: *McCurnin's clinical textbook for veterinary technicians,* ed 8, St. Louis, 2014, Saunders.)

in uncasted legs, the prognosis for survival is significantly worsened. Laminitis is less likely to occur when the casted leg is comfortable because the patient will bear more weight on the casted leg, thus providing some relief to the other legs. Still, laminitis may occur at any time, even in patients that appear comfortable on their casts. A firm distal limb wrap should always be placed on the contralateral limb to provide additional support to tendons and ligaments, and it should be reset daily to maintain firm compression. Some clinicians may also use frog supports to increase support and comfort of the opposite hoof.

Because motion and activity tend to increase the complication rate, sedation may be required to calm active or anxious horses. Most horses tolerate casts extremely well; others may require sedation or tranquilization to facilitate acceptance of the cast. Usually, a horse does not completely reject a cast, but rejection does occur, and the client should be prepared for the possibility.

Cast removal at the end of treatment is preferably done with the patient standing to avoid reinjury of the leg during recovery from anesthesia. Restraint and often sedation are necessary because horses tend to move in response to the noise and vibration of the cast saw. The cast saw is used to bivalve (score) the cast along its medial and lateral aspects. Medial and lateral scoring is preferred to prevent accidental lacerations of the superficial digital flexor tendon. The score lines are then connected by scoring across the bottom of the cast. Cast spreaders are used to open the cast in preparation for cast removal (Fig. 9-77). Bandage scissors are used to cut through the underlying stockinette and wound dressings, and the cast is removed. Once the cast is removed, the

leg should be cleansed, and a splint or heavy bandage wrap should be applied. Radiographs may be necessary after cast removal, so materials and radiographic equipment should be assembled beforehand.

> **TECHNICIAN NOTE** It is important to have radiographic equipment prepared before removing a cast because radiographs are often taken after cast removal.

HEAD AND FACE BANDAGES

Because of the anatomy of the head, it is not possible to apply firm compression bandages without compromising circulation, breathing, or vision. However, it is possible to protect wounds from environmental contamination by covering them, and sometimes light compression can be applied.

In some situations, elastic adhesive tape can be used to circle the head and secure underlying wound dressings. The tape can be applied with moderate tension, with care taken not to compromise breathing.

More commonly, an orthopedic stockinette is used to create a "head sleeve" bandage. A 4-inch stockinette can be used for foals and small equids, but a 6-inch stockinette is required for most other equine patients. The length of the stockinette should be approximately twice as long as the length of coverage desired on the head. The stockinette is rolled up into a donut shape, placed around the nose, and unrolled toward the ears. Eye and ear holes need to be cut out of the stockinette for the horse's comfort. This is best accomplished by marking the locations of these structures on the stockinette with a marking pen, removing the stockinette from the horse, and using bandage scissors to create circular 1- to 2-inch openings at each of the four marked locations. The stockinette is rolled up again, and the injured area is cleaned, medicated, and covered with a wound dressing if indicated. The stockinette is then placed back on the horse. Each of the openings can easily be enlarged for a custom fit, usually by using the fingers, to rip the material carefully. Using scissors to enlarge the openings while the stockinette is on the horse is not advisable because injury could result if the horse moves.

> **TECHNICIAN NOTE**   It is not advisable to enlarge stockinette openings with scissors because injury could result if the horse moves.

Once positioned, the stockinette wrap must be secured to keep it in place. The rostral aspect is secured directly to the skin with two to three circles of elastic adhesive tape, placed to contact the stockinette and the adjacent skin but carefully avoiding any compromise to the nasal passages. The caudal aspect of the bandage is secured by making a small slit in the stockinette between the ears. The forelock or mane hairs can be passed through this hole and secured with adhesive tape to form a securing loop of hair, which keeps the bandage from sliding down the face. If hair is not available, tape or string can be passed through the slit and around the top of the halter. Elastic adhesive tape can also be used, being cautious not to obstruct breathing or blood flow around the throat latch.

ABDOMINAL ("BELLY BAND") WRAPS AND THORACIC ("CHEST") WRAPS

These abdominal and thoracic bandages are similar with regard to materials and placement. They are used to cover wounds, incisions, and drains placed in the pleural or abdominal cavity. They can be placed to passively cover the affected area or placed with moderate tension to provide some compression or support to an area.

The basic material is 3- to 4-inch-wide, elastic adhesive tape. Multiple rolls of tape are usually necessary. The bandage is started cranially and is spiraled caudally around the patient's body to cover the desired area. Because removal of the tape tends to be painful (the tape pulls hairs out of the follicles), it is common first to cover the skin with roll gauze (or a minimal thickness of a padding material). The bandaging tape is then placed to cover the gauze completely; in addition, the gauze is anchored cranially and caudally by overlapping the tape onto the adjacent skin.

> **TECHNICIAN NOTE**   Abdominal bandages should be started cranially and spiraled caudally.

Removal of elastic adhesive tape typically pulls out hair. Short, quick pulls on the tape can help to minimize patient discomfort.

An alternative to the tape bandage just described is the spider bandage. A large, heavy cloth material (nonelastic) is cut to form a square or rectangle large enough to encircle the thorax or abdomen completely. The borders of the cloth are cut to form several extensions ("legs") of cloth that are long enough to be tied together across the back of the patient. This type of bandage is washable and reusable, which is cost saving to the client. However, it is difficult to achieve uniform, firm compression with this type of wrap.

TAIL BANDAGES AND WRAPS

Tails are bandaged for several reasons: for protection during shipping; for protection from feces, urine, or fetal fluids; and for prevention of contamination of the vulva or perineum during medical and surgical reproductive procedures. Tail bandages are used when it is impractical or impossible to have an assistant simply hold the tail out of the way. These bandages are often used during reproductive procedures.

The arterial supply to the tail is through a single major artery, the coccygeal artery, located on the tail's ventral midline. If this artery is strangulated, the entire tail can be sloughed. For this reason, it is best to avoid circling the living portion of the tail with nonelastic materials (however, these materials can be used safely on the tail hairs alone). If an elastic material is used to circle the tail, it should not be applied tightly. Tail wraps should be changed daily, and the tail should be checked closely for signs of strangulation (swelling, cool temperature, skin discoloration, loss of sensation).

> **TECHNICIAN NOTE**   If an elastic material is used to circle the tail, it should not be applied tightly.

Commercially available tail wraps are made of Neoprene rubber and are secured with hook-and-loop closure. Moisture tends to form under the rubber, so the wrap should be removed and cleaned and the tail dried daily (Fig. 9-78).

The tail can also be wrapped with roll gauze. Six-inch nonsterile gauze is ideal because it can be used to contain the tail hairs, and enough length is left to be passed around the neck and tied. With this maneuver, an assistant does not have to hold the tail out of the way while the clinician performs reproductive procedures and surgical interventions. The gauze is spiraled around the tail to a level below the vulva, with care taken not to strangulate the coccygeal artery. The gauze is seated at the base of the tail by circling it two to three times, and then the gauze is spiraled distally to the desired level. As each spiral passes over the dorsal aspect of the tail, a small loop of tail hair is grasped and pulled proximally over the gauze. This forms a series of "locking loops" of tail hairs that keeps the gauze from sliding off the tail (Fig. 9-79, *A* to *C*).

Once the desired level below the vulva is reached, a simple knot is tied to secure the wrap (distal to the coccygeal vertebrae). The gauze is passed cranially, circled around the neck once from ventral to dorsal and back, and then tied with a quick-release knot (Fig. 9-79, *D* to *H*).

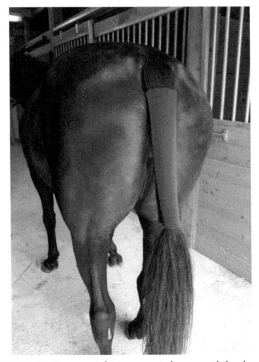

FIGURE 9-78 Commercial Neoprene tail wrap with hook-and-loop fastener.

> *TECHNICIAN NOTE* When the gauze of a tail tie is encircled around the neck, it is important to tie it with a quick-release knot.

The neck loop partially obstructs blood flow through the jugular veins, and distention is seen cranially to the loop. This will not present a problem if the loop is used for only a few minutes. However, if longer use is necessary, the person attending the horse's head should be instructed to "burp" (relieve) the jugular veins every 1 to 2 minutes by simply pulling the gauze loop away from the neck and allowing the jugular venous distention to subside (Fig. 9-80). If this step is not taken, horses can develop dyspnea from nasal swelling and can even lose consciousness (pass out) in rare instances.

> *TECHNICIAN NOTE* If the neck loop of a tail tie is to be left in place for longer than a few minutes, it is important to "burp" the jugular veins every 1 to 2 minutes by simply pulling the gauze loop away from the neck.

To remove the tail wrap, the encircling neck loop is released by pulling the quick-release knot. The tail portion of the wrap is removed by grasping the wrap at the proximal end and pulling it distally in one smooth motion (Fig. 9-81).

TAIL BAGS

Horses with conditions such as diarrhea, impending foaling, or paralysis of the tail tend to soil the tail. Soiling then requires a tail bath, which is time consuming and, in the case of infectious diarrhea such as *Salmonella,* places the technician at risk of exposure to the infectious organisms. A plastic tail bag can be useful in these cases because it prevents soiling of the tail and can be changed daily or as needed. A rectal sleeve with the hand portion removed makes an ideal plastic tail "sleeve." Removal of the hand portion is necessary to allow good air flow under the sleeve; otherwise, moisture can build and cause skin irritation.

The tail hairs are braided or taped (distal to the coccygeal vertebrae) so that they will be contained within the length of the plastic sleeve. The sleeve is then slid over the tail and is secured near the base of the tail with two to three circles of an elastic adhesive tape, by placing the tape to contact the skin adjacent to the proximal extent of the plastic sleeve. The anchoring tape should be placed passively (without applying compression) to avoid strangulation of the arterial supply (Fig. 9-82).

NERVE BLOCKS AND JOINT INJECTIONS

Equipment needed:
- Mepivacaine HCl 2%
- Needle
- Syringe
- Surgical scrub
- Alcohol

Nerve blocks are performed as a means of diagnostic local anesthesia, and they are commonly used during lameness examinations to localize the lameness to a specific area of the leg. A local anesthetic is used to deaden a nerve. If the lameness improves after application, then the painful lesion can be localized to that location or distal. Nerve blocks or joint blocks are used to localize the area of origin of the lameness. In joint injections, a steroid, hyaluronic acid, or some other drug is deposited within the joint space. These injections are often used to help treat lameness. The procedures are similar and are therefore discussed together.

Before performing a nerve block, remember that strict asepsis is extremely important, especially if the block is intended to be placed as a joint injection or joint block. A fresh bottle of local anesthetic should be used. Another consideration is that the most painful aspect of a joint injection is when the needle passes through the skin or joint capsule. Therefore, when inserting the needle, quick insertion is in your favor. Sometimes a bleb of local anesthetic in the skin can help when injection into a joint is necessary.

When you begin performing nerve blocks, you start at the most distal nerves first because you will block the nerves distally. If you started proximally, you would not be able to identify the site of origin of the lameness because you would block the whole leg to start with; therefore, by starting distally and working proximally, you are able to isolate nerves that start lower on the leg and identify where the lameness resolves as you work proximally. Something to keep in mind is never to perform a nerve block through a potentially contaminated site such as a wound or region of cellulitis because you could spread infection.

The reason that mepivacaine HCl 2% is used most commonly is that it is less irritating to the tissues compared with other local anesthetics. The toxic dose of local anesthetics is approximately 13 mg/kg or 6 mg/pound, and if this is reached, complications such as heart block, convulsions, and

bradycardia can result. After the nerve block is performed, you should wait 10 to 25 minutes for the anesthetic to take effect. With an injection into a joint, this waiting period can be 5 to 10 minutes.

To prepare the site for injection, you can clip the hair (not necessarily required unless it is a joint injection; in that case I always recommend shaving). The site should then be disinfected with 70% alcohol. For nerve injections,

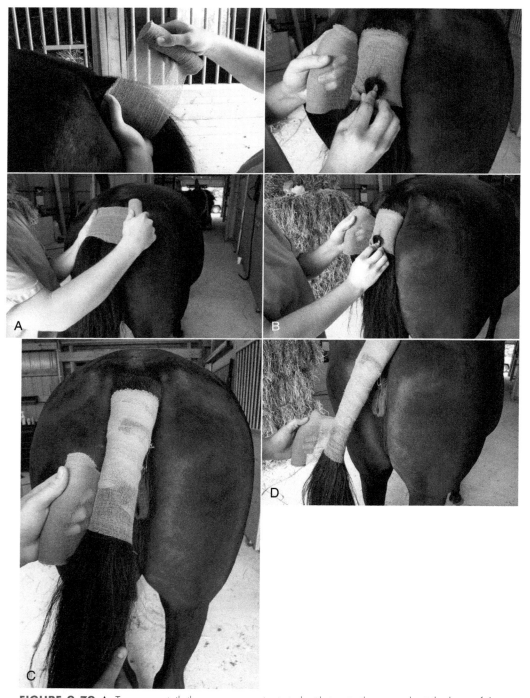

FIGURE 9-79 A, To wrap a tail, the gauze wrap is started with two to three rounds at the base of the tail. **B,** Several tail hairs are pulled proximally to form a locking loop between each pass of the gauze. **C,** For female reproductive procedures, the wrap should extend at least to the ventralmost aspect of the vulva. **D,** The wrap is commonly continued several inches below the vulva.

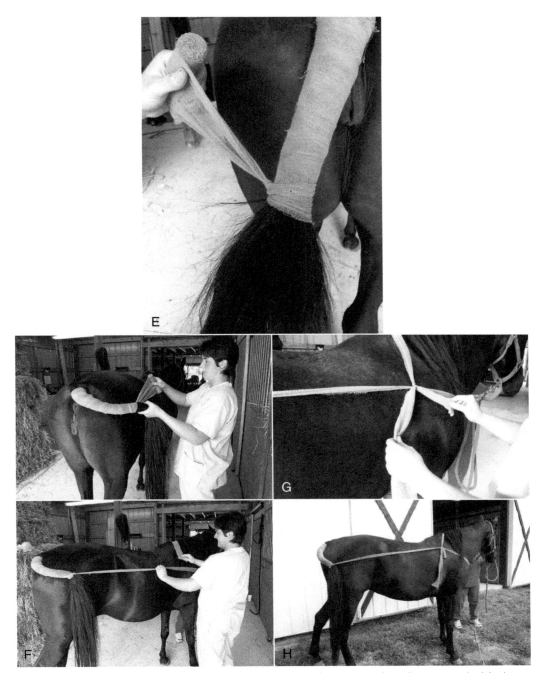

FIGURE 9-79, cont'd E, A simple knot is tied to secure the wrap. **F,** The tail is supported while the gauze is passed cranially around the neck. **G,** A quick-release knot secures the wrap around the neck. **H,** Completed tail wrap.

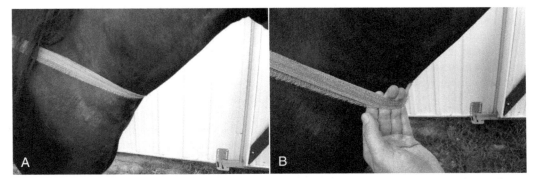

FIGURE 9-80 A, Jugular vein distention results from partial occlusion by the tail wrap. **B,** Relieving the distention by lifting the gauze away from the neck.

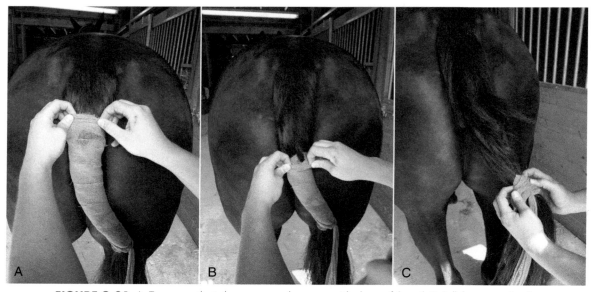

FIGURE 9-81 **A,** To remove the tail wrap, grasp the gauze at the base of the tail. **B,** Pull the gauze distally to remove it. **C,** Remove the wrap easily by sliding it off the tail.

you can then perform the injection. However, if you are performing a joint injection, the area must then have a 7- to 10-minute surgical scrub performed before the site is injected. During joint injections, sterile gloves should be worn. Figures 9-83 to 9-103 illustrate regional diagnostic anesthesia techniques relating to nerve blocks.

Ocular nerve blocks are also performed to help perform ophthalmic examinations or ophthalmic procedures. Dental nerve blocks can also be performed to help provide analgesia when performing dental procedures. The same aseptic procedures are required as with nerve blocks described earlier (Figs. 9-104 to 9-107).

PREPUTIAL AND PENILE CLEANING

The prepuce and penis may accumulate a thick, foul-smelling, dark-colored material known as smegma. *Smegma* is the combination of secretions from sebaceous glands, sweat glands, dead cells, and dirt. Smegma tends to accumulate on the surface of the glans penis and inside the prepuce, where it causes crusting and irritation of the tissues. The tip of the penis also accumulates smegma in the urethral fossa (diverticulum), which is a 1-inch-deep "pocket" that completely encircles the urethral opening (Fig. 9-108). Smegma in the urethral fossa tends to harden into round balls that horse handlers and owners refer to as "beans" (Fig. 9-109). Horses may form multiple beans, which can reach walnut size. The pocket shape of the fossa usually retains the beans and prevents them from falling out. The beans can compress the tip of the urethra and make urination difficult and painful. Because of these potential complications, part of the routine care of all male horses (castrated or not) includes cleaning the penis and prepuce; this procedure is referred to as "sheath cleaning." Some horse owners perform sheath cleaning on their own horses, but many request the

veterinarian to perform it, especially when sedation is required to make the horse cooperate.

> **TECHNICIAN NOTE**   Smegma tends to harden into round balls, called "beans," within the urethral fossa.

Sheath cleaning begins with proper restraint of the horse. Gloves (nonsterile) should be worn for the procedure. The penis is extended manually or with the aid of tranquilization. While one hand holds the penis, the other hand gently cleanses the penis and internal surface of the prepuce with either roll cotton or 4 × 4 gauze squares and warm water. Vigorous scrubbing should be avoided. Crusts are softened with water and are gently removed. The tip of the penis is examined, and a finger is inserted into the urethral fossa to remove any beans. The finger is swept 360 degrees around the fossa to ensure thorough cleaning. In cases where crust removal leaves open sores, a small amount of nonirritating antibacterial ointment applied to the lesions may be beneficial.

Mild soap may be used during the cleaning procedure, although its use is optional. Some people believe that soap alters the normal bacterial flora and predisposes the horse to infectious problems. Soap also may be irritating to the tissues (especially povidone-iodine). If soap is used, it must be completely rinsed off the area to prevent tissue irritation. Rinsing is done with clean water, never with alcohol.

The frequency of sheath cleaning varies greatly among individual male horses. Most patients benefit from cleaning several times per year, but some animals form more smegma and must be cleaned more frequently (monthly). Older males tend to form more smegma than younger males. Breeding stal-

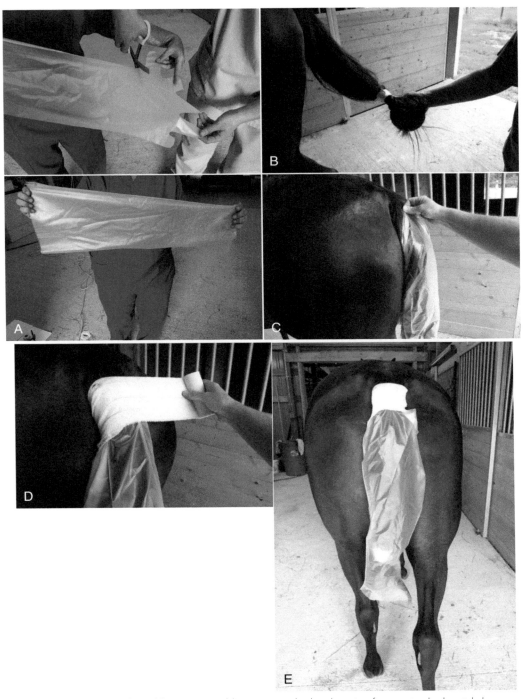

FIGURE 9-82 **A,** The tail bag is created by removing the hand portion from a standard rectal sleeve. **B,** The tail is braided or taped to a length that will be totally covered by the tail bag. **C,** The tail is placed inside the sleeve. **D,** Elastic adhesive tape is placed around the base of the tail to hold the sleeve in place. **E,** Completed tail bag.

lions are routinely cleaned before breeding or semen collection. Owners of male horses should visually observe the penis when it is extended for urination and have sheath cleaning performed as soon as smegma buildup (flakes or deposits of smegma) is observed. Sometimes the male horse does not extend the penis from the prepuce to urinate; although this may be normal for an individual, it also may indicate pain and warrants consulta-tion with a veterinarian. Similarly, preputial swelling, dribbling urine, or blood in the urine should be evaluated (Box 9-3 and Fig. 9-110).

> **TECHNICIAN NOTE** Antimicrobial ointment should be applied to open sores on the penis.

Text continued on p. 324

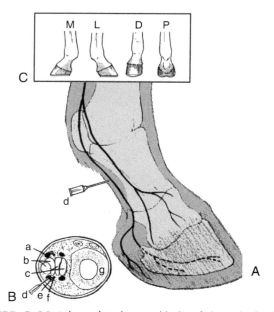

FIGURE 9-83 Palmar digital nerve blocks of the right forelimb. **A,** Lateral aspect. **B,** Cross-section. *a,* Medial palmar digital nerve; *b,* superficial flexor tendon; *c,* deep flexor tendon; *d,* lateral palmar digital nerve; *e,* vein; *f,* artery; *g,* second phalanx. **C,** Desensitized subcutaneous area. **D,** Dorsal aspect; *L,* lateral aspect; *M,* medial aspect; *P,* palmar aspect. (From Muir WW, Hubbell JAE, editors: *Equine anesthesia: monitoring and emergency therapy,* ed 2, St. Louis, 2009, Saunders.)

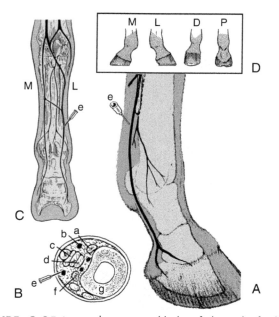

FIGURE 9-85 Low palmar nerve blocks of the right forelimb. **A,** Lateral aspect. **B,** Cross-section. *a,* Second metacarpal bone; *b,* medial palmar nerve; *c,* superficial digital flexor tendon; *d,* deep digital flexor tendon; *e,* lateral palmar nerve; *f,* fourth metacarpal bone; *g,* third metacarpal bone. **C,** Palmar aspect. **D,** Desensitized subcutaneous area. *D,* Dorsal aspect; *L,* lateral aspect; *M,* medial aspect; *P,* palmar aspect. (From Muir WW, Hubbell JAE, editors: *Equine anesthesia: monitoring and emergency therapy,* ed 2, St. Louis, 2009, Saunders.)

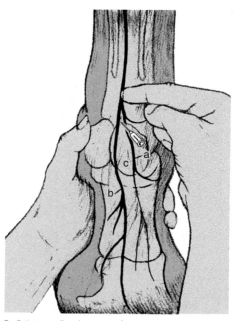

FIGURE 9-84 Needle placement for right abaxial sesamoidean nerve blocks of the right forelimb, caudolateral aspect. *a,* Dorsal digital; *b,* palmar digital nerve; *c,* right sesamoid. (From Muir WW, Hubbell JAE, editors: *Equine anesthesia: monitoring and emergency therapy,* ed 2, St. Louis, 2009, Saunders.)

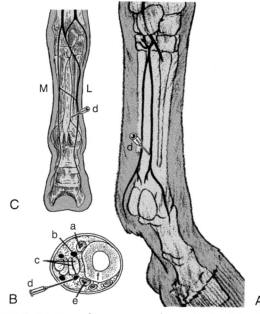

FIGURE 9-86 Low palmar metacarpal nerve blocks of the right forelimb. Needle placement to lateral palmar metacarpal nerve. **A,** Caudolateral aspect. **B,** Cross-section. *a,* Second metacarpal bone; *b,* medial palmar metacarpal nerve; *c,* deep digital flexor tendon; *d,* lateral palmar metacarpal nerve; *e,* fourth metacarpal bone; *f,* third metacarpal bone. **C,** Palmar aspect. *L,* Lateral; *M,* medial. (From Muir WW, Hubbell JAE, editors: *Equine anesthesia: monitoring and emergency therapy,* ed 2, St. Louis, 2009, Saunders.)

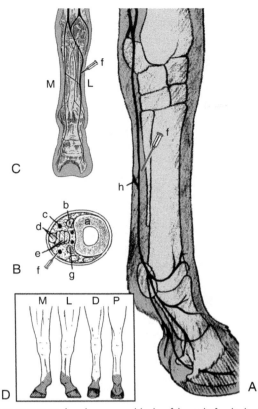

FIGURE 9-87 High palmar nerve blocks of the right forelimb. Needle placement to lateral palmar nerve. **A,** Caudolateral aspect. **B,** Cross-section. *a,* Third metacarpal bone; *b,* second metacarpal bone; *c,* medial palmar nerve; *d,* superficial digital flexor tendon; *e,* deep digital flexor tendon; *f,* lateral palmar nerve; *g,* fourth metacarpal bone; *h,* communicating branch. **C,** Palmar aspect. **D,** Desensitized subcutaneous area. *D,* dorsal aspect; *L,* lateral aspect; *M,* medial aspect; *P,* palmar aspect. (From Muir WW, Hubbell JAE, editors: *Equine anesthesia: monitoring and emergency therapy,* ed 2, St. Louis, 2009, Saunders.)

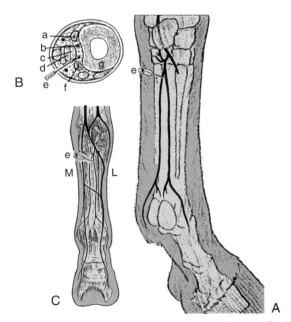

FIGURE 9-88 Proximal metacarpal nerve blocks of the right forelimb. Needle placement to lateral metacarpal nerve. **A,** Caudolateral aspect. **B,** Cross-section. *a,* Second metacarpal bone; *b,* medial palmar metacarpal nerve; *c,* suspensory ligament; *d,* accessory ligament; *e,* medial palmar metacarpal nerve; *f,* fourth metacarpal bone; *g,* third metacarpal bone. **C,** Palmar aspect. *L,* lateral; *M,* medial. (From Muir WW, Hubbell JAE, editors: *Equine anesthesia: monitoring and emergency therapy,* ed 2, St. Louis, 2009, Saunders.)

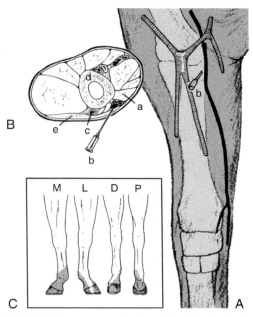

FIGURE 9-89 Median nerve blocks of the right forelimb. **A,** Craniomedial aspect. **B,** Cross-section. *a,* Flexor carpi radialis muscle; *b,* median nerve; *c,* cephalic vein; *d,* radius; *e,* superficial pectoral muscle. **C,** Desensitized cutaneous area. *D,* Dorsal aspect; *L,* lateral aspect; *M,* medial aspect; *P,* palmar aspect. (From Muir WW, Hubbell JAE, editors: *Equine anesthesia: monitoring and emergency therapy,* ed 2, St. Louis, 2009, Saunders.)

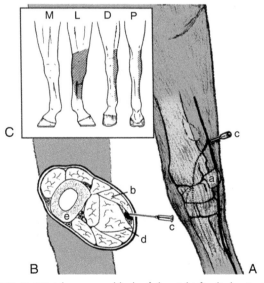

FIGURE 9-90 Ulnar nerve block of the right forelimb. **A,** Medial aspect. **B,** Cross-section. *a,* Accessory carpal bone; *b,* ulnaris lateralis muscle; *c,* ulnar nerve; *d,* flexor carpi ulnaris muscle; *e,* radius. **C,** Desensitized cutaneous area. *D,* Dorsal aspect; *L,* lateral aspect; *M,* medial aspect; *P,* palmar aspect. (From Muir WW, Hubbell JAE, editors: *Equine anesthesia: monitoring and emergency therapy,* ed 2, St. Louis, 2009, Saunders.)

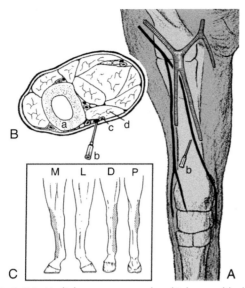

FIGURE 9-91 Medial cutaneous antebrachial nerve blocks of the right forelimb. **A,** Anteromedial aspect. **B,** Cross-section. *a,* Radius; *b,* medial cutaneous antebrachial nerve (branch of musculocutaneous nerve); *c,* cephalic vein; *d,* medial flexor carpi radialis muscle. **C,** Desensitized cutaneous area. *D,* Dorsal aspect; *L,* lateral aspect; *M,* medial aspect; *P,* palmar aspect. (From Muir WW, Hubbell JAE, editors: *Equine anesthesia: monitoring and emergency therapy,* ed 2, St. Louis, 2009, Saunders.)

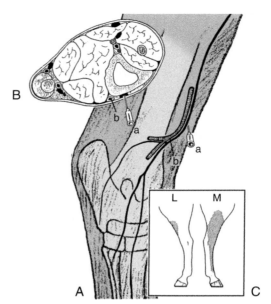

FIGURE 9-93 Saphenous nerve block of the left rear limb. **A,** Posteriomedial aspect. **B,** Cross-section. *a,* Saphenous nerve; *b,* medial saphenous vein. **C,** Desensitized cutaneous area. *L,* Lateral aspect; *M,* medial aspect. (From Muir WW, Hubbell JAE, editors: *Equine anesthesia: monitoring and emergency therapy,* ed 2, St. Louis, 2009, Saunders.)

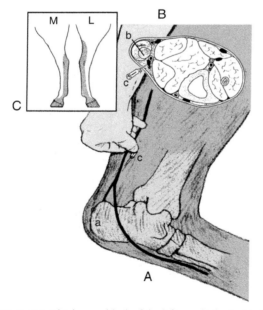

FIGURE 9-92 Tibial nerve block of the left rear limb. **A,** Medial aspect. **B,** Cross-section. *a,* Tarsus; *b,* combined tendons of gastrocnemius and superficial digital flexor tendon; *c,* tibial nerve. **C,** Desensitized cutaneous area. *L,* Lateral aspect; *M,* medial aspect. (From Muir WW, Hubbell JAE, editors: *Equine anesthesia: monitoring and emergency therapy,* ed 2, St. Louis, 2009, Saunders.)

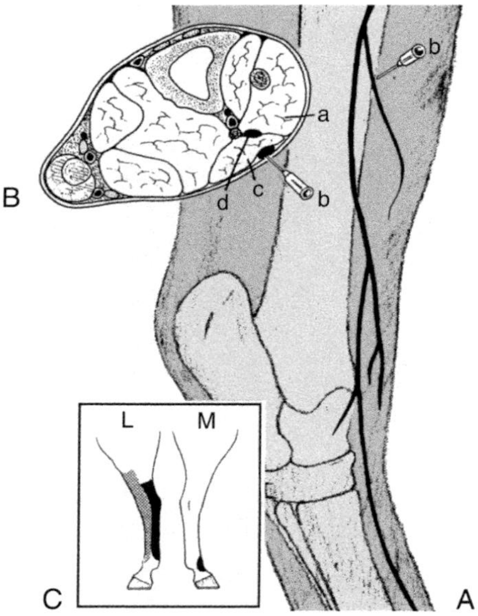

FIGURE 9-94 Superficial and deep peroneal nerve blockades of the right rear limb. **A,** Posterolateral aspect. **B,** Cross-section. *a,* Long digital extensor muscle; *b,* superficial peroneal nerve; *c,* lateral digital extensor muscle; *d,* deep peroneal nerve. **C,** Desensitized cutaneous area: *stipple,* after superficial peroneal nerve blockade; *solid,* after deep peroneal nerve blockade. *L,* Lateral; *M,* medial. (From Muir WW, Hubbell JAE, editors: *Equine anesthesia: monitoring and emergency therapy,* ed 2, St. Louis, 2009, Saunders.)

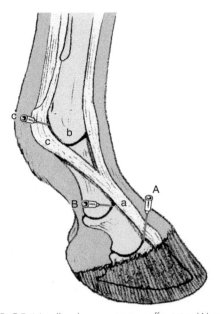

FIGURE 9-95 Needle placement into coffin joint *(A)*, pastern joint *(B)*, and lateral palmar pouch of the fetlock joint capsule *(C)*. *a*, Common digital extensor tendon; *b*, distal end of third metacarpal bone; *c*, annular ligament. (From Muir WW, Hubbell JAE, editors: *Equine anesthesia: monitoring and emergency therapy*, ed 2, St. Louis, 2009, Saunders.)

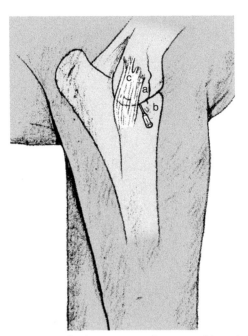

FIGURE 9-97 Needle placement into elbow joint of the right forelimb. *a*, Lateral humeral condyle; *b*, tuberosity of radius; *c*, lateral ligament. (From Muir WW, Hubbell JAE, editors: *Equine anesthesia: monitoring and emergency therapy*, ed 2, St. Louis, 2009, Saunders.)

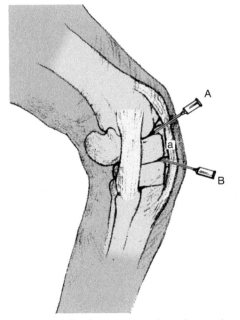

FIGURE 9-96 Needle placement into the radiocarpal joint *(A)* and intercarpal joint *(B)*. *a*, Extensor carpi radialis tendon. (From Muir WW, Hubbell JAE, editors: *Equine anesthesia: monitoring and emergency therapy*, ed 2, St. Louis, 2009, Saunders.)

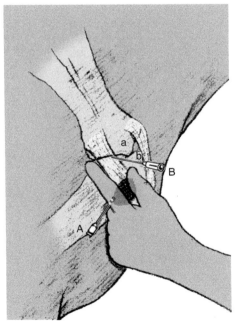

FIGURE 9-98 Needle placement into bicipital bursa *(A)* and shoulder joint *(B)* of the right forelimb. *a*, Brachial biceps tendon; *b*, anterior portion of lateral tuberosity of humerus. (From Muir WW, Hubbell JAE, editors: *Equine anesthesia: monitoring and emergency therapy*, ed 2, St. Louis, 2009, Saunders.)

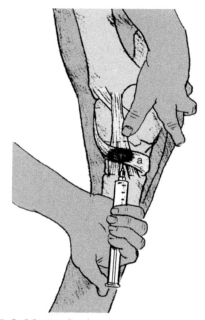

FIGURE 9-99 Needle placement into cunean bursa of the right rear limb, medial aspect. *a,* Cunean tendon. (From Muir WW, Hubbell JAE, editors: *Equine anesthesia: monitoring and emergency therapy,* ed 2, St. Louis, 2009, Saunders.)

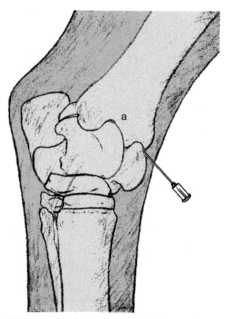

FIGURE 9-101 Needle placement into the tibiotarsal joint of the left rear limb, medial aspect. *a,* Medial malleolus. (From Muir WW, Hubbell JAE, editors: *Equine anesthesia: monitoring and emergency therapy,* ed 2, St. Louis, 2009, Saunders.)

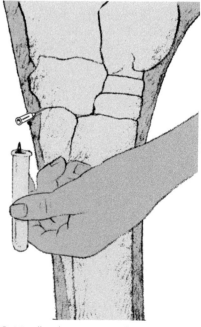

FIGURE 9-100 Needle placement into the tarsometatarsal joint of the right rear limb, posterolateral aspect. (From Muir WW, Hubbell JAE, editors: *Equine anesthesia: monitoring and emergency therapy,* ed 2, St. Louis, 2009, Saunders.)

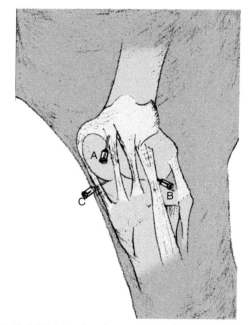

FIGURE 9-102 Needle placement into femoropatellar pouches *(A),* lateral femorotibial pouch *(B),* and medial femorotibial pouch *(C)* of the stifle joint. (From Muir WW, Hubbell JAE, editors: *Equine anesthesia: monitoring and emergency therapy,* ed 2, St. Louis, 2009, Saunders.)

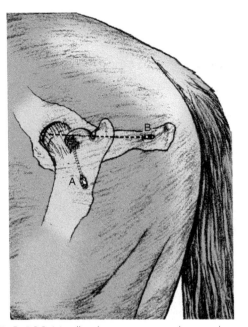

FIGURE 9-103 Needle placement into trochanteric bursa *(A)* and coxofemoral joint *(B)*. (From Muir WW, Hubbell JAE, editors: *Equine anesthesia: monitoring and emergency therapy,* ed 2, St. Louis, 2009, Saunders.)

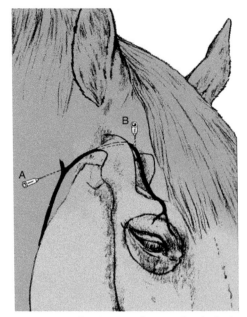

FIGURE 9-105 Needle placement for auriculopalpebral nerve block (methods *A* and *B*). (From Muir WW, Hubbell JAE, editors: *Equine anesthesia: monitoring and emergency therapy,* ed 2, St. Louis, 2009, Saunders.)

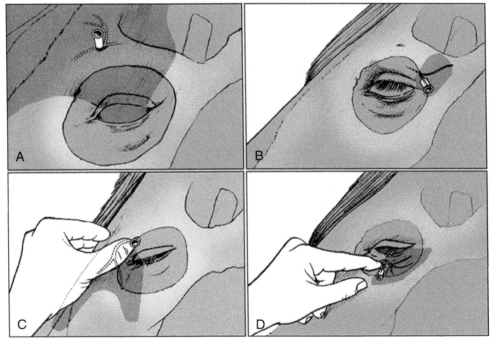

FIGURE 9-104 A, Needle placement for supraorbital (frontal) nerve block. *Stipple,* Desensitized subcutaneous area after blockade. **B,** Needle placement for lacrimal nerve block. *Stipple,* Desensitized subcutaneous area after blockade. **C,** Needle placement for infratrochlear nerve block. *Stipple,* Desensitized subcutaneous area after blockade. **D,** Needle placement for zygomatic nerve block. *Stipple,* Desensitized subcutaneous area after blockade. (From Muir WW, Hubbell JAE, editors: *Equine anesthesia: monitoring and emergency therapy,* ed 2, St. Louis, 2009, Saunders.)

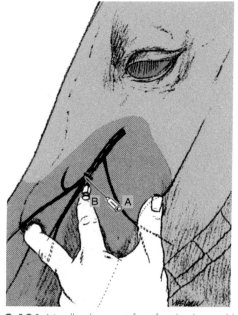

FIGURE 9-106 Needle placement for infraorbital nerve block at the infraorbital foramen *(A)* and within the infraorbital canal *(B)*. *Stipple,* Desensitized subcutaneous area after blockade. (From Muir WW, Hubbell JAE, editors: *Equine anesthesia: monitoring and emergency therapy,* ed 2, St. Louis, 2009, Saunders.)

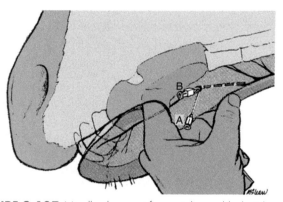

FIGURE 9-107 Needle placement for mental nerve block at the mental foramen *(A)* and mandibular alveolar nerve block within the mandibular canal *(B)*. *Stipple,* Desensitized subcutaneous area after blockade. (From Muir WW, Hubbell JAE, editors: *Equine anesthesia: monitoring and emergency therapy,* ed 2, St. Louis, 2009, Saunders.)

ELECTRONIC IDENTIFICATION

Implantation beneath the skin of a coded microchip that can be read with an electronic sensor is available for equines. The microchip, approximately the size of a rice grain, is encoded with the horse's registration or other identification number. Use of microchips is not yet common but is gaining in popularity.

The location for implantation is halfway between the withers and poll, approximately 1½ inches below the crest of the neck (Fig. 9-111). The chip is injected approximately 1 to 1½ inches beneath the skin, into the nuchal ligament. Studies in horses

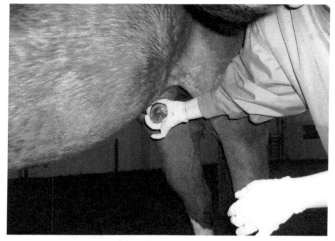

FIGURE 9-108 Tip of the glans penis. The swab is positioned at the entrance to the urethral fossa.

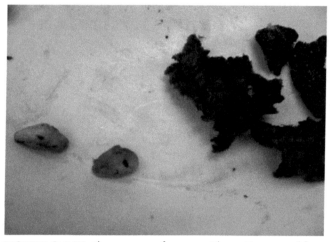

FIGURE 9-109 Three masses of smegma ("beans") recovered from the urethral fossa.

BOX 9-3	Snow and Horse Urine

Clients in colder climates commonly report seeing a red or orange color after their horses urinate on snow (especially on a sunny day) (Fig. 9-110). Although the color may result from blood in the urine, the far more likely cause is the presence of pigments called "porphyrins," which are normal components of the plants in the horse's diet. Sunlight activates the pigments in the urine, and the white snow highlights the color. Urinary tract problems are unusual in horses, so the occurrence of hematuria is uncommon. If any doubt exists, a urine sample for urine analysis and the presence of blood quickly provides an answer.

indicate that migration of the chip away from the implant site is not likely to occur. Some clients do not want the chip placed into the nuchal ligament and request the chip be placed in the same location but subcutaneously. Begin by clipping the implant location, although this is optional. Local anesthetic is optional. The injection site should be sterilely prepared. The horse is

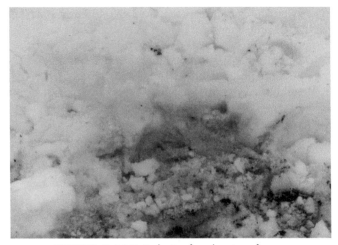

FIGURE 9-110 Red urine found on top of snow.

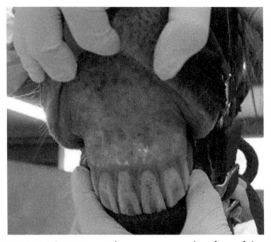

FIGURE 9-112 Tattoo on the upper mucosal surface of the equine lip. (From Sellon DC, Long MT: *Equine infectious diseases*, St. Louis, 2007, Saunders.)

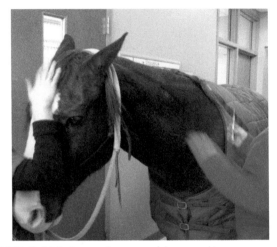

FIGURE 9-111 Proper placement of the microchip can occur at any location within the boundaries of the alcohol present in this image.

restrained as necessary. The chip is implanted by injection using a specially designed syringe and a 12-ga needle.

The injection site should be kept clean. Antibiotic ointment may be applied to the site for several days.

LIP TATTOOING

Equipment needed for lip tattooing:
- Lip clamp
- Tattoo gun
- Tattoo ink
- Alcohol
- Disinfectant

Horses can be tattooed on the mucosal side of the upper lip. Several racing authorities require lip tattoos as a method of identification. Tattoos are applied by tattoo technicians employed by the breed or racing governing bodies. The horse must be properly registered with its breed registry to receive the official tattoo. However, any horse owner can have his or her horses privately tattooed with any letter or number combination desired. Tattoo equipment is readily available from livestock supply companies.

Most official tattoos begin with a letter that corresponds to the year of birth, followed by a number sequence that matches the registration number. Thoroughbreds use all letters of the alphabet; the letter A was used in 1971, B in 1972, and so forth, until the letter A was used again in 1997. Standardbreds began a new system in 1982 (=A), but they do not use the letters I, O, Q, or U; therefore, the letter Z was used for 2003.

Horses preferably should be at least 1 year old when they are tattooed so that the lip is large enough for the tattoo gun to be applied. Once applied, the tattoo grows with the horse.

Restraint of the head is necessary; a standard lip twitch obviously cannot be applied. The upper lip is retained in a metal lip clamp that exposes and spreads the lip and helps in restraint by mimicking the effect of a twitch. Sedation may be necessary for some individuals.

After the lip clamp is applied, the area is cleaned with alcohol. The tattoo gun is checked for accuracy of the tattoo pattern and is dipped into antiseptic solution. Tattoo ink is spread across the tissue, and then the tattoo gun is applied to the lip (Fig. 9-112). The tattoo gun contains metal dies with sharp needles that make tiny punctures in the tissue and carry the ink into the tissue. The tattoo gun is applied by squeezing the handles and then is promptly removed. The fingers are used to rub the remaining ink into the perforations.

The tissue quickly heals over the punctures, capturing the ink. No special aftercare is necessary. Complications are rare.

FLUSHING OF THE NASOLACRIMAL DUCTS

Equipment needed for flushing nasolacrimal ducts:
- 20- to 22-ga lacrimal canula or 1- to 2-mm flexible catheter
- Sterile fluid
- Syringe

Like other domestic mammals, horses have a nasolacrimal duct system that functions to drain fluid from the surface of the eye to the nasal cavity. The duct system begins at the eye with two lacrimal puncta, one dorsal and one ventral, both located in the palpebral (eyelid) conjunctiva at the medial canthus (Fig. 9-113, *A*). The duct courses through the skull to open in the floor of the nasal cavity near the mucocutaneous junction of the nostril, usually in the pigmented cutaneous area (Fig. 9-113, *B*).

The duct system occasionally may become obstructed with mucus or other debris. Flushing the nasolacrimal duct is sometimes necessary to restore patency. The duct can be flushed from either end. Flushing through the lacrimal puncta can be difficult in the standing horse. Either a 20- to 22-ga lacrimal cannula or a small-diameter flexible catheter (tomcat urinary catheter) can be inserted into a punctum, and sterile fluid is injected through an attached syringe.

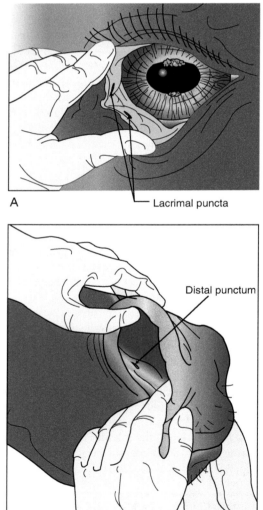

A ⌐ Lacrimal puncta

Distal punctum

B

FIGURE 9-113 A, The lacrimal puncta are located near the medial canthus of the eye. **B,** Nasal opening of the nasolacrimal duct on the floor of the nostril. (From Auer JA, Stick JA: *Equine surgery,* ed 3, St. Louis, 2006, Saunders.)

When the duct is unobstructed, fluid should flush from the nasal end of the duct.

Flushing from the nasal opening is much easier. A small 1- to 2-mm catheter is inserted into the nasal punctum, and sterile fluid is flushed. Horses usually are startled when the fluid suddenly enters the eye, and throwing the head is a common response. Personnel should be prepared for this reaction and should maintain good control of the head.

> **TECHNICIAN NOTE**   Horses are commonly startled when the fluid suddenly enters the eye during a nasolacrimal flush, and throwing the head is a common response.

SUBPALPEBRAL LAVAGE

Equipment needed for subpalpebral lavage:
- Subpalpebral lavage kit
- IV extension set
- Saline
- Cap
- Suture material
- Elastikon bandage
- Tongue depressor
- Petroleum jelly

Some ocular problems require long-term or frequent topical medication. Horses typically become resentful of ophthalmic treatments and can become difficult to handle. Occasionally, severe disease requires continual lavage of the eye. Indwelling lavage systems can be placed for reliable delivery of liquid ophthalmic solutions, except for ointments, which are too thick to be given by this method.

> **TECHNICIAN NOTE**   Horses typically become resentful of ophthalmic treatments after continuous application and can become difficult to handle.

The two main approaches for lavage systems are used: subpalpebral and nasolacrimal. Subpalpebral lavage systems are placed through one or two incisions in the upper or lower eyelid. Narrow rubber tubing is placed through the eyelid to open directly in the conjunctival sac, away from the cornea (Fig. 9-114). When preparing the skin for subpalpebral lavage, remember not to use chlorhexidine or alcohol around the eye. The tubing is sutured to the skin for stability. Usually, an IV extension set is attached to the tubing for easier access. Clinicians vary with regard to their preference for types of tubing and methods of securing tubing to the skin.

The other approach is the nasolacrimal lavage system, which uses tubing placed into the nasal punctum. A small stab incision through the nostril is often created so that the tubing can pass through the nostril and be secured to the skin. This helps protect the tubing from motion of the nostrils and possible nose rubbing by the patient.

When injecting through either type of system, the tubing should be cleaned before syringes or fluid lines are attached.

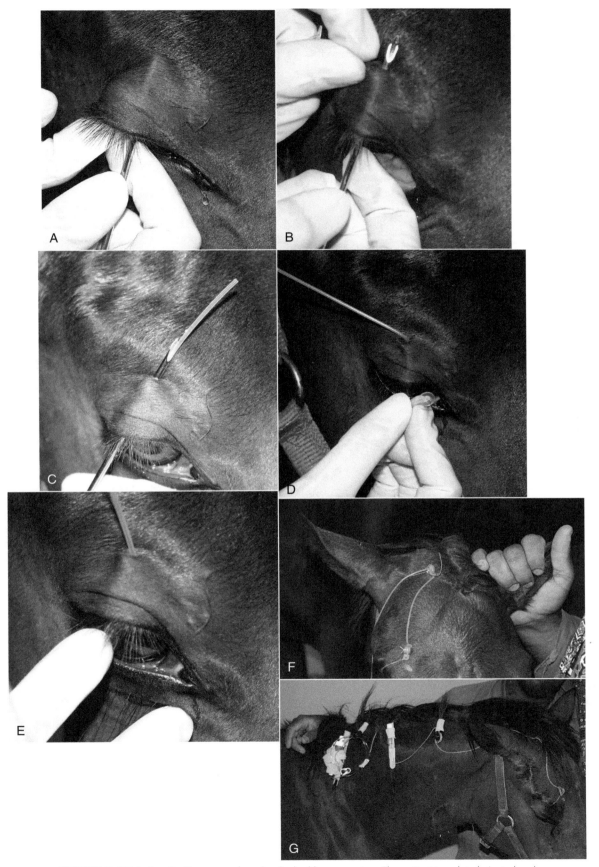

FIGURE 9-114 A to **G,** Placement of a subpalpebral lavage system. The patient is sedated. Auriculopalpebral and frontal nerve blocks are performed, and topical proparacaine (0.5 mL) is used to anesthetize the cornea and conjunctiva. From McAuliffe SB, Slovis NM: *Color atlas of diseases and disorders of the foal,* St. Louis, 2008, Saunders.)

The medication should be warm enough for the patient's comfort. The patient is often startled by the medication entering the eye, so gentle injection pressure is preferred. After a medication is injected, the catheter should be cleared with either a saline or air flush. Again, air hitting the eye can cause a patient reaction. After treatment is complete, the lavage tubing should be capped or covered to prevent debris from entering the system; an injection cap usually can serve this purpose. Excess solution flowing down the horse's face should be dried thoroughly. Continual wetness can scald the skin and cause hair loss. Applying petroleum jelly to the skin below the eye may provide some protection from "runoff."

> **TECHNICIAN NOTE** After completing a lavage tubing treatment, the catheter should be cleared with saline or air and capped or covered to prevent debris from entering the system.

SINUS TREPHINATION AND SINOCENTESIS

Equipment needed for trephination or sinocentesis:
- General anesthesia or sedation
- Clippers
- Betadine surgical scrub and alcohol
- Local anesthetic, a syringe, and needles
- Scalpel
- Jacobs hand chuck, Steinmann pin/bone drill, and stainless steel trephine
- Red rubber catheter
- Suture material and needles
- Bandage material
- Antibiotic ointment

Horses have an extensive network of paranasal sinuses, which are subject to a variety of diseases, most of which are infectious. Signs of sinus disease include nasal discharge, facial swelling, and possible malodor. The anatomy of the sinuses and their openings is complex and prevents visual examination with the endoscope and insertion of instruments through the natural internal openings. To examine and treat sinus diseases, alternate entrances directly into the sinuses through the skin must be made. *Centesis* refers to making a small-diameter hole (perforation) through bone. *Sinocentesis* refers to making a small-diameter hole through bone into a sinus. *Trephining* is the process of making a larger-diameter hole into a sinus by removing a small, circular piece of bone. Depending on the diameter of the hole, endoscopes, instruments, and tubing for flushing can be inserted for diagnostic and therapeutic purposes. Repulsion of cheek teeth can also be performed through trephine holes.

> **TECHNICIAN NOTE** Centesis refers to making a small-diameter hole through bone. Sinocentesis refers to make a small-diameter hole through bone into a sinus. Trephining is the process of making a larger-diameter hole into a sinus by removal of a small, circular piece of bone.

Sinocentesis and trephination can be performed with the patient under general anesthesia or on a standing horse by using sedation and local anesthesia.

Patient preparation for the standing procedure should be performed with appropriate physical and chemical restraint. If general anesthesia is being used, the technician should follow the anesthetic protocol.

The location depends on which sinus is to be entered (Fig. 9-115). The area is clipped and sterilely prepared. Local anesthesia (3 to 5 mL) is required if the procedure is performed on a standing animal. A stab or small incision is made through the skin with a scalpel.

The size of the intended hole determines the instrument used to penetrate the bone. Small holes (centesis) can be made with a Jacobs hand chuck and Steinmann pin or a bone drill. Larger holes are made with a stainless steel trephine (Fig. 9-116). A depth of only 2 to 3 cm is necessary to penetrate the sinus (Fig. 9-117).

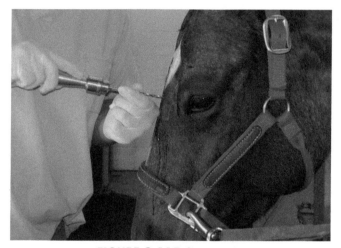

FIGURE 9-115 Sinocentesis.

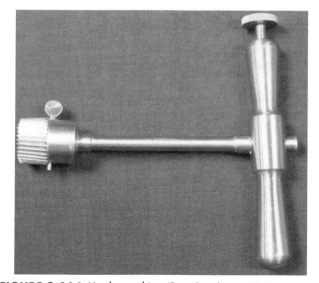

FIGURE 9-116 Horsley trephine. (From Sonsthagen TF: *Veterinary instruments and equipment: a pocket guide,* ed 2, St. Louis, 2011, Mosby.)

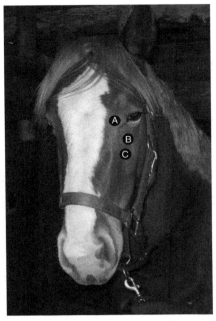

FIGURE 9-117 Location of trephine sites for the frontal sinus (A), caudal maxillary sinus (B), and rostral maxillary sinus (C).

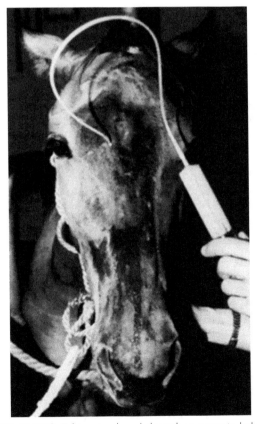

FIGURE 9-118 Tubing is placed through a centesis hole in the frontal sinus for diagnostic and treatment purposes. The tubing can be sutured to the skin for use as an indwelling catheter for sinus lavage. (From Bertone AL: The decision process: standing surgery versus general anesthesia and recumbency, *Vet Clin North Am Equine Pract* 7:485-735, 1991.)

The diagnostic or therapeutic procedure (endoscopy, sinus lavage) is then performed. Sometimes a rubber catheter or other tubing is placed through the hole and is secured to the skin for long-term flushing of the sinus (Fig. 9-118). Small stab incisions for sinocentesis can be left to heal by second intention or closed with a simple skin suture. Trephine sites can be left open to heal or the incisions can be closed, depending on the size of the trephine holes. In either case, the bone disk is discarded and not replaced. The skin can be closed with sutures or skin staples.

Open trephine holes should be covered to prevent material from entering the sinus. A head bandage using stockinette can be used to cover and protect the site. Otherwise, bandaging is optional. Pressure bandages are difficult to apply in this area, but light pressure may be possible with 4 × 4 gauze and elastic adhesive tape used to encircle the head carefully.

Aftercare includes keeping the incision clean and applying antibiotic ointment until the area heals. Sutures or staples are removed in 5 to 10 days. The area should be watched for signs of infection, including excessive swelling and discharge.

DENTISTRY

In 1995 the *American Association of Equine Practitioners (AAEP)* released a position statement on equine dentistry. It states, in part, that "Equine dentistry is the practice of veterinary medicine and should not be performed by anyone other than a licensed veterinarian or a certified veterinary technician under the employ of a licensed veterinarian."

The statement continues to define specific procedures that should be performed by veterinarians: "Any dental activity requiring sedation, tranquilization, analgesia or anesthesia and procedures which are invasive of the tissues of the oral cavity, including, but not limited to, extraction of permanent teeth, amputation of large molars, incisors and canine teeth, the extraction of first premolars (wolf teeth) and repair of damaged or diseased teeth, must be performed by a licensed veterinarian."

The role of the veterinary technician is also defined: "The rasping (floating) of molars, premolars and canine teeth and the removal of deciduous incisors and premolars *(caps)* may, provided a valid veterinary–client patient relationship exists, be performed by a certified veterinary technician under the employ of a licensed veterinarian."

The AAEP position statement should not be confused with state veterinary practice acts, and the technician should consult his or her state board of veterinary medicine for accepted veterinary practices in his or her state.

DENTAL EXAMINATION

Dental care should be part of a horse's routine health maintenance program. The oral cavity and teeth should be examined at least once per year by a veterinarian, but twice per year is a better recommendation for most horses. Horses with special dental problems may need to be checked three to four times per year. Most dental abnormalities begin with no obvious external signs and develop gradually over time.

However, the owner may report that the horse is having problems with chewing and eating, such as dropping partially chewed food from the mouth (quidding), hypersalivating, and tilting the head while eating. Foul odor to the breath often accompanies tooth root disease. Owners may also report chronic weight loss. Finding whole, undigested grain particles in the feces is not necessarily an indication of a dental problem, but it should be an indication for a complete oral examination to rule out dental abnormalities.

> **TECHNICIAN NOTE**   It is recommended that horses have their mouth inspected by a veterinarian yearly, but twice per year is even better.

The dental examination requires minimal equipment; a light source such as a penlight or flashlight and a dental speculum are all that are needed for many patients. A dose syringe to flush out the mouth is helpful. Physical restraint depends on the individual horse. Some uncooperative individuals require sedation to allow a thorough evaluation. The person performing the examination is in a vulnerable position and should stand to the side of the horse to avoid being struck by the front feet. Use of stocks or stacked hay bales may provide additional safety. Rarely, a fractious animal may require general anesthesia so that the handler can safely conduct an oral examination.

The dental examination begins with an evaluation of the incisors. The lips are separated with the hands to reveal the incisors and gums. The horse cooperates best if its breathing is not obstructed during this maneuver. The incisors are checked for number and proper occlusion (Fig. 9-119). The occlusal surfaces are checked for wear. The examiner then places the thumb into the interdental space and presses on the hard palate to encourage the horse to open the mouth (Fig. 9-120). The canines (if present) and rostral cheek teeth can be visually and manually examined, and the presence of wolf teeth (premolar 1 [PM1]) can be determined.

Full examination of the rest of the cheek teeth and oral cavity requires use of a speculum. In cooperative individuals, the tongue can be pulled laterally out of the mouth and held caudally against the commissure of the lips. In this position, the horse tends to hold the mouth open to avoid biting its own tongue (Fig. 9-121). Most individuals, however, require a mechanical mouth speculum to hold the mouth open for a thorough examination (Figs. 9-122 and 9-123). The cheek teeth are examined for number, sharp points, and occlusion.

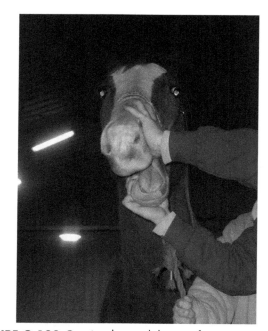

FIGURE 9-120 Opening the mouth by use of pressure against the hard palate.

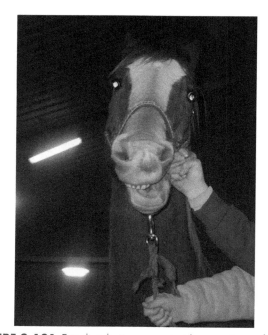

FIGURE 9-121 Extruding the tongue against the commissure of the lip encourages opening of the mouth.

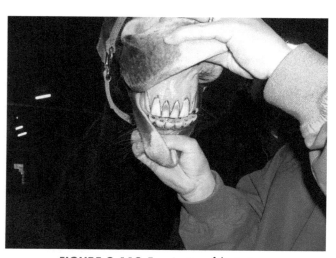

FIGURE 9-119 Examination of the incisors.

Visual examination alone may not be sufficient; manual evaluation is often necessary.

Radiographs are sometimes required as part of the dental examination, especially when involvement of tooth roots and accompanying sinus disease is suspected. Because radiographic cassettes and equipment are in close proximity to the patient's head and because of the prolonged exposure times needed for diagnostic quality films, sedation is almost always necessary. Common views include straight lateral (Fig. 9-124) and lateral oblique projections for the cheek teeth. Lateral oblique views are used to decrease superimposition and better view the cheek teeth roots. The dorsoventral projection is used less frequently for the cheek teeth but is valuable when sinus disease is suspected. Radiographs of the incisors are usually obtained with a dorsoventral (upper arcade) or ventrodorsal (lower arcade) projection. Superimposition of the incisors is alleviated by placing the film cassette between the incisors to create an intraoral or "bite plate" film. Grids are seldom necessary.

> **TECHNICIAN NOTE** Radiographs are sometimes required as part of the dental examination, especially when involvement of tooth roots and accompanying sinus disease are suspected.

The results of the dental examination should be noted in the medical record. Dental charts for equines are available and provide an excellent format to record findings and describe procedures performed. An example of an equine dental chart can be found on the Evolve website. Digital photographs can enhance documentation of pretreatment and posttreatment results. To review dental formulas and dental eruption timetables, see Chapter 8.

REMOVAL OF CAPS

The deciduous premolars ("caps") are usually present at birth or by 1 to 2 weeks of age. They are normally shed when the underlying permanent premolar teeth erupt at 2½ (PM2), 3 (PM3), and 4 (PM4) years of age (Fig. 9-125). Clients may find the caps on the stall floor or in feed buckets and may call with concern about the horse losing a tooth, or the clients may fail to recognize the "foreign object" as a tooth (Fig. 9-126).

Occasionally, the caps are not shed and are referred to as retained. Retained caps are often loose and may cause pain and reluctance to chew, swallow, or accept a bit. Retained caps should be removed. Extraction of the cap begins with adequate physical restraint. If the area is painful or the patient is uncooperative, sedation may be required. As with any dental procedure, the operator should carefully position his or her body to avoid being struck by the front legs or a violently raised head. An oral speculum facilitates the procedure. Removal is usually easily accomplished with an elevator to pry the cap loose and a grasping instrument such as cap-extracting forceps or wolf tooth forceps to remove the cap. The elevator is used to loosen any remaining tissue or tissue tags between the cap and the underlying permanent tooth. Once the cap is grasped with the forceps, the cap is gently rocked from side to side until it is removed. Bleeding is usually minimal, and no special aftercare is required.

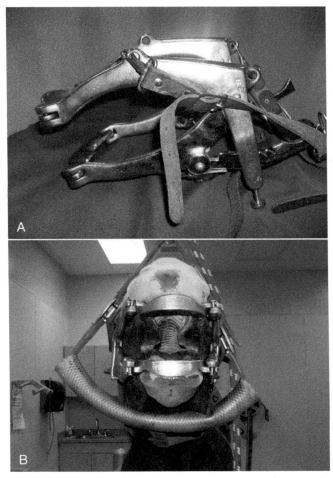

FIGURE 9-122 A and B, Full mouth speculum. Incisor plates provide leverage to hold the mouth open. The speculum is adjustable. (Courtesy Nebraska Equine.)

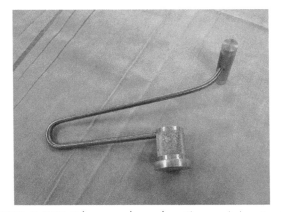

FIGURE 9-123 Schoupe oral speculum. The rounded portion is inserted between the cheek teeth on one side of the mouth. The bar is handheld outside the cheek to stabilize the speculum.

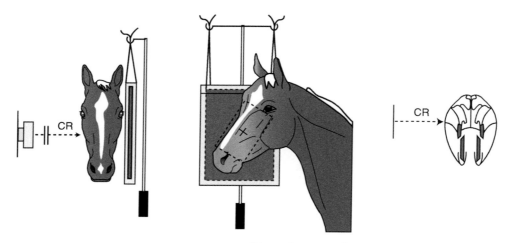

-------- Primary beam margins

FIGURE 9-124 Film cassette orientation for a straight lateral projection of the maxillary cheek teeth. *CR*, Central ray. (From Baker GJ, Easley J: *Equine dentistry,* Oxford, 2002, Saunders.)

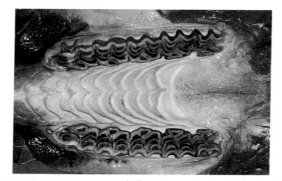

FIGURE 9-125 Transverse skull section at the level of premolar 3 (PM3) in a 3½-year-old horse. The short "caps" cover the oral aspect of each permanent PM3. (From Baker GJ, Easley J: *Equine dentistry,* Oxford, 2002, Saunders.)

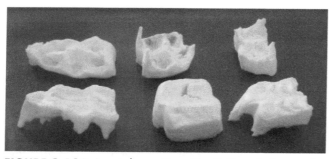

FIGURE 9-126 Assorted caps. (From Allen T: *Manual of equine dentistry,* St. Louis, 2003, Mosby.)

> **TECHNICIAN NOTE**   Caps that are not shed are referred to as retained caps.

WOLF TOOTH EXTRACTION

"Wolf tooth" is the layperson's term for the PM1. Wolf teeth are rudimentary and have no useful function. Mandibular wolf teeth are quite rare. Maxillary wolf teeth are more common

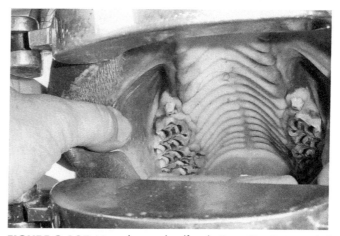

FIGURE 9-127 Normal erupted wolf teeth. (From Allen T: *Manual of equine dentistry,* St. Louis, 2003, Mosby.)

and are usually visible above the gum line immediately rostral to the second premolars (Fig. 9-127). However, they may fail to erupt ("blind" wolf teeth) and may be detected only by palpation. Many horses have no wolf teeth. Unlike the other premolars, PM1 is typically small, with a simple root. Because of its location, it may become sore from pressure from the bit and is often blamed for performance problems. Removal of wolf teeth has become a controversial subject.

> **TECHNICIAN NOTE**   Wolf tooth is the layperson's term for the first premolar.

The procedure is performed in the standing horse and involves proper physical restraint and safety precautions. Tetanus immunity status should be determined, and prophylaxis should be administered before the procedure, if necessary. Use of an oral speculum is desirable. Sedation is required; in addition, some clinicians inject 1 to 2 mL of local anesthetic into the mucosa around each wolf tooth. The instruments required are a dental elevator and a pair of extraction forceps. Wolf tooth elevators and wolf tooth forceps are made in a variety of sizes to accommodate different sizes of wolf teeth. A small scalpel blade is necessary to incise the gingiva over blind wolf teeth. The wolf tooth elevator is used to separate the gingiva and periodontal ligament from the entire circumference of the tooth, extending well below the gum line. The tooth is then grasped with the wolf tooth forceps and is gently rocked and rotated until the tooth is freed. Removal is usually straightforward, although occasionally the tooth root breaks off during extraction. This usually causes no problem and heals uneventfully. Bleeding is common after tooth removal. Typical aftercare consists of flushing the mouth with clean, warm water by using a 60-mL catheter-tip syringe several times daily for 2 to 3 days. A bit should not be placed in the horse's mouth for 3 to 5 days, to allow healing of the gingival tissue.

DENTAL FLOATING

Filing or rasping of the teeth is known as *floating*. It is the most common dental procedure in horses and is part of the routine health care program. Several factors contribute to the need for floating. The cheek teeth (premolars and molars) advance slowly from their alveoli into the mouth continuously for most of the horse's life. The occlusal surfaces are continually worn down by a natural side-to-side chewing motion, combined with sand and grit in the horse's diet, thus forming a "natural file" between opposing upper and lower teeth. However, the maxilla is approximately 30% wider than the mandible, which results in an "overhang" situation in which the upper and lower cheek teeth do not meet squarely. The buccal margin of the upper cheek teeth and the lingual margin of the lower cheek teeth are left without contact with an opposing surface. The natural file does not maintain these surfaces as well as the more central portions of the tooth, and these surfaces tend to become more prominent as the central portions are worn down. This results in formation of sharp edges, known as *points*, over time. Additionally, the upper and lower cheek teeth usually do not meet perfectly in the rostral-caudal plane. The upper cheek teeth are usually shifted slightly more rostrally, leaving the rostral margin of the upper PM2 and the caudal margin of the lower M3 without direct occlusion. Sharp points, referred to as *hooks (upper arcade)* and *ramps (lower arcade)*, tend to form along these surfaces (Fig. 9-128).

Points, hooks, and sharp edges can cause pain and discomfort to the horse and can result in ulcerations and lacerations of the tongue and oral tissues, poor performance, and problems with mastication. In severe cases, the horse may be unable to close the mouth completely. Severe cases often require cutting the teeth with special instruments to remove points before they can be filed smooth. Horses should be checked regularly for developing points and hooks, and dental floating should be performed to prevent these points and hooks from becoming problematic.

The age at which floating begins depends entirely on the individual's need for the procedure, which is determined by

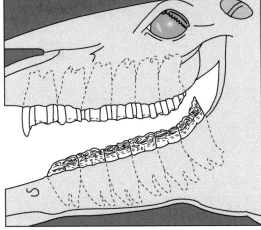

FIGURE 9-128 Hooks on the upper premolar 2 and ramps on the lower molar 3. Note the sharp points on the margins of the other cheek teeth. (From Allen T: *Manual of equine dentistry,* St. Louis, 2003, Mosby.)

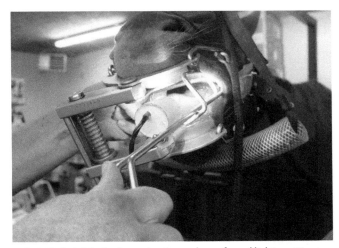

FIGURE 9-129 Oral examination and use of good lighting. (Courtesy Glenwood Veterinary Clinic.)

oral examination (Fig. 9-129). Most horses need floating by 3 to 4 years, but it is not uncommon for horses as young as 2 years old to have sharp points requiring treatment. (Note that when floating is performed in young horses, loose caps may dislodge and fall out of the mouth during the procedure.) The frequency of floating also depends on individual need. Most horses require floating at least once per year, but many need it twice yearly. Some horses, especially geriatric horses and horses with missing cheek teeth, may need floating three to four times per year.

> **TECHNICIAN NOTE**   Most horses need floating by age of 3 to 4 years.

The primary goal of floating is to remove hooks, points, and any other sharp edges from the cheek teeth, thereby restoring good occlusion and patient comfort. Floating is also used to prevent overgrowth of a tooth when the opposing tooth has been lost. Much less commonly, the canines and incisors are subject to overgrowth or prone to form sharp edges that must be filed to maintain occlusion and make the mouth comfortable.

> **TECHNICIAN NOTE**   The primary goal of floating is to remove hooks, points, and any other sharp edges from the cheek teeth, thereby restoring good occlusion and patient comfort.

The procedure is performed with the horse standing, except in intractable patients that may require general anesthesia. If horses become accustomed to the procedure at a young age and the procedure is performed by a patient operator, minimal physical restraint may be necessary. However, many horses dislike the noise and vibration associated with floating, and more aggressive physical restraint or chemical restraint must be used. The safety of personnel must be of

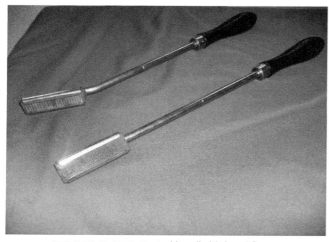

FIGURE 9-130 Typical handheld dental floats.

primary concern, especially given the vulnerable position of the operator.

A minimum amount of equipment is required for floating. A good light source is mandatory, and a mouth speculum usually is necessary. A stainless steel bucket with water and disinfectant is useful for cleaning the instruments during and after use. A dose syringe for flushing the mouth before and after the procedure also is useful.

A wide array of dental floats is available. Float handles and float blades are usually purchased separately, to allow replacement of the blade when it becomes worn or when a different blade texture (fine, medium, or coarse) is desired. Carbide blades are usually preferred over steel for their durability. Individual clinicians develop preferences for the shape and material of the handles and shafts. The basic float set includes a long, straight float handle or shaft and blade for the lower cheek teeth and a shorter, angled float handle or shaft and blade for the upper cheek teeth. Additional handles and blades with specialized shapes can be added to the basic set (Fig. 9-130). Motor-driven power floats have become popular. Floating teeth manually is a physical process that requires a good deal of stamina. Power floats save the operator some "elbow grease" and may be more effective for clinicians who lack strength. However, power floats are expensive, and horses may resent the noise they create (Fig. 9-131).

Floating is not a simple procedure. It is as much an art as it is a science and is best learned from clinicians experienced in the procedure. Seminars with wet laboratories and several good texts are available to help the technician learn proper techniques.

ELECTROCARDIOGRAM

Because the body consists primarily of water and electrolytes, similar to salt water, electrical currents are readily conducted throughout the body. It is possible to measure the changes in voltage between any two points on the surface of the body

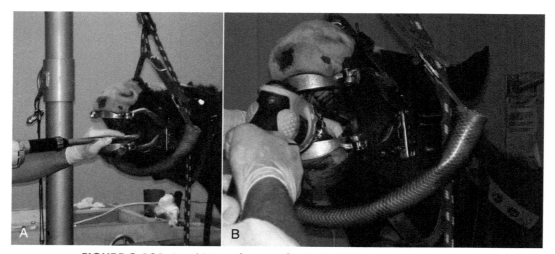

FIGURE 9-131 A and B, Use of a power floating tool. (Courtesy Nebraska Equine.)

with electrodes and record the findings on paper. This produces a trace called an electrocardiogram (ECG or EKG).

The ECG is useful for determining cardiac rate and rhythm and identifying problems with electrical conduction (arrhythmias) in large animals. However, unlike its use in small animals, it is not highly useful in calculating heart chamber enlargement in large animals because of differences in the anatomy and physiology of the Purkinje fiber system. Fortunately, echocardiography is readily available and more suitable than the ECG for assessing chamber size and myocardial function.

The standard ECG is performed on the standing animal at rest. However, some arrhythmias occur only occasionally or under special circumstances and may be missed by the standard 5- to 10-minute standing ECG. Long-term or ambulatory (Holter) ECG monitoring is readily available and is useful for detecting intermittent problems. The procedure uses flat electrodes attached to a portable monitor, which is fastened to a surcingle (chest strap) worn by the horse. The ECG is recorded onto magnetic tape and is then analyzed with computer software. Holter monitoring is useful for continuous data collection for up to 24 hours or during exercise and recovery, but it does not allow highly detailed evaluation of the waveforms. Simple heart rate monitors are available to monitor the heart rate only (no ECG trace) and are popular for race and endurance training.

PROCEDURE (STANDING ELECTROCARDIOGRAM)

The ECG machine should be plugged into a grounded circuit to prevent shocking the patient, and the ground beneath the patient should be dry (a dry rubber mat is optimal and reduces the chance of electrical interference). The ground electrode should always be attached to the patient. Patient lead cables 4 to 5 feet in length are desirable for large animal use.

> **TECHNICIAN NOTE** The ECG machine should be plugged into a grounded circuit to prevent shocking the patient, and the ground beneath the patient should be dry.

Muscle activity interferes with the accuracy of the ECG; therefore, the examination should take place in a quiet environment. The horse should stand squarely, bearing weight evenly on all four legs for the duration of each lead trace. Shivering, skin twitches, and weight shifts all decrease the quality of the trace.

The leads are attached to the animal with alligator clips, rubber straps, or adhesive pads. Alligator clips may pinch the skin too tightly for the comfort of some animals, so filing down the serrated points of the alligator clips may increase their comfort. In addition, grasping a maximal amount of skin with the clip is more comfortable than grasping a small area. The electrodes must contact the skin, not just the hair of the skin. The contact points should be moistened with an electrode gel or paste. If these products are not available, alcohol or a salt-containing solution can be substituted. However, these

products tend to evaporate rapidly and may need to be applied repeatedly to maintain effective conduction.

The ECG lead systems used in large animals are basically identical to those used in small animals and are based on Einthoven's triangle. The standard bipolar leads (I, II, III) and the augmented unipolar leads (aVR, aVL, aVF) are used most often. The chest leads (CV6LL, CV6LU, V10, CV6RL, CV6RU) are less commonly used. As with other species, lead II is used most often to calculate heart rate and assess rhythm and waveforms. Lead placement is shown in Figures 9-132 and 9-133. For the forelimb leads, the electrodes are placed over the caudal aspect of the forearm, approximately 10 to 15 cm distal to the point of the elbow (olecranon). For the hindlimb leads, the electrodes are placed over the cranial or lateral aspect of the stifle.

The base-apex lead is popular for monitoring during anesthesia because it is less affected by motion, seldom interferes with the surgical site, and produces large waveforms. The right arm (forelimb) electrode is attached to the skin over the right jugular groove in the caudal one third of the neck or just cranial to the withers on the base of the right side of the neck. The left arm (forelimb) electrode is attached to the skin of the chest wall at the level of the left olecranon, which is the area of the cardiac apex. The right leg electrode serves as the ground electrode and can be attached to the skin of the horse at any convenient location remote from the heart. The lead selector is positioned to lead I to complete the setup.

> **TECHNICIAN NOTE** The base-apex lead is popular for monitoring during anesthesia because it is less affected by motion, seldom interferes with the surgical site, and produces large waveforms.

The paper recording speed is usually 25 mm/second in large animals, although 50 mm/second can be used effectively. Sensitivity is set at 1 mV/cm. Because of the low heart rates in large animals, it is desirable to record leads for several minutes each. Labeling the tracing immediately to identify different leads is always wise.

> **TECHNICIAN NOTE** The paper recording speed is usually 25 mm/second in large animals.

Interpretation of the ECG uses the same techniques as for other species. The heart rate and rhythm are determined, and the amplitude and length of the waveforms are measured. Approximate normal ranges of waveform amplitude and duration for both horses and ponies have been published and have even been determined for some individual breeds. Several differences in waveforms should be noted in horses (versus small animals):

- The P wave in normal horses at rest is usually bifid (double peaked).
- The T wave in horses is variable and should not be overinterpreted. T-wave abnormalities seldom correlate with

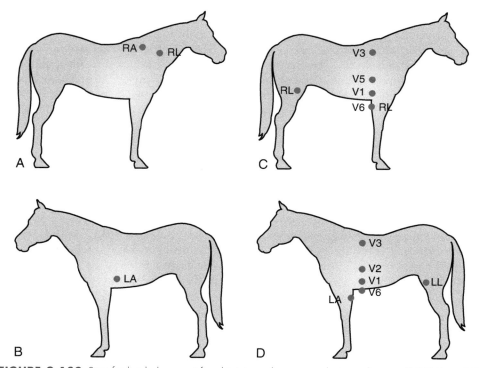

FIGURE 9-132 Sites for lead placement for obtaining a base-apex electrocardiogram (ECG) (**A** and **B**) and a complete ECG (**C** and **D**) in a horse. *Red circles* represent the site of attachment for the electrodes. **A,** Position of electrode placement on the right side of the horse for obtaining a base-apex ECG using the electrodes from lead I. **B,** Position of electrode placement on the left side of the horse for obtaining a base-apex ECG using the electrodes from lead I. **C,** Position of electrode placement on the right side of the horse for obtaining a complete ECG. **D,** Position of electrode placement on the left side of the horse for obtaining a complete ECG. *LA,* Left foreleg (left arm); *LL,* left hindleg (left leg); *RA,* right foreleg (right arm); *RL,* right hindleg (right leg); *V1,* first chest lead (CV6LL); *V2,* second chest lead (CV6LU); *V3,* third chest lead (V10); *V4,* fourth chest lead (CV6RL); *V5,* fifth chest lead (CV6RU). (From Marr C: *Cardiology of the horse,* St. Louis, 1999, Saunders.)

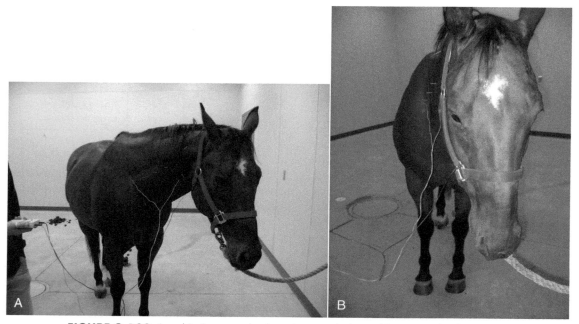

FIGURE 9-133 **A** and **B,** Base-apex lead attachment in the horse. (Courtesy Nebraska Equine.)

cardiac disease. The T wave in lead II and the base-apex lead is commonly biphasic (negative portion and positive portion).

- Wandering pacemaker (regular rhythm, with varying shapes of the P wave) is fairly common and usually is normal.
- Second-degree atrioventricular (A-V) block is present in a high percentage of horses at rest and is normal.

HOLISTIC MEDICINE

Holistic medicine is becoming more and more popular in the equine world. It is even starting to flow into some of the food production systems. Clients are becoming more accepting of these techniques, and technicians should familiarize themselves with them as well as become familiar with people in the area that are licensed to practice them. Technicians can also find that learning these techniques can make themselves more valuable to the practice and clients. Before starting to use any of these procedures, you should familiarize yourself with laws in your area and state that may affect your ability to perform these types of medicine. Several textbooks, classes, and research are available to help learn and understand the science behind these techniques:

- Massage therapy
  - Massage therapy is the manipulation of soft tissue in the body to help accomplish goals of drainage, relaxation, or stimulation. It can be helpful in situations where increased circulation is needed. It can help patients in high-stress situations and can help to speed recovery from surgical procedures and injuries.
  - Most massage sessions last from 10 to 60 minutes and can include stretches to help alleviate muscle tension.
  - Massage addresses the musculoskeletal system by increasing circulation, releasing scar tissue, balancing muscle function, and providing relaxation.
- Chiropractic therapy
  - Chiropractic therapy is a system of treating disease by manipulation of the vertebral column. Chiropractic is based on the theory that most diseases are caused by pressure on the nerves because of faulty alignment of the bones, especially the vertebrae, and that the nerves are thus prevented from transmitting to various organs of the body the neural impulses for proper functioning.
  - Acting on the theory that the pinching of nerves is the critical factor in the pathogenesis of disease, the chiropractor manipulates various parts of the spine in treating the complaint. If the patient is suffering from a displaced vertebra, the manipulation may bring relief.
- Acupuncture
  - Acupuncture is the Chinese practice of inserting needles into specific points (acupoints) along the "meridians" of the body and manipulated to relieve the discomfort associated with painful disorders, to induce surgical anesthesia, and for preventive and therapeutic purposes.
  - It is proposed that acupuncture produces its effects by the conduction of electromagnetic signals at a greater than normal rate, thus aiding the activity of pain-killing biochemicals, such as endorphins and immune system cells, at specific sites in the body.
  - Studies have also shown that acupuncture may alter brain chemistry by changing the release of neurotransmitters and neurohormones and affecting sensory perception and involuntary body functions. In recent years, the techniques have been adapted for use in veterinary medicine.
- Hydrotherapy
  - Hydrotherapy is the external use of water in the treatment of disease and injury.
  - Because of its physical properties related to the conduction of heat, buoyancy and cleansing action, water is an ideal agent for applications of heat or cold to obtain desired physiologic effects and for débridement of wounds that are extensive and are not easily cleansed by other methods.
- Herbs and oils
  - Herbology is the use of herbs for the treatment of disease or clinical signs.
  - As this practice becomes more and more popular, it is important for technicians to ask clients whether their horses are being given any herbs. Do not just ask whether the horses are receiving any medications because many people do not perceive these herbs to be medications. Clients will not offer the information unless asked whether they feed anything daily or unless they are specifically asked whether the horses take any herbs.

EQUINE EUTHANASIA

Although the general public is less likely to look on large animals as companion animals, those who work with large animals know differently. Large animals can be companions in every sense of the word, and saying good-bye to a friend is never easy. The grief and bereavement that a person may feel after the loss of a special horse, cow, sheep, goat, or pig are every bit as real as those felt for a cherished dog, cat, or bird. Even people who have a primarily economic relationship with large animals often develop a fondness for a few special individuals. However, regardless of the person's relationship with his or her animals—large or small, companion or business—it is the responsibility of humans to try to provide a humane ending when a life, for whatever reason, comes to its conclusion.

Many ways are available to euthanize a horse; however, they are not all necessarily humane. People tend to form strong opinions about which methods are acceptable and which are not. Often these opinions are based on rumors or observations made by well-meaning individuals who lack the medical knowledge to understand the response of an animal's body to the method of death. Sometimes the opinion is formed after watching a euthanasia procedure that was improperly performed or had an unexpected complication. Veterinary technicians deal with euthanasia on an almost daily basis and should not hesitate to form their own independent thoughts and opinions about the various ways to euthanize a horse. Although these opinions are (and should) be based largely on the technician's own experiences with equine euthanasia, it is wise to base these opinions on medically sound information.

It is legally advisable to have the owner or an agent for the owner sign a euthanasia consent form. These forms can be signed in advance for gravely ill horses in a hospital setting or when an owner is traveling so that a suffering animal can be promptly euthanized without waiting to contact the owner. Sometimes the veterinarian must consult with an insurance company before euthanasia is performed, although this is not necessary in an emergency situation when an animal is clearly suffering. In such an instance, the horse may be euthanized, and the insurance may be company notified as soon as possible.

> **TECHNICIAN NOTE**   It is legally advisable to have the owner or an agent for the owner sign a euthanasia consent form.

METHODS OF EUTHANASIA

When selecting an appropriate method of euthanasia, many factors must be considered (Box 9-4). According to the *2000 Report of the American Veterinary Medical Association Panel on Euthanasia,* the following are considered acceptable, humane methods for equine euthanasia:

- IV injection of barbituric acid derivatives: This is the preferred method of euthanasia for horses. Pentobarbital or pentobarbital-containing solutions are preferred. Because of the large volume of these solutions required, an IV

| **BOX 9-4** | Factors Affecting Euthanasia |

The following factors are considered when selecting the best method for euthanasia:

Patient Factors
Physical status and underlying diseases
Degree of domestication and human handling
Emergency euthanasia versus nonemergency euthanasia
Possibility of infectious disease
Patient size and weight

Human Factors
Level of training of person administering euthanasia
Availability and level of training of assistants
Safety
Owner's wishes
Aesthetics

Facility and Equipment Factors
Availability of drugs and injection supplies
Availability of equipment for physical euthanasia methods
   (captive bolt pistol, firearm)
Location of euthanasia procedure
Method and availability of restraint
Disposition of the body after euthanasia

---

catheter is suggested to facilitate the injection, although this may not always be necessary or practical. The solution should be injected rapidly, so a 14- to 16-ga needle or catheter is required. The jugular veins are the safest locations for the person administering the injection. If the veins are thrombosed or inaccessible, other large veins such as the cephalic or lateral thoracic veins can be used, with caution. Barbiturates are controlled substances, subject to U.S. Drug Enforcement Administration regulations.

- Penetrating captive bolt: This method is acceptable. It is preferred over gunshot. The person performing the procedure should be trained in the proper anatomical location and technique. The horse should be properly restrained. Loss of consciousness is extremely rapid (instantaneous), but muscle activity may continue and may be objectionable to observe.

- Inhalant anesthetics: This method is acceptable. Administration of an overdose of anesthetic gases, such as halothane, isoflurane, enflurane, or sevoflurane, is acceptable, but the large volumes required are costly and may be difficult to administer in some circumstances.

- IV injection of potassium chloride (KCl) combined with earlier general anesthesia: This method is acceptable. If the animal is in a surgical plane of anesthesia, KCl can be used to induce euthanasia. It must never be used in a conscious or lightly anesthetized animal. KCl causes cardiac arrest and is more rapid than an overdose of inhalant gas. It is considerably less expensive than barbituric acid derivatives and is not a controlled substance.

Gunshot: This method is conditionally acceptable when other methods are not available. The person performing the procedure should be trained in the use of firearms and in the proper anatomical location and technique. The horse should be properly restrained. Loss of consciousness following a properly delivered projectile is extremely rapid (instantaneous), but muscle activity may continue and may be objectionable to observe.

- IV injection of chloral hydrate: This method is conditionally acceptable, but only after sedation. Chloral hydrate affects the cerebrum slowly; therefore, earlier sedation is necessary to keep the animal restrained while the chloral hydrate takes effect.

- Neuromuscular blocking agents are absolutely condemned as euthanasia agents in all species, but they may be used in emergency situations as restraining agents to gain control of dangerous animals for euthanasia. Once the dangerous situation is under control, one of the acceptable euthanasia methods should be used as soon as possible. Neuromuscular blocking agents should not be used to perform the actual euthanasia.

Some logistical problems are related to the euthanasia of large animals. Technicians can provide valuable information to clients, who seldom are prepared to deal with the specifics of the procedure. The actual location of the procedure should be carefully selected, if time allows. For instance, euthanasia inside a stall or building creates the question of how to remove the body from the building. (This usually means dragging the body manually or with machinery such as a tractor or truck winch.) The size and weight of most large animals make removal difficult, so it is usually preferable to perform the procedure outside. This may not always be possible, especially when the animal's disease makes it impossible or dangerous to try to move it to an outdoor location.

> **TECHNICIAN NOTE** Because of the size of the animal and the difficulty of removal, most euthanasia procedures are performed outside.

When barbiturate solutions or other chemicals are used to euthanize animals, the chemical residues may be toxic to predator animals that eat the tissues of the deceased animal. If disposal of the body will be delayed, it may be prudent to cover the body with heavy plastic or tarp to discourage scavenging. This may be more of a factor when the body is outside in an open field setting, although many barns are readily accessible to dogs and other animals.

As with euthanasia of any species, the owner should be asked whether he or she wishes to be present during the procedure. Time to say goodbye should be provided. Standing equine euthanasia tends to make more of an impression on people because of the visual effect of a large animal falling to the ground, unlike small animals that can be held in the arms and cradled gently as they collapse. Given that final impression combined with the animal's possible involuntary muscle activity and reflexes that persist for several minutes, whether or not to view the procedure is a significant decision (especially when children are concerned). If the owner will view the procedure, I strongly recommend that he or she be given the opportunity to be informed beforehand about the horse's physical responses to euthanasia so that the owner is not caught off guard by the natural reflex motions and muscle activity that often accompany death. This information should not be forced on the client; rather, simply asking "Would you like me to explain the procedure—how the drugs work, and what you're likely to see?" gives the client an option. Most clients say yes, but some may find the details disturbing and not wish to hear them. If a client does wish to hear the information, keep the explanation brief and simple, and avoid excessive use of medical terms.

Because of the possible dangers associated with a large, standing animal falling to recumbency, all untrained and nonessential people—owners included—should be instructed to maintain a safe, specific distance from the procedure until an "all clear" signal is given by the veterinarian. When the animal is recumbent and limb motion has ceased, it may then be suitable for the family to approach the animal.

It is thought best for other members of a species not to witness euthanasia of their own kind because the excitement, involuntary vocalizations, and body odors associated with the procedure may be stressful. However, it is not always possible or practical to separate other equines completely. It is considered acceptable, once the procedure is complete, to allow other horses to interact with the body unless contagious disease has been diagnosed or is a possibility. This is commonly done with mares when their foal dies naturally or by euthanasia. A brief time period (45 to 50 minutes) allows the mare to observe and prod the foal's body; this interaction is thought to provide the mare a chance to better "accept" the foal's death. Of course, this has never been proved, but many horse handlers and owners believe in this practice. Because of the risk of infectious organisms, mares should not be allowed to contact or interact with aborted fetuses.

> **TECHNICIAN NOTE** Many owners believe a brief time period of 45 to 50 minutes should be allowed for the mare to inspect a dead foal's body.

Another major decision concerns disposition of the body. Technicians should be familiar with the options available in their geographic area. These options are first limited by state and local laws and then by availability. Most states have a time limit on carcass disposal after euthanasia, typically 24 to 72 hours. Burning and burial may be prohibited in some areas, or they may be allowed only if special regulations are followed. Some jurisdictions may require a special permit to burn or bury. Clients should know which options are available so that they can select the one with which they are most comfortable.

Burial requires excavation of a grave. This is usually done with a backhoe or bulldozer. It is useful to keep a list of local contractors who are willing to perform this service. Excavation may be affected by the time of year, especially in northern climates where the ground freezes in winter, making excavation difficult or impossible. Special considerations include whether the horse will be walked into the grave and euthanized there or whether the body will be pulled or pushed into the grave after death. The veterinarian likely will have a preference for his or her personal safety in each situation. Some people find it objectionable to force an animal to walk into its own grave. Others find it objectionable to watch the body being pushed into the grave by a bulldozer. Different situations call for different approaches.

General guidelines for burial include selecting a site away from any open water sources (e.g., ponds or creeks) or drinking water sources (e.g., wells). The hole should be at least 8 feet or deeper but should not penetrate within 5 feet of the water table. If the water table is less than 8 feet, then soil should be mounded above ground to produce above-ground soil coverage. At least 3 to 5 feet of dirt coverage is necessary to prevent scavenging or exposure by weather factors. Covering the body with slaked (hydrated) lime is often required by law for sanitary reasons and to speed decomposition of the body. Again, local laws should be consulted for specific burial depths, soil types, water table requirements, and carcass coverage.

If burial of the total body is not allowed or is not practical, it may be possible to offer the alternative of burying only selected body parts. Burial of the hooves and the heart is a traditional approach that may appeal to some owners. The veterinarian or technicians can remove these parts either on the farm or in the clinic (depending on where death occurs) and place them in a selected container for burial or return to the owner. Cremation of the entire body is usually not practical, but cremation of the hooves and heart is a very acceptable alternative. Cremation must usually be performed at a state-licensed incineration facility, where strict emission guidelines and temperature requirements must be followed.

If burial is not an option, then removal of the body will be necessary. The body is most often sent for rendering. Pickup is usually provided by a licensed livestock disposal hauler, which may be provided by the rendering company. If possible, euthanasia should be performed in an area with easy access for the hauler's truck. Some local regulations now require that animals euthanized with barbiturates be treated as biomedical waste, with subsequent labeling and handling requirements. Livestock disposal haulers may refuse pickup of biomedical waste if they are not certified to transport biohazardous materials. Landfills may be an alternative for disposal in some states. Landfills may accept large animal carcasses for a standard or weight-based fee. The phone numbers of rendering and hauling companies or individuals and the approximate costs for pickup should be available to clients.

Another concern related to disposition is providing clients with remembrances of their animal. Clients should be asked whether they want the halter removed for a keepsake or whether they prefer the horse to be buried with the halter. Some clients may want to have the horseshoes. A lock of mane, tail, or forelock is sometimes requested. These items are usually removed after death. The client's wishes should be respected, no matter how unusual the request, and any requested item or body part should be treated with respect.

> **TECHNICIAN NOTE**   After euthanasia of the animal, the client's wishes should be respected, no matter how unusual the request, and any requested item or body part should be treated with respect.

NECROPSY TECHNIQUES

Large animal necropsy is performed for the same reasons as small animal necropsy, and the procedures are similar. Necropsy is used to determine or confirm the cause of death and any factors that may have contributed to death. The necropsy consists of a gross visual examination and may extend to include a sample collection for special laboratory examinations, such as histopathology, toxicology, microbiology, parasitology, cytology, and chemistry.

The owner's permission should always be obtained before necropsy. Owners are not always willing to allow the procedure to be performed, and necropsy is not always necessary unless doing so will provide some necessary information. Similarly, a complete, total body necropsy procedure is not always necessary. Often the veterinarian wants to evaluate

only certain organs or tissues or collect only specific samples. The procedure may also be affected by insurance coverage, which is common in the horse industry. The insurance company may require that a necropsy be performed and may also specify the samples to be taken.

> **TECHNICIAN NOTE**   The owner's permission should always be obtained before necropsy.

The timing of the necropsy is of great importance. Autolysis (decomposition), which begins immediately following death, destroys cell architecture and alters many chemical and microbiologic findings. Autolysis is accelerated by microorganisms. The GI tract of herbivores contains incredible numbers of microbes that do not die when the herbivore dies. Other areas of the body, such as the respiratory tract and skin, also contain numerous microorganisms. Following death of the "host," the microbes can spread throughout the body without much resistance, disrupting tissues as they go. Heat, which contributes to the speed of autolysis, may come from the external environment or from internal heat created by microbial fermentation in the intestinal tract. Refrigeration of the carcass may delay (but not prevent) autolysis; however, refrigeration of large animals is available only at some clinic or hospital facilities. Therefore, most large animal necropsies must be conducted promptly after death to yield meaningful results.

> **TECHNICIAN NOTE**   Necropsies should be performed as soon after death as possible.

The location of the necropsy is important. Preferably, the procedure is performed in a setting that can be readily disinfected and can provide containment of any toxic or infectious materials. However, this ideal setting is seldom available outside of a clinic or hospital. Large animal necropsies are usually messy procedures, especially when the intestinal tract is opened. In a field setting, the procedure is ideally done in an area that can be restricted from other animals, away from water and food sources. Covering the ground with hydrated lime or saturating the ground with dilute bleach after the procedure is advised. The ability of the public to view the necropsy must be anticipated. Many laypeople may be disturbed or even offended by the sight or smell of the procedure. Blocking the view with vehicles or makeshift curtains may be helpful.

Documenting the necropsy findings is important. This should be done in the form of a written report of observations. Photographs of the necropsy findings may be advisable in certain circumstances to supplement written descriptions. The report must include an accurate description of the animal, including all identifying marks (natural and artificial). Photographs may assist the animal identification. Digital photography can facilitate the recording and storage of photographic images.

Before beginning the necropsy, all materials should be assembled. It is desirable to have supplies that are dedicated to necropsies to minimize possible spread of microorganisms. Standard dissecting equipment for necropsies is used: an assortment of scalpel blades and handles, heavy tissue (Mayo) scissors, Metzenbaum scissors, operating scissors, hemostatic forceps, boning or necropsy knives, sharpening steel, thumb tissue forceps, utility scissors, and a ruler. Special equipment for large animal necropsies may include large cutting shears (e.g., long-handled garden pruning shears) or a hand ax for opening the rib cage and a hand saw or Stryker saw for cutting bone. If the carcass is to be closed after the procedure, the closure material (suture, string, or twine) should be readily available.

If samples are to be collected, appropriate culturettes, containers, and fixatives should be gathered. Containers should be labeled before the procedure. The laboratory that will run each test should be consulted for preferred fixatives and handling procedures. Tissues for histopathologic examination are most commonly placed in 10% neutral buffered formalin for preservation. As with small animals, a ratio of 10:1 formalin-to-tissue volume should be maintained in the sample containers. Large animals do not require larger tissue samples than small animals; samples thicker than 0.5 to 0.7 cm may impede penetration of the fixative. Ideal samples are 1 cm × 1 cm × 0.5 cm; samples should not exceed 3 cm².

Protective clothing is a must, especially where zoonotic disease is a concern. Plastic arm sleeves (rectal sleeves) are recommended for exploring the abdominal and thoracic cavities. Latex examination gloves placed over the arm sleeve can provide an additional layer of protection for the hands as well as a more secure grip on instruments. Coveralls are commonly worn for large animal necropsy, and a plastic apron gives additional protection. Rubber boots or disposable shoe covers should be worn. A cap, face mask, and eye protection are important when zoonotic organisms may exist. Whatever items are worn during the necropsy should be covered, removed, or disinfected before other animals are attended.

> **TECHNICIAN NOTE** Protective clothing should be worn during necropsy procedures, especially where zoonotic disease is a concern.

EQUINE NECROPSY PROCEDURE

No single, correct technique exists for performing a necropsy. The order in which the organ systems are examined and the method of obtaining samples can be modified for individual preference and different situations. What is important is being thorough so that nothing is overlooked. Establishing a routine procedure is helpful, and checklists can help ensure that the examination and sample collection are complete. A basic necropsy examination procedure is described in the following list. In-depth methodology and techniques are well described in other sources.

1. Position: The standard body position for equine necropsy is left lateral recumbency, although the position can be modified for different situations.
2. Examine the body for external lesions, parasites, and body condition: Examine all mucous membranes and body openings, including the oral cavity. Examine any surgical incisions and veins that have been catheterized or used for injections.
3. Skin incision: Make a ventral midline incision through the skin and SC tissue from the xiphoid process extending caudally to the prepuce or mammary gland. Direct the incision toward the right inguinal canal to avoid the prepuce and penis in the male or the mammary gland in the female, return to midline, and continue to the anus. Returning to the xiphoid process, extend the skin incision to the chin along the ventral midline. Reflect the skin dorsally across the thorax and abdomen.
4. Reflect the limbs: Returning to the right inguinal canal, use a knife to incise the joint capsule of the coxofemoral joint and the ligament of the head of the femur. Reflect the hindlimb dorsally. Reflect the right forelimb dorsally by dissecting along a plane medial to the scapula.
5. Reflect the prepuce and penis or mammary gland: Dissect just deep to these structures to free them from the body wall and allow them to be reflected. The entire mammary gland can be removed if necessary for closer inspection.
6. Examine the scrotum, testicles, and spermatic cord: If necessary, the scrotum can be opened, and the testicles and spermatic cords can be examined or removed.
7. Open the abdominal cavity: Take care not to incise any abdominal organs accidentally; this is especially difficult if the abdomen is bloated. Enter the abdominal wall and peritoneum on the ventral midline, through the linea alba. Carefully make a small incision to enter the abdominal cavity through the linea alba, and then use either a hand or another instrument to form a barrier between the cutting instrument and the organs as you extend the incision cranially to the xiphoid and caudally to the pelvic brim. After completing the ventral midline incision into the abdomen, make a second incision to connect the caudal aspect of the ventral midline incision with the junction of the vertebral column and the last rib. This forms a triangular flap based along the last rib that can be reflected craniodorsally over the caudal thorax. Once the abdominal cavity is exposed, note the position of the organs as normal or abnormal, and assess the volume and appearance of the peritoneal fluid. Normally, the peritoneal fluid is clear and yellow, and the volume is approximately 200 mL. Samples of peritoneal fluid can be obtained at this time. If a urine sample is necessary, it can be aseptically aspirated from the bladder with a needle and syringe.
8. Open the thoracic cavity: Palpate the abdominal aspect of the diaphragm for defects, and then make a small puncture in the diaphragm to check for negative pressure in the thoracic cavity. The diaphragm should

collapse, and the sound of air rushing may be heard if negative pressure, which is normal, exists. Use an ax or pruning shears to cut the ribs at the costosternal junctions, with care taken not to cut the heart or lungs. Once all ribs have been cut along the sternum, cut them again approximately 6 inches lateral to the vertebral column. Sever the diaphragm on the right side along its attachment to the last rib. This frees the right rib cage so that it can be reflected dorsally. Note the position of the organs as normal or abnormal, and assess the volume and appearance of the pleural fluid. Normally, the pleural fluid is clear and yellow, and the volume is approximately 100 mL. Samples of pleural fluid can be collected at this time.

9. Remove the pluck (tongue, trachea, esophagus, heart, and lungs): These parts are removed together in one piece, en bloc. First, retract the tongue ventrally through an incision between the mandibles. Extend the neck and make an incision along the medial aspect of either mandible, while making sure that the incision is deep enough to enter the oral cavity. Evert the free portion of the tongue ventrally through the incision, between the mandibles. Sever the mandibular attachments of the tongue to allow complete eversion of the tongue. Transect the hyoid apparatus with shears to allow the tongue to be freed completely from the oral cavity and pharynx. Once freed, the tongue can be used as a "handle" to elevate and provide tension on the other organs as they are removed. Elevate the tongue, and carefully transect the soft tissue attachments on the lateral and dorsal aspects of the larynx, then the trachea and esophagus, proceeding caudally to the thoracic inlet, then through the thoracic inlet to the area of the carina. The attachments of the pleura run along the dorsal aspect of the thoracic cavity. The pluck is then attached only by the esophagus, aorta, and caudal vena cava where they penetrate the diaphragm. Cut along the thoracic aspect of the diaphragm to transect these structures where they contact the diaphragm. This will free the pluck. Remove the pluck, and examine the internal surfaces of the rib cage. Return to the head, and evaluate the pharynx, guttural pouches, and oral cavity as needed.

10. Examine the pluck:
    - Tongue: Make several transverse cuts through the tongue.
    - Pharynx: Open the pharynx and examine the tonsils.
    - Esophagus: Open the esophagus longitudinally along its entire length.
    - Thyroid glands: Observe the thyroid gland near the thyroid cartilage of the larynx.
    - Larynx, trachea, and bronchi: Open longitudinally.
    - Thymus gland (if present): Observe the thymus. The thymus is an organ that helps kick start the immune system early in an animal's life. It shrinks up and nearly disappears when the animal reaches adulthood. In a young animal the thymus is fairly large. It extends cranially from the level of the heart in the thorax up

into the neck region along both sides of the trachea, often to the level of the larynx. After puberty, however, the thymus begins to atrophy. By the time the animal reaches adulthood, it is hard or impossible to find any remnant of the thymus.

- Lungs: Palpate all lobes for deep lesions. "Book" the lung by making multiple parallel incisions through the lobes.
- Heart: Open the pericardial sac and examine the pericardial fluid for volume and appearance. Observe the surface and overall size and shape of the heart.
  - Position the apex of the heart toward you with the right side of the heart toward your right side.
  - Open the right side of the heart: Incise the right ventricle adjacent to the interventricular septum, along the right longitudinal coronary groove from its apex through the right A-V valve into the right atrium. Make a second incision along the left longitudinal coronary groove from the apex through the right A-V valve and semilunar (pulmonary) valve into the pulmonary artery.
  - Open the left side of the heart: Incise the left ventricle along the left coronary groove, continuing through the left A-V valve into the left atrium. Identify the pulmonary vein at its opening into the left atrium and open it longitudinally. Open the aorta longitudinally by inserting scissors under the medial cusp of the left A-V valve and cutting through the semilunar (aortic) valve.
  - Note the contents of each chamber. Rinse the interior surfaces with water, and examine all heart valve leaflets, chordae tendineae, papillary muscle, and endocardium.
- Lymph nodes: Evaluate the lymph nodes, which are located in the pharyngeal and tracheobronchial areas.

11. Eviscerate and evaluate the abdominal cavity:
    - Remove the omentum and spleen.
    - Identify and remove the right adrenal gland, which is located cranial and medial to the right kidney.
    - Identify and remove the pancreas, which is located in the mesentery between the base of the cecum and the duodenum, in the dorsal abdomen.
    - Remove the intestinal tract in segments (stomach, small intestine, large intestine) or remove the entire intestinal tract by transecting the root of the mesentery, the distal small colon, and the distal esophagus just caudal to the diaphragm. It may be beneficial to tie off open segments with string before transection to prevent spillage of contents.
    - Remove the liver by severing its attachments to the diaphragm.
    - Identify and remove the left adrenal gland, which is located cranial and medial to the left kidney.
    - Remove the kidneys, ureters, and urinary bladder en bloc. Dissect each kidney free, and dissect the ureter along its course to the bladder. Transect the urethra, and cut the attachments of the bladder to free the entire urinary tract.

- Remove the ovaries and uterus by pulling them cranially and transecting caudally to the cervix. If the entire female reproductive tract is to be evaluated, skip this step and proceed to open the pelvic cavity.
- Remove or evaluate male accessory sex glands and vas deferens, if necessary.
- Evaluate the abdominal aorta. Palpate it, and incise it longitudinally with scissors.

12. Open the pelvic cavity: Remove the ventral wall of the pelvis by transecting (with a handsaw) the right and left pubic bones parallel to the symphysis pubis and then continuing the cuts through the obturator foramen and ischium on each side. Evaluate the pelvic organs:
    - Rectum and anus.
    - Female reproductive tract (pelvic portion).
    - Prostate gland (males only).
13. Evaluate the abdominal and pelvic viscera:
    - Liver: Observe size, shape, and color. Palpate for deep lesions and assess consistency. Book the parenchyma, and observe for lesions.
    - Pancreas: Observe size, color, and consistency.
    - Spleen: Separate the spleen from the stomach. Palpate for deep lesions. Book the parenchyma and observe for lesions.
    - Stomach: Open the stomach along the greater curvature, including the pylorus. Observe stomach contents. Rinse gently with water and observe the gastric mucosa (excessive water pressure will alter the mucosa).
    - Intestinal tract:
      - Small intestine: Beginning with a small incision into the duodenal lumen, open the small intestine by cutting the mesenteric attachment and tensing 2 to 3 feet of intestine. Cut the intestinal wall with scissors (blunt tip inside the lumen). Evaluate the opened segment for content, then rinse and evaluate the mucosa. Repeat the procedure, opening 2 to 3 feet at a time, until the entire length of the small intestine is examined.
      - Examine the mesenteric lymph nodes located in the root of the mesentery.
      - Colonic lymph nodes: Lay out the large colon and cecum. The lymph nodes are located adjacent to the bowel, within the mesentery.
      - Large colon, cecum, transverse colon, and small colon: Open with scissors and evaluate contents, mucosa, and intestinal wall.
    - Kidneys and ureters: Observe size and shape. Open with a single sagittal incision through the entire parenchyma, from cortex to medulla to renal pelvis. Peel back the renal capsule and evaluate the outer cortical surface. Examine the renal pelvis for shape and contents. Extend incisions longitudinally to open the ureters.
    - Urinary bladder: Open and assess contents. Examine mucosa and wall thickness.
    - Adrenal glands: Section sagittally. Evaluate cortex and medulla. Handle gently to avoid creating crushing artifacts.

14. Musculoskeletal system: Incise several skeletal muscles and examine for color and consistency. Open several joints and observe synovial fluid and articular cartilage. If bone marrow is needed, the ribs are easily accessed. Use a saw to transect the bones and rongeurs or a bone curette to scoop out the marrow.
15. Superficial lymph nodes: Select several superficial lymph nodes. Examine size and consistency, and section to view the internal surfaces.

If the body is to be hauled away after the necropsy, the necropsy incisions should be closed to keep the viscera contained within the carcass. Many hauling companies do not accept a carcass unless the organs are removed or secured within the body. The incisions can be closed with heavy-gauge suture material or heavy string or twine. The closure material should pass through the skin or underlying fascia to gain adequate holding strength. The material should pass at least 1 inch away from the edges of the necropsy incision to prevent ripping through the tissues. If string or twine is used, small stab incisions must be made to pass the string or twine through these tissues. The technician must be careful when making the stab incisions to avoid self-injury.

REMOVAL OF BRAIN AND SPINAL CORD

It is occasionally desirable to remove the brain or spinal cord, or both, for evaluation of neurologic conditions. Neurologic tissue autolyzes rapidly after death. If histopathologic examination of nerve tissue is necessary, these tissues should be promptly harvested.

- Aspiration of CSF: If CSF is needed, it is aspirated from the atlantooccipital space before removing the head.
- Removal of the head: The head is disarticulated through the atlantooccipital joint, by approaching from the ventral aspect of the neck. If the brain is to be submitted for rabies evaluation, most diagnostic laboratories will accept the entire head. It should be properly packaged, labeled, and refrigerated.
- Removal of the brain: The head should be stabilized in a vice or against a solid object. The skin is incised from the angles of the mandibles dorsally across the poll and is reflected cranially. A skull cap is created by making three incisions into the bony calvarium with a handsaw.
  - Make a transverse incision across the frontal bones that connect the supraorbital foramen, just caudal to the orbits. Be sure to cut through the frontal sinus (Fig. 9-134).
  - Make two lateral incisions, from each supraorbital foramen to the occipital condyle on the same side. Be sure to cut into the foramen magnum posteriorly.
  - Loosen the skull cap with a chisel, and pry it off carefully to reveal the brain and meninges.
  - Remove the brain by incising the dura mater and reflecting it from the brain. Starting at the rostral aspect of the brain, lift the brain tissue, and sever the cranial nerves. When the entire brain can be elevated, transect the brainstem. Remove the brain, and process the tissues as necessary.

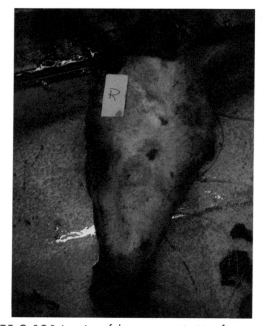

FIGURE 9-134 Location of the transverse incision for exposure of the brain.

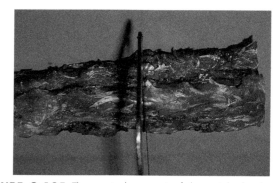

FIGURE 9-135 The cervical segment of the vertebral column has been removed. A handsaw is used to cut through the center of adjacent vertebrae to form segments. (From Colahan PT, Merritt AM, Moore JN, Mayhew IG, editors: *Equine medicine and surgery*, ed 5, St. Louis, 1999, Mosby.)

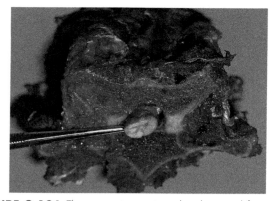

FIGURE 9-136 The segments are viewed end on, and forceps are used to grasp the dura mater so that the spinal nerves within the epidural space can be cut with scissors. (From Colahan PT, Merritt AM, Moore JN, Mayhew IG, editors: *Equine medicine and surgery*, ed 5, St. Louis, 1999, Mosby.)

- The pituitary gland will remain in the sella turcica. Use forceps to elevate the gland, and gently divide any attachments to free the gland.
- Removal of the spinal cord: Reflect the skin, musculature, and other soft tissues lateral to the dorsal spinous processes of the vertebrae. The desired segments of the vertebral column are removed intact from the carcass. The spinal cord is then removed in segments or en bloc. It is easier to remove the spinal cord in multiple small segments by cutting transversely across the middle of adjacent vertebrae to form individual segments, then grasping the dura mater and removing the spinal cord segments from the vertebral canal by severing the spinal nerves in the epidural space with scissors (Figs. 9-135 and 9-136). Each segment should be accurately labeled and packaged separately. Incising the dura mater of each segment longitudinally facilitates penetration of the fixative.
- Removing the entire spinal cord or long segments of the spinal cord in one piece is difficult. Use of hand tools (meat cleaver or axe) to split the vertebral column sagittally is possible but tends to be destructive. Power tools (especially a band saw) are preferred to perform sequential dorsal laminectomies through the vertebrae; this exposes the spinal cord. The spinal nerves must be severed to free and remove the spinal cord.

NECROPSY OF THE ABORTED FETUS

Aborted fetuses and tissues before 90 days of gestation are seldom found, especially in pasture settings. After 90 days, finding a fetus becomes more likely. When an owner finds an aborted fetus, the veterinarian is usually asked to determine the cause of death. This requires examination and diagnostic testing of the mare, the placental tissues, and the aborted fetus. The client should understand that in spite of thorough examination of the mare, placental tissues, and aborted fetus, diagnosis of the cause of an abortion is not always possible.

Aborted fetuses and placental tissues, when found, are often in advanced states of autolysis; however, this should not prevent an attempt to necropsy and obtain samples. Any aborted fetus and its associated tissues should be placed immediately in a clean plastic bag and refrigerated (not frozen). It may be possible to submit the entire refrigerated fetus to a diagnostic laboratory for full examination. If submission of the entire fetus is not feasible, a necropsy can be done to collect appropriate specimens for submission to the laboratory.

Because of the possibility that infectious organisms caused the abortion, the potential consequences of contagious disease must not be underestimated. Many contagious abortive diseases can be passed directly from mare to mare through direct or indirect contact. In addition, it is the nature of large animals to "investigate" aborted fetuses and membranes by smelling and even licking them. Whenever a mare aborts, she should be separated immediately from other pregnant mares until the cause of abortion has been determined. The ground where the abortion occurred should be disinfected and roped or fenced off to prevent access by other animals until the cause is known. If abortion occurs in a stall, the stall should be stripped and disinfected. The bedding should be handled as potentially contaminated and possibly burned if local laws allow. Isolation of the stall and areas where the mare traveled may be necessary. The veterinarian will advise the client on the best course of action. It is preferable not to open the fetus for necropsy in any area that could be accessed by other animals. The area of the necropsy should be disinfected, and all clothing, instruments, and sample containers used in the procedure must be handled appropriately.

The procedure for necropsy of the fetus is as follows:

1. Identify the sex, weigh, and measure crown-rump length (distance from poll to tail base, measured along and against the dorsal midline). Note the extent of hair growth. Note any obvious congenital or hereditary defects.
2. Place the fetus in right lateral recumbency.
3. Reflect or remove the left limbs. Skin the left body wall.
4. Incise the body wall behind the ribs into the flank area, and reflect the abdominal wall without touching the underlying viscera. Aspirate any available peritoneal fluid and place it in a serum (red top) tube.
5. Using sterile instruments and aseptic technique, sample the abdominal organs in situ. Collect pieces of spleen, liver, and kidney for viral isolation (VI) and fluorescent antibody (FA) testing. VI samples can be pooled in one container. FA samples should be kept separate, in Whirl-Pak (Nasco, Fort Atkinson, Wisc.) bags. Add enough viral transport medium to all VI and FA containers to just cover the tissues.
6. Enter the thoracic cavity through the diaphragm or by removing the left chest wall. Aspirate any available pleural fluid and place it in a serum (red top) tube.
7. Using sterile instruments and aseptic technique, sample the thoracic organs in situ. Collect pieces of lung and thymus for VI and FA testing.
8. Collect bacterial culture samples from the lung and liver. Place the tissue samples in Whirl-Pak bags. Do not add viral transport medium to the bacteriologic samples.
9. Make a small hole in the stomach wall, and sample the gastric fluid with a culturette for bacteriologic culture.
10. Once all microbiologic samples have been obtained, collect histologic samples in 10% neutral buffered formalin:
    - Liver (several sections)
    - Lung (several sections)
    - Kidney
    - Spleen
    - Heart
    - Thymus
    - Other desirable tissues: adrenal gland, stomach, small intestine, large intestine, skeletal muscle, tongue, eyelid, and brain (cerebrum, cerebellum, and brainstem)
11. If toxicologic analysis is to be performed, place a large piece of liver in a Whirl-Pak bag. Also aspirate fluid from

the anterior eye chamber and place it in a serum (red top) tube.

Promptly ship all samples to the diagnostic laboratory. Microbiologic and toxicologic samples should be shipped frozen, on ice packs. Histopathologic samples should not be frozen because freezing disrupts cell architecture.

CASE STUDY

Mrs. Reid owns champion Friesians. She has requested that the hair not be clipped for a jugular catheter because she is going to be showing the horse in a halter class in a few weeks. Should you clip the hair anyway? What should you caution the client about?

CASE STUDY

Your veterinarian is trying to perform a joint injection on a 5-year-old racing Thoroughbred owned by Mr. Frickel. As the veterinarian is preparing the injection site, the horse is shifting its weight and trying to step forward. The veterinarian tells you to keep him still. Why? How was the veterinarian preparing the injection site?

CASE STUDY

Mrs. Crook owns an 8-year-old Saddlebred mare that is undergoing a thoracocentesis today. What is a major complication of performing a thoracocentesis? What clinical signs should you monitor after a thoracocentesis? What aftercare should you provide to the mare after the procedure?

SUGGESTED READING

2000 Report of the AVMA Panel on Euthanasia, *J Am Vet Med Assoc* 218:669–696, 2001.

Allen T: *Manual of equine dentistry*, St. Louis, 2003, Mosby.

Baker GJ, Easley J: *Equine dentistry*, Oxford, 2008, Saunders.

Bassert JM, McCurnin DM, editors: *McCurnin's clinical textbook for veterinary technicians*, ed 7, St. Louis, 2010, Saunders.

Buergelt CD: Necropsy. In Colahan PT, Merritt AM, Moore JN, Mayhew IG, editors: *Equine medicine and surgery*, vol 1, ed 5. St. Louis, 1999, Mosby.

Butler KD: *The principles of horseshoeing II*, Maryville, Mo, 1985, Doug Butler Publisher.

Colahan PT, Merritt AM, Moore JN, Mayhew IG, editors: *Equine medicine and surgery*, ed 5, St. Louis, 1999, Mosby.

Davis H, Riel DL, Pappagianis M, Miguel K: Diagnostic sampling and therapeutic techniques. In Bassert JM, McCurnin DM, editors: *McCurnin's clinical textbook for veterinary technicians*, ed 7, St. Louis, 2010, Saunders, pp 585–673.

Muir WW, Hubbell JAE, editors: *Equine anesthesia: monitoring and emergency therapy*, ed 2, St. Louis, 2009, Saunders.

Hosgood G, Burba DJ: Wound healing, wound management, and bandaging. In Bassert JM, McCurnin DM, editors: *McCurnin's clinical textbook for veterinary technicians*, ed 7, St. Louis, 2010, Saunders, pp 1230–1264.

Noakes DE, Parkinson TJ, England GCW: *Veterinary reproduction and obstetrics*, ed 9, London, 2009, Saunders.

Orsini JA, Divers TJ: *Manual of equine emergencies*, ed 3, St. Louis, 2008, Saunders.

Reed SM: Neurologic diseases, *Vet Clin North Am Equine Pract* 3: 255–440, 1987.

Sirois M: *Principles and practice of veterinary technology*, ed 3, St. Louis, 2011, Mosby.

Sonsthagen T, Teeple TN: Nursing care of horses. In Sirois M, editor: *Principles and practice of veterinary technology*, ed 3, St. Louis, 2011, Mosby, pp 569–584.

Speirs VC: *Clinical examination of horses*, St. Louis, 1997, Saunders.

Stashak TS: *Adams' lameness in horses*, ed 5, Philadelphia, 2002, Lippincott Williams & Wilkins.

Stashak TS: *Equine wound management*, Ames, Iowa, 2009, Wiley-Blackwell.

Stone WC: Drains, dressings and external coaptation. In Auer JA, Stick JA, editors: *Equine surgery*, St. Louis, 1999, Saunders, pp 202–218.

Taboada J, Johnson S: The human-animal bond, bereavement, and euthanasia. In Bassert JM, McCurnin DM, editors: *McCurnin's clinical textbook for veterinary technicians*, ed 7, St. Louis, 2010, Saunders, pp 1321–1340.

Van Winkle TJ, Habecker PL: Basic necropsy procedures. In Bassert JM, McCurnin DM, editors: *McCurnin's clinical textbook for veterinary technicians*, ed 7, St. Louis, 2010, Saunders, pp 1341–1360.

White NA, Moore JN: *The equine acute abdomen*, Jackson, Wyo, 2009, Teton NewMedia.

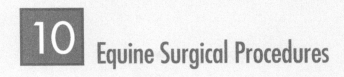 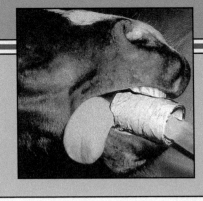

10 Equine Surgical Procedures

LEARNING OBJECTIVES

When you have completed this chapter, you will be able to

- Understand the basic differences between standing surgical procedures and general anesthesia procedures
- Prepare a patient for surgery
- Assist with or perform induction and maintenance of anesthesia
- Provide anesthetic monitoring
- Manage the patient during recovery and immediate postoperative periods
- Understand the basic risks and possible complications associated with anesthesia and surgery, and implement preventive measures when indicated

KEY TERMS

Bradycardia
Breeder's stitch
Caslick surgery
Caudal epidural
Compartment syndrome
Cryptorchidectomy

Direct blood pressure measurement
Direct tracheal intubation
False rigs
Ileus
Orchidectomy
Pneumovagina

Postanesthetic myopathy
Postanesthetic neuropathy
Proud cut
Sunken anus

KEY ABBREVIATIONS

NPO (nulla per os)
NSAID: Nonsteroidal antiinflammatory drug

EQUINE SURGERY AND ANESTHESIA

Remarkable advances in large animal anesthesia and surgical techniques have been made since the 1980s, leading to a vast array of surgical procedures currently available to the equine patient. Surgical procedures range from simple laceration repair to laser surgery and laparoscopy. Most of the instrumentation and surgical techniques have been borrowed from human surgery and adapted for veterinary use. The variety of procedures and the expertise in techniques continue to grow.

The availability of surgical procedures depends on the following considerations:
- Availability of surgical facilities
- Expertise of available surgeons
- Patients' health status
- Ability to provide aftercare and follow-up

- Prognosis
- Economic constraints

Surgical procedures can be divided into two major categories:
1. Standing surgery procedures
2. General anesthesia (recumbent) procedures

STANDING SURGERY

Most large animal surgical procedures are performed on standing, awake patients. Most of these procedures are performed for treatment and repair of traumatic injuries, such as lacerations and punctures. Other common procedures are castration, female reproductive surgery, laser and endoscopic surgery of the upper respiratory tract, and minor hoof and lower leg procedures. Less common are abdominal and thoracic procedures, ophthalmic surgery, and sinus and dental procedures. Many of these procedures can be performed on the farm, thereby saving the expense and reducing the risks associated with transportation.

Generally, the primary benefit of standing surgery is avoiding the risks associated with general anesthesia, especially recovery from general anesthesia. Recovery from general anesthesia is the single largest risk for surgical patients, even the healthy elective surgery patient. In addition, some surgical procedures are technically easier to perform on a standing patient for anatomical or physiologic reasons. It is in the patient's best interest to use a standing procedure whenever possible.

> **TECHNICIAN NOTE**   Recovery from general anesthesia is the single largest risk for large animal surgical patients.

Criteria and indications for standing surgery include the following:
- The surgical technique must be one that is safe to perform on a standing horse. This implies safety for the horse, the surgeon and other personnel, and the equipment.
- Because the risks of general anesthesia are avoided, standing surgery may be beneficial for sick, debilitated, or elderly patients.
- The risks associated with recumbency under anesthesia (e.g., compartment syndrome) are avoided; therefore, large or heavily muscled horses, such as draft breeds, should undergo standing procedures whenever possible.
- If the patient has undergone extreme stress or trauma, avoiding general anesthesia may be better for the patient.
- If the patient has a history of problems under general anesthesia or has experienced a difficult recovery, standing surgery may be preferable.
- Usually standing procedures are less expensive than comparable general anesthetic procedures. Fewer drugs, less patient monitoring, and fewer staff members are generally required, all of which reduces costs.

Standing surgery has drawbacks, however. The surgeon's comfort is often compromised, especially if operating on the lower legs (Fig. 10-1). The surgeon's visualization of the surgical field is frequently compromised because of the inability to use retractors and often poor lighting. It is very difficult to drape and maintain a sterile surgical field and to control contamination of instruments, especially under farm conditions (Fig. 10-2). Finally, because the patient is awake, the patient can move, presenting a danger to itself, personnel, and equipment. Even with heavy sedation and physical restraint, the possibility of motion must always be considered, and precautions must be taken.

Preparation for Standing Surgery

Patient preparation depends totally on the procedure and on whether it is being performed on an emergency or elective basis. If the procedure is scheduled in advance, it is preferable to restrict the patient's food intake. Most procedures

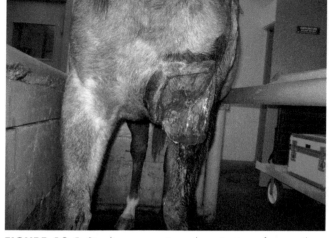

FIGURE 10-1 Standing surgery is much easier to perform on these types of lacerations. (Courtesy Nebraska Equine.)

use some form of chemical restraint. All the drugs used to produce sedation and tranquilization cause some degree of depression of gastrointestinal (GI) motility. Food restriction can reduce bulk in the intestines and reduce intake of highly fermentable foodstuffs. Clinicians have individual preferences about how to restrict food intake, but generally grain is withheld for 12 hours, and only small amounts of hay are allowed until 2 to 6 hours before the procedure. Water is not withheld. If the procedure is being performed on an emergency basis, the client should be instructed to remove all hay and grain immediately until the veterinarian arrives and evaluates the situation.

> **TECHNICIAN NOTE**   Preanesthetic fasting consists of withholding grain for 12 hours; only small amounts of hay are allowed until 2 to 6 hours before the procedure. Water is not withheld.

Optimally, the procedure should be performed in a clean, dry, dust-free area. Drafts should be prevented because they can blow dust and debris into the surgical field. Noise and motion must be minimized to prevent arousing the horse.

Surgical instruments must be available to the surgeon yet out of the way of the horse if it moves. Every attempt should be made to elevate the instruments above ground level, where contamination by dust and debris is most likely. A hay bale, stool, or overturned bucket covered with a towel is a simple way to raise instrument packs off the ground. The instrument pack can then be opened and used by surgical team members.

Restraint of the patient depends on the location of the procedure, duration of the procedure, "pain factor" of the procedure, temperament of the horse, facilities, and skill and number of available personnel. Physical restraint may range from a halter and lead shank to mechanical devices such as twitches and ropes. Chemical restraint (sedation or tranquilization) is often used; sometimes heavy sedation must be

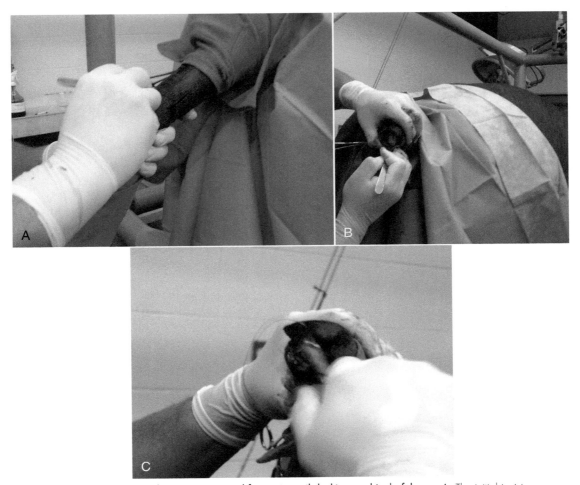

FIGURE 10-2 Standing surgery is used for equine tail docking on this draft horse. **A,** The initial incision is made to create a flap to cover the tail. **B,** The tail after removal. **C,** Suturing of the skin flap back to the tail. (Courtesy Nebraska Equine.)

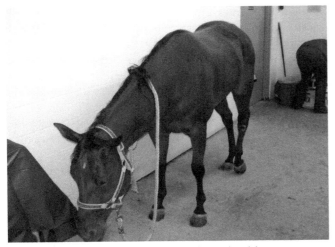

FIGURE 10-3 Characteristic stance of a sedated horse. (Courtesy Nebraska Equine.)

used (Fig. 10-3). All procedures and all patients are different; therefore, restraint must be tailored to the situation.

The pharmacology and effects of drugs used for restraint and analgesia are thoroughly discussed in numerous excellent references on anesthesia and pharmacology. The clinical effects of the most commonly used chemical restraining agents are listed in Box 10-1.

Control of Pain

Most surgical procedures either create pain, address a painful condition, or both. Analgesia must be provided to minimize the patient's discomfort. Many of the drugs used for chemical restraint have analgesic properties but are insufficient to control moderately or markedly painful procedures. Therefore, local anesthesia is usually employed for pain control.

Local anesthesia may be applied in several ways: nerve blocks, field blocks, and epidural anesthesia.

Nerve Blocks

If a nerve can be reached with a hypodermic needle, then local anesthetic drugs can be deposited over the nerve. The anesthetic diffuses into the nerve and interferes with impulse transmission for variable periods of time. The effects of blocking a nerve must be known in advance, to select the proper nerves to desensitize the surgical area and to prevent unwanted anesthesia of important structures. Anatomical and sensation "maps" for the major nerves are available and help guide the clinician in selecting which nerves to anesthetize.

BOX 10-1	Clinical Effects of Commonly Used Chemical Restraining Agents

Acepromazine (Tranquilizer)
- Peripheral vasodilation
- Tendency for hypotension, especially if animal is dehydrated or debilitated
- Tendency for mild hypothermia
- Delayed onset of action (20 to 30 minutes after IV injection)
- Long duration of action (3 to 4 hours)
- Possibly prolonged period of ataxia
- Penis possibly extended for prolonged time; subject to trauma
- Lowered seizure threshold of the brain
- Tranquilization not profound; animal still able to respond vigorously to stimuli
- No analgesic properties
- Respiratory rate decreased but tidal volume increased; net effect of relatively normal ventilation

Xylazine (Sedative-Hypnotic)
- Intramuscular route irritating to foals; owner warned of irritation and swelling at injection site; neck avoided if foal is nursing
- Rapid onset of action (≈1 to 2 minutes after IV injection)
- Good muscle relaxation; weight shifted to forelimbs, head and neck lowered
- Animal still able to respond to stimuli by kicking with hindlimbs; caution needed
- Good analgesia (for 20 to 30 minutes)
- Bradycardia, often with second-degree A-V block

- Second-degree A-V block usually transient (5 to 8 minutes)
- Dosage reduced if patient has low resting heart rate or preexisting second-degree A-V block
- Peripheral vasoconstriction
- Aid in maintaining blood pressure
- Decreased respiratory rate
- Increased urine output (up to 10 times) for 2 to 4 hours
- Sweating
- Decreased gastrointestinal motility
- Increased blood glucose up to 40%

Detomidine (Sedative-Hypnotic)
Similar to xylazine, except
- Longer duration of action (≈60 minutes)
- More potent analgesia
- More profound sedation
- Possibly more severe bradycardia

Butorphanol (Opiate)
- Opiates cannot be used alone in equids; a tranquilizer or sedative-hypnotic given first and allowed to take effect before opiate administration
- Profound sedation and excellent analgesia when used in combination with sedative-hypnotics (most often xylazine and butorphanol)
- Minimal cardiovascular effects
- Minimal or no adverse respiratory effects
- Controlled substance

A-V, Atrioventricular; *IV,* intravenous.

Local anesthetic drugs are primarily chosen according to their duration of action, matched with the anticipated length of the surgical procedure. See Chapter 9 for more specific information regarding preparation and location of nerve block placement.

Field Blocks
Field blocks are usually performed to desensitize the skin and subcutaneous tissue around a surgical area without blocking specific nerves. Rather, a line of anesthetic is deposited subcutaneously around the perimeter of the surgical area ("line block") to produce an area of desensitization. If deeper anesthesia is required, the depth of the line can be extended into underlying muscle tissue (if available). This type of block may produce small or large areas of anesthesia, depending on where the anesthetic is placed. The line block is very useful for suturing lacerations. Large field blocks are commonly used for abdominal surgical procedures performed through the flank.

Epidural Anesthesia
Caudal epidural anesthesia is routinely used for analgesia of the tail, perineum, anus or rectum, vulva, and vagina. Caudal epidural techniques are also used to decrease straining associated with obstetrical procedures for dystocias and other reproductive procedures.

Three classes of drugs can be used for caudal epidural anesthesia:
1. Local anesthetics block not only sensory fibers but also motor fibers and sympathetic fibers. Loss of motor control can cause ataxia and even collapse of the hindlimbs; this is a rare occurrence but can be disastrous if it does occur.
2. Alpha-2 agonists selectively block sensory fibers, with minimal effects on hindlimb function.
3. Opioids selectively block sensory fibers, with minimal effects on hindlimb function.

Caudal epidural anesthesia is easily performed on large animals. The site of injection is between the first and second coccygeal vertebrae, on the dorsal midline (Fig. 10-4). An estimate of this location is made by moving the tail up and down while palpating for the first movable intercoccygeal space caudal to the sacrum. The patient should be restrained, and personnel should stand to the side of the patient to avoid being kicked.

> **TECHNICIAN NOTE** Location of the caudal epidural injection site is found by lifting the tail up and down while palpating for the first movable intercoccygeal space caudal to the sacrum.

The area at the base of the tail and the caudal sacrum are clipped and surgically prepared. The anesthetist should

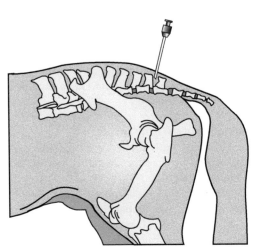

FIGURE 10-4 Location for caudal epidural in the horse. The needle is inserted in the first intercoccygeal space. (Adapted from Riebold TW: Principles and techniques of equine anesthesia, *Vet Clin North Am Equine Pract* 6:485–741, 1990.)

wear sterile gloves. The clinician inserts an 18-gauge (ga) × 1½-inch needle (large patients may require an 18-ga × 3½-inch spinal needle) at a 90-degree angle to the skin and advances it into the epidural space. Anesthetic solution is injected with a sterile syringe. Because sterile injection technique is required, the anesthetic solution should be taken from a new, previously unopened container. Sometimes the needle is left in place in case the patient needs more anesthetic later in the procedure. The needle should not be withdrawn until the clinician approves its removal because bleeding and swelling (after removing the needle) can make repeating the epidural procedure difficult. Complications are unusual, and aftercare involves simply cleaning the area and applying an antibiotic or antimicrobial ointment to the puncture site.

Epidural techniques are not performed more cranially than the first intercoccygeal space in awake patients. This is because the risk of creating ataxia and collapse of the hindlimbs increases as the site of administering the epidural moves cranially.

> **TECHNICIAN NOTE** Epidural anesthesia is not performed more cranially than the first intercoccygeal space in an awake patient because of the risk of ataxia and collapse.

Postoperative Care of the Patient

If sedation or tranquilization has been used, the patient should be "*NPO*" (Latin nulla per os, meaning "nothing by mouth") until the horse swallows normally. Water is returned first, by allowing only a few sips to ensure that the horse can swallow without coughing. Once this is determined, light hay can be returned in 1 to 2 hours. Grain is returned last, often waiting until the following day before giving full rations. The patient should be monitored closely in the first 24 hours for urine and fecal output.

Specific postoperative care depends on the nature of the surgical procedure.

GENERAL ANESTHESIA

General anesthesia can be technically simple or complex, but it is never without risk. The procedure must be respected for the risks to which both patient and staff are potentially exposed, and the risks must be carefully evaluated. Much of the risk results from patient-related factors such as size, weight, and temperament. The physiologic effects of preanesthetic and anesthetic drugs also pose certain hazards that are unique to large animal patients.

No single "correct" approach to large animal anesthesia exists. Clinicians and hospitals vary greatly with regard to all phases of administering general anesthesia: equipment, patient preparation, induction, maintenance, and recovery. Despite these variations, some generalizations can be made and are discussed in further detail here. For specific information on the pharmacology and in-depth mechanics of large animal anesthesia, the reader is referred to the many textbooks that have been written on the topic of veterinary anesthesia.

Preoperative Patient Examination and Laboratory Evaluation

The depth and extent of the physical examination and laboratory testing depend on the patient's condition and the nature of the surgical procedure. The clinician prescribes the necessary laboratory tests to be performed. At a minimum, a physical examination before any general anesthetic episode should include the following: temperature, pulse, and respiration; heart and lung auscultation; and body weight assessment. The patient's temperament and manageability also should be assessed because these individual characteristics may influence the choice of induction and recovery techniques.

Correcting Fluid, Electrolyte, and Acid-Base Imbalances Before Induction of General Anesthesia

Fluid therapy before induction of anesthesia is important to correct dehydration and other imbalances. Sometimes, the emergency nature of a case precludes complete correction of imbalances. In these cases, as much therapy as possible should be provided before induction, and the therapy should be continued once anesthesia has been successfully induced in the patient.

Preanesthetic Preparation

For preparation of an equine patient for general anesthesia, the following principles should be considered.

Ventilation Problems Under General Anesthesia

When the patient is recumbent, the weight of the intestines presses against the diaphragm and thoracic cavity and prevents the lungs from expanding normally. Oxygen levels in the blood fall, and carbon dioxide levels rise; these abnormalities worsen with time. These effects occur in lateral recumbency and are most severe in dorsal recumbency.

Ventilation may be improved by reducing the weight of the intestinal tract. Fasting the patient is the most efficient way to reduce the weight of intestinal contents. Grain and hay are usually withdrawn for at least 12 hours before general anesthesia, although clinicians vary in specifying time frames for feed withdrawal. Water is seldom withdrawn more than 2 hours before anesthesia because of the possibility of dehydrating the GI contents (and causing subsequent GI colic) and possibly dehydrating the circulatory system of the patient. Most clinicians do not withdraw water at all before premedication for the actual procedure.

Foals are allowed to nurse until approximately 30 to 60 minutes before induction of general anesthesia. This allows time for the stomach to empty, which is important because foals, unlike adults, may regurgitate after induction of anesthesia. If the foal is eating solid food, the food should be removed for 3 to 4 hours before induction. To prevent the foal's nursing from the mare, a muzzle must be used on the foal. Foal muzzles can be purchased or made from half-gallon milk cartons by cutting the carton in half. Two nostril openings are made, and the muzzle is secured behind the foal's ears with gauze or twine straps (Fig. 10-5).

> **TECHNICIAN NOTE** Water is typically not withheld before equine surgical procedures.

Anticholinergics Are Not Routinely Used for Preanesthetic Medication

Most anesthetic drugs cause some degree of depression of GI motility. Anticholinergic drugs, especially atropine, may have marked effects on depressing GI motility. The additive effect of anticholinergics and other anesthetic drugs may result in prolonged ileus, leading to GI colic. The administration of anticholinergics to decrease saliva production, as used in small animals, is not considered necessary in horses.

> **TECHNICIAN NOTE** Use of anticholinergics depresses gastrointestinal motility.

Anticholinergics are, however, very useful for treating bradycardia and second- and third-degree atrioventricular (A-V) block. These drugs should be available for emergency use. Anticholinergics are sometimes used during ophthalmic surgical procedures, when manipulation of the eyeball may create excessive vagal tone.

Minimizing Anesthetic Time

Because the risks of general anesthesia increase with time, every effort should be made to decrease anesthetic time by using the following steps.

Surgical Clipping and Preparation. Perform as much of the surgical clipping and preparing as possible before induction of anesthesia. The disposition of some patients may make this impossible; clippers should be available after induction anesthesia for these patients. Note that razors are often used for final removal of hair. However, use of razors on awake patients is difficult and often results in cuts and abrasions of the patient's skin. Therefore, if razors are necessary, they should be made available for use after induction of anesthesia.

> **TECHNICIAN NOTE** If the surgical prep requires use of a razor, it should be used after induction of anesthesia, to prevent cuts and abrasions.

Intravenous Catheterization. If intravenous (IV) catheters are to be used, they should be placed before induction.

Preparation of Equipment and Supplies. All surgical instruments and supplies should be assembled and brought to the surgical area. Equipment should be checked for proper function. Anesthetic supplies and equipment, including IV fluids, must also be anticipated. If gas anesthesia is to be used, the anesthesia machine should be checked for leaks and properly prepared.

Patient Positioning. Positioning should be discussed with the surgeon so that the operating table and patient padding and support can be set up before the induction of anesthesia.

Mouth Cleansing. The patient's mouth may harbor feed material and other debris. Feed material tends to accumulate between the cheek teeth and cheek tissue. This material may be pushed into the trachea during endotracheal intubation.

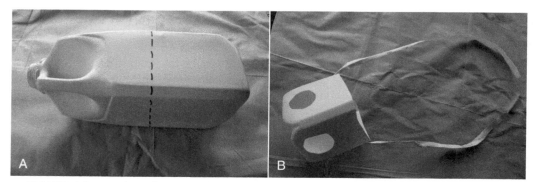

FIGURE 10-5 Foal muzzle. **A,** A half-gallon plastic carton is divided in half. **B,** Breathing holes and straps are added. The muzzle is secured to the halter or tied behind the foal's ears.

Always flush the patient's mouth with a dose syringe or water hose if endotracheal intubation is anticipated.

> **TECHNICIAN NOTE** The equine mouth should be flushed with a dose syringe or water hose if endotracheal intubation is anticipated to prevent feed material from being pushed into the trachea.

Preventing Contamination of the Surgical Room

The patient should be thoroughly cleaned to prevent contamination of the surgical room. Thorough grooming should always be performed; the patient is brushed and bathed as needed. The tail is often braided or taped to keep tail hairs out of the surgical field and to minimize contamination if the horse defecates while under anesthesia. The hooves should be cleaned and scrubbed with soapy water. If the patient is wearing horseshoes, they are usually removed at this time. The feet should be covered either before the animal enters the operating room or immediately afterward. Latex examination gloves, rectal sleeves, plastic bags, and bandaging tape are commonly used for this purpose.

Occasionally it may be desirable to leave horseshoes on, especially if they are being used to correct or treat a medical condition. In such cases, the hooves should still be cleaned, and some type of protective boot or hoof bandage should be placed over the shod hoof before anesthetic induction (Fig. 10-6).

> **TECHNICIAN NOTE** During preparation, it is important to cover the hooves before entering the operating room.

Protecting the Lower Legs During Induction and Recovery

Leg wraps or bandages should be placed on the horse to protect the tendons and ligaments of the lower legs. If removal

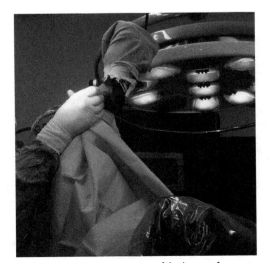

FIGURE 10-6 Appropriate covering of the hooves for surgery. (Courtesy Nebraska Equine.)

of leg protection is necessary for the surgical procedure, the wraps should be replaced for recovery from anesthesia.

> **TECHNICIAN NOTE** Leg wraps are placed to protect the legs during surgical procedures and recovery.

Protecting the Eyes

The wide-set anatomical location of the equine eyes makes them susceptible to trauma. Halters with metal buckles or billets should be removed and replaced with halters that do not have metal attachments. Padded walls or helmets can be placed to protect the eyes further. The head should be controlled during induction of anesthesia to prevent it from striking the floor or walls as the horse falls to the ground. Sharp objects and corners should be removed from the induction or recovery area or covered with padding if possible. In field settings, the lower (downward) eye should be protected from the ground surface with a towel.

> **TECHNICIAN NOTE** In a field setting, the downward eye should be protected from the ground surface with a towel.

Induction and Maintenance of General Anesthesia

General considerations for induction and maintenance of general anesthesia include the following.

Prevention of Compartment Syndrome

Compartment syndrome is not uncommon in recumbent large animals, regardless of the cause of recumbency. All recumbent animals are susceptible to compartment syndrome, and the heavy body weight of large animals exacerbates the problem. Draft horse breeds and heavily muscled individuals are predisposed to developing the condition. Muscle "compartments" refer to muscles and muscle groups in the body that are encased in a dense connective tissue called fascia, which has little elasticity. Muscles that are enclosed in these nonelastic envelopes are prevented from swelling outwardly by the fascia.

The four clinically significant muscle compartments are as follows:
1. Gluteals
2. Triceps
3. Masseters
4. Quadriceps

Normally, arteries pump blood into a muscle compartment to nourish the muscle, and veins and lymphatic vessels drain blood and tissue fluid (lymph) out of the compartment. In recumbent animals, however, the vessels may be sandwiched between the animal's own body weight pressing down from above and the ground surface below. Compartment syndrome begins with the collapse (partial or complete) of the veins and lymphatic vessels that drain the compartment. These vessels have very low pressure inside their walls, and they easily collapse when external pressure (e.g., body weight) is applied to them. Arteries, conversely, have much higher internal pressures and can resist higher compressive forces. Therefore, arteries remain open longer than do veins and lymphatic vessels.

As the arterial supply continues to pump blood into the compartment, the pressure inside the compartment starts to rise because the blood and tissue fluid cannot drain adequately through the collapsed veins and lymphatics. A vicious cycle of increasing pressure and increasing collapse of vessels inside the compartment develops. Eventually, the muscle and nerve cells in the compartment begin to suffer because they cannot receive proper nutrition or eliminate their cell waste. Various degrees of muscle and nerve dysfunction result, and the cells may even die if the condition is not successfully treated. The severity of compartment syndrome often correlates with the length of time that the conditions persist.

Compartment syndrome is the primary cause of postanesthetic myopathy (muscle dysfunction) and *postanesthetic neuropathy* (nerve dysfunction). Postanesthetic myopathy or neuropathy is the leading cause of injury and death in healthy horses undergoing elective surgical procedures. Incidence rates as high as 5% of general anesthesia cases have been reported. General anesthesia increases the risk of compartment syndrome because the drugs used to induce and maintain anesthesia usually depress the cardiovascular system and lower blood pressure. Blood pressure is the only pressure inside a vessel that resists external compression; therefore, maintaining adequate blood pressure is the primary protection against developing compartment syndrome.

> **TECHNICIAN NOTE** Postanesthetic myopathy or neuropathy is the leading cause of injury and death in healthy horses undergoing elective surgical procedures.

Compartment syndrome may affect one compartment or multiple compartments, and it may have mild, moderate, or severe effects. Clinical signs may include difficulty standing or inability to stand following general anesthesia, palpable hardening of the affected compartment, paresis or paralysis, and lameness. Acute renal failure or even complete renal shutdown occasionally may result from damage to kidney tubules from myoglobin, which is released from damaged skeletal muscle cells. Myoglobin may cause dark urine; however, dark urine is not seen in every case. The condition is quite painful, and increased heart rate, respiratory rate, sweating, and anxiety may be observed. Although the syndrome is usually observed on the patient's "down" side, it may also affect the "up" side if the limbs are not positioned properly or if prolonged hypotension is allowed to occur.

Severely affected animals may have irreversible damage to muscles, nerves, or kidneys and may cause severe damage to themselves by trying to stand on legs that cannot support their weight because of muscle or nerve damage. Euthanasia is not an uncommon ending for many affected animals; complications result in euthanasia in up to 25% of cases.

> **TECHNICIAN NOTE** Complications in 25% of compartment syndrome cases result in euthanasia.

Compartment syndrome is a serious and realistic concern and is frustrating for clinicians and anesthetists. No reliable method exists for predicting or detecting the problem while the patient is under general anesthesia, and usually the problem does not become apparent until the patient tries to stand in the recovery area. Even when all precautions to prevent the syndrome are strictly followed, some individuals develop the condition. Still, the incidence of compartment syndrome can be significantly reduced by following certain precautions:

- Minimize anesthetic time: The incidence of compartment syndrome increases with anesthesia time, especially in procedures lasting longer than 1 hour. As much prepping of the patient and setup of the surgical area as possible should be done before induction.
- Maintain anesthesia only as deeply as necessary: Blood pressure drops as the depth of anesthesia increases, thus increasing the risk to the patient.
- Use adequate padding: Facilities vary with regard to the type of padding used, but thick foam mattresses (15 to 20 cm thick), conventional mattresses, air mattresses, and waterbed mattresses can be used successfully (Fig. 10-7).
- Position the patient properly:
  - Lateral recumbency: Place the forelimbs in a "staggered" position by pulling the lower forelimb forward (cranially) to rotate the shoulder girdle. This position decreases the body weight pressing down on the triceps muscle. The hindlimbs are not staggered. Elevate the upper limbs (both forelimb and hindlimb) to a horizontal position, parallel to the ground. Do not elevate the upper limbs above this level (Fig. 10-8). Protect the masseter muscle by removing or loosening the

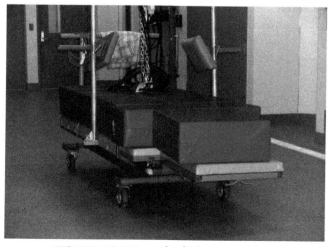

FIGURE 10-7 Example of adequate padding.

halter after induction and padding the area supporting the head.

- Dorsal recumbency: Keep the forelimbs folded naturally at the carpus. The hindlimbs are allowed to frog-leg naturally at most hospitals, but some clinicians prefer to suspend the hindlimbs in an extended position.
- Reduce carbohydrate intake: Because of the suspected relationship between a high-carbohydrate diet and post-anesthetic myositis, horses on a high-grain diet should undergo a "taper down" period of grain reduction for 1 to 2 weeks before general anesthesia.
- Maintain good systemic blood pressure during anesthesia: Correct dehydration before induction, if possible. Consider IV fluids for any procedure lasting longer than 1 hour. Research has shown that mean arterial blood pressure should be kept at more than 70 mm Hg to minimize the risk of postanesthetic myopathy or neuropathy. Blood pressure monitoring should be considered for any procedure lasting longer than 1 hour. Any hypotension should be treated promptly and aggressively.

Three Methods of Induction and Maintenance of General Anesthesia

1. Induction with injectable drugs and maintenance with injectable drugs: This is the most common method for procedures in the field and for short procedures (<1 hour). Induction must be rapid; it is desirable for the patient to lose consciousness and fall directly to the ground. If the induction drugs are not given rapidly, the patient may resist the effects of the drugs by wandering or going over backward.
2. Induction with injectable drugs and maintenance with gas anesthesia: This is the preferred method for procedures lasting longer than 1 hour. Because large animals are prone to ventilation difficulties while they are under general anesthesia and because these difficulties worsen with time, a gas anesthesia machine is valuable for its ability to

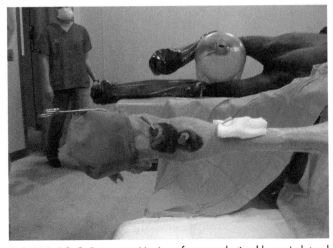

FIGURE 10-8 Proper positioning of an anesthetized horse in lateral recumbency. The "down" forelimb has been pulled cranially to "stagger" the shoulder girdle. Both upper limbs have been elevated to a horizontal position, but no higher.

provide oxygen and assist with ventilation during longer procedures.

3. Induction with gas anesthesia and maintenance with gas anesthesia: This method is generally suitable only for foals. Gas induction cannot be delivered rapidly enough to adults, thereby leading to prolonged induction with the patient resistant to the effects of the anesthetic gas. Gas induction in foals is usually done by face mask, followed by intubation through the nasotracheal or orotracheal route for maintenance.

> **TECHNICIAN NOTE** Gas induction of foals is usually done by face mask.

Induce Foals in the Company of the Mare

Unless a foal is extremely ill, it usually panics when it is are separated from its dam, and this leads to difficult induction of anesthesia. Typically, anesthesia is induced in the foal with the mare at its side; then the mare is sedated and returned to her stall or holding area. When the foal has recovered from anesthesia, the two are reunited. The mare should be observed closely during the separation because removal of the foal typically causes the mare to become frantic. Heavy sedation of the mare may be necessary.

Routes of Tracheal Intubation in Horses

As with other species, great trauma can be done to the patient if intubation is performed aggressively. Just because the animal is bigger does not mean that the larynx, pharynx, and trachea are tougher. Care must be taken during insertion of the tracheal tube and inflation of the cuff (if present).

Three routes are possible for intubation: orotracheal, nasotracheal, and direct tracheal. The route selected depends on the patient's age and size and on the surgical procedure to be performed.

Orotracheal Intubation. Orotracheal intubation is the most common method. An oral speculum must be used to maintain separation of the teeth. Oral speculums can be purchased commercially or easily made using 3- to 4-inch diameter polyvinyl chloride (PVC) pipe cut to a 2- to 3-inch length. The slick outer surface of the PVC is covered with duct tape or an adhesive tape to facilitate seating of the PVC between the incisors. The endotracheal tube is inserted through the center of the PVC speculum (Figs. 10-9 and 10-10).

Intubation can be performed with the patient in either lateral recumbency or sternal recumbency. Orotracheal intubation is performed blindly and usually is readily accomplished by following two recommendations. First, position the head and neck in the same plane, and extend the head to form a straight line from the mouth to the trachea; intubating along a crooked line is difficult. Second, grasp the patient's tongue, and pull it from the mouth to reduce the bulk of the base of the tongue, which may block the entrance to the trachea. The tube should be lubricated with sterile, water-soluble lubricating jelly.

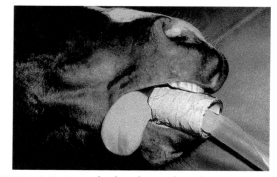

FIGURE 10-9 Orotracheal intubation through a polyvinyl chloride speculum placed between the incisors. (From Muir WW, Hubbell JAE: *Handbook of veterinary anesthesia*, ed 4, St. Louis, 2007, Mosby.)

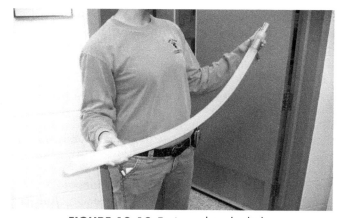

FIGURE 10-10 Equine endotracheal tube.

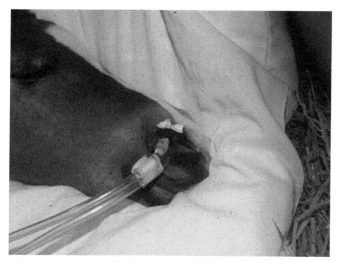

FIGURE 10-11 Foal with nasogastric and oxygen tubing in place. The nasogastric tube is sutured to the muzzle, and the oxygen tubing is taped to the nasogastric tube. If oxygen tubing alone is being used, then it should be sutured directly to the muzzle. (From McAuliffe SB, Slovis NM: *Color atlas of diseases and disorders of the foal*, St. Louis, 2008, Saunders.)

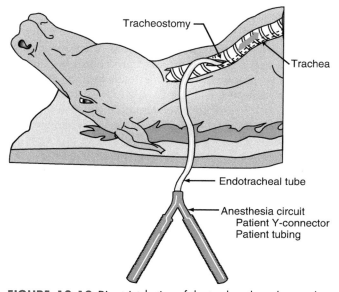

FIGURE 10-12 Direct intubation of the trachea through a tracheostomy.

Nasotracheal Intubation

Nasotracheal intubation is used primarily for foals and small individuals (<100 kg). Because of the small diameter of nasotracheal tubes, providing adequate movement of anesthetic gases and oxygen may be difficult or impossible in adult horses. Anesthesia is usually induced in foals with a face mask or injectable drugs; the foals are then intubated by the nasotracheal route. Although inducing anesthesia in foals through the nasotracheal tube is possible, the foals may resist intubation while they are conscious; local anesthetic may be added to the lubricating jelly to decrease the patients' sensitivity of the nasal cavity. As with orotracheal intubation, the head and neck should be aligned and the head extended to straighten the course of intubation. The tube should be well lubricated with sterile, water-soluble lubricating jelly (Fig. 10-11).

Direct Tracheal Intubation

Direct tracheal intubation is uncommonly performed. It is reserved for procedures where orotracheal or nasotracheal tubes would interfere with the surgical procedure; this situation occurs primarily with procedures of the larynx and pharynx. The intubation procedure is accomplished by first performing a tracheostomy and then inserting a standard, cuffed endotracheal tube directly through the tracheostomy into the trachea (Fig. 10-12). Care should be taken not to

advance the tube so far that it enters a primary bronchus. This would lead to gas delivery to only one lung, with negative consequences. Care must also be taken not to bend the endotracheal tube at a sharp angle, which would decrease the diameter of the tube and compromise ventilation. The endotracheal tube should be the same diameter as would be used for orotracheal intubation. A cuffed tracheostomy tube can be used in place of standard endotracheal tubes (Fig. 10-13).

After the surgical procedure, the endotracheal tube is withdrawn and replaced with a standard tracheostomy tube. This allows the patient to breathe while laryngeal and pharyngeal swelling from the surgical procedure subside (usually over several days). When the patient can breathe adequately

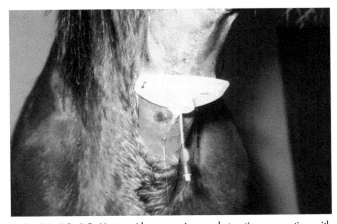

FIGURE 10-13 Horse with upper airway obstruction presenting with severe dyspnea requiring placement of tracheostomy tube. (From Sellon DC, Long MT: *Equine infectious diseases*, St. Louis, 2007, Saunders.)

BOX 10-2	Emergency Tracheostomy Pack

1. Local anesthetic
2. 20- to 25-gauge syringe needles
3. 3- or 6-mL syringes
4. Disposable scalpel blade (no. 10) and handle
5. Metzenbaum scissors
6. Mosquito hemostats
7. J-type, self-restraining, or cuffed tracheostomy tube

through the normal route, the tracheostomy tube is removed, and the site is managed as a healing tracheostomy.

Tracheotomy and Tracheostomy

Tracheostomy may be performed as an emergency or elective procedure (Box 10-2). Obstructions of the upper airway, such as swelling resulting from snake bite, compression or blockage by tumors, and lymph node swelling, may create life-threatening compromise to breathing. Elective tracheostomy is performed whenever severe postoperative swelling is anticipated following surgical procedures in the nasal, pharyngeal, or laryngeal regions. Elective tracheotomy or tracheostomy is also performed to administer gas anesthesia when an orotracheal or nasotracheal tube would interfere with surgical access to the mouth, nose, or throat.

Rarely, permanent tracheostomy is required. Patients with permanent tracheostomy lose the natural defense mechanisms of the upper airways (filtration and humidification) because these defenses are essentially bypassed, thus making these animals susceptible to lower respiratory tract infections. These patients should be maintained in a dust-free environment and watched closely for signs of disease. Daily cleaning of the site is necessary to remove secretions.

Tracheostomy is usually performed with the horse standing, but it may be performed with the patient under general anesthesia. The usual location is the junction of the cranial and middle third of the neck.

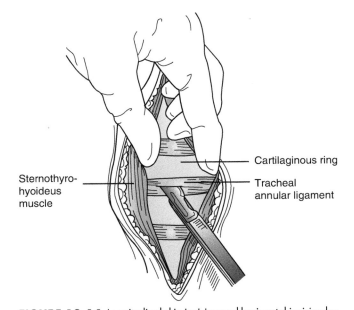

FIGURE 10-14 Longitudinal skin incision and horizontal incision between tracheal rings for tracheotomy. (From Orsini JA, Divers TJ: *Manual of equine emergencies*, ed 3, St. Louis, 2008, Saunders.)

Appropriate physical and chemical restraint is applied. The neck should be positioned in a straight line, regardless of whether the patient is standing or recumbent.

If possible, the area over the trachea should be clipped and sterilely prepared. In an emergency situation, complete sterile preparation may not be possible. The trachea is penetrated with a sharp object, and any tube available is used to provide an airway. Local anesthesia (3 to 5 mL) is required if the procedure is performed on a conscious patient.

A longitudinal 5- to 10-cm incision is made directly on the ventral midline through the skin and subcutaneous tissue. The muscle bellies of the sternothyrohyoideus muscles are divided on the ventral midline to expose the trachea. Two tracheal rings are identified, and an incision is made in the tissue between them by rotating the scalpel blade 90 degrees and "stabbing" the blade through the tissue. This horizontal stab incision is then extended approximately 2 cm to either side. Care is taken not to cut the cartilage rings (Fig. 10-14). When the incision is complete, a tracheostomy tube or endotracheal tube is inserted, depending on the patient's needs.

While the tracheostomy tube is in place, it should be inspected frequently for proper positioning and possible obstruction by secretions. It should be removed once or twice daily and replaced or cleaned in an antiseptic solution. The tracheostomy site is cleaned with a sterile dilute antiseptic solution (e.g., dilute povidone-iodine) before the tracheostomy tube is replaced. Discharge from the skin wound often occurs and may scald the skin. Petroleum jelly applied to the "runoff" area ventral to the tracheostomy site helps to prevent skin scald.

TECHNICIAN NOTE Application of petroleum jelly applied to the "runoff" area ventral to the tracheostomy site helps prevent skin scald.

After the tracheostomy tube is removed, the incision is left to heal by second intention. Healing is usually complete in approximately 3 weeks. The site is cleaned once or twice daily with sterile dilute antiseptic solution, and an antibacterial ointment is applied to the healing skin edges, with care taken not to place ointment inside the wound, where it could accidentally enter the trachea.

> **TECHNICIAN NOTE**   Healing of the incision from a tracheostomy is by second intention and takes approximately 3 weeks.

Subcutaneous emphysema may develop adjacent to the tracheostomy site. This complication is recognized by swelling and a crepitant or "bubble wrap" texture on palpation. No specific treatment exists. The body gradually reabsorbs the subcutaneous air.

Large Animal Anesthesia Machines

Large animal anesthesia machines contain the same basic components as small animal anesthesia machines. However, many of the components of large animal anesthesia machines are larger than those of small animal anesthesia machines (Fig. 10-15). Large animals require larger volumes of carbon dioxide absorber, larger reservoir bags, and larger-diameter patient tubing (Table 10-1). The large volume of rubber surfaces in large animal anesthesia circuits tends to absorb fairly large quantities of anesthetic gas. Absorption of gas by rubber makes the concentration of gas in the circuit lower than the desired concentration on the anesthetic vaporizer. This effect continues until the rubber becomes saturated with anesthetic gas, typically requiring at least 10 to 15 minutes. Achieving surgical

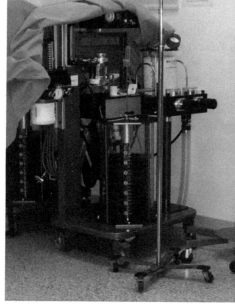

FIGURE 10-15 Typical large animal anesthesia machine and ventilator.

anesthesia depth during this time may be difficult because the rubber competes with the patient for absorption of the gas. Therefore, the circuit should be "preloaded" with anesthetic gas before the patient is attached to the machine. Preloading allows time for the rubber to become saturated and denitrogenates the circuit as well. Preloading can be accomplished by plugging or covering the patient connector of the Y-tubing with duct tape and then turning on the anesthetic gas to moderate levels for at least 10 to 15 minutes before attaching the patient. Preloading is part of the routine preparation of the anesthesia machine and circuit (Fig. 10-16).

Patient Monitoring

Monitoring of the patient is essential. Anesthetic records should always be kept, regardless of the length of the procedure. Large animal anesthetic records are similar to small animal records. An example of an anesthetic record can be found on the Evolve website. The primary concerns for equine patients under anesthesia are hypothermia, hypoventilation, hypotension, and bradycardia (Table 10-2).

Basic parameters such as temperature, pulse rate, and rhythm; respiratory rate and depth; capillary refill time; and mucous membrane color should always be monitored. Additional monitoring may include the following.

Body Temperature. Body temperature is measured rectally. Hypothermia may develop during long procedures, especially in cold environments or air-conditioned operating rooms. A rectal temperature lower than 35.6° C (96° F) has been associated with increased ataxia during the recovery period. Efforts to warm the patient should be instituted before the body temperature reaches this level. Fluid bags warmed in a microwave oven can be packed adjacent to the patient's body, and exposed skin outside the operating field can be covered with clean blankets. Care should be taken that fluid bags warmed in a microwave are not hot enough to cause skin burns.

TABLE 10-1	Large Animal Gas Anesthesia Machine and Circuit Components	
Carbon dioxide absorber (soda lime)	2 pounds	Foal
	5 pounds	Pony, small adult
	10 pounds	Adult
Reservoir bag	5 L	Foal
	15 L	Pony, small adult
	30 L	Adult
Patient Y-tubing	2 cm	Foal
	5 cm	Adult
Endotracheal tubes (inner diameter)	10–16 mm	35–135 kg body weight
	16–20 mm	135–250 kg body weight
	20–25 mm	250–350 kg body weight
	25–30 mm	350–450 kg body weight
	30 mm	≥450 kg body weight

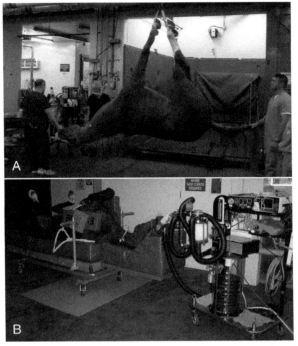

FIGURE 10-16 A, Once the horse is intubated and is confirmed to be stable by the anesthetist, the animal is hoisted for placement on the operating table. The anesthetist controls and supports the head while the patient is on the hoist. **B,** The horse is positioned on a thick foam pad to prevent muscle damage. Side paddles are used to keep the horse in dorsal recumbency on the table, and smaller foam pads support the large muscles of the upper forelimbs. Once the horse is positioned, it is connected to a large animal anesthesia machine. (From Bassert, JM, Thomas J, editors: *McCurnin's clinical textbook for veterinary technicians,* ed 8, St. Louis, 2014, Saunders.)

> **TECHNICIAN NOTE**   Care should be taken that fluid bags warmed in a microwave are not hot enough to cause skin burns.

Hyperthermia. Hyperthermia is rare in large animal patients under anesthesia, but malignant hyperthermia syndrome has been reported in horses under gas anesthetic. When this condition is identified, treatment must be aggressive—cool the patient and terminate anesthesia as soon as possible.

Electrocardiogram Monitoring. Electrocardiogram monitoring of cardiac activity is highly desirable for all general anesthesia procedures. The base-apex lead attachment is useful for electrocardiogram monitoring during surgical procedures. Aside from using longer lead wires, no special equipment is required for monitoring large animal patients.

> **TECHNICIAN NOTE**   The base-apex lead attachment is useful for electrocardiogram monitoring during surgical procedures.

Blood Pressure Monitoring. Blood pressure monitoring is recommended for any procedure lasting longer than 1 hour. Palpating the strength of arterial pulses is an unreliable indictor of blood pressure and is discouraged; mechanical measurements are preferred. Blood pressure can be measured directly or indirectly:

Direct blood pressure measurement is performed with an intraarterial catheter and a pressure transducer. The most common arteries used are the transverse facial artery (located caudal to the lateral canthus of the eye, below the zygomatic arch) and the dorsal metatarsal artery (located on the lateral

TABLE 10-2	Guidelines for Treating Common Complications of General Anesthesia in Adult Horses		
COMPLICATION	**RECOGNITION**	**COMMENTS**	**TREATMENT CONSIDERATIONS**
Hypothermia	Rectal temperature <36.6° C (<96° F)	Best to begin treatment before temperature reaches this level	Warm with warm water bags, blankets Increase temperature in room
Hypotension	Mean arterial pressure <70 mm Hg*	Begin treatment	Decrease vaporizer setting Increase intravenous fluid rate Administer cardiovascular stimulants (especially sympathomimetics)
Hypoventilation	Respiratory rate <6/min Decreased tidal volume <10 mL/kg	Best assessed by arterial blood gas (especially carbon dioxide) measurement; respiratory rate, mucous membrane color, and depth of breathing can be misleading	Decrease vaporizer setting Institute assisted or controlled ventilation
Bradycardia	Heart rate < 30/min Heart rate < 25/min	Consider treatment Emergency	Decrease vaporizer setting Administer anticholinergic or sympathomimetic drugs If surgical procedure is causing increased vagal tone, stop procedure temporarily until heart rate responds to treatment (most likely with gastrointestinal and ocular surgery)

*Mean arterial pressure = 0.33 (systolic pressure − diastolic pressure) + diastolic pressure.

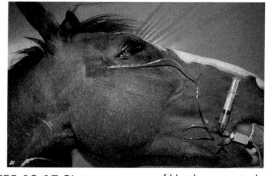

FIGURE 10-17 Direct measurement of blood pressure in the transverse facial artery. The intraarterial catheter is connected to a pressure transducer with heparinized saline-filled plastic tubing. (From Trim CM: Principles of chemical restraint and general anesthesia. In Colahan PT, Mayhew IG, Merritt AM, Moore JN, editors: *Equine medicine and surgery,* ed 5, St. Louis, 1999, Mosby.)

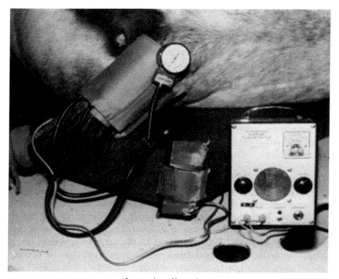

FIGURE 10-18 Use of a tail cuff and Doppler ultrasound unit for indirect measurement of blood pressure. (From Riebold TW: Principles and techniques of equine anesthesia, *Vet Clin North Am Equine Pract* 6:485–741, 1990.)

aspect of each hindlimb, between metatarsals 3 and 4). Direct measurement is technically more difficult to perform but yields more accurate results than indirect measurement (Fig. 10-17).

Indirect blood pressure measurement is usually performed using a Doppler ultrasound unit and an inflatable tail cuff (sphygmomanometer) over the coccygeal artery (Fig. 10-18). Alternatively, a rear leg artery can be used. For accurate readings, the cuff should be at the same level as the heart.

Alternative instruments are available that use oscillometry with an inflatable tail cuff to take pulse and blood pressure readings, as well as calculate mean arterial pressure. These instruments are convenient but expensive and are sensitive to vibrations and motion. They are less reliable when the heart rate is low (especially when second-degree A-V block is present).

For adults, blood pressures from 100 to 120 mm Hg systolic/70 to 80 mm Hg diastolic (70 to 60 mm Hg for foals, although this is highly variable), or mean arterial pressures greater than 70 mm Hg, are desirable. Treatment of hypotension may be necessary if pressures fall to less than these levels.

Because of the tendency for hypotension under general anesthesia, the use of IV fluids is recommended to support compromised patients or whenever the procedure is anticipated to last more than 1 hour. Lactated Ringer's solution is typically given at 10 mL/kg/hour for the first hour, and then the rate is reduced to 5 mL/kg/hour for the remainder of the procedure. The rate can be increased if necessary to treat hypotension or hypovolemia from blood loss.

Hypertension (mean arterial pressure > 90 mm Hg) is usually related to light anesthesia and often corresponds to the amount of pain produced by the surgical procedure. Increasing delivery of anesthetic to return the patient to an appropriate level of anesthesia is required.

Oxygenation and Ventilation. Oxygenation and ventilation are best assessed by arterial blood gas sampling. Arterial blood can be rapidly analyzed for oxygen and carbon dioxide levels, as well as blood pH. This information is invaluable to the anesthetist for assessing adequacy of ventilation and

acid-base imbalances. The equipment for analysis is usually found only at larger hospitals and clinics and currently is not practical in field situations.

An alternative for measuring oxygen levels in the blood is the pulse oximeter. In large animals, the transducer is placed on the tongue. The thickness of the tongue and motion may interfere with the accuracy of this instrument. Hemoglobin oxygen saturation levels higher than 90% are critical for proper oxygenation of the blood. However, the oxygen must still be delivered to the tissues. Low blood pressure or bradycardia, or both, can lead to decreased cardiac output and may interfere with oxygen delivery, even when the blood is well saturated.

Ideally, adults should maintain a respiratory rate between 8 and 12 breaths/minute (>20 for foals). A respiratory rate of less than 6 breaths/minute warrants immediate assistance. Note that respiratory rate is not the only factor needed for adequate ventilation; each breath must also exchange a sufficient tidal volume of air (tidal volume of 10 mL/kg is ideal for spontaneous breathing under general anesthesia). In other words, an adult breathing at the desired rate of 12 breaths/minute may be severely hypoventilating if the breaths are shallow and are not exchanging enough air. Another factor that adds to hypoventilation is ventilation/perfusion mismatch. This condition occurs when the parts of the lungs that are well oxygenated do not correspond to the parts of the lungs that are well perfused with blood (Fig. 10-19). Ventilation/perfusion mismatch is accentuated in large animals because of the size and weight of the lungs. Atelectasis (collapse) of the lower (dependent) portions of the lungs begins quickly once the animal becomes recumbent. This position results in poor ventilation in the lower portions of the lung as the alveoli collapse under the weight. However, the effects of gravity also tend to "pull" more blood into the lower regions

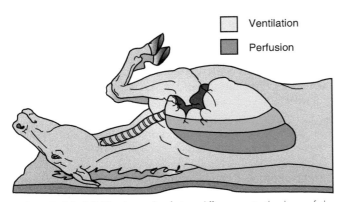

☐ Ventilation
■ Perfusion

FIGURE 10-19 Ventilation/perfusion differences in the lung of the anesthetized horse in dorsal recumbency. Similar effects are seen in lateral recumbency. (Adapted from Greene SA, Keegan RD: Special considerations in the management of equine anesthesia. In Auer JA, editor: *Equine surgery,* St. Louis, 1992, Saunders.)

of the lung. The net effect is more blood and less oxygen and anesthetic gases in the lower lung areas. The ultimate result is poor exchange between gases and the blood, regardless of the patient's rate or depth of breathing. For these reasons, respiratory rate alone cannot be relied on to indicate the patient's respiratory status.

It is standard practice to "sigh" the animal by squeezing the reservoir bag once every 1 to 2 minutes to expand the chest visibly. This practice is thought to reopen collapsed airways and alveoli, thereby helping to maintain ventilation. "Sighing" is not the same as intermittent positive-pressure ventilation, or "bagging," which is treatment for hypoventilation. Sighing is intended to help maintain normal ventilation, not treat hypoventilation, and it should not be used for that purpose.

Pulse Rate. Pulse rate can be assessed by palpation, without any special equipment. Ideally, adults should maintain a pulse rate of at least 30 to 50 per minute (minimum of 80 to 100 in foals). If the pulse rate falls to less than these ranges, treatment for bradycardia should be instituted.

Depth of Anesthesia. Depth of anesthesia is best assessed through eye position and reflexes. A slow palpebral reflex is desirable, and a prompt, strong corneal reflex should always be present. With inhalant (gas) maintenance, the eye rotates from a central position to a rostral position as the horse progresses from light to moderate anesthesia. The eye returns to a central position when anesthesia is excessively deep. Note that ketamine, an agent commonly used for inducing or maintaining anesthesia, tends to keep the eye in a central position as long as its effects persist (≈20 to 30 minutes).

Light anesthesia is signaled in several ways. Nystagmus usually indicates that anesthesia is too light. Respiratory rate, heart rate, and blood pressure also increase. Patients may begin to move the limbs, sometimes violently, when anesthesia becomes too light. The anesthetist should be alert to the signs of light anesthesia and treat it promptly by increasing the vaporizer gas concentration, improving delivery of gas anesthetic with assisted ventilation (if hypoventilation is contributing to the problem), and possibly adding supplemental injectable anesthetics until the proper anesthetic depth is achieved.

If the surgical procedure has begun, the anesthetist may request that the surgeon temporarily halt the procedure to minimize stimulation of the patient until the proper depth of anesthesia can be restored. Motion of the patient presents a real danger to personnel and equipment.

Changing Position of Patient

Rolling patients that are under general anesthesia presents unique ventilation concerns. Uncommonly, a patient needs to be rolled from one recumbency to another in a single surgical procedure, and for some procedures the surgeon can approach only in this fashion. As discussed earlier, when a patient is in lateral recumbency, the "down" or lower lung tends to partial collapse from the weight of the upper lung and intestinal contents. This lung does not exchange air as well as the "top" or upper lung. If the patient is rolled rapidly to the opposite lateral recumbency, the partially collapsed and congested lower lung quickly becomes the upper lung but is not immediately capable of normal gas exchange. In addition, the formerly upper lung has now become the downward lung and immediately begins to collapse. The patient may suffer extreme hypoventilation during this time. Still, rolling can be performed safely by allowing some time for the lungs to adjust to their new positions. The patient is first slowly rolled from lateral to dorsal recumbency and is held there for several minutes to allow the congestion or collapse of the previously lower lung to improve. Then, the roll is slowly completed. The patient should be monitored for hypotension during any rolling procedure.

> **TECHNICIAN NOTE** Rolling the equine patient during surgical procedures can cause hypoventilation.

Additional Considerations

Control of bleeding during surgical procedures is obviously necessary for patients' health but also is necessary for the surgeon's visualization of the surgical field. One popular method of maintaining a "bloodless" surgical field for procedures on the distal limbs is temporary occlusion of blood flow to the area by using a tourniquet. Properly applied tourniquets prevent inflow of arterial blood but also prevent venous drainage. This venous blood can exit through a surgical incision and can block the surgeon's vision. Therefore, before a tourniquet is activated, it is common first to try to "push" as much blood out of the distal limb as possible with an Esmarch bandage (also known as an Esmarch tourniquet).

A tourniquet is first positioned at the desired level, proximal to the surgical area. The tourniquet can be made from surgical rubber tubing, or a pneumatic tourniquet cuff can be used. If tubing is used, minimal foam or cloth padding should be placed beneath the tubing to protect tendons and other underlying structures. If a pneumatic cuff is used, gauze rolls are placed over the major vessels to maximize occlusion when the cuff is inflated. The tourniquet is positioned but is not yet "activated" at this time.

The Esmarch bandage is then applied. The Esmarch bandage is a long strip of latex or other rubber material that is wrapped around the leg with as much tension as possible, beginning just below the coronary band. The wrapping proceeds proximally, by overlapping each preceding layer by half, until the level of the tourniquet is reached. The Esmarch bandage essentially forces blood proximally, out of the distal limb. Once the level of the tourniquet is reached, the tourniquet is activated (tied or inflated). The Esmarch bandage is then removed, and the surgical area is prepared for the surgical procedure (Fig. 10-20).

Tourniquets are painful. If the patient has not reached a surgical plane of anesthesia or had received local anesthesia in the area, lightening of anesthesia may occur. Increases in heart rate and blood pressure may also result. Tourniquets are generally safe to use for up to 2 hours, although tissue damage may begin to occur as early as 30 minutes after activation. The anesthetist should note on the anesthetic record the time of activation and should periodically notify the surgeon of the amount of time that the tourniquet has been in place. The tourniquet should be removed as soon as possible, and the time of removal should be noted in the record.

> **TECHNICIAN NOTE** The anesthetist should periodically notify the surgeon of the amount of time that the tourniquet has been in place.

Recovery
Before the Horse Is Standing

In small animal species, recovery is usually the time when most anesthetic danger has passed and the anesthetist can relax somewhat. Most small animals recover from general anesthesia with minimal assistance and monitoring. In contrast, recovery from general anesthesia in large animals is perhaps the most nerve-racking part of the whole procedure. Recovery poses more risk to the equine patient than does induction or maintenance. The "nature of the beast" is primarily responsible for the risk. Horses are a species of prey, so they resist being recumbent unless by their own choice. Their natural instinct on awakening from anesthesia is to get up, now. Unfortunately, horses almost always regain consciousness faster than the anesthetic drugs are metabolized, thus leaving a brain that says "stand" to legs that are not yet capable of standing. In some patients, compartment syndrome may contribute to the inability to stand. Some patients struggle violently in their attempts to rise and can cause damage to themselves, creating lacerations, fractures, and other trauma that may be severe enough to require euthanasia.

> **TECHNICIAN NOTE** During recovery from anesthesia, some patients struggle violently to stand.

One anesthetic combination that is an exception is xylazine with ketamine. This is the drug combination most commonly used to induce and maintain general anesthesia in horses, primarily for short procedures (20 to 35 minutes). Horses tend to have uneventful recoveries from this drug combination, especially when they are allowed sufficient time to remain recumbent, and most stand on the first attempt with a minimum of difficulty.

Even when standard recommendations for allowing horse to recover from general anesthesia are followed, some patients have a rough recovery. Therefore, emergency drugs and equipment should be readily available. More than one staff member should be available in case an assisted recovery is necessary. To provide the best conditions for a successful recovery, these recommendations should be followed:

- Allow horses to recover in lateral recumbency. If the surgical procedure was performed with the patient in lateral recumbency, allow the patient to recover in the same recumbency unless an underlying orthopedic or neurologic condition makes it unwise to do so. If the patient must be rolled to allow for recovery, follow the same precautions for rolling (discussed earlier).
- Do not encourage the patient to try to stand before the drugs have had sufficient time to wear off. The time necessary depends on the type of drugs used, the amount used, and the patient's underlying physical condition. Recovery usually proceeds best when the horse is allowed to rest quietly until it decides to rise on its own. Therefore, during the recovery period, avoid external stimuli such as bright lights, loud noise, and excessive physical manipulation, especially when consciousness begins to return. If the patient is recovering under field conditions, cover

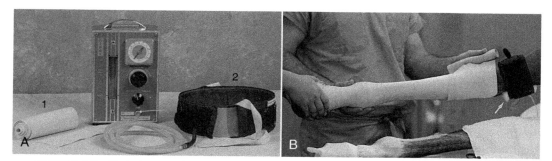

FIGURE 10-20 A, An Esmarch tourniquet *(1)* and a pneumatic tourniquet *(2)* are used for occluding blood flow in a limb. **B,** Application of an Esmarch tourniquet around the limb to the level of the pneumatic tourniquet. Gauze rolls are placed over vascular pressure points under the tourniquet *(arrow)*. (From Auer JA, Stick JA, editors: *Equine surgery*, ed 2, St. Louis, 1999, Saunders.)

the eyes to prevent stimulation from sunlight. Some individuals try to stand well before they are able. Low doses of a sedative such as xylazine may encourage the horse to lie quietly, thus allowing more time for metabolism of the primary anesthetic drugs. Conversely, some horses remain recumbent long after the effects of anesthesia have worn off. Prolonged recumbency can contribute to compartment syndrome and should be discouraged. It is a judgment call to determine when sufficient time has passed and when the horse should actually be encouraged to stand.

- Supplemental oxygen is desirable during recovery, especially if the procedure lasted longer than 1 hour. Humidified oxygen should be used if possible. Oxygen lines can be placed in the endotracheal tube and inserted into a nostril or nasotracheal tube (if used), and oxygen can be administered at a rate of approximately 15 L/minute. This treatment can boost blood oxygen levels by as much as 30%. Oxygen demand valves, hand activated intermittently by the anesthetist for 1 to 2 seconds, can be useful for intubated patients that fail to breathe spontaneously at an adequate rate or depth.

- If the horse was intubated for the procedure, a staff member should remain with the patient until attempts to swallow are observed. At that time, the tracheal tube can be withdrawn. Swallowing also signals that return to consciousness is not far away—at this time, it becomes dangerous for personnel to stay in the immediate area where the horse is recovering.

- Do not leave the patient unobserved during any phase of recovery. The patient is attended closely until swallowing occurs. At that time, if the patient is in a recovery stall or other enclosure, leave the enclosure. The risks of being crushed or pinned during the horse's attempts to stand are too great. No one should stay inside an enclosed area with an actively recovering horse. In an open field recovery, all unnecessary personnel should be instructed to clear the area. Typically, only one person remains with the horse to control the head during recovery, and this person should have training in equine anesthesia techniques.

- Continue to observe the patient even after the animal has left the recovery room. Observation can be made either from outside the stall or with video cameras. The patient may experience trauma or become cast (pinned and unable to rise) against a wall, in a corner, or under mattresses and pads. Compartment syndrome and other painful conditions may make it difficult for the horse to stand. These problems must be identified and addressed promptly; frequently, the animals require assistance. If unusual difficulty in rising is observed, an assisted recovery using head, leg, or tail ropes may be necessary (Figs. 10-21 and 10-22).

> **TECHNICIAN NOTE** Continue to observe the patient during recovery. Use of video cameras can be helpful.

- Always closely attend foals during all phases of recovery. Foals should never be left alone. Two people typically stay with the foal; one person attends the head, and another person holds the tail to assist the foal in standing. The risk to personnel is minimal during recovery of a foal, but the staff should position themselves safely out of reach of the hooves.

- Occasionally, after extubation, the patient may make a loud rattling or snorting noise, especially during inspiration. This noise is usually caused by edema of the nasal turbinates (less commonly laryngeal spasm or edema), which develops during anesthesia. However, the condition cannot be recognized until extubation returns the horse to being an obligate nose breather. Nasal turbinate edema may severely compromise breathing and warrants immediate treatment when identified. Elevate the head, with the nose tilted slightly higher than the rest of the head. A nasotracheal tube (15- to 25-mm inner diameter endotracheal tube) should be placed in one nostril so that the tube enters the trachea, thus

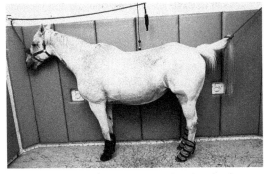

FIGURE 10-21 Assisted recovery using head and tail ropes passed to personnel outside the recovery stall. The horse must still provide the effort to stand, but the ropes can provide some lift and help to steady the horse. (From Trim CM: Principles of chemical restraint and general anesthesia. In Colahan PT, Mayhew IG, Merritt AM, Moore JN, editors: *Equine medicine and surgery*, ed 5, St. Louis, 1999, Mosby.)

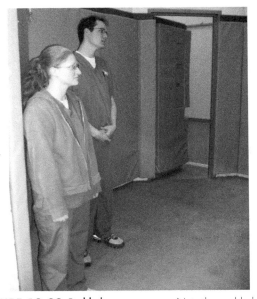

FIGURE 10-22 Padded recovery room. Note the padded floor.

ensuring a patent airway (Fig. 10-23). Firmly secure naso-tracheal tubes with tape or straps to the halter or muzzle of the horse to prevent aspiration of the tube into the trachea. Intranasal 1% phenylephrine (Neo-Synephrine, 3–5 mL in each nostril) may help reduce the nasal swelling, but this treatment is not a substitute for establishing a patent airway when it is needed. Once the patient is standing, the nasotracheal tube can be removed. Resolution of the edema usually proceeds without complication. To minimize the incidence of nasal turbinate edema, the head ideally should not be positioned lower than the heart during the anesthetic period.

> **TECHNICIAN NOTE**   Occasionally, after extubation, the patient may make a loud rattling or snorting noise, especially during inspiration, caused by edema of the nasal turbinates.

> **TECHNICIAN NOTE**   The head should not be positioned lower than the heart during the anesthetic period.

After the Horse Is Standing

Once the horse is standing, staff may quietly reenter the area. The horse should be checked closely for trauma, and IV catheters should be checked and flushed. The horse should be allowed to stand quietly as long as necessary until its legs are stable enough to walk safely. The horse can then be moved to its stall or paddock, with caution. At this stage, many horses are still slightly ataxic and do not negotiate corners well, especially with the hindquarters. The horse should

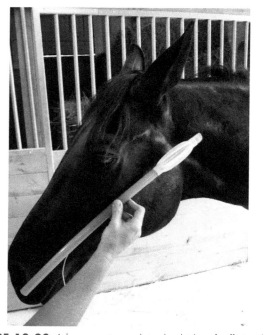

FIGURE 10-23 A large canine endotracheal tube of sufficient length to reach the trachea can be used for nasotracheal intubation. Inflation of the cuff is not necessary unless assisted ventilation is needed.

be led in a wide arc around corners and carefully through doorways. A sharp blow to the point of the hip (tuber coxae), even at a walk, can produce a fracture, but this is easily avoided if precautions are followed. Often, a second person is useful to help guide the patient's hindquarters around these obstacles.

Horses should not be allowed to eat or drink immediately after general anesthesia. Some horses are so hungry that they will eat their stall bedding; these patients should be either placed in a stall without bedding or muzzled. Some horses are talented at eating through or around muzzles, so muzzled horses should be watched closely.

> **TECHNICIAN NOTE**   Some horses are talented at eating through or around muzzles.

The clinician will determine whether oral intake is allowed, based on the patient's underlying condition. Water is returned first, with only a few sips allowed to ensure that the patient can swallow without coughing or refluxing from the nostrils. Larger volumes of water are returned gradually over several hours, and then a handful of grass or grass hay can be offered (usually after 2 hours). If the swallowing reflex appears coordinated, small amounts of hay or grass can be given. High-carbohydrate feedstuffs and larger volumes of solid food are usually not returned until the following day. Intestinal motility and bowel movements should be closely monitored in the initial hours following general anesthesia. The risk of postanesthetic colic is increased by the depressive effects of anesthetic drugs on GI motility. Foals should be muzzled for 1 hour after their return to the mare, to allow time for normal swallowing reflexes to return.

PAIN MANAGEMENT

Pain management is a key component of proper surgical procedure, but it is also important for diseases or injuries that occur in our patients. Several drugs are available to help alleviate pain in large animals. Many drugs used for control of pain in animals are used off-label, used extralabel, or cannot be used in large animal at all. All drugs must be prescribed by a licensed veterinarian, so it is important to remember as a technician that you do not have the authority to use these drugs without a veterinarian's permission. The veterinarian should be the person who selects the drug, dose, and route.

Pain can be graded on a scale by signs of pain, including groaning, squealing, bellowing, bruxism, tucking up of the abdomen, lying down, not wanting to lie down, being agitated, being depressed, anorexia, having decreased fecal production, thrashing, hiding, hyperesthesia, head hanging low to the ground, leaning on objects, limping, non–weight bearing, showing decreased mobility, having unusual stances (including wide stance), and dog sitting.

On physical examination, tachycardia, tachypnea, fever, and hypertension can all be indications of pain.

Nonsteroidal Antiinflammatory Drugs

All nonsteroidal antiinflammatory drugs (NSAIDs) appear to be effective analgesics for somatic (musculoskeletal) pain. Some have visceral pain inhibition properties. Some have the ability to decrease fevers, and some can decrease inflammation. Because most NSAIDs are administered by mouth, they require 30 to 40 minutes to take effect.

NSAIDs work by inhibiting prostaglandin synthesis. Prostaglandins are important in the pain pathway but are also part of the normal GI, reproductive, renal, and ophthalmologic function. Most NSAIDs prevent pain and inflammation by inactivating the enzyme cyclooxygenase (COX), which is responsible for helping make prostaglandins. The two types of COX enzymes are COX-1 and COX-2. Inhibition of both COX isoenzymes, but particularly COX-2, has been linked to analgesic effects. Most NSAIDs inhibit both COX-1 and COX-2, although the ratio of COX-1 to COX-2 inhibitory effects of individual NSAIDs varies considerably. Drugs that are COX-2 selective (carprofen, meloxicam, deracoxib) or specific (firocoxib) are less likely to interfere with intestinal barrier function and produce GI ulceration; however, all NSAIDs have the potential to be nephrotoxic.

Because of the need for prostaglandins in normal physiologic function, care should be taken when these drugs are used in patients with renal, hepatic, hematologic, or GI diseases (Table 10-3).

Alpha-2 Agonists

Alpha-2 agonists are often used for sedation, but they do have some pain-relieving properties. They work by promoting alpha-2 receptor activity. Although alpha-2 receptors are part of the sympathetic nervous system, alpha-2 agonists cause sedative effects. Care should be taken when using these medications because loud noises can cause animals treated with these drugs to rise from a perceived sleep. Most of the side effects of alpha-2 agonists occur when these drugs are given by the IV route, but side effects can occur with any route of administration. Adverse reactions include temporary behavior changes, profound cardiovascular depression, respiratory depression, increased urination, intestinal bloat, colic, gastric distention, premature parturition, sweating in horses, seizures, and collapse. Although the effects of this group of drugs can be reversed, remember that if you reverse these effects in a patient, you are also reversing the analgesic properties of the drug (Table 10-4).

Opioids

Opioids are compounds derived from opium poppy alkaloids and synthetic drugs with similar pharmacologic properties. These drugs produce analgesia and sedation (hypnosis) while reducing anxiety and fear. Narcotic effects are produced in combination with opiate receptors at deep levels of the brain (e.g., thalamus, hypothalamus, limbic system). Side effects can include panting, flatulence, personality changes, increased sound sensitivity, and bradycardia. Overdose may cause severe depression of the central nervous system, respiratory system, and cardiovascular system (Table 10-5).

Other Drugs

Ketamine and gabapentin also have some analgesic properties. Ketamine is a dissociative agent that induces a cataleptic state, which can inhibit the sensation of pain. Gabapentin is used to control neuropathic pain (Table 10-6).

TABLE 10-4	Alpha-2 Agonists in Equine Pain Management		
	DOSE	CONCENTRATION	ROUTE
Xylazine	0.2–1 mg/kg q30–60min	100 mg/mL	IV, IM, SC
Detomidine	0.02–0.04 mg/kg q1–2h	10 mg/mL	IV or IM

IM, Intramuscular; *IV*, intravenous; *SC*, subcutaneous.

TABLE 10-3	Nonsteroidal Antiinflammatory Drugs in Equine Pain Management		
	DOSE	CONCENTRATION	ROUTE
Flunixin meglumine	1.1 mg/kg q12–24h	50 mg/mL	IV, IM, SC, PO
Phenylbutazone	4.4–8.8 mg/kg q12h	IV: 200 mg/mL PO: 100-mg tablets 6-g tube 12-g tube	IV or PO Do not give by the IM route
Ketoprofen	2.0–2.5 mg/kg q24h	100 mg/mL	IV or IM
Carprofen	0.7–1.4 g/kg q12–24h	IV: 50 mg/mL PO: 25-, 50- and 100-mg tablets	
Meloxicam	0.6 mg/kg q12–24h	5 mg/mL	
Acetylsalicylic acid (aspirin)	5–20 mg/kg q12–24h	240-g bolus 480-g bolus	PO
Naproxen	5 mg/kg IV 10 mg/kg PO q24h for up to 14 days	IV bolus slowly	IV or PO

IM, Intramuscular; *IV*, intravenous; *PO*, oral; *SC*, subcutaneous.

TABLE 10-5	Opioids in Equine Pain Management		
	DOSE	**CONCENTRATION**	**ROUTE**
Morphine	0.05–0.1 mg/kg q4–6h	0.5–50 g/mL	IV or IM
Butorphanol	0.01–0.04 mg/kg q2–4h	10 mg/mL	IV, IM or SC
Buprenorphine	0.006–0.02 mg/kg q6–8h	0.3 mg/mL	IV, IM or SC
Meperidine	0.2–1 mg/kg q4–6h	100 mg/mL	IV or IM

IM, Intramuscular; *IV*, intravenous; *SC*, subcutaneous.

TABLE 10-6	Other Drugs in Equine Pain Management		
	DOSE	**CONCENTRATION**	**ROUTE**
Ketamine	1–2 mg/kg q4–6h	100 mg/mL	IV or IM
Gabapentin	2–5 mg/kg q8–12h	100 mg tablet 300 mg tablet	PO

IM, Intramuscular; *IV*, intravenous; *PO*, oral.

SURGICAL PROCEDURES

CASTRATION

> **TECHNICIAN NOTE**   Equipment needed for castration:
> - Field anesthetic agent, syringes, and needles
> - Local anesthetic agent, syringes, and needles
> - Ropes
> - Towels
> - Bandage material for a tail wrap if standing
> - Surgical scrub and alcohol
> - Scalpel blade and handle
> - Emasculator
> - Suture material (in case it is needed)

Castration (orchidectomy or gelding) is the most commonly performed equine surgical procedure. Chemical castration, as performed in ruminants, currently is not available for equines. Removal of the testicles reduces or prevents sexual behavior and aggressive behavior and prevents reproduction by individuals judged to have inferior or undesirable genetic traits. Castration may also be necessary to treat certain malignant diseases, testicular trauma, or inguinal or scrotal hernias. The procedure can be performed on animals at any age but is seldom done before 6 months. Most commonly, the procedure is performed in horses between 1 and 2 years old, when puberty begins and the accompanying behavior becomes objectionable. Some owners believe that castration at a young age retards the horse's skeletal and muscular growth; others believe that castration before puberty results in greater growth in

height. Some owners wait to see whether the horse has a future as a breeding stallion and the castrate the horse later in its life.

> **TECHNICIAN NOTE**   Castration is the most commonly performed equine surgical procedure, usually performed in horses between 1 and 2 years old.

The procedure is almost always performed in the field. However, some owners prefer that the procedure be done in a hospital setting for cleanliness and in case of complications during or after the procedure. When the procedure is performed in the field, the operative area should be clean and free of wind or drafts. Noise and other distractions should be minimized. When the procedure is performed with the patient under general anesthesia, grassy areas usually are preferable to dirt surfaces. If a dirt surface is the only option, a large tarp or blanket should be placed beneath the hind end of the patient to minimize ground contamination.

> **TECHNICIAN NOTE**   A grassy area usually is preferable to a dirt surface for performing castrations in the field setting.

The basic prerequisite for castration is the presence of two fully descended testicles. Because a simple visual assessment is unreliable, the veterinarian palpates the horse to ensure that both testicles are accessible before the surgical procedure is begun. Equines have a high incidence of retained testicles. Failure of one or both testicles to descend fully into the scrotal sacs is abnormal; such an animal is referred to as a cryptorchid. Testicles may be retained in the abdomen (abdominal cryptorchid) or in the inguinal canal (inguinal cryptorchid; "high flanker"). Retained testicles in general do not produce sperm because the temperature adjacent to or within the body is too high. However, retained testicles produce testosterone efficiently, with resultant stallion-like behavior. Retained abdominal testes may become tumorous. For these reasons, it is advisable to locate and remove retained testicles.

The surgical strategy for castrating a cryptorchid (cryptorchidectomy) is different from routine castration, and general anesthesia usually is necessary. Retained testicles may be difficult to locate and difficult to remove surgically, especially if they are retained in the abdomen. The use of laparoscopy to locate and remove abdominally retained testes has been advocated.

> **TECHNICIAN NOTE**   Equines have a high incidence of retained testicles, which may become tumorous.

Castration is almost always performed using an instrument called an emasculator. Several styles of emasculator are available. Some of these instruments crush and cut the spermatic cord at the same time with one set of jaws (Serra and White emasculators); others have a two-jaw system (Reimer emasculator) that crushes the spermatic cord

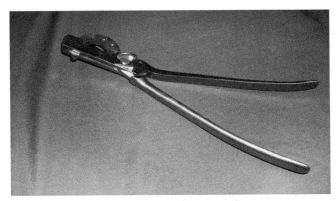

FIGURE 10-24 White emasculator.

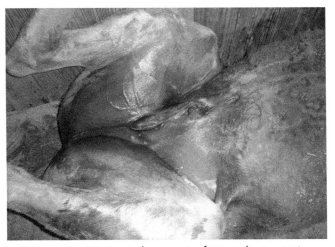

FIGURE 10-25 Surgical preparation for recumbent castration.

with one handle and cuts the spermatic cord with the other (Fig. 10-24). Surgeons usually develop preferences for a particular style of emasculator. The success of the surgical procedure depends in part on sharp, tight emasculators. To prepare the emasculators for use, first disassemble and clean them. Disassembly is necessary to clean the recesses of the instrument jaws thoroughly. A wing nut located on the instrument must be unscrewed to take the instrument apart. After the instrument is cleaned, it is reassembled, wrapped, and sterilized in an autoclave. Reassembly must be accurate, with the handles and jaws in proper orientation to the wing nut. The surgeon uses the wing nut to orient the emasculators when applying the instrument to the spermatic cord.

Patient Position

Castration can be performed with the horse standing or recumbent. A standing procedure may be preferable to avoid the risks of anesthetic recovery or when patient-related factors such as large body size or a history of anesthetic problems increase the risks of general anesthesia. The standing procedure is performed with a combination of heavy sedation and local anesthetic (deposited directly into the scrotal skin, testes, and spermatic cord). Because the horse is capable of responding to stimuli, including pain, the risk of injury to both the clinician and the horse is increased. The procedure is often performed with the horse standing next to a wall, to limit its ability to move. The surgeon and horse handler should stand on the same side of the horse. The tail should be wrapped or braided to keep it from contaminating the surgical field.

> TECHNICIAN NOTE During a standing castration, the tail should be wrapped or braided to keep it from contaminating the surgical field.

The recumbent procedure requires general anesthesia. Because the procedure is fairly quick (15 to 30 minutes), short-acting IV anesthesia usually is adequate. The basic anesthetic protocol is heavy sedation with an alpha-2 agonist (xylazine or detomidine), followed by induction of anesthesia with ketamine or a ultrashort-acting thiobarbiturate. Clinicians may add acepromazine or butorphanol to the

sedative "cocktail." Some add the muscle relaxant guaifenesin to the induction agent. Many drug combinations are possible in an attempt to improve overall analgesia and muscle relaxation, as well as duration of anesthesia. Some surgeons supplement general anesthesia with local anesthesia of the spermatic cord. Positioning for the recumbent procedure may be lateral or dorsal. In lateral recumbency, the upper hindlimb must be pulled cranially or flexed dorsally to give access to the scrotum. This is usually accomplished by placing a rope around the pastern and either tying the rope around the neck or having an assistant hold the rope for the duration of the procedure. In dorsal recumbency, the horse's body must be stabilized between hay bales or other supports. Clinicians have preferences for patient positioning.

Patient Preparation

The horse should have limited access to food before the surgical procedure, in anticipation of depressed GI motility caused by the sedative and anesthetic drugs. IV catheterization for administration of anesthetic drugs is recommended but not essential. The patient should receive tetanus prophylaxis before (preferred) or immediately after the procedure. Some veterinarians give antibiotics routinely before the procedure; this is done for prophylaxis and is not mandatory. The patient should be groomed well before the procedure.

> TECHNICIAN NOTE It is common for the equine patient to receive tetanus prophylaxis at the time of castration.

Procedure

Clipping is not usually necessary for routine castration. Surgical preparation of the skin is performed with surgical scrub and alcohol or clean water rinses of the prepuce and scrotum (Fig. 10-25). The inner thighs should be included in the scrub area. Draping is not performed for the standing procedure and is seldom performed for recumbent castrations in the field.

The surgical procedure involves two scrotal incisions, one over each testicle. The veterinarian exteriorizes a testicle and as much of its spermatic cord as possible and then applies emasculators to crush and cut the spermatic cord (Fig. 10-26). The procedure is repeated for the other testicle. It is sometimes necessary to ligate the spermatic cord with suture material. After emasculation, the spermatic cord is checked for hemorrhage. Excess tissue and fat in the scrotal sac are removed because they tend to hang from the incisions and serve as "fly food." The scrotal incisions may be sutured closed, but the common method is to enlarge (stretch) the incisions manually and leave them open to allow drainage.

Aftercare

The most common complications of castration are hemorrhage and excessive swelling. Hemorrhage occurs commonly, and the source is usually skin vessels in the scrotum. This bleeding is not life-threatening and stops within several hours. However, life-threatening hemorrhage may occur from the stump of the severed spermatic cord. Ligation, application of hemostatic clamps, or repeat emasculation is required to stop the hemorrhage and prevent possible death. After castration, the horse should be observed frequently during the first 24 hours for hemorrhage. A good rule of thumb for the bleeding horse is that if the drops of blood can be counted, the condition probably is not a life-threatening hemorrhage; the veterinarian should be alerted to the situation. However, if the bleeding occurs in a continuous stream or if the drops occur so rapidly that they cannot be counted, the situation requires urgent veterinary attention. Stall rest for the first 24 hours after castration is recommended to allow the severed blood vessels time to form adequate clots and to allow full recovery from anesthesia. Excessive activity in this initial postoperative period may dislodge clots that are trying to form.

Drainage from the incisions is expected after the surgical procedure, as is mild swelling of the scrotum and prepuce. The client is instructed on when and how to exercise the

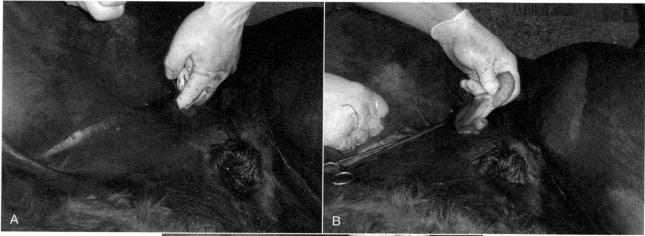

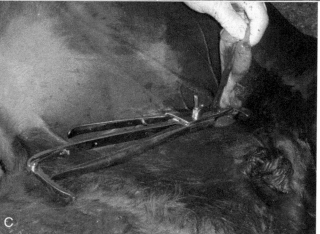

FIGURE 10-26 A, Surgical incision. B, Location of the testicle. C, Emasculation of the spermatic cord.

horse; exercise is thought to facilitate drainage and minimize swelling. Exercise is usually advised after the initial 24-hour postoperative period. Excessive swelling blocks the incisions and prevents external drainage, which leads to extreme swelling of the scrotum and prepuce, and the retained fluid is predisposed to infection. The veterinarian may need to inspect and manually reopen incisions that are not draining.

> **TECHNICIAN NOTE** After castration, exercise is usually advised after an initial 24-hour period of stall rest.

Hydrotherapy of the surgical area is sometimes prescribed to decrease edema in the scrotum and prepuce. Water should never be directed into the incisions; this risks driving debris and organisms into the scrotal sac (the abdominal cavity has a direct communication with the inside of the spermatic cord). The water stream should be carefully applied to the sides of the prepuce and scrotum.

> **TECHNICIAN NOTE** Hydrotherapy of the surgical area is sometimes prescribed to decrease edema after the castration procedure.

Because of the communication of the spermatic cord (through the vaginal process) with the abdominal cavity, evisceration of intestines may occur after the surgical procedure. This complication is rare but potentially fatal. Evisceration is most likely in the first 4 hours after the procedure but may occur up to 6 days postoperatively. The owner should inspect the surgical site with the veterinarian immediately after the surgical procedure to observe the normal postoperative appearance. Later, if any tissue protrudes from the incision that was not seen immediately after the surgical procedure, the veterinarian should be notified immediately.

Horses castrated after onset of puberty should not have contact with mares for several weeks after the surgical procedure, to avoid arousal. It takes approximately 30 days for testosterone levels to subside following the procedure. Persistent stallion-like behavior may occur in geldings and is more likely when males are castrated later in life. Such individuals are referred to as *"false rigs,"* and blame is usually placed on poor surgical technique by the veterinarian for failing to remove the epididymis or enough spermatic cord *("proud cut")*. However, the epididymis and spermatic cord cannot produce testosterone, and increased testosterone levels in false rigs are seldom documented. More likely, the persistent "sexual" behavior was learned before castration or is part of the normal social interaction of horses (unrelated to sexual stimulation). Healing of the scrotal incisions is usually complete in 3 to 4 weeks.

CASLICK SURGERY

> **TECHNICIAN NOTE** Equipment needed for Caslick surgery:
> - Rectal sleeve and nonsterile lubricant
> - Tail wrap or bandaging material
> - Sterile surgical gloves
> - Local anesthetic, 6- or 12-mL syringe, small-gauge needle (22- to 25-ga)
> - Nonabsorbable suture, 2-0 (usually on reel), with or without nonabsorbable suture, 0-0, or sterile umbilical tape, for breeder's stitch
> - Standard "laceration pack":
>   - Needle holders
>   - Thumb tissue forceps
>   - Operating scissors
>   - Surgical scissors (Metzenbaum and Mayo)
>   - Scalpel handle and no. 10 surgical blade
>   - Sterile 4 × 4 gauze squares
>   - Surgical needles, cutting or reverse cutting

The vulva forms an important protective seal for the vagina. Normally, when a female defecates, the fecal material and liquid fall directly to the ground. This is possible because the anus and vulva are aligned in a vertical plane. However, in some females, the anus is located more cranially than the vulva ("sunken anus"), resulting in a sloping perineum (Fig. 10-27). In extreme cases, a vulvar "shelf" exists below the anus. These abnormal conformations result in abnormal contact with fecal material when it is voided, and if the lips of the vulva do not form a perfect seal, the material can easily enter the vagina. Because the vagina leads to the cervix and thereby the uterus, contaminants in the vagina can enter the uterus and cause uterine infection; this is one of the most common causes of uterine infections.

The lips of the vulva also guard against involuntary aspiration of air into the vagina. When air enters the vagina (pneumovagina or "windsucking"), it may carry dust, dirt, fecal matter, and other contaminants with it. Faulty conformation of the vulva and vulvar lips may result in pneumovagina.

Abnormal vulvar conformation may be inherited and is apparent at a young age. A sunken anus may be acquired later in life and is a normal occurrence in old mares. Thin females also tend toward this conformation. Breeding and foaling injuries may tear the vulva and result in scarring, which prevents the lips from meeting and forming an effective seal.

Caslick surgery is the most common reproductive surgical procedure performed on female horses. It is performed to treat pneumovagina and prevent contamination of the vagina. It is also commonly performed on racehorses when they enter race training because of the widely held belief that females running at top speeds aspirate air, even if the vulva has a good conformation.

> **TECHNICIAN NOTE** Caslick procedures are commonly performed in females to treat pneumovagina and in mares entering race training.

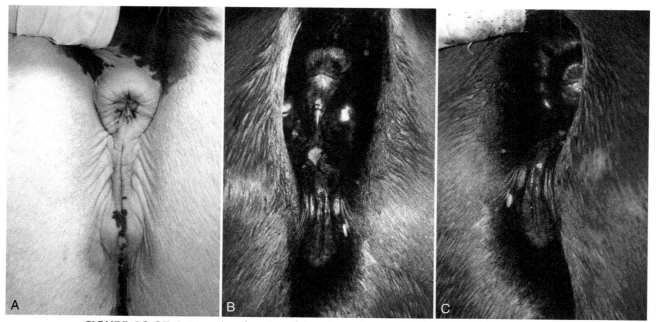

FIGURE 10-27 **A,** Normal conformation of the vulva in the mare. **B,** Abnormal conformation with parting of the vulvar lips at the dorsal commissure. **C,** Sunken anus. (From Sellon DC, Long MT: *Equine infectious diseases,* ed 2, St. Louis, 2014, Saunders.)

Patient Preparation

Tetanus immunization status should be confirmed. The procedure is performed using local anesthesia of the vulva. The horse will need to be restrained, usually with a twitch; some horses require tranquilization. The surgeon may perform a rectal examination to remove feces from the rectum. The tail is wrapped and secured out of the surgical field, and the perineum is prepared with surgical scrub soap and clean water. The surgeon anesthetizes the vulvar lips with several milliliters of local anesthetic, and a final scrub of the site is performed.

Procedure

A strip of vulvar mucosa is either split with a scalpel blade or removed with surgical scissors; this is done only across the dorsal aspect of the vulva. The ventral aspect must be left open so that the horse can urinate normally. The veterinarian uses several anatomical landmarks to determine the proper length of tissue to remove. The bleeding tissue edges are brought together with suture, to form a side-to-side bridge of tissue that will heal with scar tissue.

Sometimes a single additional heavy-gauge suture is placed across the most ventral aspect of the suture line. This single stitch, known as a "breeder's stitch," protects the integrity of the surgical site while it heals. Breeding or performing vaginal procedures on the female with the breeder's stitch in place is possible.

Aftercare

Antibiotic ointment may be placed on the incision line. The owner is instructed to keep the area clean. If material accumulates on the sutures, it can be gently removed by picking with clean gauze squares; however, wiping or scrubbing directly across the sutures should be avoided. Sutures are removed in 10 to 21 days.

If a pregnant mare has been "sewn down," the tissue should be "released" before foaling. If foaling occurs through the tissue bridge, the tissue may tear severely and lead to more disfigurement of the vulva. Release of the site is done by cleansing the area and using scissors or a scalpel to separate the tissue on midline. Because the tissue is scar tissue, it is devoid of nerves and therefore does not require desensitization. However, as with any reproductive procedure, the horse should be properly restrained.

> **TECHNICIAN NOTE**   Sutures placed during a Caslick procedure are removed in 10 to 21 days.

ABDOMINAL SURGERY

Abdominal surgical procedures in the horse may be performed for the diagnosis and treatment of colic. Standing surgery through a flank incision can be used to treat some abdominal problems but usually is not possible or feasible. Most abdominal surgical procedures are performed with the horse under general anesthesia, in dorsal recumbency. The surgical team usually consists of at least four staff members: a primary surgeon, an assistant surgeon, a circulating operating room nurse, and an anesthetist. Teamwork is essential, especially in the preparation and induction phases of anesthesia, operating room setup, and patient positioning and surgical preparation. Because of the critical and involved nature of the anesthesia, the anesthetist must be able to be totally devoted to the task of anesthesia, without distraction.

The surgical approach is usually through a ventral midline incision, which may reach 30 to 40 cm in length. Although clipping the patient preoperatively is preferable, often the emergency nature of the case does not allow time, and clipping is done on the operating table. The standard clip is from xiphoid

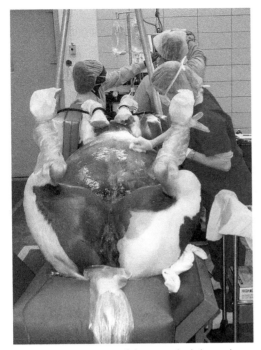

FIGURE 10-28 Preparation of the ventral abdominal area for abdominal surgery in a horse with colic that is under general anesthesia and is positioned in dorsal recumbency. (From Bassert, JM, Thomas J, editors: *McCurnin's clinical textbook for veterinary technicians*, ed 8, St. Louis, 2014, Saunders.)

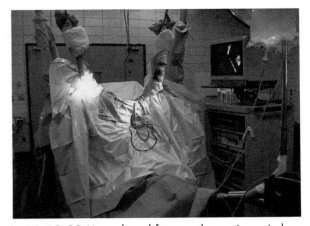

FIGURE 10-30 Horse draped for an arthroscopic surgical procedure of the carpi. Adhesive, impervious drapes are placed around the carpi to reduce surgical wound contamination from the skin. (From Bassert, JM, Thomas J, editors: *McCurnin's clinical textbook for veterinary technicians*, ed 8, St. Louis, 2014, Saunders.)

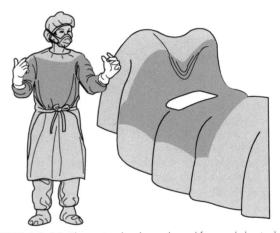

FIGURE 10-31 The patient has been draped for an abdominal surgical procedure. *Shaded areas* indicate the sterile surgical field, which extends to include scrubbed personnel. (From Auer JA, Stick JA, editors: *Equine surgery*, ed 2, St. Louis, 1999, Saunders.)

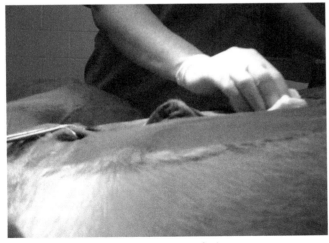

FIGURE 10-29 Preparation for hernia repair.

to the udder or prepuce, lateral to each flank fold (Figs. 10-28 and 10-29). Additionally, the incisional area is usually shaved. The penis in males must be prevented from extending from the prepuce during the procedure; therefore, either a pursestring suture or several towel clamps commonly are placed to close the prepuce. Before the prepuce is closed, an absorbent material, such as a stack of gauze 4 × 4 squares, is placed inside the prepuce to absorb any urine that may be passed.

The principles of asepsis and sterile surgery are no different from those in any other species and should be followed in every hospital or clinic performing equine surgical procedures (Figs. 10-30 to 10-32). However, facilities

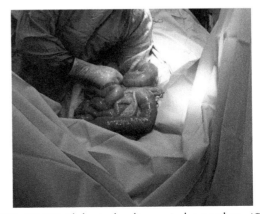

FIGURE 10-32 Abdominal colic surgical procedure. (Courtesy Nebraska Equine.)

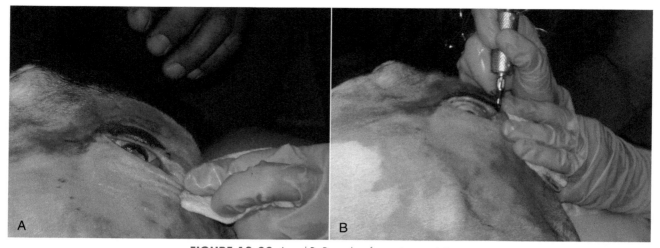

FIGURE 10-33 A and B, Procedure for equine eye tattoos.

differ considerably in their methods of anesthesia and recovery, patient preparation, surgical instruments and materials, and operating room protocol. The technician at any hospital or clinic will need to "learn the ropes." Flexibility and patience are desirable traits for everyone on the surgical team.

CASE STUDY

A 3-year-old Paint mare is experiencing squinting and extreme weeping from her blue eye, which is surrounded by white pigmented skin, especially during the summer. Another Paint horse owner suggested to Mrs. Petersen that she have eye tattoos applied to the horse's eye to aid in prevention of sun damage and to decrease the weeping (Fig. 10-33). Mrs. Petersen has arrived at the veterinary clinic and would like to have the procedure performed. In her mind, the procedure is elective. The mare is extremely well muscled and in great condition. If the horse were to be placed under general anesthesia for the procedure, what common complication in heavily muscled healthy equine patients should you warn Mrs. Petersen about? What preventive measures will you tell Mrs. Petersen the veterinarian will take to prevent this complication?

CASE STUDY

Mrs. Olsen has made an appointment for her yearling stud to be castrated. The procedure is scheduled as a farm call. When you arrive at Mrs. Olsen's farm, you see a clean grassy area adjacent to the barn. The driveway is made of limestone rock. The horses are kept in a dry lot, and there is an empty dry lot on the other side of the barn. Where should you take the equipment for the procedure? The veterinarian palpates the stud to identify the location of both testicles. On palpation, the veterinarian informs Mrs. Olsen that the horse is a unilateral cryptorchid. What does this mean? Mrs. Olsen informs the veterinarian that she would like to continue the procedure, removing just one of the testicles. If the other testicle is not removed, what are some possible complications?

SUGGESTED READING

Bassert JM, McCurnin DM: In *McCurnin's clinical textbook for veterinary technicians*, ed 7, St. Louis, 2010, Saunders.

Brown M: Veterinary anesthesia, analgesia, and anesthetic nursing. In Sirois M, editor: *Principles and practice of veterinary technology*, ed 3, St. Louis, 2011, Mosby, pp 387–420.

Colahan PT, Mayhew IG, Merritt AM, Moore JN: In *Equine medicine and surgery*, ed 5, St. Louis, 1999, Mosby.

Muir WW, Hubbell JAE, Skarda RT, Bednarski RM: *Handbook of veterinary anesthesia*, ed 3, St. Louis, 2006, Mosby.

Noakes DE, Parkinson TJ, England GCW: *Arthur's veterinary reproduction and obstetrics*, ed 9, London, 2009, Saunders.

Orsini JA, Divers TJ: *Manual of equine emergencies*, ed 3, St. Louis, 2008, Saunders.

Reed SM: Neurologic diseases, *Vet Clin North Am Equine Pract* 3:255–440, 1987.

Riebold TW: Principles and techniques of equine anesthesia, *Vet Clin North Am Equine Pract* 6:485–741, 1990.

Speirs VC: *Clinical examination of horses*, St. Louis, 1997, Saunders.

Stashak TS: *Adams' lameness in horses*, ed 5, Philadelphia, 2002, Lippincott Williams & Wilkins.

Thomas JA, Lerche P: Veterinary anesthesia. In Bassert JM, McCurnin DM, editors: *McCurnin's clinical textbook for veterinary technicians*, ed 7, St. Louis, 2010, Saunders, pp 887–939.

Thomas JA, Lerche P: *Anesthesia and analgesia for veterinary technicians*, ed 4, St. Louis, 2011, Mosby.

White NA: *The equine acute abdomen*, Philadelphia, 1990, Lea & Febiger.

11 Common Equine Diseases

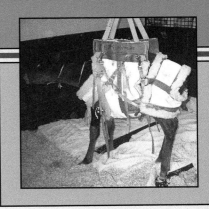

LEARNING OBJECTIVES

After studying this chapter, you will be able to

- Describe and recognize clinical signs associated with specific diseases
- Understand the etiology of the diseases
- Understand and describe common treatments for disease
- Know the common scientific names of parasites associated with this species
- Know the common *vaccinations* and their schedules associated with this species

KEY TERMS

Abscess
Anaerobic
Anorexia
Antemortem
Antibiotic
Antioxidant
Antitoxin
Ataxia
Atrophy
Coccoid
Direct contact
Dyspnea
Fomite

Gram-negative
Gram-positive
Incubation period
Indirect contact
Morbidity
Mortality
Mucopurulent
Myoglobinuria
Paired serum samples
Paralysis
Petechiae
Polydipsia
Polyuria

Postmortem
Pyrexia
Serology
Spirochete
Sporocysts
Thrombocytopenia
Vaccination
Viral antigen
Viral nucleic acid detection
Virus isolation
Warm-blooded

KEY ABBREVIATIONS

AGID: Agar gel immunodiffusion (test)
COPD: Chronic obstructive pulmonary disease
EIA: Equine infectious anemia

ELISA: Enzyme-linked immunosorbent assay
EPM: Equine protozoal myeloencephalitis
EPSM: Equine polysaccharide storage myopathy

HYPP: Hyperkalemic periodic paralysis
NSAID: Nonsteroidal antiinflammatory drug
PCR: Polymerase chain reaction

Veterinary technicians are *not* allowed to diagnose. The purpose of these disease-related chapters is to help educate technicians about the common diseases seen in each species. Having a basic understanding of these diseases will help technicians to provide high-quality client education and have a more thorough understanding of the practices and principles applied to clinical prevention measures and clinical procedures. Most often if we understand why we are doing something we are more likely to perform at our best. The other advantage of discussing common diseases is to understand further why we vaccinate for many of the diseases present in each species. Many times owners will ask and technicians should be able to explain what each vaccination is for and why it is important. However, technicians should remember that it is *not* their job to recommend a vaccination protocol, to diagnose, or to prescribe.

> **TECHNICIAN NOTE** Technicians should not recommend vaccination protocols, diagnose, or prescribe.

BACTERIAL DISEASES

ANTHRAX

- Etiology: *Bacillus anthracis*
- Gram-positive bacillus
- Sudden death and septicemia
- Reportable disease
- Vaccine in the presence of an outbreak

Anthrax can affect all *warm-blooded* animals, including humans, and it is discussed in Chapter 15.

BOTULISM

- Etiology: *Clostridium botulinum*
- Gram-positive rod
- Sudden death and muscle necrosis
- Vaccine

Botulism is caused by the bacteria *C. botulinum*. It is a gram-positive, spore-forming, *anaerobic* bacterium that survives in soils, freshwater sediments, and marine sediments. Infection is often the result of ingestion of the toxin through contaminated feed. Toxicoinfectious botulism can be seen in horses and especially foals in the eastern United States. This type of infection, known as "shaker foal syndrome," results when the horse or foal has the organism growing in its gastrointestinal tract and the organism is producing the toxin. Eight types of botulism are recognized. Large animals are most often infected with types B, C, and D. Horses are not the only large animal that can be infected with *C. botulinum*. Cattle and sheep can also become infected. The toxin prevents the release of acetylcholine at the neuromuscular junction, thus resulting in *paralysis*, especially of the cranial nerves.

Clinical signs include creeping paralysis that usually begins at the head and moves caudally (Fig. 11-1). Veterinarians diagnose botulism with identification of *C. botulinum*

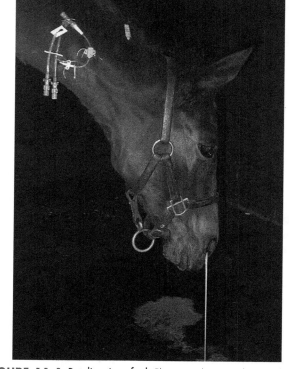

FIGURE 11-1 Botulism in a foal. Pharyngeal paresis has resulted in an inability to swallow. Note the milk coming from the nostrils soon after nursing. (From McAuliffe SB, Slovis NM: *Color atlas of diseases and disorders of the foal*, Oxford, 2008, Saunders.)

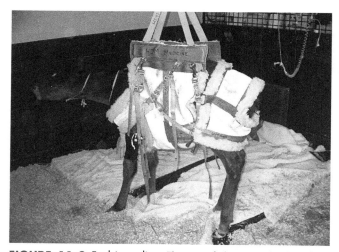

FIGURE 11-2 Foal in a sling. The use of slings can be beneficial in rehabilitating botulism foals, treating milder cases of botulism, or rehabilitating after any neurologic disorder that has resulted in prolonged recumbency. (From McAuliffe SB, Slovis NM: *Color atlas of diseases and disorders of the foal*, Oxford, 2008, Saunders.)

in the feces, blood, or feed that was ingested. Treatment is generally supportive but may include attempts to flush the toxin from the gastrointestinal tract by using gastric lavage or purgatives. *Mortality* is often high as a result of respiratory paralysis (Fig. 11-2).

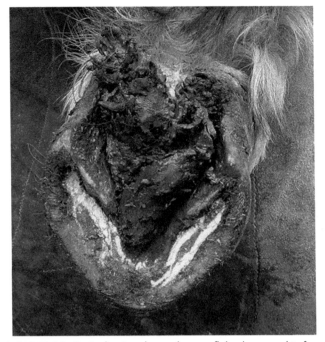

FIGURE 11-3 Canker in a horse shows a flaky, hypertrophic frog. (From Auer JA, Stick JA: *Equine surgery,* ed 3, St. Louis, 2006, Saunders.)

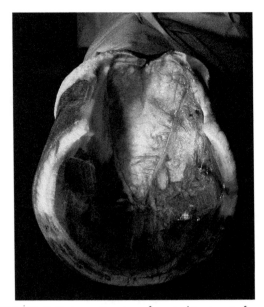

FIGURE 11-4 Postoperative view of surgical treatment of canker after removal of the entire frog. (From Auer JA, Stick JA: *Equine surgery,* ed 3, St. Louis, 2006, Saunders.)

CANKER

- *Fusobacterium necrophorum* and one or more *Bacteroides* species
- Gram-negative bacillus
- Odorous sole debris and lameness

Equine canker is a chronic hypertrophic, moist pododermatitis of the epidermal tissues of the foot (Fig. 11-3). The most commonly isolated agents include *F. necrophorum* and one or more *Bacteroides* species. The disease is often seen in the South and the Midwest. The exact cause of canker is unknown, but most horses affected by canker have a history of being housed in wet areas year round. Lameness usually does not manifest until the corium is involved. Equine canker has a characteristic odor. The frog usually is very friable and resembles cottage cheese. Treatment often involves superficial débridement and topical antimicrobial agents (Fig. 11-4).

LYME DISEASE

- Etiology: *Borrelia burgdorferi*
- Gram-negative spirochete
- General malaise and lameness

Lyme disease is caused by at least three strains of *B. burgdorferi,* a *gram-negative,* unicellular *spirochete* with flagellar projections. *B. burgdorferi* does not live long outside its host. The bacterium follows a 2-year enzootic life cycle that involves ixodid ticks and mammals (Fig. 11-5). The primary vector for the disease is the deer tick. The female tick is the most likely competent vector. Other ticks associated with the disease include the black-legged tick and the western black-legged tick. Infection of the horse occurs when a tick attaches to a horse for longer than 24 hours. For successful transmission of the bacteria, the tick must be attached for at least 24 hours and

sometimes up to 48 hours. The organism lives in the tick's gut and is transferred as the tick feeds on the blood of the horse.

Lyme disease is most prevalent in regions of high humidity and dense vegetation (Fig. 11-6). Although Lyme disease can occur during any time of the year, most cases occur from May through August in the North Central and Pacific Coast states.

Clinical signs include low-grade *pyrexia,* depression, stiffness, lameness, loss of appetite, joint swelling, and eye problems. However, when high fevers and leg edema are present, the condition most often is the result of *Anaplasma phagocytophilum* because many ticks are infected with both *A. phagocytophilum* and *Borrelia.*

Diagnosis of Lyme disease usually is accomplished with *enzyme-linked immunosorbent assay (ELISA)* or immunofluorescent antibody testing.

Treatment of Lyme disease includes tetracycline and oral doxycycline. Doxycycline cannot be administered intravenously to horses because of the potential side effects. Tetracycline should not be administered orally to horses because of the low bioavailability and the risk that active drug may reach the colon and cause diarrhea. Prevention should include use of an insecticide, use of antimicrobials if early exposure to *Ixodes* ticks is known to have occurred, and vaccination.

POTOMAC HORSE FEVER

- Etiology: *Neorickettsia risticii*
- Gram-negative cocci
- General malaise and lameness
- Vaccine available

Potomac horse fever is caused by the bacterium *N. risticii,* formerly known as *Ehrlichia risticii.* It is a gram-negative obligate intracellular bacterium with an attraction to monocytes.

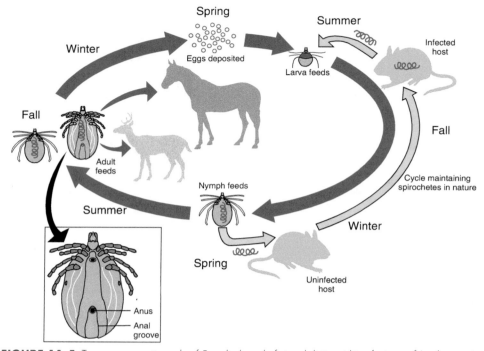

FIGURE 11-5 Two-year enzootic cycle of *Borrelia burgdorferi* and distinguishing features of *Ixodes* species ticks. *Inset,* Female ventral abdomen. (From Sellon DC, Long MT: *Equine infectious diseases,* ed 2, St. Louis, 2014, Saunders.)

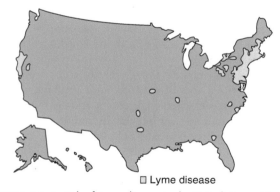

FIGURE 11-6 Risk of Lyme disease in the United States. (Courtesy Centers for Disease Control and Prevention, Atlanta. From Sellon DC, Long MT: *Equine infectious diseases,* St. Louis, 2007, Saunders.)

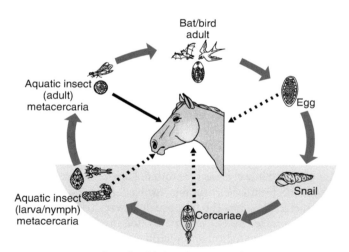

FIGURE 11-7 Life cycle of helminthic vector of *Neorickettsia risticii* and natural route of transmission. The *solid red arrow* indicates the demonstrated route of transmission with adult aquatic insects. *Dashed black arrows* indicate possible routes of infection with trematode eggs, free cercariae, or larval or nymphal aquatic insect stages. (From Sellon DC, Long MT: *Equine infectious diseases,* St. Louis, 2007, Saunders.)

N. risticii lives inside trematodes (flukes) that infect snails. When the trematodes release their larvae and enter a water environment, the larvae are infected with *N. risticii*. The larvae of the caddis and mayfly, which also live in water, consume the infected trematode larvae and become infected with *N. risticii* themselves. When the caddis and mayfly larvae hatch, they are infected with *N. risticii*. If a horse then accidentally eats one of the flies, the horse becomes infected (Figs. 11-7 and 11-8). The bacteria will begin to replicate inside the gastrointestinal tract of the horse and cause the clinical signs of depression, diarrhea, fever, toxemia, abortion in pregnant mares, and sometimes laminitis.

A definitive diagnosis requires identification of *N. risticii* in the feces or blood of the infected horse. A *polymerase chain reaction (PCR)* test is available for detection of *N. risticii*.

Treatment often involves oxytetracycline if the disease is diagnosed early, and it most often resolves clinical signs within 3 days. Fluid therapy and *nonsteroidal antiinflammatory drugs (NSAIDs)* may be provided as supportive treatments.

RAIN ROT/*DERMATOPHILUS* INFECTION

- Etiology: *Dermatophilus congolensis*
- Gram-positive actinomycete
- Skin lesions

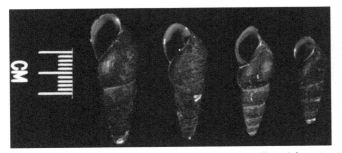

FIGURE 11-8 *Juga yrekaensis* pleurocerid snails collected from Potomac horse fever–endemic region in northern California (bar = 1 cm). (From Sellon DC, Long MT: *Equine infectious diseases,* ed 2, St. Louis, 2014, Saunders.)

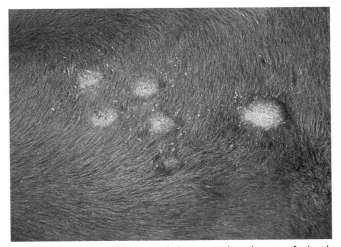

FIGURE 11-9 Circular areas of alopecia with scaling in a foal with dermatophytosis. (From McAuliffe SB, Slovis NM: *Color atlas of diseases and disorders of the foal,* Oxford, 2008, Saunders.)

Rain rot is caused by *D. congolensis,* a gram-positive, non–acid-fast, facultative anaerobic actinomycete. *D. congolensis* also infects cattle, sheep, goats, pigs, cats, and dogs. Rain rot often manifests in areas with high temperatures and high humidity. Animals that are wet for prolonged periods of time often develop the disease.

The condition can affect animals of all ages and manifests as crusty scabs or matted tufts of hair. The lesions are usually found on the head, neck, and chest (Fig. 11-9). Yellow or green pus can be found underneath larger scabs. A definitive diagnosis is made from culture and identification of *D. congolensis.*

Treatment includes antimicrobial therapy. In horses, the lesions should be soaked and removed. In food-producing animals, lime sulfur can be used as a more cost-effective treatment.

SALMONELLA INFECTION

- Etiology: several *Salmonella* species
- Gram-negative rod
- Diarrhea

Several *Salmonella* serotypes can cause diarrhea in adult horses. Five of the most common serotypes are *Salmonella agona, Salmonella newport, Salmonella anatum, Salmonella Krefeld,* and, possibly the most pathogenic, *Salmonella typhimurium.*

Horses infected with *Salmonella* can have one of three types of infection: carrier, mild clinical, or acute clinical. Carrier horses are subclinical carriers that intermittently shed the organism. If a carrier horse is stressed, the horse may develop clinical signs. Horses that develop the mild clinical form of the disease develop pyrexia, *anorexia,* depression, and soft and watery diarrhea (Fig. 11-10). Horses with this form of *Salmonella* infection often display clinical signs for 4 to 5 days but shed the organism in their feces for days to months after the infection. The third form of the disease, acute clinical infection, causes watery and foul-smelling diarrhea, abdominal pain, severe depression, anorexia, and pronounced neutropenia. Horses with this form of infection often dehydrate quickly, with resulting electrolyte imbalances and, with prolonged diarrhea, enterocolopathy and bacteremia. Horses left untreated with the acute clinical form of the disease have an increased likelihood of death.

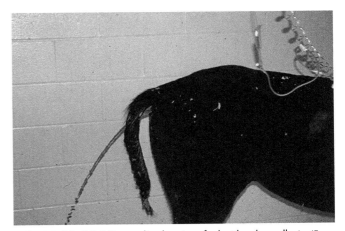

FIGURE 11-10 Watery diarrhea in a foal with salmonellosis. (From McAuliffe SB, Slovis NM: *Color atlas of diseases and disorders of the foal,* Oxford, 2008, Saunders.)

Diagnosis of the disease is based on clinical signs, neutropenia, and fecal cultures. *Salmonella* cannot be consistently cultured from fecal material because it requires multiple fecal samples to be collected and cultured throughout the day. Culturing a rectal biopsy can increase the chances of identifying the organism, but this approach is not without risk to the patient. Another alternative to culture is the PCR test available for *Salmonella* identification. Horses that are subclinical carriers can be very difficult to identify because of the intermittent shedding.

Salmonella infections, both the mild clinical and acute clinical forms, should be treated with intravenous fluid and electrolyte replacement. The use of gastrointestinal protectants and *antibiotics* is controversial. NSAIDs are given to help counteract the effects of endotoxins and to control pain. In severe causes, administration of equine plasma may be indicated to correct hypoproteinemia. The plasma may also provide specific antibodies to the endotoxin and

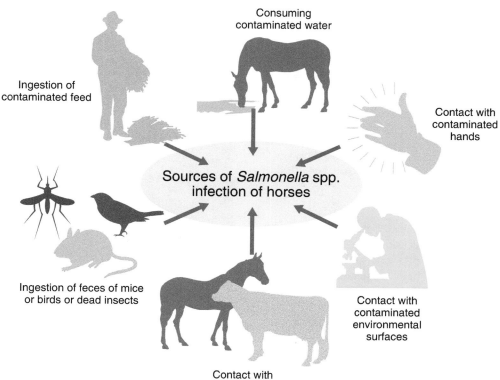

FIGURE 11-11 Examples of the multiple potential sources for *Salmonella* exposure to equids. (From Sellon DC, Long MT: *Equine infectious diseases,* ed 2, St. Louis, 2014, Saunders.)

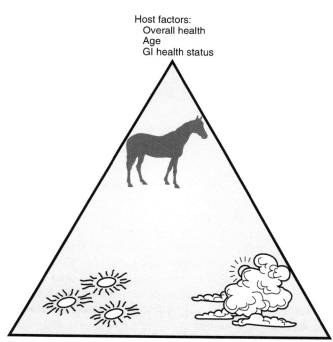

FIGURE 11-12 Triad of disease factors resulting in *Salmonella* infection. *GI,* Gastrointestinal. Disease results when multiple risk factors come together, including those associated with the host, the agent, and the environment. (From Sellon DC, Long MT: *Equine infectious diseases,* ed 2, St. Louis, 2014, Saunders.)

coagulation factors. Because of the zoonotic risk and the risk of contamination of other horses with *Salmonella,* clients and other facility staff must be educated on the importance of quarantine. Prevention of *Salmonella* can be difficult because *Salmonella* is present in the environment (Figs. 11-11 and 11-12).

> **TECHNICIAN NOTE**   Because of the zoonotic risk and the risk of contamination of other horses with *Salmonella,* it is extremely important to educate clients and other facility staff of the importance of quarantine.

STRANGLES

- Etiology: *Streptococcus equi*
- Gram-positive cocci
- Lymph node abscessation
- Vaccine available

Strangles (distemper) is caused by the bacterium *S. equi. S. equi* is a *gram-positive coccoid* often transmitted through the nasal discharge produced from an infected horse. The transmission can occur by *direct contact* or *indirect contact.*

A horse with strangles often presents with a sudden fever, *mucopurulent* nasal discharge (Fig. 11-13), and abscessation of the submandibular and retropharyngeal lymph nodes

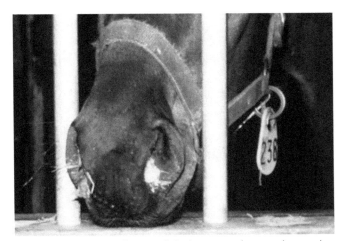

FIGURE 11-13 Purulent nasal discharge in a horse with strangles. (From Sellon DC, Long MT: *Equine infectious diseases*, ed 2, St. Louis, 2014, Saunders.)

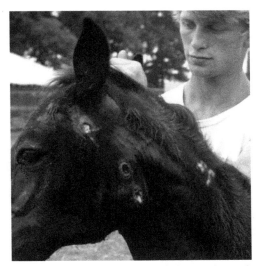

FIGURE 11-15 Multiple rupture sites of abscessed retropharyngeal and submandibular lymph nodes in a foal with strangles. (From Sellon DC, Long MT: *Equine infectious diseases*, ed 2, St. Louis, 2014, Saunders.)

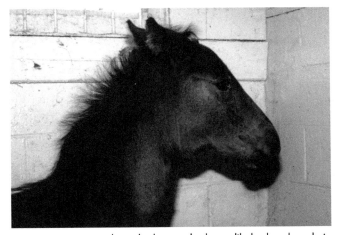

FIGURE 11-14 Enlarged, abscessed submandibular lymph node in a foal with strangles. (From Sellon DC, Long MT: *Equine infectious diseases*, ed 2, St. Louis, 2014, Saunders.)

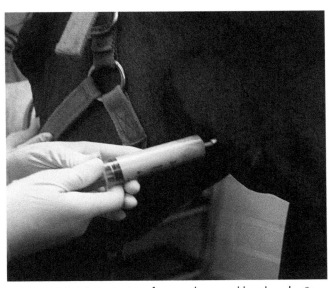

FIGURE 11-16 Aspiration of a retropharyngeal lymph node. *Streptococcus equi* var. *equi* was cultured from the aspirate. (From McAuliffe SB, Slovis NM: *Color atlas of diseases and disorders of the foal*, Oxford, 2008, Saunders.)

(Figs. 11-14 and 11-15). Younger horses are more likely to develop more severe lymph node abscessation, which extends the recovery period. The submandibular and retropharyngeal abscesses may make it difficult for the horse to swallow. Some horses may become listless or anorexic.

If the disease spreads throughout the body, the disease is often termed "metastatic strangles" or "bastard strangles." The fatality rate of horses with bastard strangles increases greatly. Common sites of abscessation include the kidney, spleen, liver, mesentery, lung, and brain.

TECHNICIAN NOTE If the abscesses spread throughout the body, the disease is often called metastatic strangles or bastard strangles.

Diagnosis of strangles is performed with culture of nasal swabs, pus from an *abscess* (Fig. 11-16), or nasal washes. Other forms of diagnosis can include PCR and *serology*.

Veterinarians are divided on the form of therapy to use. Some veterinarians think antibiotic therapy should be administered, and others think it should not. When drug therapy is used, penicillin is often the drug of choice. Most horses will recover from the disease with rest and palatable food. Warm compresses can be used to mature the abscesses. Once the abscesses have ruptured or have been lanced, they should be flushed daily with povidone-iodine solution. If the farm has multiple horses, the horses with abscesses should be isolated. All other horses should have their temperature taken twice a day, and any horse with a fever should be isolated. Prevention of the disease includes vaccination and quarantine of new horses.

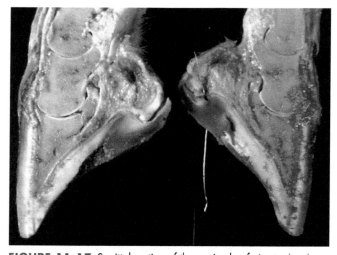

FIGURE 11-17 Sagittal section of the equine hoof. A wire has been placed through the area of subsolar abscessation responsible for introduction of *Clostridium tetani.* (From Sellon DC, Long MT: *Equine infectious diseases,* St. Louis, 2007, Saunders.)

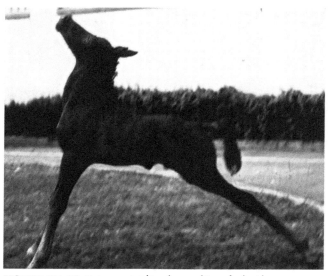

FIGURE 11-18 Extensor rigidity observed in a foal with tetanus secondary to umbilical abscess. (Courtesy College of Veterinary Medicine, North Carolina State University. From Sellon DC, Long MT: *Equine infectious diseases.* St. Louis, 2007, Saunders.)

TETANUS

- Etiology: *Clostridium tetani*
- Gram-positive bacillus
- Severe stiffness
- Vaccine available

Tetanus is caused by endotoxins produced by the bacterium *C. tetani. C. tetani* is a motile, anaerobic, gram-positive bacillus. The most common cause of infection is contamination of wounds (Fig. 11-17). Puncture wounds that contain rusty metal, dirt, or manure are particularly likely to cause infection. Contaminated surgical incisions and umbilical structures may also lead to tetanus.

> **TECHNICIAN NOTE** Puncture wounds that contain rusty metal, dirt, or manure are particularly likely to cause tetanus.

The *incubation period* of tetanus ranges from 1 to 60 days but usually averages between 7 and 10 days. The disease begins with generalized stiffness. With mild infections, the stiffness may remain localized in the head and neck. Stiffness leads to the characteristic stance known as the "sawhorse appearance" (Fig. 11-18), in which the head, neck, back, and legs are stiff and the tail head is elevated. In some more severe cases, the horse may even be recumbent, and *dyspnea* may be seen. Diagnosis is often based on clinical signs.

Treatment should include placing the horse in a quiet, dark area. Water and feed should be placed high in the stall so that the horse does not have to lower its head to eat and drink. Some horses may need body support to prevent them from falling. The wound should be cleaned, and tetanus *antitoxin* can be infiltrated around the wound. Sedatives and muscle relaxants can be used to control the muscle stiffness. The mortality rate is often 50%. Horses that survive the disease usually stabilize within 2 to 7 days, with gradual recovery over a few weeks.

> **TECHNICIAN NOTE** Feed and water should be placed high in the stall of a patient with tetanus so that the horse does not have to lower its head to eat and drink. Prevention should include an injection of tetanus antitoxin after wounds have occurred.

THRUSH

- Etiology: *Fusobacterium necrophorum*
- Gram-negative bacillus
- Hoof soreness and degeneration

Thrush is a degenerative condition of the frog involving the central and lateral sulci. The condition is caused by several organisms, but the most commonly isolated bacterium is *F. necrophorum.* Unsanitary conditions often cause the infection of one or multiple frogs.

Clinical signs often involve a characteristic odor and black discharge (Fig. 11-19). Lameness may result if sensitive structures of the hoof are involved. Diagnosis is made from clinical signs. Treatment involves cleaning away the affected area of the frog and treating with an antiseptic.

OTHER MICROBIAL DISEASES

Equine Protozoal Myeloencephalitis

- Etiology: *Sarcocystis neurona*
- Neurologic disease
- Reportable disease

Equine protozoal myeloencephalitis (EPM) is most commonly caused by the protozoan *S. neurona,* but it also can be caused by the protozoan *Neospora hughesi. S. neurona* is the most common cause of EPM. In the United States the

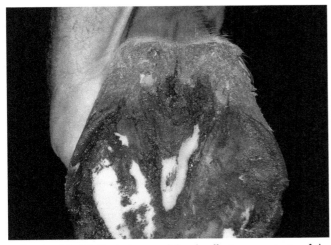

FIGURE 11-19 Typical case of thrush affecting a majority of the frog. (From Floyd A, Mansmann R: *Equine podiatry*, St. Louis, 2007, Saunders.)

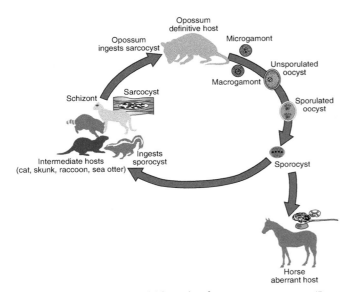

FIGURE 11-20 Proposed life cycle of *Sarcocystis neurona*. (From Sellon DC, Long MT: *Equine infectious diseases*, ed 2, St. Louis, 2014, Saunders.)

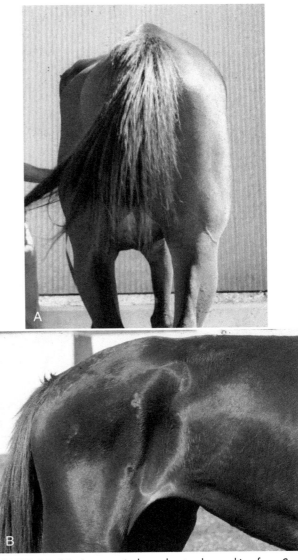

FIGURE 11-21 Asymmetrical muscle atrophy resulting from *Sarcocystis neurona* infection. **A,** Atrophy of left gluteal muscles. **B,** Atrophy of right quadriceps, tensor fasciae latae, and biceps femoris. (Courtesy Dr. Robert MacKay. From Sellon DC, Long MT: *Equine infectious diseases*, ed 2, St. Louis, 2014, Saunders.)

only definitive host for *S. neurona* is the opossum, although armadillos, raccoons, cats, and skunks have been identified as natural intermediate hosts. Transmission of the disease occurs when horses consume *sporocysts* in opossum feces (Fig. 11-20).

Clinical findings of EPM vary greatly, depending on the localization of the parasite. Asymmetrical muscle *atrophy* is a common clinical sign of EPM that often affects the quadriceps and gluteal muscles (Fig. 11-21). The horse may show signs of cranial nerve abnormalities, such as atrophy of the tongue, self-mutilation of the tongue, and recumbency (Fig. 11-22).

A definitive diagnosis requires identification of characteristic lesions and parasites within the central nervous system on necropsy. *Antemortem* tests include evaluation of serum and cerebrospinal fluid, but these tests are not considered definitive.

Treatment involves antiprotozoal drugs and supportive therapy such as NSAIDs, and many veterinarians think that horses should be supplemented with vitamin E as an *antioxidant*. Prevention should involve reducing access by opossums to horse feeds and pastures.

TECHNICIAN NOTE Prevention of equine protozoal myeloencephalitis involves reducing access by opossums to horse feeds and pastures.

PIROPLASMOSIS

- Etiology: *Babesia equi* and *Babesia caballi*
- Protozoan
- General malaise and anemia
- Reportable disease

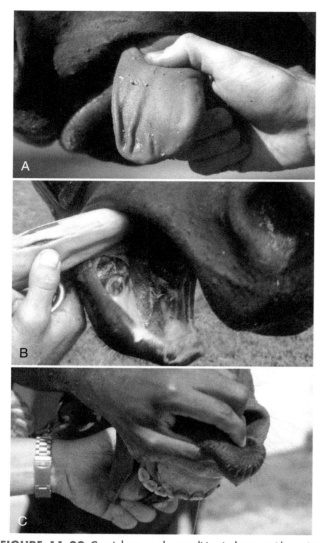

FIGURE 11-22 Cranial nerve abnormalities in horses with equine protozoal myeloencephalitis. **A,** Unilateral atrophy of tongue caused by impaired hypoglossal nerve (cranial nerve XII). **B,** Self-mutilation of tongue secondary to loss of trigeminal nerve (cranial nerve V) sensory function. **C,** Deviation of mandible to the right secondary to a loss of trigeminal nerve motor function. (Courtesy Dr. Robert MacKay. From Sellon DC, Long MT: *Equine infectious diseases*, ed 2, St. Louis, 2014, Saunders.)

Piroplasmosis is a tick-borne protozoal disease caused by one of two protozoans that invade red blood cells: *B. equi* and *B. caballi.* These protozoans are transmitted primarily by ixodid ticks. The ticks are found worldwide, but the disease is most common in tropical, subtropical, and temperate regions.

The life cycle of *B. caballi* begins when an infected tick feeds on a naïve horse. The most common tick for transmittal of *B. caballi* is *Dermacentor nitens.* The sporozoites immediately invade the erythrocytes, and within the erythrocytes the parasites develop from a small anaplasmoid body (trophozoites) into a large pyriform body (merozoites). The cycle then continues when a naïve tick feeds on the horse and ingests the infected erythrocytes. Most of the trophozoites are destroyed in the midgut of the tick, but the merozoites

survive, thus allowing the new tick to infect another horse. The life cycle of *B. equi* is similar to that of *B. caballi,* except for transovarial transmission within the tick and the possible addition of a preerythrocytic stage within lymphocytes (Figs. 11-23 and 11-24).

Clinical signs of piroplasmosis include pyrexia, depression, anemia, thirst, and eye problems (Fig. 11-25). The urine is yellow to reddish in color. The mortality rate is 10% to 15%. Prevention involves tick control and sterilization of needles and medical instruments between uses. Never reuse needles in horses.

Diagnosis of piroplasmosis can be accomplished with blood smears, complement fixation tests, indirect immunofluorescent antibody tests, ELISA, PCR, or in vitro organism cultivation.

Treatment of adult horses with acute clinical signs involves administration of imidocarb dipropionate, diminazene, amicarbalide, euflavine, and/or tetracyclines. Prevention of the disease should include restriction of movement of infected horses and tick feeding prevention (Fig. 11-26).

DERMATOPHYTOSIS

- Etiology: *Trichophyton* and *Microsporum* species
- Fungus
- Skin lesions

Dermatophytosis is also known as ringworm. It is a common superficial cutaneous fungal infection caused by keratinophilic fungi that invade the stratum corneum of the skin and other keratinized structures. *Trichophyton equinum* is the most common agent that causes ringworm in horses (Fig. 11-27). Other agents include *Trichophyton verrucosum, Trichophyton mentagrophytes, Microsporum canis, Microsporum equinum,* and *Microsporum gypseum.* Ringworm is highly contagious and is spread by direct or indirect contact. Indirect contact includes sharing tack, stalls, feed and water containers, and insects. The fungus can survive on equipment for up to 12 months. Clinical signs include small, round lesions covered with small scales (Fig. 11-28). The hair often breaks off just above the skin level. Older lesions may heal in the center, but the edges are quite active.

Identification of ringworm may be made with a Wood lamp or by culture or histologic examination (Fig. 11-29). However, you must remember that not all fungi light up with the Wood lamp, so a negative test does not mean that the fungus is not present.

Ringworm can be treated with povidone-iodine, thiabendazole ointment, sulfur dip, miconazole, ketoconazole, fluconazole, or captan. The environment can be treated with diluted bleach (1:40) and by elimination of infected tack.

WHITE LINE DISEASE

- Etiology: bacteria, fungus, or yeast
- Lameness

White line disease is caused by the invasion of bacteria, fungus, or yeast into the inner horn. When the infection results from fungus, it is also called "onychomycosis." The affected area of the hoof fills with a cheesy material and air

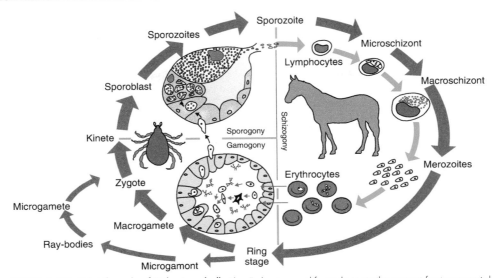

FIGURE 11-23 Life cycle of *Babesia caballi.* The *Babesia equi* life cycle is similar except for transovarial transmission within the tick and the possible addition of a preerythrocytic stage within lymphocytes. (From Sellon DC, Long MT: *Equine infectious diseases,* ed 2, St. Louis, 2014, Saunders.)

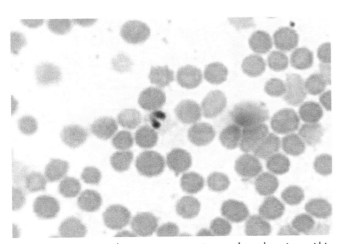

FIGURE 11-24 *Babesia equi* merozoites and trophozoites within erythrocytes. (From Sellon DC, Long MT: *Equine infectious diseases,* ed 2, St. Louis, 2014, Saunders.)

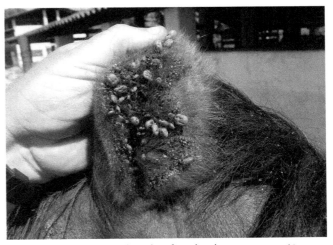

FIGURE 11-26 Horse heavily infected with *Dermacentor (Anocentor) nitens.* This parasite is one of the most common ticks capable of transmitting *Babesia caballi.* (From Sellon DC, Long MT: *Equine infectious diseases,* St. Louis, 2007, Saunders.)

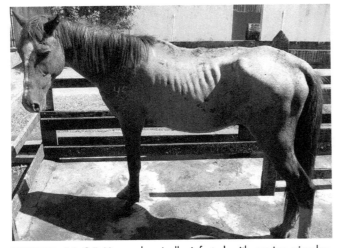

FIGURE 11-25 Horse chronically infected with equine piroplasmosis. (From Sellon DC, Long MT: *Equine infectious diseases,* St. Louis, 2007, Saunders.)

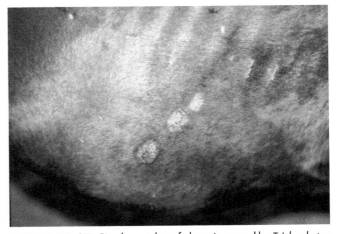

FIGURE 11-27 Circular patches of alopecia caused by *Trichophyton equinum* on the shoulder of a horse. In this case, pruritus was present and lesions were excoriated. (From Sellon DC, Long MT: *Equine infectious diseases,* St. Louis, 2007, Saunders.)

pockets that are often packed with debris (Figs. 11-30 and 11-31). The infection starts at the ground and, if left untreated, can migrate to the coronary band. Clinical signs are often similar to those of laminitis. The horse may be lame, or its sole may be warm to the touch. Sometimes the pockets are filled with a black, foul-smelling substance similar to that seen in thrush. Treatment involves resection of the underlying hoof wall and topical application of an antiseptic.

VIRAL DISEASES

ENCEPHALOMYELITIS

- Etiology: alphaviruses
- Neurologic disease

- Vaccine available
- Reportable diseases

Eastern equine encephalomyelitis, western equine encephalomyelitis, and Venezuelan equine encephalomyelitis are caused by equine alphaviruses.

Eastern equine encephalomyelitis and western equine encephalomyelitis both are found throughout North America. Venezuelan equine encephalomyelitis is most commonly found in the southern United States and in countries farther south. Encephalomyelitis is transmitted by mosquitoes. Common clinical signs include fever, *ataxia*, anorexia,

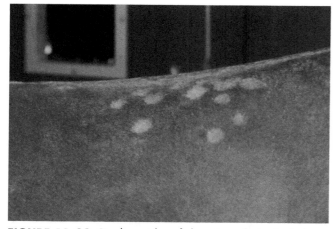

FIGURE 11-28 Circular patches of alopecia on the back of a horse that were most likely caused by a contaminated saddle pad. Lesions showed minimum inflammation. No pruritus was present. (From Sellon DC, Long MT: *Equine infectious diseases*, St. Louis, 2007, Saunders.)

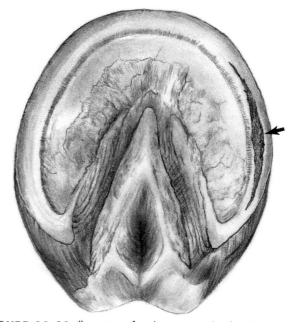

FIGURE 11-30 Illustration of a characteristic hoof-wall defect in a horse with white line disease (ground surface view). (From Robinson NE: *Current therapy in equine medicine*, ed 6, St. Louis, 2009, Saunders.)

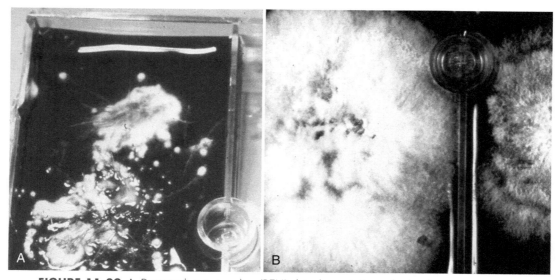

FIGURE 11-29 **A,** Dermatophyte test medium (DTM) plate demonstrating red color change in conjunction with growth of *Trichophyton*. **B,** Nondermatophyte fungal growth on DTM agar. (From Sellon DC, Long MT: *Equine infectious diseases*, St. Louis, 2007, Saunders.)

paralysis, circling, head pressing, and hyperexcitability (Fig. 11-32).

Diagnosis is presumptive before death. No known treatments for encephalomyelitis exist. Treatment should be supportive. Prevention should include vaccination.

EQUINE VIRAL ARTERITIS

- Etiology: equine arteritis virus
- Flulike illness and abortion
- Vaccine available
- Reportable disease

Equine viral arteritis is caused by equine arteritis virus (EAV). EAV causes flulike symptoms, abortion, and, in very young horses, pneumonia. The disease is transmitted through respiratory particles or by venereal routes (Fig. 11-33). Even though horses can transmit the disease through bodily fluids (e.g., urine), aborted fetuses, and aerosol, infected semen is the primary source of infection. Semen from infected stallions can be chronically or acutely infected with the virus. The stallion is the natural reservoir for the virus. The incubation period is 2 to 14 days.

> **TECHNICIAN NOTE**   Semen from infected stallions can be chronically or acutely infected with equine arteritis virus.

Horses are often subclinical carriers of the virus. Clinical signs that manifest in adults often include abortion, respiratory signs, and fever. In foals, clinical signs can include pneumonia and enteritis.

The disease has many possible differential diagnoses. To confirm a case of equine arteritis, *virus isolation, paired serum samples, viral antigen,* or *viral nucleic acid detection* should be used.

Treatment of horses with severe infections includes NSAIDs, fever-reducing drugs, diuretics, and rest. Most adult horses recover uneventfully. No effective treatment exists for foals with pneumonia or for carrier stallions.

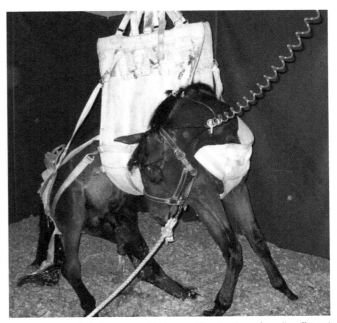

FIGURE 11-32 Two-year old Thoroughbred colt profoundly affected with eastern equine encephalomyelitis virus. This horse had clinical signs for approximately 36 hours. Initial signs consisted of fever and depression. The horse rapidly deteriorated and by 24 hours after onset could not be aroused. This horse also had persistent priapism, a common clinical sign in male horses with encephalitis. (From Sellon DC, Long MT: *Equine infectious diseases,* ed 2, St. Louis, 2014, Saunders.)

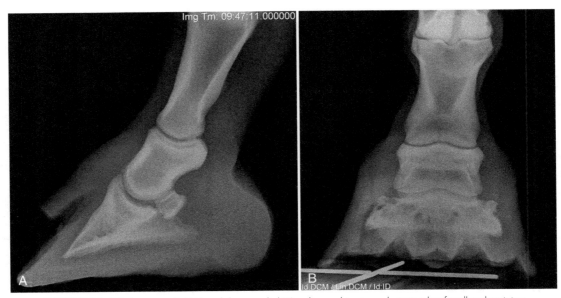

FIGURE 11-31 Lateromedial (**A**) and dorsomedial (**B**) radiographic views depicting hoof wall undermining associated with white line disease. Notice in **A** that the distal portion of the separated hoof wall was removed before radiographic examination. (From Robinson NE: *Current therapy in equine medicine,* ed 6, St. Louis, 2009, Saunders.)

Stallions that carry the virus should be surgically castrated. Prevention of the disease includes vaccination.

> ### TECHNICIAN NOTE
> Stallions that carry the equine arteritis virus should be surgically castrated.

EQUINE INFECTIOUS ANEMIA

- Etiology: lentivirus
- Subclinical to general malaise to neurologic disease
- Coggins test
- Reportable disease

Equine infectious anemia (EIA; swamp fever) is caused by equine infectious anemia virus (EIAV). EIAV is a lentivirus of the Retroviridae family. The disease is transmitted through blood-sucking insects.

Clinical signs of EIA vary, depending on the virus strain and the susceptibility of the horse. Acute EIA is caused by a virulent strain of EIA. The incubation period ranges from 5 to 30 days. When clinical signs manifest, the horse often develops a fever, becomes lethargic, and is anorexic (Fig. 11-34). The mucous membranes appear pale and may have *petechiae*. The animal may be icteric, and neurologic signs may develop (Fig. 11-35). Blood analysis reveals *thrombocytopenia* and anemia.

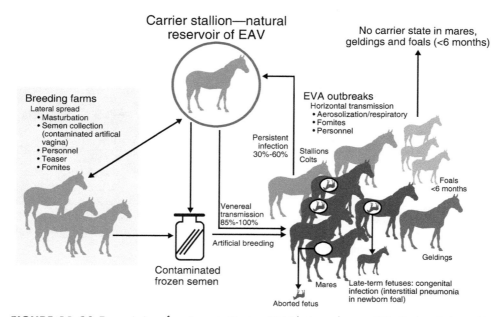

FIGURE 11-33 Transmission of equine arteritis virus (EAV) between horses. *EVA,* Equine viral arteritis. (From Sellon DC, Long MT: *Equine infectious diseases,* St. Louis, 2007, Saunders.)

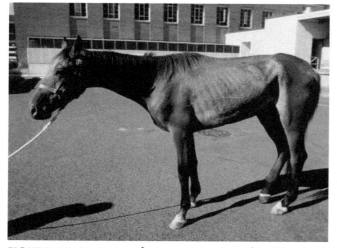

FIGURE 11-34 Equine infectious anemia virus–infected horse with clinical signs of chronic equine infectious anemia. (From Sellon DC, Long MT: *Equine infectious diseases,* ed 2, St. Louis, 2014, Saunders.)

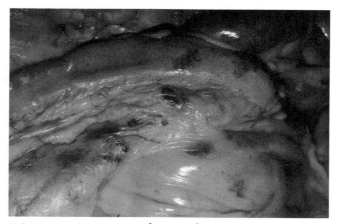

FIGURE 11-35 Necropsy of equine infectious anemia virus–infected horse with acute equine infectious anemia. Note the icteric mesentery and the numerous serosal and mesenteric hemorrhages. (From Sellon DC, Long MT: *Equine infectious diseases,* St. Louis, 2007, Saunders.)

Diagnosis of the disease is made by serologic testing known commonly as Coggins testing.

> **TECHNICIAN NOTE**   Diagnosis of equine infectious anemia is made by serologic testing known commonly as Coggins testing.

Four serologic tests are accepted by the U.S. Food and Drug Administration: the *agar gel immunodiffusion test (AGID)*, cELISA, and synthetic antigen ELISA.

No specific therapy is available for horses diagnosed with EIA. The disease is reportable in the United States. Most often the horse is recommended for euthanasia. If the owner elects not to euthanize, the animal must be quarantined from other horses, the horse cannot undergo interstate travel, and supportive therapy is recommended (Fig. 11-36).

> **TECHNICIAN NOTE**   Equine infectious anemia is a reportable disease in the United States.

EQUINE INFLUENZA

- Etiology: Orthomyxoviridae virus
- Influenza (flu)
- Vaccine available

Equine influenza A is caused by a virus of the Orthomyxoviridae family. Influenza is a common respiratory condition of the horse. The disease often affects horses that intermingle with other horses, such as occurs at rodeos and horse shows. The disease has high *morbidity* and low mortality.

> **TECHNICIAN NOTE**   Equine influenza A often affects horses that intermingle with other horses, such as occurs at rodeos and horse shows.

The disease has a short incubation period of approximately 48 hours. The virus targets the lower respiratory tract and affects the epithelial cells, particularly those of the trachea and bronchial tree. Replication of the virus causes cellular death. The loss of epithelial cells causes inflammation of the columnar ciliated cells, and this predisposes the horse to secondary bacterial infections. If secondary bacterial infections can be prevented, the epithelial damage will resolve within 3 weeks.

Clinical signs of equine influenza include a fever often in excess of 106° F, anorexia, and weight loss. After the horse develops a fever, the animal also often has a mucopurulent nasal discharge, an increased respiratory rate, and sometimes retropharyngeal lymphadenopathy (Fig. 11-37). Clinical signs often resolve in 1 or 2 weeks, but coughing may persist for approximately 3 weeks.

Diagnosis is often presumptive, based on the short incubation period and clinical signs. Definitive diagnosis requires one of the following tests: virus isolation, immunoassay, immunofluorescence, PCR, or antibody detection (Fig. 11-38).

Treatment is supportive. The horse should rest, remain hydrated, and, if necessary, be given NSAIDs. If the disease does not clear within 10 days, antimicrobial therapy should be considered for any possible secondary bacterial infections. Prevention should include vaccination.

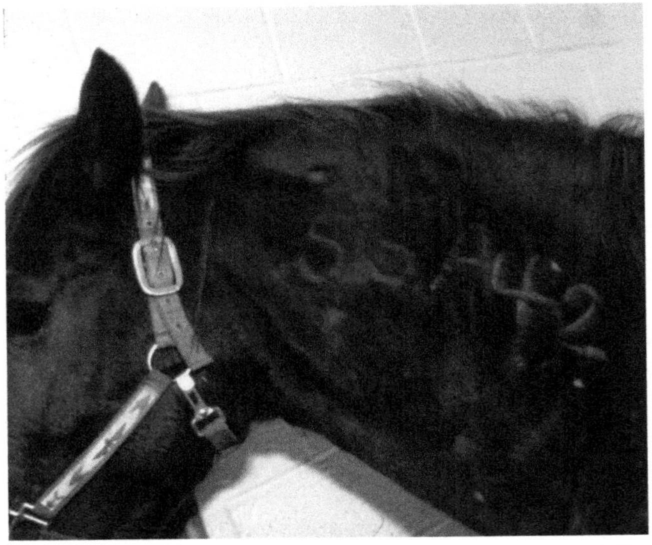

FIGURE 11-36 Branded equine infectious anemia "reactor." The number "55" is the individual horse identification number, the letter "A" designates the horse as an equine infectious anemia virus reactor, and the number "42" designates the state in which the horse was identified. (From Sellon DC: Equine infectious anemia. In Colahan PT, Merritt AM, Moore JN, Mayhew IG, editors: *Equine medicine and surgery*, ed 5, St. Louis, 1999, Mosby.)

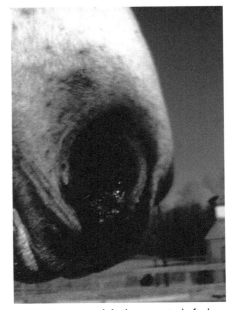

FIGURE 11-37 Serous nasal discharge typical of a horse with acute influenza virus infection. (Courtesy College of Veterinary Medicine, North Carolina State University. From Sellon DC, Long MT: *Equine infectious diseases*. St. Louis, 2007, Saunders.)

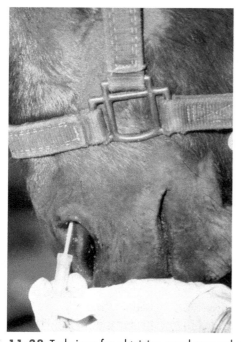

FIGURE 11-38 Technique for obtaining nasal mucosal swab for antigen detection or virus isolation. Short, polyester-tipped (non–cotton-tipped) swab is appropriate for sample collection. Virus isolation from a nasal mucosal swab is most sensitive for detection of equine influenza virus if obtained during the first 24 to 48 hours of fever. (From Sellon DC, Long MT: *Equine infectious diseases*, ed 2, St. Louis, 2014, Saunders.)

RABIES

- Etiology: rhabdovirus
- Neurologic disease
- Vaccine available
- Reportable disease (to state officials)

Rabies is caused by an enveloped ribonucleic acid rhabdovirus. The disease causes lethal polioencephalomyelitis and ganglionitis in infected animals. The virus is transmitted to horses through bites from other infected animals, such as skunks, raccoons, foxes, and bats (Figs. 11-39 and 11-40). The virus enters the horse's body through the saliva of the infected animal.

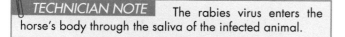

TECHNICIAN NOTE The rabies virus enters the horse's body through the saliva of the infected animal.

Horses that present with rabies often show clinical signs related to the gastrointestinal system, cerebral and cranial nerves, and spinal cord, for example, ataxia, lameness, and loss of bladder control. The disease is progressive. As time passes, the clinical signs worsen. Horses infected with rabies often progress into either a depressed or an aggressive form of the disease (Fig. 11-41).

Diagnosis is unreliable without diagnostic examination of the brain and spinal cord. Rabies has no treatment. Prevention includes vaccination and wildlife management practices.

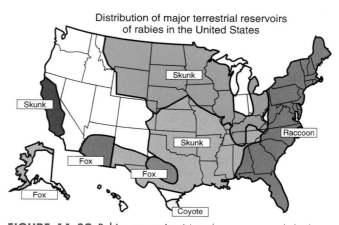

FIGURE 11-39 Rabies reservoirs. Note the raccoon and skunk rabies present in the central (skunk) and mid-Atlantic to northeastern (raccoon) distribution in the continental United States. (Courtesy Centers for Disease Control and Prevention, Atlanta.)

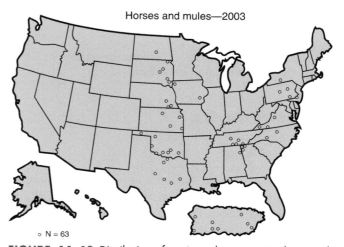

FIGURE 11-40 Distribution of equine rabies cases in the United States and Puerto Rico in 2003. Note the central and mid-Atlantic to northeastern distribution in the continental United States. Most cases are caused by the local reservoir type, that is, central (skunk) and mid-Atlantic to northeastern (raccoon). (Courtesy Centers for Disease Control and Prevention, Atlanta.)

RHINOPNEUMONITIS

- Etiology: herpesvirus
- Respiratory disease and abortion
- Vaccine available
- Reportable disease (if neurologic)

Rhinopneumonitis is caused by equine herpesvirus type 1 (EHV-1) and equine herpesvirus type 4 (EHV-4). These viruses cause respiratory conditions, abortion, and neurologic conditions in horses.

The virus affects the upper respiratory tract and causes mucopurulent nasal discharge, lymphadenopathy, and coughing (Figs. 11-42 and 11-43). EHV-1 is most often responsible for abortion storms in mares, but EHV-4 can also cause abortion. Stallions with EHV-1 may develop scrotal edema, loss of libido, and reduced sperm quality. Myeloencephalopathy caused by equine herpesvirus is rare but can occur.

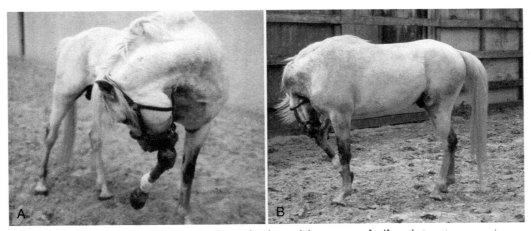

FIGURE 11-41 A and **B,** Arabian stallion with rabies exhibiting signs of self-mutilation. Aggressive biting behavior led to human injury and rabies virus exposure, with subsequent human prophylactic treatment. (From Sellon DC, Long MT: *Equine infectious diseases,* ed 2, St. Louis, 2014, Saunders.)

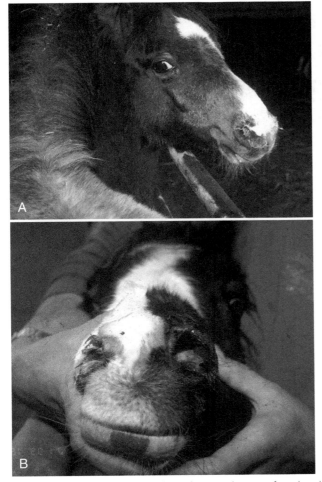

FIGURE 11-42 A and **B,** Foals and young horses infected with equine herpesvirus type 1 may develop clinically apparent respiratory disease. Nasal discharge initially is serous but quickly becomes mucopurulent. (From Sellon DC, Long MT: *Equine infectious diseases,* ed 2, St. Louis, 2014, Saunders.)

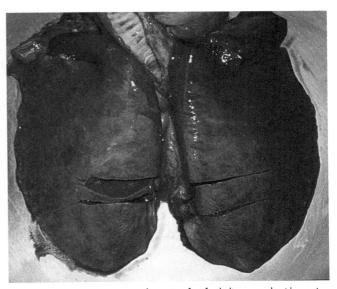

FIGURE 11-43 Severe atelectasis of a foal diagnosed with equine herpesvirus type 1. Note the small, white, necrotic foci of the lung parenchyma. Histopathologic examination confirmed equine herpesvirus lung inclusion bodies. (From McAuliffe SB, Slovis NM: *Color atlas of diseases and disorders of the foal,* Oxford, 2008, Saunders.)

Neurologic signs often include ataxia, fever, loss of anal tone, paralysis of the tail, urinary incontinence, and recumbency (Fig. 11-44).

Diagnosis is often accomplished by *postmortem* PCR.

Treatment involves isolation of horses infected with the respiratory form of equine herpes because these horses are contagious. All other cases of EHV infection should be treated with supportive care.

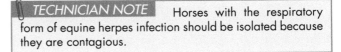

TECHNICIAN NOTE Horses with the respiratory form of equine herpes infection should be isolated because they are contagious.

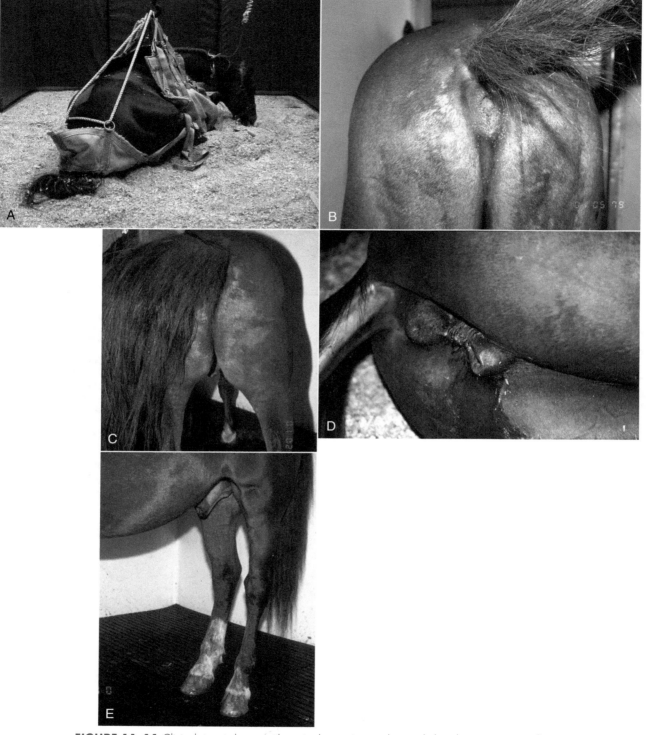

FIGURE 11-44 Clinical signs in horses with equine herpesvirus myeloencephalopathy vary in severity from mild ataxia and proprioceptive deficiency to severe ataxia and recumbency requiring extensive supportive care (**A**). Other clinical signs may include loss of anal tone (**B**), flaccid paralysis of the tail (**C**), and urinary incontinence (**D**) with secondary urine scald on the hindlegs (**E**). (**A**, Courtesy Dr. Chris Sanchez, University of Florida. From Sellon DC, Long MT: *Equine infectious diseases*, ed 2, St. Louis, 2014, Saunders.)

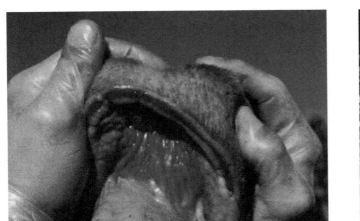

FIGURE 11-45 Ulceration of oral mucosa at the mucocutaneous junction in a horse caused by vesicular stomatitis virus infection. (From Sellon DC, Long MT: *Equine infectious diseases*, ed 2, St. Louis, 2014, Saunders.)

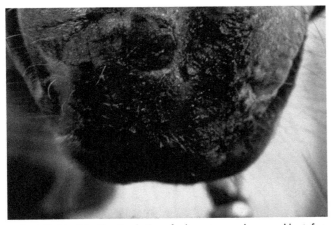

FIGURE 11-46 Crusting lesion of a horse's muzzle caused by infection with vesicular stomatitis virus serotype New Jersey. (From Sellon DC, Long MT: *Equine infectious diseases*, ed 2, St. Louis, 2014, Saunders.)

VESICULAR STOMATITIS

- Etiology: Rhabdoviridae family
- Vesicles
- Reportable disease

Vesicular stomatitis is caused by a virus of the Rhabdoviridae family. The virus is transmitted through insects such as the black fly, sand fly, mosquito, and housefly. The incubation period of the virus is 3 to 7 days. The horse initially has a fever and excessive saliva production. The horse develops fluid-filled white areas on the oral mucosa. The white vesicles rupture quickly and leave ulcerations (Figs. 11-45 and 11-46). As the disease progresses, vesicles and lesions may develop in other areas of the body, including the coronary band, belly, muzzle, prepuce, and udder (Fig. 11-47).

Diagnosis is through antibody detection, detection of viral genetic material, and viral isolation.

Treatment is often limited because most horses recover within 7 to 14 days, but in more severe cases supportive care may be needed.

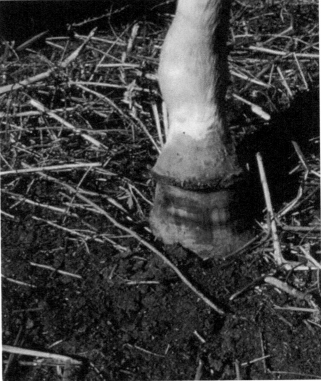

FIGURE 11-47 Coronitis caused by infection with vesicular stomatitis virus serotype New Jersey. (From Sellon DC, Long MT: *Equine infectious diseases*, ed 2, St. Louis, 2014, Saunders.)

WEST NILE VIRUS INFECTION

- Etiology: Flaviviridae family
- General malaise and neurologic disease
- Vaccine available
- Reportable disease (if neurologic)

West Nile virus infection is caused by a virus of the Flaviviridae family. The disease is spread by mosquitoes. The mosquito first bites an infected bird and then bites a horse, thus passing on the virus (Figs. 11-48 and 11-49).

Clinical signs of the disease include a low-grade fever, lack of appetite, depression, colic, personality changes that range from hyperexcitability to apprehensiveness, unresponsiveness, and coma. Some horses develop paralysis and have to be euthanized; others die spontaneously. Many horses start to show signs of recovery within 3 to 7 days and complete a full recovery within 1 to 6 months.

West Nile virus infection is diagnosed using immunoglobulin M (IgM)–capture ELISA (MAC-ELISA) of serum or cerebrospinal fluid, plaque reduction neutralization test (PRNT) of serum or viral isolation, and PCR performed on brain tissue.

Treatment is often supportive, and vaccination is the best prevention. Control of the environment and removal of stagnant water from a property can help keep down the mosquito population.

CUTANEOUS PAPILLOMAS

- Etiology: *Equus caballus* papillomavirus type 1
- Cutaneous papillomas

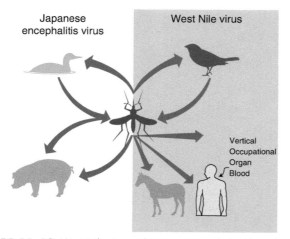

FIGURE 11-48 West Nile virus and Japanese encephalitis life cycle in which the primary transmission cycle occurs between avian or porcine reservoirs and mosquitoes. Horses and humans are aberrant hosts. (From Sellon DC, Long MT: *Equine infectious diseases*, ed 2, St. Louis, 2014, Saunders.)

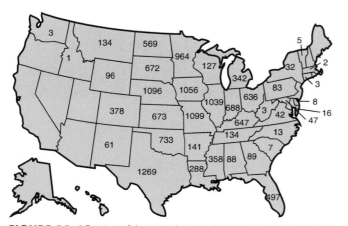

FIGURE 11-49 Map of the United States depicting the numbers of reported cases of West Nile virus encephalomyelitis in horses during 2002, the largest epizootic year since encroachment in 1999. (From Sellon DC, Long MT: *Equine infectious diseases*, St. Louis, 2007, Saunders.)

Cutaneous papillomas are known as warts. They are caused by an infection of *E. caballus* papillomavirus type 1. Warts frequently appear around the lips and muzzles of horses, but they also can appear on the eyelids, prepuce, inner thighs, and distal limbs (Fig. 11-50). The virus is spread by direct contact with other horses, usually where horses gather, such as horse shows or sales, or during breeding. The virus can also be spread by *fomites*. These papillomas usually are harmless unless they are irritated by tack. Most lesions spontaneously disappear within 3 to 4 months if they are not treated. Lack of resolution within 6 to 9 months may indicate an underlying immune deficiency. If removal is necessary, chemical cautery or cryosurgery can be performed. Prevention includes isolation of infected horses.

VACCINATION SCHEDULES

Vaccination schedules recommended by the American Association of Equine Practitioners are listed in Table 11-1.

NONINFECTIOUS DISEASES

CHOKE

Choke occurs when feedstuffs become lodged in the equine esophagus. Common causes of choke include inadequate water intake, large feed particles, quick eating habits, and food that is too dry. Feeding things such as whole apples, carrots, and ears of corn can predispose horses to choke. Prevention of choke includes encouraging adequate water intake, soaking feeds before feeding, and using methods to slow eating.

CHRONIC OBSTRUCTIVE PULMONARY DISEASE

Chronic obstructive pulmonary disease (COPD) is also known as heaves, broken wind, and chronic alveolar emphysema. COPD is a noninfectious respiratory disease. Some controversy exists over the causes of COPD, but the most commonly recognized cause is exposure to air pollutants

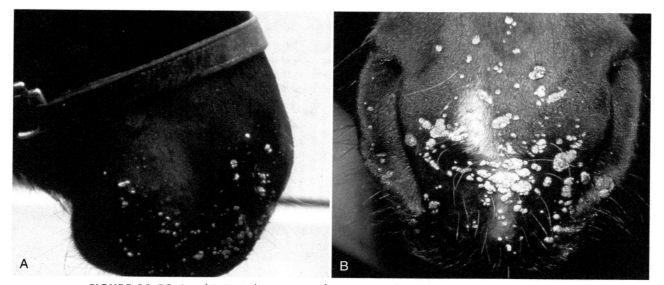

FIGURE 11-50 A and **B**, Typical appearance of warts on muzzle and lips of a young horse. (Courtesy Dr. Melissa Hines. From Sellon DC, Long MT: *Equine infectious diseases*, St. Louis, 2007, Saunders.)

TABLE 11-1 | American Association of Equine Practitioners Guidelines for Vaccination of Horses*

The following schedule is a suggested vaccination schedule provided by the AAEP and is based on generally accepted veterinary practices. These guidelines are neither regulations nor directives for all situations and should not be interpreted as such. It is the responsibility of attending veterinarians, through an appropriate veterinarian-client-patient relationship, to use this information coupled with available products to determine the best professional care for their patients. For complete discussion of vaccination guidelines, please see the AAEP resource guide "Guidelines for Vaccination of Horses."

DISEASE/ VACCINE	FOALS/WEANLINGS	YEARLINGS	PERFORMANCE HORSES	PLEASURE HORSES	BROODMARES	COMMENTS
West Nile virus	First dose: 3–4 months Second dose: 1 month later (plus third dose at 6 months in endemic areas)	Annual booster, before expected risk. Vaccinate semiannually or more frequently (every 4 months), depending on risk	Annual booster, before expected risk. Vaccinate semiannually or more frequently (every 4 months), depending on the risk	Annual booster, before expected risk. Vaccinate semiannually or more frequently (every 4 months), depending on the risk	Annual, 4–6 weeks prepartum	Annual booster is after primary series. In endemic areas, booster as required or warranted by to local conditions conductive to disease risk. Vaccinate semiannually or more frequently (every 4 months), depending on risk
Tetanus toxoid	**From nonvaccinated mare:** First dose: 3–4 months Second dose: 4–5 months **From vaccinated mare:** First dose: 6 months Second dose: 7 months Third dose: 8–9 months	Annual	Annual	Annual	Annual, 4–6 weeks prepartum	Booster at time of penetrating injury or surgery if last dose not administered within 6 months
Encepha- lomyelitis (EEE, WEE, VEE)	**EEE (in high-risk areas):** First dose: 3–4 months Second dose: 4–5 months Third dose: 5–6 months **WEE, EEE (in low-risk areas) and VEE:** **From nonvaccinated mare:** First dose: 3–4 months Second dose: 4–5 months Third dose: 5–6 months **From vaccinated mare:** First dose: 6 months Second dose: 7 months Third dose: 8 months	Annual, spring Annual, spring	Annual, spring Annual, spring	Annual, spring Annual, spring	Annual, 4–6 weeks prepartum Annual, 4–6 weeks prepartum	In endemic areas, booster EEE and WEE every 6 months; VEE needed only when threat of exposure exists; VEE may be available only as a combination vaccine with EEE and WEE

Continued

TABLE 11-1   American Association of Equine Practitioners Guidelines for Vaccination of Horses*—cont'd

DISEASE/VACCINE	FOALS/WEANLINGS	YEARLINGS	PERFORMANCE HORSES	PLEASURE HORSES	BROODMARES	COMMENTS
Influenza	**Inactivated injectable: From nonvaccinated mare:** First dose: 6 months Second dose: 7 months Third dose: 8 months, then at 3-month intervals **From vaccinated mare:** First dose: 9 months Second dose: 10 months Third dose: 11–12 months, then at 3-month intervals	Every 3–4 months	Every 3–4 months	Annual, with added boosters before likely exposure	At least semiannual, with one booster 4–6 weeks prepartum	Series of at least three doses is recommended for primary immunization of foals. Not recommended for pregnant mares until data are available. Use inactivated vaccine for prepartum booster. If first dose is administered to foals <11 months of age, administer second dose at or after 11 months
	Intranasal modified live virus: First dose: 11 months (has been safely administered to foals <11 months)	Every 6 months	Every 6 months	Every 6 months	Annual before breeding (see comments)	
Rhinopneumonitis (EHV-1 and EHV-4)	First dose: 4–6 months Second dose: 5–7 months Third dose: 6–8 months, then at 3-month intervals	Booster every 3–4 months up to annually	Booster every 3–4 months up to annually	Optional: Semiannual if elected	Fifth, seventh, and ninth months of gestation (inactivated EHV-1 vaccine); optional dose at third month of gestation	Vaccination of mares before breeding and 4–6 weeks prepartum is suggested. Breeding stallions should be vaccinated before the breeding season and semiannually
Strangles	**Injectable:** First dose: 4–6 months Second dose: 5–7 months Third dose: 7–8 months (depending on product used) Fourth dose: 12 months **Intranasal:** First dose: 6–9 months Second dose: 3 weeks later	Semiannual	Optional: Semiannual if risk is high	Optional: Semiannual if risk is high	Semiannual, with one dose of inactivated M-protein vaccine 4–6 weeks prepartum	Vaccines containing M-protein extract may be less reactive than whole-cell vaccines. Use when endemic conditions exist or risk is high. Foals as young as 6 weeks of age may safely receive the intranasal product. Third dose should be administered 2–4 weeks before weaning
Rabies	**Foal born to nonvaccinated mare:** First dose: 3–4 months Second dose: 12 months **Foal born to vaccinated mare:** First dose: 6 months Second dose: 7 months Third dose: 12 months	Annual	Annual	Annual	Annual, before breeding	Vaccination recommended in endemic areas. Do not use modified live virus vaccines in horses
Potomac horse fever	First dose: 5–6 months Second dose: 6–7 months	Semiannual	Semiannual	Semiannual	Semiannual, with one dose 4–6 weeks prepartum	Booster during May to June in endemic areas

Disease						Comments
Botulism	**Foal from vaccinated mare:** Three-dose series of toxoid at 30-day intervals starting at age 2–3 months **Foal from nonvaccinated mare:** See comments	Consult your veterinarian	Consult your veterinarian	Consult your veterinarian	Initial three-dose series at 30-day intervals, with last dose 4–6 weeks prepartum Annually thereafter, 4–6 weeks prepartum	Only in endemic areas. Third dose administered 4–6 weeks after second dose may improve response of foal to primary immunization. Foal from nonvaccinated mare may benefit from (1) toxoid at age 2, 4, and 8 weeks; (2) transfusion of plasma from vaccinated horse; or (3) antitoxin. Efficiency requires further study
Equine viral arteritis	**Intact colt intended to be breeding stallion:** One dose at age 6–12 months	Annual for colt intended to be breeding stallion	Annual for colt intended to be breeding stallion	Annual for colt intended to be breeding stallion	Annual for seronegative open mares before breeding to carrier stallion; isolate mare for 21 days after breeding to carrier stallion	Annual for breeding stallions and teasers, 28 days before start of breeding season. Virus may be shed in semen for up to 21 days. Vaccinated mares do not develop clinical signs even though they become transiently infected and may shed virus for a short time
Rotavirus A	Little value in vaccinating foal because of insufficient time to develop antibodies to protect during susceptible age	Not applicable	Not applicable	Not applicable	Vaccinate mare at 8, 9, and 10 months of gestation, each pregnancy. Passive transfer of colostral antibodies aids in preventing rotaviral diarrhea in foal	Check concentrations of immunoglobulins in foal to ensure no failure of passive transfer

Adapted from www.aaep.org/pdfs/AAEP_vacc_guide.pdf.
AAEP, American Association of Equine Practitioners; *EEE,* eastern equine encephalomyelitis; *EHV-1,* equine herpesvirus type 1; *EHV-4,* equine herpesvirus type 4; *VEE,* Venezuelan equine encephalomyelitis; *WEE,* western equine encephalomyelitis.
*As with administration of all medications, the label and product insert should be read before administration of all vaccines. Schedules for stallions should be consistent with the vaccination program of the adult horse population on the farm and modified according to risk.

such as dust and molds. Some conditions that may predispose the horse to COPD include diet, possible genetic linkage, and a history of respiratory tract infections. The disease most commonly affects horses more than 6 years old.

Clinical signs of COPD include difficult breathing, abdominal breathing, nasal discharge, coughing, and lack of stamina. Some horses display hyperpnea only at rest. Most horses initially experience episodes of difficult breathing. Conditions that may initiate an episode include feeding of certain types of roughages, being stabled, and exercise. Some horses have what is known as summer pasture–associated COPD and experience dyspnea episodes only when they are out to pasture. As the disease progresses, episodes may occur more frequently, and the condition may become chronic. Because of the increased effort of the abdominal muscles to encourage breathing, some horses develop a "heave line" (a ridge along the costal arch). The clinical signs of the disease may lead to bronchiolitis, emphysema, and structural changes to the alveolar walls and interstitial tissues.

Diagnosis of the disease is usually made from the history and clinical signs. Endoscopy may be used to identify tracheobronchial exudate. Fluid collected from bronchoalveolar lavage (BAL) or a tracheal wash can be used in the diagnosis and usually shows neutrophils with normal morphology. Even though allergies are thought to be responsible for COPD, eosinophils are not commonly found in the samples collected. Culture of the sample often reveals opportunistic bacterial infections.

Treatment often involves removing respiratory irritants from the horse's environment. This includes trying to decrease dust within the stable, feeding cubed forages instead of loose forages, and soaking feeds before feeding. Changing the stall bedding to paper or wood chips can improve dust levels within the environment. Most horses improve with changes to the environment. However, if the horse shows only slight improvement with the changes in environment, then permanent damage to the respiratory tract may have occurred and is irreversible.

COLIC

Colic is defined as abdominal pain. The four general causes of colic are (1) distention of the gut, (2) pulling at the root of the mesenteric artery, (3) ischemia or infarction, and (4) enteritis or ulcerations. Distention of the gut can be caused by fluid, sand, gas, ingesta leading to impaction, lack of water or fiber in the diet, overeating of concentrate, overconsumption of water, spasms, or paralysis (Figs. 11-51 to 11-53). Pulling at the root of the mesenteric artery is caused by torsion (twisting of the gut in response distention), hernia, or a tumor. Ischemia or infarction can be caused by torsion or thrombus from strongyles. Enteritis or ulceration is caused by inflammation of the gastrointestinal tract by factors such as stress, disease, salmonellosis, or parasites (Fig. 11-54).

Clinical signs include repeated standing and lying down, rolling, kicking at the abdomen, pawing, looking at the abdomen, grunting, sweating, distention of the abdomen, positioning as if to urinate, straining to defecate, decreased bowel movements, rapid breathing, flared nostrils, abnormal behavior, and lack of appetite (Figs. 11-55 to 11-57).

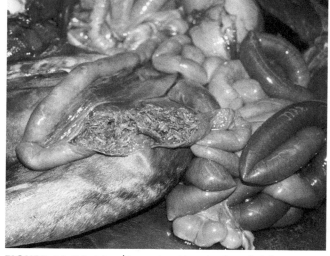

FIGURE 11-51 Jejunal impaction. Note the distended, firm jejunum. (From McAuliffe SB, Slovis NM: *Color atlas of diseases and disorders of the foal,* Oxford, 2008, Saunders.)

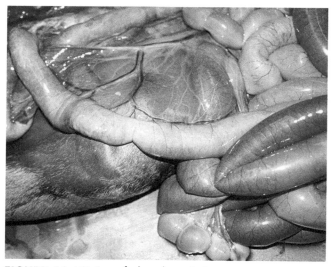

FIGURE 11-52 Same foal as shown in Figure 11-51. Note the impacted feed material within the jejunum. (From McAuliffe SB, Slovis NM: *Color atlas of diseases and disorders of the foal,* Oxford, 2008, Saunders.)

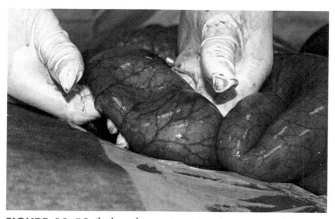

FIGURE 11-53 Ileal sand impaction. Note the impression left on the bowel after application of finger pressure. (From McAuliffe SB, Slovis NM: *Color atlas of diseases and disorders of the foal,* Oxford, 2008, Saunders.)

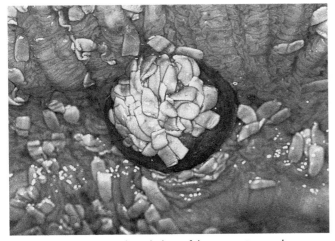

FIGURE 11-54 *Anoplocephala perfoliata* parasites on the mucosa of the ileocecal junction and cecum. The parasites caused recurrent colic by inducing ileal impaction. (Courtesy C.J. Proudman. From Robinson NE: *Current therapy in equine medicine*, ed 6, St. Louis, 2009, Saunders.)

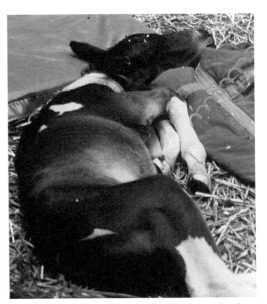

FIGURE 11-56 Marked abdominal distention and colic in a foal with impending enteritis. (From McAuliffe SB, Slovis NM: *Color atlas of diseases and disorders of the foal*, Oxford, 2008, Saunders.)

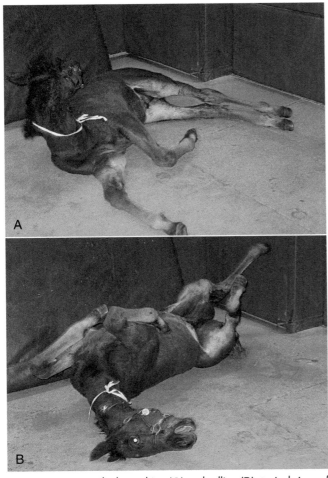

FIGURE 11-55 Flank watching (**A**) and rolling (**B**), typical signs of colic. (From McAuliffe SB, Slovis NM: *Color atlas of diseases and disorders of the foal*, Oxford, 2008, Saunders.)

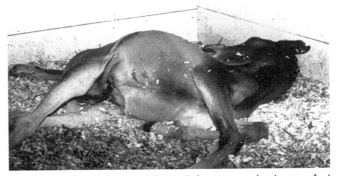

FIGURE 11-57 Marked abdominal distention and colic in a foal with colon torsion. (From McAuliffe SB, Slovis NM: *Color atlas of diseases and disorders of the foal*, Oxford, 2008, Saunders.)

Diagnosis of colic is based on clinical signs gathered from a physical examination. The physical examination should include auscultation of borborygmi, abdominal palpation, observation of mucous membranes, heart rate, respiration rate, rectal temperature, passing a nasogastric tube for observation of reflux, and abdominocentesis.

It is important to obtain a thorough history. Having clients gather information about some of the clinical signs, including the appearance of mucous membranes, heart rate, respiration rate, capillary refill time, and rectal temperature, can be valuable. Some clients are readily able to supply this information to you. However, others may not have the equipment or knowledge, and you may have to inform clients about how to obtain these vital measurements. This information can be useful to the veterinarian before the horse's arrival or before the veterinarian's arrival at the farm or stable. Communication with clients is extremely important. It is essential to let clients know that they should not give pain medication before the veterinarian's approval. Some clinical signs of colic can be masked if pain medication is given, thus making diagnosis more difficult. Clients should be informed to remove the horse from access to food and water. Clients should be instructed to prevent the horse from rolling if it is attempting to do so. This goal can often be accomplished by hand walking. The client should continue these practices until the veterinarian evaluates the patient.

Treatment of mild colic often includes placement of a nasogastric tube for administration of mineral oil, pain medication, hand walking, and continued monitoring. Treatment of severe colic often involves intravenous fluids (shock doses if necessary) and sometimes even abdominal surgical procedures. Horses with heart rates great than 70 beats per minute, horses that are unresponsive to pain medication, and horses with an abnormal rectal temperature are often classified as having severe colic.

Prevention of colic includes the following steps:

- Establishing and adhering to a set daily routine
- Feeding a high-quality forage as the primary component of the diet
- Avoiding excessive grain and energy-dense supplements
- Taking precautions to prevent access to feed rooms and feed storage bins
- Dividing rations into smaller, frequent meals
- Routine deworming
- Providing daily exercise or turnout
- Making gradual feed and exercise changes
- Avoiding medications unless prescribed by a veterinarian (some medications can cause ulcers or decrease peristaltic movement)
- Inspecting feedstuffs for toxic substances such as blister beetles and toxic plants
- Inspecting feeds for foreign indigestible materials
- Providing fresh clean water
- Reducing stress
- Feeding horses in feeders that are not on the ground
- Cooling horses that have been exercised before stalling or turnout
- Offering only small sips of lukewarm water to "hot" horses
- Monitoring horses prepartum and postpartum for clinical signs of colic
- Keeping accurate records

CUSHING DISEASE

Cushing disease is also referred to as hyperadrenocorticism or cortisol excess. In horses the disease is usually secondary to adenoma or hyperplasia.

Clinical signs often include the following: *polydipsia* and *polyuria;* long, thick, curly hair coats; failure to shed in the spring; dull hair coats; development of a sway back and pot belly; laminitis; fat deposition in the supraorbital fossae; weight loss; increased appetite; depression; increased sweating, possibly in patches; and loss of muscle tone over the back. The horses may be diabetic, often are immunocompromised, and are at greater risk for developing laminitis.

The disease can be diagnosed using blood tests that measure levels of adrenocorticotropic hormone (ACTH), cortisol, insulin, and glucose.

Treatment consists of a drug such as cyproheptadine or pergolide mesylate. Treatment can be extremely expensive.

EXERCISE-INDUCED PULMONARY HEMORRHAGE

Exercise-induced pulmonary hemorrhage (also known as EIPH or bleeders) is hemorrhage that originates from small pulmonary vessels associated with strenuous exercise. Female horses are thought to be at a slightly higher risk of the disease, as are older horses doing strenuous work. When horses undergo strenuous exercise, they have very high pulmonary and atrial pressures. The smaller vessels in the lungs are then damaged. The blood from the damage to the alveoli then makes its way up the trachea.

Diagnosis includes observation of blood by endoscopy and BAL for enumeration of erythrocytes in the BAL fluid.

Treatments are variable: rest to allow the pulmonary lesions to heal, furosemide, nasal strips, nitric oxide, bronchodilators, procoagulants, antiinflammatory agents, and omega-3 fatty acids.

EXERTIONAL MYOPATHIES

Exertional myopathy causes cramping, fatigue, and muscle pain in horses and is most often associated with exercise. One common result of exertional myopathy that is especially associated with exercise is necrosis of the striated skeletal muscle. Necrosis of the striated skeletal muscle is also known as exertional rhabdomyolysis. Other terms for exertional rhabdomyolysis are azoturia, cording up, and tying up. Exertional rhabdomyolysis can be divided into two categories: sporadic exertional rhabdomyolysis and chronic rhabdomyolysis.

Sporadic Exertional Rhabdomyolysis

Sporadic exertional rhabdomyolysis occurs most commonly when a horse is asked to perform for long periods of time or perform heavy exercise when it is not in a condition to do so. For example, taking a horse that has been in the pasture all winter and going on an endurance ride for 8 hours could cause sporadic exertional rhabdomyolysis. Deficiencies of vitamin E, selenium, sodium, or calcium can also cause exertional rhabdomyolysis.

Clinical signs associated with exertional rhabdomyolysis include muscle cramping, refusal to move, increased respirations, increased heart rate, and excessive sweating.

When a veterinarian diagnoses a horse with sporadic exertional rhabdomyolysis, the horse usually has increased serum creatine kinase (CK) and aspartate aminotransferase (AST). Obtaining a good history is important because the veterinarian will want to know whether this is the first time such an episode has occurred and what the horse's exercise schedule has been. Horses with sporadic exertional rhabdomyolysis most likely will not have a history of the disease or the clinical signs.

Treatment of exertional rhabdomyolysis typically consists of stall rest. All exercise should cease. The horse should be provided fresh water and a hay diet for a few days following an incident. With severe exertional rhabdomyolysis, the renal system can become compromised by ischemia and by the nephrotoxic effects of *myoglobinuria* and dehydration. It is extremely important to correct the fluid balance in these horses. Use of diuretics is contraindicated in horses not receiving intravenous fluid therapy. Prevention includes feeding a balanced diet and conditioning a horse for the level of exercise it will be asked to perform.

Chronic Exertional Rhabdomyolysis

Polysaccharide storage myopathy (PSSM), recurrent exertional rhabdomyolysis, and hyperkalemic periodic paralysis (HYPP) all are types of exertional rhabdomyolysis in which horses have recurrent episodes, sometimes even during light exercise.

Equine Polysaccharide Storage Myopathy

Equine polysaccharide storage myopathy (EPSM), also known as PSSM, is commonly seen in draft horses, Quarter Horse–related breeds, and warm bloods. The disease is inherited.

Horses often display clinical signs when they are exercised after a few days of rest. Clinical signs include a camped-out stance, sweating, hindlimb stiffness, abnormal gait, and reluctance to move. In draft horses, signs include loss of muscle mass, difficulty backing, difficulty standing when lifting a hindlimb, and progressive weakness.

Veterinarians often diagnose EPSM based on increased CK and AST levels, as well as the clinical signs associated with the disease, but some draft horses have normal CK and AST values. Other tests that may be requested include complete blood count (CBC), urinalysis, exercise testing, blood vitamin C and selenium levels, periodic acid–Schiff staining for glycogen, and muscle biopsy.

Treatment often includes feeding the horse a diet of forage at 1.5% to 2% of its body weight while limiting the horse's starch intake to less than 10% and increasing the fat in the diet to meet the horse's digestible energy requirements. This diet is recommended for most horses because horses with EPSM are more sensitive to insulin, which results in absorption of higher levels of glucose. The horse should gradually be introduced to exercise and turnout.

Recurrent Exertional Rhabdomyolysis

Recurrent exertional rhabdomyolysis is commonly seen in Thoroughbreds, Arabians, and Standardbreds. The disease is most commonly caused by an autosomal dominant trait in Thoroughbreds. In other breeds it is most likely the result of improper regulation of intracellular calcium in the skeletal muscle. Clinical signs include muscle stiffness, sweating, and refusal to move.

Veterinarians often request a CBC, chemistry panel, urinalysis, exercise testing, blood vitamin C and selenium levels, or muscle biopsy to help diagnose the condition.

Treatment of the disease involves trying to reduce anxiety in the horse. Some methods that may be effective include regular exercise, turnout or use of a hot walker, feeding this horse before others, or providing a barn friend (e.g., a goat or another horse). Horses with recurrent exertional rhabdomyolysis often need a higher caloric intake than other horses. Dantrolene or phenytoin has been used for treatment of these horses; however, treatment can be expensive.

Hyperkalemic Periodic Paralysis

Hyperkalemic periodic paralysis (HYPP) is an autosomal dominant trait associated with Quarter Horses, Quarter Crosses, Appaloosas, and American Paints. Horses can be homozygous or heterozygous for the trait. Homozygous horses tend to be identified earlier than heterozygous horses. Most horses are identified as HYPP positive between birth and 3 years of age.

Horses with HYPP may not present with clinical signs; however, those that do present with signs most often display episodes of muscle weakness or twitching. In more severe episodes, the horse may sit like a dog, stagger, have periodic obstruction of the upper respiratory system, or even be recumbent. Most of these horses recover uneventfully.

Horses of impressive descent (e.g., Quarter Horse stallion) would be suspected of having this condition. During the beginning of an HYPP episode, some owners administer light exercise, corn syrup, or grain to induce insulin-mediated movement of potassium across the cell membrane. With severe episodes, calcium gluconate or sodium bicarbonate, or both, may be administered. In the event of period obstruction of the upper respiratory system, a veterinarian may request placement of a tracheostomy tube.

To decrease the incidence of episodes in horses with HYPP, clients should decrease dietary potassium. Some feeds that should be avoided include beet or sugar molasses, alfalfa, brome hay, soybean oil or meal, and canola oil. The following feeds are lower in potassium and may be good choices for horses with HYPP: beet pulp, corn, oats, barley, and late cuts of Bermuda grass or Timothy hay. Commercial diets are available for horses with HYPP. Horses should receive several smaller meals throughout the day. If dietary changes are not successful in regulating HYPP episodes, a veterinarian may choose to administer acetazolamide or hydrochlorothiazide, although clients should be aware that some breed organizations restrict both the use of these drugs during competition and the breeding of horses with HYPP.

HABRONEMIASIS

Cutaneous habronemiasis is also known as summer sores. It is characterized by granulomatous lesions caused by the larvae of *Draschia megastoma, Habronema muscae,* and *Habronema microstoma.* The condition is often seasonal, and this season correlates with fly populations. Infections are common in areas of high heat and humidity. Poor sanitation is another factor contributing to increased incidence. Diagnosis is based on the location and characteristics of the lesions. Time of year and environment also contribute to a diagnosis.

Lesions are commonly located on the glans penis or urethral process. Within these lesions, caseous material composed of eosinophils and larvae is often seen. It is important to differentiate these lesions from sarcoids and squamous cell carcinoma. Confirmatory diagnosis is easily made with histopathologic evaluation (Fig. 11-58).

Treatment of habronemiasis consists of killing the parasites, decreasing inflammation, and treating the secondary bacterial infections. Larvae are eliminated with diethylcarbamazine, organophosphates, and ivermectin.

HERNIA

A hernia is any protrusion of an internal organ through the wall of its containing cavity. Often the intestine passes through an opening in the abdominal wall. Umbilical and scrotal or inguinal hernias are fairly common in young foals (Fig. 11-59; see also Box 11-2). Hernias usually correct themselves; if they do not, surgical treatment is often delayed until the foal is weaned.

HYPOTHYROIDISM

Hypothyroidism is caused by low levels of triiodothyronine (T_3) and thyroxine (T_4). Clinical signs of hypothyroidism include slow shedding or the absence of shedding in the spring, long and rough hair coat, intolerance to cold, depression, weakness, lack of muscle tone, tying up, laminitis, infertility, irregular heat cycles, and lack of milk production. Weight can be a poor indicator of hypothyroidism. Some horses are heavy, easy keeps with a crested neck, whereas others are underweight or are losing weight.

Congenital hypothyroidism can occur in foals. Congenital hypothyroidism is often caused by consumption of a low-iodine diet by the mare during pregnancy or consumption of goitrogens by the mare while grazing during pregnancy. Foals with congenital hypothyroidism often have goiter (Fig. 11-60).

Hypothyroidism in adults can be difficult to diagnose and can be misdiagnosed. Diagnosis is often accomplished with a CBC, serum chemistry panel, and thyroid-stimulating hormone stimulation test. It is important to remember that high-protein diets and some medications can cause low levels of T_3 and T_4.

Treatment of hypothyroidism consists of supplemental T_3 and T_4 through feed additives.

LAMENESS

Lameness is not a disease; it is a clinical sign. Lameness is one of the most common clinical signs that can affect a horse. A horse that is lame fails to travel in a regular and sound manner. The irregular gait can result from a structural or functional disorder of one or more limbs or of the trunk. Most often lameness is associated with pain, but not always. Nervous disorders can cause lameness without pain.

Lameness can be classified in several different ways: weight bearing, non–weight bearing, mixed lameness, and complementary or compensatory. In weight-bearing lameness, the animal tries to decrease the weight being placed on the affected leg by taking shorter steps, leaving the leg

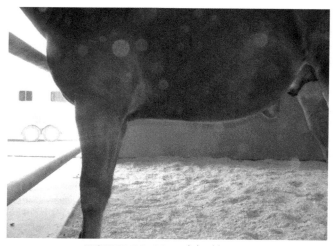

FIGURE 11-59 Umbilical hernia.

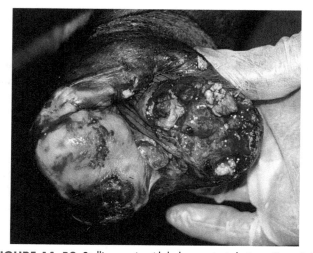

FIGURE 11-58 Stallion penis with habronemiasis lesions. (From Sellon DC, Long MT: *Equine infectious diseases*, ed 2, St. Louis, 2014, Saunders.)

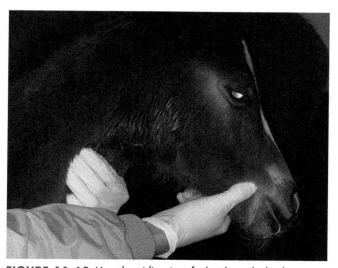

FIGURE 11-60 Hypothyroidism in a foal with marked enlargement of the thyroid gland. (From McAuliffe SB, Slovis NM: *Color atlas of diseases and disorders of the foal*, Oxford, 2008, Saunders.)

on the ground for a shorter period of time, and elevating the body while the animal steps onto the affected limb. Weight-bearing injuries are often associated with injuries to the motor nerves, ligaments, tendons, bones, and feet. Non–weight-bearing lameness is also known as swinging leg disorder. Non–weight-bearing injuries are seen as the animal brings the limb forward; they are often associated with joints, muscles, extensor tendons, bursas, and tendon sheaths. Mixed lameness affects both the weight-bearing phase of the gait and the swinging phase. Complementary or compensatory lameness develops as a compensation for the originally affected limb. For example, if the original injury occurred in the left forelimb, the right forelimb develops complementary lameness from compensation.

Another way to classify lameness is according to a predisposing or inciting cause of lameness. Lameness classified as predisposing indicates that lameness results from a factor that predisposed the horse to lameness. Predisposing causes of lameness include poor shoeing, systemic disease, faulty conformation, poor condition, immaturity, and poor hoof care. Lameness classified as inciting indicates the lameness is the result of trauma. Some causes of inciting lameness include trailer accidents, being kicked by another horse, and incoordination (the horse cross-fires).

In large animals, the most common location for lameness is the forelimb, except in Standardbreds. Young horses show a higher incidence of lameness, especially if they are in extensive training.

Diagnosis of lameness requires a thorough history and examination of the horse at rest and in motion. Sometimes the following tests are indicated when evaluating lameness: local anesthesia (nerve blocks or intraarticular anesthesia), radiographs, ultrasound, bone scintigraphy, magnetic resonance imaging, arthroscopy, synovial fluid analysis, clinical pathologic examination, electromyography, muscle biopsy, gait analysis using high-speed cinematography, and thermography.

Identification of the lame limb can be accomplished by watching the horse in motion. Forelimb identification involves watching the head. When the lame limb is bearing weight, the horse's head will rise. If lameness is bilateral, head position may not indicate the lame limb. The horse will most likely not bear as much weight on the affected limb, and the stride will most likely be shorter. Identification of the lame hind limb involves watching the croup. When the limb that is affected is bearing weight, the croup on the affected side will in general be raised. When both hind limbs are lame, the horse will be reluctant to move, and when it does, the movement will be stiff and restricted, as if the horse had a back injury.

The conditions discussed in the following subsections are common causes of lameness in horses.

Laminitis

Laminitis is inflammation of the sensitive laminae of the foot. Proposed causes of laminitis include endotoxin-induced microthrombosis, alterations in vascular flow to the laminae, vasoconstriction, and activated lamellar enzyme destruction. Predisposing conditions include grazing during certain months of the year, grain overload, inflammatory conditions of the gastrointestinal tract, metritis, retained placenta, endotoxemia, sepsis, pleuropneumonia, Cushing disease, prolonged weight bearing on one limb, and exposure to black walnut wood shavings. Ponies seem to be particularly susceptible to laminitis.

Acute laminitis is subdivided into three categories: subacute, acute, and refractory. Subacute laminitis is a mild form of the disease. Causes include riding on hard surfaces, hooves that are trimmed too short, and exposure to black walnut shavings. Clinical signs often resolve quickly without permanent laminar damage. Rotation of the coffin bone usually does not occur. Acute laminitis is more severe. The disease does not respond as rapidly to treatment, and coffin bone rotation is more likely. Refractory laminitis is a form of acute laminitis that does not respond or responds minimally within 7 to 10 days of treatment. Clinical signs of acute laminitis include increased digital pulses, lifting of the feet every few seconds, lameness, a camped-out stance, and pain.

Chronic laminitis is a continuation of the acute stage. It begins at the first signs of coffin rotation (Figs. 11-61 and 11-62). Chronic laminitis can be divided into three phases: early chronic, chronic active, and chronic stable. Early chronic laminitis begins with rotation of the coffin bone. The rotation may take days to months. The chronic active stage occurs when the coffin bone is rotated but unstable and could penetrate the sole. Rotation of the coffin bone may result in separation of the coronary band over the extensor process region, and serum oozes out through this separation. Seedy toe may develop when the white line separates during laminitis.

Diagnosis of laminitis is based on clinical signs, radiographs, and sometimes local anesthesia.

Treatment of acute laminitis involves trying to prevent chronic laminitis, antiendotoxin therapy, vasodilator therapy, anticoagulant therapy, corrective trimming, and surgical treatment. Laminitis is considered an emergency, and treatment should be started immediately.

Bruised Sole, Corns, and Abscesses

Corns are bruises of the soft tissue underlying the sole of the foot that cause development of a reddish discoloration underneath the affected area. Working on hard surfaces, having flat soles, or stepping on small objects all can cause corns. Most horses recover with rest, but chronic lameness can result when new bone growth has occurred on the distal phalanx. Sometimes bruises develop into abscesses with pockets of pus. Abscesses must rupture to relieve the pressure (Fig. 11-63, *A*). Sometimes abscesses rupture out the coronary band, and at other times they can be encouraged to rupture on the palmar surface of the hoof by soaking the hoof in Epsom salts (Fig. 11-63, *B*). Treatment includes drying the abscess and preventing infection.

Navicular Syndrome

Navicular syndrome is a complex condition with no known cause. The best definition is a syndrome that

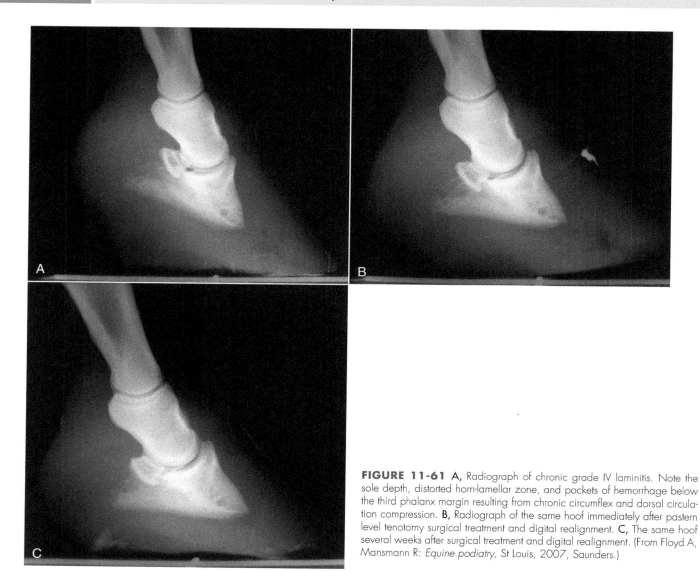

FIGURE 11-61 A, Radiograph of chronic grade IV laminitis. Note the sole depth, distorted horn-lamellar zone, and pockets of hemorrhage below the third phalanx margin resulting from chronic circumflex and dorsal circulation compression. **B,** Radiograph of the same hoof immediately after pastern level tenotomy surgical treatment and digital realignment. **C,** The same hoof several weeks after surgical treatment and digital realignment. (From Floyd A, Mansmann R: *Equine podiatry,* St Louis, 2007, Saunders.)

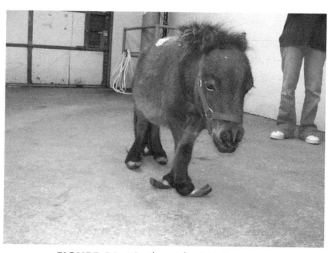

FIGURE 11-62 Chronic laminitis in a pony.

causes clinical signs associated with the navicular region (Fig. 11-64). Predisposing conditions include hard work, small feet, trimming of the heels too low, and upright pasterns. Navicular syndrome causes intermittent lameness in horses that are between 4 and 15 years old. Clinical signs include a short, choppy stride and pointing of the affected toe while standing. Treatment often involves special shoeing, but this is not always effective. When special shoes are not effective, some owners opt to have the navicular nerve cut. However, these horses cannot be used for hard work and can be dangerous to ride because they cannot feel the ground. Some horses that have been "nerved" have remained useful. To determine whether a horse has been nerved, look for ½- to 1-inch scars above the bulbs of the front feet.

Quittor

Quittor is a deep-seated sore that drains at the coronet. It has many causes, primary causes are corns and puncture

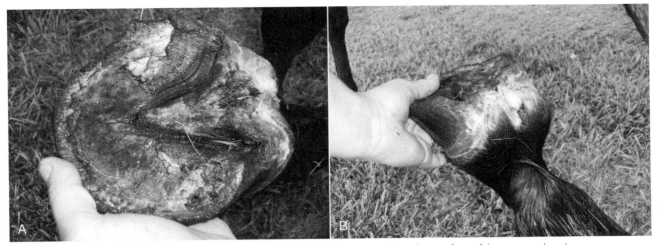

FIGURE 11-63 A, Hoof abscess. B, Rupture of the abscess out the palmar surface of the coronary band.

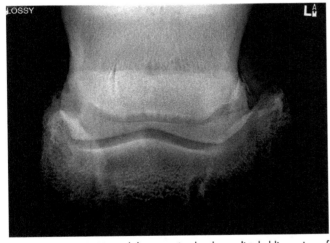

FIGURE 11-64 Normal dorsoproximal-palmarodistal oblique view of navicular bone. (From Floyd A, Mansmann R: *Equine podiatry*, St. Louis, 2007, Saunders.)

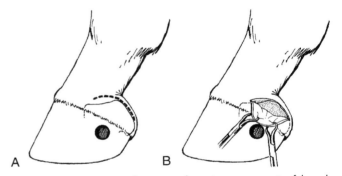

FIGURE 11-65 Surgical treatment for quittor, or necrosis of the collateral cartilage. A and B, A slightly curved incision beginning just dorsal to the coronary band over the diseased collateral cartilage produces a skin flap, which allows removal of the proximal part of the necrotic cartilage. A hole drilled in the hoof wall is required for adequate drainage if infection and necrosis extend distal to the coronary band. (From Auer JA, Stick JA: *Equine surgery*, ed 3, St. Louis, 2006, Saunders.)

wounds. Quittor can also result from chronic inflammation of the collateral cartilage of the distal phalanx (Fig. 11-65).

Sand Cracks, Toe Cracks, Quarter Cracks, and Heel Cracks

Sand cracks are also known as toe cracks and quarter cracks. They are vertical cracks in the hoof wall. Quarter cracks are located in the quarter part of the hoof. Toe cracks are located in the toe region of the hoof (Fig. 11-66). Heel cracks are located in the heel region of the hoof. Cracks result from dryness and brittleness of the hoof, injury to the coronet band, and long hoof walls. Treatment of cracks involves burning a crescent at the tip of the crack or filing a groove across the tip. Corrective shoeing can be performed to treat severe cracks. In addition, commercial sealants can help keep the crack from expanding and contracting during movement. Cracks can be prevented by keeping the hooves moist with hoof dressing and regular trimming.

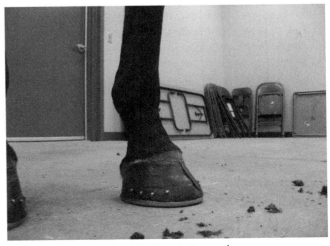

FIGURE 11-66 Toe crack.

Grease Heal

Grease heal is also known as dermatitis verrucosa and scratches. Grease heal is a chronic seborrheic dermatitis of the plantar surface of the fetlock or pastern. It usually is found on the hindlimbs, but it can affect the palmar surface of the fetlock on the forelimb. The lesion is often greasy and foul smelling. Lameness may or may not be present. Grease heal can be prevented by keeping good housing conditions. Horses housed in muddy conditions may develop the condition. Treatment involves clipping the hair of the region, cleaning it with soap and water, and applying an antiseptic. If cellulitis develops, it will require systemic antibiotic therapy and tetanus prophylaxis.

Seedy Toe

Seedy toe is also known as hollow wall or dystrophia ungulae. Seedy toe is a condition of the hoof wall in the toe region. It often occurs secondary to laminitis. The palmar surface of the hoof may look normal on initial examination, but a hollow space is found on dressing. The space can be small, or it can involve the entire palmar surface of the hoof. A mealy substance is present inside. The area should be cleaned and packed with juniper tar and oakum.

Side Bone

Side bones are ossified lateral cartilages located proximal to the rear quarter of the hoof head (Fig. 11-67). Side bones often occur on the forelimbs. They can occur on one or both legs and on either side or both sides of the hoof. The causes are not known but are suggested to include riding on hard surfaces, injury to the cartilage, and poor conformation that increases concussion. The horse may become lame during ossification but usually recovers after the ossification. Treatment often involves rest and administration of NSAIDs.

Bucked Shins

Bucked shins are usually diagnosed in horses that are 2 to 3 years old and are involved in intense training. The temporary unsoundness usually occurs during the first few weeks of training. The unsoundness originates at the dorsal surface of the cannon bone and causes inflammation of the periosteum. The horse often becomes lame and exhibit pains when pressure is applied to the dorsal aspect of the cannon bone. Treatment of bucked shins involves rest for 30 to 60 days. Most horses recover. If the horse fails to recover within 30 to 60 days, fractures should be considered. Prevention of the unsoundness involves gradual increases in exercise.

Splints

Splints comprise abnormal or new bone growth that occurs on the splint bones or cannon. Splints are caused by strain or trauma to the interosseous ligament between the splint bones and cannon. Some splint injuries are the result of conformation faults, such as bench knees. The new growth occurs because of influx of blood supply to the area after the strain or trauma. Splints are common in young horses that are overworked, resulting in excess strain to the medial splint

bones. Clinical signs usually begin as subtle lameness, possibly seen in only one of the horse's gaits. As the unsoundness progresses, the horse may show lameness in more of its gaits, such as walking. This is usually followed by pain and heat at the palmar surface of the cannon. The lameness often subsides, the splint calcifies to the cannon, and a lump develops. At this point, the splint injury is considered more of a blemish than an unsoundness.

Sweeney

Sweeney refers to any group of atrophied muscles, although this definition varies within the equine community. With atrophy of the shoulder muscles, the atrophy is usually associated with damage to the nerve over the shoulder crossing the spinal cord. Sweeney has no known treatment. Some dishonest horse traders have injected irritants into the atrophied area to fill the area with scar tissue and hide the unsoundness.

Shoe Boil or Capped Elbow

Shoe boil is a soft swelling at the elbow caused by irritation. The two common causes are an injury from a long heel on a front shoe or the heel calk of the shoe and an injury from contact with the surface on which the horse is lying. Early treatment is best and often involves applying an irritant such

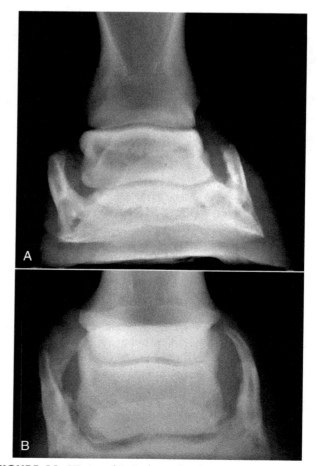

FIGURE 11-67 A and B, Radiographically apparent ossification of the collateral cartilages (side bone). (From Floyd A, Mansmann R: *Equine podiatry*, St. Louis, 2007, Saunders.)

as tincture of iodine daily and using a shoe boil boot or roll. The roll prevents the heel of the foot or shoe from pressing on the elbow while the horse is lying down. Prevention involves never leaving long heels on front shoes.

Bone Spavin

The best description of a bone spavin is distal tarsal osteoarthritis. A bone spavin is a new bone growth on the medial and proximal end of the third metatarsal, third tarsal, and central tarsal bones, leading to arthritis. Bone spavins are caused by faulty conformation, such as sickle hocks, or stress on the hock. Large bone spavins are known as "jack spavins." Clinical signs include pain when the horse flexes the hock, a

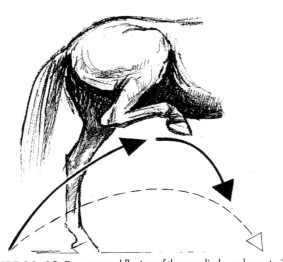

FIGURE 11-68 Exaggerated flexion of the rear limb, a characteristic sign in horses with stringhalt. (From Auer JA, Stick JA: *Equine surgery,* ed 3, St. Louis, 2006, Saunders.)

tendency to roll the hip during movement, and dragging the toe. Treatment involves surgical intervention, but full recovery is not always possible.

Curb

Curb is a fullness of the plantar surface distal to the hock that is caused by an enlarged plantar ligament. Anything that increases ligament stress can cause curb, which thickens the ligament. Poor conformation, such as sickle hocks and cow hocks, predispose a horse to curb. Hard stops or long sliding stops can cause curb.

Stringhalt

Stringhalt is an involuntary flexion of the hock during forward movement (Figs. 11-68 and 11-69). It may affect one or both of the hindlimbs. The true cause is unknown, but nerves are thought to degenerate, causing the problem. Some horses show jerking of the leg toward the abdomen with movement. The signs are usually exaggerated while the horse is turning and after the horse has had a rest. Treatment involves surgical intervention to remove part of the tendon of the lateral digital extensor. If stringhalt is untreated, the horse will often worsen with age. Most cases show improvement after surgical treatment.

Ringbone

Ringbone is new bone growth that occurs on the proximal, middle, or distal phalanx (Fig. 11-70). Ringbone most commonly occurs on the forelimbs, but it can occur on the hindlimbs. Horses may develop ringbone for several reasons, including poor conformation (horses that are toed in or toed out or have straight pasterns), heavy work sustained over the years, excessive pulling on the ligaments of the pastern joints

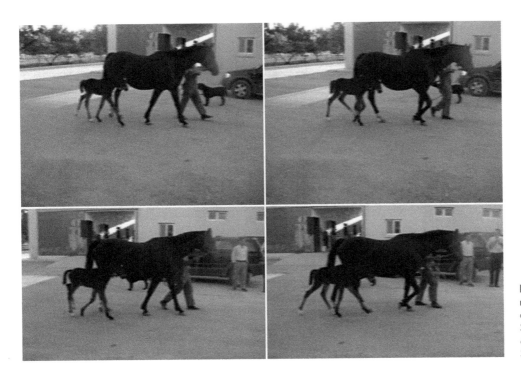

FIGURE 11-69 Stringhalt in a neonatal foal. Note the exaggerated lifting of the hind leg. (From McAuliffe SB, Slovis NM: *Color atlas of diseases and disorders of the foal,* Oxford, 2008, Saunders.)

or coffin bones, or constant work on hard surfaces. Any of these conditions can result in disruption of the periosteum, which causes new bone growth on either side of the bone or all the way around the bone.

Ringbone can be classified in two ways: by its location on the bone or by the joints involved. High ringbone appears on distal end of the first phalanx and/or the proximal end of the second phalanx. Low ringbone occurs on the distal end of the second phalanx and/or the upper end of the third phalanx. Articular ringbone involves the joint surface of the pastern or coffin joints. Periarticular ringbone occurs around the joint but does not involve the joint surface. Clinical signs vary, depending on the location and joint involvement. Some ringbone may go unnoticed; however, articular ringbone always causes lameness.

Sesamoiditis

Sesamoiditis is inflammation of the proximal sesamoid bones. The horse does not extend the fetlock to a normal level. On palpation, the fetlock shows inflammation, and the horse often flinches in pain. In chronic cases, the horse undergoes periosteum damage, and new bone growth occurs.

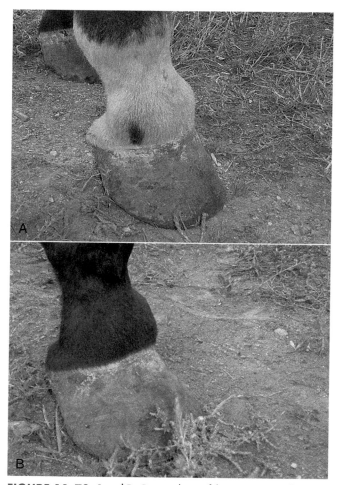

FIGURE 11-70 A and **B,** Osteoarthritis of the pastern or coffin joints is called ringbone. (From Bertone JJ: *Equine geriatric medicine and surgery,* St. Louis, 2006, Saunders.)

Osselets

Osselets involve inflammation around the fetlock joint. They are the result of strain or concussion on immature bones. Upright pasterns are a predisposing factor. On palpation, the inflamed area feels like putty as a result of hemorrhage and fluid that collects beneath the periosteum, and the area may be warm. The horse usually moves with a short, choppy stride indicative of pain in the fetlock joint. Osselets usually affect horses for years because the condition is arthritic.

Windpuffs

Windpuffs are also known as wind galls or "puffs." Windpuffs involve enlargement of the fluid sacs located immediately around the pastern or fetlock joints. Windpuffs can occur on the forelimbs or hindlimbs. Windpuffs are usually caused by hard work or by hard work on hard surfaces. Windpuffs are often treated with cold packs over the "puff" and a liniment applied to the area; however, the puff reappears when the horse is exercised. Windpuffs are not serious, and treatment does not result in permanent benefits. These lesions indicate only that the horse has been worked hard at some point in its life.

Bog Spavin

Bog spavin is a filling of the natural depression of the dorsal surface of the hock, a chronic distention of the joint capsule. Usually, two smaller swellings are located on the plantar surface of the hock. The swellings are lower than the swelling associated with a thoroughpin. A bog spavin is smaller than a blood spavin. Bog spavins are caused by faulty conformation. When horses are too straight in the hock joint, the joint suffers from concussion and trauma. Other horses may develop bog spavins from trauma, such as from quick stops and quick turns.

Carpal Hygroma

Carpal hygroma, also known as "popped knees," is traumatic bursitis of the carpus. It is an inflammatory condition of the knee. Carpal hygroma is usually characterized by sudden onset and is caused by a sprain or strain on the ligaments that hold the carpal bones of the knee in place. It can also be caused by damage to the joint capsule. After the initial injury, fluid often fills the area. Trauma can cause carpal hygroma. Poor conformation can predispose a horse to the condition. Popped knees should not be confused with a hygroma, which is a fluid-filled swelling over the front surface of the knee caused by trauma. The fluid is not located within the joint capsule.

Capped Hock

Capped hock is traumatic bursitis of the hock. Capped hock is an enlargement at the point of the hock that is caused by bruising when the horse kicks a hard surface. The condition is a cosmetic concern but has few limiting capabilities. During early treatment, tinctures of iodine can be applied to reduce the size. Capped hock will not subside if the area undergoes continued agitation.

Bowed Tendon

Bowed tendons are the result of severe strain on the superficial flexor tendon or deep flexor tendon, or both. The tendon sheath separates from the tendon, and this separation causes hemorrhage inside the tendon sheath. In some cases, the tendon itself undergoes some tearing. Bowed tendons usually occur in fatigued horses asked to distribute their weight onto one leg at high speeds. Most bowed tendons occur on forelimbs, but injuries to the hindlimbs can occur.

One indication that a horse has a bowed tendon is a thickened palmar surface of the cannon. Most horses can recover but are unable to perform heavy work without reinjuring the tendon.

Thoroughpin

Tenosynovitis of the tarsal sheath is also called thoroughpin. Thoroughpin is a soft, puffy area of the hock caused by trauma or tendon strain. Excess synovial fluid forms and accumulates in the tarsal synovial sheath. When pressed, the soft area moves to the opposite side of the leg. Treatment involves pressure and massage of the area, but it is not always effective.

Patellar Luxation

Patellar luxation is also known as stifle. Patellar luxation occurs when the stifle is displaced. The patella usually moves upward and to the inside, but it can be placed back in normal position. Young horses can recover with age, but older horses tend to remain unsound.

Physitis

Physitis is also referred to as epiphysitis. It is a disease characterized by enlargement of the growth plates of certain long bones. The disease affects young, rapidly growing foals; the highest incidence of the disease occurs in foals that are between 4 and 8 months old. The cause is unknown. Clinical signs most often include enlargement of the distal radius, tibia, and third metacarpal and third metatarsal bones. Treatment often consists of changing the foal's ration, limiting exercise, and administering NSAIDs.

Subchondral Cystic Lesions

Subchondral cystic lesions are also known as bone cysts or osseous cystlike lesions. Subchondral cystic lesions can be articular or nonarticular. They do not always produce lameness and can go unnoticed. Normal bone remodeling may resolve the defect. Most horses that develop subchondral cystic lesions are less than 3 years old. The most common sites include the stifle, pastern, coffin, elbow, and pastern joints. Treatment involves intraarticular medication or surgical débridement.

MELANOMAS

Melanomas are benign growths that occur on the tail and anus and on the head of gray horses (Figs. 11-71 and 11-72). These growths are rare in horses 6 to 7 years old but occur in approximately 80% of gray horses that are more than 15 years old. Melanomas start out the size of BB shot and gradually increase in size. Some can be surgically removed. They can become malignant and invade vital organs, thus causing death. The major problem is the interference with tack that these growths may cause.

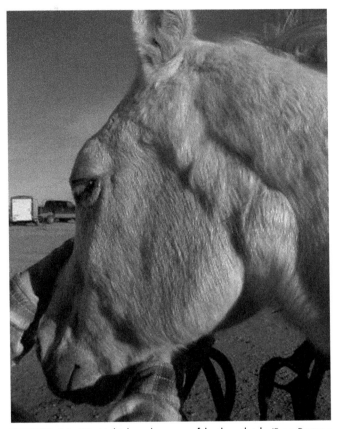

FIGURE 11-71 Multiple melanomas of the throatlatch. (From Bertone JJ: *Equine geriatric medicine and surgery*, St. Louis, 2006, Saunders.)

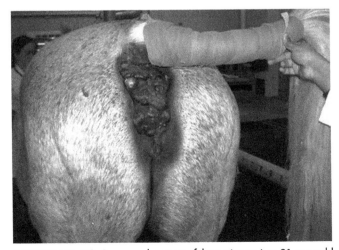

FIGURE 11-72 Severe melanomas of the perineum in a 21-year-old mare. (From Robinson NE: *Current therapy in equine medicine*, ed 6, St. Louis, 2009, Saunders.)

RECURRENT UVEITIS

Recurrent uveitis is also known as equine recurrent uveitis, periodic ophthalmia, recurrent iridocyclitis, and moon blindness. Recurrent uveitis can lead to blindness in horses through recurrent inflammation of the uveal tact (iris, ciliary body, choroid) in one or both eyes. Causes of moon blindness include bacterial or viral infections, parasites, and trauma. Leptospirosis is the most common implicated infectious disease. The *Onchocerca cervicalis* microfilaria is the most common implicated parasite. Appaloosas may be predisposed to the condition, and Standardbreds may have a reduced risk.

Clinical signs include blepharospasm, conjunctival and ciliary injection, lacrimation, vascularization, hypopyon or hyphema, swollen dull iris, vitreal inflammation, hypotonia, photophobia, peripheral corneal edema, aqueous flare, miosis, and retinal vasculitis or peripapillary inflammation (Fig. 11-73). Secondary conditions that may result from uveitis include anterior and posterior synechiae, lens luxation, pigment changes in the iris, peripapillary retinal scars, retinal detachments, vitreal debris, and cataracts. The most common causes of blindness from secondary conditions are cataracts and pupillary seclusion. Uveitis is the most common cause of cataracts in horses.

Diagnosis is often made from clinical signs. Diagnosing the cause may be more difficult and should include serum for leptospiral titration and any other organism suspected by the veterinarian. If *O. cervicalis* is suspected because of conjunctival granulomas or keratoconjunctivitis at the temporal quadrant of the cornea, conjunctival biopsies or wet mounts may be indicated.

Inflammation must be reduced quickly to prevent secondary conditions. Topical and systemic antiinflammatory therapy is usually prescribed. Most often the use of topical corticosteroids is indicated because other types of antiinflammatory agents do not effectively reduce inflammation in the uveal tract. Sometimes systemic antibiotics are indicated, depending on the cause of the uveitis and the presence of a fever. Horses with cataracts caused by uveitis are poor candidates for surgical treatment. Prognosis is variable, and prevention should include vaccination for *Leptospira pomona*.

ROARING/LARYNGEAL HEMIPLEGIA

Animals that whistle or wheeze when respiration is increased, such as during exercise, are known as "roarers." The noise is often associated with inspiration, not expiration. It can be caused by broken rings in the trachea or, as in most cases, paralysis of the muscles that control vocal cord tension. Approximately 90% of cases can be surgically corrected (Fig. 11-74).

WOBBLER SYNDROME

A wobbler is a horse with a condition of the spinal cord that affects the horse's coordination. A true wobbler has compression of the spinal cord in the neck region. Most wobblers are identified between birth and 4 years of age. Most often the incoordination begins in the hindlimbs and progressively becomes worse. The condition can be so severe that the horse actually falls down when asked to change direction. These horses are unsafe to ride, and true wobblers will not

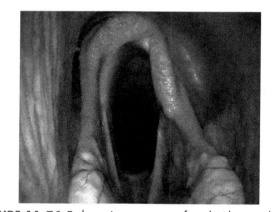

FIGURE 11-74 Endoscopic appearance of grade 4 laryngeal hemiplegia. (From Auer JA, Stick JA: *Equine surgery*, ed 3, St. Louis, 2006, Saunders.)

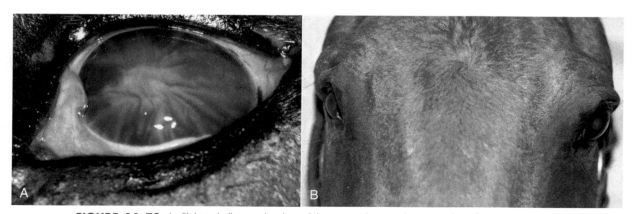

FIGURE 11-73 A, Phthisis bulbi, or shrunken globe, secondary to chronic ocular inflammation associated with equine recurrent uveitis. **B,** Phthisis bulbi of the horse's right eye, front view. (**A,** Courtesy Dr. Stacy Andrew; **B,** Courtesy Dr. David Wilkie. From Gilger B: *Equine ophthalmology*, St. Louis, 2005, Saunders.)

improve. The condition may be genetic. These horses should not be used for breeding. Some wobblers are candidates for surgical correction. Equine degenerative myeloencephalopathy is a degenerative disease of the nervous system that can cause wobbling symptoms. The condition is linked to deficiencies of vitamin E during rapid growth phases.

SARCOIDS

Sarcoids are cutaneous tumors of fibroblastic origin. Sarcoids have been linked to exposure of bovine papillomavirus (BPV) type 1 and, less commonly, type 2. Although this link is unclear, it has been made. The tumors can develop anywhere on the body, and the appearance varies with the type of sarcoid. Six types are recognized. Sarcoids on the distal limbs and periorbital region have the worst prognosis.

Diagnosis of sarcoids includes histopathologic examination. Many treatment options are available, with variable success. Surgical excision is an option, but recurrence is likely. Imiquimod, chemotherapy, and irradiation have all been attempted.

TOXINS

Equine toxicities are listed in Table 11-2.

PARASITES

Major equine parasites are described and shown in Table 11-3.

PROBLEMS SPECIFIC TO FOALS

Issues specific to foals include persistent patent urachus (Box 11-1), umbilical hernia (Box 11-2), neonatal bacterial septicemia (Box 11-3), prematurity (Box 11-4), and neonatal maladjustment syndrome (Box 11-5).

TABLE 11-2	Common Equine Toxins		
TOXICITY OR AGENT	**SCIENTIFIC NAME**	**TOXIN**	**SYMPTOMS**
Ionophore toxicity	Ionophores	Ionophore	Neurologic, musculoskeletal, cardiac, or smooth muscle abnormalities
Yew poisoning	*Taxus brevifolia*, multiple others	Taxine alkaloids	Conduction disturbances of the heart
Poison hemlock	*Conium maculatum*	Piperidine alkaloids	Muscular weakness, trembling, ataxia, slobbering, tachycardia, dilated pupils, polyuria and polydypsia
Red maple leaf	*Acer rubrum*	Unknown	Nonspecific depression and anorexia. Rarely peracute death from severe methemoglobinemia and tissue anorexia
Oleander toxicosis	*Nerium oleander*	Cardiac glycosides	Death, colic
Blister beetles	*Epicauta*; others of the family Meloidae	Bicyclic terpenoid vesicant	Colic
Bracken fern	*Pteridium aquilinum*	Ptaquiloside	Acute onset of fever, lethargy, loss of appetite, and hemorrhage
Yellow star thistle	*Centaurea solstitialis*	Neurotoxin	Neurological
Tansy ragwort	*Senecio jacobaea*	Pyrrolizidine alkaloid	Acute liver failure, anorexia, depression, icterus, visceral edema, ascites

TABLE 11-3	Equine Parasites			
COMMON NAME/ ILLUSTRATION*	**SCIENTIFIC NAME**	**IMPORTANCE**	**DIAGNOSIS**	**COMMON TREATMENTS**
Large Strongyle 	*Strongylus vulgaris*	Larval migration can result in blockage of intestinal circulation leading to death; adults can cause anemia	Eggs in fecal flotation or identification using Baermann apparatus	Ivermectin, moxidectin, fenbendazole

Continued

TABLE 11-3	Equine Parasites—cont'd			
COMMON NAME/ ILLUSTRATION*	**SCIENTIFIC NAME**	**IMPORTANCE**	**DIAGNOSIS**	**COMMON TREATMENTS**
Small Strongyle 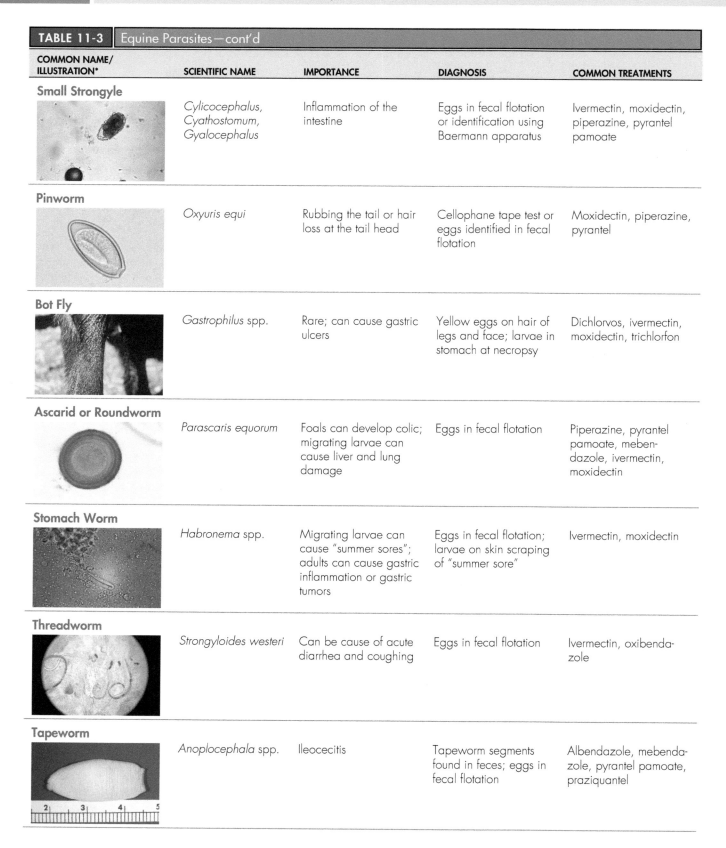	Cylicocephalus, Cyathostomum, Gyalocephalus	Inflammation of the intestine	Eggs in fecal flotation or identification using Baermann apparatus	Ivermectin, moxidectin, piperazine, pyrantel pamoate
Pinworm	Oxyuris equi	Rubbing the tail or hair loss at the tail head	Cellophane tape test or eggs identified in fecal flotation	Moxidectin, piperazine, pyrantel
Bot Fly	Gastrophilus spp.	Rare; can cause gastric ulcers	Yellow eggs on hair of legs and face; larvae in stomach at necropsy	Dichlorvos, ivermectin, moxidectin, trichlorfon
Ascarid or Roundworm	Parascaris equorum	Foals can develop colic; migrating larvae can cause liver and lung damage	Eggs in fecal flotation	Piperazine, pyrantel pamoate, mebendazole, ivermectin, moxidectin
Stomach Worm	Habronema spp.	Migrating larvae can cause "summer sores"; adults can cause gastric inflammation or gastric tumors	Eggs in fecal flotation; larvae on skin scraping of "summer sore"	Ivermectin, moxidectin
Threadworm	Strongyloides westeri	Can be cause of acute diarrhea and coughing	Eggs in fecal flotation	Ivermectin, oxibendazole
Tapeworm	Anoplocephala spp.	Ileocecitis	Tapeworm segments found in feces; eggs in fecal flotation	Albendazole, mebendazole, pyrantel pamoate, praziquantel

TABLE 11-3	Equine Parasites—cont'd			
COMMON NAME/ ILLUSTRATION*	**SCIENTIFIC NAME**	**IMPORTANCE**	**DIAGNOSIS**	**COMMON TREATMENTS**
Apicomplexa 	*Babesia* spp.	Fever, anemia, spleno-megaly, icterus	Blood smear evaluation	Phenamidine
Lice 	*Bovicola* spp. (biting louse) *Haematopinus asini* (sucking louse) *Microthoracius* spp. (sucking louse)			Sprays, dusts, oral, injectable, pour-on
Flies A B	*Musca domestica* (house fly) *Musca autumnalis* (face fly) *Siphona (Haemato-bia)* (horn fly) *Stomoxys calcitrans* (stable fly) *Tabanus* and *Chrys-ops* spp. (horse fly/ deer fly) Mosquitoes *Hypoderma* spp. (cattle grubs)			Sprays, dusts, oral, injectable, pour-on
Mites 	*Sarcoptes scabiei* (dry mange) *Psoroptes equi* (scale and wet mange) *Chorioptes bovis* (tail and hock mange) *Demodex* spp. (nodu-lar mange)			Sprays, dusts, oral, injectable, pour-on
Ticks 				Sprays, dusts, oral, injectable, pour-on

*Illustrations from Hendrix CM, Robinson E: *Diagnostic parasitology for veterinary technicians*, ed 4, St. Louis, 2012, Mosby.

BOX 11-1	Persistent Patent Urachus

Common Complaint

The foal appears to dribble or stream urine from the umbilicus. It may urinate from the urethra at the same time, thus producing two separate streams of urine. The umbilical area is constantly moist.

Etiology

Patent urachus. The urachus is usually patent at birth and closes naturally within 48 hours as the umbilical stump withers and dries.

When It Is a Problem

If urine passes through the umbilicus after 48 hours of age, this is referred to as a persistent patent urachus. A veterinarian should be consulted.

Treatment

- Keep the umbilicus clean and dry. Continue application of antiseptics.
- Monitor rectal temperature two to three times daily.
- Prophylactic antibiotics may be prescribed.
- Assist closure of the urachus. Usually chemical cautery is tried first, using silver nitrate, tincture of iodine, phenol, or other cauterizing agent.
- If the foal does not respond after several days of treatment or if signs of local or systemic infection are seen, surgical resection of the umbilicus with ligation of the urachus may be recommended.

BOX 11-2	Umbilical Hernia

Clinical Signs

Soft, fluctuant swelling at the umbilicus. Rarely, the swelling appears to change size, depending on the contents of the hernia, which may shift in and out of the hernia sac. A hard, firm swelling may indicate strangulation of the hernia contents.

Etiology

The natural opening in the abdominal wall for the umbilical cord should close down after birth as the umbilical cord atrophies. If the opening fails to close completely, a defect up to 3 to 4 inches long may remain. Segments of bowel or omentum may slide through this "hole" and come to rest beneath the skin but outside the body wall. The presence of these contents outside the body wall is referred to as an *umbilical hernia*. The abnormal contents may slip back into the abdomen, only to reappear later. This cycle may continue for months, perhaps years in some cases. Umbilical hernias are always palpable and are usually visible, especially when intestine or omentum is located within the hernia sac.

When It Is a Problem

- Occasionally, the contents become strangulated in the hernia sac (strangulating hernia); this is an emergency situation. Strangulating hernias are recognized by colic and usually increasing size and firmness of the hernia as the strangulated tissues swell.
- Some owners may find the visual appearance of a nonstrangulating hernia to be an unacceptable cosmetic problem.

Treatment

- Treatment depends on the size of the hernia ring, the presence or likelihood of strangulation, the age of the foal, and the ability of the owner to monitor the foal closely. Many small hernia rings (<2 inches) close spontaneously if abnormal contents are kept out of the ring. Hernia rings less than 1 inch in diameter have the best chance for spontaneous closure. Experienced horse owners can be instructed on how to reduce the hernia and monitor the foal for signs of bowel entrapment. Closure may continue until 6 to 12 months of age, after which complete closure is unlikely.
- Historically, hernia clamps have been used to "treat" umbilical hernias. After the contents are reduced, the clamp is placed over the hernia sac like a large "chip clip," causing strangulation necrosis of the skin and underlying hernia sac. The clamp falls off in 2 to 3 weeks. However, whether this method produces true closure of the abdominal wall defect is questionable, and risk of infection from the necrosis exists. Hernia clamps may improve the cosmetic appearance of small hernias. Generally, they are not commonly used.
- Surgical closure (umbilical herniorrhaphy) is intended for cases of confirmed strangulation, cases where strangulation is likely, cases where the owner does not want to risk strangulation, cases with large (>2 inches) hernia rings, or cases where the cosmetic appearance is objectionable to the owner.

Comments

- Umbilical hernias are the second most common congenital defect in horses. Some veterinarians believe that individual horses have a genetic predisposition to the condition and advise against breeding these animals.
- Predicting whether a hernia will lead to strangulation and, if so, when, is impossible. Client education can be challenging!

BOX 11-3 | Neonatal Bacterial Septicemia ("Septic Foal")

Significance

Neonatal bacterial septicemia is the most common cause of morbidity and mortality in foals from birth to 7 days of age. The mortality rate is approximately 75%. Failure of passive transfer of antibodies is the leading risk factor for the development of septicemia.

Etiology

Neonatal bacterial septicemia is caused by blood-borne bacteria and their toxins. It usually is caused by one species of bacteria, but mixed infections are possible. The foal may acquire the infection before birth (through uterine infections or by transmission through the placenta) or after birth (through the respiratory system, gastrointestinal [GI] system, umbilicus, or wounds). Gram-negative bacteria, especially *Escherichia coli*, are most often cultured. *Streptococcus* and *Staphylococcus* are also possible. Anaerobes may also contribute to mixed infections.

Clinical Signs

Clinical signs depend entirely on where in the body the bacteria establish infection. Clinical signs may range from one location/body system to multiple locations and body systems. Septicemic shock and death are not uncommon.

Early Clinical Signs (Often Vague)

- Weakness, lethargy
- Decreased appetite, decreased suckling strength
- Dehydration (sunken eyes, entropion, capillary refill time > 2 seconds)
- Increased time spent in recumbency (naps)
- Febrile (temperature > 102° F), elevated heart rate

Later Clinical Signs

- Febrile (temperature > 102.0° F) or possibly hypothermic (<99.0° F) if in shock; may briefly have a normal temperature as body temperature passes from fever to hypothermia with developing shock
- Elevated heart rate, weak pulses
- Elevated respiratory rate
- Abnormal mucous membrane color: pale, brick red, or cyanotic; petechiae may be seen if disseminated intravascular coagulation develops
- Specific organ system signs depending on localization of bacteria; joints, bones, lungs, central nervous system, GI organs, and kidneys may be affected in any combination

Diagnosis

Diagnosis is made by blood culture. Submit at least 10 mL of blood, collected aseptically. Both aerobic and anaerobic cultures should be submitted (minimum 5 mL in each culture medium).

Treatment

- Specific therapy is provided by systemic antibiotics on the basis of blood culture results. Most affected foals have inadequate antibody levels, which must be supplemented by transfusion of plasma or plasma substitutes.
- The risk of GI ulcers is extremely high; antiulcer medication is routinely given. Nutritional support is also often necessary.
- Other treatment depends on the individual case. Laboratory analysis of blood and other body fluids, radiographs, and diagnostic ultrasound are used to identify problems and guide treatment. Every case is different.

BOX 11-4 | Premature Foals

Definition

Equine gestation averages 330 to 345 days. Prematurity is usually defined as delivery before gestational age of 320 days; however, the presence of clinical signs may occur at gestational ages older than 320 days. These cases are properly referred to as *dysmature*.

Clinical Signs

- Small size and body weight
- Generalized weakness
- Delayed time to stand
- Poor suckling reflex
- Silky hair coat
- Floppy ears
- Prominent forehead (normal in miniature horses)
- Hyperextension of fetlocks (flexural limb deformity)

Clinical Significance

Premature foals are at high risk for respiratory, metabolic, musculoskeletal, and infectious problems.

Treatment

No specific therapy exists. Provide nursing care as needed for the foal's individual problems. Closely monitor foals (temperature, pulse, and respiration and physical examination) and provide a clean, dry, warm environment. Adequate antibody levels should be confirmed with a blood test and treated if deficiency is found.

BOX 11-5 | Asphyxia (Neonatal Maladjustment Syndrome, "Dummy" Foals)

Common Complaint

These foals are usually born without apparent difficulty and act normally for the first hours of life. However, by 24 hours, they appear to lose the suckling reflex and affinity for the mare. They may wander aimlessly, appear blind, become recumbent, and possibly have seizures.

Etiology

The cause of peripartum asphyxia syndrome is not yet confirmed, but it is believed to be a derangement in cerebral blood circulation and blood pressure, combined with low oxygen levels, during birth. Histopathologic examination shows cerebral edema and hemorrhages.

Clinical Signs

Clinical signs are primarily neurologic and develop after birth. Because infection is not part of the syndrome, temperature, pulse, and respiration and complete blood count are usually normal. If the foal is febrile, a separate infectious process (e.g., septicemia) should be suspected in addition to peripartum asphyxia syndrome.

Treatment

No specific therapy exists; provide supportive care as needed. A high level of supportive care may be necessary for recumbent foals. If the disorder is not complicated by infectious processes, at least 50% of foals recover with proper supportive care, and recovery is usually complete.

CASE STUDY

A 3-month-old foal arrives at your clinic with abscessation of the throatlatch. Where should you keep the foal until Dr. Kruger can diagnose the condition? Why would you want to limit the contact this foal has with other horses at your clinic? What equipment will you want to prepare for treatment if *Streptococcus equi* infection is confirmed?

CASE STUDY

A 13-year-old Percheron arrives at the clinic for gastrointestinal upset. Dr. Fitzwater is running late, so you decide to groom the horse to improve the client's perception of your clinic. On grooming the front legs, you find yellow specks randomly distributed over the legs. Should you tell the veterinarian about your findings? Could your finding possibly be related to the horse's gastrointestinal upset?

SUGGESTED READING

Auer JA, Stick JA: *Equine surgery*, ed 3, St. Louis, 2006, Saunders.

Bertone J: *Equine geriatric medicine and surgery*, St. Louis, 2006, Saunders.

Evans JW: *Horses*, ed 3, College Station, Tex, 2005, Owl Books.

Floyd A, Mansmann R: *Equine podiatry*, St. Louis, 2007, Saunders.

Foreyt WJ: *Veterinary parasitology reference manual*, ed 5, Ames, Iowa, 2007, Iowa State Press.

Gilger B: *Equine ophthalmology*, ed 2, St. Louis, 2011, Saunders.

Hendrix CM, Robinson E: *Diagnostic parasitology for veterinary technicians*, ed 3, St. Louis, 2006, Mosby.

Kahn CM, Line S: *The Merck veterinary manual*, ed 10, Whitehouse Stanton, NJ, 2010, Merck & Co.

McAuliffe SB, Slovis NM: *Color atlas of diseases and disorders of the foal*, Oxford, 2008, Saunders.

Robinson NE: *Current therapy in equine medicine*, ed 6, St. Louis, 2008, Saunders.

Sellon DC, Long MT: *Equine infectious diseases*, St. Louis, 2007, Saunders.

Stashak TS: *Adams' lameness in horses*, ed 5, Baltimore, 2002, Lippincott Williams & Wilkins.

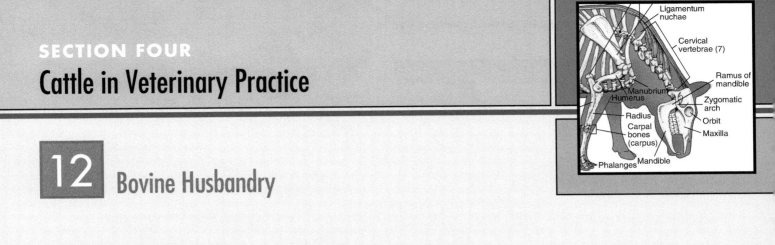

Ligamentum nuchae
Cervical vertebrae (7)
Ramus of mandible
Manubrium
Humerus
Zygomatic arch
Radius
Orbit
Carpal bones (carpus)
Maxilla
Phalanges Mandible

12 Bovine Husbandry

OUTLINE

LEARNING OBJECTIVES

When you have completed this chapter you will be able to

- Know and understand the zoologic classification of the species
- Know and be able to proficiently use terminology associated with this species
- Know normal physiologic data for the species and be able to identify abnormal data
- Identify and know the uses of common instruments relevant to the species
- Describe prominent anatomical or physiologic properties of the species
- Identify and describe characteristics of common breeds
- Describe normal living environments and husbandry needs of the species
- Understand and describe specific reproductive practices of the species
- Understand specific nutritional requirements of the species

KEY TERMS

Atresia ani
Atresia coli
Atresia recti
Bull
Bull calf
Calf
Calving
Challenge feeding

Cow
Creep feeding
Dental pad
Heifer
Heifer calf
Horned
Marbling
Milk fat

Omphalophlebitis
Patent urachus
Polled
Steer
Superovulation
Synchronized
Umbilical hernia

ZOOLOGIC CLASSIFICATION

Kingdom	Animal
Phylum	Chordata
Class	Mammalia
Order	Artiodactyla
Family	Bovidae
Genus	*Bos*
Species	*Taurus*
	Indicus

TERMINOLOGY AND PHYSIOLOGIC DATA

Box 12-1 lists common terminology used to describe the age and breeding status of cattle. Table 12-1 lists normal physiologic data for cattle.

COMMON BOVINE INSTRUMENTS

Visit the Evolve website for pictures and descriptions of common bovine instruments.

BOX 12-1	Cattle Terminology
Cow	Mature female
Bull	Mature male
Steer	Castrated male
Heifer	Immature female
Calf	Neonate
Heifer calf	Neonate female <1 year of age; can be called first, second, third, or fourth calf heifer
Bull calf	Neonate male <1 year of age
Calving	Act of parturition

TABLE 12-1	Normal Physiologic Data for Cattle
Temperature	100° F–102.5° F
Pulse rate	40–80/min
Respiratory rate	10–30 breaths/min
Adult weight	Varies by breed

ANATOMICAL TERMS

Figures 12-1, 12-2, and 12-3 will help you review the terms for body parts and areas of cattle, as well as the names of bones and joints.

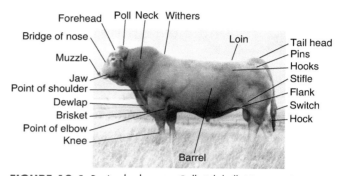

FIGURE 12-1 Bovine body parts: Gelbvieh bull. (Courtesy American Gelbvieh Association, Westminster, Colo.)

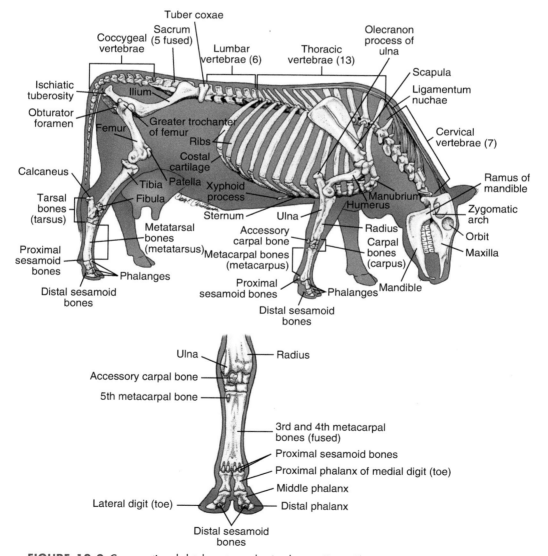

FIGURE 12-2 Comparative skeletal anatomy: bovine bones. (From Christenson DE: *Veterinary medical terminology*, ed 2, St. Louis, 2008, Saunders.)

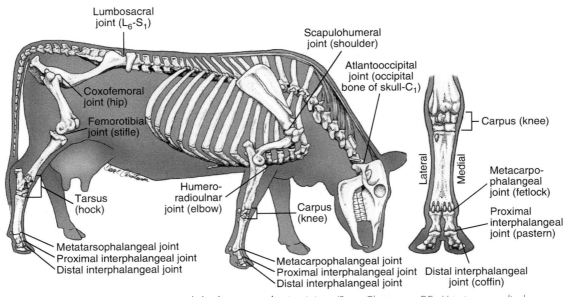

FIGURE 12-3 Comparative skeletal anatomy: bovine joints. (From Christenson DE: *Veterinary medical terminology*, ed 2, St. Louis, 2008, Saunders.)

BREEDS OF CATTLE

COMMON BREEDS OF BEEF CATTLE

American Salers
Color: Dark mahogany red
Average cow weight: 1200 to 1500 pounds
Breed association: American Salers Association
Website: http://www.salersusa.org/

The Salers ("Sa-Lair") breed of cattle is native to the Auvergne region of south central France. The Salers is a *horned* breed. Salers cattle are a dark mahogany red. One strain of Salers is naturally *polled,* and some strains are black. Salers *cows* are noted for their ease of calving and their good maternal ability. Other desirable characteristics of Salers cattle include good foraging ability on poor range, high weaning weights, and excellent carcass quality that meets current market demand for beef. American Salers cattle can be registered with the American Salers Association (Fig. 12-4).

Angus
Color: Black
Average cow weight: 1200 to 1600 pounds
Breed association: American Angus Association
Website: http://www.angus.org/

The official name of the Angus breed is the Aberdeen-Angus. The breed originated in Scotland in the shires of Aberdeen and Angus. Angus cattle are black. They have a smooth hair coat and are polled. They are an alert and vigorous breed. Angus cattle perform well in the feedlot. They produce a desirable carcass of high-quality meat with extensive *marbling.* Nearly all Angus cattle are pure for the dominant polled gene. When the Angus is used in crossbreeding programs, nearly all the

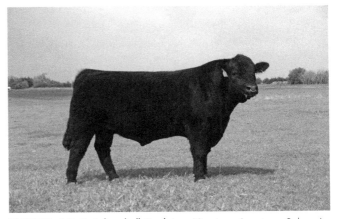

FIGURE 12-4 Salers bull Predator. (Courtesy American Salers Association.Parker, Colo.)

calves are polled. A few Angus cattle carry a red recessive gene for red color. Sometimes, a red *calf* is born to black parents. The red calf is not eligible for registry in the American Angus Association. Angus cattle crossbred to Hereford cattle will produce what is known as a black baldy, which is a black calf with a white face. Another possible coloration is a black brockle-faced calf, which is a black calf with a white face, but the face has a black pattern throughout it (Fig. 12-5).

TECHNICIAN NOTE Registered purebred Angus cattle are black.

Beefmaster
Color: Varies
Average cow weight: 1300 to 1500 pounds
Breed association: Beefmaster Breeders United
Website: http://www.beefmasters.org/

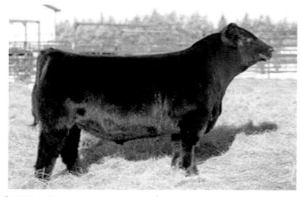

FIGURE 12-5 Angus. (Courtesy of Dennis Garwood. Atkinson, Nebr.)

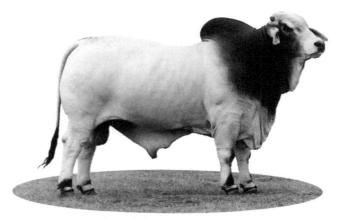

FIGURE 12-7 Brahman bull. (Courtesy Australian Brahman Breeders' Association Limited. Rockhampton, Queensland, Australia.)

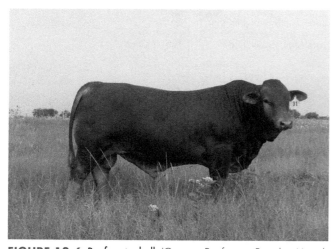

FIGURE 12-6 Beefmaster bull. (Courtesy Beefmaster Breeders United. San Antonio, Tex.)

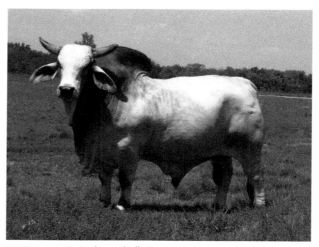

FIGURE 12-8 Brahman bull. (Courtesy American Brahman Breeders Association, Houston, Tex.)

The Beefmaster breed began in Texas. The breed is the result of crosses among Herefords, Shorthorns, and Brahmans. The breed has a variety of colors. Reds and duns are more common than other colors. Some of the cattle are horned and some are polled. The cattle have drooping ears and loose hide. Selection has been mainly for good disposition, fertility, gain, conformation, hardiness, and milk production. The three breed associations for this breed are Beefmaster Breeders Universal, the Foundation Beefmaster Association, and the National Beefmaster Association (Fig. 12-6).

Brahman
Color: Varies
Average cow weight: 1200 to 1500 pounds
Breed association: American Brahman Breeders Association
Website: http://www.brahman.org/

The Brahman breed was developed in the southwestern part of the United States from *Bos indicus*–type cattle imported from India. Brahman cattle vary from very light gray or red to almost black. The *bulls* have dark areas on the neck and shoulders. They have drooping ears, loose hide, a pendulous sheath, and a hump over their shoulders. The major use of Brahman

cattle in the United States is crossing with other breeds. The resulting hybrids have proved to be desirable beef animals. Cattle of this breed can be registered with the American Brahman Breeders Association (Figs. 12-7 and 12-8).

Brangus
Color: Black or red
Average cow weight: 1300 to 1500 pounds
Breed association: International Brangus Breeders Association
Website: http://gobrangus.com/

The Brangus breed was developed in the United States by crossing Brahman and Angus cattle. Brangus cattle are solid black and polled. They have drooping ears and loose hide. Bulls have a small hump over the shoulders. They are adaptable to different climates. They have good mothering ability and feed efficiency, and they produce desirable carcasses. Cattle of this breed must undergo an inspection to determine conformation and breed character before the animals can be registered with the American Brangus Breeders Association (Fig. 12-9).

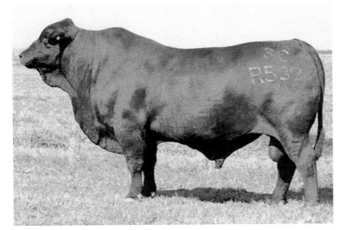

FIGURE 12-9 Brangus bull TCB Catawba Warrior R532. (Courtesy Spitzer Ranch. Fairplay, S.C.)

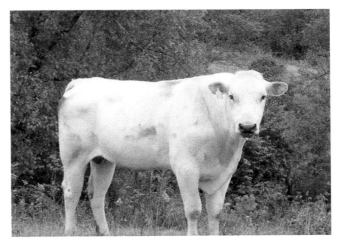

FIGURE 12-11 Chianina bull. (Courtesy Champagne Farm, Sharpsburg, Ky.)

The Chianina breed of cattle originated in the Chiana Valley in Italy. The original Chianina cattle were white with a black switch. The skin pigment is black. They have high heat tolerance and a gentle disposition. Chianina probably are the largest breed of cattle. Mature bulls can grow to 6 feet at the withers and weigh as much as 4000 pounds. Mature cows can grow to 5 feet at the withers and can weigh up to 2400 pounds. They are popular in crosses for a number of reasons. They improve the growth rates of their offspring, they are good foragers and good mothers, they have a high degree of tolerance to insects and diseases, and they are well adapted to hot and cold climates. Chianina cattle can be registered with the American Chianina Association (Fig. 12-11).

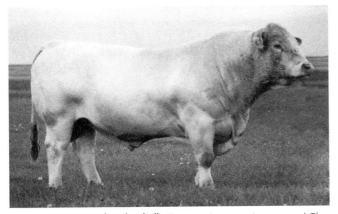

FIGURE 12-10 Charolais bull. (Courtesy American International Charolais Association, Kansas City, Mo.)

Charolais

Color: Light straw color
Average cow weight: 1500 to 1800 pounds
Breed association: American International Charolais Association
Website: http://www.charolaisusa.com/

The Charolais breed originated in France. Charolais cattle are white to light straw color with pink skin. They are large and heavily muscled. Mature bulls weigh 2000 to 2500 pounds, and mature cows weigh 1500 to 1800 pounds. Most are naturally horned. Their horns are white, slender, and tapered. Charolais have a high feed efficiency. They are well adapted to many areas and are used in many crossbreeding programs. Naturally polled Charolais can also be registered. Cattle of this breed can be registered with the American International Charolais Association (Fig. 12-10).

Chianina

Color: White to gray with a black switch
Average cow weight: 1600 to 2400 pounds
Breed association: American Chianina Association
Website: http://www.chicattle.org

Gelbvieh

Color: Reddish to russet
Average cow weight: 1200 to 1400 pounds
Breed association: American Gelbvieh Association
Website: http://www.gelbvieh.org/

The Gelbvieh breed was developed in West Germany. They are a reddish-gold to russet color with dark skin pigment and dark hooves. They are of a medium weight and size, have good milking ability, and produce a very acceptable carcass (Fig. 12-12). Gelbvieh cattle can be registered with the American Gelbvieh Association.

Horned and Polled Herefords

Color: White face, dewlap, underline, flank, and switch with red bodies
Average cow weight: 1200 pounds
Breed association: American Hereford Association
Website: http://www.hereford.org

The Hereford breed originated in England. Hereford cattle have white faces and red bodies, ranging from yellow to dark red. They have white on the dewlap, underline, flank, and switch. Herefords can be polled or horned. They have a docile nature and are easily handled. They have a superior

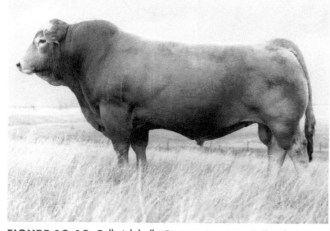

FIGURE 12-12 Gelbvieh bull. (Courtesy American Gelbvieh Association, Westminster, Colo.)

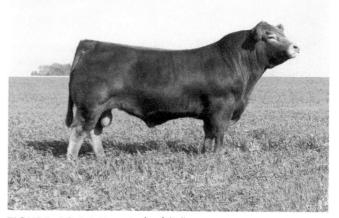

FIGURE 12-14 Limousin beef bulls. (Courtesy Tammy Mikkelson [Wulf Cattle].)

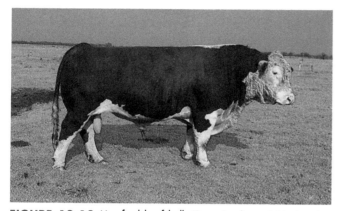

FIGURE 12-13 Hereford beef bull. (From Sambraus HH: *A colour atlas of livestock breeds*, London, 1992, Mosby-Wolfe.)

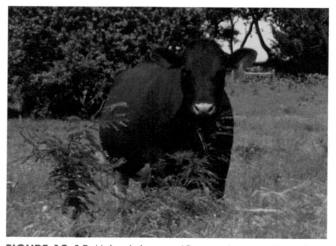

FIGURE 12-15 Maine-Anjou cow. (Courtesy American Maine-Anjou Association, Platte City, Mo.)

foraging ability, vigor, and hardiness. They produce more calves under adverse conditions than do many other breeds. When Herefords are used in crosses, the white color pattern tends to be dominant. Mature bulls weigh approximately 1800 pounds, and mature females weigh approximately 1200 pounds. Horned Herefords can be registered with the American Hereford Association. Polled Herefords are eligible for registration with both the American Hereford Association and the American Polled Hereford Association (Fig. 12-13).

Limousin
Color: Mahogany red to gold with a light tan underline, muzzle, and legs
Average cow weight: 1350 pounds
Breed association: North American Limousin Foundation
Website: http://www.nalf.org/

Limousin cattle originated in France. They have a mahogany red to gold color with a light tan underline, muzzle, and legs. The skin is free of pigmentation. The spread of horns is horizontal, then forward and upward. The Limousin head is small and short with a broad forehead. The neck is also short. Mature bulls weigh from 2000 to 2400 pounds, and

mature cows weigh approximately 1350 pounds. Limousin cattle are noted for their carcass leanness and large loin areas (Fig. 12-14). Limousin cattle can be registered with the North American Limousin Foundation.

Maine-Anjou
Color: Dark red with white undermarkings and patches of white on the body
Average cow weight: 1500 to 1900 pounds
Breed association: American Maine-Anjou Association
Website: http://www.maine-anjou.org/

The Maine-Anjou originated in France. They are dark red with white undermarkings and patches of white on the body. Some cattle are roan. They are large and have lightly pigmented skin. They are a horned breed with medium-sized horns that curve forward. They are considered docile and easily handled. These cattle are fast growing and have a well-marbled carcass. Mature bulls weigh approximately 2750 pounds (Fig. 12-15). Maine-Anjou cattle can be registered with the American Maine-Anjou Association.

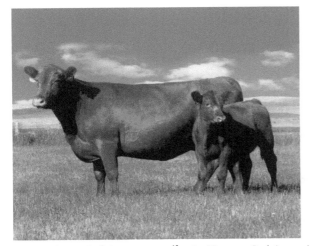

FIGURE 12-16 Red Angus cow-calf pair. (Courtesy Red Angus Association of America, Denton, Tex.)

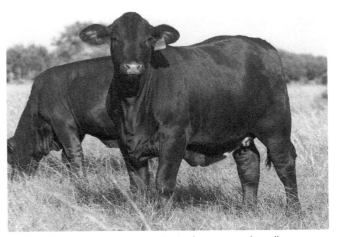

FIGURE 12-17 Santa Gertrudis heifer PB Female–Gill. (Courtesy Santa Gertrudis Breeders International, Kingsville, Tex.)

Red Angus

Color: Red
Average cow weight: 1150 pounds
Breed association: Red Angus Association of America
Website: http://redangus.org/

Red Angus herds began in the United States in approximately 1945. The herds developed from crossing red with the red from Black Angus cattle. Because the red gene is recessive, the offspring of the red crosses are always red. Red Angus cattle can be registered with the Red Angus Association of America. Because red absorbs less heat than black, Red Angus cattle can tolerate warmer temperatures than Black Angus. Red Angus cattle have many of the same characteristics of Black Angus, except their color (Fig. 12-16).

Santa Gertrudis

Color: Cherry red with occasional white markings
Average cow weight: 1540 pounds
Breed association: Santa Gertrudis Breeders International
Website: http://santagertrudis.com/

The Santa Gertrudis breed was developed on the King Ranch in Texas. The breed is a result of crosses of Brahman bulls with Shorthorn cows. The cattle are cherry red with occasional white markings. They have drooping ears. The cattle also have loose skin. The hair grows short and straight in warm climates and long in colder climates. Most of the animals are horned, although some are polled. Santa Gertrudis cattle are eligible for registration with the Santa Gertrudis Breeders International. They produce desirable carcasses with little waste fat. They also have a tendency to resist diseases and insects (Fig. 12-17).

Shorthorn

Color: Red, white, or roan
Average cow weight: 1300 pounds
Breed association: American Shorthorn Association
Website: http://www.shorthorn.org/

The Shorthorn breed originated in England. They are red, white, or roan. They have small horns that curve inward or are polled. They are easily handled and have good dispositions. Mature bulls weigh up to 2400 pounds, and mature cows weigh up to 1500 pounds. Shorthorns are adaptable to many climates. They have excellent crossing ability with other breeds. They are good mothers with excellent milking ability. Shorthorns produce a desirable carcass. Cattle of this breed can be registered with the American Shorthorn Association (Fig. 12-18).

Simmental

Color: Varies
Average cow weight: 1450 to 1800 pounds
Breed association: American Simmental Association
Website: http://www.simmental.org

Simmental cattle originated in the Simmen Valley of Switzerland. Simmental cattle can be red and white, yellow and white, black and white, gray and white, or solid. They are a horned breed with medium-sized horns. The Simmental is a large-bodied animal and is noted for being docile. Mature bulls weigh from 2300 to 2600 pounds, and mature cows weigh approximately 1450 to 1800 pounds. They have extremely rapid growth rates, are thickly muscled, and produce a carcass without excess fat. They are adaptable to a wide variety of climates. Cattle of this breed can be registered with the American Simmental Association (Fig. 12-19).

Texas Longhorn

Color: Varies
Average cow weight: 1000 pounds
Breed association: Texas Longhorn Breeders Association of America
Website: http://www.tlbaa.org/

The Texas Longhorn developed in Spain. They have many shades and combinations of colors. They have horns that curve upward and spread to 4 feet or more. Their legs are

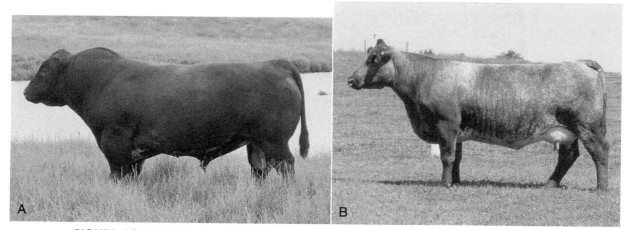

FIGURE 12-18 A, Shorthorn bull. **B,** Shorthorn cow. (Courtesy of the American Shorthorn Association, Omaha, Nebr.)

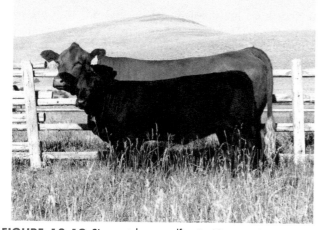

FIGURE 12-19 Simmental cow–calf pair. (Courtesy American Simmental Association, Bozeman, Mont.)

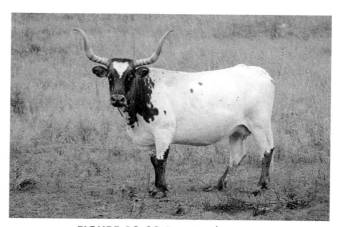

FIGURE 12-20 Texas Longhorn cow.

long, and their shoulders are large and high. They have a large head with small ears and long hair between their horns. Their neck is short and stocky. They are slow to mature, have high fertility, are resistant to many diseases and parasites, and are well adapted to harsh environments. They have the ability to survive on sparse rangeland. They are noted for their easy *calving* ability, hardiness, and longevity (Fig. 12-20). Texas Longhorns can be registered with the Texas Longhorn Breeders Association of America.

COMMON BREEDS OF DAIRY CATTLE
Ayrshire
Color: Red, mahogany, or brown
Average cow weight: 1200 pounds
Breed association: Ayrshire Cattle Society
Website: http://www.ayrshirescs.org

The Ayrshire breed originated in the county of Ayr in the southwestern part of Scotland. The Ayrshire may be any shade of cherry red. Other colors are mahogany, brown, or white but may be mixed with red, mahogany, or brown. Each color should be clearly defined. The preferred colors are

black or brindle. The horns curve up and out. They are of medium length, small at the base, and tapered toward the tips. These cattle have straight lines and well-balanced udders. The udders are attached high at the caudal aspect and extend forward. The teats are medium in size. Ayrshires are vigorous and strong and have excellent grazing ability. Mature cows weigh approximately 1200 pounds, and mature bulls weigh approximately 1800 pounds. Ayrshires rank third among the dairy breeds in average milk production per cow at 11,700 pounds. They average approximately 4% *milk fat* and rank fourth among the five dairy breeds in average milk fat produced per cow (Fig. 12-21). Ayrshire cattle can be registered with the Ayrshire Cattle Society.

Brown Swiss
Color: Solid brown
Average cow weight: 1500 pounds
Breed association: Brown Swiss Association
Website: http://www.brownswissusa.com

The Brown Swiss originated in Switzerland. Brown Swiss are solid brown, ranging from light to dark. White and off color spots are objectionable colors. The nose and tongue are black. The horns incline forward and slightly upward. They are of

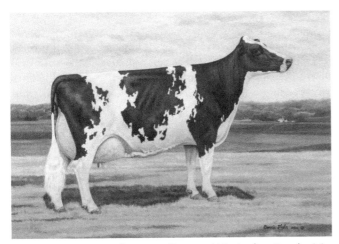

FIGURE 12-21 Ayrshire cow. (Courtesy U.S. Ayrshire Breeders' Association, Columbus, Ohio.)

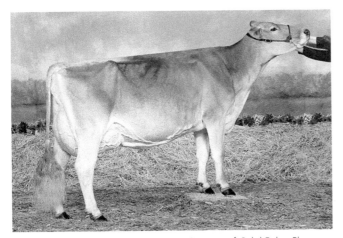

FIGURE 12-22 Brown Swiss cow. (Courtesy of Cybil Fisher Photography and Brown Swiss Cattle Breeders' Association of the USA, Beloit, Wis.)

medium length and taper toward black tips. Brown Swiss are large-framed cattle. Mature cows weigh approximately 1500 pounds, and mature bulls weigh 2000 pounds. The *heifers* mature more slowly than other breeds. Brown Swiss cattle have a quiet, docile temperament. They are considered good grazers and have high heat tolerance. Brown Swiss cows rank second among the dairy breeds in average milk production per cow at 12,100 pounds. They average approximately 4.1% milk fat and rank third among the dairy breeds in average milk fat produced per cow. Cattle of this breed can be registered with the Brown Swiss Cattle Breeders' Association of the USA (Fig. 12-22).

Guernsey

Color: Any shade of fawn with white markings
Average cow weight: 1100 pounds
Breed association: American Guernsey Association
Website: http://www.usguernsey.com/

The Guernsey originated on the Isle of Guernsey, which is located in the English Channel off the coast of France. The Guernsey may be any shade of fawn with white markings.

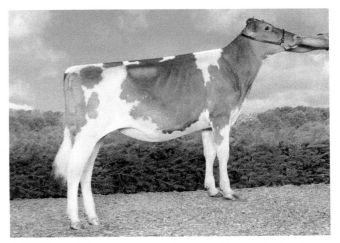

FIGURE 12-23 Guernsey cow. (Courtesy Monument View Farms, Greenwich, N.Y.)

Black and brindle colors are objectionable. The skin is yellow. A clear or buff muzzle is preferred over smoky or black. The horns curve outward and to the front. They are medium in length, small and yellow at the base, and taper toward the tips. These cattle are an early maturing breed. They are adaptable and gentle. Mature cows weigh approximately 1100 pounds, and mature bulls weigh approximately 1800 pounds. Guernseys rank fourth among the dairy breeds in average milk production per cow at 10,600 pounds. They average approximately 5% milk fat and rank second among the dairy breeds in average milk fat produced per cow. Guernseys produce milk that is golden (Fig. 12-23). Guernsey cattle can be registered with the American Guernsey Association.

Holstein-Friesian

Color: Black and white or red and white
Average cow weight: 1500 pounds
Breed association: Holstein Association USA
Website: http://www.holsteinusa.com

The Holstein-Friesian originated in the Netherlands. Holsteins are black and white. A recessive gene occasionally causes the appearance of a red and white color. The switch has white on it. Solid black or solid white animals are not registered with the Holstein-Friesian Association of America. Off colors include black on the switch, solid black belly, one or more legs encircled with black that touches the hoof at any point, and black and white intermixed to give gray spots. The horns incline forward and curve inward. They are of medium length and taper toward the tips. Holsteins are the largest of the dairy breeds. Mature cows weigh approximately 1500 pounds, and bulls weigh approximately 2200 pounds. They have large udders. Holsteins have excellent grazing ability and a large feed capacity. The cows are generally quiet, but the bulls can be aggressive and dangerous. Holsteins are adaptable to a wide range of conditions. Holsteins rank first among the dairy breeds in average milk production per cow at 14,500 pounds. They average approximately 3.5% milk fat and rank fifth among the dairy breeds in average milk fat produced per cow (Fig. 12-24).

Jersey

Color: Cream, light fawn, or almost black
Average cow weight: 1000 pounds
Breed association: American Jersey Cattle Association
Website: http://www.usjersey.com/

The Jersey breed originated on the Isle of Jersey, which is located in the English Channel off the coast of France. Jerseys can be cream, light fawn, or almost black. Some animals have white markings. The muzzle is black. The switch and tongue may be black or white. The Jersey is the smallest of the dairy cattle breeds. Mature cows weigh approximately 1000 pounds, and bulls weigh approximately 1600 pounds. The horns curve inward and are inclined forward. They are of medium length and taper toward the tips. Jersey cattle have excellent udders that are well attached. They are adaptable and efficient users of feed. Jerseys have excellent grazing ability even on poor pastures. The cows may be somewhat nervous, and the bulls can be aggressive. Jerseys are early maturing and have excellent dairy type. Jerseys rank fifth among the dairy breeds in average milk production per cow at 10,000 pounds. They average approximately 5.4% milk fat and rank first among the dairy breeds in average milk fat produced per cow (Fig. 12-25). Jersey cattle can be registered with the American Jersey Cattle Association.

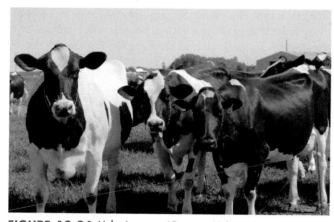

FIGURE 12-24 Holstein cows. (Courtesy Holstein Association USA, Brattleboro, Vt.)

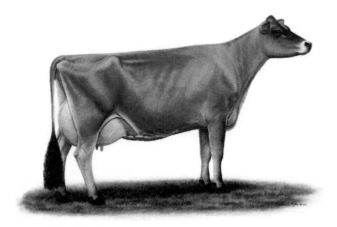

FIGURE 12-25 Jersey cow. (Painting by Bonnie Mohr. Copyright owned by the American Jersey Cattle Association, Reynoldsburg, Ohio, and used with permission.)

REPRODUCTION

The normal reproductive course for any large animal species is discussed in Chapter 3. The reproductive procedures discussed here are variations that exist among cattle. Table 12-2 lists breeding information for cattle. Figure 12-26 shows the bovine estrous cycle.

TABLE 12-2	Cattle Breeding Information
Male Reproductive Parameters	
Age of male at puberty	7–18 mo
Length of spermatogenesis	61 days
Length of copulation	1–3 sec
Site of semen deposition	Vagina
Ejaculate volume (mL)	3–5
Total sperm ($\times 10^{-9}$)	4–5
Motile sperm (%)	30
Morphologically normal sperm (%)	70
Scrotal circumference bull age (mo)	Size (cm)
≤15	30
15–18	31
18–21	32
21–24	33
>24	34
Female Reproductive Parameters	
Type of estrous cycle	Year-round polyestrous
Age of female at puberty	7–18 mo
Time of first breeding	13–15 mo
Estrous cycle frequency	21 days
Duration of estrus	18 hr
Time of ovulation	12–18 hr after estrus
Optimal time of breeding	12 hr after standing heat
Maternal recognition of pregnancy in days	15–16 days as a result of IFN-t
Source of progesterone during days of gestation	0–150: CL 150–250: placenta >250: CL and placenta
Type of placenta	Placentomes
Gestation period	283 days (276–295 days)
Birth weight	60–100 pounds
Litter size	1–2
Weaning age	Dairy cattle 3 mo, beef cattle 4–6 mo
Pregnancy Diagnosis in Days After Ovulation	
Ultrasound	>14 days
Transrectal palpation	>30 days
Progesterone	20–24 days
Estrone sulfate	>100 days
PSPB	>15 days
IEPF	1 day

CL, Corpus luteum; *IEPF,* immunosuppressive early pregnancy factor; *IFN-t,* interferon-tau; *PSPB,* pregnancy-specific protein B.

SEMEN COLLECTION

Electroejaculation is the method most commonly used for semen collection in the bull. Vocalization during the procedure is common, and extension of the hindlegs may occur. While the penis is extended, it can be examined as described in the reproductive examination. Trained bulls may allow collection using a female in estrus and an artificial vagina.

ARTIFICIAL INSEMINATION

For artificial insemination of cattle, semen is deposited directly into the uterus, just beyond the cervix. This is accomplished using an intrauterine transcervical approach. Insemination of the cow should take place 12 hours after the first detection of estrus. Therefore, it is common to perform heat detection twice a day. Those cows that are observed in heat in the morning are inseminated that evening, and those observed in the evening are inseminated the following morning. The cow is restrained in the standing position. The inseminator uses one hand that is lubricated and covered with an obstetrical sleeve to enter the rectum; this hand is used to locate and stabilize the cervix and extend the vagina. The other hand operates the insemination pipette, by passing it through the vagina to enter the cervix and gently manipulating it through the cervix until the tip is approximately ¼ inch (0.5 cm) into the uterus. The semen is slowly deposited at this location (Fig. 12-27). The gun is removed from the vagina slowly, and the arm in the rectum is removed.

EMBRYO TRANSFER

Embryo transfer in cattle has been available since the late 1970s. The development of this procedure has allowed accelerated proliferation of genetic material from the dam as well as the sire. The ability to freeze and transport bovine embryos around the world has made embryo transfer an extremely useful form of technology for disease control and biosecurity programs and for genetic salvage of valuable individuals; it has also helped to develop new lines and breeds of cattle. The typical protocol for embryo transfer collection in cattle is as follows.

1. *Superovulation* of the donor is the first step of embryo transfer in cattle. It is the least predictable step. First, the donor should have an ultrasound scan performed to evaluate the reproductive tract. Then, twice-daily injections of follicle-stimulating hormone (FSH) are used to perform superovulation. Tables 12-3 and 12-4 give two different superovulation protocols commonly used in cattle. Accurate estrus detection of the donor is of great importance. It helps to determine the proper time of insemination and also the degree of synchronization present between the donor and recipients.

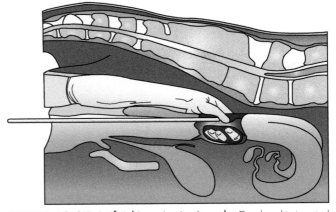

FIGURE 12-27 Artificial insemination in cattle. One hand is inserted in the rectum to stabilize the cervix and confirm passage of the artificial insemination pipette into the uterus. (Modified from Noakes DE, Parkinson TJ, England GCW: *Veterinary reproduction and obstetrics,* ed 9, London, 2009, Saunders.)

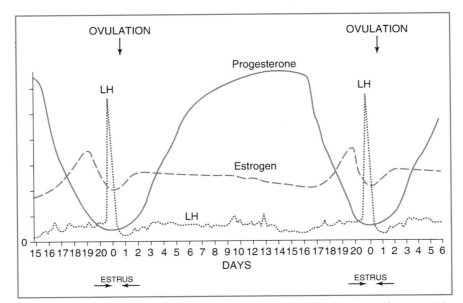

FIGURE 12-26 Bovine estrous cycle. Estrus is 12 to 18 hours long, and luteinizing hormone (LH) peaks during estrus. Diestrus lasts until approximately day 17, and progesterone levels are high throughout diestrus. If a pregnancy signal is not secreted by the early embryo by day 16 or 17, prostaglandin is released from the uterus, goes to the corpus luteum, and causes luteolysis (luteal death). The cycle then starts over. (From Bassert JM, McCurnin DM, editors: *McCurnin's clinical textbook for veterinary technicians,* ed 7, St. Louis, 2010, Saunders.)

TABLE 12-3	Superovulation Protocol Commonly Used in Cattle*	
TREATMENT DAY	**TREATMENT 1**	**TREATMENT 2**
−27	25 mg (5.0 mL) $PGF_{2\alpha}$	25 mg (5.0 mL) $PGF_{2\alpha}$
−17	25 mg (5.0 mL) $PGF_{2\alpha}$	25 mg (5.0 mL) $PGF_{2\alpha}$
−14	Estrus	Estrus
−4: am	80 mg (4.0 mL) FSH	50 mg (2.5 mL) FSH
−4: pm	80 mg (4.0 mL) FSH	50 mg (2.5 mL) FSH
−3: am	60 mg (3.0 mL) FSH	50 mg (2.5 mL) FSH
−3: pm	60 mg (3.0 mL) FSH	50 mg (2.5 mL) FSH
−2: am	40 mg (2.0 mL) FSH 35 mg (7.0 mL) $PGF_{2\alpha}$	50 mg (2.5 mL) FSH 25 mg (5.0 mL) $PGF_{2\alpha}$
−2: pm	40 mg (2.0 mL) FSH 25 mg (5.0 mL) $PGF_{2\alpha}$	50 mg (2.5 mL) FSH 25 mg (5.0 mL) $PGF_{2\alpha}$
−1: am	20 mg (1.0 mL) FSH	50 mg (2.5 mL) FSH
−1: pm	20 mg (1.0 mL) FSH	50 mg (2.5 mL) FSH
0	Estrus and AI	Estrus and AI
7	Embryo recovery, transfer, and freezing	Embryo recovery, transfer, and freezing

From Youngquist RS, Threlfall WR: *Current therapy in large animal theriogenology*, ed 2, St. Louis, 2007, Saunders.
AI, Artificial insemination; *FSH*, follicle-stimulating hormone; *PGF$_{2\alpha}$*, prostaglandin $F_{2\alpha}$.
*If the donor does not come into estrus, FSH treatment may be continued for 1 additional day at the dosage level of the last scheduled day. AI of donor at 4 to 6 hours after onset of estrus, repeated once 10 to 12 hours later.

TABLE 12-4	Superovulation Protocol Commonly Used in Cattle
TREATMENT DAY	**TREATMENT**
0	CIDR inserted vaginally
2: pm	100 μg GnRH
4: pm	60 mg (3.0 mL) FSH
5: am	60 mg (3.0 mL) FSH
5: pm	60 mg (3.0 mL) FSH
6: am	50 mg (2.5 mL) FSH
6: pm	50 mg (2.5 mL) FSH
7: am	40 mg (2.0 mL) FSH
7: pm	40 mg (2.0 mL) FSH, 35 mg (7.0 mL) $PGF_{2\alpha}$
8: am	40 mg (2.0 mL) FSH, 35 mg (7.0 mL) $PGF_{2\alpha}$ CIDR out
9: am	Estrus and AI
9: pm	Estrus and AI
16	Embryo recovery, transfer, and freezing

From Youngquist RS, Threlfall WR: *Current therapy in large animal theriogenology*, ed 2, St. Louis, 2007, Saunders.
AI, Artificial insemination; *CIDR*, controlled internal drug release; *FSH*, follicle-stimulating hormone; *GnRH*, gonadotropin-releasing hormone; *PGF$_{2\alpha}$*, prostaglandin $F_{2\alpha}$.

2. Insemination of the donor cow is the next step. Artificial insemination is performed twice with a 10- to 12-hour interval beginning 4 to 6 hours after the onset of estrus. This covers the range of time over which the ovulations may occur.

3. Next comes collection of embryos: Fertilized eggs take at least 4 days to reach the uterus. Embryos usually are recovered 6 to 8 days after artificial insemination. Nonsurgical methods of embryo recovery are preferred. The most common method is placement of a three-way Foley-type balloon catheter into the uterus or a uterine horn. The balloon is inflated, and the uterus is flushed with a special liquid medium (modified phosphate-buffered saline). The catheter allows simultaneous injection of the medium and backflow collection of the medium into a special container or Petri dish. The container can be fitted with a commercially available embryo filter to "strain" the embryos into a smaller volume of medium.

4. Identification and selection of embryos: A stereoscopic (dissecting) microscope is used to examine the medium and identify embryos. The magnification should be 50× to 100×. The embryos are assessed for stage of development, which should be compatible with the number of days since insemination. Embryos are also rated for quality and classified as good, moderate, or poor. Degenerated or defective embryos are discarded. A micropipette is used to aspirate and transfer the embryos to holding dishes or containers filled with modified phosphate-buffered saline solution. They can be used fresh for up to 8 hours, stored cooled (4° C) for up to 3 days, or cryopreserved for long-term use after special preparation for freezing.

5. Embryo transfer: The embryos are transferred to recipient cows that have been hormonally manipulated to prepare the reproductive tract to receive an embryo. The recipient is usually *synchronized* so that her estrous cycle matches that of the donor cow. Recipients can be prepared in three ways. In the first method, you can select six to eight recipients from a large pool of cycling females. This strategy limits the number of embryos and time when embryos can be collected. Approximately 5% of the herd will be in heat on any given day. In the second method, estrous cycles of any number of recipients can be synchronized with prostaglandin $F_{2\alpha}$ ($PGF_{2\alpha}$) or its analogues, or with controlled internal drug release (CIDR) devices, to exhibit heat the same day as or just ahead of the donor. In the third method, a timed embryo transfer, analogous to timed artificial insemination (Ov-Sync), can also be used. The importance of close synchrony between the age and stage of development of the embryo and the endocrine status of the endometrium of the recipient must be emphasized. Pregnancy rates following embryo transfer are best when the recipient is in estrus from 36 hours before to 12 hours after the donor. The selected embryo is aspirated into a small-gauge intravenous (IV) catheter with a 1-mL

syringe. The syringe is used to "inject" the embryo into the recipient. Alternatively, the embryos can be loaded into a plastic insemination straw and deposited with an insemination gun. Methods of transfer can be nonsurgical or surgical. Surgical transfer is performed in the standing cow through a flank incision or flank laparoscopy. The uterus is identified and penetrated with a blunt needle, a catheter is attached, and the embryo is injected directly into the lumen of the uterus. Nonsurgical transfer is performed similarly to the technique used for artificial insemination, but the insemination pipette is inserted more deeply into the uterus, and the embryo is injected there.

UTERINE CULTURE, BIOPSY, AND INFUSION

Preparation of the female for any uterine procedure is similar to that described for the horse. The tail is tied or held out of the way, and the vulva and perineum are washed thoroughly with warm water and disinfectant scrub. The clinician's preference dictates the specific materials and equipment used for the procedures.

Uterine infusion and lavage are often used for treatment of uterine infections. Lavage is performed to "wash out" the uterus by instilling large volumes of fluid and then siphoning out the fluid and debris. To accommodate the fluids and debris, large-bore tubing such as an equine stomach tube is often used. This is not a sterile procedure, but it should be performed as cleanly as possible. Similarly, uterine infusion is used to place liquid medications into the uterus, generally in smaller volumes that are intended to remain in the uterus to maximize contact time with the bacteria. Antibiotic solutions are most often used for infusions. Infusion and lavage fluids should be warm.

CLINICAL SIGNS OF IMPENDING PARTURITION

Clinical changes associated with impending parturition are softening of the muscles and ligaments of the hindquarters and tail head, thus giving the tail head an elevated appearance 24 to 48 hours before labor. Other signs include swelling of the vulva, thick mucous discharge from the vulva, anxiousness, separation from the herd, abdominal straining, enlargement of the udder, and distention of the teats. The cow may tend to separate from the herd and become defensive of her "personal space." A slight fall in rectal temperature (0.6° C) is reported to occur as early as 54 hours before birth but is not a reliable predictor of labor.

PARTURITION

Stage 1
Stage 1 typically lasts 2 to 6 hours. During this time, the mother displays restlessness and little interest in food and occasionally may kick at the belly and strain.

Stage 2
Stage 2 occurs in 30 minutes to 4 hours; the average is approximately 75 minutes. Heifers generally take longer than

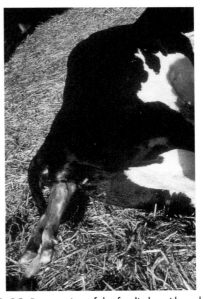

FIGURE 12-28 Presentation of the forelimbs with no head presenting. (From Blowey RW, Weaver AD: *Color atlas of diseases and disorders of cattle*, ed 3, Oxford, 2012, Mosby.)

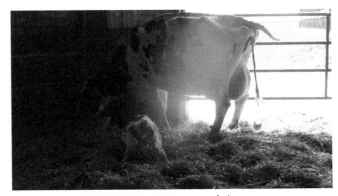

FIGURE 12-29 Passage of placenta.

cows to deliver the fetus. Because the placenta detaches slowly, the fetus can continue to receive oxygen for much longer than the equine fetus, and live deliveries may occur up to 6 to 8 hours after stage 2 begins. If no progress is made after 1 hour of straining to deliver or if abnormal fetal posture is observed, the delivery should be treated as dystocia, and immediate veterinary consultation is advisable (Fig. 12-28).

Stage 3
Stage 3 involves slow detachment from the uterine wall. Cows typically take approximately 4 to 6 hours to expel the placenta, and up to 12 hours is not uncommon. If the fetal membranes are not passed within 24 hours, veterinary assistance is warranted. Cows may eat the afterbirth (Fig. 12-29).

DYSTOCIA

Dystocia is fairly common in cattle. Procedures for addressing this situation are outlined in Chapter 3 (Fig. 12-30).

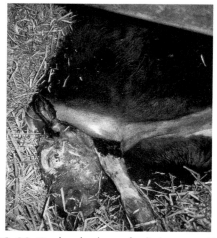

FIGURE 12-30 Head and only one forelimb present. (From Blowey RW, Weaver AD: *Color atlas of diseases and disorders of cattle*, ed 3, London, 2012, Mosby.)

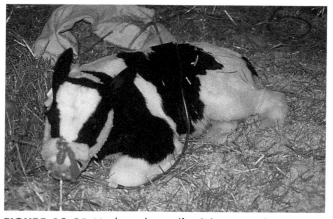

FIGURE 12-31 Newborn clone calf with hypoxemia being treated with intranasal oxygen. (From Divers TJ, Peek SJ: *Rebhun's diseases of dairy cattle*, ed 2, St. Louis, 2008, Saunders.)

RUMINANT NEONATAL CARE

The neonatal period is a time of significant losses to the producer through morbidity and mortality. Neonates are susceptible to various conditions as they adapt to their new environment. Starvation and hypothermia are among the leading causes of mortality in the first 3 days of life. Caring for the very young involves not only knowledge of routine care but also recognition of abnormalities. Early identification and treatment of problems offer the best chance for success.

ROUTINE CARE OF THE NEONATAL CALF

Once delivery is complete, the following needs of the newborn must be addressed:
1. Oxygenation and pulse assessment
2. Temperature regulation
3. Care of umbilical cord and umbilicus
4. Nutrition (nursing)
5. Bonding of cow and calf
6. Passage of meconium
7. Adequacy of passive transfer of antibodies
8. Physical examination of the calf

Oxygenation and Pulse Assessment

The most immediate need is ensuring that the airway is cleared of fetal membranes and fluid. The fetal membranes can be manually removed if they are blocking the nostrils. A bulb syringe or suction tubing can be used to aspirate liquid from each nostril. Most of the fluid in the lungs will be reabsorbed gradually by the lymphatic system. Suspending the calf by the hindlimbs to assist drainage is unnecessary, and suspending the calf may interfere with normal function of the diaphragm. Breathing can be stimulated by placing the calf in sternal recumbency and briskly rubbing the body with towels. A piece of straw or a swizzle stick (the kind found in bar drinks) can be used to stimulate the nasal mucosa of the calf by causing it to sneeze, which will help

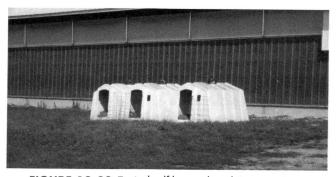

FIGURE 12-32 Typical calf hut used on dairy operations.

remove fluid from the lungs. Calves normally take the first breath within 30 seconds of birth and develop an irregular rate that gradually becomes regular at 45 to 60 breaths per minute (Fig. 12-31).

The pulse should be assessed for rate and quality. A heart rate of 90 to 110 beats per minute (bpm) is normal in neonatal calves. The pulse should be strong and have regular rhythm.

Mucous membranes should be moist and pale pink to pink. Capillary refill time should be less than 2 seconds.

Temperature Regulation

All neonates are susceptible to hypothermia in the postnatal period. Drying the animal and providing a draft-free area, deep bedding, and supplemental heat sources when the environmental temperature is low help maintain body heat (Fig. 12-32). Following an initial period of low rectal temperature immediately after birth, the temperature of the newborn calf should be 37° C to 38° C (100° F to 102° F).

Care of Umbilical Cord and Umbilicus

The umbilical cord usually ruptures naturally without complication. Excessive hemorrhage is uncommon but can be controlled by placing hemostatic clamps across the bleeding stump for several hours. If the cord must be manually cut

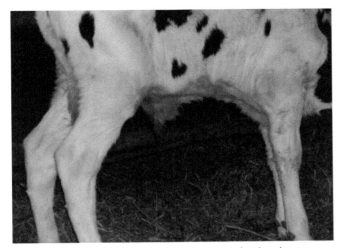

FIGURE 12-33 Umbilical stump treated with iodine.

or ruptured, the same methods as described for foals should be used (see Chapter 6). Topical treatment of the umbilical stump with 3% povidone-iodine solution or dilute chlorhexidine solution (1:4) is recommended. Continued treatment once or twice daily for the first several days of life is desirable but is not always practical in a farm setting (Fig. 12-33).

The umbilicus should be observed for swelling, discharge, moisture, and pain. *Umbilical hernia, omphalophlebitis,* and umbilical abscessation are conditions that require medical or surgical treatment, or both, and should be evaluated by a veterinarian. Umbilical herniation is the most common congenital defect in cattle. Umbilical infections usually develop in the first 2 weeks of life. *Patent urachus* is common in foals but is uncommon in cattle.

Nutrition (Nursing)

Calves typically achieve sternal recumbency several minutes after birth and try to stand within 15 to 30 minutes. Most calves are standing and nursing within 1 to 2 hours (range, 1 to 4 hours). The average time to nursing is 81 minutes in beef breeds; dairy breeds typically take longer. Calves may have some difficulty locating and nursing teats on large, distended udders where the teat ends are close to the ground. Observing the newborn from a distance to assess and confirm nursing behavior is important.

As with other species, colostrum ingestion and absorption are essential for natural passive transfer of antibodies. As a general guideline, the newborn should ingest 10% to 15% of its body weight in colostrum within the first 12 to 24 hours of life. However, this recommendation is affected by the concentration of immunoglobulin G (IgG) in the colostrum and assumes that the colostrum is of good quality (adequate IgG level). Colostrum quality can be assessed with a colostrometer; a specific gravity greater than 1.050 corresponds to an adequate IgG level in the colostrum of approximately 50 g/L. The concentration of IgG in the colostrum of dairy breeds is considerably lower than in beef breeds, and more volume of colostrum from dairy cows compared with beef cows may be needed to achieve adequate levels of protection in the calf.

A common recommendation is for calves to receive at least 4 L of colostrum (dairy cow origin) before 12 hours of age compared with 1 to 2 L for beef cow colostrum.

If the calf's nursing intake is in question, colostrum can be bottle fed or tube fed by dividing the desired total colostrum volume into smaller portions given every 2 hours, preferably within the first 12 hours of life. Some farms routinely administer colostrum by stomach tube several hours after birth to ensure adequate intake (Fig. 12-34). To avoid overdistention of the abomasum, no more than 2 L of liquid should be given per feeding. Sick neonates may not tolerate this feeding volume and may require more frequent feedings of smaller amounts. Note that sick neonates metabolize IgG faster and therefore may require more IgG for protection than healthy calves.

Nutritional management of beef and dairy calves is vastly different. Beef calves normally remain with the dam and suckle naturally until they are weaned at several months of age. Dairy calves, however, typically are separated from the dam after they suckle colostrum or are removed sometime in the first few days of life. They are fed twice daily on bucket-fed or bottle-fed milk or, more commonly, milk replacers (powders reconstituted with water). The general recommendation is to feed milk replacer at 5% to 6% of body weight twice daily, although different milk replacer formulations may have different feeding recommendations. Always consult the product label. The composition of milk replacement products has been the subject of much research and debate, especially with regard to the amount, digestibility, and source of protein (milk derived versus plant derived versus animal derived) used in the formulation.

The maintenance and growth energy requirements for healthy calves have been estimated. The maintenance requirement is approximately 50 kcal/kg/day. The growth requirement is approximately 300 kcal/100 g of body weight gain. These requirements are expected to be significantly higher for sick neonates. Whole milk contains approximately 70 kcal/100 mL; an average calf would need to consume 3 L for daily maintenance, as well as an additional 4 to 5 L to gain 1 kg of body weight.

Hypoglycemia is a life-threatening condition and may develop rapidly (within hours), especially in sick or weak neonates that are unable to nurse normally. Hypoglycemia alone causes weakness and depression as early clinical signs. Blood (serum) glucose level can be measured and ideally should range from 90 to 120 mg/dL; portable glucometers are convenient for field use. Treatment with supplemental oral or parenteral glucose solutions is indicated when glucose levels fall to less than 90 mg/dL; a level lower than 60 mg/dL is immediately life-threatening.

Bonding of Cow and Calf

Human interference should be minimized in the neonatal period to allow maternal bonding to occur (Fig. 12-35). Rejection of calves is uncommon but is more likely to occur with first-calf heifers, twin births, and calves delivered by cesarean section.

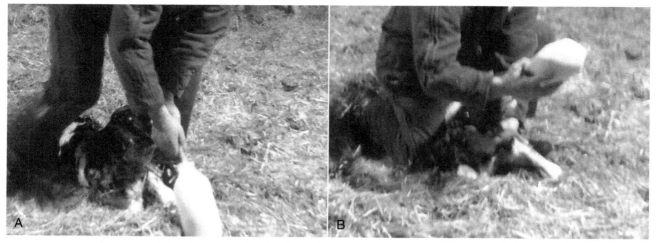

FIGURE 12-34 A, Placement of oral calf drencher. **B,** Administration of colostrum through the oral calf drencher.

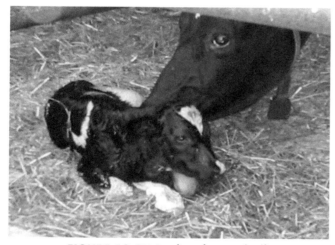

FIGURE 12-35 Bonding of cow and calf.

Passage of Meconium

Meconium, the first feces, typically is dark and may range in consistency from hard to pasty. It should be passed in the first 24 hours of life. If the meconium is not passed or if colic signs are observed, veterinary consultation for meconium impaction is recommended. If digital examination of the rectum or insertion of a rectal thermometer is not possible, or if only mucus is present in the rectum, a genetic defect of the intestinal tract such as incomplete colon, rectum, or anus (*atresia coli, atresia recti,* and *atresia ani,* respectively) should be considered in the differential diagnosis.

> **TECHNICIAN NOTE**   Meconium should be passed within the first 24 hours of life.

Adequacy of Passive Transfer of Antibodies

Routine testing of blood antibody levels is seldom performed in ruminants, primarily because of the economic costs associated with testing and treatment. Even if testing confirms a low level of antibodies in the calf, treatment with IV plasma transfusion is seldom economically justified. However, in valuable calves, blood may be analyzed for immunoglobulins with a serum IgG level, radial immunodiffusion, refractometry using serum, or latex agglutination tests performed at approximately 24 hours of age. Although it is still the subject of some debate, most clinicians consider a minimum serum IgG level of 1000 mg/dL to be adequate (sample drawn between 24 and 48 hours of age). After 24 hours of age, when the gastrointestinal tract can no longer absorb orally administered IgG, failure of passive transfer (<1000 mg/dL IgG) may be treated only with IV plasma products or IV hyperimmune serum. Commercially prepared bovine plasma is available but expensive. Alternatively, fresh plasma can be collected on the farm, preferably from the dam or other animal on the same farm so that immunity to the local environmental microorganisms is high.

Physical Examination of the Calf

A complete physical examination begins with observation from a distance. The neonate is observed for mental alertness and behavior, suckling activity, and gait. Respiratory rate and effort are also best observed from a distance because the rate and effort usually increase with restraint. After the visual examination, the calf is restrained for the "hands-on" examination, which may range from a simple check of temperature, pulse, and respiration to a thorough evaluation using a body systems approach (Table 12-5).

IDENTIFICATION AND CARE OF THE SICK NEONATAL CALF

Many conditions that affect neonatal foals also affect neonatal calves. Neonatal bacterial septicemia is a similar disease in both species, with failure of passive transfer of colostral antibodies being the primary risk factor. Environmental conditions and management practices also play a role. As with foals, initial clinical signs are vague and often include

TABLE 12-5	Normal Physical Examination Parameters for Calves	
PARAMETER	**NORMAL**	
Cardiovascular System		
Mucous membrane color	Pale pink to pink; no petechiae or icterus	
Capillary time	<2 sec	
Pulse rate	90–110 bpm	
Heart auscultation	Absence of murmurs	
Respiratory System		
Respiratory rate	40–60 breaths/min	
Respiratory effort	Absence of nostril flare	
Respiratory noise	Regular	
Respiratory rhythm	Regular	
Lung auscultation	Moist sounds immediately after birth	
	Easier to hear sounds than in adults	
	Audible sounds over all lung fields	
Gastrointestinal System		
Suckling reflex	Vigorous	
Oral cavity	Absence of cleft palate	
Gastrointestinal auscultation	Borborygmus in all quadrants	
	Absence of tympany (pings)	
Passage of meconium	Within 24 hr of birth	
Abdominal contour	Absence of distention	
Urinary System		
Urination	Within 12 hr of birth	
	Volume >34 mL/kg/day	
	Absence of straining	
Umbilicus		
Appearance	Dry, nonpainful, small	
Ophthalmic System		
Corneas	Clear	
Sclera	Bilateral hemorrhages normal	
Eyelids	Absence of entropion	
Musculoskeletal System		
Gait	No lameness	
Joints	No effusion	
Limbs	Straight or mild carpal valgus	
Ribs	Absence of fractures, crepitus	
Neurologic System		
Mental attitude	Bright, alert, responsive	
Gait	Lacks coordination in initial attempts to stand	
Stance	Initial base-wide stance after birth	
Head carriage	Absence of head tilt	

depression, dehydration, and diarrhea. Lethargy, decreased suckling, weakness, and increased recumbency time may also occur. As the disease progresses, signs depend on the organ systems that are affected. Mortality without treatment is high. Gram-negative bacteria account for most cases of septicemia, and *Escherichia coli* is most often isolated.

Specific therapy for neonatal septicemia involves administration of antibiotics, with blood culture and other body fluid samples to confirm bacterial identity and sensitivity to antimicrobial drugs. Other therapy is supportive based on the organ systems affected. IV fluid therapy, parenteral nutrition, respiratory support, management of recumbency issues, control of seizures, and treatment of failure of passive transfer all are possible in neonatal calves. Methods are similar to those described in Chapter 6 for foals. However, such measures are seldom economically feasible, and the veterinarian must communicate with the client to find the best solutions to the animal's problems. Blood work and diagnostic imaging studies, which are highly desirable clinical tools, are not essential for low-level "practical" management of the disease. Broad-spectrum antibiotics, minimal fluid therapy through a stomach (ororumen) tube or drenching, administration of colostrum, and keeping the calf warm and dry can often be successful if instituted early in the course of disease. Recumbent animals with involvement of multiple organ systems have a poor prognosis, even with aggressive treatment.

Diarrhea may occur in the absence of septicemia, especially in calves more than 4 days old. "Calf scours" is a common condition of calves that may have a high morbidity with significant fatalities. Scours has numerous causes, including the following:

- Bacteria: *E. coli*, *Salmonella*, *Clostridium perfringens* type D
- Viruses: rotavirus, coronavirus, bovine viral diarrhea
- Protozoa: *Cryptosporidium*, *Eimeria*
- Nutrition: milk replacers, milk "overload"
- Management: overcrowding and stress

Because the etiologic agents usually are infectious, it is common to have a herd problem with the disease. Multiple factors may be involved. The veterinarian must work closely with the owner to identify risk factors and management factors, identify the specific cause, and plan treatment and prevention strategies. The most common causes of death in calves with diarrhea are dehydration and associated metabolic acidosis. The cornerstones of treatment are correcting and preventing further dehydration through use of oral (stomach tube) or parenteral fluids; bicarbonate is often added to fluids to correct acidosis. Hypoglycemia and electrolyte imbalances may also require treatment by fluid therapy. Total removal of milk from the diet during the diarrheal episode has historically been a common recommendation but now is currently debated. Research has demonstrated improved survival and less weight loss when milk feedings are continued and alternated with oral electrolyte and bicarbonate fluids. Segregation of sick calves in a "sick pen" or barn is recommended, along with proper cleaning and disinfection procedures. All personnel should remember that *Salmonella* and *Cryptosporidium* are zoonotic etiologic agents and

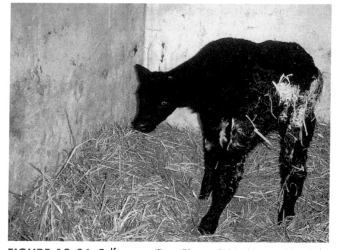

FIGURE 12-36 Calf scours. (From Blowey RW, Weaver AD: *Color atlas of diseases and disorders of cattle*, ed 2, London, 2003, Mosby.)

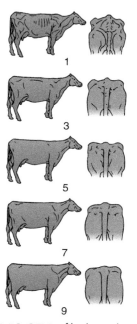

FIGURE 12-37 Beef body condition score.

should take precautions to prevent possible human infections (Fig. 12-36).

Calf pneumonia is primarily a disease of calves more than 4 weeks old and is a common condition in this age group. It is caused by a combination of management factors (stress, overcrowding), environmental factors (temperature, stress, poor ventilation), and infectious (bacterial, viral, or mycoplasmal) agents. High morbidity with some mortality is typical. Treatment relies on early identification of the sick individual, segregation of affected animals, and antibiotic therapy. High fever (>104.0° F), depression, tachypnea, and a soft, moist cough are the hallmarks of the disease.

In contrast, neonatal pneumonia in calves less than 4 days old is uncommon. When it occurs, neonatal pneumonia is more likely the result of neonatal septicemia or bacteremia. Neonatal pneumonia is uncommon as a primary disease but may be caused by several of the viruses that affect bovines (bovine respiratory syncytial virus, infectious bovine rhinotracheitis virus, bovine viral diarrhea virus, bovine coronavirus). *Mycoplasma* species may also cause neonatal pneumonia.

NUTRITION

Figure 12-37 shows body condition scoring for beef cattle and dairy cattle. Figure 12-38 shows the dentition of ruminants. Cattle are ruminants. Ruminants are herbivores and are able to convert products such as cellulose in plants into meat products for human consumption. Cattle do not have upper incisors, but they do have a *dental pad* (Fig. 12-39 and Table 12-6).

The rumen (paunch) of a cow can hold approximately 42.5 gallons and is responsible for microbial digestion with bacteria and protozoans. During fermentation, poor-quality forage and nonprotein nitrogen such as urea are used to produce volatile fatty acids, amino acids, vitamins B and K, methane, and carbon dioxide. The methane and carbon dioxide are eructated, and the other products of fermentation are used by the body. Cattle also synthesize their own vitamin C. Rumen pH should remain between 6.2 and 7.2, although the

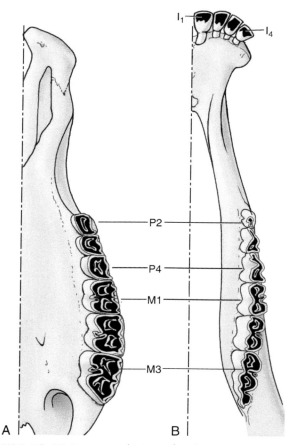

FIGURE 12-38 Permanent dentition of cattle. Upper (A) and lower (B) teeth. (From Dyce KM, Sack WO, Wensing CJG: *Textbook of veterinary anatomy*, ed 4, St. Louis, 2010, Saunders.)

approximately 2.5 gallons. The large intestine is approximately 33 feet long and can hold 7.5 gallons.

FEEDING CONSIDERATIONS BY AGE AND USE

Cattle should be provided water ab libitum. Healthy, mature cattle drink between 10 and 14 gallons of water per day. Dairy cows require 3 to 5 gallons of water to produce 1 gallon of milk. A cow at peak lactation may need up to 45 gallons of water per day.

Medicated feeds are feed products intended to be a substantial source of nutrients in the diet of an animal. The term includes products commonly referred to as supplements, concentrates, premix feeds, and base mixes. Producers should only use those products approved by the U.S. Food and Drug Administration (FDA) and administer them as directed on the label. All directions for the use of a medicated feed additive are on the label attached to the bag or are supplied with a bulk order. No one, including a veterinarian, can legally prescribe the use of any feed additive other than as directed on the product label. Extra-label drug use does not apply to feed additives or feed medications. Veterinary feed directives do not apply for extra-label drug use.

> **TECHNICIAN NOTE** Cattle cannot be fed additives off label.

Cows in good condition can be fed good-quality hay or pasture until 2 weeks before calving. During the last trimester, cows should gain the amount of weight anticipated to be lost during calving. Obese cows are just as undesirable as underweight cattle. Obesity can cause reproductive problems and predispose the cow to ketosis and other problems.

Energy requirements are greatest for cattle during lactation. For lactating cattle, a fully balanced ration with proper dry matter intake (DMI) is essential for optimum milk production. Concentrates supply the highest level of energy, but these concentrates must be balanced with roughages to avoid problems such as obesity, digestive problems, and decreased milk production.

Challenge feeding is often the basis on which cattle are fed. Cow size does not seem to have much effect on the efficiency of milk production, so cattle are often fed based on the level of production of which they are capable.

Beef calves should be creep fed, which is feeding small amounts of grain in a location to which the dam does not have access. This aids in lowering weaning stress and enables the calves to start to digest foodstuff they will be eating in their postweaning life stage. *Creep feeding* generally shows a 50-pound weight advantage at weaning.

Feeding of cattle for slaughter is discussed in Chapter 1.

Cattle and other ruminants should not be fed material derived from mammalian sources, such as meat, bone meal, and other animal by-products. This rule was established in August 1997 by the FDA to minimize the potential of spreading transmissible spongiform encephalopathy. Tallow, blood

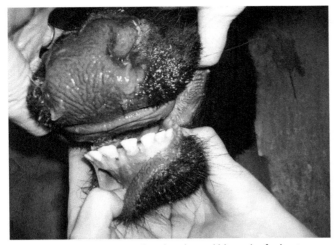

FIGURE 12-39 Dental pad and mandible teeth of a bovine.

TABLE 12-6	Bovine Dental Formulas and Dental Eruption Table

Deciduous: Dental Formula: 2(I0/3 C0/1* PM3/3) = 20 Total

Permanent: Dental Formula: 2(I0/3 C0/1* PM3/3 M3/3) = 32 Total

Eruption	I1	Birth–2 wk
	I2	Birth–2 wk
	I3	Birth–2 wk
	C	Birth–2 wk
	PM2 (first cheek tooth)	Birth–2 wk
	PM3 (second cheek tooth)	Birth–1 wk
	PM4 (third cheek tooth)	Birth–1 wk
Eruption	I1	2 yr
	I2	3 yr
	I3	4 yr
	C	5 yr
	PM2 (first cheek tooth)	2 yr
	PM3 (second cheek tooth)	1–2 yr
	PM4 (third cheek tooth)	3 yr
	M1 (fourth cheek tooth)	5–6 mo
	M2 (fifth cheek tooth)	1 yr
	M3 (sixth cheek tooth)	2 yr

*The canine tooth is in line with the incisors and adjacent to them. It is shaped like an incisor, giving the false appearance of four incisors; however, it is common practice to refer to the canine tooth as the fourth incisor (I4).

rumen may be more acidic in livestock fed diets high in grain. Dietary fiber is required to keep these microorganisms alive. The honeycomb reticulum can hold 2.5 gallons and is responsible for regurgitation of food during rumination. The omasum (manyplies) holds approximately 4 gallons and is thought to squeeze fluid out of the ingested food. The abomasum (true, glandular stomach) can hold approximately 5 gallons and is the beginning of peptic digestion of proteins. The small intestine of cattle is approximately 150 feet long and can hold approximately 16 gallons. The cecum is 3 feet long and can hold

TABLE 12-7	Nutritional Requirements for Cattle			
AGE	**CRUDE PROTEIN (%)**	**CALCIUM (%)**	**PHOSPHORUS (%)**	**DIGESTIBLE ENERGY (Mcal)**
Growing dairy cow (200–1,399 pounds)	6.5–17.1	0.19–0.98	0.12–0.32	0.45–1.04
Lactating dairy cow (800–1,800 pounds)	0.70–0.99	0.029–0.062	0.024–0.044	7.16–10.89
Dairy bull (1,000-2,900 pounds)	20.3–28.6	0.98–1.5	0.14–0.59	14.3–32.1
Growing beef (300–1,300 pounds)	0.34–2.4	10–42	6–24	3–8.4
Yearling beef (700–1,400 pounds)	6.8–14.8	19–28	14–24	8–12
Lactating beef cow or heifer (800–1,400 pounds)	2–2.3	23–42	19–26	9.3–13.3
Breeding beef bull (1,300–2,100 pounds)	2–2.3	23–33	22–33	9.3–13.3

by-products, gelatin, and milk products are excluded from regulation and are acceptable for use in ration formulation.

Table 12-7 details the nutritional requirements of cattle by age and use.

MINERALS

Sodium and chloride should be fed free choice to cattle. Feeding iodized salt will help prevent deficiencies of iodine, which most commonly occur in pregnant animals. Deficiencies of iodine can lead to increases in stillbirths.

Calcium deficiencies may occur with high-grain diets and are often corrected with the use of limestone.

Phosphorus availability is influenced by the phosphorus content of the soil. In young animals, phosphorus deficiency results in poor appetite, slow growth, and unthriftiness. In lactating animals, bones may become fragile and cows may have a poor appetite.

Because only small amounts of cobalt are stored in the body, deficiencies may occur rapidly. Cobalt deficiencies can cause listlessness, ocular discharge, anemia, ketosis, abortions, decreased milk production, and decreased appetite; for these reasons, cobalt should be fed with trace mineralized salt. Feeding too much cobalt can lead to cobalt toxicity. Signs include decreased growth rates, incoordination, and elevated hemoglobin and packed cell volume levels.

Copper deficiency includes signs of neurologic disorders, lameness, anemia, and diarrhea. Signs of copper toxicity include liver and kidney disease, increased incidence of respiratory disease in calves, hemorrhagic diarrhea, and gastroenteritis.

Selenium levels vary in the soil. Selenium should be fed in a trace mineralized salt. Growing cattle that are fed low-protein diets require more selenium and vitamin E in the diet to prevent deficiencies. Selenium deficiencies predispose cattle to reproductive problems and immunosuppression. Cows deficient in selenium may give birth to calves that have white muscle disease.

Zinc should be added to trace mineralized salt. Signs of zinc deficiency include reduction in growth, reduced conception rates, reduced immune response, bone irregularities, decreased appetite, decreased wound healing, and hoof problems. Young male animals require higher levels of zinc for normal testicular development.

Iron is an essential component of hemoglobin. Iron deficiencies rarely occur in adults but may be an issue in calves

fed an all-milk diet. Treatment of deficiencies includes iron dextran injections in calves.

CASE STUDY

Mr. Jarrett would like to start milking cows. He has arrived at the clinic to look for information on dairy cattle. He has just asked you what the differences are among the main dairy breeds and has asked you to rank them in terms of milk production and milk fat. He is going to use the information to help him determine which breed he should purchase for his operation. Please answer the questions he asked you.

CASE STUDY

Mr. Duncan is feeding cattle in southern Kansas, where he has recently seen an increase in white muscle disease within his beef herd. He is coming in for a consultation with the attending veterinarian. What records should you ask him to bring along? When he arrives, what information would you pull to the top for your veterinarian to review?

CASE STUDY

Mr. Nocita owns a cow/calf operation in western Nebraska. He raises purebred Angus cattle. This year his prize cow gave birth to a red calf. He would like to know if his neighbor's bull jumped the fence. What should you tell him?

SUGGESTED READING

Gillespie JR, Flanders FB: *Modern livestock and poultry*, ed 8, Clifton Park, NY, 2010, Delmar Cengage Learning.

Hafez ESE, Hafez B, editors: *Reproduction in farm animals*, ed 7, New York, 2000, Wiley-Blackwell.

Hunt E: Neonatal disease and disease management. In Howard JL, Smith RA, editors: *Current veterinary therapy: food animal practice*, ed 4, St. Louis, 2008, Saunders, pp 70–77.

Noakes DE, Parkinson TJ, England GCW: *Veterinary reproduction and obstetrics*, ed 9, St. Louis, 2009, Saunders.

Smith BP: *Large animal internal medicine*, ed 4, St. Louis, 2008, Mosby.

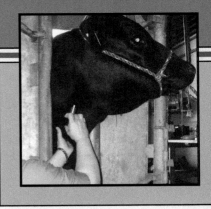

OUTLINE

LEARNING OBJECTIVES

When you have completed this chapter, you will be able to

- Understand the basic natural instincts of cattle and how they affect the handling and restraint of cattle
- Set up and prepare the patient for each procedure, perform the procedure (when appropriate), or assist the clinician in performing diagnostic sampling and medication procedures
- Properly insert and maintain an intravenous catheter and monitor the catheter for complications
- Explain the rationale and indications for each of the clinical procedures described
- Set up materials and equipment and prepare the patient as needed for the procedure
- Perform or assist in necropsy and sample collection procedures and maintain a safe environment during these procedures

KEY TERMS

Balling gun
Drenching
Foot rot
Frick speculum
Hemal processes

Hematoma
Hoof block
Injection site lesion
Mastitis
Ororumen

Rumenocentesis
Subclinical mastitis
Suburethral diverticulum
Titillating

KEY ABBREVIATIONS

BQA Beef Quality Assurance
CMT California mastitis test

SCC Somatic cell count
WBC White blood cell

WMT Wisconsin mastitis test

DIAGNOSTIC SAMPLING

VENOUS BLOOD SAMPLING

Collection of blood for diagnostic testing is one of the most common procedures performed in cattle. Blood is usually submitted to a state or federal diagnostic laboratory for disease screening, which is especially important for herd health and control of disease in animals producing food (meat or milk) for human consumption. Blood can also be used to diagnose and guide treatment of individual animal diseases.

The location of venipuncture depends on the amount of blood needed and the type of restraint to be used. Although theoretically any accessible vein can be used, several locations are preferred for anatomical and safety reasons.

To begin, the animal should be properly restrained. Cattle tend to resist venipuncture, and it should never be attempted on an unrestrained animal. Simply placing a halter on the animal is not enough. The body must be restricted in movement, usually in a chute or head catch gate. Even when the animal is properly restrained, the technician should be prepared for a response by the animal when the needle penetrates the skin. The technician avoid standing or kneeling where he or she may be injured. If kneeling is necessary, you should only ever kneel on one leg to allow for a quick rise and then the ability to step back from the situation quickly.

The venipuncture site should always be cleaned before a blood sample is drawn. Disinfection of the site with 70%

435

isopropyl alcohol is sufficient. A common error is simply wiping off the hair. The site, including the skin, should be wiped down. The area should be well soaked with the disinfectant. A simple check is to apply the disinfectant repeatedly and discard the applicator (gauze or cotton swabs) after each "scrub" until the applicator material remains white. Soaking the site with alcohol also helps visualization of the vein.

Jugular Vein

Equipment needed for jugular venipuncture:
- Alcohol and 4×4 gauze pads
- 16- or 18- gauge (ga) × 1½-inch needle
- Syringe or Vacutainer (BD, Franklin Lakes, N.J.) system
- Appropriate blood tubes

The jugular vein is one of the most common locations for venipuncture (Fig. 13-1). It is the largest-diameter and most accessible vein and is safest for the technician when the head is properly restrained. Preferably, the head is pulled up and slightly to the opposite side from the technician; this requires use of a halter or nose tongs. A head that is pulled extremely to the side may make distention of the vein difficult to see.

Young calves may be restrained standing or placed in lateral recumbency. If a calf is standing, the head needs to be held tightly against the restrainer's body, with care taken not to wrap the arms around the neck where they may interfere with access and distention of the jugular vein. If the blood draw is to be performed in a recumbent animal, care should be taken not to injure the eyes.

After the site is cleaned, the vein is distended by placing all the fingers or a fist firmly into the jugular groove. The diameter of the jugular vein is quite large (1 to 2 inches), and the vein cannot be completely occluded using just one finger or one thumb (Fig. 13-2). One should allow enough time for the vein to fill so that it can be readily seen. While one hand maintains distention, the other hand places a 16- or 18-gauge (ga), 1½-inch needle through the skin and into the vein at a 45-degree angle to the skin surface. This should be done in one swift, committed motion, noting that bovine skin may be somewhat thicker than expected. The needle can be placed in either direction (cranially or caudally) for withdrawal of blood, depending on personal preference. Similarly, depending on preference, the needle can be placed alone and then the syringe attached when placement in the vein is confirmed, or both can be placed as a single unit.

> **TECHNICIAN NOTE**   Distention of the vein should be performed with the fist or with all the fingers.

Distention of the vein is maintained while blood is collected into an attached syringe or Vacutainer (BD) tube. Once the sample is collected, the distention is released, and the needle is withdrawn. Digital pressure is applied directly to the site for 15 to 30 seconds to discourage *hematoma* formation. The head restraint may then be released.

Coccygeal (Tail) Vein

Equipment needed for coccygeal venipuncture:
- Alcohol and 4×4 gauze pads
- 18-, 19-, or 20-ga, 1- to 1½-inch needle
- Syringe or Vacutainer (BD) system

The tail vein is another common location for blood collection because it is easily accessed if the animal has limited side-to-side mobility and the technician can be safely positioned to avoid a kick. Cattle are generally more tolerant of venipuncture in the tail than in the neck. Tail restraint is applied with one hand, by using the vertical tail hold or "jack." This also positions the tail for venipuncture (note that

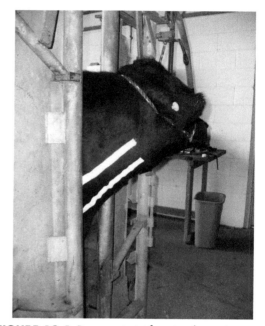

FIGURE 13-1 Proper restraint for a jugular venipuncture.

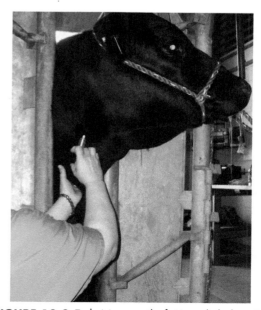

FIGURE 13-2 Technician uses the fist to occlude the vein.

venipuncture cannot be performed with the tail twisted). The other hand is used to clean the site with alcohol and perform the venipuncture. Without proper cleaning of this site, fecal contamination of the sample is inevitable.

> **TECHNICIAN NOTE** Cattle are generally more tolerant of tail venipuncture than neck venipuncture.

Because the diameter of the tail vein is considerably smaller than that of the jugular vein, needles larger than 18 ga should not be used. An 18-, 19-, or 20-ga, 1- to 1½-inch needle is used. Usually, the syringe is left attached during the procedure (Fig. 13-3). The procedure is best performed in the proximal third of the tail, directly on the ventral midline of the tail. The coccygeal vertebrae in this area have hemal processes (arches), which are bony canals on the ventral aspect of the vertebral bodies. The hemal processes protect the coccygeal artery and vein, which run through the canal; therefore, venipuncture must be done between the vertebrae, where no hemal

processes are present. The hemal processes are easily felt on the ventral midline as firm, bony protrusions (Fig. 13-4).

The soft space between any two hemal processes is palpated, and the needle is directed into the space at a 45- to 90-degree angle to the skin. The needle is advanced while aspirating gently on the syringe; the vessels are generally encountered ½ to 1 inch beneath the skin. If the needle contacts bone, slowly retract the needle and continue to aspirate. Once the needle bevel is in the lumen of the vein, maintain the position while withdrawing the blood sample (Fig. 13-5).

The needle is withdrawn, and the tail is lowered. Digital pressure is kept over the site for approximately 15 seconds to discourage hematoma formation. Occasionally, the coccygeal

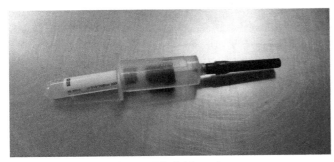

FIGURE 13-3 Vacutainer.

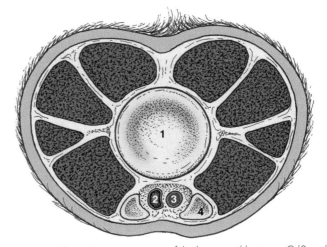

FIGURE 13-4 Transverse section of the bovine tail between Cd3 and Cd4. *1*, Intervertebral disk; *2*, median caudal vein; *3*, median caudal artery; *4*, hemal process. (From Dyce KM, Sack WO, Wensing CJG: *Textbook of veterinary anatomy*, ed 4, St. Louis, 2010, Saunders.)

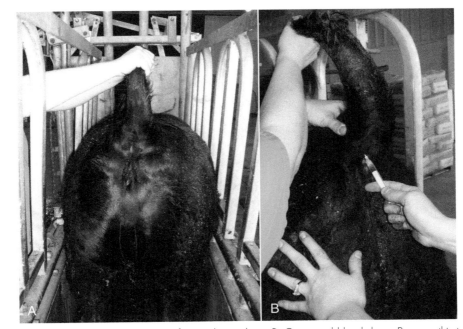

FIGURE 13-5 A, Proper positioning for a tail vein draw. **B,** Coccygeal blood draw. Because this tail is slightly twisted, the needle should be removed and replaced.

artery is entered accidentally during the procedure; this usually presents no problem other than hematoma formation. If the artery is entered, digital pressure over the site should be maintained for 45 to 60 seconds.

> **TECHNICIAN NOTE**   If the artery is entered, digital pressure should be applied to the site for 45 to 60 seconds.

Subcutaneous Abdominal (Milk) Vein

The right and left milk veins course along the ventrolateral body wall of the thorax and abdomen. They provide major venous drainage of the udder, especially during lactation. They are easily identified as large-diameter tubular structures just beneath the skin, with a pronounced tortuous (twisty) course (Fig. 13-6).

The milk veins appear inviting for venipuncture because of their large size; however, they are very prone to prolonged (sometimes pronounced) bleeding and large hematoma formation and should be used for blood sampling only when no other vein is available or suitable for sampling.

> **TECHNICIAN NOTE**   Even though milk veins are easily identified, they should be used only when no other vein is available or suitable for sampling. They are prone to prolonged bleeding and large hematoma formation.

Numerous other texts describe blood analysis in great detail and should be used as references for complete analysis. Table 13-1 lists normal complete blood count values. Table 13-2 lists normal blood chemistry values for cattle, and Table A2-3 in Appendix 2 is a guide to white blood cell (WBC) identification.

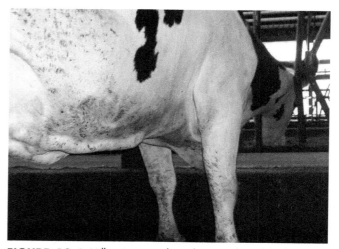

FIGURE 13-6 Milk vein seen along the ventrolateral body wall of the abdomen.

TABLE 13-1	Normal Complete Blood Count Values	
Packed cell volume (PCV) (%)	Increased with polycythemia, dehydration, stress, in neonates, and high globulin levels; decreased with anemia, bleeding, overhydration, and in weanlings	24–46 (35)
Hemoglobin (g/dL)	Increased with polycythemia; decreased with anemia	8–15 (12)
Red blood cell count ($\times 10^6/\mu L$)	Increased with polycythemia and dehydration; decreased with anemia, overhydration	5–10 (7)
Total protein (g/dL)	Increased in dehydration and in lipemic samples; decreased with overhydration	6–8
White blood cell count ($\times 10^3/\mu L$)	Increased with acute local inflammation, toxicity, and bacterial infections; decreased with marrow diseases, radiation, drug therapy, and certain viruses	4–12 (8)
Platelets ($\times 10^5/\mu L$)	Decreased in DIC, toxicities, bovine viral diarrhea	1–8 (5)
Mean corpuscular volume (MCV) (fL)	Increased with vitamin B_{12} and folic acid deficiency; decreased with iron deficiency	40–60 (52)
Mean corpuscular hemoglobin (MCH) (pg)	Increased with hemolysis; decreased with iron deficiency	14.4–18.6
Mean corpuscular hemoglobin concentration (MCHC) (g/gL)	Increased with hemolysis, lipemia, and Heinz bodies.	30–36 (32.7)
Bone marrow myeloid-to-erythrocyte (M:E) ratio		0.31–1.85:1 (0.71:1)
Differential, Absolute		
Segs		15%–45% 600–4000 (7000)
Bands		0%–2% 0–120 (20)
Lymphocytes		45%–75% 2500–7500 (4500)
Monocytes		2%–7% 25–840 (400)
Eosinophils		2%–20% 0–2400 (700)
Basophils		0%–2% 0–200 (50)

DIC, Disseminated intravascular coagulation.

ARTERIAL BLOOD SAMPLING

Arterial sampling is difficult in awake animals, even when they are well restrained. Blood can be drawn from the brachial and femoral arteries on the limbs or from the auricular (ear) arteries. The auricular arteries and palpable peripheral limb arteries may be accessible in anesthetized patients.

ABDOMINOCENTESIS

Equipment needed for abdominocentesis:
- Clippers
- Surgical scrub and alcohol
- 18- to 20-ga × 1½- to 3-inch needle or canula
- Red top tube

Abdominal (peritoneal) fluid is collected from the most dependent portion of the ventral abdomen. However, the procedure in adults is performed slightly to the right of ventral midline (3 to 5 cm) to avoid the rumen. Sometimes the location of the procedure is altered based on the suspected abdominal disease; in these cases, the clinician will indicate where the abdomen should be prepared.

The site should be clipped and sterilely prepared. A needle or cannula at least 1½ to 3 inches long must be used to penetrate the abdominal wall of cattle. Needle diameter may range from 18 to 20 ga. The milk veins (subcutaneous abdominal veins) must be avoided (Fig. 13-7).

RUMEN FLUID COLLECTION

Equipment needed for rumen fluid collection:
- Clippers
- Surgical scrub and alcohol
- 18- to 20-ga × 1½- to 3-inch needle or canula
- Red top tube

Rumen fluid analysis can aid in the diagnosis of diseases of the forestomachs. The sample can be obtained by the orogastric (otherwise known as *ororumen*) route, by passage of an orogastric tube, or directly through the lower left abdominal wall by *rumenocentesis*.

Rumenocentesis is performed with a 14-ga needle through a site caudal to the xiphoid process and left of ventral midline. The site should be clipped and sterilely prepared. The clinician inserts the needle through the skin, into the rumen, and aspirates the rumen fluid with a syringe.

Rumen fluid may be analyzed for color, pH, odor, identification, and assessment of microbial organisms and numbers, and electrolyte levels. Normal rumen fluid is green, has a "sweet pungent" fermented odor, and should contain a mixed population of actively motile protozoa. The pH generally ranges from 6.5 to 7.5.

TABLE 13-2	Normal Blood Chemistry Values	
VALUE	**COMMENTS**	**RANGE**
Blood urea nitrogen (mg/dL)	Increased with kidney disease, azotemia, and uremia	7.8–24.6
Creatinine (mg/dL)	Increased with kidney disease	0.6–1.8
Glucose (mg/dL)	Decreased in fatty liver disease; increased with diabetes and stress	42.1–74.5
Albumin (g/dL)	Increased with dehydration; decreased with brucellosis, chronic liver disease, glomerular disease, hyperglobulinemia, hypertension, malnutrition, and malabsorption	2.8–3.9
Total bilirubin (mg/dL)	Increased in animals with liver disease, bile duct obstruction, jaundice, or hemolytic anemia	0–0.8
Aspartate aminotransferase (AST) (μg/L)	Increased in liver disease or with muscle damage; can be increased after exercise	45.3–110.2
γ-Glutamyltransferase (GGT) (μg/L)	Increased with hepatocellular and cholestatic liver disease, hepatocyte necrosis, and cholestasis	4.9–25.7
Creatine kinase (μg/L)	Increased with muscle disease	14.4–107
Alkaline phosphatase (μg/L)	Increased with liver disease and cholestasis, steroids, and growth	17.5–152.7
Lactate dehydrogenase (LDH) (μg/L)	Increased with hepatocyte damage, muscle damage, and hemolysis	308.6–938.1
Sodium (mEq/L)	When increased can cause neurologic disorders and hypertension; decreases can be caused by *Escherichia coli*, polyuria or polydipsia, weight loss, and anorexia	134.5–148.1
Potassium (mEq/L)	Increases can be caused by severe metabolic acidosis; decreases can be caused by anorexia, increased renal excretion, abomasal stasis, intestinal obstruction, enteritis, and weight loss	4–5.8
Chloride (mEq/L)	Increased during displaced abomasums	95.7–108.6
Calcium (mg/dL)	Increased with kidney stones, renal failure, and some cancers; decreased in milk fever, renal disease, and bone disease	8.4–11
Phosphorus (mg/dL)	Increased in renal failure; decreased with osteomalacia, rickets, and tetany	4.3–7.8
Magnesium (mg/dL)	Decreased in milk fever, grass tetany, fever, and hypersalivation	1.7–3

From Aiello SE: *The Merck veterinary manual*, ed 8, Whitehouse Station, N.J., 1998, Merck & Co.

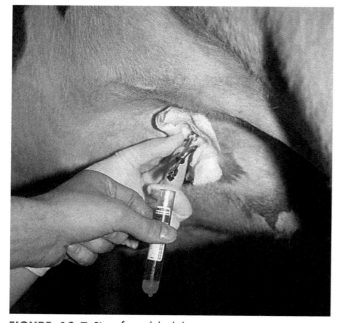

FIGURE 13-7 Site of caudal abdominocentesis. (From Smith BP: *Large animal internal medicine*, ed 4, St. Louis, 2008, Mosby.)

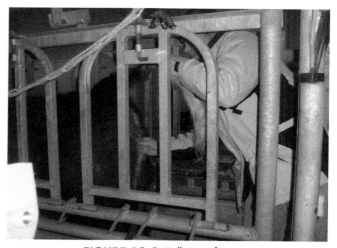

FIGURE 13-8 Titillation of a cow.

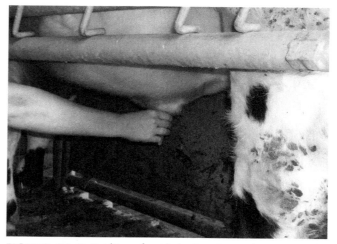

FIGURE 13-9 Catching of voided urine. Some clinicians use the threads of a capped tube to rub the inside of the sheath, thus stimulating urination in males.

URINE COLLECTION

The technician should be on high alert once an animal is in the chute. Urination may occur at any time in the chute, and you may miss the opportunity to catch some urine if you are not paying attention. Cows can be stimulated to urinate, but volume is the problem if they have already urinated. Steers and bulls have no real reliable method of stimulation, and sometimes you must just wait for the opportunity so save yourself some time and just catch some urine if it presents itself. Urine is collected either by catching a voided sample or by bladder catheterization through the urethra. Cystocentesis is possible in calves but is seldom performed.

> **TECHNICIAN NOTE** Cystocentesis is possible in calves but is seldom performed.

Voided Urine Sampling
Sterile Collection Container

In cattle, females may be encouraged to urinate by "*titillating*," which is a method of stimulating the perineal area (Fig. 13-8). The skin beneath the vulva is lightly stroked with the fingers or with straw until urination occurs. The tail should not be held during the procedure so as not to distract the cow. If at all possible it is best not to touch the cow anywhere other than the perineal area. If this method does not work, repeated parting of the lips of the vulva may be effective. The initial urine stream is not collected because it contains more "contaminants" (debris and bacteria). A midstream sample is preferred and is collected into a clean container. If bacterial culture is to be performed, the container should be sterile.

Urine stimulation in males is difficult. Manual stimulation of the prepuce is sometimes effective. This can be done by running your finger on the inside of the sheath. A capped tube with threads is rubbed on the inside of the sheath to stimulate urination in males (Fig. 13-9).

> **TECHNICIAN NOTE** Some clinicians have success obtaining a voided sample from males by rubbing the inside of the sheath with the threads of a capped tube.

Bladder or Urethral Catheterization
Female Catheterization

Equipment needed for female urethral catheterization:
- Warm water
- Surgical scrub
- Sterile gloves
- Sterile lubricating jelly

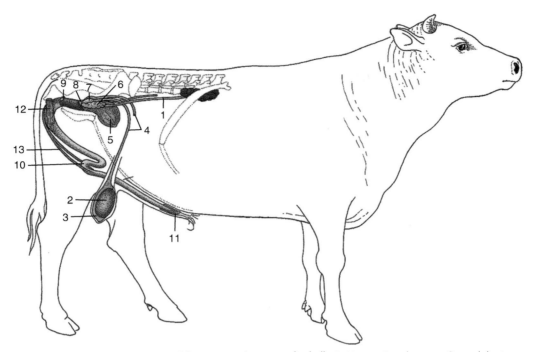

FIGURE 13-10 Disposition of the urogenital organs of a bull. *1,* Ureter; *2,* right testis; *3,* epididymis; *4,* deferent duct; *5,* bladder; *6,* vesicular gland; *7,* ampulla of deferent duct; *8,* body of prostate; *9,* bulbo-urethral gland; *10,* sigmoid flexure of penis; *11,* glans penis; *12,* ischiocavernosus; *13,* retractor penis. (From Dyce KM, Sack WO, Wensing CJG: *Textbook of veterinary anatomy,* ed 4, St. Louis, 2010, Saunders.)

- Urinary catheter, 12 to 20 French
- Sterile collecting container

The procedure for catheterization of the female urethra is similar to that in the mare and is performed in the most sterile manner possible. The animal must be properly restrained. The tail must be held or tied out of the way for the entire procedure. The vulva is prepared with warm water and antiseptic soap or solution. The clinician wears sterile gloves and uses sterile lubricating jelly to pass a hand or the fingers into the vestibule of the vagina. The urethral opening is generally within 5 to 10 cm of the vulva (depending on the size of the animal) and opens on the ventral midline. A suitable catheter is placed into the urethral entrance and is advanced into the bladder.

Female ruminants have a small blind "sac" extending from the ventral aspect of the urethra *(suburethral diverticulum)* that will prevent passage of the catheter if it accidentally enters the sac. If resistance is encountered, simply withdraw the catheter slightly and redirect it in a more dorsal direction. Once the catheter is in the bladder, urine can be collected by gravity flow or by aspirating with a sterile syringe.

> **TECHNICIAN NOTE** Female ruminants have a small blind "sac," called the suburethral diverticulum, that extends from the ventral aspect of the urethra.

Adult cows can be catheterized with a rigid or a flexible urinary catheter. A 12- to 20-French diameter is suitable. Urinary catheters should always be sterile.

> **TECHNICIAN NOTE** If a urine cup is not available, the outside casing of a 60-mL syringe can easily be used to hold a urine sample. The cap can be replaced and taped in place.

Male Catheterization

Bladder catheterization in male cattle is virtually impossible by the urethral route because cattle have a sigmoid flexure and the urethra is extremely long (Fig. 13-10).

FECAL COLLECTION

> **TECHNICIAN NOTE** Equipment needed for fecal collection:
> - Glove
> - Lubrication

Fecal collection should be performed with a gloved hand. The technician should either take samples from the ground if not contaminated or lubricate the hand and obtain a sample from the rectum (Fig. 13-11, *A*). To obtain a sample from the rectum, lubricate the gloved hand and place the fingers together so that all the fingers and thumbs are touching. Gently insert the hand into the rectum. Never use extreme force to gain entrance to the rectum. It is not necessary to enter the rectum at great lengths; enter just enough to wipe the rectum wall with the fingers. Never separate the fingers. Just scope the rectum and remove the hand. It is common to turn the glove inside out and tie the top

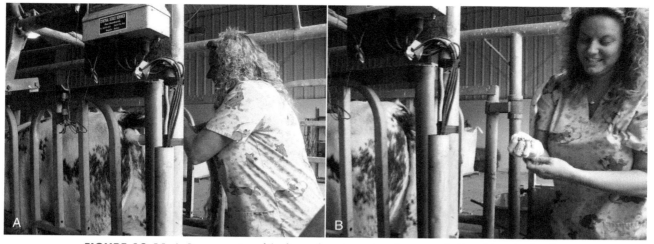

FIGURE 13-11 **A,** Proper position of the fingers for entrance into the rectum. **B,** Use of the other hand to grab the inside of the glove and begin turning it inside out.

of the glove to keep the sample until return to the clinic or until the sample arrives at the laboratory (Fig. 13-11, *B*).

Tritrichomonas foetus collection
Equipment needed for *Tritrichomonas foetus* sampling:
- *Tritrichomonas* collection tube
- 20- or 30-mL syringe
- Sterile water
- Tritrichomonas testing media tube

Tritrichomonas foetus sampling is performed on bulls to determine whether the organism is present in the smegma or preputial fluid. Collection from the uterine or vaginal fluid is possible from cows, but because the organism is transient in the female, collection from the bull is more common. After collection of the sample, the organisms can be observed by direct microscopic examination, by examination of culture media inoculated with infected material, or by polymerase chain reaction.

The preferred sample is from the glans penis. To collect the sample, the sterile *Tritrichomonas* sample pipette is inserted into the sheath of the bull, and a vigorous back and forth scraping motion is performed along the glans while applying negative pressure to a 20- or 30-mL syringe. Some laboratories prefer that you use sterile water to help flush the smegma from the area and then use negative pressure to collect the sample. Make sure you check with your laboratory or instructions on your testing media.

Testing from the female is from the cervical mucus or uterine secretions. These samples are collected by inserting a sterile insemination pipette and applying negative pressure using a 20- or 30-mL syringe. The material collected is then inoculated into the appropriate medium.

The two most common media are the InPouch medium (BioMed Diagnostics, White City, Ore.) and the TF transit tubes (BioMed Diagnostics). When using InPouch medium, at least 5 mm of sample should be placed in the bottom of the bag. For samples collected using TF transit tubes, the sample volume should be between 0.5 and 1.0 mL of smegma scrapings.

For instructions following collection, contact your diagnostic laboratory. Many laboratories will have you incubate the samples before sending. Special instructions and their preferences can be obtained from the laboratory to which you are submitting samples.

CEREBROSPINAL FLUID SAMPLING
Equipment needed for cerebrospinal fluid collection:
- Sedative, needles, and syringes
- Clippers
- Surgical scrub and alcohol
- Rope if recumbent
- 18- to 20-ga needle × 3-inch spinal needle
- Syringe
- Red top tube

Cerebrospinal fluid samples can be collected from either the atlantooccipital space (i.e., cisterna magna) or the lumbosacral space, using the same landmarks as described for horses (Fig. 13-12). The animal must be heavily sedated or under general anesthesia for use of either location. The atlantooccipital space is accessed only with the animal in lateral recumbency, with the head ventroflexed as much as possible. The lumbosacral space is also accessed in lateral recumbency with the spine ventroflexed. In older calves and adult cattle, the lumbosacral tap can be performed in a standing, sedated animal if very secure restraint is available.

Regardless of patient positioning, attention must be given to keeping the spine in a straight alignment, because any lateral deviations make the procedure difficult. Needle diameter for either location can be either 18 or 20 ga. The lumbosacral space is not as deep as in the horse; a 3½-inch length spinal needle is suitable for most ruminants (including adult cattle).

MILK SAMPLING
Equipment for milk sampling:
- Predip solution
- Paper towels

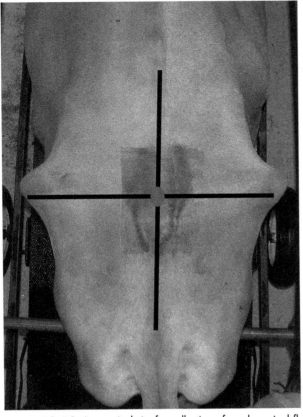

FIGURE 13-12 Anatomical site for collection of cerebrospinal fluid (CSF) at the lumbosacral space. The spinal needle is slowly inserted perpendicular to the point where a line drawn between the caudal aspects of the two tuber coxae intersects the midline (between L6 and S1 vertebrae). The animal may react (twitching) when the spinal needle passes through the interarcuate ligament and penetrates the extradural space. At this time, a loss of resistance is felt. The needle is further inserted to reach the subarachnoid space. A gentle negative pressure can be applied to withdraw the CSF into a syringe. (From Anderson DE, Rings DM: *Current veterinary therapy: food animal practice,* ed 5, St. Louis, 2008, Saunders.)

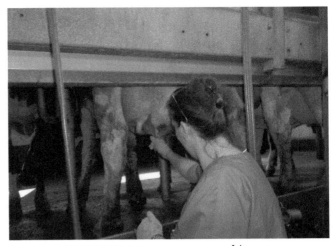

FIGURE 13-13 Proper stripping of the teats.

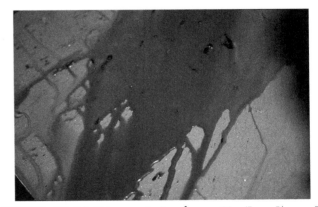

FIGURE 13-14 Strip examination for mastitis. (From Blowey R, Weaver A: *Color atlas of diseases and disorders of cattle,* ed 3, St. Louis, 2012, Mosby.)

- Sterile collection container
- Postdip solution

Milk sampling is often performed in dairy cattle suspected of having *mastitis.* Milk sampling for mastitis is done by hand milking.

The basic procedure for hand milking is as follows:

1. Palpate the udder and teats. The classic clinical sign of mastitis is a hard, hot, and often painful quarter.
2. Wash teats with a sanitizing solution.
3. Dry teats thoroughly with individual paper towels for each teat.
4. Grasp the teat at its base by gently but firmly "pinching" it between the thumb and first or second finger (Fig. 13-13).
5. While maintaining the "pinch," slide the pinch down the teat, toward the teat end. Any milk in the teat canal has only one way out—the teat orifice—because the finger pinch prevents it from moving backward.
6. The "sliding pinch" can be repeated as many times as needed to collect the desired volume of milk. The pinch must be totally released when the fingers are returned to the base of the teat.

Mastitis Tests
Strip Cup (Plate) Examination
Equipment for strip cup examination:
- Strip cup

The strip cup is a special milk collection cup with a black lid (see Fig. 15-19 in Chapter 15). The first milk that is expressed from the teat, called the foremilk, should be squirted onto the black lid and observed for abnormalities and odor. Normal milk should be watery, chalky colored, and free of solid clumps; it should not have a sour or fetid odor. Clumps (see Fig. 15-20 in Chapter 15), clots, flakes, abnormal color, blood (Fig. 13-14), and bad odor all are indicators of possible mastitis. Strip cup examination is an important screening test but detects only "clinical mastitis" (obvious clinical signs); it does not detect *subclinical mastitis* (without visible clinical signs). Further testing is necessary to confirm the disease. Some studies indicate that in any given herd, 90% to 95% of the cows or heifers will test positive for subclinical mastitis.

Somatic Cell Counts

Equipment for somatic cell counts:
- Milk cell counter
- Milk collection container

Leukocytes and epithelial cells enter the mammary gland as a result of damage secondary to inflammation caused by mastitis. The amount of mammary inflammation can be indirectly measured through a somatic cell count (SCC). A milk cell counter stains the cells with a fluorescent dye and then rapidly counts the number of cells. Measurements are taken from each quarter, each cow, or the bulk tank. The SCC is not a direct test for mastitis because several other factors (e.g., stress and antibiotics) can affect the SCC.

California Mastitis Test

Equipment for the California mastitis test:
- California mastitis test kit
- Paddle
- Reagent

The California mastitis test (CMT) is one of the most commonly used field tests to identify individual cows affected with mastitis. The test specifically identifies which quarters (or halves) are affected. This is important because mastitis seldom involves an entire udder; more commonly, only one or two quarters will be diseased. The test is sensitive enough to detect subclinical mastitis and roughly quantifies the severity of inflammation. Inflammation in the udder stimulates migration of WBCs into the affected gland and causes the death of some of the epithelial (milk-producing) cells of the affected gland. These sloughed epithelial cells and WBCs, referred to as "somatic cells," enter the milk, where they may be detected. The CMT basically uses detergent chemicals to lyse somatic cells in the milk, a process that releases their DNA. The test then detects the released DNA by changes in the consistency of the tested milk. The consistency reflects the SCC of the milk; the higher the count, the more severe the inflammation.

The test uses a white plastic test "paddle" with four cups labeled A to D (Fig. 13-15). The test should not be performed on the foremilk, which typically contains higher SCCs, even in normal milk. The udder is cleaned, and the foremilk is discarded. Then, each quarter is milked into a separate paddle cup. Only enough milk to cover the bottom of the cup is necessary (2 to 3 mL). One way to ensure the proper volume of milk is to fill all the cups with several squirts of milk, then briefly tilt the paddle vertically so that excess milk spills from the cup. The test reagent is then added, using an equal volume of reagent as milk in each cup (see Fig. 15-24 in Chapter 15). The paddle is kept horizontal and is gently moved in a circular path to produce swirling of the cup contents. The test is read after about 10 seconds of mixing while the technician continues to swirl the paddle. Interpretation must be prompt because mild positive reactions tend to disappear after 20 to 30 seconds.

Accurate recording of the results is important for identifying which quarters are affected and require treatment. The paddle has a handle, which should be consistently pointed in the same direction (relative to the cow) so that the technician can always be sure which teats correspond to which sample cup. For instance, if the handle is always pointed toward the cow's head, then the results can be accurately recorded no matter which side of the cow the technician stood on to take the samples.

Interpretation of the CMT involves two variables: changes in consistency and changes in color. Consistency changes correspond to the SCC and are placed into one of five possible categories (Fig. 13-16 and Tables 13-3 and 13-4). Color changes correspond to the pH of the mixture. The test reagent contains bromcresol purple, a pH indicator that remains purple in alkaline conditions and turns yellow in acidic conditions (pH 5.2). A grade of "+" is given for alkaline milk and "Y" for acidic milk. Acidic milk is unusual. Normal milk has a pH of 6.4 to 6.8.

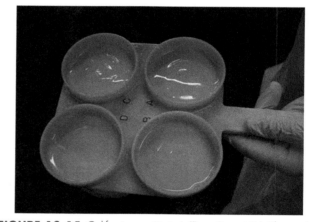

FIGURE 13-15 California mastitis test. (From Bassert JM, Thomas JA, editors: *McCurnin's clinical textbook for veterinary technicians,* ed 8, St. Louis, 2013, Saunders.)

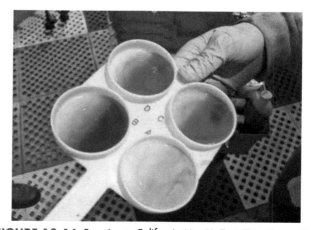

FIGURE 13-16 Reaction to California Mastitis Test. (From Bassert JM, Thomas JA, editors: *McCurnin's clinical textbook for veterinary technicians,* ed 8, St. Louis, 2013, Saunders.)

To interpret results of the California mastitis test, technicians observe the consistency and color changes that occur within the sample.

False-positive CMT results may occur in late lactation, during estrus, and when the foremilk is tested; the SCC tends to be naturally high in all these situations. In addition, trauma to the udder or teat elevates the SCC, thereby indicating inflammation but not necessarily infection.

Positive quarters usually are treated with oxytocin and a thorough milk-out or intramammary infusion.

Wisconsin Mastitis Test

Equipment for the Wisconsin mastitis test:
- Milk collection container
- Wisconsin mastitis test

The Wisconsin mastitis test (WMT) is commonly used by milk receiving plants to measure the quality of the farm bulk tank milk sample picked up by the milk hauler. The principle of the WMT is the same as that of the CMT. Instead of a subjective rating, in the WMT the amount of gel that forms is measured in millimeters that remain in a calibrated tube. The WMT is conducted under more precise procedures and standard temperature conditions.

Milk Culture and Sensitivity

Equipment for milk culture and sensitivity testing:
- Sterile glass tubes with screw caps

Milk culture is seldom necessary to confirm the diagnosis of mastitis, but it may be helpful for screening a herd for subclinical cases or identifying the bacteria in cases that are severe or refractory to routine antibiotic therapy. Samples may be collected individually from each quarter, or all four quarters may be pooled together for a screening sample for each animal.

Samples should be collected into sterile tubes; glass tubes with screw caps are preferred. Tubes should be labeled and paperwork finished before the procedure. Box 13-1 details the sample collection process.

MEDICATION TECHNIQUES

ORAL MEDICATION

Some oral medications can be placed in the water source or mixed with food. This can be done for individual animals or on a herd basis. However, this is not a reliable method of delivering most medications. When delivery of medication to individual animals or control doses for each animal must be ensured, medication administration techniques for individuals must be used.

TECHNICIAN NOTE Placing medications in food or water is not a reliable method of delivering most medications.

TABLE 13-4	California Mastitis Test: Interpretation of Results
TEST SCORE	**INTERPRETATION IN CATTLE**
N	Normal (0–200,000 cells/mL)
T	Normal (150,000–500,000 cells/mL)
1	Suspicious (500,000–1,500,000 cells/mL)
2	Mastitis (1,500,000–5,000,000 cells/mL)
3	Mastitis (>5,000,000 cells/mL)

TABLE 13-3	California Mastitis Test: Grading Test Reactions		
SYMBOL	**SUGGESTED MEANING**	**DESCRIPTION OF VISIBLE REACTION**	**"QUICKIE" DESCRIPTION**
N	Negative	Mixture remains liquid with no evidence of formation of a precipitate.	Water
T	Trace	Slight precipitate forms and is best seen by tipping the paddle back and forth and observing the mixture as it flows over the bottom of the cup. Trace reactions tend to disappear with continued movement of the fluid.	Slime
+1	Weak positive	Distinct precipitate forms, but there is no tendency for gel formation. The precipitate may disappear with continued movement of the paddle.	Thick slime
+2	Distinct positive	Mixture thickens immediately with some suggestion of gel formation. As the mixture is swirled, it tends to move and twirl the center of the cup, leaving the bottom of the outer edge of the cup exposed. When the motion is stopped, the mixture levels out again and covers the bottom of the cup.	Gel
+3	Strong positive	Gel is formed, causing the surface of the mixture to become convex. Usually a central peak projects above the main mass after motion of the paddle has stopped. Viscosity is greatly increased so that the mass tends to adhere to the bottom of the cup.	Jelly

1. Wash hands thoroughly, and put on examination gloves to reduce the chances of environmental contamination.
2. Wash teats in a sanitizing solution, and dry teats with individual paper towels.
3. Strip and discard one to two squirts of milk from each teat.
4. Dip teats in germicidal teat dip, and allow 30 seconds of contact time. Dry each teat with an individual paper towel.
5. Thoroughly clean the teat orifice with a cotton swab soaked in alcohol. Begin with the far teats, then the near teats (prevents contaminating the near teats when reaching across to swab the far side).
6. Open the sterile tube, and hold it at a 45-degree angle so that debris cannot fall into the tube. Do not allow anything to touch the opening of the tube. Collect one to two squirts from each quarter. Begin with the near teats, then collect the far teats.
7. Cap the tube immediately.
8. Tubes should be refrigerated (4° C [39° F]), not frozen, until they can be processed in the laboratory. Processing should occur within 24 hours by swabbing on a blood agar plate and should be followed by routine microbial culture methods. In rare cases when processing cannot be done within 24 hours, the samples should be frozen as soon as possible.

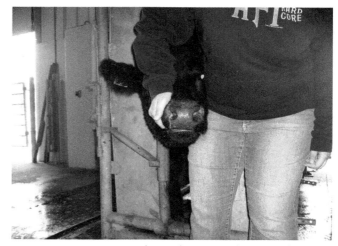

FIGURE 13-17 Proper technique for opening the mouth of cattle for balling gun insertion.

Balling Gun

The *balling gun* is an instrument used to deliver medication that is in capsule or bolus (large tablet) form. Balling guns are available in different sizes and are made of metal, plastic, or a combination of metal with a plastic tip. The instrument should be checked for sharp edges before it is used. Severe trauma (laceration, abscessation) to the pharynx, epiglottis, and oral cavity of the animal may result from poor technique.

> **TECHNICIAN NOTE**   Poor use of a balling gun can result in severe trauma to the pharynx, epiglottis, and oral cavity.

Head restraint is essential. Cattle are best placed in a head catch. With cooperative cattle, the operator can stand next to the head and can face in the same direction as the animal. Place one arm across and over the bridge of the animal's nose, and use the hand on that arm to reach in the interdental space to place pressure on the hard palate or to grasp the nostrils (Fig. 13-17). It has been my experience that grasping the nostrils upsets animals more than helps your cause. Use the other hand to operate the balling gun. The head of any species should not be elevated beyond a natural position (nose should not be higher than top of the head) to decrease the risk of accidental aspiration of medication into the trachea. If the animal is reluctant to open the mouth, pressing on the hard palate through the interdental space or putting

a finger or thumb in each nostril and elevating the nose may provide encouragement.

The balling gun (loaded with medication) is introduced into the side of the mouth through the interdental space, above the tongue. It is then redirected caudally and is advanced over the base of the tongue. Failure to deliver the medication over the tongue base will likely cause the animal to spit it out (Fig. 13-18). However, the gun should not be placed so far back that it wedges in the pharynx or larynx, where it can cause significant damage. The plunger of the instrument is pressed to "eject" the tablet into the mouth, and the balling gun is carefully removed with a smooth motion. Care should be taken not to slam on the plunger because you can cause severe damage to the pharynx and larynx. Attempts to hold the mouth shut until swallowing occurs can be attempted. I have found it is best just to hold up on the lower jaw. The animal is observed to ensure that all medication is swallowed.

The balling gun is not a suitable instrument for very young animals or for horses.

> **TECHNICIAN NOTE**   The balling gun is not a suitable instrument for very young animals or for horses.

Drenching

Delivery of liquid oral medication directly into the oral cavity is referred to as *drenching*. Liquid medications can be delivered with an oral dose syringe or 60-mL catheter-tip syringe by using a technique similar to passage of the balling gun. The tip of the syringe should be positioned over the base of the tongue to prevent spillage from the mouth (Fig. 13-19). The tip of the nose should not be held higher than the top of the head to minimize the risk of aspiration into the trachea. The liquid should not be injected with unnecessarily high pressure because this could "shoot" medication into the trachea. Rather, deliver the liquid slowly, and allow the animal time to swallow. If the animal coughs, stop the procedure until the animal has a chance to "clear its throat" and settle down.

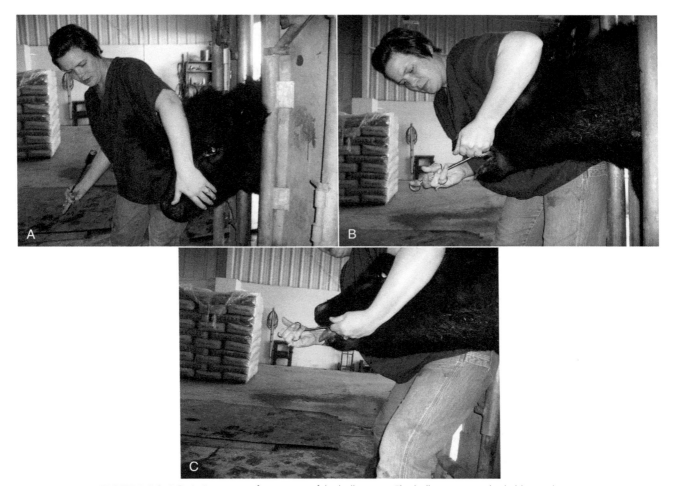

FIGURE 13-18 A, Preparation for insertion of the balling gun. The balling gun must be held tipped up to prevent the pill from falling out. **B,** Insertion of the balling gun into the oral cavity. **C,** Administration of medication by depressing the plunger.

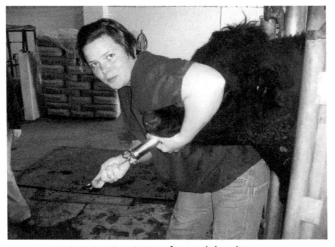

FIGURE 13-19 Use of an oral drenching gun.

> **TECHNICIAN NOTE**   The tip of the nose should never be held higher than the top of the head during drenching.

Frick Speculum

The *Frick speculum* is a rigid metal tube that can be used as an oral or vaginal speculum in cattle. It is placed in the mouth in exactly the same fashion as a balling gun. Held in this position, it can be used to deliver boluses and liquids or assist passage of an orogastric (stomach) tube (Figs. 13-20 and 13-21).

The stainless steel construction allows the Frick speculum to be disinfected and sterilized.

Rumen (Gastric) Intubation

Large quantities of fluids can be delivered directly into the rumen or reticulum by passage of a stomach tube. Intubation is also used to relieve rumen bloat and can be used to withdraw samples of rumen fluid for analysis or transfer to other animals (rumen inoculation). The tube can be placed through the nasogastric or orogastric (ororumen) route. The nasogastric route is used in horses but is not commonly used in ruminants. The nasal passages of cattle are of smaller diameter than those in horses, which significantly limits the tube diameter that can be used. Therefore, the oral route is used most often (Fig. 13-22).

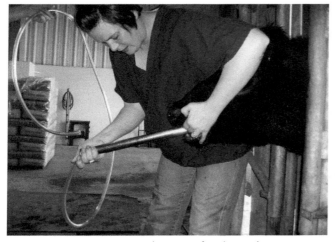

FIGURE 13-20 Placement of Frick speculum.

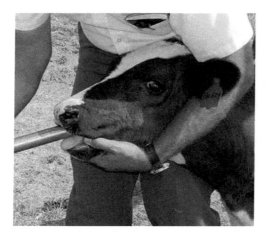

FIGURE 13-21 Frick speculum has been placed to allow passage of a stomach (ororumen) tube. (From Bassert JM, McCurnin DM, editors: *McCurnin's clinical textbook for veterinary technicians*, ed 7, St. Louis, 2010, Saunders.)

TECHNICIAN NOTE   The ororumen route is more popular in cattle than is the nasogastric route used in horses.

The mouth must first be held open with a speculum to keep the animal from damaging the tube. Various speculums are available commercially, and many can be easily homemade. In cattle, the Frick speculum is popular.

The stomach tube must be sized appropriately for length and diameter. The length of most commercially available tubes is sufficient to reach the rumen. The necessary length can be estimated by holding the tube outside the animal and simulating the distance from the mouth to the rumen. The outer diameter of the tube should be approximately ⅝ to 1 inch for adult cattle. A small or medium foal stomach tube is suitable for calves.

The tip and first portion of the tube should be lubricated with either water or a water-soluble lubricant. The speculum is placed and may need to be held by an assistant. The stomach tube is placed through the speculum and is advanced to the pharynx. Once the tube reaches the back of the pharynx, resistance is felt. The animal usually swallows at this time, and the tube is advanced into the esophagus with the swallow. It may be necessary to withdraw the tube slightly, rotate it slightly, and advance it again if the initial attempt fails. Coughing often indicates entry into the trachea, but this is not always 100% reliable. Feeling air pass out of the tube when the animal exhales may also indicate improper placement in the trachea, although this is also not always reliable. Proper placement in the esophagus is confirmed by palpating or observing the tube in the esophagus and feeling mild resistance as it is passed. The tube's location in the rumen is finally confirmed by noting the strong smell of rumen gas, aspirating rumen fluid, or having an assistant listen with a stethoscope over the rumen (left paralumbar fossa) while the operator blows air through the tube. The assistant should hear a gurgling sound with

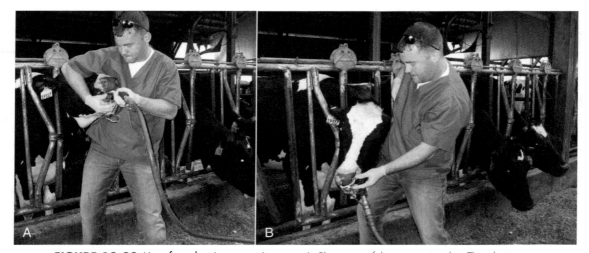

FIGURE 13-22 Use of an electric orogastric pump. **A,** Placement of the orogastric tube. The tube is covered with stainless steel rings to prevent the animal from chewing on the tube. **B,** Confirmation of placement by palpation of the neck.

the stethoscope. No material should be delivered through the tube until you are absolutely certain that the tube has reached the rumen.

Liquids can be given by gravity flow through a funnel, by dose syringe, or with a stomach pump. Water or air is then used to "clear" residual medication from the tube. Before the tube is removed, the end should be kinked off or occluded to prevent accidental spillage of its contents into the trachea and nasal passages as the tube is withdrawn. Removal should be done in a single, smooth motion.

> **TECHNICIAN NOTE** Proper placement of an oro-gastric tube is confirmed by palpation of the tube in the esophagus. If the tube cannot be felt, it most likely is in the trachea and is being protected by the cartilage rings.

Ruminants are capable of regurgitation. Passage of the tube may stimulate regurgitation. Regurgitation may occur through and around the stomach tube. Aspiration of the regurgitated liquid into the lungs is a real concern. For this reason, the head should not be forced into an elevated position during passage of the tube or while the tube is in the rumen. When it is time for tube removal, the end of the tube should be capped with your finger or the tube bent in half to prevent the aspiration of the tube content because it would drain out of the tube if the tube was not bent or capped. The tube should not be pulled out like a whip but rather pulled hand over hand.

PARENTERAL INJECTION TECHNIQUES
Intramuscular Injections

Research has shown that intramuscular (IM) injections usually cause scar tissue formation at the injection site. The scar tissue is visible and causes toughness in the meat, which may extend as much as 3 inches from the injection site. There is also the risk of abscessation. These "injection site blemishes" must be trimmed out of the meat when it is processed, thus decreasing the value of the carcass (Fig. 13-23). According to Beef Quality Assurance (BQA), in 2000, based on each steer

or heifer slaughtered, $3.59 per head was lost as a result of injection site lesions. In 2000, 30.31 million head of cattle were slaughtered. This resulted in a trend of avoiding IM injections into the muscles that yield valuable cuts of meat (hindlegs) and the development of subcutaneously injectable drugs (when possible) to replace IM medications.

BQA is a national program that provides guidelines for beef cattle production. The program raises consumer confidence through offering proper management techniques and a commitment to quality within every segment of the beef industry. Any question about withdrawal times when medications or vaccines are administered can be answered by contacting the Food Animal Residue Avoidance Databank (FARAD).

Producers have embraced BQA because it is the right thing to do, but they have also gained through increased profitability. As an educating program, BQA helps producers identify management processes that can be improved.

> **TECHNICIAN NOTE** Intramuscular injections cause injection site lesions that must be trimmed out of the meat during processing, thus reducing profits.

Table13-5 shows proper needle selection.

> **TECHNICIAN NOTE** Beef Quality Assurance guidelines should be followed for all livestock handling.

Injection guidelines include the following:
1. Use subcutaneous (SC) products whenever possible, instead of IM products (must be approved by the U.S. Food and Drug Administration for SC administration).
2. Use sharp, single-use, sterile 16- to 20-ga, 1- to 1½-inch-long needles (depending on size of animal, size of muscle, and "thickness" of medication). Generally, cattle require a 16- to 18-ga needle; calves require an 18- to 20-ga needle.

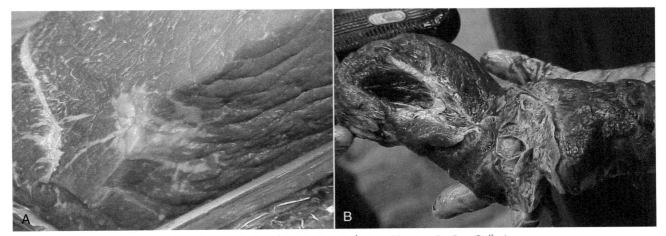

FIGURE 13-23 A and **B,** Injection site lesions. (Courtesy Dr. Dee Griffin.)

TABLE 13-5	Beef Quality Assurance Route of Administration Guidelines*								
	SUBCUTANEOUS ½-¾ INCH NEEDLE			INTRAVENOUS 1½ INCH NEEDLE			INTRAMUSCULAR 1-1½ INCH NEEDLE		
	CATTLE WEIGHT			CATTLE WEIGHT			CATTLE WEIGHT		
	<300	300–700	>700	<300	300–700	>700	<300	300–700	>700
Thin Measurements in gauge	18	18–16	16	18–16	16	16–14	20–18	18–16	18–16
Thick Measurements in gauge	18–16	18–16	16	16	16–14	16–14	18	16	16

Data from Beef Quality Assurance.
*Select the smallest gauge needle that will allow injection without bending.

3. Do not inject more than 10 mL per IM injection site in cattle.
4. Keep IM injection sites separated by at least 4 inches.
5. The preferred IM injection site is in front of the shoulder (lateral cervical area).
6. Avoid injecting through wet or dirty skin.
7. Do not use chemical disinfectants in syringes when using live virus product because these disinfectants decrease the effectiveness of the product.
8. Replace needles immediately after they bend or become burred, are contaminated with dirt or feces, and after every 10 to 15 head. Ideally, needles should be changed after each animal. Needles should be changed after use on each animal with a known blood-borne infectious disease. Under no circumstances can an animal carrying a broken needle be sold or sent to a packer. The needle can travel to consumable product areas and become lodged and enter the food supply. Animals with foreign needles are destroyed rather than sold.
9. Never mix products because doing so could extend the withdrawal time, reduce the effectiveness, or cause tissue damage.
10. Keep records of all injections, the amount, and the location.

Intramuscular Injection Sites

IM injection locations and techniques are similar to those used in the horse. Appropriate restraint should always be applied before injection. The site should always be cleaned (down to and including the skin) with 70% alcohol or other suitable antiseptic.

> **TECHNICIAN NOTE**   Whenever possible, injections should be given in the lateral cervical area. Other areas would compromise more valuable cuts of meat.

All IM injections should be made in the lateral cervical muscles to avoid valuable cuts of meat is the lateral cervical muscles. This site should be used whenever possible. To create the triangle, the slope of the shoulder, the nuchal ligament, and the vertebrae are used as boundaries (Fig. 13-24).

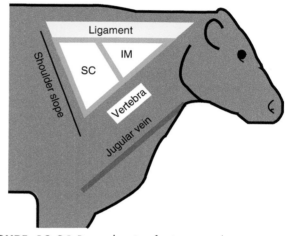

FIGURE 13-24 Proper location for intramuscular injections. The head of this animal is on the left. (Courtesy Dr. Dee Griffin.)

Intravenous Injections

The jugular vein is the preferred site to administer intravenous (IV) medications and fluids. Preparation for jugular IV injections is the same as for IV blood collection (Fig. 13-25). Some argument exists among veterinarians about which direction the needle is facing during an injection. Many believe that the needle should point toward the heart. However, others say that the direction of the needle does not matter.

After insertion of the needle, a bell IV setup can then be used to attach a bottle of medication to the IV needle and administer large volumes of medication.

The cephalic vein, caudal auricular vein, and coccygeal (tail) vein may also be used for small volumes of drugs. The coccygeal vein should not be used for any drug that causes irritation if accidentally given perivascularly. The coccygeal artery, which is the only arterial supply to the tail, lies adjacent to the vein; any tissue reaction (swelling, scarring) could compromise blood flow and possibly result in necrosis and sloughing of the tail.

Subcutaneous Injections

SC injections can be given anywhere that skin can be lifted with the fingers. In ruminants, the common locations

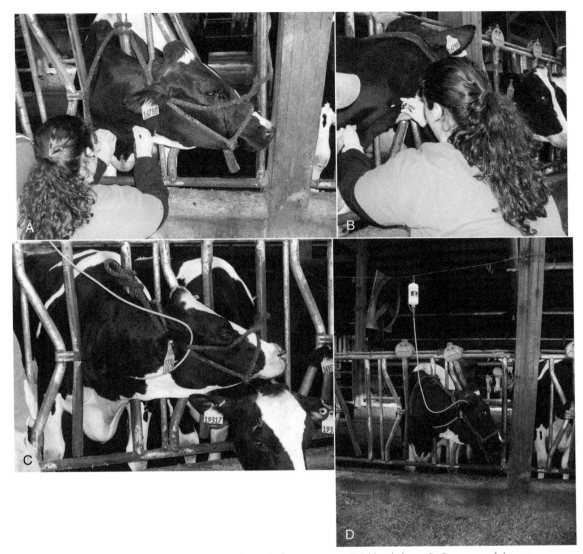

FIGURE 13-25 A, Proper direction of needle for intravenous (IV) blood draw. **B,** Distention of the vein and blood return from the needle after proper placement. **C,** Attachment of a bell IV line for administration of medication. **D,** Complete bell IV setup for administration of IV fluids.

are over the lateral cervical region, over the thorax several inches caudal to the shoulder, in the axilla, in the ventral aspect of the flank ("flank fold"), and in the pectoral area (brisket). The area over the scapula, just caudal to the scapular spine, is less often used. Injections into the back area are possible but are usually avoided because doing so devalues the hide.

Maximum injection volume is determined by location. Injected volumes usually are small, but up to 250 mL can be given at one site in adult cattle and up to 50 mL in calves. The use of large volumes tends to cause some leakage of the medication through the needle hole after the needle is withdrawn. Pinching or putting pressure over the needle hole may minimize this occurrence.

Restraint depends on the species and the location of the injection and should always be maximized to ensure that the technician does not inject himself or herself. As a general guideline, when giving injections to beef cattle, have only one hand in the chute. This allows the free hand to access chute release mechanisms in the event that you become pinned. Figure 13-26 illustrates the SC injection technique used to avoid tenting the skin in this type of system. When restraining calves in lateral recumbency, it is acceptable and expected for the technician to tent the skin.

Care of Automatic Dosing Syringes and Vaccines

Inadequate syringe care results in localized infections. Disposable multiple-dose syringes can be purchased and are ideal. If nondisposable syringes are used, the external portion of the syringe should be cleaned with soap and water. The syringe should then be rinsed with distilled or deionized water near boiling point (>180° F). The water should be squirted through the syringe at least three to five times. The syringe should be completely disassembled, and all the connectors, rings, and tubes should be cleaned. Do not use soap

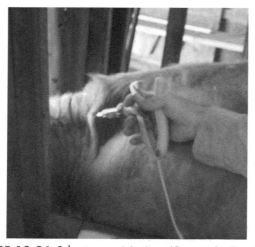

FIGURE 13-26 Subcutaneous injections. (Courtesy Dr. Dee Griffin.)

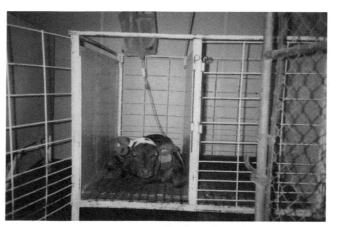

FIGURE 13-27 Calf with jugular catheter.

on internal components because the residues may kill modi-fied live virus (MLV) vaccines. The syringes should be dried and completely cool before they are used. Heat can kill MLV vaccines. Store the syringes in a dust-free, dry, low-humidity environment.

Vaccines should always be transported in a closed refrig-erated container. It is important to ensure that vaccines do not freeze. They should be kept cool while cattle are being processed. When mixing up vaccine, mix up the amount of vaccine that will be used in 1 hour.

Intradermal Injections

Injections into the dermis are more often used for diagnostic, rather than treatment, purposes. In ruminants, tuberculosis testing is the primary indication for intradermal (ID) injec-tions. The standard location for routine tuberculosis testing is the caudal tail fold. The right and left caudal tail folds are best seen by elevating the tail. This maneuver puts tension on the tail folds, which are located at the base of the tail. ID skin testing for allergic reactions is performed in the lateral cervical or flank area.

> **TECHNICIAN NOTE**   Intradermal injections are most commonly used for routine tuberculosis testing.

Hair, if present, must be clipped before injection. ID in-jections are performed by first cleaning the skin. Depend-ing on the material to be injected, antiseptics may or may not be used. Antiseptic residues may cause tissue reaction if injected intradermally, which can confuse proper interpreta-tion of skin tests. The skin should be allowed to dry before injection is given.

A 25- or 26-ga needle is used for the injection, although a 22- or 23-ga needle may be necessary in cattle for the thicker skin of the neck and flank. The skin is pinched firmly; the needle bevel should face outward toward the operator. The needle is held parallel to the pinched skin and is advanced into the dermis. Injection should produce a small bleb within

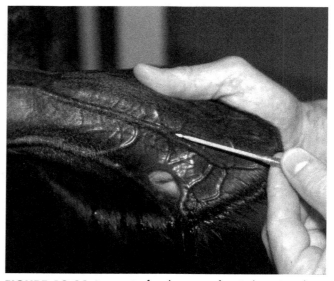

FIGURE 13-28 Proper site for placement of auricular vein catheter in the ear of a cow. To avoid kinking, the vein is entered distally so that the tip is at least 3 cm from the base of the ear when the entire catheter is inserted. (From Fubini S, Ducharme N: *Farm animal surgery,* St. Louis, 2004, Saunders.)

(not beneath) the skin. If a bleb is not seen, the needle likely is placed too deeply, and the injection procedure should be repeated.

Intravenous Catheterization

The jugular vein is the preferred site for IV catheterization in all ruminant species (Fig. 13-27). If the jugular veins are not usable, the cephalic veins can be used. The caudal au-ricular vein (ear vein) in adult cattle may accept a small-gauge catheter but is rarely feasible because of difficulties in stabilizing a catheter at that location (Fig. 13-28). The sub-cutaneous abdominal veins (milk veins) are not suitable for indwelling IV catheters. Catheter diameter may be 10 to 14 ga for cattle (18 to 20 ga for the ear vein), and 14 to 18 ga for calves. For small individuals, catheters 2 to 3 inches long can be used.

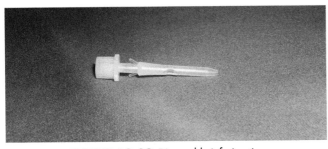

FIGURE 13-29 Disposable infusion tip.

> **TECHNICIAN NOTE** The jugular vein is the preferred site for intravenous catheterization.

Insertion technique and principles of maintaining the catheter are identical to those described for horses (see Chapter 9). Head restraint with a halter and nose tongs is desirable for catheterizing the ear vein.

Intramammary Infusion

Medications can be deposited (infused) into individual teats for treatment or prevention of diseases of the mammary glands. Antibiotics are by far the most common type of medication given by the intramammary route. They are most commonly used to treat active cases of mastitis in lactating cows ("wet cow treatment") or for treatment or prevention of mastitis in cows that are completing a lactation cycle ("dry cow treatment"). Mastitis primarily affects dairy cows, but all milk-producing females are susceptible.

> **TECHNICIAN NOTE** Antibiotics are by far the most common type of medication given by intramammary infusion.

Mammary infusions are usually purchased in disposable plastic syringes that are designed to treat a single teat and its associated gland. The syringe may come with an attached infusion tip, or a teat cannula or disposable plastic infusion tip may need to be placed on the end of the syringe (Fig. 13-29). Infusion tips, cannulas, or catheters should never be used on more than one teat unless they have been thoroughly cleaned and sterilized. Single-use, disposable plastic infusion tips are preferred and are inexpensive.

The standing position is preferred for all species. Dairy animals usually require minimal restraint, but occasionally the pain associated with mastitis causes the animal to resent handling of the affected gland. Applying a tail hold may be helpful in these cases. Nondairy animals should be approached with caution and require more secure restraint, typically using some form of chute restraint for cattle. The technician should not sit or be in a position where he or she could be injured by a kick.

> **TECHNICIAN NOTE** The technician should not sit or be in a position where he or she could be injured by a kick.

Because contact time must be maximized for the antibiotics to have their best effect, treatment is usually done after milking. Expressing all the milk in the affected gland also helps the infusion to distribute within the gland. "Mastitis milk" is contaminated with bacteria and should be collected in a container and then safely discarded to prevent environmental contamination.

Infusion of any material into the udder must be done as cleanly as possible. The hands should be washed with soap and water before the procedure. The teats and udder are washed with warm water and mild antiseptic soap, and each teat is dried with an individual cloth towel or paper towel (preferred) to prevent cross-contamination of the teats. Any residual milk is stripped from the teat. Each teat to be treated is dipped in a liquid germicidal teat dip and allowed 30 seconds of contact time before drying with an individual towel. Each teat orifice to be treated is then thoroughly cleaned with a cotton swab soaked in alcohol. Cranial teats should be swabbed first (to prevent contamination by the technician's arms when reaching across the udder). The alcohol is allowed to air dry. Infusion is performed in reverse order from cleansing (i.e., treat the near teats first, then reach across to treat the far teats) to prevent contaminating the clean teat ends.

> **TECHNICIAN NOTE** When cleaning teats for infusion, the cranial teats should be cleaned first. The infusion should take place in the caudal teats first. This helps prevent contamination of the teats by the technician's arms.

With one hand stabilizing the end of the teat, insert the infusion tip through the teat orifice. Driving the tip deeply into the teat canal is not necessary, and attempting to do so may cause injury and increase risk of contamination. Simply advance the tip just beyond the teat opening (⅛ to ¼ inch). Then use the stabilizing hand to gently pinch the teat orifice closed around the infusion tip, to prevent leakage of medication. Slowly depress the plunger to deliver the medication. After delivering the desired volume, withdraw the syringe and tip, and gently squeeze the teat end closed with one hand. Use the other hand to gently massage the medication up into the associated gland to help its distribution. Dip the teat again in a germicidal teat dip and allow it to air dry.

Whenever antibiotics or other medications are delivered by intramammary infusion, the milk is subject to a withdrawal time to allow for clearance of drug residues. The required withdrawal time varies with different antibiotics and should be printed on the package insert and on the individual infusion syringes. Placing a temporary marking on all treated animals is common practice to prevent accidental milking and contamination of the milk supply destined for human consumption.

Intranasal Administration

Some vaccines and a small number of medications are available for intranasal administration. They are administered by a method similar to that used in small animals. Head restraint is necessary. The nasal passage to be used should be cleared of any nasal exudates. The nose should be slightly elevated. The medication syringe (without needle!) is inserted just inside the nostril, and the plunger is depressed in one rapid motion. A common response of the animal is to throw its head upward; therefore, the technician should avoid positioning his or her body anywhere above the animal's head. Another common response of the animal is to sneeze, which expels some of the medication. This is usually of little consequence because pharmaceutical companies compensate for response by adding extra volume to the dose syringes.

> **TECHNICIAN NOTE**   A common response of cattle to intranasal injection is to throw their heads upward, so the technician should take care to avoid a head strike.

HOOF TRIMMING

Ruminants have cloven hooves, meaning that each limb has two weight-bearing digits, each with its own individual hoof (Fig. 13-30). The digits are commonly referred to as "claws." Hooves grow continuously during the life of the animal; the bovine hoof wall grows an average of 5 mm per month. Because of the difference in anatomy, cattle bear weight differently from horses. The difference in weight bearing leads to differences in types of lameness and how the hooves are trimmed. Normal movement of the animal wears away the hoof wall at various rates, depending on the nature of the ground surface and the activity level of the animal. Cattle bear most of their weight on the front feet, and the front medial claw bears the most weight. In the back feet, the lateral claw bears the most weight. Overgrowth may occur and require trimming to prevent potentially harmful deviations of the hoof, such as "corkscrew claws" and "scissor claws." Uneven growth can cause friction between the digits in the interdigital cleft, with resulting sores and abscesses and the possible development of foot rot.

Hoof trimming can be done on an as-needed basis or as part of a regular herd health program. Trimming may also be an essential part of the treatment of certain diseases such as foot rot. Cattle seldom allow the legs to be manually lifted and manipulated, and restraint can be a major problem. Cattle usually must be restrained in a chute and the legs lifted with ropes (see Chapter 2). Alternatively, they can be placed on a special mechanical or hydraulic "tilt table," which elevates the cattle off the ground and tips them into varying degrees of lateral recumbency. If none of these methods is available, a final option is to cast the animal with ropes.

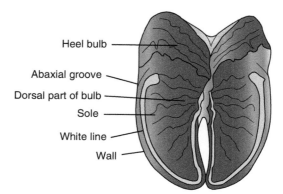

FIGURE 13-30 Ground surface of the hooves of the bovine forefoot. (Modified from Dyce KM, Sack WO, Wensing CJG: *Textbook of veterinary anatomy,* ed 3, St. Louis, 2002, Saunders.)

Various hoof knives, rasps, hoof nippers, hoof trimming shears, and curettes for trimming hooves are available. Motorized rotary burrs may be helpful; however, motorized equipment must be used carefully to prevent excessive heating of the internal tissues in the hoof. Instruments should be disinfected between animals to prevent spreading infectious bacterial and fungal organisms.

> **TECHNICIAN NOTE**   Motorized equipment must be used carefully during hoof trimming to prevent excessive heating of the internal tissues in the hoof.

The goal of hoof trimming is to provide a flat, level, weight-bearing surface on both digits of each foot so that the digits bear weight evenly between them. In cattle, unlike horses, the entire palmar or plantar surface of the hoof should bear weight evenly. After the bottom of the foot is cleaned off, any excessive toe is removed. The outer wall of each hoof is trimmed to parallel the coronary band; no portion of the wall should overlap or cover the sole. The inner hoof wall of each digit should be trimmed similarly but slightly shorter than the outer hoof wall. Heels seldom need trimming unless they are overgrown. The hooves should be inspected for bruising and lesions around the coronary bands and lesions and growths in the interdigital cleft, such as interdigital fibroma (hyperplasia or "corns") (Figs. 13-31 and 13-32). The clinician should be alerted if these lesions are seen. Use of hoof blocks may be necessary. Hoof blocks are placed on the healthy toe to provide elevation to the entire foot. Placing the hoof block on the good toe shifts the weight off the good toe and allows the hoof time to heal it also keeps the compromised claw off the ground.

EUTHANASIA

The euthanasia methods that are available for ruminants are similar to those for horses, and most of the same factors must be considered (see Chapter 9). Food consumption affects the methods for euthanasia that can be safely used because chemical residues must be avoided. Sometimes animals must

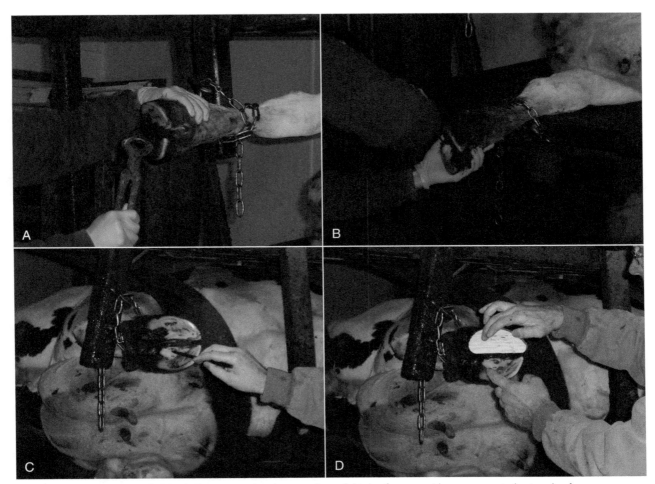

FIGURE 13-31 A, Tapping on the plantar surface of this hoof can provide responses similar to a hoof tester if an underlying condition is present. **B,** Trimming the interdigital space. **C,** Common lesions seen in dairy cattle. **D,** Use of a hoof block.

be euthanized on the farm as a result of emergency or severe medical conditions and therefore will not enter the human food supply. However, if these farm-euthanized animals are to be sent for rendering, the rendering company may have residue restrictions. It is advisable to investigate the local rendering operations and become familiar with their restrictions and policies.

Some owners may be emotionally attached to their ruminant animal and elect a more typical "companion animal" euthanasia and burial. The veterinary practice should be familiar with local laws and regulations concerning cremation and burial options.

According to the American Veterinary Medical Association Panel on Euthanasia (2000), the following euthanasia methods are considered acceptable for ruminants:

- IV injection of barbituric acid derivatives: Tissue residues are toxic and prevent use of this method in animals intended for animal or human consumption. Carcass disposal should preclude scavenging by other animals.
- IV injection of potassium chloride (KCl) is performed in conjunction with general anesthesia.

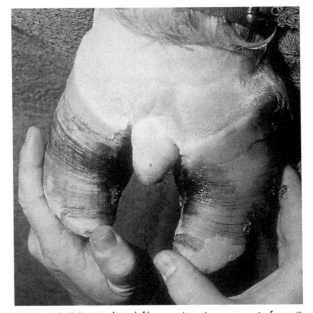

FIGURE 13-32 Interdigital fibroma (corn) on a cow's foot. (From Bassert JM, McCurnin DM, editors: *McCurnin's clinical textbook for veterinary technicians,* ed 8, St. Louis, 2014, Saunders.)

- Penetrating captive bolt: This should be delivered by trained personnel. Because no chemical residues are involved, this is the method most often used in slaughterhouses.

The following euthanasia methods are considered conditionally acceptable:

- IV injection of chloral hydrate, after sedation, can be performed.
- Gunshot, to the head only: Use only when other methods are not available.
- Electrocution: This is applied directly to the head or brain (one-step procedure) or applied after the animal is rendered unconscious by another method (two-step procedure).

NECROPSY TECHNIQUES

Many of the considerations discussed for the horse (see Chapter 9) must be given to ruminant necropsy. The importance of history taking as part of the complete examination must not be overlooked and is especially important for herd situations. Failure to recognize or diagnose infectious diseases, toxicities, or nutritional problems can have implications for all animals in a herd and may have disastrous economic consequences.

RUMINANT NECROPSY PROCEDURE

The importance of personal protective equipment cannot be overemphasized when conducting necropsies on any species. The basic procedure for equine necropsy may be followed, with a few variations. Following are some of the procedural methods used for ruminants.

Position

Ruminant necropsy is usually performed with the animal in left lateral recumbency. This positions the rumen on the downward side, where it interferes minimally with abdominal exploration and visualization.

> *TECHNICIAN NOTE* Ruminant necropsy is usually performed with the animal in left lateral recumbency to minimize interference with the rumen, which is located on the left side.

Gastrointestinal Tract

The rumen or reticulum often is markedly distended with gas from microbial fermentation that continues after death (postmortem bloat or tympany). The distention may be severe enough to cause postmortem rectal or vaginal prolapse, or both. Gas can be relieved by inserting a large-bore needle or by making a small stab incision through the rumen wall directly over the gas cap. Note that incising directly over fluid contents will release them and contaminate the adjacent tissues.

> *TECHNICIAN NOTE* Making a stab incision over fluid in the rumen will release contents onto the adjacent tissue and may contaminate them.

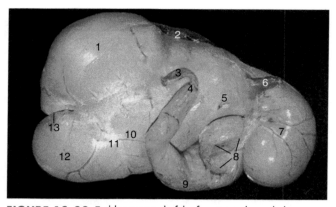

FIGURE 13-33 En bloc removal of the forestomachs and abomasum of a sheep, viewed from the right side. The esophagus (6) and proximal duodenum (3) have been transected. The reticulum (7), omasum (8), and abomasum (9) are easily seen. Everything else is rumen and its various compartments. (From Clayton HM, Flood PF: *Color atlas of large animal applied anatomy*, London, 1996, Mosby-Wolfe.)

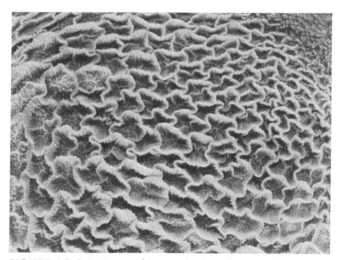

FIGURE 13-34 Mucosa of the reticulum has a honeycomb shape that tends to trap foreign objects. (From Clayton HM, Flood PF: *Color atlas of large animal applied anatomy*, London, 1996; Mosby-Wolfe.)

The ruminant forestomachs and abomasum may be removed en bloc by first tying off the distal esophagus and the proximal duodenum with one to two string ligatures and then transecting them. The attachments of the rumen are cut across the dorsal aspect of the abdominal cavity. The forestomachs and abomasum are then rolled out of the abdomen. Each organ should be individually opened and examined (Fig. 13-33).

The contents of the rumen and reticulum should be examined for foreign bodies, especially in the reticulum, where the honeycomb-shaped mucosa tends to trap sharp objects (Fig. 13-34). The rumen mucosa undergoes autolysis fairly rapidly and may slough easily during the necropsy examination. Submission of rumen contents for laboratory analysis may be necessary in some cases.

> *TECHNICIAN NOTE* The reticulum should be examined for foreign objects such as metal.

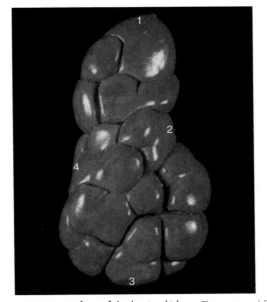

FIGURE 13-35 Surface of the bovine kidney. The perirenal fat and renal capsule have been removed. *1,* cranial pole; *2,* depression in dorsal surface close to hilus; *3,* caudal pole; *4,* ventral border. (From Clayton HM, Flood PF: *Color atlas of large animal applied anatomy,* London, 1996, Mosby-Wolfe.)

Ruminants, unlike horses, have gallbladders. The gallbladder is removed with the liver. Bile duct patency should be checked before the gallbladder is removed. This is done by incising into the lumen of the duodenum, applying pressure on the gallbladder, and observing bile flowing from the bile duct into the duodenum. After the liver and gallbladder are removed, the gallbladder should be opened and evaluated.

Urinary Tract

The kidneys of the cow normally are multilobulated, resembling a large bunch of grapes on the capsular surface (Fig. 13-35).

> *TECHNICIAN NOTE* Cattle normally have lumpy kidneys.

NECROPSY OF ABORTED FETUSES

Abortion diagnosis is commonly done in ruminants because of the economic impact of abortions and the need to prevent them whenever possible. A certain number of fetal losses to stillbirth and abortion is expected in livestock production operations. The veterinarian and farm owner must decide when expected losses may be excessive and which individual cases and circumstances may warrant a thorough diagnostic workup. The cost of laboratory diagnostics must be carefully considered.

The technician should be familiar with the diagnostic laboratory and its sample submission procedures so that samples are handled and shipped properly. This helps ensure valid and timely test results. The basic fetal necropsy procedure is described in Chapter 9.

CASE STUDY

You are riding with Dr. Heath to a farm call. On the way, the veterinarian tells you he needs to go treat a calf with diarrhea on the north side of the farm. He asks you to go to the south side of the farm and prepare for a calf necropsy, to save time. What tools should you take with you? In what position should you place the calf when you get there?

CASE STUDY

You are going to Schneider's dairy to draw blood samples from the entire herd. The dairy is equipped with head gates in each pen. From which anatomical location will you most likely draw blood?

SUGGESTED READING

Anderson DE, Rings DM: *Current veterinary therapy: food animal practice,* ed 5, St. Louis, 2008, Saunders.

Bassert JM, McCurnin DM: *McCurnin's clinical textbook for veterinary technicians,* ed 7, St. Louis, 2010, Saunders.

Bentz AI, Gill MS: Large animal medical nursing. In Bassert JM, McCurnin DM, editors: *McCurnin's clinical textbook for veterinary technicians,* ed 7, St. Louis, 2010, Saunders, pp 713–768.

Cebra ML, Cebra CK: Food animal medicine and surgery. In McCurnin DM, Bassert JM, editors: *McCurnin's clinical textbook for veterinary technicians,* ed 6, St. Louis, 2006, Saunders, pp 1056–1092.

Davis H, Riel DL, Pappagianis M, Miguel K: Diagnostic sampling and therapeutic techniques. In Bassert JM, McCurnin DM, editors: *McCurnin's clinical textbook for veterinary technicians,* ed 7, St. Louis, 2010, Saunders, pp 585–673.

Fubini SL, Ducharme NG: *Farm animal surgery,* St. Louis, 2004, Saunders.

Hafez ESE, Hafez B, editors: *Reproduction in farm animals,* ed 7, New York, 2000, Wiley-Blackwell.

Noakes DE, Parkinson RJ, England GCW: *Veterinary reproduction and obstetrics,* ed 9, London, 2009, Saunders.

Sheldon CC, Sonsthagen TF, Topel JT: *Animal restraint for veterinary professionals,* St. Louis, 2007, Mosby.

Sirois M: *Principles and practice of veterinary technology,* ed 3, St. Louis, 2011, Mosby.

Smith BP: *Large animal internal medicine,* ed 4, St. Louis, 2008, Mosby.

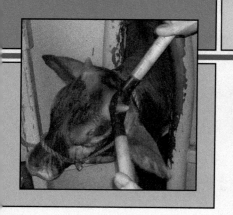

14 Bovine Surgical Procedures

LEARNING OBJECTIVES

When you have completed this chapter, you will be able to

- Understand the basic differences between standing surgical procedures and general anesthesia procedures
- Prepare a patient for surgical procedures
- Assist and/or perform induction and maintenance of anesthesia
- Provide anesthetic monitoring
- Manage the patient during the recovery and immediate postoperative periods
- Understand the basic risks and possible complications associated with anesthesia and surgery, and implement preventive measures when indicated

KEY TERMS

Bladder marsupialization
Casting
Celiotomy
Cosmetic dehorning
Cystotomy
Dehorning

Hemostasis
Horn button
Lithotripsy
Marcenac approach
Myiasis
Scur

Supernumerary teats
Tipping
Urethrostomy
Urethrotomy

KEY ABBREVIATION

FARAD: Food Animal Residue Avoidance and Depletion (program)

RUMINANT SURGERY AND ANESTHESIA

The advances in large animal surgical and anesthetic procedures are not limited to horses. Essentially all the technology available to equines—surgical lasers, endoscopy and laparoscopy, arthroscopy, and internal fixation—are available to ruminants. However, the economic value of these animals seldom justifies the expenses involved in surgical treatment of many diseases. The production animal usually must be able to "pay its way." Notable exceptions are high-producing dairy females and registered breeding stock of all species, which may have considerable value. In addition, pet animals often engage an owner's emotions, and the bond formed between them may increase the likelihood of paying for costly procedures.

> **TECHNICIAN NOTE** The decision to perform a surgical procedure is often based on the value of the animal.

As with equines, surgical procedures can be divided into two main categories:
1. Standing surgery procedures
2. General anesthesia (recumbent) procedures

A third option that is sometimes used in ruminants is a combination of heavy sedation with forced recumbency (*casting*). This method is often used to treat conditions of the limbs and feet and is often used when performing a vasectomy.

STANDING SURGERY

Most surgical procedures in ruminants are performed in with the animal in the standing position, and they use a combination of sedation or tranquilization and local or regional anesthesia. Cattle generally seem to tolerate standing procedures better than do horses. Standing procedures are often used to repair traumatic injuries such as lacerations and punctures. Castration, cesarean section (C-section), correction of gastrointestinal (GI) tract abnormalities, enucleation, *dehorning*, and treatment of distal limb injuries are some of the more common standing surgical procedures. The indications and considerations for standing surgery in ruminants are identical to those in horses (see Chapter 10).

Surgical procedures may be accompanied by medications such as antibiotics, antiinflammatory drugs, local anesthetics, and muscle relaxants. The practitioner always has concern for drug residues. Pregnancy status of females must be determined in order to anticipate possible drug effects on the fetuses. Information for all medications should be carefully recorded, including dose, route of administration, location of administration, and any instructions or advice given to the client regarding drug use. No anesthetic agents are approved for use in food-producing animals. So after selection of drugs it is important to contact the Food Animal Residue Avoidance and Depletion program (FARAD) for appropriate use and withdrawal times in livestock.

Preparation

Preparation (prepping) for standing surgery usually is straightforward. Ideally, the location where the procedure is to be performed should be clean, dry, and free of drafts; however, field situations usually are less than ideal. When this occurs, you must improvise to try and create the best possible conditions for the given situation.

Equipment and supplies should be assembled beforehand. Preferably, the surgical instruments should be kept elevated above ground level; they should be convenient to the surgeon but out of reach of the animal if it moves.

The form of restraint depends entirely on the following factors: facilities available; personnel availability and experience; expected duration of the procedure; and patient-related factors, such as species, age, temperament, anatomical location of the procedure, anticipated level of pain, and general health of the animal.

If sedation or tranquilization is to be used in adult ruminants, withholding food and water before administration of these drugs may be preferable, especially for intraabdominal procedures. Sedatives and tranquilizers depress GI motility, which increases the risk of rumen tympany (bloat). Additionally, ruminants occasionally regurgitate when they are heavily sedated and risk aspiration of the regurgitated material. Decreasing the volume of rumen contents may reduce these risks. Food can be safely withheld for up to 12 to 24 hours before the procedure and water for up to 6 hours. Because many standing procedures are performed on an emergency basis, without time for fasting, equipment should be available to deal with these complications should they occur.

> **TECHNICIAN NOTE** If withholding of food from ruminants is indicated, food should be withheld for 12 to 14 hours. Water should be withheld only for up to 6 hours.

Control of Pain

Local anesthesia is used alone or to supplement the analgesic effects of some sedatives and tranquilizers (Table 14-1). Lidocaine, mepivacaine, and bupivacaine are the most commonly used local anesthetic drugs. Because lidocaine is the least expensive and least toxic (comparatively) of these drugs, it is most commonly used in farm animals. However, none of the local anesthetic drugs are approved for use in food animals in the United States, and clients must be advised of withdrawal times. Sometimes, large volumes of these drugs are injected to produce large areas of desensitized tissue, and toxic doses may be reached. Lidocaine has a toxic (total) dose of 13 mg/kg body weight in cattle. Signs of toxicity from this family of local anesthetics (amides) include hypotension, drowsiness or sedation, muscle

TABLE 14-1	Pain Management*					
	DOSE	**CONCENTRATION**	**ROUTE**	**MEAT WITHDRAWAL TIME**	**MILK WITHDRAWL TIME**
Flunixin meglumine	1.1-2.2 mg/kg q12–24h	50 mg/mL	IV	4 days	36 hr
Ketoprofen	3 mg/kg/day for up to 3 days	12.5-, 25-, 50-, 75-mg tablets 100 mg/mL	IV, IM	7 days	24 hr
Meloxicam	0.5 mg/kg q24h	5 mg/ml	IV, IM, SC, PO	15 days	5 days
Acetylsalicylic acid (aspirin)	50–100 mg/kg q12h	240 gr bolus 480 gr bolus	PO	24 hr	24 hr
Xylazine	0.1–0.2 mg/kg IM 0.03–0.1 mg/kg IV	100 mg/mL	IV, IM	10 days	120 hr
Ketamine	1–2 mg/kg q4–6h	100 mg/mL	IV or IM	3 days	48 hr

IM, Intramuscularly; *IV*, intravenously; *PO*, orally; *SC*, subcutaneously.
*For an explanation of drug categories please see Chapter 10.

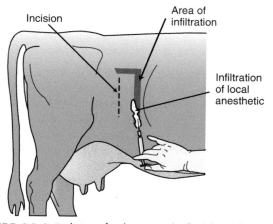

FIGURE 14-1 Technique for the inverted L flank block for standing abdominal surgery.

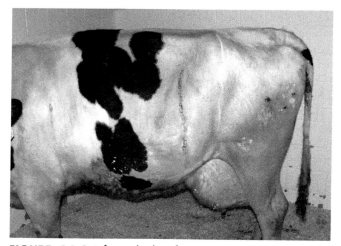

FIGURE 14-2 Left paralumbar fossa incision (cesarean section). (From Fubini SL, Ducharme NG: *Farm animal surgery*, St. Louis, 2004, Saunders.)

twitching, respiratory depression, and possibly convulsions. Treatment is supportive because no specific antidote exists. Intravenous (IV) fluids, respiratory support, and anticonvulsants can be given as needed. To minimize the risk of toxicity, the local anesthetic concentration should be no stronger than 2%.

Local anesthesia in ruminants can be performed in several ways. Usually, the anatomical location and expected level of pain dictate the method of local anesthesia used. Specific nerve blocks and field blocks may be used, similar to those described for equines. Common techniques used in ruminants are described in the following subsections.

L Block

Equipment for L block:
- Clippers
- Surgical scrub and alcohol
- Water
- Local anesthetic agent
- 18-gauge (ga) × 1½- to 3-inch needle
- Syringe

The L block is a type of field block used to desensitize the flank for standing flank laparotomies. Local anesthetic is deposited in an inverted L configuration in the flank (Fig. 14-1). A line block may also be performed using the same procedure, except that the area where the local anesthetic agent is deposited is in a dorsoventral line. The part of the L that runs cranially to caudally is not placed. The anesthetic agent must be deposited in several layers (i.e., subcutaneous tissue and all muscular layers of the abdominal wall). Large volumes of local anesthetic are required; often up to 100 mL of 2% solution is necessary in adult cattle. The anesthetic agent is deposited with an 18-gauge (ga) × 1½- to 3-inch needle. Before beginning the surgical procedure, allow at least 10 to 15 minutes for the anesthetic to diffuse and take effect. The inverted L essentially forms a wall of anesthesia that protects the surgical field (Fig. 14-2). It is the simplest technique for desensitizing the flank and therefore is commonly used.

Paravertebral Block

Equipment for the paravertebral block:
- Clippers
- Surgical scrub and alcohol
- Water
- 16- to 8-ga × 3- to 6-inch needle
- 14- × 1-inch needle
- Syringes
- Local anesthetic agent

This technique uses multiple specific nerve blocks to create a large region of flank anesthesia. Innervation of the flank arises from the spinal nerves of the T13, L1, and L2 spinal segments. These nerves can be blocked near their exit from the vertebral column at a "paravertebral" location. The two main ways to approach these nerves are from (1) a dorsal approach near the intervertebral foramina (Cambridge, Farquharson, or proximal paravertebral method) or (2) a lateral approach near the tips of the transverse processes of the lumbar vertebrae (Magda, Cornell, or distal paravertebral method) (Fig. 14-3). Cattle require a 16- to 18-ga × 3- to 6-inch needle for the proximal paravertebral (dorsal) approach. However, some clinicians prefer to place a 14-ga × 1-inch needle first as a trocar through the skin and muscle layers and then insert an 18-ga needle through the 14-ga needle to actually deliver the anesthetic agent. Up to 20 mL of anesthetic is necessary for each of the three injection sites in cattle.

For the distal paravertebral (lateral) approach, an 18-ga × 1½- to 3-inch needle is sufficient for cattle. From 10 to 20 mL of anesthetic agent is deposited at each of the three injection sites.

The paravertebral block desensitizes all layers of the flank, from the skin down to the peritoneum. With the proximal paravertebral approach, once the block takes effect, paralysis of the longissimus muscle along the spine may cause temporary lateral curvature of the spine (bowing or scoliosis) toward the side of the block. This curvature may create some gaping of the skin incision, thus making suture closure more difficult. The distal paravertebral approach should not create scoliosis.

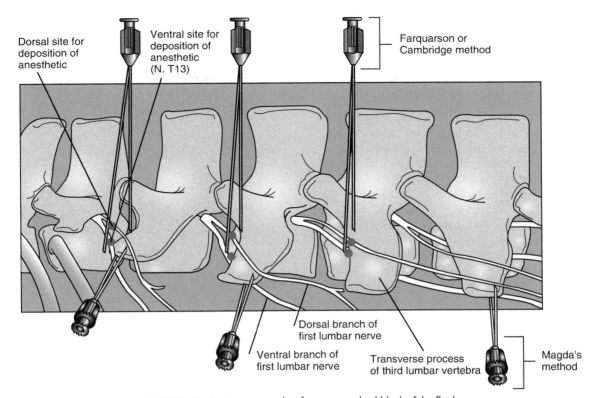

Dorsal site for deposition of anesthetic

Ventral site for deposition of anesthetic (N. T13)

Farquarson or Cambridge method

Dorsal branch of first lumbar nerve

Ventral branch of first lumbar nerve

Transverse process of third lumbar vertebra

Magda's method

FIGURE 14-3 Two approaches for paravertebral block of the flank.

Cornual Nerve Block

Equipment for the cornual nerve block:
- Clippers
- Surgical scrub and alcohol
- 18- to 20-ga × 1- to 1½-inch needle
- Syringe
- Local anesthetic agent

The cornual nerve block is used for desensitization of the horn and horn base for dehorning surgical procedures.

Cattle have a single nerve supply to each horn. The cornual nerve emerges from the orbit and ascends toward the base of the horn just below the temporal ridge of the frontal bone. A local anesthetic agent (≈3 to 5 mL in calves, 5 to 10 mL in adults) is deposited with an 18- to 20-ga × 1- to 1½-inch needle just ventral to the temporal ridge at a site approximately halfway between the horn base and the lateral canthus of the eye. The nerve is covered only by skin and a thin layer of muscle at this location; depth of needle penetration is 1 cm in calves to 2.5 cm in large adults (Fig. 14-4).

Adult cattle with well-developed horns may require a second injection of several milliliters of anesthetic agent at the base of the horn, along the caudal aspect, just beneath the skin.

Another type of block that can be used as an adjunct to the corneal nerve block is a ring block where the lidocaine is deposited in a complete circle around the base of the horn. This is often performed for cosmetic dehorning.

Intravenous Regional Analgesia (Bier Block)

Equipment for intravenous regional analgesia:
- Sedative, syringes, and needles

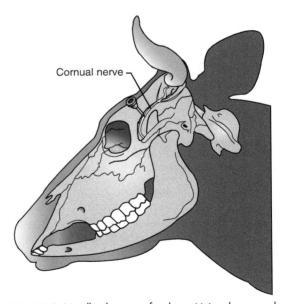

Cornual nerve

FIGURE 14-4 Needle placement for desensitizing the cornual nerve in the bovine. The cornual nerve follows the temporal ridge to the base of the horn. (Modified from Muir WW 3rd, Hubbell JAE, Skard R, et al: *Handbook of veterinary anesthesia,* ed 3, St. Louis, 2000, Mosby.)

- Restraint ropes or a tilt table
- Clippers
- Surgical scrub and alcohol
- Tourniquet
- Cotton or foam padding
- Local anesthetic agent
- 18- to 20-ga × 1-inch needle

IV analgesia is considered superior to specific nerve blocks and ring blocks for most surgical procedures on the distal limbs. The technique uses an IV injection of a local anesthetic agent, distal to a previously placed tourniquet. The anesthetic diffuses out of the veins and blocks the nerves in the area. Although this block is seldom performed on standing animals, it is a common method of local analgesia for surgical procedures on awake, sedated animals in lateral recumbency.

The animal is restrained, sedated, and cast (placed in recumbency) for administration of this form of regional anesthesia. A tourniquet is applied at the desired level on the limb, which is determined by the location of the surgical procedure. For procedures on the feet, the tourniquet is placed at midcarpus or midtarsus. For more proximal procedures, the tourniquet is placed just proximal to the carpus or tarsus. Rubber tubing or other elastic strapping material is suitable for the tourniquet. Cotton or foam padding should be used beneath the tubing for additional protection of underlying tissues, especially where the tourniquet crosses superficial tendons. Proximal to the tarsus, the grooves in front of the common calcaneal tendon should be "filled in" on both sides of the leg with roll gauze or other soft padding before placing the tourniquet. This step is necessary to achieve complete arterial occlusion.

Any large superficial vein can be used, but generally the dorsal metacarpal (metatarsal) or palmar (plantar) metacarpal (metatarsal) veins are used (Fig. 14-5). The site should be clipped and prepared. Lidocaine without epinephrine (2%) or mepivacaine (2%) is injected by the IV route, with the needle directed distally; the backpressure creates some resistance to injection. Up to 30 mL can be administered. After the needle is withdrawn, digital pressure should be placed over the injection site for longer than normal to prevent hematoma formation.

> **TECHNICIAN NOTE**   Cotton or foam padding should be placed beneath a tourniquet to protect the underlying tissues.

Anesthesia is sufficient for the surgical procedure in 10 to 15 minutes and persists as long as the tourniquet is kept in place. A tourniquet may cause complications such as tissue necrosis, pain, and swelling if it is left in place longer than 2 hours. The tourniquet should be released gradually to prevent a bolus release of local anesthetic drug into the general circulation and possible resulting hypotension. The anesthetic effects on the distal limb disappear rapidly within 5 to 10 minutes after the tourniquet is the released.

Caudal Epidural Analgesia

Equipment for caudal epidural analgesia:
- Clippers
- Surgical scrub and alcohol
- 25 ga-needle and syringe
- Local anesthetic agent
- 18-ga × 1½- to 2-inch needle

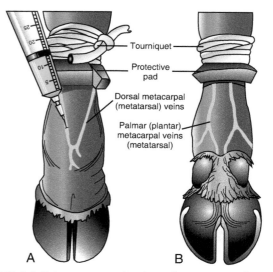

FIGURE 14-5 Intravenous regional anesthesia. **A,** Dorsal aspect of the distal limb. **B,** Palmar (plantar) aspect.

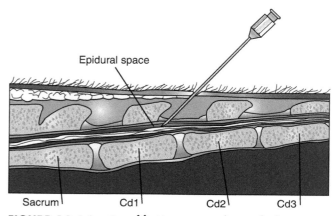

FIGURE 14-6 Location of first intercoccygeal space for bovine caudal epidural anesthesia.

Caudal epidural analgesia is commonly used in ruminants, especially for obstetrical procedures and treatment of prolapses of the uterus, vagina, and rectum. When the epidural procedure is properly performed, the anus, perineum, vulva, caudal vagina, and caudal aspects of the thighs are desensitized, which decreases pain and straining by the animal. Motor control of the hindlegs is usually retained, but occasionally hindlimb ataxia occurs if excessive anesthetic diffuses cranially.

The technique is similar to that described in horses. The procedure is performed through the dorsal aspect of the tail base, at the first intercoccygeal space (the sacrococcygeal space is another possibility but is more difficult to identify and is less commonly used). To identify the first intercoccygeal space, manipulate the tail up and down while palpating the dorsal aspect of the tail base for the first obviously movable articulation (joint) caudal to the sacrum (Fig. 14-6). The area is clipped and prepared in sterile fashion, and aseptic technique is used for the procedure. In general, blocking the skin and subcutaneous tissue is not necessary, but a small

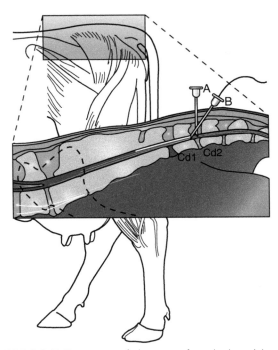

FIGURE 14-7 Comparison of placement of standard caudal epidural (A) and continuous caudal epidural (B) in cattle. (Modified from Muir WW 3rd, Hubbell JAE, Skard R, et al: *Handbook of veterinary anesthesia,* ed 3, St. Louis, 2000, Mosby.)

bleb of subcutaneous anesthetic can be placed with a 25-ga needle if desired. For placement of the epidural anesthetic agent, cattle require an 18-ga × 1½- to 3-inch needle. The needle enters on dorsal midline at a 45-degree angle, and anesthetic is deposited into the epidural space. Lidocaine 2% without epinephrine is most commonly used (1 mL/100 kg body weight, or ≈5 to 6 mL in adult cattle). Mepivacaine 2% also is suitable, and xylazine (Rompun) can be combined or used as the sole agent.

The anesthetic agent generally takes effect in 10 to 20 minutes and lasts 1 to 2 hours on average. If prolonged anesthesia is necessary, a small-diameter epidural catheter (commercially available) or similar sterile medical tubing can be placed into the epidural space to provide continuous caudal epidural anesthesia. The catheter is placed and threaded cranially along the epidural space as in horses (Fig. 14-7). The catheter is placed and maintained aseptically. The end of the catheter is protected with an injection cap, and the exposed portion of the catheter should be secured to the skin. Small doses of lidocaine can be given every few hours as needed for pain or straining. A protective gauze bandage is advisable between uses. This technique spares the discomfort and tissue trauma from repeated standard epidural procedures. Disadvantages include kinking of the catheter and plugging of the tip with tissue or fibrin. Continuous caudal epidural anesthesia is also used successfully in equines.

Cranial epidural analgesia is generally avoided in cattle. It is performed at the lumbosacral space, using landmarks similar to lumbosacral cerebrospinal fluid centesis.

Cranial epidural procedures are technically more difficult to perform and have more potential complications than do caudal epidural procedures, including accidental injection into the subarachnoid space or cerebrospinal fluid. Posterior paralysis, including the hindlimbs, occurs and produces recumbency. Animals may require assistance standing as the anesthesia begins to wear off. They are prone to "splay-legged" recoveries with overabduction of hindlimbs and resulting damage to the pelvis and inner thigh muscles.

GENERAL ANESTHESIA

Most surgical procedures in ruminants can be performed as standing procedures. General anesthesia is required when the technical or anatomical aspects of the procedure or the ability to control pain and motion exceed the capability of sedative drugs and local anesthesia. The techniques used to perform general anesthesia in ruminants are similar to those used in horses. However, some important differences exist: (1) the physiologic features of ruminants create the potential for several unique complications during the induction and maintenance phases of anesthesia; and (2) in sharp contrast to horses, ruminants tend to have uneventful recoveries that seldom require special assistance.

Anesthetic Risks for Ruminants

For preparation and administration of general anesthesia to the ruminant patient, the following risks should be considered.

Regurgitation

Ruminants are prone to regurgitation. The contents of the rumen or reticulum may be regurgitated during heavy sedation or general anesthesia. Aesthetic drugs relax the smooth muscle sphincters that normally protect both ends of the esophagus, thus making regurgitation more likely. The amount of regurgitated material often is voluminous. In adult cattle, gallons of rumen liquid may be expelled in a matter of seconds. The primary risk associated with regurgitation is aspiration of this material into the trachea and lungs, leading to aspiration pneumonia.

To minimize the risk of regurgitation, the most important principles are to reduce the size of the rumen and decrease pressure inside the organ. In adult cattle, food is withheld for 12 to 36 hours, and water is withheld for 6 to 12 hours before general anesthesia. In calves that are consuming solid food material, fasting for 2 to 4 hours is sufficient (withhold food only; water is permitted).

> **TECHNICIAN NOTE**　　To minimize the risk of regurgitation, the most important principles are to reduce the size of the rumen and decrease pressure inside the organ. In adult cattle, food is withheld for 12 to 36 hours, and water is withheld for 6 to 12 hours before general anesthesia. In calves that are consuming solid food material, fasting for 2 to 4 hours is sufficient (withhold food only; water is permitted).

In very young ruminants, the rumen or reticulum has little function, and the risk of regurgitation is minimal. Fasting of neonates may cause hypoglycemia and is not recommended.

Other precautions include the following:

- A cuffed endotracheal tube is essential to protect the trachea from aspiration. It should be inserted as soon as possible after anesthetic induction. Endotracheal intubation should be the priority of the anesthetic team at this time. Materials for intubation (oral speculum, appropriately sized endotracheal tube, sterile lubricant, laryngoscope, air syringe) should be assembled beforehand and be readily available.
- Stimulation of the pharynx and larynx, which occurs during intubation, may induce a gag reflex and cause regurgitation, especially in light planes of anesthesia. Intubation technique should be rapid and minimize stimulation of this area. The cuff should be inflated as soon as the tube is properly inserted.
- Ruminants should never be rolled while they are under anesthesia unless a cuffed endotracheal tube is in place.

Bloat

Ruminants are prone to distention of the rumen (bloat) during general anesthesia. The combined effects of drug-induced depression of GI motility and the ongoing fermentation in the rumen or reticulum create gas, which may accumulate and cause bloat. The distention of the rumen may press on the diaphragm and lungs and contribute to hypoventilation. Some degree of bloat is expected in all anesthetized ruminants; the key is to minimize it. Precautions include the following:

- Institute fasting to decrease the contents and weight of the rumen.
- Be prepared to treat bloat, especially after the procedure. A stomach tube, oral speculum, or rumen trocar should be readily available in the surgical and recovery areas.

Hypoventilation

Ruminants, like horses, are prone to hypoventilation and inadequate arterial oxygenation. The size and weight of the rumen or reticulum and other GI organs compress the lungs and compromise diaphragm function. Aesthetic drugs depress the respiratory centers in the brain. The combined effect is likely to produce hypoventilation. Fasting is essential to reduce the size and weight of the GI tract. Aesthetic depth should not exceed what is necessary for the surgical procedure.

Compartment Syndrome

Ruminants are at risk for development of compartment syndrome. Large body weight places adult cattle at greatest risk for developing postanesthetic myopathy and neuropathy; small ruminants are at considerably less risk. The risk factors and preventive measures are similar to those described in horses (see Chapter 10). Proper patient positioning and padding during general anesthesia are essential (Figs. 14-8 and 14-9).

Preanesthetic Preparation and Anesthetic Management
Preanesthetic Evaluation

A basic physical examination should always be performed. The extent of blood work and other laboratory tests depends on the health status of the animal and the nature and length of the procedure.

Preanesthetic Drugs

Most of the anesthetic drugs used in ruminants are not approved for use in food animals. Drug residues must be considered and the client advised accordingly. Withdrawal times may not be established for many of these drugs because their use is "extra label." The FARAD databank (www.farad.org or 888-USFARAD) is a valuable resource for current information on pharmacokinetics and withdrawal recommendations. Many combinations of these drugs are used for sedation and anesthesia in livestock. Some of the drugs in use include those discussed in the following subsections.

Acepromazine. Acepromazine helps calm nervous cattle but does not have a strong tranquilizing effect at recommended

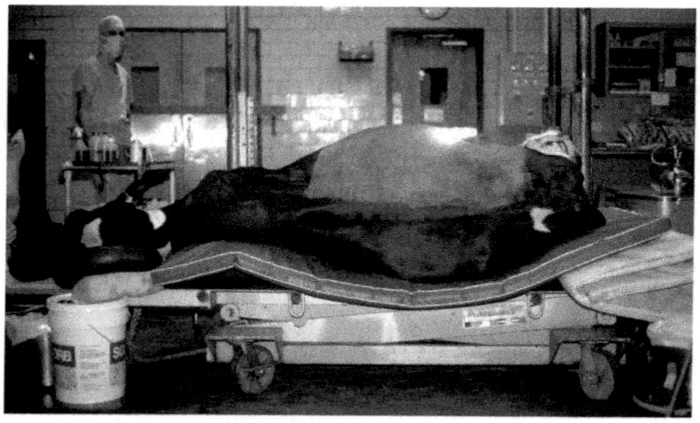

FIGURE 14-8 Cow in lateral recumbency under general anesthesia. Placing appropriate pads under the cow's shoulder and hip creates a cavity that supports the distended rumen. (From Smith DF: Bovine intestinal surgery: part 1. *Mod Vet Pract* 65:853–857, 1984.)

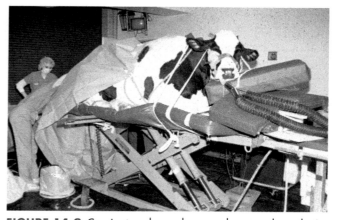

FIGURE 14-9 Cow in sternal recumbency under general anesthesia. (From Fubini SL, Ducharme NG: *Farm animal surgery*, St. Louis, 2004, Saunders.)

doses. Males experience a prolonged period of penile relaxation, which increases risk of injury to the penis. The tranquilization effects last 2 to 4 hours, and the prolonged time of drug elimination may be undesirable. Acepromazine should be avoided in dehydrated patients because of its tendency to produce hypotension by dilation of peripheral blood vessels.

Xylazine. Xylazine is the most commonly used preanesthetic sedative drug. It is useful for casting animals for recumbent procedures and for sedation during standing surgical procedures. Low doses (0.05 to 0.1 mg/kg by the IV route, 0.1 to 0.5 mg/kg by the intramuscular [IM] route) provide excellent sedation. Moderate doses may result in recumbency.

It is very important to be aware that ruminants are highly sensitive to xylazine. Approximately one tenth of a "horse dose" produces similar sedative effects in cattle. Some breeds such as Herefords and Brahmas may be even more sensitive, and goats and sheep may be more sensitive than cattle. To prevent accidental overdosing, only low-concentration xylazine (20 mg/mL) should be used in ruminants.

> **TECHNICIAN NOTE** To prevent accidental overdosing of xylazine, only low-concentration xylazine (20 mg/mL) should be used in ruminants.

Clinical effects include the following:
- Bloat: often develops from depression of rumen motility
- Bradycardia (dose-dependent cardiovascular depression)
- Decreased ventilation (dose-dependent respiratory depression)
- Hyperglycemia: leads to increased urine output
- Uterine contractions: may cause premature labor in late pregnancy
- Passes, unchanged, into milk: may affect nursing neonates

The sedation, cardiovascular, respiratory, and muscle relaxation effects can be reversed with either yohimbine or tolazoline. Rapid IV injection of alpha-2 antagonists should be avoided.

Detomidine or Medetomidine. The clinical indications, effects, and sensitivity of detomidine or medetomidine are similar to those of xylazine.

Anticholinergics (Atropine, Glycopyrrolate). Ruminants produce copious amounts of saliva and continue to do so while they are under anesthesia. However, anticholinergic drugs do not significantly reduce saliva production and are not used for this purpose in ruminants. Patient positioning with the nose below the level of the pharynx and use of a cuffed endotracheal tube are used to prevent aspiration of saliva (a "spit bucket" under the patient's mouth is useful). Anticholinergic agents increase the incidence of bloat because of their depressant effects on GI motility.

Induction
Induction Drugs
Many anesthetic induction and maintenance drug regimens are possible. As with horses, injectable drugs can be used for induction and maintenance, or injectable drugs can be used for induction, followed by inhalant gases for maintenance.

Inhalant Gases. In animals weighing less than 150 pounds, face mask induction is possible. Oxygen (3 to 5 L/minute) is given for 1 to 2 minutes before the anesthetic gas is introduced. Recommended gas concentrations are halothane 3% to 4%, isoflurane 3%, and sevoflurane 4% to 6%. Intubation is performed as soon as depth of anesthesia allows.

Thiobarbiturates. Thiobarbiturates are not for use in animals less than 3 months old. Thiobarbiturates can cross the placenta and cause adverse effects on the fetus.

Ketamine. Ketamine is used in combination with a sedative such as xylazine or acepromazine.

Guaifenesin. Guaifenesin is combined with thiobarbiturates, xylazine, or ketamine for induction and sometimes for maintenance. It is used for its muscle relaxant effects and to decrease required doses of other anesthetic drugs. Guaifenesin can immobilize an animal, but it is not an anesthetic or analgesic drug. It is given by the IV route "to effect." Solutions for IV use in ruminants should not exceed 5% because significant hemolysis may occur at stronger concentrations.

> **TECHNICIAN NOTE** Solutions of guaifenesin for intravenous use in ruminants should not exceed 5% because significant hemolysis may occur at stronger concentrations.

One popular guaifenesin combination is the "triple drip or GKX," a mixture of xylazine, guaifenesin, and ketamine that is given by the IV route (note that ruminant triple-drip formulations are different from equine triple-drip doses because of ruminants' sensitivity to xylazine; they should never be substituted for each other). An initial loading dose is given to produce recumbency, and then the infusion rate is decreased for maintenance anesthesia. However, the potential for excessive cardiovascular and respiratory depression exists. An alternative "double-drip" formulation, using only IV guaifenesin with ketamine, is a safer alternative for induction of anesthesia in calm or sedated animals and can be used effectively for maintenance of anesthesia for 1 to 2 hours.

> **TECHNICIAN NOTE** Ruminant triple-drip combinations are different from equine triple-drip combinations, and the two should never be substituted for each other.

Telazol. Telazol (tiletamine and zolazepam) can be used for induction of anesthesia in calves. It also can be used for maintenance of short-term surgical anesthesia.

Propofol. Propofol can be used for induction in calves. A single dose produces approximately 10 minutes of surgical anesthesia, which facilitates intubation and other short procedures. A continuous drip can be used to maintain anesthesia for slightly longer periods of time.

Endotracheal Intubation

After induction of anesthesia, rapid intubation and inflation of the cuff are essential. All necessary intubation equipment should be assembled before anesthesia is induced, and appropriately sized cuffed endotracheal tubes should be selected and lubricated with sterile lubricating jelly. Two common methods of intubation are used.

Direct Visualization. A long-blade laryngoscope is useful for calves (Fig. 14-10). Intubation is easiest to accomplish with the patient in sternal recumbency, with the head and neck held in extension. Tubes less than 12 mm in internal diameter may be easier to insert using a long plastic or metal stylet as a guide. The stylet is placed inside the endotracheal tube such that 15 to 20 cm of the stylet tip will be exposed at the distal end of the tube. The laryngoscope is placed in the mouth, and the epiglottis is visualized. The tip of the scope is used to depress the epiglottis. The stylet tip is placed just beyond the larynx into the trachea. With the stylet held steady in this position, the endotracheal tube is passed over the stylet into the trachea, and the cuff is inflated. The stylet is withdrawn.

Palpation. This method is suitable only for adult cattle. An oral speculum is positioned to open the mouth. The head and neck should be extended so that the trachea, throat, and nose form a straight line. Sternal recumbency is preferred but not essential. One hand is cupped over the end of the endotracheal tube and is inserted into the mouth and pharynx. The epiglottis is palpated and depressed with one or more fingers while the tip of the tube is manually guided into the trachea. The arm is withdrawn, and the cuff is inflated. This method allows rapid identification of the tracheal entrance and insertion of the tube, rather than making repeated attempts to pass the endotracheal tube blindly, which may stimulate regurgitation before the tube has been successfully inserted. Be sure to remove all your jewelry before performing this technique (Fig. 14-11).

As with other species, appropriate endotracheal tube size is estimated by palpation of tracheal diameter through the skin of the neck (Table 14-2).

Maintenance of Anesthesia

Anesthesia can be maintained with injectable drugs or with inhalant gases. Generally, inhalation anesthesia is preferred for longer (>60 minutes) procedures. Small animal anesthesia machines can be used for animals weighing up to approximately 150 kg (Table 14-3).

> **TECHNICIAN NOTE**   In general, inhalation anesthesia is used for procedures lasting longer than 60 minutes.

Nitrous oxide gas is not recommended for use in ruminants, primarily because of its poor solubility in blood. This property creates a tendency for nitrous oxide to diffuse out of

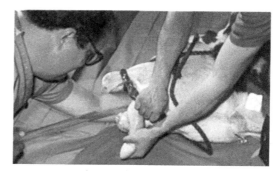

FIGURE 14-11 Intubation of an adult cow by palpation of the larynx. A mouth speculum is used to keep the mouth open. (From Hubbell JAE, Hull BL, Muir WW: Perianesthetic considerations in cattle. *Compend Contin Educ Pract Vet* 8:F92–F102, 1986.)

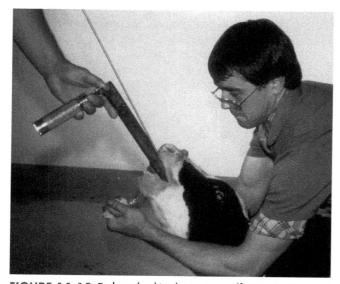

FIGURE 14-10 Endotracheal intubation in a calf. Note that the head and neck are extended perpendicular to the body. A long (18-inch) laryngoscope blade can be used to visualize the larynx and deflect the epiglottis ventrally to provide a clear view of the opening to the trachea. (From Fubini SL, Ducharme NG: *Farm animal surgery*, St. Louis, 2004, Saunders.)

TABLE 14-2	Approximate Endotracheal Tube Sizes (Internal Diameter)
TUBE SIZE (mm)	**RUMINANT**
10–14	Calves
15–18	Older calves (×200 kg)
20–25	Cows
25–30	Bulls

TABLE 14-3	Percentage of Gas Anesthesia for Ruminants	
INHALANT GAS	**INDUCTION PERCENTAGE (%)**	**MAINTENANCE PERCENTAGE (%) (SURGICAL ANESTHESIA)**
Halothane	3–5	1–2
Isoflurane	2–4	1.5–2.5
Sevoflurane	4–6	3–4

the blood and into gas-filled organs such as the rumen, thus contributing to the development of bloat.

> **TECHNICIAN NOTE** Nitrous oxide gas is not recommended for use in ruminants, primarily because of its poor solubility in blood.

Monitoring of Anesthesia

Aesthetic monitoring is similar to that used for horses. An anesthetic record should be maintained for each anesthetic episode. As with horses, hypotension, hypoventilation, and bradycardia are the most commonly encountered complications. The following parameters may be monitored.

Depth of Anesthesia.

- Ocular reflexes: As with other species, the corneal reflex should always be present. The palpebral reflex may be delayed but should be present.
- Eyeball position: The eye tends to roll ventromedially in light surgical anesthesia and returns to a central position in deep surgical anesthesia (Fig. 14-12).
- Pupil size: The pupils dilate when an overdose of inhalant gas occurs. A central eyeball position with dilated pupils usually indicates that excessive anesthesia has been administered, and immediate evaluation and action are indicated to prevent possibly severe complications.
- Muscle movement: Lack of muscle movement in response to the surgical procedure should be monitored.

Ventilation.

- Respiratory rate and depth (tidal volume): Respiratory rate of 20 to 40 breaths/minute is desirable in adult ruminants.
- Mucous membrane color
- Blood gas monitoring

Circulation.

- Peripheral pulse strength: can be taken at the coccygeal, median, median auricular, or femoral arteries. This finding is subjective and may be misleading.
- Mucous membrane color

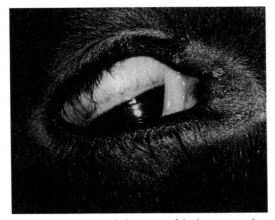

FIGURE 14-12 Ventromedial rotation of the bovine eye during light anesthesia. (From Muir WW 3rd, Hubbell JAE, Skard R, et al: *Handbook of veterinary anesthesia*, ed 3, St. Louis, 2000, Mosby.)

- Capillary refill time
- Heart rate: depends largely upon the anesthetic drugs used. In general, desirable heart rates to maintain under anesthesia are 60 to 120 beats/minute.

Blood Pressure Monitoring.

- Indirect: Place the cuff over the coccygeal artery.
- Direct: Place the catheter in the median auricular artery.
- Mean arterial pressure should be maintained at more than 70 mm Hg. Mean arterial pressure lower than 60 mm Hg indicates hypotension requiring immediate treatment.

Body Temperature.

- Body temperature is especially important in young animals.

Intravenous Fluids

IV fluids are recommended for systemically sick animals, for procedures in which significant hemorrhage occurs, and for routine procedures lasting longer than 1 hour. Placement of an IV catheter before any general anesthetic episode is advisable for emergency access and fluid administration if needed. Lactated Ringer's solution is most often used at a rate of 5 to 10 mL/kg/hour. Neonates may require a dextrose solution (5% dextrose) or addition of a glucose-containing solution to supplement IV fluids.

Oxygen Supplementation

When anesthesia is maintained with injectable anesthetic agents, delivery of supplemental oxygen may be desirable or necessary. Ambu-bags are helpful in assisting breathing in small ruminants. Supplemental oxygen can also be delivered directly from a gas anesthesia machine or directly from an oxygen tank by placing insufflation tubing into the endotracheal tube.

Recovery

Ruminants are allowed to breathe 100% oxygen from the anesthesia machine for as long as possible before they are disconnected from the device. After patients are disconnected from the anesthesia machine, oxygen from a tank source can be given in the recovery area by placing insufflation tubing into the endotracheal tube while it is in place.

Ruminants are allowed to recover in sternal recumbency if possible. This position improves ventilation and facilitates eructation (necessary to alleviate the bloat that usually develops to some degree during anesthesia). They can be propped sternally between support pads or hay bales. The front legs are folded beneath the chest. If lateral recumbency is necessary, right lateral recumbency is less likely to cause regurgitation (less weight on the rumen).

Regurgitation and aspiration still are possible during recovery. Leaving the endotracheal tube in place with the cuff at least partially inflated is important until the swallowing reflex is observed. The tube should be removed with the cuff partially inflated. The head should be placed so that any regurgitated material can flow freely from the mouth; this requires that the head be slightly "downhill."

Equipment for treatment of bloat should be readily available. An oral speculum, stomach tube, rumen trocar, and skin preparation materials are recommended.

Cattle are generally "sensible" in the recovery stall and seldom try to stand prematurely. Assistance is not often required. However, the recovery period should still be closely observed, and personnel should be available to assist should an emergency occur.

COMMON SURGICAL PROCEDURES

CASTRATION

Castration is one of the most commonly performed surgical procedures in ruminants. Although it can be done at any age, the complication rate and difficulty of the procedure increase with age; therefore, early castration usually is in the best interest of the animal. Preferably, castration is performed at a time of year when flies and other insects are at a minimum. The environment should be clean and dry. Tetanus prophylaxis must be provided either with protection from the dam's colostrum or by injection of tetanus antitoxin or tetanus toxoid.

Castration may be performed with strict attention to aseptic technique and anesthesia. Sterile gloves and instruments may be used and the skin prepared properly. In reality, however, adhering to these surgical "principles" requires extra time and expense, and these principles are not often followed in field situations. In these settings, instruments should always be cleaned of blood and debris and disinfected between use in different animals. Skin preparation is minimized to a brief but thorough scrub. The operator's hands should be washed and disinfected thoroughly between animals. Despite appearances, these field methods have been used successfully for many years.

An animal can be castrated in a variety of ways. Castration methods are selected on the basis of species, age, management, and environmental factors. Although all methods have been used successfully, some are used less often because of associated complications. The common practice of performing castration without local anesthesia or sedation has become controversial. However, the immature metabolism of very young animals limits the selection of drugs that can be safely used, and the restraint and pain caused by injecting local anesthetic drugs may be as stressful and painful as the castration itself. Use of drugs also increases the time and cost of the procedure. However, as animal welfare awareness increases, the use of anesthesia will also undoubtedly increase. The most recent advance is the finding that meloxicam given to calves before castration is actually cost effective. This drug is an excellent analgesic, and calves that received it before castration were shown to have better average daily gains after castration than in calves that did not receive meloxicam. The U.S. Food and Drug Administration (FDA) has also allowed meloxicam use legally through the Animal Medicinal Drug Use Clarification Act (AMDUCA). The dosage that has been found to be effective is 1 mg/kg, and a one-time dose has been found to be effective for 3 to 5 days.

TECHNICIAN NOTE   Meloxicam use for castration and dehorning is legal under the Animal Medicinal Drug Use Clarification Act (AMDUCA), and this drug is effective as an analgesic for calves.

The two basic categories of castration methods are open and closed. Both techniques are used in ruminants. Open castration methods involve incision through the skin of the scrotum to expose the testicles. The incisions are left open to drain and heal by second intention. Although closure of the incisions with suture is surgically possible, it is hardly ever done because closure prevents drainage from the wound and requires more time and expense to perform. Closed castration techniques are performed without skin incision. Closed techniques usually are bloodless when performed correctly, which is an advantage during insect season. However, closed techniques are not without potential complications. (Closed castration [without skin incision] is never used in horses. In horses, the terms "open" and "closed" refer to whether the *vaginal tunic* is incised. Thus, the use of these terms may be confusing.)

Before any castration procedure, the presence of both testicles in the scrotum should be confirmed. Cryptorchidism does occur in cattle, and removal of only one descended testicle should be avoided.

Calves less than 1 month old typically are held in lateral recumbency because they are too small for cattle chutes. Older calves are candidates for standing castration in a cattle chute or stocks, with tail restraint. The commonly used methods of castration in the bovine include the following.

Surgical "Knife" Castration

This procedure is most commonly performed before or at the time of weaning, at approximately 3 to 4 months of age. However, it can be performed at any age. The first step of the procedure is scrotal incision to expose the testicles. A scalpel blade or castrating knife is used to cut laterally across and remove the entire bottom third of the scrotum, which exposes the testicles. Another method of incising the scrotum is with a Newberry knife, which is placed in the middle of the scrotum and is pulled quickly, distally, to produce a vertical scrotal incision between the testicles (Fig. 14-13).

TECHNICIAN NOTE   Surgical "knife" castration is most commonly performed at the time of weaning.

The second step of the procedure is removal of the testicles. A testicle is grasped and pulled out of the scrotum to expose the spermatic cord. In young calves, the testicle can simply be pulled until the cord stretches and ruptures. The separation causes the smooth muscle in the wall of the testicular blood vessels to spasm shut ("vasospasm"), thereby providing *hemostasis*. Alternatively, in older animals with more development of the spermatic cord, the cord can be ligated with absorbable suture and then cut to remove the testicle.

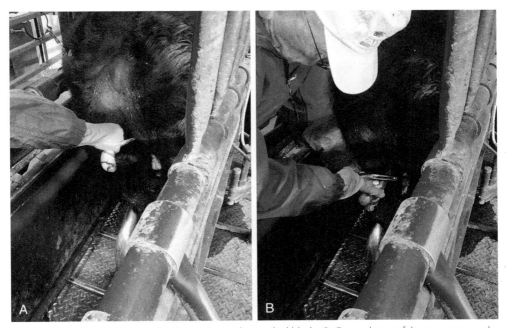

FIGURE 14-13 A, Incision into the scrotum with a scalpel blade. **B,** Emasculation of the spermatic cord.

The procedure is repeated on the other testicle. The scrotal incision is left open for drainage and heals as an open wound. After the procedure, antiseptic or antibiotic spray is usually applied to the scrotal incisions. During insect season, insect repellent should be applied directly to the areas around the incision but not in the incision itself.

Emasculators

The use of emasculators is necessary for animals with more developed spermatic cords, to provide more reliable hemostasis. The scrotum is incised as described for surgical knife castration. After the testicle and spermatic cord are exposed, emasculators are applied across the spermatic cord. The emasculators simultaneously crush and sever the spermatic cord (Fig. 14-14). The emasculators are left in place for a brief time, depending on the size of the spermatic cord. The procedure is repeated on the other testicle. Antiseptic or antibiotic topical medications and insect repellent are used as described for surgical knife castration.

Emasculatome (Burdizzo)

This "bloodless" castration method is popular for castration during fly season. The emasculatome is a crushing "pincer"-type instrument that is used to crush the spermatic cord above the testicle, through the skin, without an incision. The spermatic cord is identified beneath the skin by palpation, and the instrument is applied across it (usually two applications, 1 to 2 cm apart). The procedure is repeated for the other spermatic cord. The instrument is never applied across the entire width of the scrotum, to preserve some blood flow to the scrotum and allow it to survive. The testicles subsequently atrophy within the scrotum but usually do not slough. This method is less reliable because it is performed "blindly" through the skin. Incomplete destruction of the spermatic cord may result.

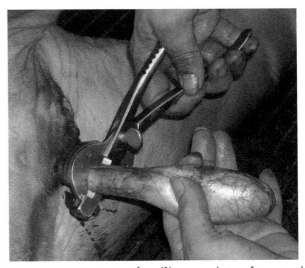

FIGURE 14-14 Castration of a calf by emasculation after removal of the bottom half of the scrotum. (From Bassert JM, McCurnin DM, editors: *McCurnin's clinical textbook for veterinary technicians,* ed 8, St. Louis, 2014, Saunders.)

Elastrator

"Banding" is a procedure in which an instrument is used to apply a special rubber band around the base of the scrotum, proximal to (above) the testicles. The band is so tight that it acts as a tourniquet, resulting in necrosis and sloughing of the testicles and scrotum in 2 to 3 weeks. Although no incision is used, the necrotic tissue may attract insects, so insect repellent must be used during insect season. Clostridial disease is a serious issue with elastrator band use, and vaccination for clostridial diseases should always be performed at the same time as banding.

Chemical Castration

Chemical castration has been used for very young males weighing less than 150 pounds. Each testicle is injected with a castration solution containing a chemical that gradually destroys the testicular tissue and a local anesthetic for pain relief. The method is bloodless, and normally no tissue sloughing occurs. Castration is complete in 60 to 90 days. Proper injection technique is essential for the success of the procedure; otherwise, incomplete castration and other complications may result. The commercial availability of the solution has not been reliable.

Vaccination

A vaccine against gonadotropin-releasing hormone (GnRH) has been recently developed.

Complications of Castration

Hemorrhage and infection are the primary postoperative complications of castration. Hemorrhage is a complication of open (incisional) castration methods. Animals should be observed for hemorrhage for 24 hours after open castration procedures. Infections usually occur from 5 to 15 days after open castration and are often associated with failure of the incisions to drain. Common clinical signs are marked swelling, fever, and inappetence. Some clinicians administer antibiotics prophylactically in the hope of reducing postoperative infections.

DEHORNING (CORNUECTOMY)

Ruminants may be horned or polled (genetically lacking horns), depending on species, breed, and sex. Horns grow continuously throughout the life of the animal unless the horns are removed at their base. Horns are often removed for several reasons. Horns are potentially dangerous weapons, even potentially fatal to humans and to other animals. Great damage can be caused by fighting using the horns. Feedlots typically pay less money for horned animals because of the additional expense of having the horns removed before the animals can be safely placed in a drylot group. Horned animals are more likely to cause damage to facilities and require more space in transportation vehicles and at the feedbunk. Horns may become tangled in fences, branches, and other objects, with resulting great trauma to the animal, including death by hanging. Dehorning is a common procedure in cattle.

It is in the animal's best interest to remove the horns at the earliest possible age. Removal of mature horns has a higher complication rate, including increased hemorrhage, risk of infection (sinusitis and possible brain abscessation), and incomplete removal. Removal also requires more sedation and local anesthesia and greater technical skill. Removal of horns at an early stage is greatly preferred.

In horned animals, each horn grows from a separate horn bud *(horn button),* located on top of the head between the ears. The horn buds may be present at birth, or they may become palpable as two hard lumps under the skin in the first couple of weeks. An irregular whorl of hair often covers each developing horn bud. Removal of the horn buds, before actual horn growth begins, is referred to as "disbudding." At this early stage, the horn buds are not yet attached to the skull, so the frontal sinus is not exposed when the horns are removed. Disbudding can be accomplished using several methods.

Chemical Cautery

Various chemical pastes are available to cauterize and kill the germinal epithelium that eventually generates the horn. Best results are obtained if the procedure is performed in the first week of life, generally from day 3 to 7. Clipping the hair around the horn bud may increase contact with the paste and produce a more reliable result. Applying a liberal petroleum jelly "ring" around the area before treatment may help prevent the chemicals from running into the eyes and other tissues and possibly causing severe trauma. The chemicals are caustic to the tissues of other animals and humans, so great care must be taken with their use. The paste should be allowed to dry completely before the animal is allowed to nurse. This method is not highly reliable in completely killing the germinal tissue and often results in a small, deformed, partial horn growth or "*scur*" that must be removed later by other methods. This procedure seems to cause more persistent pain than other methods, and the animal may rub the area in response, thus possibly spreading the paste to other areas and causing damage. The animal should be kept out of the rain for several days. Because of the potential risks, chemical cautery cannot be highly recommended for disbudding.

Heat Cautery

Heat cautery can be performed in young calves to cauterize the horn bud. This procedure is further described in Chapter 18. In the Midwest, the procedure is often done to control bleeding after use of the Barnes dehorner at weaning.

Several dehorning methods are available. They are generally selected according to the size of the horns.

Surgical Removal

Surgical excision of the horn buds is possible. General anesthesia may be used.

After several weeks of age, horn growth has begun, and removal is then referred to as "dehorning." Dehorning usually is performed on a conscious, sedated animal with local anesthesia used for control of pain. Sedation with xylazine and local anesthesia with a cornual nerve block or ring block at the base of the horn is most often used for these procedures. The animal must be physically restrained and the head securely held or tied. General anesthesia may be used, especially for adult animals with large horns. Clipping and surgical preparation of the skin are performed before the procedure. Tetanus vaccination status should be confirmed, and tetanus prophylaxis should be provided as needed.

Surgical Saws

Large horns are removed by making a circular skin incision around the base of the horn and then removing the horn and

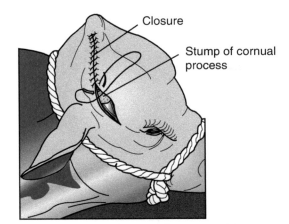

FIGURE 14-15 Primary closure used in cosmetic dehorning surgery.

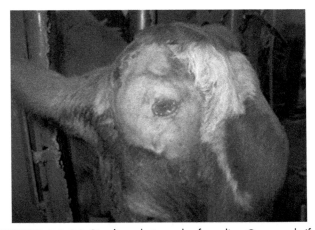

FIGURE 14-16 Standing photograph of yearling Guernsey heifer with frontal deformation caused by fluid-filled sinus several months after dehorning. The dehorning site never completely healed over and periodically produced exudate. At the time of initial evaluation, the animal was reluctant to have the skull examined and demonstrated marked unilateral dullness on percussion and deformation of the right side of the skull. This photograph was taken several days after a cornual opening was débrided and a ventral trephine hole was produced to facilitate drainage. Material continued to drain from the sinus despite daily saline lavage. (From Anderson DE, Rings DM: *Current veterinary therapy: food animal practice*, ed 5, St. Louis, 2008, Saunders.)

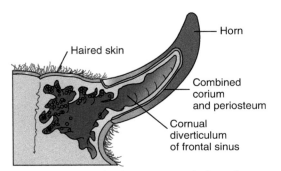

FIGURE 14-17 Longitudinal cross-section of a horn showing extension of the frontal sinus of the skull into the horn. Dehorning, which is performed at the base of the horn, may expose the sinus.

the horn base with either a dehorning saw or a Gigli wire saw. An assistant is useful to stabilize the animal's head while the sawing is performed. Hemorrhage occurs and must be controlled. Sometimes the surgeon can close the skin over the exposed sinuses with sutures ("*cosmetic dehorning*"), but this is rarely possible with large horns (Fig. 14-15).

Complications of dehorning must be considered, and owners must be well informed. Hemorrhage from removal of developed horns is expected and may be considerable. The frontal sinus develops within the horn base and is exposed by dehorning; the resulting hole may be impressively large (Fig. 14-16 and 14-17). This exposure makes bacterial infection and parasitic invasion (*myiasis*—infection by fly maggots) of the sinus possible. Rarely, infections extend through

the sinus and calvarium into the meninges and brain tissue. To minimize complications, blood clots should be removed from the exposed sinuses. Antibiotic ointment can be applied to the skin edges, and bandages can be applied to the head to cover the open sinuses. Bandages can be made from small stacks of sterile 4 × 4 gauze squares and held in place with elastic tape placed carefully in a figure-of-eight configuration around the head and ears. Some clinicians do not advocate the use of bandages and instead prefer to allow the area to heal as an open wound.

Antibiotic sprays and powders placed directly into the sinus may be irritating and delay healing, although historically they have been used successfully. Use of insect repellent is essential if dehorning is performed during fly season. Some clinicians advocate systemic antibiotics and nonsteroidal antiinflammatory drugs. Healing normally occurs in 6 to 8 weeks for smaller horns. Large horns may require several months for healing and occasionally may fail to heal completely.

Some owners may request removal of only the tips of the horns (*"tipping"*). The procedure should be performed beyond the extent of the frontal sinus within the horn to prevent creating a permanent opening. Radiographs may be taken to confirm the extent of the frontal sinus. Wire or dehorning saws can be used to remove the tip. Tip removal does not prevent the continual growth of the horn.

Tube or Spoon Dehorners
Very small horns can be removed with tube or spoon dehorners. These small handheld "gouges" are placed over the developing horn and are twisted in a circular motion to cut away the horn and horn base. Bleeding is minimal and can be controlled with pressure.

Lever-Type Dehorners
The Barnes dehorner is the most popular style of scoop-type dehorner for small and medium horns. It consists of two long handles, each with an extremely sharp metal cutting edge. The handles are held together while the circular opening is placed over the horn and the horn base. Spreading the handles apart actually closes the cutting edges together, thus producing a scooping-type cutting action that cuts under and removes the horn and its base

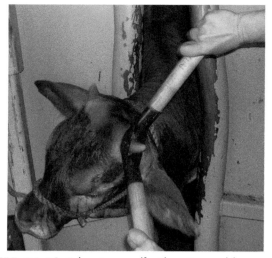

FIGURE 14-18 Dehorning a calf with a Barnes dehorner. (From Bassert JM, McCurnin DM, editors: *McCurnin's clinical textbook for veterinary technicians*, ed 8, St. Louis, 2014, Saunders.)

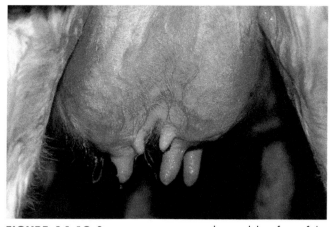

FIGURE 14-19 Supernumerary teats on the caudal surface of the bovine mammary gland. (From Blowey RW, Weaver AD: *Color atlas of diseases and disorders of cattle*, ed 3, St. Louis, 2012, Mosby Ltd.)

in one piece (Fig. 14-18). Different size instruments are available for different sizes of horns.

The Keystone dehorner is a larger instrument for larger horns. Pulling the lever handles together closes the cutting jaws of the instrument and removes the horn. Hemorrhage often is considerable and must be controlled by pulling the cornual arteries or cautery. Skull fractures are more likely to occur with this method than with others.

TAIL AMPUTATION (TAIL DOCKING)

Amputation of the tail can be done as an elective procedure but sometimes is a necessary procedure following severe injury. Elective tail amputation is sometimes performed in dairy cattle and is referred to as *tail docking.*

In dairy cattle, tail docking historically has been done to facilitate udder hygiene and improve the comfort and health of milking personnel (by reducing getting "swatted" with urine- and feces-soaked tails). However, neither the beneficial health claims to personnel nor the claims of improved udder and milk hygiene have been substantiated. Potential animal welfare issues have been identified, such as pain and discomfort related to the procedure and especially the animal's inability to remove flies from the hindquarters. The American Veterinary Medical Association (AVMA) Animal Welfare Committee released the following position statement in 2004:

> *The AVMA opposes routine tail docking of cattle. Current scientific literature indicates that routine tail docking provides no benefit to the animal, and that tail docking can lead to distress during fly seasons. When medically necessary, amputation of tails must be performed by a licensed veterinarian.*

Injury to the tail may be severe enough to necessitate amputation in any species. Depending on the animal and the circumstances, the procedure may be done using general anesthesia or with sedation and local anesthesia (caudal epidural or subcutaneous ring block).

The tail is clipped and prepared in a sterile manner. A tourniquet at the base of the tail may be used for hemostasis. The clinician decides on the level of amputation, depending on the injury. The skin is pushed forward as much as possible to allow for skin to cover the wound. The vertebral column usually is severed through an intervertebral space, with enough skin left to suture over the remaining stump. Medication for pain control, antibiotics, and insect repellent may be necessary after the surgical procedure.

SUPERNUMERARY TEATS

Supernumerary teats are extra or accessory teats are found occasionally in ruminants. They usually are small and may arise directly from the udder or from the side of a main teat. The most common location is caudal to the main teats (Fig. 14-19). They typically communicate with their own small, but functional, mammary gland tissue. Extra teats may interfere with proper fit of the milking machine cups and may become affected with mastitis; therefore, they are commonly amputated.

Tetanus prophylaxis should be provided. The amputation technique depends on the age of the female. Methods include use of an emasculatome (Burdizzo) or an emasculator to crush the base of the extra teat (for hemostasis) in animals more than 6 months old. In older (mature) animals with more developed teats and gland tissue, removal requires sedation and local anesthesia, skin incision, and dissection of the teat and its associated gland tissue. The incision is closed in layers with suture.

URETHROSTOMY FOR UROLITHIASIS

Several surgical treatments have been used for treatment and management of the condition urolithiasis. Surgical procedures are designed to prevent recurrent obstruction and its associated life-threatening complications. However, the procedures do not prevent stone formation; they only attempt to provide better channels for elimination of stones. Clients must understand the difference between preventing stone obstruction and preventing stone formation when considering surgical intervention. Any attempt to prevent stone formation must involve changes in nutritional management.

Perineal *urethrostomy* has historically been the surgical procedure of choice. It may be performed using general anesthesia or with heavy sedation with anesthesia provided by an epidural procedure. The patient's position may be standing or dorsal or lateral recumbency. The perineal area is clipped and surgically prepared. The surgeon makes a midline incision between the anus and scrotum to expose the penis (Fig. 14-20). Dissection is continued to incise the penis and open the urethra. The exposed urethra is carefully sutured to the skin to produce a permanent, new urethral opening in the perineal area (as clients frequently observe, "He pees like a girl"), so the layperson's term for perineal urethrostomy is "heifering." A Foley catheter is placed for several days to maintain the new opening during the initial postoperative period. Because the new opening is proximal to the sigmoid flexure and is wider than the distal penile urethra, stones should theoretically void with less risk of obstruction. Unfortunately, a high incidence of stricture formation is associated with the procedure; the procedure also prevents breeding by intact males. Urine scalding of the thighs is common after the procedure. At present, perineal urethrostomy is considered a salvage procedure.

Currently, *cystotomy* and tube cystostomy are preferred surgical procedures. Long-term survival is better, and breeding function can be preserved. General anesthesia is required. The patient is positioned in dorsal recumbency, and the ventral abdomen is clipped and surgically prepared. A right paramedian incision is made to enter the abdomen. The bladder is identified and opened; this allows the surgeon to remove all bladder calculi and to lavage the bladder. A catheter then can be passed through the bladder into the urethra to allow flushing of any stones in the urethra. When the bladder and urethra are cleared, the incisions in the bladder and the abdominal wall are closed. In some cases, urethral obstructions may not be cleared completely by this approach; these patients are candidates for tube cystostomy. For tube cystostomy, a Foley catheter is placed in the bladder and exits through a stab incision in the abdominal wall. This allows continual drainage of urine and gives the obstructed, inflamed urethral tissue a chance to rest and heal. The hope is that the urethral stones will pass as the swelling subsides. The Foley catheter should be examined regularly for proper placement and patency, and it should be kept clean. The skin incisions should be monitored for signs of infection and kept clean of debris and exudates. The catheter is eventually clamped to force urination through the urethra. After normal, full-stream, pain-free urination through the urethra is confirmed for 1 to 2 days, the Foley catheter is deflated and removed. The bladder generally seals and heals rapidly, without complication.

Other surgical procedures such as *urethrotomy*, combined perineal urethrostomy with cystotomy, *bladder marsupialization* (permanently attaching the bladder to the abdominal

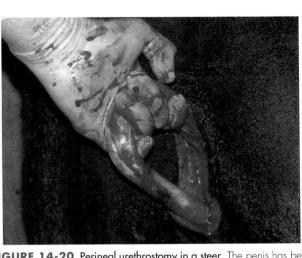

FIGURE 14-20 Perineal urethrostomy in a steer. The penis has been mobilized and brought to the incision with good mobility, allowing for a tension-free fixation. (From Anderson DE, Rings DM: *Current veterinary therapy: food animal practice*, ed 5, St. Louis, 2008, Saunders.)

wall and creating a permanent opening for urine to void), penile amputation, and urethroscopy with laser *lithotripsy* have been described and used variably in different ruminant species. Some of these procedures are used only to salvage individuals intended for slaughter.

Considerations for Any Incision Into the Abdominal Cavity

Theoretically, an incision can be made anywhere, in any direction, and be of any length. However, the anatomy and biomechanics of the abdominal wall, such as the fascia, tension lines, and direction of muscle fibers, dictate the best locations and directions for incisions. When selecting a surgical approach, the surgeon must also consider the location of the organs or structures that need to be accessed.

CELIOTOMY
Ventral Celiotomy

Ventral abdominal approaches usually require general anesthesia, with the patient in dorsal recumbency. The following are standard locations of ventral *celiotomy* incisions (Fig. 14-21):

- Ventral midline approach: This incision is made directly on the midline, in a craniocaudal direction, with entry into the abdominal cavity through the linea alba. The incision may be of any length or location between the xiphoid process and the pelvis. It is the most common ventral approach; it assists thorough exploration of the abdomen.
- Ventral paramedian approach: This incision is made either to the right or the left of the ventral midline and parallel to the ventral midline.
- Inguinal approach: This incision is directly over an inguinal canal.
- Transverse abdominal approach: This is rarely used for entry into the pelvic cavity. It begins caudal to the umbilicus and extends transversely no farther than the fold of the flank.

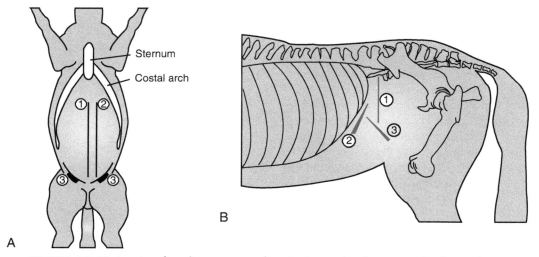

FIGURE 14-21 Locations for celiotomy approaches. **A,** *1,* ventral midline approach; *2,* ventral paramedian approach; *3,* inguinal approach (right and left). **B,** *1,* paralumbar fossa approach; *2,* paracostal approach; *3,* Marcenac approach.

Flank Celiotomy

In flank celiotomy, an incision is made through the flank into the abdomen. "Laparotomy" is a synonym for flank celiotomy. Laparotomy is performed with the patient either standing or in lateral recumbency. The incision may be made high, low, or in the middle of either flank. The following are several standard locations for laparotomy incisions:

*   Paralumbar fossa approach: This is the most common flank approach. The paralumbar fossa is the large depression between the last rib and the tuber coxae. The skin incision is made in a dorsoventral direction. The deeper incisions through the muscle layers may be made either dorsoventrally through all the muscles or parallel to the direction of the muscle fibers of each muscle ("grid" incision).
*   Paracostal approach: This angled incision parallels the last rib.
*   *Marcenac approach:* This low oblique flank incision is made in a craniodorsal to caudoventral direction. It is used occasionally for C-section.
*   Caudal rib resection: This procedure is used to approach structures that are in the dorsal abdomen that cannot be exteriorized through more ventral approaches (kidney or spleen). Portions of the caudal one or two ribs are removed with a Gigli wire saw to expose the peritoneum. The procedure opens the caudalmost aspect of the thoracic cavity en route to the abdominal cavity. Entering the thoracic cavity may cause respiratory difficulty, so the anesthetist should be prepared to assist ventilation.

Vaginal Celiotomy

In vaginal celiotomy, an incision is made through the cranial portion of the vaginal wall into the abdomen. "*Colpotomy*" is a synonym for vaginal celiotomy. Colpotomy is usually performed with the patient standing. It is most often used to remove ovaries. Often this is performed through a line block in the left flank.

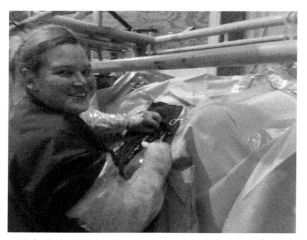

FIGURE 14-22 Cesarean section. Note the sterile field.

Cesarean Section

The preparation for a C-section is similar to that for all other celiotomy procedures. The location of the incision varies among veterinarians, and the technician should make sure to be familiar with the veterinarian's preferences before preparing the patient for the procedure. Often, caudal epidural anesthesia is performed as well as the celiotomy. The technician should be prepared to gown and glove in the event assistance with removing the calf from uterus is needed (Fig. 14-22).

Left or Right Displacement of the Abomasum

Left displacement of the abomasum refers to relocation of the abomasum to the left side of midline between the rumen and the left body wall. This displacement can be medically managed. In addition, several minimally invasive closed procedures are available, including rolling, blind tack, toggle pin, and laparoscopy-assisted toggle pin. The final option is to perform a celiotomy with abomasopexy.

Right displacement is less common and occurs when the abomasum relocates to the right side of the midline. It also can be medically managed and surgically corrected; however, it is usually associated with a less favorable prognosis.

Prolapses

Treatment of prolapses starts with placement of caudal epidural anesthesia. After the epidural anesthesia is in effect, the prolapse should be thoroughly cleaned using a povidone-iodine (Betadine) or chlorhexidine solution. All necrotic tissue should be removed. All folds and depressions should be thoroughly cleaned. The clinician will then replace the organ. The technician should be prepared to administer the antibiotics or other drugs of the clinician's choice.

CASE STUDY

You have been sent to the clinic pharmacy to obtain xylazine for use as a preanesthetic. When you arrive at the pharmacy, you notice two different concentrations of xylazine. You know that your patient is a 4-year-old Holstein. Which concentration of xylazine should you bring to the veterinarian?

CASE STUDY

It is midsummer, and you are going to Mr. Fritz's home to dehorn 500 head of weanling Hereford calves. Mr. Fritz lives 60 miles from the clinic. Which methods of dehorning could the veterinarian choose to use? Which method will he most likely use? What equipment will you want to make sure is inside the pickup truck before you leave?

SUGGESTED READING

Anderson DE, Rings DM: *Current veterinary therapy: food animal practice*, ed 5, St. Louis, 2008, Saunders.

Bentz AI, Gill MS: Large animal medical nursing. In Bassert JM, McCurnin DM, editors: *McCurnin's clinical textbook for veterinary technicians*, ed 7, St. Louis, 2010, Saunders, pp 713–768.

Fubini SL, Ducharme NG: *Farm animal surgery*, St. Louis, 2004, Saunders.

Hafez ESE, Hafez B, editors: *Reproduction in farm animals*, ed 7, New York, 2000, Wiley-Blackwell.

Mitchell CF, Moore RM, Gill MS: Large animal surgical nursing. In Bassert JM, McCurnin DM, editors: *McCurnin's clinical textbook for veterinary technicians*, ed 7, St. Louis, 2010, Saunders, pp 1056–1092.

Muir WW 3rd, Hubbell JAE, Skard R, et al.: *Handbook of veterinary anesthesia*, ed 3, St. Louis, 2000, Mosby.

Noakes DE, Parkinson RJ, England GCW: *Veterinary reproduction and obstetrics*, ed 9, London, 2009, Saunders.

Sonsthagen TF, Teeple TN: Nursing care of food animals, camelids, and ratites. In Sirois M, editor: *Principles and practice of veterinary technology*, ed 3, St. Louis, 2011, Mosby, pp 585–611.

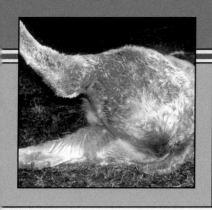

15 Common Bovine Diseases

OUTLINE

LEARNING OBJECTIVES

When you have completed this chapter, you will be able to

- Describe and recognize clinical signs associated with all common bovine diseases
- Understand the etiology of the diseases
- Understand and describe common treatments for bovine disease
- Know the common scientific names of parasites associated with cattle
- Know the common vaccinations and their schedules associated with cattle

KEY TERMS

Clinical mastitis
Complement fixation tests
Contagious mastitis
Corkscrew claw
Environmental mastitis
Epididymitis

Free-gas bloat
Frothy bloat
Gangrenous mastitis
Iceberg concept
Milk ring tests
Orchitis

Placentomes
Rose Bengal test
Scissor claw
Slipper foot
Subclinical mastitis

KEY ABBREVIATIONS

BRD: Bovine respiratory disease (complex)
BSE: Bovine spongiform encephalopathy
BVD: Bovine virus diarrhea

CF: Complement fixation
IBR: Infectious bovine rhinotracheitis
LDA: Left displacement of the abomasum
PEM: Polioencephalomalacia

RDA: Right displacement of the abomasum
TB: Tuberculosis

BACTERIAL DISEASES

ANTHRAX

- Etiology: *Bacillus anthracis*
- Gram-positive bacillus
- Sudden death and septicemia
- Reportable disease
- Vaccine in the presence of an outbreak

Anthrax is also known as splenic fever. Anthrax is caused by *Bacillus anthracis,* which is a gram-positive, nonmotile, spore-forming bacterium. Cattle are often infected through contaminated pastures or by eating contaminated feedstuffs. The anthrax bacillus is commonly found in soils that have neutral or alkaline pH. In these types of soils, the bacteria often multiply. As the bacteria multiply, they rise to infectious levels, which explains the several years between outbreaks. Outbreaks often occur after flooding in endemic areas. During an outbreak, insects can spread the disease from animal to animal.

Anthrax can affect all warm-blooded animals, including humans. The disease is acute, febrile, and characterized by septicemia. Cattle with anthrax are often found dead. The death frequently is sudden and occurs in an otherwise seemingly healthy animal. If animals do not present as deceased, clinical signs include ataxia and bleeding from the orifices (nose, mouth, vulva, and anus). The blood often is dark and fails to clot. The incubation period of anthrax is 1 to 14 days (average, 3 to 7 days). Other clinical signs include localized swelling of subcutaneous tissue, especially in areas of the neck, shoulders, and thorax. Another major clinical sign is the absence of rigor mortis. Death often results within a few days of infection.

> **TECHNICIAN NOTE**   Bleeding from the orifices and the absence of rigor mortis are clinical signs of anthrax.

If the veterinarian suspects anthrax in a deceased animal, a necropsy should not be performed. When the bacteria are exposed to oxygen from an open carcass, they form spores that are resistant to extreme temperatures and chemical disinfectants. The diagnosis should be based initially on a blood smear. The disease can be confirmed by laboratory tests and growth of *B. anthracis* on an agar plate. The differential diagnosis includes bloat, clostridial disease, lightning strike, anaplasmosis, and bacillary hemoglobinuria. When necropsy is performed, the characteristic finding is an enlarged, dark, and soft-textured spleen (Fig. 15-1).

If anthrax is identified in the early stages, aggressive systemic penicillin or oxytetracycline therapy may be useful. Vaccination should be practiced in endemic areas. Efforts should be made to control the disease as quickly as possible. Anthrax is a reportable disease, and the state veterinarian should be contacted immediately. The cattle in question should be quarantined. Any materials that were contacted by the dead animal and the dead animal itself should be cremated and buried deep within the earth. Producers should disinfect all livestock areas, use insect repellents, control rodents and wild animals, and practice good sanitary conditions for themselves.

> **TECHNICIAN NOTE**   Anthrax is a reportable disease.

BLACKLEG

- Etiology: *Clostridium chauvoei*
- Gram-positive rod
- Sudden death and muscle necrosis
- Vaccine

Blackleg is caused by *Clostridium chauvoei,* which is a large, anaerobic, spore-forming, rod-shaped organism. The development of blackleg is often sporadic. Infected animals harbor the bacteria in their muscles. When the infected animal develops an open wound or undergoes bruising, the area provides an anaerobic environment in which the bacteria thrive.

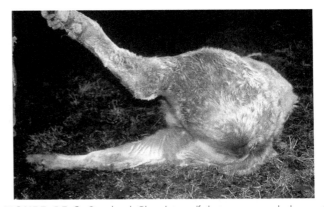

FIGURE 15-1 Characteristic, soft-textured spleen of a calf infected with anthrax. (From Blowey RW, Weaver AD: *Color atlas of diseases and disorders of cattle,* ed 3, London, 2012, Mosby Ltd.)

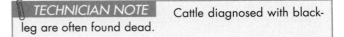

FIGURE 15-2 Crossbred Charolais calf that was severely lame at pasture has massive gluteal swelling of the left leg. (From Blowey RW, Weaver AD: *Color atlas of diseases and disorders of cattle,* ed 2, London, 2003, Mosby.)

> **TECHNICIAN NOTE**   Cattle diagnosed with blackleg are often found dead.

The disease often manifests in feedlot cattle. Although most animals are found dead in the absence of clinical signs, animals with cases caught early can present acutely with depression and lameness (Fig. 15-2). At necropsy, necrotic muscle can be isolated. The necrotic muscle has a distinct, rancid smell. Often the affected muscle lies adjacent to normal tissue. The diagnosis is frequently made based on these characteristic necrotic lesions (Fig. 15-3), and it is confirmed by fluorescent antibody staining.

The differential diagnosis includes malignant edema, anthrax, and lightning strike. Prevention of blackleg includes vaccination on enzootic farms. Cattle caught in the early stages of the disease should be treated with penicillin and nonsteroidal antiinflammatory drugs.

BOVINE RESPIRATORY DISEASE COMPLEX

- Etiology: various causes
- Respiratory disease
- Vaccine with limitations

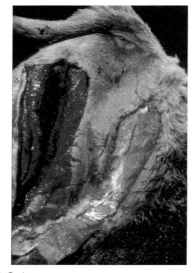

FIGURE 15-3 At postmortem examination, necrotic tissue was found in the left gluteal muscle compared with none in the right gluteal muscle. (From Blowey RW, Weaver AD: *Color atlas of diseases and disorders of cattle,* ed 3, London, 2012, Mosby Ltd.)

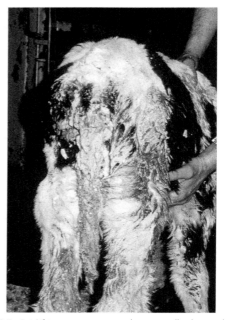

FIGURE 15-4 White scours occurs when partially digested white milk is passed in the feces. (From Blowey RW, Weaver AD: *Color atlas of diseases and disorders of cattle,* ed 2, London, 2003, Mosby.)

Bovine respiratory disease complex is known as BRD. The disease has a multifactorial etiology. The disease is caused by stress and interactions of the environment such as crowding, poor ventilation, dust, transport, and commingling. Many bacteria and viruses are involved in the pathologic process, and often infection with one pathogen allows for colonization of another. The purpose of the place of BRD here in this chapter is to familiarize technicians with the complex because its name is often used to imply multiple causes.

BRUCELLOSIS

- Etiology: *Brucella abortus*
- Gram-negative rod
- Abortion
- Reportable disease
- Vaccine with limitations

Brucellosis is also known as Bang disease and contagious abortion. Brucellosis is caused by *Brucella abortus,* but it also can be caused by *Brucella melitensis* or *Brucella suis. Brucella* species are gram-negative rods that grow best in a carbon dioxide–enriched aerobic environment. The infection occurs when cattle ingest infected placenta, feedstuffs, fetuses, tissue, milk, or uterine discharge. Congenital infection may occur. Much of the United States is free of *B. abortus,* but some wild animals still carry the infection and could infect cattle. Infection results in abortion between 7 and 8 months of gestation. Most cows abort only once and then become carriers. Carriers shed the organism in the milk, fetus, placenta, and uterine discharge.

> **TECHNICIAN NOTE**   Brucellosis causes abortion in cattle between 7 and 8 months of gestation.

The major clinical sign of brucellosis infection within a herd is an abortion storm. Infected cows may be more prone to retained placentas, endometritis, and infertility. Bulls may develop *orchitis* and *epididymitis.* Synovitis (hygromas) may occur, and fistulous withers may be seen in horses.

The differential diagnosis includes trichomoniasis, leptospirosis, neosporosis, and infectious bovine rhinotracheitis (IBR). A diagnosis can be confirmed through blood agglutination tests (card tests), *milk ring tests,* and *complement fixation (CF) tests.* The *Rose Bengal test* can be used as a rapid screening test.

Screening for the disease is possible and is carried out, especially in endemic areas. When a positive animal is identified, the entire herd should be tested, and positive animals should be slaughtered. Heifer calves can be vaccinated against the disease. The vaccine is often called Bang vaccine. Some states require vaccination of heifer calves 4 to 8 months of age. Bull calves and steer calves should not be vaccinated for fear of causing a chronic infection in reproductive organs. The disease is zoonotic and is called "undulant fever" in humans. Pasteurization of milk kills the bacteria, although consumption of unpasteurized milk products is dangerous for the human population because of the increased risk of infection.

> **TECHNICIAN NOTE**   Brucellosis causes undulant fever in humans.

CALF ENTERITIS

- Etiology: multiple causes, bacteria, viruses, and parasites
- General malaise, diarrhea, and dehydration
- Some vaccines

Calf enteritis is also known as scours (Fig. 15-4). Calf scours is a major cause of death in the first few weeks of life.

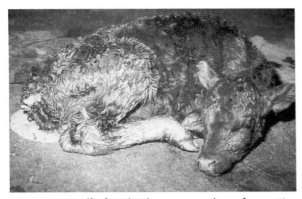

FIGURE 15-5 Calf infected with *Cryptosporidium* infection. The calf shows signs of dehydration and has sunken eyes. The calf has a dry muzzle, hyperemia of the nares, and purulent nasal discharge. (From Blowey RW, Weaver AD: *Color atlas of diseases and disorders of cattle*, ed 2, London, 2003, Mosby.)

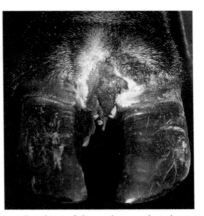

FIGURE 15-6 Sloughing of skin in the interdigital space. The necrotic tissue was cleaned off before this photograph was taken. (From Blowey RW, Weaver AD: *Color atlas of diseases and disorders of cattle*, ed 2, London, 2003, Mosby.)

Calves infected in the first few days of life are often infected with bacteria (e.g., *Escherichia coli* and *Clostridium perfringens*). When taking a history in these cases it is important to gather husbandry conditions, the age of the calf, and the color and consistency of the feces, as well as the possible presence of fecal blood. Cattle infected between 10 to 14 days of life are often infected with viruses (e.g., rotavirus and corona virus). Another type of infection that occurs in this age bracket is *Cryptosporidium* (Fig. 15-5). *Salmonella* infection may manifest at any age.

> **TECHNICIAN NOTE**   Calf scours is a major cause of death in the first few weeks of life.

The major clinical sign is diarrhea leading to dehydration. Management of calf scours should include good hygiene, proper passive transfer through colostrum, vaccinations, and good feeding practices.

> **TECHNICIAN NOTE**   Dehydration is a major side effect of diarrhea associated with scours.

FOOT ROT

- Etiology: *Fusobacterium necrophorum, Dichelobacter nodosus*
- Gram-negative bacillus
- Lameness
- Vaccine

Infectious foot rot is a contagious and common disease of cattle. Animals of all ages are susceptible, but the very young are rarely afflicted. The condition is painful, and animals in pain do not thrive. Major economic losses result from weight loss, low production, and costs of treatment.

> **TECHNICIAN NOTE**   Foot rot can cause economic losses as a result of weight loss, low production, and costs of treatment.

Foot rot is often caused by a mixed infection involving two primary bacterial organisms. *Dichelobacter* (formerly *Bacteroides*) *nodosus* is an anaerobic bacterium that has the ability to destroy keratin. *Fusobacterium necrophorum* is an anaerobic bacterium thought to be necessary for *D. nodosus* to invade, by causing dermatitis between the claws, which *D. nodosus* then can use as an entry point. *Corynebacterium (Actinomyces) pyogenes* may be involved, especially in the formation of deep abscesses.

> **TECHNICIAN NOTE**   The two primary agents of foot rot are *Dichelobacter nodosus* and *Fusobacterium necrophorum*.

The development of foot rot is largely influenced by management and environmental factors. The organisms favor moist or wet ground conditions. Trauma to the interdigital area from lacerations, abrasions, punctures, or softening from continual moisture allows the organisms to cause disease. Foot rot is uncommon in dry environments and in animals with healthy, intact skin in the interdigital cleft. Infected animals shed the organism directly from wounds into the soil, where other animals can pick it up by foot contact with the soil. Untreated animals can be a source of herd infections for months to years.

One or more feet may be affected. Cattle may be mild or moderately lame, but severe lameness affecting multiple individuals in a herd is the common presentation. Inflammation and necrotic tissue are present in the affected interdigital clefts and often produce an exudate and characteristic bad odor. Local swelling is common and may cause the claws to spread apart. A skin fissure often develops, with swollen, necrotic skin edges and purulent exudate (Fig. 15-6). The infection may extend to undermine the hoof walls in the areas adjacent to the interdigital infection (Fig. 15-7). The pain causes lameness, with the animal limping or holding the leg up in an attempt to avoid bearing weight. Fever may develop, especially with deep tissue infection. Deep abscesses

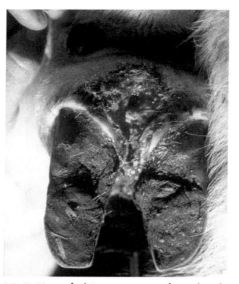

FIGURE 15-7 "Super foul," a severe case of interdigital necrobacillosis that extends onto the heel skin. (From Blowey RW, Weaver AD: *Color atlas of diseases and disorders of cattle*, ed 2, London, 2003, Mosby.)

and infection of the coffin and pastern joints and associated tendons may develop.

Foot rot is most commonly diagnosed from clinical signs. Gram stain of exudates may demonstrate the organisms, but this test usually is not necessary. Culture of the primary organisms is difficult.

The most important treatments are débridement of affected skin and hoof trimming to remove as much infected tissue as possible and "open up" infected areas to contact with air. Topical antibacterial agents, either antibiotics or antiseptics/astringents (copper sulfate, zinc sulfate, or 4% to 5% formalin), are commonly applied to all affected areas after trimming and débriding. Temporary bandages may be necessary after extensive débridement is performed. Foot baths can be strategically placed so that animals must travel through them; these may help provide long-term treatment of a herd. Zinc sulfate is preferred for foot baths because it does not stain like copper sulfate and does not irritate and burn tissue like formalin. Systemic antibiotics are sometimes used and are always indicated in cases of deep-seated infection. Drug residues must be considered.

Management practices must be assessed, especially with the goal of eliminating conditions of constant moisture. Affected animals should be separated from the herd as soon as the disorder is noticed, to prevent further contamination of the environment.

Regular hoof trimming, regular use of foot baths, and management to eliminate moist ground conditions are the most important preventive measures. Vaccinations against foot rot have been developed; however, the short duration of protection and the incidence of local injection site reactions have led to limited use of the vaccines. Still, in herds where foot rot is a continual problem, vaccination may reduce the

number and severity of infections. Chronically infected animals should be culled.

JOHNE DISEASE

- Etiology: *Mycobacterium avium* subspecies *paratuberculosis*
- Gram-positive organism
- Subclinical to chronic diarrhea and malaise
- Reportable disease

Johne disease is also known as paratuberculosis. Johne disease is caused by *Mycobacterium avium* subspecies *paratuberculosis*. Although the incidence of clinical disease in herds is only approximately 1% annually, no treatment exists. The disease is contracted through contact with infected animals by the fecal-oral route. Infection of most animals occurs at approximately 30 days of age. Clinical signs usually do not occur until 3 to 5 years of age but have been seen in cattle as young as 12 to 18 months.

The four stages of Johne disease are silent, subclinical, clinical, and advanced clinical infection. Johne disease begins with a silent infection usually between 30 days and 2 years of age. Animals with silent infection shed the bacterium but do not show clinical signs. Cattle in the subclinical stage of the disease are also known as carrier animals. These animals are spreading the disease but are still not showing clinical signs. Only approximately 15% to 25% of these animals will test positive for paratuberculosis on fecal culture. If the animal is identified, it can be culled at this time, but most of these animals move onto the clinical stage of the disease while they remain in the herd. Because these animals are still shedding the pathogen but cannot be identified, Johne disease is difficult to remove from herds completely. The clinical stage of the disease is the first time that infected animals may show signs of the disease. The problem with Johne disease is the tip of the iceberg concept *(Iceberg concept)*. The iceberg concept states that for every animal with clinical signs born in the herd, another 15 to 20 animals are infected, and fewer than half of these infections will be detected by a sensitive fecal culture. When the disease worsens, the animal is considered to have moved to the advanced clinical stage.

> **TECHNICIAN NOTE**   Johne disease is difficult to remove from herds.

Clinical signs include continuous or intermittent profuse watery diarrhea and sometimes weight loss (Fig. 15-8). The most important aspect of Johne disease is the economic loss associated with decreased production. Decreases in production can be associated with reduced feed efficiency, decreased milk production, reduced slaughter weights, increased incidence of mastitis, and premature culling.

At necropsy, pale, enlarged intestinal lymph nodes are often found. Another common clinical finding is thickened rugal folds within the intestine. The differential diagnosis includes salmonellosis, parasites, and bovine virus diarrhea (BVD). Care should be taken when handling infected

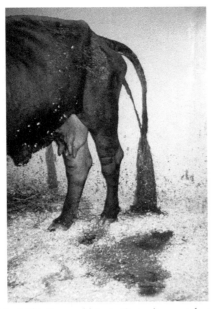

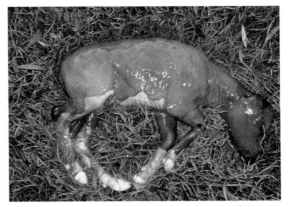

FIGURE 15-9 Aborted fetus, possibly the result of leptospirosis. (From Blowey RW, Weaver AD: *Color atlas of diseases and disorders of cattle*, ed 3, London, 2012, Mosby Ltd.)

FIGURE 15-8 This 8-year-old Santa Gertrudis cow infected with Johne disease has profuse watery diarrhea. (From Blowey RW, Weaver AD: *Color atlas of diseases and disorders of cattle*, ed 2, London, 2003, Mosby.)

livestock because of potential zoonosis. Whether Johne disease can cause Crohn disease in humans is debated.

Johne disease has no effective treatment. The diagnosis is made from biopsy and histopathologic examination of the intestinal lymph nodes. Cattle should be tested, and animals found to be positive should be culled. Prevention includes culling of all heifers from infected cows, good hygiene, and pasteurization of pooled colostrums. Producers should purchase cattle only from herds certified as free of *Mycobacterium* subspecies *paratuberculosis;* these herds are essential sources of noninfected cattle. Segregation of calves from cows until they are more than 1 year old may also help control Johne disease. Several programs are designed to control Johne disease. Depending on your state, a specific protocol may exist; otherwise, a national protocol is available.

LEPTOSPIROSIS

- Etiology: *Leptospira* species
- Gram-negative spirochete
- Abortion
- Vaccine
- Reportable disease

Leptospirosis is caused by the bacterium *Leptospira interogens. Leptospira* is a spirochete. Common serovars are *Leptospira pomona, Leptospira hardjo,* and *Leptospira grippotyphosa.* The disease is contracted through urine or the urine-contaminated environment (e.g., contaminated wildlife and water). Leptospirosis can be found worldwide but is most commonly found in wet, warm climates. *Leptospira* can persist in water-saturated soil for 183 days.

The disease often manifests as an abortion storm (Fig. 15-9). Stillbirths, loss of milk production, septicemia,

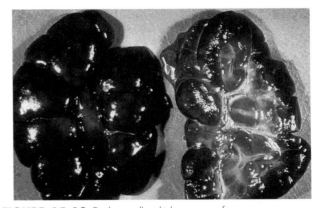

FIGURE 15-10 Dark, swollen kidneys are often seen on necropsy of an infected cow with leptospirosis. (From Blowey RW, Weaver AD: *Color atlas of diseases and disorders of cattle*, ed 3, London, 2012, Mosby Ltd.)

hemoglobinuria, weak neonates, and reduced fertility can be seen within infected herds. Periodic ophthalmia (recurrent uveitis) may be seen in an infected horse. Even after resolution of clinical signs, animals can spread leptospirosis in the urine for 10 to 118 days.

> **TECHNICIAN NOTE** Leptospirosis often manifests as an abortion storm during the last trimester.

At necropsy, animals infected with *L. pomona* have swollen, dark kidneys (Fig. 15-10). Diagnosis of the disease is often accomplished by paired serum samples or histopathologic examination.

Prevention of the disease should include vaccination and purchase of leptospirosis-free livestock. Prompt vaccination and antibiotic therapy, if performed early, may be beneficial. Leptospirosis is zoonotic, and care should be taken to prevent contraction of the disease.

> **TECHNICIAN NOTE** Leptospirosis is zoonotic.

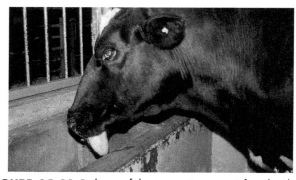

FIGURE 15-11 Prolapse of the tongue in a cow infected with listeriosis. (From Blowey RW, Weaver AD: *Color atlas of diseases and disorders of cattle*, ed 3, London, 2012, Mosby Ltd.)

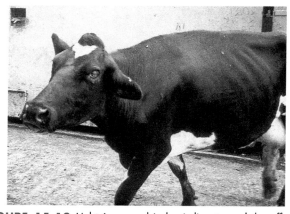

FIGURE 15-12 Holstein compulsively circling toward the affected side as a result of listeriosis infection. (From Blowey RW, Weaver AD: *Color atlas of diseases and disorders of cattle*, ed 2, London, 2003, Mosby.)

LISTERIOSIS

- Etiology: *Listeria monocytogenes*
- Gram-positive coccobacillus
- Neurologic disease and abortion

Listeriosis is caused by the bacterium *Listeria monocytogenes,* which is a small, motile, gram-positive, non–spore-forming, extremely resistant coccobacillus. *L. monocytogenes* can survive in a wide range of temperatures. The organism is most commonly contracted from the consumption of contaminated silage. Moldy silage or silage with a high pH is more likely to be contaminated with the bacterium.

> **TECHNICIAN NOTE**   Listeriosis is often contracted through contaminated silage, although mice and rats can contaminate feed as well.

Clinical signs of the disease include fever, facial nerve paralysis, tongue hanging from the mouth (Fig. 15-11), circling (Fig. 15-12), drooping ears, blindness, and abortion. The uterus can also become infected with *L. monocytogenes,* causing metritis, abortion, stillbirth, neonatal death, and possibly carrier animals.

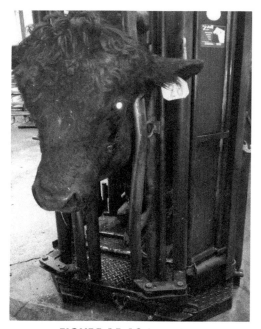

FIGURE 15-13 Lumpy jaw.

The differential diagnosis includes rabies, poisoning, botulism, and bacterial meningitis. Treatment should include penicillin and nonsteroidal antiinflammatory drugs. Prevention should include proper management of silage feeds.

LUMPY JAW

- Etiology: *Actinomyces bovis*
- Gram-positive rod
- Granulomatous mass

Lumpy jaw is also known as actinomycosis. Lumpy jaw is caused by the bacterium *Actinomyces bovis,* a gram-positive rod. The bacteria often gain access to the body through the oral cavity when the animal consumes coarse hay or sticks that penetrate the mucosa and allow entrance of the bacteria. Another common entrance point for the bacteria is skin punctures that occur around the head. The bacteria then travel through the soft tissue to the adjacent bone and develop into granulomatous masses (Fig. 15-13).

Clinical signs include mass formation on the mandible or maxillary jaw (Figs. 15-14 and 15-15). The animal is often unaffected until the mass interferes with mastication. Once mastication is affected, the animal often loses weight quickly and is culled.

Treatment is often ineffective, although attempts can be made with antibiotics and débridement.

MALIGNANT EDEMA

- Etiology: *Clostridium septicum*
- Gram-positive cocci
- Malaise and edema
- Vaccine

Malignant edema is caused by the bacterium *Clostridium septicum,* which is a large, spore-forming rod. The bacteria are found in soil and in the gastrointestinal (GI) tracts

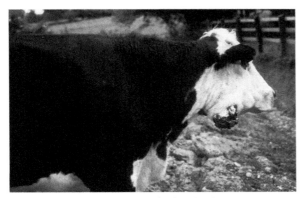

FIGURE 15-14 Crossbred Hereford with "lumpy jaw." A large, fist-sized mass lies over the angle of the mandible. (From Blowey RW, Weaver AD: *Color atlas of diseases and disorders of cattle*, ed 2, London, 2003, Mosby.)

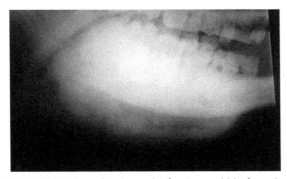

FIGURE 15-15 Lateral radiograph of a 2-year-old heifer with mandibular actinomycosis shows massive periosteal new bone formation and cavitation. (From Blowey RW, Weaver AD: *Color atlas of diseases and disorders of cattle*, ed 2, London, 2003, Mosby.)

of some animals. The disease is contracted most commonly through superficial contaminated wounds. The head and neck are most often infected, although infection can occur anywhere on the body.

Clinical signs include the formation of an edematous lesion; gas lesions are less common. The animal loses weight and develops a fever, and then toxemia develops.

Treatment includes penicillin and nonsteroidal antiinflammatory drugs. Vaccinations are available, but the disease is often sporadic, and vaccination may be needed only in endemic areas.

MASTITIS

- Etiology: multiple causes
- Inflammation of the mammary gland
- Vaccine for some animals

Mastitis (inflammation of the mammary gland) causes an estimated loss of more than $1 billion to the dairy industry in the United States each year (Fig. 15-16). The diagnosis and treatment of mastitis are critical for the health of dairy animals and for the successful production of milk that is safe for human consumption. Nondairy animals may also develop mastitis and suffer from the related pain and inflammation (Fig. 15-17). Mastitis is almost always caused by bacterial infection (septic mastitis), but inflammation without infection

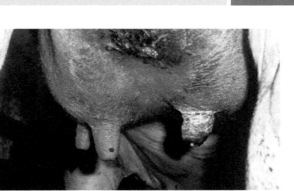

FIGURE 15-16 Distention of the udder from mastitis. Left untreated, this infection could possibly burst through the udder wall. (From Blowey RW, Weaver AD: *Color atlas of diseases and disorders of cattle*, ed 3, London, 2012, Mosby Ltd.)

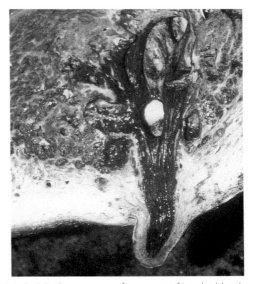

FIGURE 15-17 Cross-section of a mastitis-infected udder shows deep red inflammation of the teat cistern and teat canal mucosa. (From Blowey RW, Weaver AD: *Color atlas of diseases and disorders of cattle*, ed 3, London, 2012, Mosby Ltd.)

may occur if a teat or udder is traumatically injured (e.g., lacerated, kicked, or stepped on).

Approximately 95% of mastitis cases are caused by two organisms: *Streptococcus agalactiae* and *Staphylococcus aureus*. These bacteria tend to cause local infections of the mammary glands and seldom cause systemic illness. Both these bacteria can be spread from cow to cow *(contagious mastitis)*. *S. agalactiae* is relatively easy to treat with antibiotics and good sanitation practices. *S. aureus* tends to form microabscesses that resist penetration by antibiotics, thus making infection difficult to treat.

> **TECHNICIAN NOTE** The two most common agents of mastitis are *Streptococcus agalactiae* and *Staphylococcus aureus*.

Other causes of mastitis include coliforms (especially *E. coli*, *Klebsiella* species, *Enterobacter aerogenes*). They release endotoxins, which enter the bloodstream and can cause endotoxemia and even death. Acute septic mastitis is characterized by fever, anorexia, rumen atony, dehydration, and diarrhea. The affected milk is watery and looks like Gatorade. Treatment involves systemic antibiotics, nonsteroidal antiinflammatory drugs, possible fluid therapy, and stripping of all milk every 2 to 4 hours (Fig. 15-18).

Corynebacteria can also cause mastitis. The milk is thick and creamy, sometimes called "mayonnaise mastitis."

Mastitis from corynebacteria infection is difficult to impossible to treat successfully. Mastitis caused by leptospirosis results in milk that is thick but contains no clots or blood, and affected quarters are not hard and hot. The condition is sometimes called "cold mastitis." *Leptospira* is a fastidious bacterium that is difficult to culture. *Mycoplasma* rarely causes mastitis, but if it does, it has no cure and most animals are culled. Environmental streptococci (e.g., *Streptococcus uberis, Streptococcus bovis,* and *Streptococcus dysgalactiae*) and *Enterococcus* species all can cause mastitis. Some cases of mastitis can even be caused by fungus.

Mastitis is divided into two major categories based on clinical signs. *Clinical mastitis* has clinical signs that need no special equipment for detection, for example, palpation of a hard, hot mammary gland or visualization of abnormal milk (clumps of exudates or foul odor) (Figs. 15-19 to 15-22). *Subclinical mastitis* has no obviously visible clinical signs in the udder or in the milk and must be detected by special diagnostic testing. Definitive diagnosis of mastitis is made through sampling and testing of milk (Figs. 15-23 to 15-25 and Box 15-1).

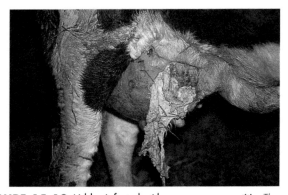

FIGURE 15-18 Udder infected with gangrenous mastitis. The overlying skin of the infected quarter has sloughed off over a 1- to 2-month period. (From Blowey RW, Weaver AD: *Color atlas of diseases and disorders of cattle,* ed 3, London, 2012, Mosby Ltd.)

METRITIS

- Etiology: multiple causes
- Variable
- Inflammation of the uterus

Uterine infections are common in cattle after calving because of the high incidence of retained placentas and dystocia.

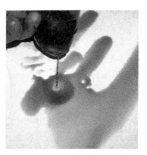

FIGURE 15-21 Brown serous discharge from a mastitis-infected quarter. (From Blowey RW, Weaver AD: *Color atlas of diseases and disorders of cattle,* ed 2, London, 2003, Mosby.)

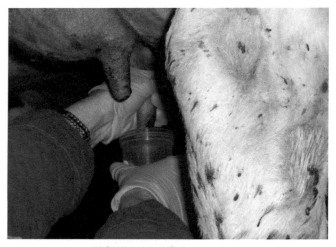

FIGURE 15-19 Strip cup test.

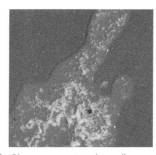

FIGURE 15-20 Clumps present in this milk sample indicate mastitis. (From Blowey RW, Weaver AD: *Color atlas of diseases and disorders of cattle,* ed 2, London, 2003, Mosby.)

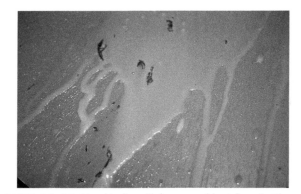

FIGURE 15-22 Blood in the milk from an udder infected with mastitis. Some milk can be almost red. (From Blowey RW, Weaver AD: *Color atlas of diseases and disorders of cattle,* ed 2, London, 2003, Mosby.)

The most common type of uterine infection is endometritis, an infection of the lining of the uterus. It is characterized by a whitish to yellowish mucopurulent vaginal discharge in a cow that has recently given birth (Figs. 15-26 and 15-27). Because the infection is superficial, cows generally show no signs of systemic disease. Occasionally, bacterial infections extend into the deeper layers of the myometrium (metritis), where access to blood vessels is possible. Bacteria and bacterial toxins may be absorbed into the bloodstream, with resulting septicemia, endotoxemia, and associated severe systemic illness and shock. Cows with metritis require intensive medical therapy to survive. Chronical bacterial endometritis may develop into pyometra, with accumulation of purulent exudates in the uterus.

> *TECHNICIAN NOTE* Uterine infections are commonly associated with dystocia and retained placentas.

Common organisms causing uterine infections are *Actinomyces (Corynebacterium) pyogenes*, streptococci, staphylococci, coliforms, and gram-negative anaerobes; mixed infections are common. Uterine culture is seldom performed in cases of endometritis. Aerobic cultures often grow a "mixed bag" of organisms that may or may not be actual pathogens, and anaerobic culture is difficult to perform. Uterine biopsy is also rarely used. However, both procedures can be done in cattle, by using the same instruments and methods as those used in the horse.

PINKEYE

- Etiology: *Moraxella bovis*
- Gram-negative organism
- Eye inflammation and irritation
- Vaccine

Pinkeye is also known as infectious bovine keratoconjunctivitis and infectious ophthalmia. Pinkeye is caused by *Moraxella bovis*, a gram-negative bacterium. Bright sunlight, irritants, stress, and dry, dusty environments often exacerbate the disease.

> *TECHNICIAN NOTE* Dry, dusty environments can exacerbate pinkeye.

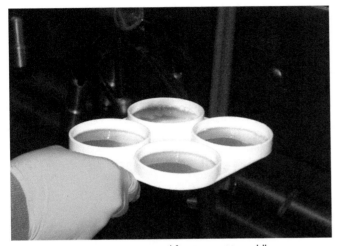

FIGURE 15-23 California mastitis paddle.

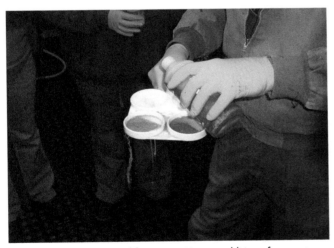

FIGURE 15-24 California mastitis test, addition of reagent.

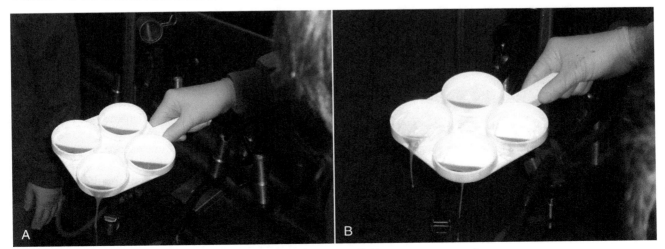

FIGURE 15-25 A and B, Positive California mastitis test result.

BOX 15-1	Types of Mastitis

Contagious mastitis: Spread can occur directly from cow to cow, usually at milking time (milking machines or contaminated hands or towels).

Environmental mastitis: Spread to individual cows occurs through environmental contamination of bedding, soil, standing water, or feces.

Gangrenous mastitis: Severe infection results in destruction of the affected quarter, with necrosis and sloughing. Severe *Staphylococcus* infections and wounds that allow *Clostridium* species to become established may result in gangrenous mastitis.

Clinical mastitis: Visible signs of disease are present in the milk or the affected quarter, or both.

Subclinical mastitis: No visible signs of disease are present. This disorder causes the greatest economic loss to dairy farmers because of lowered production. It requires special diagnostic testing of the milk for diagnosis.

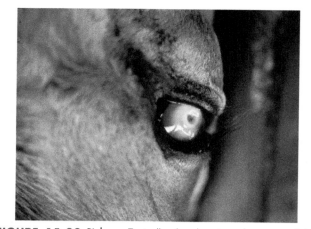

FIGURE 15-28 Pinkeye. Typically, the ulcer is in the center of the cornea and may be superficial or erode deeply into the stroma in more advanced cases, such as this one. (From Blowey RW, Weaver AD: *Color atlas of diseases and disorders of cattle*, ed 3, London, 2012, Mosby Ltd.)

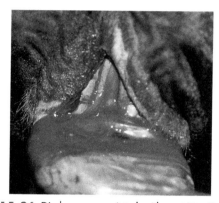

FIGURE 15-26 Discharge associated with metritis. (From Blowey RW, Weaver AD: *Color atlas of diseases and disorders of cattle*, ed 3, London, 2012, Mosby Ltd.)

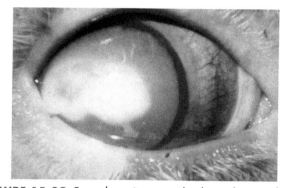

FIGURE 15-29 Corneal opacity seen with advanced stages of pinkeye. (From Blowey RW, Weaver AD: *Color atlas of diseases and disorders of cattle*, ed 2, London, 2003, Mosby.)

which all are factors predisposing to pinkeye. Treatment often consists of antibiotic therapy and isolation of infected animals. Vaccinations for pinkeye are available but controversial.

SHIPPING FEVER

- Etiology: multiple causes
- Variable
- Respiratory disease

Shipping fever is also known as pasteurellosis. Pasteurellosis is caused by *Mannheimia (Pasteurella) haemolytica* and sometimes *Pasteurella multocida. Pasteurella* species are gram-negative bacteria. *Haemophilus somnus* is also another causative agent of shipping fever. These bacteria are normal flora of the upper respiratory system and often become overabundant after stress or viral infection.

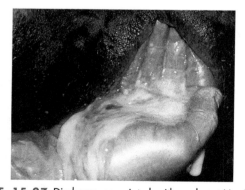

FIGURE 15-27 Discharge associated with endometritis. This discharge is mixed with blood. (From Blowey RW, Weaver AD: *Color atlas of diseases and disorders of cattle*, ed 3, London, 2012, Mosby Ltd.)

Clinical signs include blepharospasm, lacrimation, photophobia, keratitis, conjunctivitis, and corneal opacity and ulceration (Figs. 15-28 and 15-29).

The diagnosis is often made based on clinical signs. Prevention of pinkeye should include low stocking rates, fly prevention, and attempts to control dust and bright sunlight,

Clinical signs often include depression, low head carriage, wet cough, open-mouth breathing, weight loss, fever, and wheezing or cracking noises on auscultation of the lungs (Fig. 15-30).

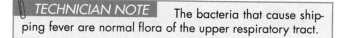

TECHNICIAN NOTE   The bacteria that cause shipping fever are normal flora of the upper respiratory tract.

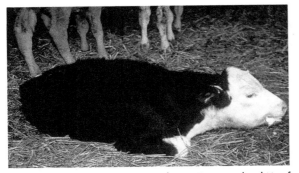

FIGURE 15-30 Severe respiratory distress in a crossbred Hereford. (From Blowey RW, Weaver AD: *Color atlas of diseases and disorders of cattle*, ed 3, London, 2012, Mosby Ltd.)

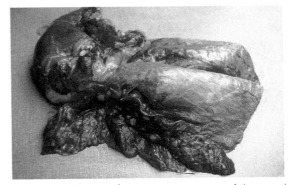

FIGURE 15-32 Shipping fever. Pneumonic areas of the apical and cardiac lobes showing scattered, pale yellow abscesses. (From Blowey RW, Weaver AD: *Color atlas of diseases and disorders of cattle*, ed 2, London, 2003, Mosby.)

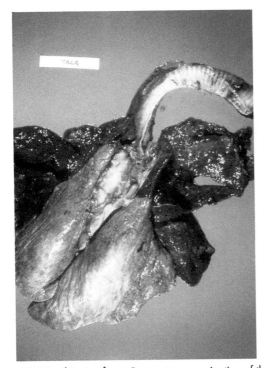

FIGURE 15-31 Shipping fever. Postmortem examination of the lungs showing froth in the major bronchi. The apical and cardiac lobes are dark red, slightly swollen, and firm and contain microabscesses. (From Blowey RW, Weaver AD: *Color atlas of diseases and disorders of cattle*, ed 3, London, 2012, Mosby Ltd.)

At necropsy, the lungs often are dark red and swollen (Fig. 15-31). Abscesses may be present (Fig. 15-32). The diagnosis depends on bacterial culture from necropsied lung tissue.

Treatment should include antimicrobial therapy and non-steroidal antiinflammatory drugs in advanced cases. Prevention is possible with *Pasteurella* toxoid vaccines.

TUBERCULOSIS

- Etiology: *Mycobacterium bovis*
- Acid-fast bacillus
- Respiratory disease
- Reportable disease

Tuberculosis (TB) is caused by *Mycobacterium bovis* in cattle. TB is a granulomatous disease caused by an acid-fast bacillus of the genus *Mycobacterium*. The disease is often chronic and debilitating. All the *Mycobacterium* species can produce infection in host species other than their own. TB is contracted through infected droplets spread by the lungs, although contaminated milk can spread the disease. In rare occasions, intrauterine or coital transmission of infection has been documented. The disease causes emaciation, weakness, anorexia, low-grade fevers, and lethargy. Sometimes the lesions within the lung can be heard by auscultation. Because clinical signs are often difficult to detect, TB testing is important.

The single most important diagnostic test for TB is the intradermal tuberculin test; purified protein derivatives (PPD) prepared from the culture filtrate of *M. bovis* or *M. avium* can be used. The main method of control involves testing and slaughter. In an affected herd, testing every 3 months is recommended.

VIBRIOSIS

- Etiology: *Campylobacter fetus* subspecies *venerealis* or *Campylobacter fetus* subspecies *fetus*
- Gram-negative organism
- Early embryonic loss
- Vaccine

Vibriosis is caused by the gram-negative curved or spiral polar flagellated bacterium *Campylobacter fetus* subspecies *venerealis* or *Campylobacter fetus* subspecies *fetus*. The disease is transmitted venereally. Other forms of contraction include contaminated instruments, infected semen, and contaminated bedding. The bacteria cause early embryonic death, an extended calving season, infertility, and occasionally abortion.

Clinical signs of the disease in cows are often absent. The only indication of vibriosis may be an extended calving season resulting from early embryonic losses and irregular estrous cycles. Most cases of infertility are limited to replacement heifers.

The diagnosis of the disease requires culture of the organism from vaginal mucus, reproductive discharges, aborted fetuses (lung and stomach contents), or sheath aspirates from bulls. Vaccinations are available, and antibiotic-treated semen should be used.

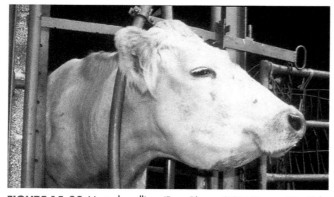

FIGURE 15-33 Ventral swelling. (From Blowey RW, Weaver AD: *Color atlas of diseases and disorders of cattle*, ed 3, London, 2012, Mosby Ltd.)

WOODEN TONGUE

- Etiology: *Actinobacillus lignieresii*
- Gram-negative coccobacillus
- Tumorous abscess of the tongue

Wooden tongue is also known as actinobacillosis. Wooden tongue is caused by the bacterium *Actinobacillus lignieresii*, a gram-negative coccobacillus. When the bacteria gain access to the oral cavity, they cause a hard, tumorous abscess of the tongue (hence the name wooden tongue).

> **TECHNICIAN NOTE** Wooden tongue causes abscesses on the tongue that result in swelling of the ventral jaw.

Clinical signs include abscessation of the tongue and possible swelling of the ventral jaw (Figs. 15-33 and 15-34). The bacterium, part of the normal flora of the upper GI tract, can also cause cutaneous actinobacillosis if other areas of the body are infected (Fig. 15-35).

Treatment consists of systemic antibiotics for 7 to 10 days. Suggested antibiotics include tetracyclines, erythromycin, or tilmicosin.

OTHER MICROBIAL DISEASES

BOVINE SPONGIFORM ENCEPHALOPATHY

- Etiology: prion
- Neurologic disease
- Reportable disease

Bovine spongiform encephalopathy (BSE) is caused by an abnormal protein called a prion. By many lay people, it is known as mad cow disease. The disease causes neurologic disease in adult cattle that progresses to death, usually around 3 months after infection. Transmission in cattle is through ingestion of infected meat and bone meal. The disease is similar to scrapie in sheep.

In the early stages, clinical signs often include nose licking, teeth grinding, head tossing, and snorting. As the disease progresses, the animal begins to become bothered

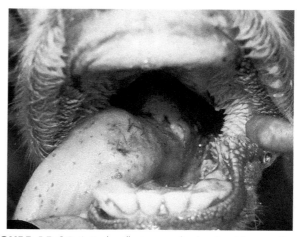

FIGURE 15-34 Actinobacillosis caused a localized firm swelling of the dorsum in this dairy cow. (From Blowey RW, Weaver AD: *Color atlas of diseases and disorders of cattle*, ed 3, London, 2012, Mosby Ltd.)

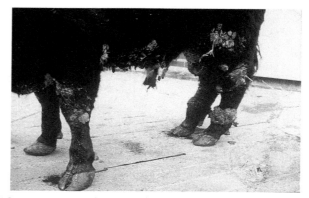

FIGURE 15-35 Other areas of the body can develop cutaneous actinobacillosis. (From Blowey RW, Weaver AD: *Color atlas of diseases and disorders of cattle*, ed 3, London, 2012, Mosby Ltd.)

by small external stimuli of the integumentary system. For example, brushing the fine hairs of the cow's ears may cause the animal to throw its head violently; it exhibits an exaggerated response. In later stages of the disease, the animal stands staring off into the distance with a low head carriage. If the animal attempts to walk, it will often be ataxic, have muscle tremors, or may even fall (Fig. 15-36). Cattle often sit like a dog during the more advanced stages of BSE (Fig. 15-37).

The brain must be examined for a confirmed diagnosis. The differential diagnosis includes rabies, listeriosis, and hypomagnesemia.

No treatment exists for BSE. Prevention is achieved through control of by-product feeding. According to U.S. Food and Drug Administration regulations, the animals cannot be fed mammalian-derived protein sources; however, this rule has some exceptions. Producers still can feed cattle "nonprohibited materials," such as pure porcine or equine protein, blood and blood products, gelatin, inspected meat products that have been cooked and offered for human food, meat products that have been further heat processed for animal feed use, milk products (milk and milk proteins), and protein derived from poultry, marine, and vegetable sources.

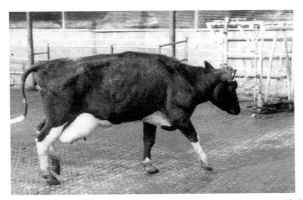

FIGURE 15-36 Characteristic stance associated with a cow with bovine spongiform encephalopathy that is trying to maintain its balance. (From Blowey RW, Weaver AD: *Color atlas of diseases and disorders of cattle*, ed 2, London, 2003, Mosby.)

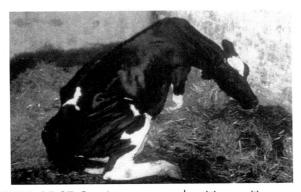

FIGURE 15-37 Cow in a common dog-sitting position seen in animals with bovine spongiform encephalopathy. (From Blowey RW, Weaver AD: *Color atlas of diseases and disorders of cattle*, ed 2, London, 2003, Mosby.)

> **TECHNICIAN NOTE** Political and economic losses make prevention of BSE outbreaks extremely important.

DERMATOPHYTOSIS

- Etiology: *Trichophyton verrucosum*
- Skin lesions

Dermatophytosis (ringworm) is commonly caused by *Trichophyton verrucosum*, but it also can be caused by *Microsporum* species. Ringworm is a fungal infection of the skin and hair.

Ringworm often affects calves but can affect adults. The lesions are frequently found on the head and neck and consist of encrusted circles of thickened skin (Fig. 15-38). Ringworm is irritating, and animals often scratch themselves on their surroundings (feed bunks, water troughs, posts). When the animals scratch themselves, they leave spores behind on the object being used. These spores can survive in the environment for as long as 4 years.

> **TECHNICIAN NOTE** Ringworm often causes encrusted circular lesions on the head and neck.

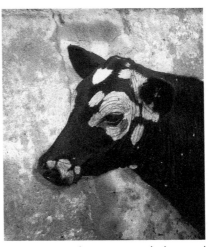

FIGURE 15-38 Common lesions seen with dermatophytosis. (From Blowey RW, Weaver AD: *Color atlas of diseases and disorders of cattle*, ed 3, London, 2012, Mosby Ltd.)

The infection often resolves spontaneously. However, if animals are of high value (e.g., 4-H calves), they can be treated with antifungal drugs, either topically or orally.

TRICHOMONIASIS

- Etiology: *Tritrichomonas foetus*
- Early embryonic loss
- Vaccine
- Reportable disease

Trichomoniasis is caused by *Tritrichomonas foetus*, a protozoan that causes venereal diseases in cattle. Transmission occurs when uninfected cattle are bred to infected bulls. Once infected, bulls are infected for life, unlike cows, which often are free of infection 3 months after contracting the protozoan. Transmission is possible through artificial insemination because the protozoan does survive the freezing process.

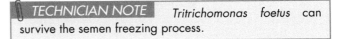

> **TECHNICIAN NOTE** *Tritrichomonas foetus* can survive the semen freezing process.

The most common clinical finding is embryonic death, although late-term abortion is possible. Diagnosis is made from culture of *Trichomonas*.

Treatment consists of separating cows that are more than 5 months pregnant and culling all bulls. The bulls then should be replaced with virgin bulls.

VIRAL DISEASES

BOVINE RESPIRATORY SYNCYTIAL VIRUS INFECTION

- Etiology: Paramyxoviridae
- Respiratory disease
- Vaccine

Bovine respiratory syncytial virus infection is caused by an RNA virus of the Paramyxoviridae family. The infection is seen primarily in young cattle. The virus often replicates in the lower respiratory tract and predisposes the lungs to secondary bacterial infections. Morbidity is high, and mortality can be 0% to 20%.

The disease is characterized by fever (104° F to 108° F), anorexia, depression, increased respiratory rates, and nasal and ocular discharge.

The disease can be diagnosed through virus isolation. Paired serum samples may be useful in diagnosis. Paired serum samples should be taken 2 to 3 weeks apart.

Vaccines to prevent the disease are available. During a disease outbreak, the primary focus is treatment of secondary bacterial infections using antibiotics. Supportive therapy can include nonsteroidal antiinflammatory drugs or fluid therapy, or both.

BOVINE VIRUS DIARRHEA

- Etiology: Flaviviridae
- Several manifestations

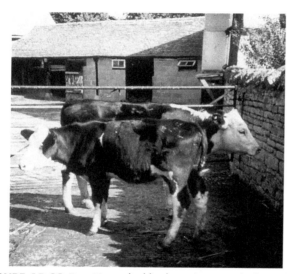

FIGURE 15-39 Two 18-month-old calves. The nearer heifer, with an abnormal rust-colored coat, is stunted as a result of chronic persistent infection (antigen positive, antibody negative) from material infection with bovine virus diarrhea early in pregnancy. (From Blowey RW, Weaver AD: *Color atlas of diseases and disorders of cattle,* ed 3, London, 2012, Mosby Ltd.)

- Vaccine
- Reportable disease

BVD is caused by a virus of the Flaviviridae family. BVD is transmitted in the secretions and excretions of infected cattle.

BVD also can be transmitted from cow to calf in the first 4 months of fetal development. If infection of the calf occurs at this time, the result usually is fetal reabsorption. During a necropsy of the calf at this time, cerebral hypoplasia may be seen.

> **TECHNICIAN NOTE**   Because of carriers, elimination of bovine virus diarrhea is difficult.

A calf that is infected in utero during the second trimester will be born and become a carrier of the disease for life. Clinical signs manifest between the ages of 3 and 30 months (Fig. 15-39) and include oral erosion (Fig. 15-40), intestinal ulceration, and some respiratory involvement (Fig. 15-41).

The differential diagnosis includes paratuberculosis, salmonellosis, and other causes of oral ulceration.

BVD can be identified by virus isolation from whole blood (buffy coat) or other tissues, immunohistochemistry staining of viral antigen in skin biopsy samples (e.g., ear tissue obtained with ear notch pliers), antigen-capture enzyme-linked immunosorbent assay, polymerase chain reaction methods, and microtiter virus isolation (immunoperoxidase monolayer assay) from serum.

FOOT AND MOUTH DISEASE

- Etiology: Picornaviridae
- Vesicular disease
- Reportable disease

Foot and mouth disease is caused by a virus from the Picornaviridae family. Foot and mouth disease is a highly contagious, foreign, and sometimes fatal disease of cloven-hoofed animals. The incubation period for the virus causing foot and mouth disease ranges from 2 to 12 days. The disease is transmitted by the following means: through the air;

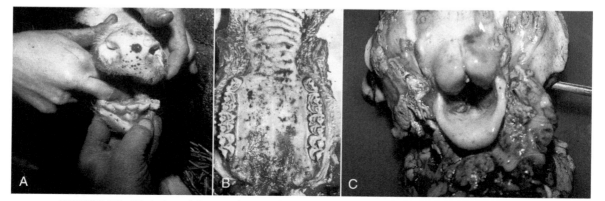

FIGURE 15-40 A, B, and C, Typical erosive lesions associated with bovine virus diarrhea. (From Blowey RW, Weaver AD: *Color atlas of diseases and disorders of cattle,* ed 2, London, 2003, Mosby.)

by contaminated animals; by contaminated facilities, cloths, and vehicles; by feeding raw or improperly cooked garbage containing infected meat or animal products; and through semen.

Cattle infected with foot and mouth disease often present with drooling because of the major erosion of oral tissue caused by lesions on the tongue and hard palate (Figs. 15-42 and 15-43). The animals often are not eating and are depressed. Cattle may appear lame as a result of coronary band lesions (Fig. 15-44), although lesions of the coronary band often are not as prevalent in cattle as in swine.

The differential diagnosis includes vesicular stomatitis, bovine papular stomatitis, and digital dermatitis.

No treatment exists for foot and mouth disease. Most affected animals recover but are left debilitated by the disease. It causes severe losses in the production of meat and milk. Because the disease spreads widely and rapidly and because of the extreme economic loss, prevention of foot and mouth disease is extremely important in the United States.

> *TECHNICIAN NOTE* It has been estimated that if a foot and mouth disease outbreak were to occur in the United States, the economic losses could be in the billions of dollars within 1 year.

INFECTIOUS BOVINE RHINOTRACHEITIS

- Etiology: bovine herpes virus I
- Respiratory disease
- Vaccine
- Reportable disease

IBR (also called red nose) is caused by bovine herpes virus I. Clinical signs often affect the respiratory system,

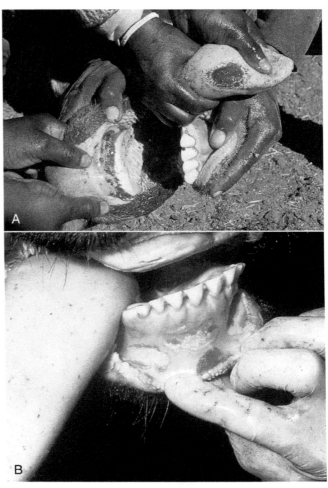

FIGURE 15-42 A and B, Ruptured foot and mouth disease vesicles in the oral cavity. (From Blowey RW, Weaver AD: *Color atlas of diseases and disorders of cattle,* ed 2, London, 2003, Mosby.)

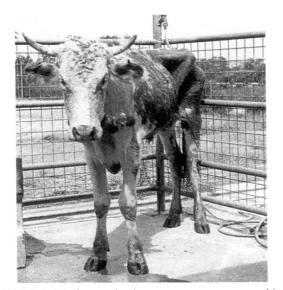

FIGURE 15-41 This crossbred steer is a constant source of bovine virus diarrhea (BVD) to susceptible animals and is emaciated as a result of chronic and persistent infection with BVD. (From Blowey RW, Weaver AD: *Color atlas of diseases and disorders of cattle,* ed 2, London, 2003, Mosby.)

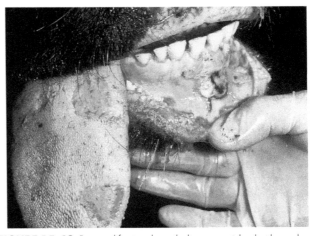

FIGURE 15-43 Ruptured foot and mouth disease vesicles that have developed a secondary bacterial infection. (From Blowey RW, Weaver AD: *Color atlas of diseases and disorders of cattle,* ed 2, London, 2003, Mosby.)

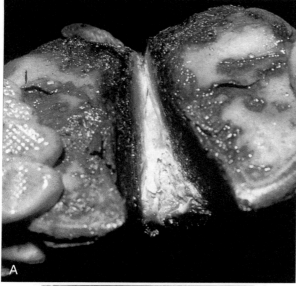

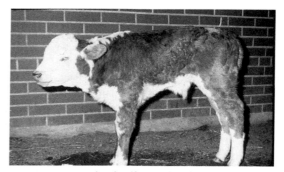

FIGURE 15-45 Crossbred calf severely infected with infectious bovine rhinotracheitis. (From Blowey RW, Weaver AD: *Color atlas of diseases and disorders of cattle*, ed 3, London, 2012, Mosby Ltd.)

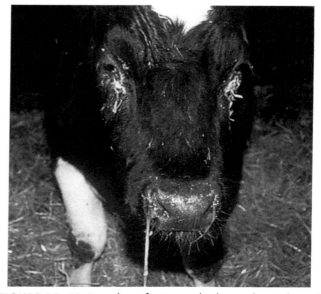

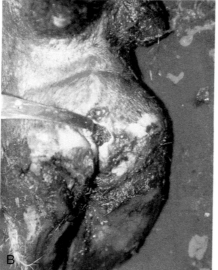

FIGURE 15-44 A and **B,** Ruptured foot and mouth disease vesicles of the coronary band and interdigital space. (From Blowey RW, Weaver AD: *Color atlas of diseases and disorders of cattle*, ed 2, London, 2003, Mosby.)

FIGURE 15-46 Secondary infection may lead to purulent oculonasal discharge. (From Blowey RW, Weaver AD: *Color atlas of diseases and disorders of cattle*, ed 3, London, 2012, Mosby Ltd.)

although abortion and genital tract infections can be seen. Respiratory signs include fever, ocular discharge, mucopurulent nasal discharge, conjunctivitis, depression, cough, and dyspnea (Fig. 15-45). IBR is also known as red nose because of the inflamed nostrils often associated with the disease. Secondary bacterial infections are common (Fig. 15-46). In addition to causing respiratory disease, the virus can cause conjunctivitis, abortions, encephalitis, and generalized systemic infections.

At necropsy, necrosis and hemorrhage of the larynx and trachea are seen (Fig. 15-47).

The diagnosis of IBR is made based on clinical signs, and in large outbreaks virus isolation can be attempted. Treatment of secondary bacterial infections should be attempted. Prevention should include vaccination (Table 15-1).

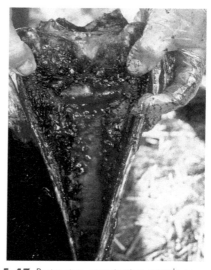

FIGURE 15-47 Postmortem examination reveals severe necrotizing and hemorrhagic laryngotracheitis. (From Blowey RW, Weaver AD: *Color atlas of diseases and disorders of cattle*, ed 3, London, 2012, Mosby Ltd.)

NONINFECTIOUS DISEASES

FATTY LIVER DISEASE

- Etiology: animals going off feed
- General malaise

Fatty liver disease often develops before or after parturition and occurs most commonly in cattle that are overconditioned at parturition. Cows should enter the dry period with an average body score of 3 to 3.5 (on a scale of 1 to 5). The disease begins when blood concentrations of nonesterified fatty acids (NEFAs) are increased. Uptake of NEFAs by the liver is equal to that of blood concentrations. The liver is responsible for converting NEFAs to triglycerides that are exported as lipoproteins or stored. The problem is that ruminants do not export these lipoproteins quickly, and triglycerides accumulate in the liver (Fig. 15-48). The condition worsens when the animal has low blood glucose levels because insulin suppresses fat mobilization from adipose tissue. Fatty liver disease can occur 24 hours after the animal goes off feed.

> **TECHNICIAN NOTE** Cows should have a body condition score of 3 to 3.5 on a five-point scale before calving.

Cows often do not have clinical signs. Cattle with fatty liver are more prone to developing ketosis, but ketosis does not necessarily mean that the animal is suffering from fatty liver disease. Animals that should be suspected of having the disease are cows that are slow to increase milk production and feed intake after calving and downer cows.

The diagnosis usually is made after the cow is off feed or has died of another complication. Prevention of fatty liver disease should be attempted through proper condition scores before calving. Cows with a body condition score less than 2.5 should be provided additional energy by feeding during the dry period to improve their condition. However, overconditioned cows should not be encouraged to lose weight during the dry phase because this mobilizes fat and

TABLE 15-1	Bovine Vaccinations*				
DISEASE OR VACCINATION	**CALVES**	**REPLACEMENTS**	**FEEDLOT CATTLE**	**ADULTS**	**COMMENTS**
Anthrax	In the presence of outbreak, by state or federal permission	In the presence of outbreak, by state or federal permission	In the presence of outbreak, by state or federal permission	In the presence of outbreak, by state or federal permission	
Bang vaccination	Heifer calves 3–12 mo old				Depending on local and state laws
Bovine respiratory syncytial virus	Weaned calves	Heifers and bulls	Feedlot cattle		
Bovine virus diarrhea type 1 and 2	Calves >2 wk old, weaned calves	Heifers and bulls		Cows and bulls	Killed bovine virus diarrhea vaccine must be used in pregnant cows and nursing calves
Clostridial bacteria	Calves >10 days old, weaned calves	Heifers and bulls	Feedlot cattle	Cows and bulls	Known as 5-, 7-, or 8-way vaccines
Infectious bovine rhinotracheitis	Calves >2 wk old, weaned calves	Heifers and bulls		Cows	
Leptospirosis		Heifers and bulls		Cows and bulls	
Parainfluenza 3 virus	Calves >2 wk old, weaned calves	Heifers and bulls	On arrival	Cows	
Pasteurella	Weaned calves		Feedlot cattle		
Pinkeye	Calves >30 days old		Feedlot cattle		
Salmonella	Calves >2 wk old		Feedlot cattle		Entire dairy herd in the presence of an outbreak
Scour vaccine				Cows 30 days before calving	
Somnus		Heifers and bulls	Feedlot cattle		
Trichomonas				Cows and bulls before breeding	
Vibrio		Heifers and bulls		Cows and bulls before breeding	

*Vaccination protocols should be designed specific to producers by veterinarians.

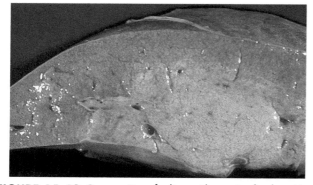

FIGURE 15-48 Cross-section of a liver with massive fat deposition. (From Blowey RW, Weaver AD: *Color atlas of diseases and disorders of cattle*, ed 2, London, 2003, Mosby.)

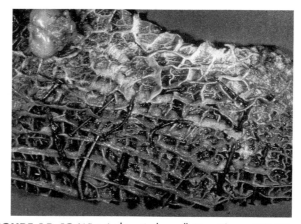

FIGURE 15-49 Wires in the reticular wall. (From Blowey RW, Weaver AD: *Color atlas of diseases and disorders of cattle*, ed 3, London, 2012, Mosby Ltd.)

increases the NEFA concentration. Fatty liver disease has no proven treatment, but animals with early cases may benefit from intravenous (IV) glucose solutions and parenteral glucocorticoids.

HARDWARE DISEASE

- Etiology: foreign body penetration of abomasum
- Endocarditis

Hardware disease is also known as traumatic reticuloperitonitis or traumatic gastritis. The disease is more common in dairy cattle than in beef cattle, but it can occur in either type. Hardware disease is caused by consumption of a foreign body. Cattle do not completely chew their food before swallowing, so they are prone to foreign body consumption. Feeding silage can increase the risk of hardware disease when the animals accidently consume metal, often nails or wire. The nails or wires either drop into the reticulum or pass into the rumen and subsequently are carried over the ruminoreticular fold into the reticulum by rumen contractions. As the reticulum contracts, the foreign body often penetrates the wall (Fig. 15-49). Pregnancy, "riding behavior," and parturition increase the chances of penetration. If the foreign body pierces the wall, the metal can migrate to other areas of the body, such as the spleen, liver, or heart (Fig. 15-50). Penetration of the diaphragm by the foreign body often causes pericarditis, followed by myocarditis, endocarditis, and septicemia (Figs. 15-51 and 15-52). Once penetration occurs, the peritoneal cavity is contaminated with ingesta and bacteria, resulting in peritonitis.

Clinical findings often include decreases in milk production and fecal output. Physical examination shows a slightly increased rectal temperature, a normal or slightly elevated heart rate, dehydration, and often rapid and shallow respiration. The animal will walk with an arched back and step lightly and carefully. Sudden forced movement may cause grunting. Grunting can also be heard by pressing on the ventral thorax and then pinching the thoracic spinous processes while listening to the trachea with a stethoscope. If the disease has progressed to pleuritis or pericarditis, the animal often will present with depression, a fever, and a heart rate greater than 90 beats per minute (bpm). A washing machine murmur may be heard on auscultation of the heart.

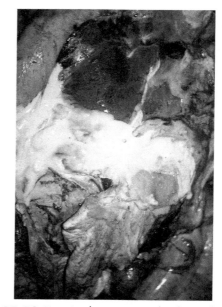

FIGURE 15-50 Hepatic abscessation in hardware disease. (From Blowey RW, Weaver AD: *Color atlas of diseases and disorders of cattle*, ed 3, London, 2012, Mosby Ltd.)

The diagnosis is often based on history and clinical findings. Frequently, an increase in neutrophils with a left shift is seen, and fibrinogen and total plasma protein levels may be high.

Treatment consists of surgical removal of the foreign body early in the course of the disease or administration of antibiotics and use of a magnet (Fig. 15-53). Prevention of the disease includes proper management of feeds and housing to prevent consumption of foreign bodies. Administration of magnets is performed as a form of prevention.

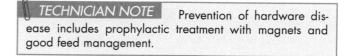

TECHNICIAN NOTE   Prevention of hardware disease includes prophylactic treatment with magnets and good feed management.

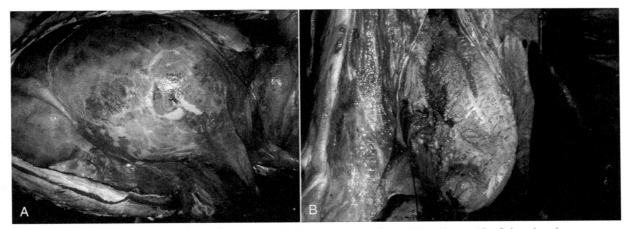

FIGURE 15-51 Hardware disease. **A** and **B,** Peritonitis. (From Blowey RW, Weaver AD: *Color atlas of diseases and disorders of cattle,* ed 3, London, 2012, Mosby Ltd.)

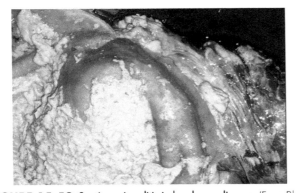

FIGURE 15-52 Septic pericarditis in hardware disease. (From Blowey RW, Weaver AD: *Color atlas of diseases and disorders of cattle,* ed 3, London, 2012, Mosby Ltd.)

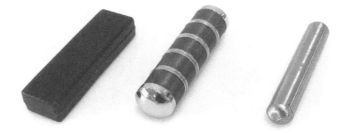

FIGURE 15-53 Magnets used in the treatment and prevention of hardware disease. (From Sonsthagen TF: *Veterinary instruments and equipment: a pocket guide,* ed 2, St. Louis, Mosby, 2011.)

HYPOCALCEMIA

- Etiology: decreased calcium
- Down cow

Hypocalcemia is also known as milk fever or postparturient paresis. Hypocalcemia is caused by low levels of circulating calcium in the bloodstream. The loss of calcium is associated with milk production. It is often seen in prepartum or postpartum dairy cows. Milk fever can occur in cows of any age but most commonly affects high-producing cows more than 5 years old. The Jersey breed seems to have a higher incidence of the disease.

Clinical signs include sternal or lateral recumbency, muscle twitching, tachycardia, an S shape to the neck (thought to be caused by the animal trying to maintain sternal recumbency), or the head resting on the hindquarters (Figs. 15-54 and 15-55). The animal may be hyperexcitable or ataxic, display head bobbing, shuffle the feet while walking, have cold extremities, or display bloat. The animal usually shows signs of GI stasis, such as the lack of defecation. Auscultation of the heart reveals tachycardia sometimes approaching 120 bpm. The heart sounds are often faint.

TECHNICIAN NOTE Although suggested by the name "milk fever," fever is not a clinical sign of hypocalcemia.

The diagnosis is often made based on assessment of the animal's history and clinical signs.

Treatment involves the replacement of calcium, usually through IV treatment. Some veterinarians also use dextrose, magnesium, and phosphorus in their treatments. Proper body scores before parturition can help decrease the incidence of milk fever. Increased calcium in the ration during phase 4 also can help to prevent hypocalcemia.

HYPOMAGNESEMIC TETANY

- Etiology: hypomagnesemia
- Down cow

Hypomagnesemic tetany is also known as grass tetany or grass staggers. Hypomagnesemia is caused by low levels of magnesium in the blood and cerebrospinal fluid. Hypomagnesemia can be seen in animals grazing lush pastures, dairy cows after parturition, animals after reduction of feed intake resulting from inclement weather, and cattle fed silage diets.

Clinical signs include convulsions, stiffness, hyperexcitability, dilated pupils, frothing at the mouth, muscle spasms, and death (Fig. 15-56). Death can occur within hours or progress over a period of 2 to 3 days. Auscultation of the heart shows tachycardia and loud heart sounds.

TECHNICIAN NOTE Animals that are found dead may show indications of convulsions before death, such as disruption of the dirt around them.

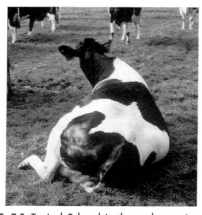

FIGURE 15-54 Typical S bend in the neck associated with hypocalcemia. (From Blowey RW, Weaver AD: *Color atlas of diseases and disorders of cattle,* ed 3, London, 2012, Mosby Ltd.)

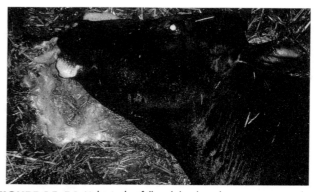

FIGURE 15-56 Holstein that fell and developed extensor spasm when it was brought in for milking. Note the "staring eye," dilated pupil, frothing at the mouth, and sweaty coat. (From Blowey RW, Weaver AD: *Color atlas of diseases and disorders of cattle,* ed 2, London, 2003, Mosby.)

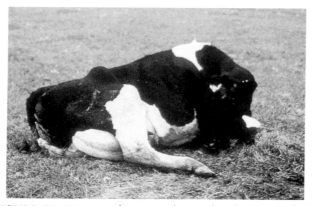

FIGURE 15-55 Hypocalcemic cow lying with its head on its flank. (From Blowey RW, Weaver AD: *Color atlas of diseases and disorders of cattle,* ed 3, London, 2012, Mosby Ltd.)

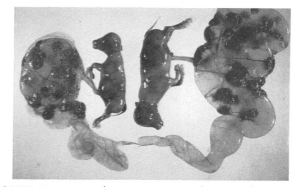

FIGURE 15-57 Twin bovine pregnancy with conjoined circulations. Freemartinism is possible. (From Blowey RW, Weaver AD: *Color atlas of diseases and disorders of cattle,* ed 3, London, 2012, Mosby Ltd.)

Treatment involves sedation to control convulsions and administration of magnesium and calcium (hypocalcemia often is a component of the disease). Prevention should include supplemental magnesium in the diet. During inclement weather, it is important to provide supplemental feed to livestock to encourage feed consumption.

INTERSEXUALITY

Intersexuality implies an individual with genital anatomical features of both sexes (hermaphrodite). Intersex conditions occur rarely in cattle and sheep and more often in goats.

Freemartinism
- Etiology: heifer and bull calf twins
- Infertility

In cattle the most common form of intersexuality is freemartinism. A freemartin is a female born twin to a male, with normal-appearing external female genitalia but grossly abnormal internal genitalia. The condition results when the fetal membranes of the twins form blood vessel communications (vascular anastomoses) between them, thus allowing testosterone and other hormones from the male to influence development of the female. Reports indicate that the condition

affects 92% of females born twin to a male. A persistent hymen, prominent clitoris, and abnormally small (hypoplastic) ovaries are common, as are various degrees of development of testicles, epididymis, vesicular glands, and other internal male structures. The condition manifests internally in many ways, but the result is a sterile individual. Freemartins can be diagnosed in several ways based on clinical signs and chromosome analysis (karyotyping), but measuring vaginal length between 1 and 4 weeks of age and confirming the absence of a cervix are inexpensive and often used. Freemartins have an abnormally short vagina (Fig. 15-57).

> **TECHNICIAN NOTE**   Freemartins have an abnormally short vagina.

KETOSIS
- Etiology: decreased food intake
- General malaise

Ketosis, also known as acetonemia or ketonemia, affects dairy cattle in the first 6 weeks following parturition. Ketosis can result whenever the animal goes off feed and is commonly seen in dairy cows fed for high milk production. The disease is most often seen between the third and fourth weeks of lactation. The condition is more prominent in stabled

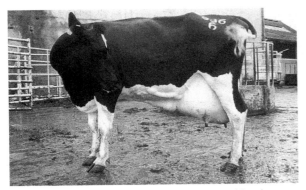

FIGURE 15-58 Biting at the flanks by a 5-year-old Holstein. (From Blowey RW, Weaver AD: *Color atlas of diseases and disorders of cattle,* ed 2, London, 2003, Mosby.)

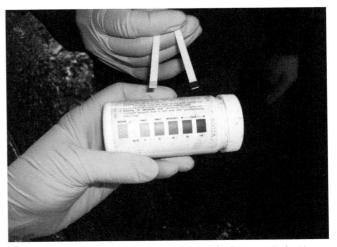

FIGURE 15-59 *Left,* Ketone stick negative for ketones. *Right,* Ketone stick positive for ketones.

dairy cattle improperly fed during the dry phase or phase 1 of lactation. When energy requirements are not met by food consumption, the animal uses its fat reserves. Ketones are a by-product of fat metabolism. If too many ketones are present, the animal will begin to show clinical signs. Metritis, mastitis, left displacement of the abomasum (LDA), right displacement of the abomasum (RDA), fatty liver, retained placenta, and stress all predispose cows to ketosis.

Clinical signs include weight loss, depression, arched back, decreased milk production, sweet-smelling breath, constipation, and sometimes nervous licking and biting of the body or surroundings (Fig. 15-58). Cows often seek out nonconsumable products such as twigs, coarse hay, and straw to eat rather than their provided ration. In advanced cases, head pressing and ataxia may be seen.

> **TECHNICIAN NOTE** Sweet-smelling breath is often a clinical sign of ketosis.

The diagnosis is often based on clinical signs and confirmation of excess ketone production with the Rothera test or with urine ketone sticks (Fig. 15-59). The Rothera test is performed on milk and is more accurate than urine ketone determinations.

Treatment involves replacement of quick, usable energy and often administration of IV glucose. The animals are often given long-term energy sources, such as propylene glycol, through a gastric tube. Glucocorticoid administration may also be a component of ketosis treatment. Many cows require a follow-up treatment within 24 hours. Cows with adequate body scores (3.5 on a five-point scale) before parturition are less likely to develop ketosis. Cows should not be fat. Cows should be provided with a small amount of the concentrate ration they will receive during lactation 2 weeks before parturition. The amount of concentrate should be increased gradually until parturition. Cows that have been affected by ketosis in the past are more likely to develop ketosis during subsequent lactations.

LAMENESS

Lameness in cattle is important because it significantly decreases production. Lameness examinations performed on horses

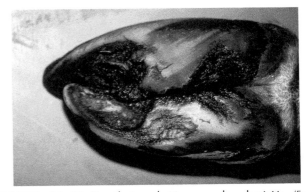

FIGURE 15-60 Growth irregularities secondary laminitis. (From Blowey RW, Weaver AD: *Color atlas of diseases and disorders of cattle,* ed 2, London, 2003, Mosby.)

are similar to those for cattle. Lameness can be caused by ulcers, foreign bodies, white line disease, fractures, spondylosis, degenerative joint disease, tarsal bursitis, dislocations, paresis, sand cracks, carpal hygroma, arthritis, frostbite, and ergot. Prevention of lameness includes regular trimming of the hooves.

Corkscrew Claw

Corkscrew claw occurs when the claw (usually the lateral claw) of both hindlimbs is twisted spirally throughout its length (Fig. 15-60).

Scissor Claw

Scissor claw occurs when one toe grows across the other (Fig. 15-61).

Slipper Foot

Slipper foot occurs when the claw is flat and curls upward to form a square end.

Laminitis

Laminitis is also known as lactic acid acidosis and founder. Laminitis is any change to the corium of the hoof. Laminitis

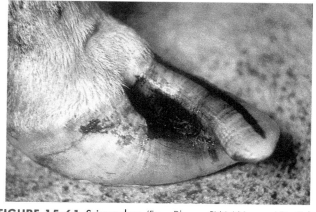

FIGURE 15-61 Scissor claw. (From Blowey RW, Weaver AD: *Color atlas of diseases and disorders of cattle*, ed 2, London, 2003, Mosby.)

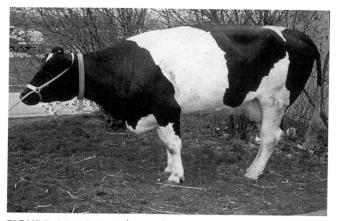

FIGURE 15-63 Typical acute laminitis stance. (From Blowey RW, Weaver AD: *Color atlas of diseases and disorders of cattle*, ed 2, London, 2003, Mosby.)

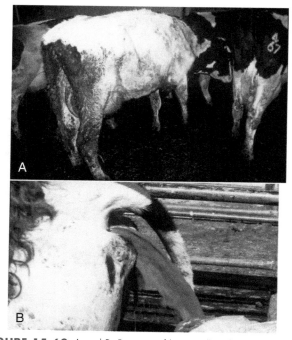

FIGURE 15-62 A and **B,** Passage of loose yellow feces that contain grain particles may be seen with rumen acidosis. (From Blowey RW, Weaver AD: *Color atlas of diseases and disorders of cattle*, ed 3, London, 2012, Mosby Ltd.)

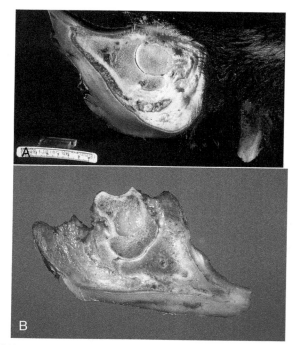

FIGURE 15-64 A, Longitudinal section through the foot of a 6-year-old Shorthorn bull with early chronic coriosis (laminitis). The sole laminae are thickened and hemorrhagic, and pink striations indicate the presence of blood in the sole horn, particularly at the toe. **B,** At a later stage, the line of hemorrhage in the sole horn beneath the pedal bone is easily recognizable. (From Blowey RW, Weaver AD: *Color atlas of diseases and disorders of cattle*, ed 2, London, 2003, Mosby.)

can occur for several reasons, including trauma, metabolic disease, infection, and dietary disturbances. The causes of laminitis are similar to those in horses. One theory is that high carbohydrate intake results in an increase in *Streptococcus bovis* and *Lactobacillus* species, leading to an acidotic state in the rumen (Fig. 15-62). Because these bacteria do not survive in the rumen, they die, causing release of an endotoxin. The endotoxins have a vasoactive effect that damages the laminae. Another theory is that epidermal growth factor (EGF) found in the corium of the claw inhibits the differentiation of keratinocytes.

Clinical signs often include small and careful steps, hemorrhages in the sole, and edema of the coronary band (Figs. 15-63 and 15-64).

LEFT OR RIGHT DISPLACEMENT OF THE ABOMASUM AND ABOMASAL VOLVULUS

- Etiology: unknown
- General malaise

LDA and RDA have no definitive cause. In LDA, the abomasum moves from its normal position (suspended over the greater and lesser omenta) to the left. In RDA, the abomasum moves from its normal position to the right. Abomasal volvulus can occur if RDA is not corrected, but RDA is not always necessary for abomasal volvulus to be present.

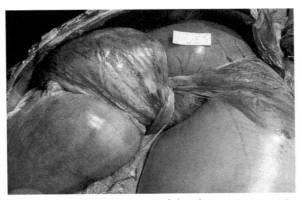

FIGURE 15-65 Complex torsion of the abomasum. (From Blowey RW, Weaver AD: *Color atlas of diseases and disorders of cattle*, ed 3, London, 2012, Mosby Ltd.)

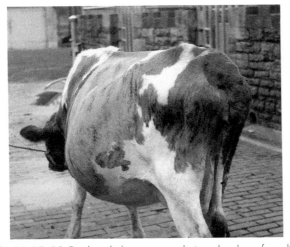

FIGURE 15-66 Displaced abomasum results in a slow loss of condition resulting from partial inappetence; the bulge of the abomasum may then become more obvious in the left flank. (From Blowey RW, Weaver AD: *Color atlas of diseases and disorders of cattle*, ed 3, London, 2012, Mosby Ltd.)

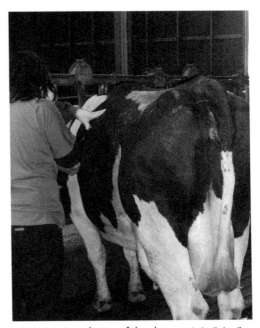

FIGURE 15-67 Auscultation of the characteristic "ping" associated with left displaced abomasum.

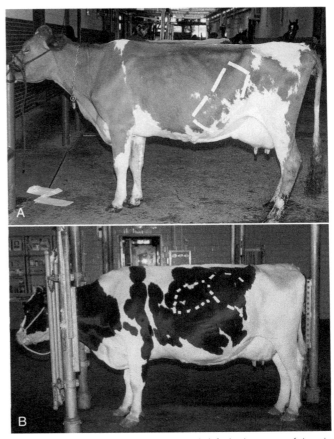

FIGURE 15-68 A, Guernsey cow with left displacement of the abomasum in caudal location. **B,** Coexisting left displaced abomasum and ruminal gas (ping) in a cow. (From Divers TJ, Peek SM: *Rebhun's diseases of dairy cattle*, ed 2, St. Louis, 2007, Saunders.)

In abomasal volvulus, the abomasum rotates on its mesenteric axis (Fig. 15-65). LDA is more common than RDA. Approximately 80% of displaced abomasums occur within 1 month of parturition, but they can occur at any time.

Clinical signs include the animal going off feed, decreased milk production, and decreased fecal output. The cranial aspect of the abdomen just behind the rib cage may appear "sprung" on the affected side (Fig. 15-66).

The diagnosis is commonly made based on history and the presence of a characteristic "ping" on either the left or right side (LDA on the left, RDA on the right). The "ping" can be heard when auscultating and using percussion along the side of the animal (Figs. 15-67 to 15-69).

> **TECHNICIAN NOTE** Left or right displacement of the abomasum produces a characteristic "ping" on the affected side.

Treatment is most effective with surgical replacement of the abomasum in the correct position. Replacement of the

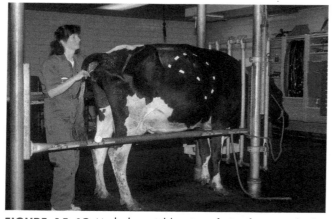

FIGURE 15-69 Marked cranial location of ping from a right displaced abomasum and omental tear. (From Divers TJ, Peek SM: *Rebhun's diseases of dairy cattle*, ed 2, St. Louis, 2007, Saunders.)

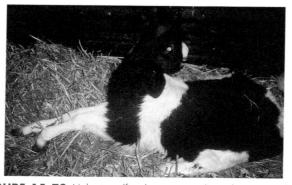

FIGURE 15-70 Holstein calf with pronounced opisthotonos and extensor spasm of the front legs. (From Blowey RW, Weaver AD: *Color atlas of diseases and disorders of cattle*, ed 2, London, 2003, Mosby.)

abomasum often requires removal of gas and fluid buildup within the abomasum before it can be replaced.

POLIOENCEPHALOMALACIA

- Etiology: thiamine deficiency
- Neurologic disease

Polioencephalomalacia (PEM) is a metabolic condition that causes neurologic signs in cattle around the world. The incidence of PEM is increased in cattle in the feedlot and in animals receiving pasture-fed grain supplements. PEM most commonly occurs in young, rapidly growing animals, but it can affect any age group. The disease can be caused by an induced thiamine deficiency caused by products of abnormal rumen fermentation (thiaminases). Other causes of the disease include feeding dietary urinary acidifiers and sulfur toxicity. Sulfur toxicity has been seen when high levels of wet corn gluten are fed because sulfur products are used to refine corn into the by-product wet corn gluten and distillers' grains.

PEM implies a loss of cerebral neurons. Clinical signs associated with the disease include depression, head pressing, ataxia, cortical blindness, tremors, tetany, opisthotonos, convulsions, and paddling. As the disease progresses,

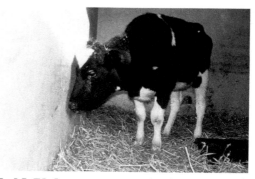

FIGURE 15-71 Depression, ataxia, head pressing, and cortical blindness are clinical signs of polioencephalomalacia. (From Blowey RW, Weaver AD: *Color atlas of diseases and disorders of cattle*, ed 2, London, 2003, Mosby.)

the animal most likely will become recumbent (Figs. 15-70 and 15-71).

> **TECHNICIAN NOTE**   Animals may act enraged and display violent actions, such as running through fences.

The diagnosis of PEM is often based on clinical signs and is presumptive on a favorable response to intensive parenteral therapy with thiamine hydrochloride. At necropsy of the brain, bilateral cortical necrosis is often seen.

Treatment of the disease includes multiple IV injections of thiamine HCl within the first few hours of clinical signs. Other treatments may include diuretics or dexamethasone, or both. Mortality can be 50% or more in untreated animals.

PROLAPSES

- Etiology: multiple causes
- Organ prolapse

Vaginal, uterine, and rectal prolapses are periparturient problems that are common in ruminants.

Vaginal Prolapse

Vaginal prolapse is fairly common in cows (Fig. 15-72). It usually occurs during the last 2 to 3 weeks of gestation. The cause is unknown, although many factors have been implicated. Obesity, estrogen-containing legumes and feeds, estrogen growth implants, persistent coughing, short tail docking, multiple fetuses, hypocalcemia, hormonal imbalances, and overconsumption of low-quality forage all have been theorized to cause vaginal prolapse. Beef breeds are more commonly affected than are dairy breeds.

The condition is recognized by protrusion of the vagina from the vulva. Varying degrees of prolapse from minimal protrusion to complete eversion are possible. The condition typically is progressive. It often begins with mild prolapse that is seen when the animal lies down but disappears when the animal stands up. This progresses to failure to disappear when the animal stands, with increasing swelling and irritation.

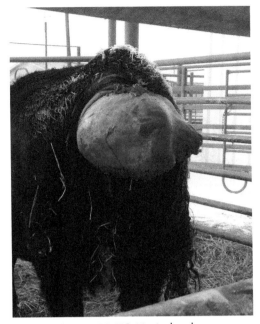

FIGURE 15-72 Vaginal prolapse.

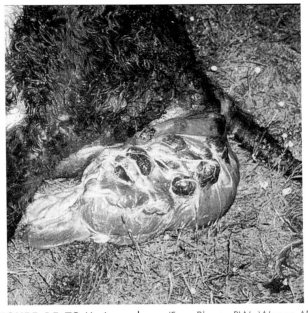

FIGURE 15-73 Uterine prolapse. (From Blowey RW, Weaver AD: *Color atlas of diseases and disorders of cattle*, ed 3, London, 2012, Mosby Ltd.)

The animal begins to strain in response to the irritation, thus leading to more prolapse of the organ and creating a "vicious cycle" of progressive prolapse, inflammation, and straining. If the blood supply is compromised, necrosis may begin, and absorption of toxins can cause severe systemic signs.

Treatment depends on the severity of the condition. In most cases, the goal is replacement of the organ, followed by a method to keep the organ in the retained position. Caudal epidural analgesia is often used to prevent straining and desensitize the perineum. Sedation may be necessary. The prolapsed organ is gently washed with mild antiseptic soap and thoroughly rinsed. Next, the organ is coated with a water-soluble lubricant and is carefully massaged back into its normal position. If swelling is excessive, various mixtures of salts or sugars have been used topically to "draw" water out of the exposed tissue.

Several methods can be used to retain the vagina once it has been replaced. Heavy suture material or umbilical tape has been used to suture the vulva partially closed so that the vagina cannot prolapse but urine can be voided. The Buhner method of placing a subcutaneous pursestring suture is popular and simple to perform, and it gives the best results of the available suture patterns. The suture material should be removed just before parturition to prevent ripping and tearing of the vulva. Buhner suture can be used in all species.

Surprisingly, vaginal prolapse rarely affects pregnancy or causes dystocia. The animal may have an inherited predisposition for vaginal prolapse, and the condition tends to recur in subsequent pregnancies. Affected females usually are culled or removed from the breeding herd.

Uterine Prolapse

Prolapse of the uterus generally occurs immediately after or within a few hours of parturition. The condition is unusual after 24 hours post partum. Dairy cows are most often affected. As with vaginal prolapse, the cause is unknown, but many factors have been associated. Many animals are hypocalcemic, which results in a flaccid, atonic uterus. During and immediately after giving birth, the cervix is dilated, and the flaccid uterus may be expelled by straining or any activity that causes an "abdominal press" by the female. Dystocia and traction on the fetus or a retained placenta may increase the incidence of uterine prolapse.

The prolapse is visible as a large mass protruding from the vulva, often hanging down below the animal's hocks. It typically develops progressively rather than being expelled in one large motion. The uterus can be distinguished from the vagina by the bumpy caruncles on the endometrial lining of the uterus; the vaginal lining is smooth (Fig. 15-73). Various degrees of additional trauma, such as lacerations, may occur while the organ is exposed.

Treatment is similar to that described for vaginal prolapse. Caudal epidural analgesia decreases straining and desensitizes the perineum; sedation may be indicated. The clinician decides on the position of the patient, which may be standing or recumbent. In either case, it may be helpful to have the female positioned on an incline with the hindquarters elevated so that gravity works in favor of the clinician. The exposed uterus is cleansed, and any lacerations are repaired. The organ is lubricated and gently replaced. Assistants may be necessary to elevate and support the uterus, as well as keep it clean and moist, while the clinician replaces it. A tray, towel, or surgical drape can be used like a hammock to support the uterus. Ancillary treatment with oxytocin to encourage uterine tone and involution usually is indicated after replacement. Hypocalcemia must be corrected either orally or with parenteral calcium-containing solutions.

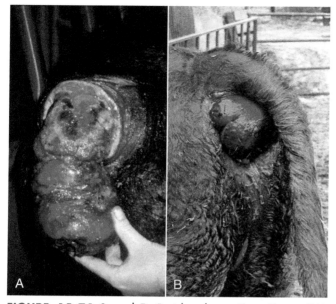

FIGURE 15-74 A, and B, Rectal prolapse. (From Blowey RW, Weaver AD: *Color atlas of diseases and disorders of cattle,* ed 3, London, 2012, Mosby Ltd.)

Once the organ has been repositioned, closure of the vulva is controversial. Closure does not prevent the organ from inverting again; it merely prevents the inverted organ from being exteriorized. If the uterus is completely and fully replaced all the way to the tips of the uterine horns and uterine tone is corrected by oxytocin and calcium administration, the prolapse is unlikely to recur. When closure is elected, Buhner suture usually is used.

The prognosis depends on the amount of trauma and contamination of the prolapsed tissue. Early replacement of a minimally damaged organ has a good prognosis. The condition does not tend to recur with subsequent deliveries, and most females are able to conceive again. However, when the organ is markedly traumatized, heavily contaminated, or necrotic, the prognosis is poor. Hemorrhage, bacterial toxemia, and septicemia may occur, leading to shock and death. A technique for surgical amputation of the uterus is sometimes used to try to salvage the animal's life in these cases. Uterine prolapse does not appear to be hereditary.

Rectal Prolapse

Rectal prolapses in cattle may be associated with uterine or vaginal prolapse or dystocia (Fig. 15-74). Other causes of rectal prolapse include diarrhea, excessive "riding" behavior, traumatic injury, neoplasia of the rectum, and urolithiasis.

Clinical findings include an elongated tube protruding from the anus. Treatment of rectal prolapse consists of replacing the rectum. An epidural analgesic procedure is often performed to reduce further straining, permit surgical correction, and replace the prolapse. A pursestring suture is often placed, using umbilical tape and a Buhner needle, and the anus is closed, leaving about a finger and half opening in the rectum.

RETAINED PLACENTA

- Etiology: failure of placenta to separate

Retained fetal membranes are common in cattle. The attachments of the ruminant placenta to the uterus (*placentomes*) separate gradually, and normally the placenta is passed within several hours after the fetus is delivered. This delayed separation has a positive effect during dystocia, by allowing the fetus to continue receiving oxygen for a prolonged time and increasing its chances for surviving the dystocia. The negative aspect of delayed separation is the high incidence of retained placentas after delivery and the related clinical problems that may result. Fetal membranes provide an ideal "culture medium" for bacteria, which can enter and colonize the uterus, with resulting uterine infection. In some cases, bacterial toxins enter the bloodstream and cause severe systemic illness (septicemia, toxemia) and possibly death.

> **TECHNICIAN NOTE** Retained fetal membranes are common in cattle.

Several risk factors have been associated with retained placentas. Retained placentas are more likely to occur following dystocia, cesarean section, and abortion. Dietary deficiencies of selenium and vitamin A have been implicated. Hypocalcemia may be involved in some cases. Age and breed of the dam may also play a role.

Retained fetal membranes are easy to observe in cattle. They are seen protruding from the vulva and are often several feet in length (Fig. 15-75).

The placenta in ruminants should be passed within 6 to 8 hours. If the female shows no sign of systemic illness, it usually is safe to wait 12 to 18 hours post partum before providing veterinary treatment. Treatment usually includes medication to stimulate contractions and involution of the uterus; oxytocin and prostaglandin $F_{2\alpha}$ are most often used. Antibiotics are often given systemically and less commonly by intrauterine infusions or boluses; intrauterine treatments currently are controversial. Experienced clinicians may attempt manual removal of the placenta in cattle. Although manual removal may seem like an obvious choice for treatment, it is not a simple procedure, and many potential complications are associated with it. Considerable trauma to the uterus may occur, including tearing away of the uterine lining and prolapse of the uterus. Small pieces of the membranes may tear off and be left in the uterus, thus causing uterine infection. Manual removal typically is the last resort when medical methods and time have failed.

Clients should never be encouraged to pull on the membranes or tie solid objects or weights to the membranes. The tetanus prophylaxis status of the animal should be determined, especially in small ruminants. Veterinary consultation is advised in all cases.

RICKETS

- Etiology: lack of calcium, phosphorus, or vitamin D
- Weak skeletal system

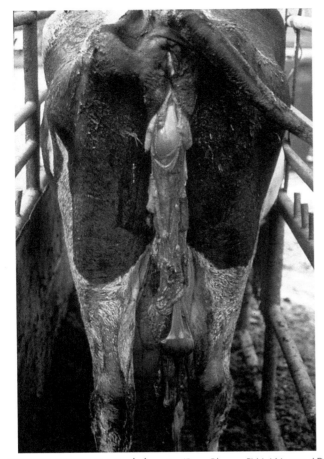

FIGURE 15-75 Retained placenta. (From Blowey RW, Weaver AD: *Color atlas of diseases and disorders of cattle*, ed 3, London, 2012, Mosby Ltd.)

Rickets is a condition of improper calcification of the organic matrix in bone. The improper calcification causes soft, weak bones that lack density. The disease affects young animals and is caused by a lack of calcium, phosphorus, or vitamin D. An abnormal calcium-to-phosphorus ratio is the most likely cause.

Clinical signs include swollen, tender joints, enlargement of the epiphysis, bowed limbs, stiffness, beads on the ribs, and arched back (Fig. 15-76).

Treatment includes correction of the diet. Exposure to sunlight may increase the production of vitamin D. The prognosis is good if permanent damage to the bone or fracture has not occurred.

RUMINAL DISTENTION

- Etiology: multiple causes
- Rumen distention

Ruminal distention is a clinical sign, not a specific disease. The rumen may distend with fluid, gas, or both. Gas distention is also referred to as ruminal tympany or bloat. Fluid distention is sometimes referred to as "splashy rumen." Causes of ruminal distention are numerous and include the following:

- Dietary: inadequate roughage, overconsumption of grain ("grain overload"), ingestion of foreign bodies, toxin ingestion

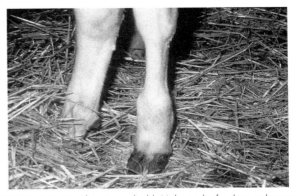

FIGURE 15-76 This 6-month-old Holstein heifer has enlargement of the fetlock joint secondary to widening of the distal metatarsal joint caused by rickets. (From Blowey RW, Weaver AD: *Color atlas of diseases and disorders of cattle*, ed 3, London, 2012, Mosby Ltd.)

- Mechanical: esophageal obstruction that prevents eructation, stenosis of outflow tracts from the rumen or reticulum or the abomasum
- Derangement of motility: dysfunction of the vagus nerve, hypomotility or atony secondary to many other diseases, drugs, and advanced pregnancy

The often used term "vagal indigestion" is somewhat confusing ("vague indigestion"). It has been used as a synonym for chronic indigestion from any disease that disturbs outflow from the forestomachs or abomasum. Outflow disturbance may be caused by a variety of conditions, including true dysfunction of the vagus nerve. However, primary vagus nerve problems are uncommon; emptying defects of the forestomachs are more prevalent than vagus nerve disease. Emptying defects may be caused by mechanical obstructions (foreign bodies, such as sheets of plastic or placentas), anatomical obstructions (pyloric stenosis, compression by tumors or abscesses), or physiologic alterations in motility.

Bloat (ruminal tympany) is the term properly used to refer to distention of the rumen with the gases of fermentation. Gas may exist in two forms: free gas and foamy gas (froth). Ruminants produce large amounts of gas as a result of fermentation of plant material in the rumen or reticulum. Rumen gas can exit only by one route—the cardia and esophagus—by the process of eructation. Ruminants have the capability to eructate several times more gas than can be produced in the rumen; therefore, overproduction of gas is not the problem. The real problem is inability of the gas to exit the rumen, either because something is interfering with eructation or the gas is trapped inside bubbles (foam).

Bloat is classified as frothy bloat or free-gas bloat. Passage of a stomach (ororumen) tube usually is necessary to differentiate them. *Frothy bloat* is often associated with legume pastures or green chop, especially when they are lush. Legumes contain high levels of soluble proteins that tend to form foam with "stable" bubbles that cannot be eructated and are not easily broken down. Accumulations of "non-bubble" gas are referred to as *free-gas bloat*. Free-gas bloat has many possible causes, such as obstruction of the esophagus (choke), obstructions of the cardia (abscesses, tumors, foreign bodies, fluid buildup in the rumen above the level of the cardia), hypomotility (from hypocalcemia, hyperacidity of rumen contents, or drugs), and positioning in lateral recumbency. Bloat is more common in cattle than in small ruminants.

> **TECHNICIAN NOTE** Bloat is classified as frothy bloat or free-gas bloat.

Ruminal distention may be mild, moderate, or severe and may occur acutely or chronically. The diagnosis is made by observation of the abdominal contour (silhouette), abdominal auscultation, ballottement of the rumen, and rectal examination. The rumen occupies most of the left side of adult ruminants, and distention tends to cause enlargement on the left side of the animal. Gas distention produces primarily distention of the upper left abdominal quadrant (especially visible in the left paralumbar fossa). Fluid distention produces primarily distention of the lower left abdominal quadrant. Severe fluid distention can enlarge the rumen such that the distention also affects the right lower abdominal quadrant (Fig. 15-77).

Auscultation typically reveals hypomotility or complete atony of the rumen, although hypermotility may occur early in the disease in some cases. If a gas cap develops in the rumen, it may be detected by percussion ("pinging") over the upper left abdominal quadrant; however, LDA may also produce a "ping" in this area, so this test is not specific for bloat. Rumen ballottement can be used to count rumen contractions and assess the ruminal fluid content. Rectal examination in large ruminants is useful for assessing rumen size and contents. Radiographs may be helpful in identifying metallic foreign bodies.

Distention can produce other clinical signs. Anorexia is common. Discomfort is often indicated by the animal's repeatedly rising and lying down. Heart rate tends to increase as distention increases. Severe distention may press on the thoracic cavity, thereby compromising lung expansion and resulting in shallow, rapid, frequently open-mouth breathing. Severe distention may also compromise venous blood flow returning to the heart, with development of shock.

Treatment options are medical and surgical, depending on the cause and severity of ruminal distention. Mild cases often resolve on their own. Keeping the animal up and moving may help. In contrast, acute severe gas bloat can be life-threatening within 1 to 4 hours because of the respiratory and cardiovascular compromise. Decompression can be life-saving and is the most critical treatment. Passage of a stomach (ororumen) tube is the simplest and quickest method of decompression. It is effective for free gas, but foam does not readily exit through or around the tube. When a tube cannot relieve gas, an exit for the gas must be created through the abdominal wall. This may be achieved using a trocar or surgical incision into the rumen.

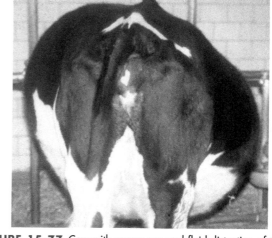

FIGURE 15-77 Cow with severe gas and fluid distention of the rumen. The left upper, left lower, and right lower abdominal quadrants are distended in a classic "papple"-shaped abdomen caused by vagal indigestion. (From Fubini SL, Ducharme NG: *Farm animal surgery*, St. Louis, 2004, Saunders.)

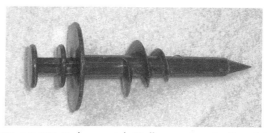

FIGURE 15-78 Corkscrew-style (Buff rumen screw) self-retaining rumen trocar. (From Fubini SL, Ducharme NG: *Farm animal surgery*, St. Louis, 2004, Saunders.)

Trocarization of the rumen may be done with a large-bore hypodermic needle or with commercially available rumen trocars. The site for trocarization is determined by auscultation and "pinging" of the left side of the abdomen for the point of maximal tympany, typically at a location in the left paralumbar fossa. The thoracic cavity must be avoided. The site is clipped and sterilely prepared (prepped). Local anesthetic may be deposited in the subcutaneous and muscle layers of the abdomen. The clinician wears sterile gloves and places the trocar through the skin into the rumen. Some of the larger trocars may require a stab incision through the skin and abdominal wall. Most trocars are used to alleviate the gas and medicate the rumen and then are withdrawn. A few trocars are designed to be indwelling for longer periods of time and may be self-retaining (Fig. 15-78).

Surgical rumenotomy or rumenostomy may be necessary to decompress the rumen, explore the rumen, or remove rumen contents and foreign objects. Rumen surgical procedures are usually performed in the standing animal through a left flank approach, by using sedation and local anesthesia. Use of a rumen board assists rumenotomy. The rumen board is designed to support a portion of the rumen outside the abdomen so that any spillage of contents from the open rumen

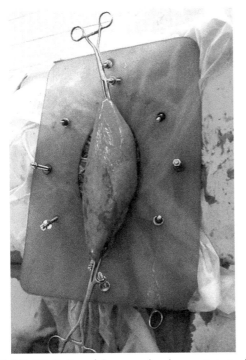

FIGURE 15-79 Portion of the rumen has been exteriorized through the left flank and stabilized with a rumen board. The rumen can be safely opened with a vertical incision. (From Fubini SL, Ducharme NG: *Farm animal surgery*, St. Louis, 2004, Saunders.)

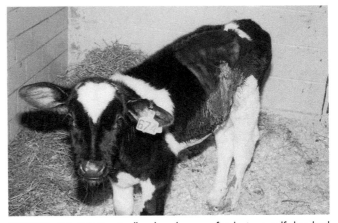

FIGURE 15-80 Surgically placed rumen fistula in a calf that had chronic free-gas bloat. The ingesta spilling down the side of the abdomen cause no problem. (From Divers TJ, Peek SM: *Rebhun's diseases of dairy cattle*, ed 2, St. Louis, 2007, Saunders.)

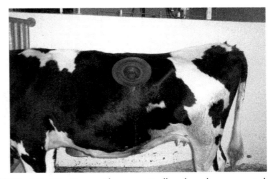

FIGURE 15-81 Cow with a surgically placed commercial rumen fistula. (From Fubini SL, Ducharme NG: *Farm animal surgery*, St. Louis, 2004, Saunders.)

does not contaminate the abdominal cavity (Fig. 15-79). After evacuation and exploration of the rumen through the rumenotomy, the rumen incision is closed and returned to the abdomen. Closure of the abdominal wall is performed in several layers.

A permanent opening of the rumen through the abdominal wall, called a rumenostomy (also known as *rumen fistula*), may be surgically created for selected cases. This technique is helpful for chronic bloaters. The opening of the rumenostomy is protected by a commercially available plastic, lightweight fistula with a removable cover (Figs. 15-80 and 15-81).

When frothy bloat is detected, various oral medications may be used to try to break up the foam bubbles. These antifoaming medications are primarily surfactants, which reduce the surface tension of the bubbles and encourage their breakup. They may be given through a stomach tube or, if rumen trocarization is performed, given directly into the rumen through the trocar. Poloxalene and dioctyl sodium sulfosuccinate are popular surfactants. Mineral oil is also used in some cases. Animals should be removed from the offending pasture or feeds.

UROLITHIASIS

- Etiology: dietary
- Stones in the urinary tract

Urolithiasis (water belly, urinary calculi) is the formation of urinary stones (calculi). Urinary stones are composed of various types and amounts of minerals and mucoproteins. Obstructive urolithiasis occurs when the urinary stones

become lodged in the urinary tract and produce partial or complete obstruction to the passage of urine. The disease is somewhat similar to that seen in felines. Both males and females may form urinary stones, but females are much less likely to experience obstruction of the urinary tract because the female urethra is wider, shorter, and straighter, which facilitates passage of the stones.

Urinary tract obstruction is seen most often in male animals being fitted for shows and in feedlot animals. A definite nutritional role exists in the development of urinary calculi, which are composed primarily of calcium salts and phosphate compounds. The typical diet of affected animals is high in concentrates (grain), low in roughage, improperly balanced (low) in the calcium-to-phosphorus ratio, and often high in magnesium. The high-grain diets commonly fed to pet, show, and feedlot animals are largely responsible for the imbalances associated with the condition. Other compounds, such as oxalates (from plants) or silica in the soil, may play a role in some parts of the country. Limited access to water may lead to concentrated urine and therefore contribute to the problem. A hereditary predisposition may also be involved.

Uroliths may form in any part of the urinary tract. Clinical signs depend on the size and location of the stones and

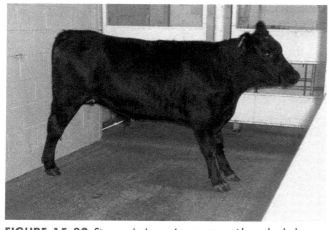

FIGURE 15-82 Stranguria in an Angus steer with urethral obstruction caused by a urolith. (From Smith BP: *Large animal internal medicine*, ed 4, St. Louis, 2008, Mosby.)

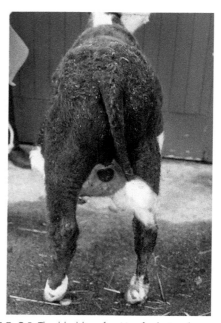

FIGURE 15-84 The bladder of a Hereford steer has ruptured as a result of urethral obstruction, and the urine has gathered in the ventral abdominal cavity, thus causing progressive swelling and distention of the flanks. (From Blowey RW, Weaver AD: *Color atlas of diseases and disorders of cattle*, ed 2, London, 2003, Mosby.)

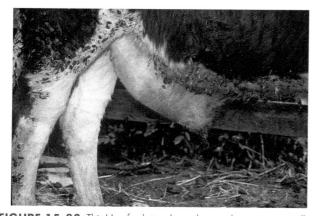

FIGURE 15-83 This Hereford steer has a large subcutaneous swelling containing urine as a result of urethral rupture in the sigmoid region. (From Blowey RW, Weaver AD: *Color atlas of diseases and disorders of cattle*, ed 2, London, 2003, Mosby.)

most commonly include stranguria and dysuria with frequent posturing to urinate (Fig. 15-82). Swishing the tail indicates discomfort. Hematuria and abdominal pain may be seen. Complete obstruction of the urinary tract may occur in the kidney, ureters, bladder neck, or most commonly the urethra. Pressure necrosis and rupture of the urinary tract may occur if complete obstructions are not relieved. Ruptures allow leakage of urine internally. Bladder ruptures allow urine to empty directly into the abdominal cavity (uroperitoneum), and urethral ruptures allow subcutaneous accumulation of urine. Systemic absorption of the "leaked" urine can lead to uremia and eventually death if untreated (Figs. 15-83 and 15-84).

The most common locations of urethral obstruction are the sigmoid flexure of the penis and the urethral process at the tip of the penis. The sigmoid flexure of the male ruminant penis provides two hairpin turns where stones may have difficulty passing. Early castration has been associated with failure of the male urethra to reach maximal diameter, thus possibly contributing to the likelihood of

urethral obstruction. However, castration (at any age) has no effect on the physiologic processes that lead to stone formation.

The diagnosis usually begins with extension of the penis and palpation of the urethral process in small ruminants. Acepromazine sedation is often used to facilitate relaxation of the retractor penis muscle. Xylazine is not recommended because of its diuretic effect. Abdominal palpation may be possible in small ruminants and may reveal bladder distention. Rectal examination and palpation of the bladder may be possible in larger animals. In cases of urethral rupture, subcutaneous swelling may be palpable, usually in the area of the sigmoid flexure. The swelling typically is large and fluctuant. Diagnostic ultrasound can be a valuable tool for visualizing the kidneys, ureters, bladder, and urethra. Plain film abdominal radiographs in smaller individuals may demonstrate calcium-containing stones. Contrast studies may be necessary to visualize the location and full extent of urinary stones. Blood work is important in cases of complete obstruction and may reveal elevations of blood urea nitrogen and creatinine, electrolyte abnormalities, and evidence of dehydration.

Treatment depends on the location, severity, and duration of the clinical signs. Perineal urethrostomy is shown in Figure 15-85 and is discussed in Chapter 14. Sheep and goats usually are sedated (most commonly with acepromazine intravenously) and positioned on the rump. The penis is exteriorized for examination by pulling the sheath caudally with one hand while extending the sigmoid flexure with the other hand to force the penis cranially. The glans is grasped with dry gauze and pulled to

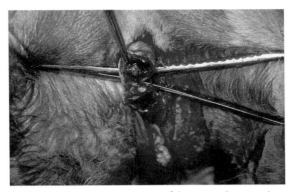

FIGURE 15-85 Intraoperative view of the perineal region shows the dilated urethra proximal to the sigmoid flexure and the obstructing calculus. (From Blowey RW, Weaver AD: *Color atlas of diseases and disorders of cattle*, ed 2, London, 2003, Mosby.)

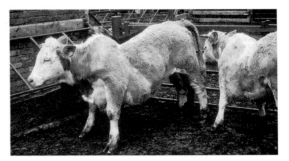

FIGURE 15-86 Flying scapula in two beef steers. (From Blowey RW, Weaver AD: *Color atlas of diseases and disorders of cattle*, ed 3, London, 2012, Mosby Ltd.)

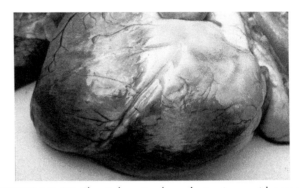

FIGURE 15-87 Chronic hypertrophy and extensive grayish areas on the heart of a calf with white muscle disease. (From Blowey RW, Weaver AD: *Color atlas of diseases and disorders of cattle*, ed 2, London, 2003, Mosby.)

full extension. If the obstruction is confirmed to be at the urethral process, the process can be easily amputated at its base along the glans penis. Amputation does not prevent the animal from breeding in the future. Amputation of the urethral process is necessary to introduce a urethral catheter in these species.

Catheterization of the urethra and retrograde flushing may relieve the obstruction in some cases; however, the anatomy of the male ruminant urethra makes catheterization difficult and limits its usefulness. In addition, passage of a catheter and flushing with pressure may cause ruptures if the urethral tissue has been devitalized by the calculi.

Regardless of the treatment, clients must be educated to prevent recurrences. Nutritional management is essential for prevention. Laboratory analysis of stones from the patient can identify the principal components of the stones, to allow better nutritional management of each individual. Similarly, nutritional analysis of the diet can be a valuable tool for formulation of a diet that is not likely to induce stone formation.

Nutritional management generally includes free access to fresh, clean water. Sodium chloride is often added to the diet to improve water consumption, but salt also has beneficial effects on preventing the actual formation of stones. Various oral additives such as ammonium chloride may be given to acidify the urine; a urine pH of 6.8 or less is desirable. Clients can be instructed to monitor voided urine one to two times weekly by using pH paper or urine dipsticks. Toxicity is possible with ammonium chloride, and signs include anorexia, depression, and diarrhea. Foodstuffs high in cations, such as legumes (alfalfa or clover) and molasses, should be avoided because they tend to encourage alkaline urine pH. Pelleted feeds have also been associated with an increased incidence of calculi. Grass hay should be the primary roughage source.

Balancing the calcium-to-phosphorus ratio is essential; a 2:1 ratio is recommended and may require calcium additives to achieve this balance. Cereal grains such as corn and oats are low in calcium and high in phosphorus and should be minimized or eliminated. Legumes tend to be high in calcium and low in phosphorus and may adversely affect the calcium-to-phosphorus ratio. Legumes also may be high in estrogen compounds and protein, both of which can contribute to stone formation. High-protein diets should be avoided. Magnesium should not exceed 0.6% of the diet in any animal.

WHITE MUSCLE DISEASE

- Etiology: lack of selenium and vitamin E
- Clinical signs vary

White muscle disease is also known as enzootic muscle dystrophy. It can cause "flying scapula" (Fig. 15-86). White muscle disease commonly occurs in young animals and is caused by vitamin E or selenium deficiency. The disease often manifests during the spring, after turnout of cattle onto pasture. The animals need to use their muscles more readily but lack the ability to do so because of deficient diets fed throughout the winter.

Clinical signs include uncoordinated movement, lameness, paralysis of the hindlimbs, dyspnea, and sudden death. In response to the loss of muscle function, the scapula often rises above the level of the spine. At necropsy, the heart is pale and lobed (Fig. 15-87). White lesions may be seen on the diaphragm and in the skeletal muscle.

> **TECHNICIAN NOTE** White muscle disease can lead to flying scapula.

Treatment should include parenteral injection of vitamin E and selenium. Prevention should include adequate amounts of vitamin E and selenium in diets.

FORMULARY

When veterinarians select drugs for use in food-producing animals, they must use caution. Several drugs are prohibited from use in food animals. Other drugs must be used only as the label indicates. As a veterinary technician, it is important to know these rules so you can help communicate effectively with your clients. Other concerns that must be taken into consideration when a veterinarian is selecting drugs to be used in food-producing animals are withdrawal times. The withdrawal time is the time from when the animal was last treated with the drug to when the animal can be slaughtered for food or the animal's milk can go to market. To find up-to-date information about dosages, uses, concentrations, and withdrawal times, you should consult www.farad.org, the website of the Food Animal Residue Avoidance and Depletion program (FARAD). A convenient application (app) for telephones and tablets is also available. Producers should be provided with these withdrawals. Recommendations are to print these times on invoices and to document them in the patient's record. The information in Box 15-2 was taken directly from the FARAD website in March of 2014.

PARASITES

Major bovine parasites are listed in Table 15-2.

TOXINS

Common cattle toxins are listed in Table 15-3.

BOX 15-2	Provisions of the American Medicinal Drug Use Clarification Act

Groups I and II

Under provisions of the American Medicinal Drug Use Clarification Act (AMDUCA) and 21 CFR part 530, FDA can prohibit use of an entire class of drugs in selected animal species if FDA determines that: (I) an acceptable analytical method needs to be established and such a method has not or cannot be established; or (II) the extra-label use of the drug or drug class presents a public health risk. FDA can also limit the prohibition on extra-label use to specific species, indications, dosage forms, routes of administration, or a combination of these.

The first group of drugs has NO allowable extra-label use in any food-producing animal species. This means under no circumstances can these drugs be used in food-producing animals.
- Chloramphenicol
- Clenbuterol
- Diethylstilbestrol (DES)
- Any drugs from the fluoroquinolone class
- Glycopeptides—all agents, including vancomycin
- Medicated feeds
- Nitroimidazoles—all agents, including dimetridazole, ipronidazole, metronidazole, and others
- Nitrofurans—all agents, including furazolidone, nitrofurazone, and others

The next group of drugs has restricted extra-label uses in food-producing animal species. This means they can only be used in certain circumstances.
- Adamantane and neuraminidase inhibitors in all poultry, including ducks—these agents are approved for treatment or prevention of influenza A
- Cephalosporin-class antibiotics **except** cephapirin in all classes of cattle, chickens, pigs, and turkeys—ELDU restrictions apply to **all production classes of major food-animal species.**
  1. No ELDU for purpose of disease prevention
  2. No ELDU that involves unapproved dose, treatment duration, frequency, or administration route
  3. Agent must be approved for that species and production class—ELDU restrictions DO NOT APPLY to minor-use food animal species.
- Indexed drugs—some exceptions for minor-use species
- Phenylbutazone—in female dairy cattle (20 months of age or older)
- Sulfonamide-class antibiotics—in lactating dairy cattle—approved uses are allowed for sulfadimethoxine, sulfabromomethazine and sulfaethoxypyridazine

GROUP III. Drugs With Special Restrictions for Grade "A" Dairy Operations

Based upon recommendations by the National Conference on Interstate Milk Shipments (NCIMS), the FDA publishes a set of minimum standards and requirements for the production of Grade "A" milk. These standards, which are published collectively as the Grade A Pasteurized Milk Ordinance (Grade "A" PMO), provide applicable CFR references and can be used as an inspectional guide to cover specific operations in the dairy industry, including pasteurization equipment, packaging, quality control, and record keeping requirements. Although the PMO does not have the force of regulations, it provides procedures and standards of general applicability that are acceptable to FDA. Owing to human food safety concerns, certain drugs are not to be used or not to be stored on dairy operations or administered to lactating dairy cattle. These restrictions include:
- Non–medical grade dimethylsulfoxide (DMSO)—no use or storage allowable
- Dipyrone—no use allowable
- Colloidal silver—no use or storage allowable
- Systemically acting drugs that are applied topically (including fenthion, famphur and xylene, phosmet, levamisole, and all ivermectins and avermectins)—no use allowable

From Food Animal Residue Avoidance and Depletion program: www.farad.org/
CFR, Code of Federal Regulations; ELDU, extra-label drug use; FDA, Food and Drug Administration.

TABLE 15-2	Bovine Parasites and Parasitic Diseases			
COMMON NAME AND PHOTOGRAPH	**SCIENTIFIC NAME**	**IMPORTANCE**	**DIAGNOSIS**	**TREATMENT**
Brown Stomach Worm*	*Ostertagia ostertagi*	Larval destruction of gastric glands causes severe diarrhea and weight loss Type I: produces eggs Pre-type II: not clinically apparent, fourth-stage larvae inhibited in gastric glands Type II: eggs often not found in feces	Fecal flotation and identification at necropsy	Fenbendazole, doramectin, eprinomectin, ivermectin, morantel tartrate, moxidectin
Bankrupt Worm or Small Stomach Worm*	*Trichostrongylus axei*	Loss of weight, dehydration, diarrhea, bottle jaw Prepatent period of 3 wk	Eggs in fecal flotation and identification at necropsy	Ivermectin, doramectin, eprinomectin, fenbendazole, moxidectin, morantel tartrate
Nodular Worm*	*Oesophagostomum radiatum*	Possible diarrhea Prepatent period of 40 days	Eggs in fecal flotation and identification at necropsy	Moxidectin, morantel tartrate, levamisole, eprinomectin, doramectin
Cattle Bankrupt Worm*	*Cooperia pectinata* *Cooperia punctata* *Cooperia spatulata* *Cooperia mcmasteri (surnabada)*	Decreased growth, anorexia	Eggs in fecal flotation and identification at necropsy	Doramectin, ivermectin, moxidectin, eprinomectin, albendazole, fenbendazole, levamisole, morantel tartrate
Hookworm*	*Bunostomum phlebotomum*	Loss of weight, diarrhea, anemia, death in young animals	Eggs in fecal flotation and identification at necropsy	Ivermectin, moxidectin, doramectin, eprinomectin, fenbendazole

Continued

TABLE 15-2	Bovine Parasites and Parasitic Diseases—cont'd			
COMMON NAME AND PHOTOGRAPH	**SCIENTIFIC NAME**	**IMPORTANCE**	**DIAGNOSIS**	**TREATMENT**
Whipworm* 	*Trichuris ovis*	Extreme infections can cause fatal hemorrhage into cecum Prepatent period of 2 mo	Eggs in fecal flotation Adults in cecum and large intestine at necropsy	Ivermectin, fenbendazole, eprinomectin
Capillary Worm† 	*Capillaria* spp.	Egg may be confused with *Trichuris* spp. Prepatent period of 6 wk	Eggs in fecal flotation	Ivermectin, doramectin, eprinomectin, fenbendazole
Threadworm* 	*Strongyloides papillosus*	Prepatent period of 1–2 wk	Larvated eggs or larvae in fecal flotation	Eprinomectin
Hair Worm, Black Scour Worm† 	*Trichostrongylus colubriformis*		Eggs in fecal flotation Adults in small intestine at necropsy	Levamisole, morantel tartrate, doramectin, eprinomectin, fenbendazole, moxidectin
Barber's Pole or Wire Worm* 	*Haemonchus placei*	Prepatent period of 17–21 days Eggs not able to larvate after 4–5 days of refrigeration	Fecal flotation Adults in abomasum at necropsy	Levamisole, ivermectin, albendazole, doramectin, morantel tartrate, moxidectin, eprinomectin, tetramisole
Lungworm† 	*Dictyocaulus viviparous*	Respiratory symptoms (e.g., cough, cyanosis, dyspnea) Prepatent period of 4 wk	Baermann technique for larvae from feces Fecal flotation Adults in lung at necropsy	Ivermectin, doramectin, eprinomectin, moxidectin, levamisole, fenbendazole
Common Liver Fluke 	*Fasciola hepatica*	Anemia, weight loss, decreased performance, hepatitis, death Prepatent period of 10–12 wk	Eggs in fecal sedimentation Flukes in liver and bile ducts at necropsy Enzyme-linked immunosorbent assay	Clorsulon, nitroxynil, rafoxanide

TABLE 15-2	Bovine Parasites and Parasitic Diseases—cont'd			
COMMON NAME AND PHOTOGRAPH	**SCIENTIFIC NAME**	**IMPORTANCE**	**DIAGNOSIS**	**TREATMENT**
Tapeworm†	*Moniezia benedeni*	Prepatent period of 40 days	Proglottids in feces Fecal flotation Adults in small intestine at necropsy	Fenbendazole, albendazole, dichlorophen, lead arsenate, niclosamide
Beef Cysticercosis, Measles†	*Taenia saginata*	Carcass condemnation or trimming Transmission from eggs in human feces orally consumed by cattle	Serologic tests and confirmation on necropsy	None that are economically justified
Rumen Fluke†	*Paramphistomum* spp.	Diarrhea	Fecal sedimentation	Oxyclozanide, niclosamide
Babesia or Pyroplasma†	*Babesia bigemina*	Texas cattle fever, anemia, splenomegaly, fever Incubation period variable (14–70 days)	Stained blood smear	Berenil, phenamidine, acriflavine
Thin-Necked Intestinal Worm: Sheep and Cattle†	*Nematodirus filicollis, Nematodirus battus, Nematodirus spathiger*	*N. battus* is especially dangerous Prepatent period of 14–21 days	Fecal flotation Adults in small intestine at necropsy	Eprinomectin, ivermectin, moxidectin, albendazole, fenbendazole, levamisole, morantel tartrate
Coccidia†	*Eimeria bukidnonensis, Eimeria aubemensis, Eimeria bovis, Eimeria cylindrica, Eimeria alabamensis, Eimeria zurnii, Eimeria ellipsoidalis*	Coccidiosis, bloody diarrhea, decreased performance, death Prepatent period of 12–18 days	Fecal flotation Hemorrhagic intestines with white raised lesions on necropsy	Sulfaguanidine, monensin, lasalocid
Cryptosporidium†	*Cryptosporidium* spp.	Diarrhea in calves 2–4 wk old Zoonotic to humans	Fecal flotation	Supportive care
Esophageal Worm†	*Gongylonema pulchrum*		Eggs in fecal flotation	None available

Continued

TABLE 15-2	Bovine Parasites and Parasitic Diseases—cont'd

COMMON NAME AND PHOTOGRAPH	SCIENTIFIC NAME	IMPORTANCE	DIAGNOSIS	TREATMENT
Brisket Worm† 	Stephanofilaria stilesi	Lesions on ventral abdomen Prepatent period of 6–8 wk	Deep skin scrapings	Control of horn flies
Skin Nodular Worm† 	Onchocerca spp.	Keratitis or iritis Possibility of condemned carcass Prepatent period of 6–12 mo	Microfilaria identification in skin sample from near skin nodule	None
Abdominal Worm† 	Setaria cervi	Possible cerebral nematodiasis Prepatent period variable	Microfilaria in the blood	None
Common Cattle Bot Fly and Northern Cattle Bot Fly* 	Hypoderma lineatum Hypoderma bovis	Reduction in weight gain, decreased hide value Migration to esophagus or spinal column causing warbles Life cycle of 10–12 mo	Warbles	Pour-on ivermectin, trichlorfon, famphur, organophosphates, coumaphos, fenthion, moxidectin
Screwworm† 	Cochliomyia hominivorax	Reportable disease in United States Highly pathogenic, high mortality Maggots penetrating through broken skin Life cycle of 3 wk	Larvae from wounds should be sent to the state diagnostic laboratory	Ivermectin, organophosphates
Face Fly† 	Musca autumnalis	Possible predisposition to bacterial keratoconjunctivitis (pink eye) Possible transmission of eye worms (Thelazia spp.), infectious bovine rhinotracheitis Life cycle variable, ~10–14 days	Identification of flies	Pour-ons, dips, sprays, dusts, back rubbers, orals, injectables, feed additives
Horn Fly* 	Siphona (Haematobia) irritans	Production loss Life cycle of ≥3 wk	Identification of adult fly Smaller than house fly and usually feeds with head down	Pour-ons, dips, sprays, dusts, back rubbers, orals, injectables, feed additives

TABLE 15-2 | Bovine Parasites and Parasitic Diseases—cont'd

COMMON NAME AND PHOTOGRAPH	SCIENTIFIC NAME	IMPORTANCE	DIAGNOSIS	TREATMENT
House Fly* Arista / Palp / Labellum	*Musca domestica*	Production loss Life cycle of 10–14 days	Identification of flies	Pour-ons, dips, sprays, dusts, back rubbers, orals, injectables, feed additives
Stable Fly† 	*Stomoxys calcitrans*	Production loss Life cycle of ≥4 weeks	Identification of adult fly Size of house fly	Pour-ons, dips, sprays, dusts, back rubbers, orals, injectables, feed additives
Horse Fly† 	*Tabanus* spp.	Transmission of anaplasmosis Production loss Bites possibly causing stampedes; very painful	Identification of adult fly	Pour-ons, dips, sprays, dusts, back rubbers, orals, injectables, feed additives
Biting Louse† 	*Bovicola (Damalinia) bovis*	Production loss Most common in fall and winter Usually on neck, brisket, head, and between legs in cattle Life cycle of ~4 wk	Identification of eggs, nymphs, adult lice	Pour-ons, dips, sprays, dusts, back rubbers, orals, injectables, feed additives
Sucking Louse* 	*Linognathus vituli* (long-nosed or blue cattle louse) *Haematopinus eurysternus* (short-nosed cattle louse)	Production loss Possible anemia Life cycle of ~4 wk	Identification of eggs, nymphs, adults	Pour-ons, dips, sprays, dusts, back rubbers, orals, injectables, feed additives
Mange Mite or Scab Mite† 	*Psoroptes* spp.	Reportable disease in some states Dramatic weight loss Life cycle of ~3 wk	Skin scrapings	Pour-ons, dips, sprays, dusts, back rubbers, orals, injectables, feed additives
Mange Mite† 	*Sarcoptes scabiei*	Reportable disease in some states Life cycle of ~3 wk	Skin scrapings	Pour-ons, dips, sprays, dusts, back rubbers, orals, injectables, feed additives

Continued

TABLE 15-2	Bovine Parasites and Parasitic Diseases—cont'd			
COMMON NAME AND PHOTOGRAPH	**SCIENTIFIC NAME**	**IMPORTANCE**	**DIAGNOSIS**	**TREATMENT**
Mange Mite[†]	*Chorioptes* spp.	Reportable disease of cattle in some states Tail or foot mange Life cycle of ~3 wk	Skin scrapings	Pour-ons, dips, sprays, dusts, back rubbers, orals, injectables, feed additives
Ticks[†]	*Dermacentor variabilis* (American dog tick), *Dermacentor andersoni* (Rocky Mountain wood tick), *Dermacentor albipictus* (winter tick), *Dermacentor occidentalis* (Pacific Coast tick), *Ixodes scapularis* (black-legged tick), *Amblyomma americanum* (lone star tick), *Amblyomma maculatum* (Gulf Coast tick), *Boophilus annulatus* (cattle tick), *Boophilus microplus* (southern cattle tick), *Otobius megninii* (spinose ear tick), *Ornithodoros coriaceus* (pajaroello tick)	Possible transmission of anaplasmosis		Pour-ons, dips, sprays, dusts, back rubbers, orals, injectables, feed additives
Mange Mite[†]	*Demodex bovis*			Pour-ons, dips, sprays, dusts, back rubbers, orals, injectables, feed additives

Note: Some photographs are not of the exact species listed but are of similar species.
*From Bowman DD: *Georgis' parasitology for veterinarians,* ed 10, St. Louis, 2014, Saunders.
†From Hendrix CM, Robinson E: *Diagnostic parasitology for veterinary technicians,* ed 4, St. Louis, 2012, Mosby.

TABLE 15-3	Common Cattle Toxins
TOXIN	**EFFECTS IN CATTLE**
Nitrate	Retarded growth, lowered milk production, vitamin A deficiency, goitrogenic effects, abortions, fetotoxicity, and death
Urea	Ruminal tympany, jugular pulses, twitching, tetanic spasms, abnormal CNS behavior, and death
Lead	Blindness, salivation, spastic twitching of the eyelids, jaw champing, bruxism, muscle tremors, convulsions, and death
Mycotoxins	Reduced feed intake, reproductive failure, immunosuppression
Alkaloids	Liver disease, edema of the abomasum, anorexia, hindleg weakness, knuckling, excessive salivation, pollakiuria, and death
Cyanogenic	Dyspnea, salivation, lacrimation, muscle fasciculation, and death
Photosensitizing agents	Dermatologic signs
Saponins	Vomiting, abdominal pain, diarrhea, convulsions, and death
Tannins	Anorexia, depression, emaciation, ammonia smell to the breath, ocular and nasal discharge, icterus and constipation, liver disease, and death

CNS, Central nervous system.

CASE STUDY

A technician is on a farm call with the veterinarian to Mr. Savich's ranch on December 17. The farm call was warranted by a phone call from Mr. Savich reporting large numbers of aborted fetuses. His herd is not due to calve until the middle of February. The veterinarian would like you to collect necropsy samples from the aborted calves with him. What disease or diseases could cause these abortions? What precautions will you take when collecting the aborted fetal tissue samples, and why?

CASE STUDY

Mr. Goracke owns 50 head of cattle on his ranch in southeast Nebraska. His cattle have developed round, encrusted lesions on their heads and necks. The veterinarian has diagnosed the lesions as dermatophytosis. What is the common name for this condition? Mr. Goracke would like to turn a profit on these calves and would like to know what the most cost-effective treatment would be, if any. What will the veterinarian most likely tell Mr. Goracke?

SUGGESTED READING

Anderson DE, Rings DM: *Current veterinary therapy: food animal practice,* ed 5, St. Louis, 2008, Saunders.

Blowey RW, Weaver AD: *Color atlas of diseases and disorders of cattle,* ed 2, London, 2003, Mosby.

Bowman DD: *Georgis' parasitology for veterinarians,* ed 9, St. Louis, 2008, Saunders.

Divers TJ, Peek SJ: *Rebhun's diseases of dairy cattle,* ed 2, St. Louis, 2007, Saunders.

Foreyt WJ: *Veterinary parasitology reference manual,* ed 5, Ames, Iowa, 2007, Iowa State University Press.

Hendrix CM, Robinson E: *Diagnostic parasitology for veterinary technicians,* ed 3, St. Louis, 2006, Mosby.

Kahn CM, Line S: *The Merck veterinary manual,* ed 10, Whitehouse Station, NJ, 2010, Merck & Co.

Radostits O, Gay CC, Hinchcliff KW, et al: *Veterinary medicine: a textbook of the diseases of cattle, horses, sheep, pigs and goats,* ed 10, Oxford, 2007, Saunders.

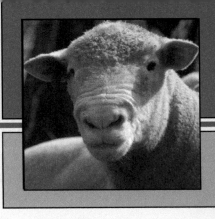

16 Ovine and Caprine Husbandry

OUTLINE

LEARNING OBJECTIVES

When you have completed this chapter, you will be able to

- Know and understand the zoologic classification of the species
- Know and be able to proficiently use terminology associated with this species
- Know normal physiologic data for the species and be able to identify abnormal data
- Identify and know the uses of common instruments relevant to the species
- Describe prominent anatomical or physiologic properties of the species
- Identify and describe characteristics of common breeds
- Describe normal living environments and husbandry needs of the species
- Understand and describe specific reproductive practices of the species
- Understand specific nutritional requirements of the species

KEY TERMS

Ad libitum
Beard
Billy
Buck
Buck kid
Cashmere
Crutching
Dewlap
Doe

Doe kid
Electroejaculation
Ewe
Ewe lamb
Facing
Jugs
Kid
Kidding
Lamb

Lambing
Nanny
Ram
Ram lamb
Wattles
Wether
Wether lamb
Yearling doe
Yearling ewe

KEY ABBREVIATION

USDA AIPL: U.S. Department of Agriculture Animal Improvement Programs Laboratory

ZOOLOGIC CLASSIFICATION

SHEEP

Kingdom	Animal
Phylum	Chordata
Class	Mammalia
Order	Artiodactyla
Family	Bovidae
Genus	*Ovis*
Species	*Aries*

GOATS

Kingdom	Animal
Phylum	Chordata
Class	Mammalia
Order	Artiodactyla
Family	Bovidae
Genus	*Capra*
Species	*Hircus*

TERMINOLOGY AND PHYSIOLOGIC DATA

Table 16-1 lists common terminology used to describe the age and breeding status of sheep and goats. Table 16-2 lists normal physiologic data for sheep and goats.

COMMON OVINE AND CAPRINE INSTRUMENTS

Visit the Evolve website to find pictures and descriptions for common ovine and caprine instruments.

ANATOMICAL TERMS

Figures 16-1 and 16-2 detail the terms for body parts and areas of sheep and goats, including the bones and joints.

TABLE 16-1	Terminology	
	SHEEP	**GOATS**
Adult female	Ewe	Doe/nanny
Adult male	Ram	Buck/billy
Castrated male	Wether	Wether
Immature female	Yearling ewe	Yearling doe
Neonate	Lamb	Kid
Castrated neonate	Wether lamb	
Intact male neonate	Ram lamb	Buck kid
Female lamb	Ewe lamb	Doe kid
Act of parturition	Lambing	Kidding

BREEDS OF SHEEP

FINE WOOL BREEDS
Merino
- Color: White face and legs with white wool
- Breed association: American & Delaine-Merino Record Association
- Website: www.countrylovin.com/admra/

Merino sheep originated in Spain. The three types of Merinos are A, B, and C. The A and B types have wrinkled skin. Type A is more wrinkled than type B. Type A and B Merinos are called American Merinos. The type C Merino, called the Delaine Merino, has very little wrinkle to the skin. The Delaine Merino tends to be more popular in the United States. It is a medium size and has an angular body. The Delaine Merino has a white face and legs with white wool on the head

TABLE 16-2	Physiologic Data	
	SHEEP	**GOATS**
Temperature	101° F –104° F	101° F –104° F
Pulse rate	70–90/min	70–90/min
Respiratory rate	12–25 breaths/min	12–30 breaths/min
Adult weight	Varies by breed	Varies by breed

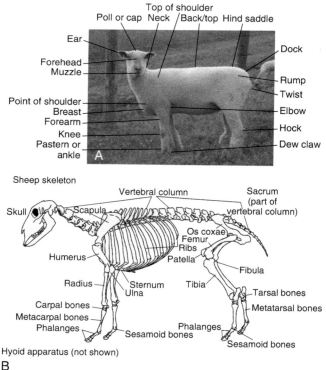

FIGURE 16-1 Anatomy of the sheep. **A,** External parts. **B,** Skeleton.

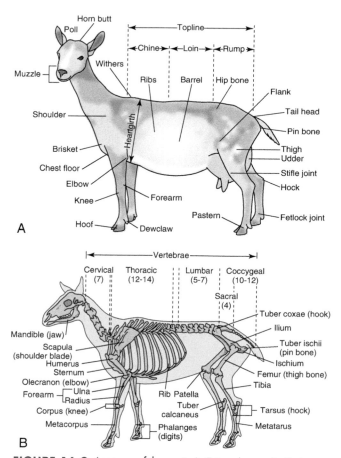

FIGURE 16-2 Anatomy of the goat. **A,** External parts. **B,** Skeleton.

and legs. The skin is pale. The rams are horned, and the ewes are polled (Fig. 16-3).

Rambouillet
- Color: White face and legs with white wool
- Breed association: American Rambouillet Sheep Breeders Association
- Website: www.countrylovin.com/arsba/

The Rambouillet originated in France and was developed from the Spanish Merino. The breed is known for its large, angular, blocky body type. It has a white face and legs with white wool on the head and legs. The Rambouillet has pale skin. The rams are polled or horned. All ewes are polled. The breed is primarily raised for wool production and is common in the western United States (Fig. 16-4).

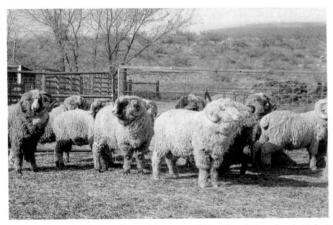

FIGURE 16-3 Merino sheep. (Courtesy of Bliss Ranch, Loveland, Colo.)

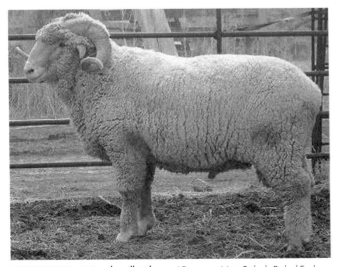

FIGURE 16-4 Rambouillet sheep. (Courtesy Matt Rabel, Rabel-Forbes-McGivney Rambouillets, Kaycee, Wyo.)

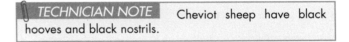

MEDIUM WOOL BREEDS
Cheviot
- Color: White face and legs with black hooves and black nostrils
- Breed association: American Classic Cheviot Sheep Association
- Website: www.cheviots.org/

The Cheviot originated in northern England and southern Scotland. It has a small, blocky body type. It has a white face and legs with black hooves and black nostrils. The head and legs are free of wool, and the skin is pink. The breed is polled and has small, erect ears (Fig. 16-5).

Corriedale
- Color: White face, ears, and legs with wool on the head and legs
- Breed association: American Corriedale Association
- Website: www.americancorriedale.com/

The Corriedale originated in New Zealand. It was the result of crossing Lincoln and Leicester rams with Merino ewes. The Corriedale has a white face, ears, and legs with wool on the head and legs. The body size is medium to large, with a blocky appearance. The breed is polled (Fig. 16-6).

Dorset
- Color: White ears, nose, face, and legs with wool on the head and legs
- Breed association: Continental Dorset Club
- Website: www.dorsets.com/

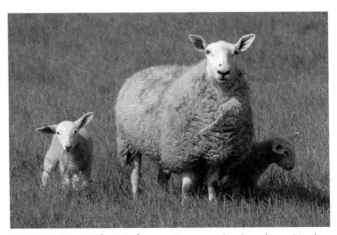

FIGURE 16-5 Cheviot sheep. (Courtesy John Seraphine, Heatherhope Farm, Sycamore, Ill.).

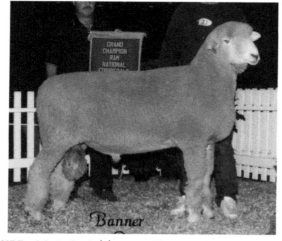

FIGURE 16-6 Corriedale ram. (Courtesy American Corriedale Association/Corriedale Extra.)

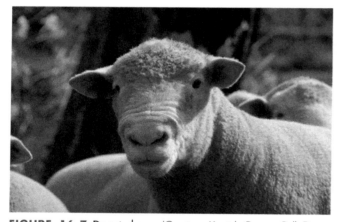

FIGURE 16-7 Dorset sheep. (Courtesy Kentish Downs Poll Dorset Stud, Holbrook, New South Wales, Australia.)

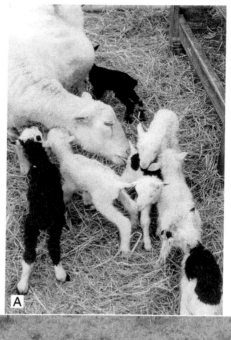

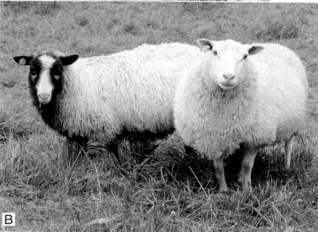

FIGURE 16-8 A and B, Finnish sheep. (Courtesy of Elizabeth H. Kinne Gossner/Stillmeadow Finnsheep, DeRuyter, N.Y.)

The Dorset originated in southern England. The Dorset is of medium size and has a blocky body type. The ears, nose, face, and legs are white, with wool on the head and legs. The skin of this breed is pink. The strains are both polled and horned. The ewes will breed out of season, so fall lambs can be produced (Fig. 16-7).

> **TECHNICIAN NOTE**   Dorset ewes will breed out of season.

Finnsheep
- Color: White ears, nose, face, and legs with wool on the head and legs
- Breed association: International Finnsheep Registry
- Website: www.internationalfinnsheepregistry.org/

Finnsheep originated in Finland. Finnish sheep are a medium-sized breed used for fleece and meat. The breed is commonly used in crossbreeding programs to increase lambing crops. Finnish ewes commonly have triplets, and many have four to six lambs yearly. One of the most notable characteristics is the naturally short tail. The tail should never be docked and should be covered with hair at the end. When this sheep is crossbred, the tail is noticeably longer. The breed has white ears, nose, face, and legs, with the head and legs free of wool. The skin is pink. Although the breed is predominately white, other natural occurring colors are seen. The breed is considered polled, although some rams may have horns (Fig. 16-8).

> **TECHNICIAN NOTE**   Finnish sheep commonly have three to six lambs per year.

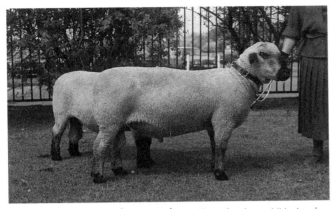

FIGURE 16-9 Hampshire meat sheep. (From Sambraus HH: *A colour atlas of livestock breeds*, London, 1992, Mosby-Wolfe.)

Hampshire

- Color: Black face, legs, ears, and nose, with wool on the head and legs
- Breed association: American Hampshire Sheep Association
- Website: www.hampshires.org/

The Hampshire breed originated in southern England. The Hampshire is large and has a blocky body type. The face, legs, ears, and nose are black. It has wool on the head and legs. The head of a Hampshire has a slight Roman nose. The skin has a dark pigment, and the ears are held horizontally to the head. The breed is polled. Hampshires are one of the more popular breeds in the Midwest (Fig. 16-9).

Montadale

- Color: White, face, ears, and legs, with the head and legs free of wool
- Breed association: Montadale Sheep Breeders Association
- Website: www.montadales.com/

The Montadale originated in the United States. It is a medium to large breed with a blocky body type. The breed has a white face, ears, and legs. The head and legs are free of wool. The skin is pink. The ears are medium size and are carried somewhat erect. This breed is polled (Fig. 16-10).

Oxford

- Color: Brown-gray face and legs, with wool on the legs and head that extends over the poll down to the eyes
- Breed association: American Oxford Sheep Association
- Website: www.americanoxfords.org/

The Oxford breed originated in England. It has a large frame with a brown-gray face and legs. It has wool on the legs and head that extends over the poll down to the eyes. Its skin is pink, and its short ears are set horizontal to the heads. The breed is polled (Fig. 16-11).

Polypay

- Color: White face and legs, with wool on the head and legs

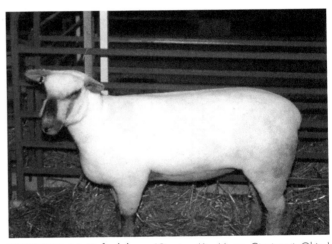

FIGURE 16-10 Montadale sheep. (Courtesy Kim Myers, Cincinnati, Ohio.)

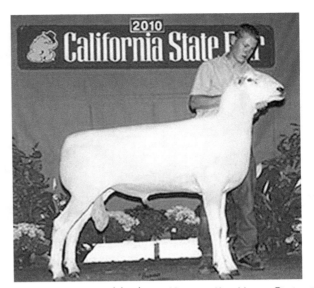

FIGURE16-11 Oxford sheep. (Courtesy Kim Myers, Cincinnati, Ohio.)

- Breed association: American Polypay Sheep Association
- Website: www.countrylovin.com/polypay/index.html

The Polypay was developed in the United States. It has a white face and legs, with wool on the head and legs. The skin is pink (Fig. 16-12).

Romanov

- Color: Mottled face, with head and legs free of wool
- Breed association: North American Romanov Sheep Association
- Website: www.narsa-us.com/

The Romanov originated in the former Soviet Union. It has a smaller body type than other medium wool breeds. It has a mottled face, and the head and legs are free of wool. The breed also has darkly pigmented skin. This breed of sheep is particularly known for its prolificacy and maternal strengths, and it commonly produces litters of four to six lambs (Figs. 16-13 and 16-14).

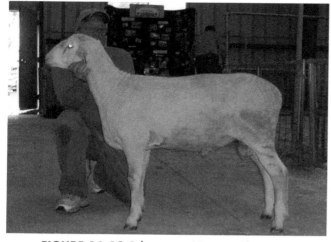

FIGURE 16-12 Polypay ram. (Courtesy Glen Jones.)

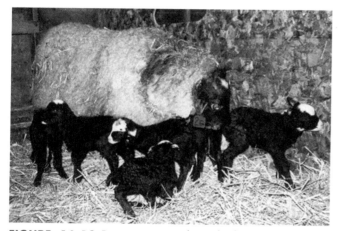

FIGURE 16-13 Romanov ewe with six lambs. (Courtesy Ileana Wenger, DVM, Ontario, Canada)

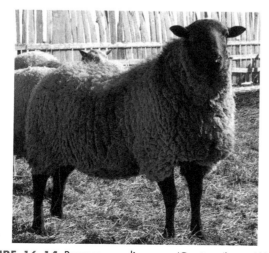

FIGURE 16-14 Romanov yearling ram. (Courtesy Ileana Wenger, DVM, Ontario, Canada)

> **TECHNICIAN NOTE** The Romanov is known for its maternal strengths.

Shropshire
- Color: Brown to dark brown face and legs, with heavy covering of wool on the head and legs
- Breed association: American Shropshire Registry Association
- Website: www.shropshires.org/

The Shropshire originated in England. It has a smaller frame with a blocky body type and is polled. It has a brown to dark brown face and legs, with a heavy covering of wool on the head and legs. The ears are medium size and are carried slightly erect (Fig. 16-15).

Southdown
- Color: Light brown face and legs, with wool on the head and legs
- Breed association: American Southdown Breeders Association
- Website: www.southdownsheep.org/

The Southdown originated in England. It is a moderately framed sheep with well-balanced confirmation. Yearling rams in moderate flesh weigh 225 to 250 pounds. Yearling ewes typically weigh between 160 and 200 pounds. The Southdown breed has a light brown face and legs, with wool on the head and legs. The breed also has medium ears that are carried slightly erect. The breed is polled (Fig. 16-16).

Suffolk
- Color: Black face, ears, and legs
- Breed association: United Suffolk Sheep Association
- Website: www.u-s-s-a.org/

The Suffolk breed originated in southern England. The Suffolk has a large, blocky body type. The face, ears, and legs are black. The breed is polled and has no wool on the head or legs.

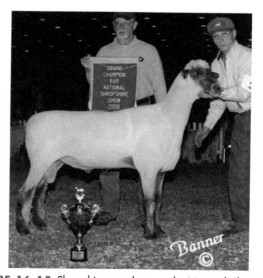

FIGURE 16-15 Shropshire ram that was the National Champion in 2008. (Courtesy American Shropshire Registry Association, Leyden, Mass.)

It has a large, drooping ear, with pink to gray skin and a slight Roman nose. The Suffolk is popular for producing market lambs in the United States (Fig. 16-17).

> 📎 *TECHNICIAN NOTE* The Suffolk is popular for producing market lambs in the United States.

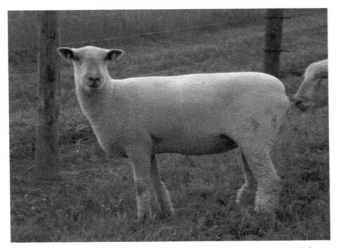

FIGURE 16-16 Southdown ewe. (Courtesy American Southdown Breeders Association, Fredonia, Tex.)

LONG WOOL BREEDS
Cotswold
- Color: White face and legs
- Breed association: Cotswold Breeders Association
- Website: www.cotswoldbreedersassociation.org/

The Cotswold is an old breed of sheep that originated in England. It has a large, blocky body type that is firm and solid to the touch. The body is covered with thick, long, lustrous wool composed of wavy curls that extend to the legs. The head is wide between the eyes and is distinguished by a fine tuft of wool on the forehead. The face and legs are white, although a grayish-white color is not objectionable. Dark spots may occur on the face and legs. The breed is polled (Fig. 16-18).

> 📎 *TECHNICIAN NOTE* The Cotswold has a fine tuft of wool on the forehead.

Lincoln
- Color: White with white face and legs
- Breed association: National Lincoln Sheep Breeders Association
- Website: www.lincolnsheep.org/

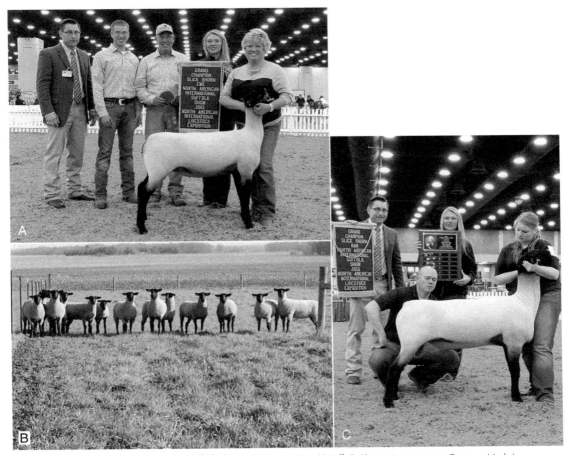

FIGURE 16-17 A to **C,** Suffolk sheep. (Courtesy United Suffolk Sheep Association, Canton, Mich.)

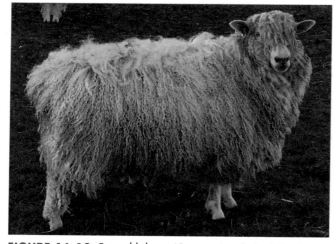

FIGURE 16-18 Cotswold sheep. (Courtesy Angela Reid, Dorchester, Oxfordshire, United Kingdom.)

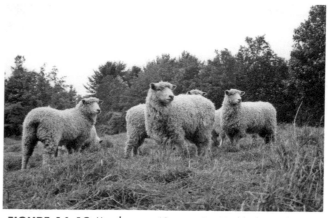

FIGURE 16-19 Lincoln ewes. (Courtesy Joe Haddock, Jericho, Vt.)

The Lincoln originated in England. The Lincoln is large and has a blocky body type. It is white, with a white face and legs. The wool covers part of the head and legs. The breed is polled and produces long, lustrous, ringlets of wool. This breed is commonly used in crossbreeding programs (Fig. 16-19).

> **TECHNICIAN NOTE** The Lincoln has long ringlets of wool.

Romney
- Color: White face, with black or mottled gray nostrils
- Breed association: American Romney Breeders Association
- Website: www.americanromney.org/

The American Romney traces its beginnings to Kent, England. The Romney is a versatile white-faced breed that has the ability to produce high-quality meat and wool under diverse climate conditions and management systems. It has a relatively broad face, large and clear eyes, and alert, thickly felted ears. White ears are desirable, but minor black spots are acceptable. The nostrils should be black or dark, mottled gray. The poll should be free of horns and hair. The back is smooth, blending from the neck and ending at a square rump. Black hooves are desirable. Sheep of this breed can be registered with the American Romney Breeders Association (Fig. 16-20).

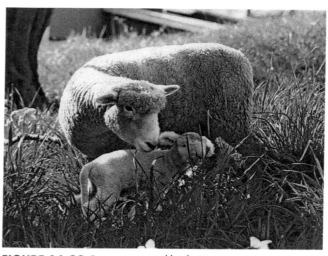

FIGURE 16-20 Romney ewe and lamb. (Courtesy American Romney Breeders Association, Coquille, Ore., and Kim Myers.)

The Boer goat originated in the Eastern Cape province of South Africa in the early 1900s. Current breed standards require a white body with a red head and a white blaze. A few red patches are allowed, and a pigmented skin is preferred. The breed is horned and has a Roman nose. Polled individuals occur occasionally. Mature females weigh 200 to 265 pounds. The breed is prolific, with a common kidding rate of 200%. Because Boer goats have an extended breeding season, three kiddings every 2 years are possible (Fig. 16-21).

> **TECHNICIAN NOTE** Current breed standards for the Boer goat require a white body with a red head and a white blaze.

BREEDS OF GOAT

COMMON MEAT BREEDS

Boer Goats
- Color: White, with a red head and a white blaze
- Breed association: American Boer Goat Association
- Website: http://www.abga.org/

Pygmy Goats
- Color: Various colors
- Breed association: National Pygmy Goat Association
- Website: http://www.npga-pygmy.com/

The Pygmy goat that is found in United States came from the French Cameroons, an area of Africa, and it was originally

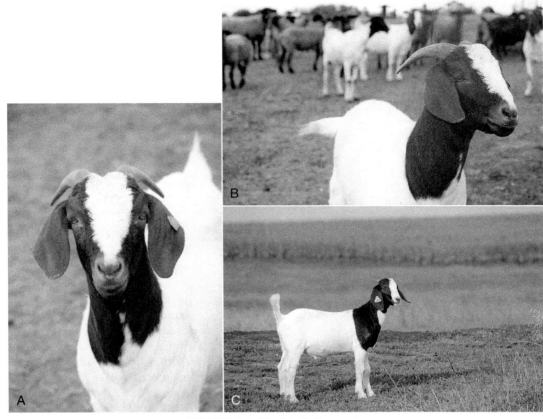

FIGURE 16-21 A to **C,** Boer goats.

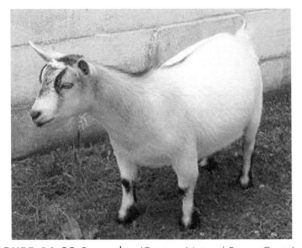

FIGURE 16-22 Pygmy doe. (Courtesy National Pygmy Goat Association, Snohomish, Wash.)

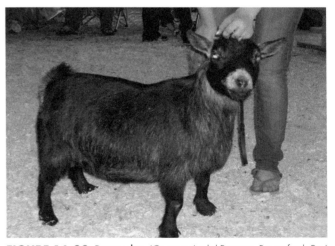

FIGURE 16-23 Pygmy doe. (Courtesy Lynbil Pygmys. Royersford, Pa.)

called the Cameroon dwarf goat. The legs and head are relatively small compared with the body. Genetically polled animals are not acceptable for registry in the National Pygmy Goat Association. Pygmy goats may be any color; preferred colors are white, although gray and black in a grizzled (agouti) pattern can be seen. Breed standards include the following (except for black goats): The muzzle, forehead, eyes, and ears are accented in lighter tones than the body, and the front and rear hooves, cannons, and dorsal stripe are darker than the body color. Goats that are caramel colored must have light vertical stripes on the front sides of darker socks. Some limited random markings are acceptable. Female goats may have no *beard* or one that is sparse or trimmed. Male goats should have a full, long, flowing beard. Pygmy goats are also used for milk production. They are easily handled because of their small size and make good pets (Figs. 16-22 and 16-23).

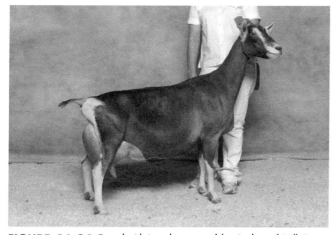

FIGURE 16-24 French Alpine doe owned by Redwood Hill Farm, Jennifer Lynn Bice. (Courtesy Redwood Hill Farm, Sebastopol, Calif.)

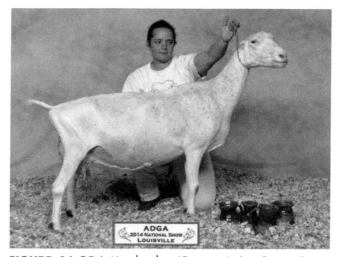

FIGURE 16-25 LaMancha doe. (Courtesy Andrea Forrest, Forrest-Pride Dairy Goats.)

COMMON DAIRY BREEDS

French Alpine
- Color: Various colors
- Breed association: Alpines International Club
- Website: http://www.alpinesinternationalclub.com/

The French Alpine goat originated in France from Swiss foundation stock. The breed ranges in color from pure white to black, with many other varied color patterns. Color shades include fawn, brown, gray buff, and red. It has erect ears and short hair. It does not have a *dewlap* and can be bearded but does not have to be. The breed has polled and horned goats. Bucks weigh 170 to 180 pounds, and does weigh 125 to 135 pounds (Fig. 16-24).

LaMancha
- Color: Various colors
- Breed association: American LaMancha Club
- Website: http://www.lamanchas.com/ears.htm

The American LaMancha is a newly developed breed. It was developed by crossing a short beard Spanish breed with several of the purebred breeds in United States. A LaMancha goat may be any color. It has straight face with short hair. The breed has two different types of ears. The gopher ear is 1 inch or less long, with little or no cartilage, and the end is turned upward or downward. The elf ear may be 2 inches long, cartilage shaping is allowed, and the end must be turned upward or downward. Bucks must have a gopher ear to be eligible for registration (Fig. 16-25).

> **TECHNICIAN NOTE**   LaMancha goats have either a gopher ear or an elf ear.

Nubian
Color: Various colors
Breed association: International Nubian Breeders Association
Website: http://www.i-n-b-a.org/

The Nubian goat originated in Africa. Nubians may be any color or combination of colors. Common shades include black, gray, cream, white, tan, and reddish brown. It has short hair, drooping ears, a Roman nose, and no fringe along the spine. Most Nubians are polled, although some have horns. The doe is beardless. Bucks weigh 175 to 180 pounds, and does weigh 130 to 135 pounds (Fig. 16-26).

Saanen
- Color: White or cream
- Breed association: National Saanen Breeders Association
- Website: http://nationalsaanenbreeders.com/

Saanens have a majestic air about them, which, coupled with their milk-producing ability, identifies the does as "Queens of the Diary Goats." People are drawn to the all-white or cream Saanen breed because of their large size, vitality, herd compatibility, and "eager to please" temperament. The largest part of the breed's popularity, however, is its milking ability. The latest figures furnished by the U.S. Department of Agriculture Animal Improvement Programs Laboratory (USDA AIPL) shows the Saanen breed as one of the leaders in the industry. Saanen goats are represented through the National Saanen Breeders Association (Fig. 16-27).

Toggenburg
- Color: Light fawn to dark chocolate brown, with two white stripes down the face
- Breed association: National Toggenburg Club
- Website: http://www.nationaltoggclub.org/

The Toggenburg goat originated in Switzerland. The color varies from light fawn to dark chocolate brown. The ears are white, with dark spots in the middle. This breed has two white stripes down the face from the eye to the muzzle. The legs and rump are white. The Toggenburg has short to medium-length hair that lies flat. The ears are erect. It may or may not have *wattles*. Toggenburgs usually are polled, although

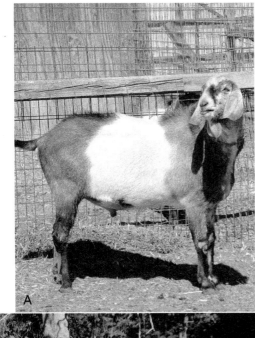

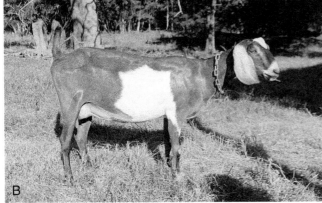

FIGURE 16-26 A and **B,** Nubian goats. (Courtesy International Nubian Breeders Association, Franklin, Tex.)

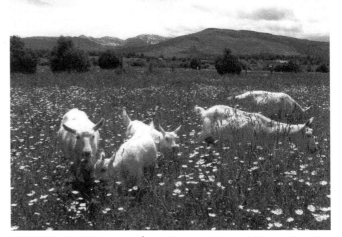

FIGURE 16-27 Saanen does. (Courtesy National Saanen Breeders Association, Dallas.)

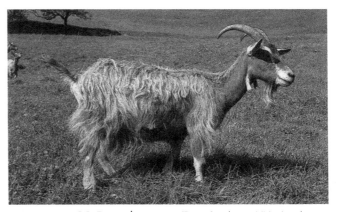

FIGURE 16-28 Toggenburg goat. (From Sambraus HH: *A colour atlas of livestock breeds,* London, 1992, Mosby Wolfe.)

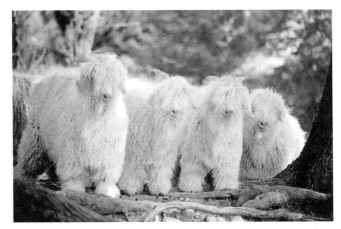

FIGURE 16-29 Angora goats. (Courtesy American Angora Goat Breeders, Rocksprings, Tex.)

some may have horns. Bucks weigh 150 to 175 pounds, and does weigh 100 to 135 pounds (Fig. 16-28).

COMMON FIBER BREEDS
Angora Goats
- Color: White
- Breed association: American Angora Goat Breeders Association
- Website: http://www.aagba.org/

The Angora goat is an ancient breed. It originated in Turkey in the province of Angora. Angoras are horned, although some individuals are polled. The breed has long, thin drooping ears. The Angora is white and open faced. Mature bucks weigh 125 to 275 pounds, and mature does weigh 80 to 90 pounds. The fleece of the Angora goat is called mohair. Older goats produce coarser fleece. Therefore, kid fleece is more valuable. Average mohair production is 6 to 7 pounds per head per year (Fig. 16-29).

Cashmere
Cashmere refers to the soft down or winter undercoat of fiber produced by most breeds of goats, except the Angora. No true genetic breed of cashmere goat and no breed registry for goats that produce cashmere fiber exist.

> *TECHNICIAN NOTE*   No true genetic breed of cashmere goat exists.

TABLE 16-3 | Breeding Information for Sheep

Age of male at puberty*	6–9 mo
Length of spermatogenesis	47 days
Length of copulation	1–2 sec
Site of semen deposition	External cervical os
Ejaculate volume (mL)	0.8–1.0
Total sperm (×10⁹)	3–4
Motile sperm (%)	30
Morphologically normal sperm (%)	70
Scrotal Circumference Ram by Weight (kg)	Size (cm)
<45	23–27
45–70	27–33
70–90	30–36
90–115	31–37
115–135	33–38
135–160	36–40
Ram by Age in Months	
6–12	30
12–18	33

Female Reproductive Parameters

Age of female at puberty*	6–9 mo
Type of estrous cycle	Seasonally polyestrous, short-day breeders, breed dependent
Time of first breeding	12–19 mo
Estrous cycle frequency	13–19 days (average, 17 days)
Duration of estrus	18–48 hr (average, 30 hr)
Time of ovulation	24–30 hr after onset of estrus
Optimal time of breeding	Every 12 hr when in estrus
Maternal recognition of pregnancy	13–14 days as a result of IFN-t
Source of progesterone by day of gestation	0–50: CL >50: placenta
Type of placenta	Placentomes
Gestation period	148 days
Birth weight	7–12 pounds
Litter size	1–3 in most breeds
Weaning age	9–12 wk

Pregnancy Detection in Days After Ovulation

Ultrasound	>18 Doppler: >60
Progesterone	20–24
Estrone sulfate	>70
PSPB	>18

CL, Corpus luteum; *IFN-t,* interferon-tau; *PSPB,* pregnancy-specific protein B.
*Variable depending on breed and body condition. In sheep, the time of year when born has a marked effect. Females born late may not mature in time for the year's breeding season and therefore will not begin cycling until the following year's breeding season.

REPRODUCTION

The normal reproductive course for any large animal species is discussed in Chapter 3. Tables 16-3 and 16-4 list specific breeding information for sheep and for goats, respectively. The following reproductive procedures are variations that exist among species.

TABLE 16-4 | Breeding Information for Goats

Male Reproductive Parameters

Age of male at puberty	3 mo
Length of spermatogenesis	48 days
Length of copulation	1–2 sec
Site of semen deposition	Vagina
Ejaculate volume (mL)	0.6–1.0 mL
Total sperm (×10⁹)	2–3
Motile sperm (%)	70
Morphologically normal sperm (%)	80
Total sperm (10⁹)	1
Scrotal Circumference: Age in Months	cm
5	14
8	20
21	26
36	30

Female Reproductive Parameters

Type of estrous cycle	Varies by breed
Age of female at puberty	3 mo
Time of first breeding	7–18 mo
Estrous cycle frequency	12–30 days (average, 22 days)
Duration of estrus	2–3 days
Time of ovulation	24–30 hr after onset of estrus
Optimal time of breeding	Every 12 hr when in estrus
Maternal recognition of pregnancy in days	13–14 because of IFN-t
Source of progesterone by day gestation	Corpus luteum
Type of placenta	Placentomes
Gestation period	140–160 days (average, 151 days)
Birth weight	Breed dependent
Litter size	1–3
Weaning age	3 mo

Pregnancy Detection in Days After Ovulation

Ultrasound	>20 days Doppler: >40 days
Abdominal palpation	>28 days
Progesterone	20–24 days
Estrone sulfate	>50 days
PSPB	>24 days
PAG	>21 days

IFN-t, Interferon-tau; *PAG,* pregnancy-associated glycoprotein; *PSPB,* pregnancy-specific protein B.

RUT

Rut is the mating period of male goats, and it coincides with the doe's heat. Rut is characterized by decreased appetite and extreme interest in does; bucks exhibit a flehmen response and urinate on their face and forelegs. During this time the buck develops a strong odor, both as a result of its behavior and from the sebaceous scent glands at the base of the horns. These scent glands are important to attract does.

SEMEN COLLECTION

Electroejaculation is the most commonly used method of semen collection. The semen is collected with the ram standing or placed in lateral recumbency. The penis is manually extended from the prepuce. The collection container should be prepared and held ready because some males may ejaculate at this time. If not, the rectum is cleared, and the lubricated electroejaculator probe is inserted and is used to massage the accessory sex glands and apply a brief electrical current. The procedure is repeated until ejaculation occurs. The tip of the glans penis and urethral process should be held within the margins of the collection container, with sterile gauze pads used to handle the penis. Vocalization and muscle contractions are typical during the procedure. Trained rams may be collected using an artificial vagina; the ram mounts a female in estrus or a mounting dummy.

> **TECHNICIAN NOTE** In sheep and goats, electroejaculation is the most commonly used method for semen collection.

In bucks, a semen collection technique using massage of the glans penis through the prepuce has been described. Otherwise, electroejaculation with the buck standing is used. The buck is placed in a chute or is pressed against a wall for restraint. The electroejaculation technique is the same as described for a ram (Fig. 16-30).

ARTIFICIAL INSEMINATION

In sheep and goats, semen may be deposited in the vagina, in the cervix, or directly into the uterus by a transcervical or laparoscopic method. Insemination timing can vary, but it is most commonly 12 hours after the first estrous detection. Because of herd size, this procedure is often accomplished with the use of estrous synchronization. Insemination doses vary with technique used. For vaginal insemination, the dose is often 300 to 400 million viable sperm. The cervical insemination dose is often 100 to 200 million viable sperm. Transcervical insemination doses are often 50 to 100 million viable sperm, and laparoscopic insemination doses are often 20 to 40 million viable sperm. Although conception rates tend to increase as the depth of semen deposition into the reproductive tract increases, the technical difficulty of the insemination also increases. Vaginal and cervical insemination may be done with the female standing; elevating

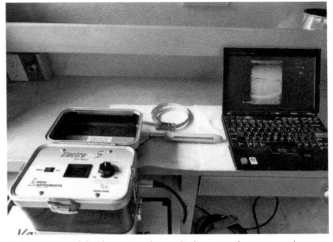

FIGURE 16-30 Electroejaculators. Both contain batteries and require no external power source. Other models are available. Artificial vagina. (From Pugh DG, Baird AN: *Sheep and goat medicine*, ed 2, St. Louis, 2012, Saunders.)

the hindquarters facilitates the cervical procedure. A light source and vaginal speculum are necessary for visualization of the cervix. The cervix of the ewe is tortuous and has several cervical rings that make cervical entry difficult. In goats, semen may be deposited in the vagina, in the cervix, or directly into the uterus. Transcervical insemination should be performed with the animal in the standing position. It is often not rewarding to deposit frozen semen into the vagina.

> **TECHNICIAN NOTE** A light source and vaginal speculum are needed to visualize the cervix in sheep.

Depositing semen directly into the uterus may be done "naturally" through the cervix or surgically through laparoscopy. Transcervical insemination into the uterus requires a light source, vaginal speculum, and special equipment for opening and penetrating the cervix. In goats, the cervix is identified, and the vaginal speculum is locked in the lumen by using slight pressure. In sheep, the cervix is retracted using Bozeman forceps. Next, the insemination pipette is advanced through the cervix. Semen is deposited into the uterine body at a depth of 32 to 38 mm. In sheep, an angled-tip insemination pipette can help with passage through the cervix. Sheep usually are restrained on their backs in a V-shaped cradle. The anatomy of the ewe's cervix makes this method technically challenging.

> **TECHNICIAN NOTE** Transcervical insemination is difficult because of the presence of numerous cervical rings.

Laparoscopic insemination involves sedation of the female and restraint in dorsal recumbency, often using a cradle with the head angled downward at a 40-degree

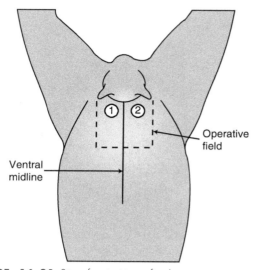

FIGURE 16-31 Sites for incisions for laparoscopic insemination (1, 2). The laparoscope is placed through one incision and the insemination instruments through the other. The surgical field is outlined. (Modified from Pugh DG, Baird AN: *Sheep and goat medicine*, ed 2, St. Louis, 2012, Saunders.)

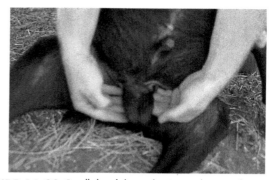

FIGURE 16-32 Small, hard, hypoplastic testicles on a homozygous polled yearling buck. (From Pugh DG: *Sheep and goat medicine*, St. Louis, 2002, Saunders.)

angle. The female should be held off feed and water for 24 hours before the procedure. The abdomen is clipped and prepared in sterile fashion for the surgical procedure. The laparoscopic incisions are performed using local anesthesia (Fig. 16-31).

The surgeon places the laparoscope in the abdomen, identifies the uterus, and inserts a needle into the uterine lumen. Semen is injected with an insemination pipette or special insemination "gun." The incisions are closed with suture, and the skin is covered with antibiotic ointment. The female is placed in a quiet area for recovery and is kept quiet for several hours. The surgical procedure is quick, and complications are rare. The procedure can be repeated in subsequent years.

EMBRYO TRANSFER

The recovery and transfer of embryos in small ruminants must usually be achieved by surgical methods because the anatomy of the female's cervix makes nonsurgical approaches difficult, especially in ewes. The surgical methods require general anesthesia, dorsal recumbency, and either a ventral midline incision or a laparoscopy approach just cranial to the udder.

Recovery of embryos usually occurs between 5 and 6 days after estrus, and the embryos are handled as described in cattle (see Chapter 12). An average of 8 to 10 suitable embryos can be obtained from each flush of a donor female.

> **TECHNICIAN NOTE** The average collection of embryos is 8 to 10.

Commonly, two embryos are transferred to each recipient female because sheep are naturally capable of supporting twin pregnancies should both transferred embryos survive. The necessity of surgical methods increases the risk and cost of the procedure; therefore, embryo transfer in sheep has not achieved the same popularity as in cattle.

> **TECHNICIAN NOTE** Embryo transfer has not reached the same level of popularity in sheep as in cattle.

POLLED INTERSEX

In goats of many European breeds, infertility and the intersex condition are linked to the polled (hornless) genotype. The gene for polledness is dominant in these breeds; unfortunately, an infertility gene (autosomal recessive) is linked to the polled gene. Therefore, goats may have one of three possible genetic combinations (H is the polled gene, and h is the horned gene):

- HH: polled
- Hh: polled (H is dominant)
- Hh: horned

Homozygous polled (HH) males are not intersex, but they have up to a 35% infertility rate resulting from abnormalities of the testicles or epididymis, or both (Fig. 16-32). Homozygous polled (HH) females are intersex (male pseudohermaphrodites), with various degrees of development of both male and female reproductive organs and testosterone-producing tissue, usually in the form of hypoplastic testicles. They are sterile. They often show male behavior from testosterone production, including aggression and increased odor during breeding season; however, they do not produce sperm.

Heterozygotes have normal fertility. Although they do not produce horns, they may be recognized by prominent frontal "bumps" where the horns would have been. These bumps typically are oval and lie close together in a V-shaped formation.

Infertility is not an issue for people not interested in breeding goats, but it is a major concern for producers and purebred breeders. To prevent homozygous polled offspring and the associated intersex or infertility, one of the breeding pair should be genetically horned (hh). Surgical removal of horns does not change the genetic makeup of an individual. Polled intersexes are extremely rare in Angora and Nubian goats, thus indicating a different heritability of the traits. The presence or absence of horns has no relationship with the occurrence of freemartinism.

CLINICAL SIGNS OF AND PREPARATION FOR IMPENDING PARTURITION

Approximately 3 to 4 weeks before lambing, *crutching* is commonly performed. Crutching, the shearing of wool from the vulva and udder, is important because it allows the farmer to observe swelling of the vulva and udder, helps control passage of infectious fecal organisms to lambs, and helps the lambs find the udder. *Facing,* the shearing of wool from around the eyes in breeds with facial wool, is also done to improve the dam's vision of her newborn lambs. Vaccination of the ewe to boost clostridial antibody levels is also done at this time, as is deworming.

Twins and triplets are more common than singleton births in goats. Approximately 4 weeks before birth, the doe is vaccinated and dewormed. Dairy does are commonly moved into special pens for kidding, and the hair around the udder and perineum may be clipped. Goats that give birth in the field should have access to a shelter or a sheltered area. In natural conditions, does typically hide their kids after they are born. The doe leaves her kids hidden while she browses for food; however, she remains within an audible distance and responds to distress calls from the kids. Whether the doe is in a pen or in the field, it is important to provide an area for the doe to "hide" her kids. Small boxes can be constructed in pens for artificial cover.

TECHNICIAN NOTE Does hide their kids after they are born.

In both goats and sheep, the clinical signs of approaching parturition include swelling of the vulva, mucoid vulvar discharge, relaxation of the pelvic ligaments, and enlargement of the udder. Ewes are often moved to lambing pens or stalls (known as *"jugs"*) when these signs are seen. Most births occur during daytime hours.

PARTURITION
Stage 1
In stage 1 of labor, the ewe becomes restless, may urinate frequently, and may lie down repeatedly as contractions begin. She may separate from the flock if she has not already been segregated into a designated lambing area. Stage 1 usually lasts approximately 1 to 4 hours. Goats tend to separate from the herd, become restless, paw, and show nesting behavior. Stage 1 may last up to 12 hours in goats, especially in first-time (primiparous) mothers.

TECHNICIAN NOTE Stage 1 usually lasts 1 to 4 hours in sheep but can last up to 12 hours in goats.

Stage 2
The duration of stage 2 is variable, but it typically lasts 1 to 3 hours, depending on the size of the fetus and its presentation. Most births (95%) occur in anterior "head-diving" presentation, with the head and front legs appearing first. However, successful breech births are possible, especially if the fetus is small and the hind feet are presented first. Twin births are common in sheep, and triplets are not unusual. The interval between delivering each fetus in a multiple birth varies from several minutes to an hour. Straining for an hour without producing a fetus is an indication for assistance. In goats, stage 2 usually is completed within 2 hours. If obvious contractions fail to produce a fetus in 30 to 60 minutes, dystocia may be occurring, and veterinary assistance should be sought. Most births occur in anterior presentation.

TECHNICIAN NOTE Assistance during birth may be warranted if a fetus is not produced after 30 to 60 minutes of obvious contractions.

Stage 3
Stage 3 usually occurs within 2 to 3 hours but may take up to 6 hours after delivery. If the ewe shows no signs of toxemia or septicemia, no treatment is necessary until 12 hours post partum. Stage 3 should be complete within 4 hours for goats.

TECHNICIAN NOTE Treatment for retained placenta usually is not necessary until 12 hours post partum.

DYSTOCIA

Dystocia is common in sheep but is uncommon in goats. Fetal malposition is a common cause of dystocia in both species. A fetotomy is rarely needed in sheep but may be performed if deemed necessary; generally, removal of only the head is necessary. The procedure is described in more detail in Chapter 3.

TECHNICIAN NOTE Most kids are born in anterior presentation.

Dystocia of small ruminants can be identified by forceful straining without the appearance of a fetus at the vulva within 1 hour. If one fetus has been delivered, only 20 minutes should be given between fetuses before dystocia is considered. Dystocia should also be considered if parturition is not complete within 2 hours of rupture of the amniotic sac.

ROUTINE CARE OF THE NEONATE
Routine care of newborn lambs and kids is similar to that of calves. The immediate needs of the newborn include those discussed in the following sections.

Oxygenation and Pulse Assessment

Fetal membranes, fluid, and mucus should be cleared from the nostrils. Briskly rubbing the lamb with towels helps stimulate breathing and dries the body. Sternal recumbency facilitates breathing. If spontaneous breathing does not occur within 20 to 30 seconds after birth, artificial respiration through the mouth or nostril may be attempted. A respiratory resuscitation rate of approximately 20 breaths/minute is desirable.

> **TECHNICIAN NOTE** The respiratory resuscitation rate should be approximately 20 breaths/minute, and resuscitation should be started if the animal does not begin to breathe within 20 to 30 seconds after birth.

The heart rate should be 90 to 150 beats/minute (bpm). If a pulse cannot be palpated, cardiac massage can be performed by compressing the lamb's ventral chest wall just behind the elbows, by using the thumb and two to three fingers. Return of a palpable pulse and improvement in mucous membrane color indicate that effective resuscitation has occurred, and chest compressions can be stopped. Close monitoring of the cardiovascular and respiratory systems is essential following any resuscitation effort.

> **TECHNICIAN NOTE** Resuscitation efforts can be stopped once a palpable pulse has returned and the mucous membranes are pink.

Temperature Regulation

Lambs and kids are especially susceptible to hypothermia in the first 36 hours of life. Heat lamps and other devices can be used if environmental temperatures are cold. Lambs with rectal temperatures lower than 100° F should be warmed immediately. Heat lamps, blow dryers, blankets, and warm water bottles are useful.

> **TECHNICIAN NOTE** Lambs and kids are especially susceptible to hypothermia in the first 36 hours of life.

Care of the Umbilical Cord and Umbilicus

Treatment of the navel with iodine or chlorhexidine solutions is advised. The umbilicus should be observed for signs of infection (heat, pain, swelling, exudates), which is most likely to occur in the first 2 weeks of life.

> **TECHNICIAN NOTE** Umbilical infections are most likely to occur within the first 2 weeks of life.

Nutrition (Nursing)

Lambs may attempt to stand as soon as 10 to 15 minutes after birth, and most stand successfully in approximately 30 minutes. Successful nursing should occur within 1 to 2 hours (average, 90 minutes). Lambs may need assistance in finding the udder. Palpation of the abdomen for "fullness" after observing the kid on the doe's teat may help to confirm that nursing has successfully occurred. Commercial goat milk replacers are available but are not substitutes for colostrum. Normal kids are strong and vigorous, especially in their efforts to nurse.

> **TECHNICIAN NOTE** Nursing should occur within 1 to 2 hours after birth.

Maternal Bonding

Does and ewes vigorously lick the newborn and usually eat the fetal membranes. This behavior is considered essential for maternal bonding. Fetal fluids comprise a crucial element in recognition and bonding of the ewe with her lambs. Maternal bonding is mediated by the sense of smell, with an olfactory attraction to the amniotic fluid. The maternal bonding period is short, and the first 6 to 12 hours are most critical. Minimal human interference is advisable during this time. It is usual to manually assist ewes that are having difficulty delivering and to clear membranes from the newborn's nostrils, but further contact is minimized unless an emergency situation occurs.

Does should not be frightened or disturbed during the critical first hour after birth. Dairy kid management, like dairy calf management, often involves removal of the kids shortly after birth and hand raising them. Under these circumstances, maternal bonding is not of concern.

Passage of Meconium

Meconium should be passed within 24 hours.

Adequacy of Passive Transfer of Antibodies

Lambs and kids should consume a total of 10% to 15% of their body weight in colostrum in the first 24 hours of life. It is important to provide colostrum soon after birth. If nursing intake is questionable, a goal of 50 mL/kg in the first 2 to 4 hours is desirable. Bottle or tube feeding may be necessary to ensure ingestion of colostrum. Species-specific colostrum is preferred, but in lambs, goat colostrum may be substituted. Cow colostrum has questionable efficacy. Commercial "colostrum substitutes" typically are unacceptably low in immunoglobulins.

> **TECHNICIAN NOTE** Lambs and kids should consume a total of 10% to 15% of their body weight in colostrum in the first 24 hours of life.

Physical Examination of the Lamb

Examination of the lamb by using a body systems approach is possible and is indicated, especially in any sick or weak lamb. The same approach as described in calves is used (see Chapter 12), with initial observation from a distance, followed by restraint and a hands-on systemic evaluation.

IDENTIFICATION AND CARE OF THE SICK NEONATE

Starvation and diarrhea are the primary causes of neonatal death on most farms. Starvation occurs when neonates fail to ingest sufficient calories. Rejected and weak neonates (as a result of hypothermia, prenatal or postnatal infections, prematurity, or congenital defects) are most susceptible. Diarrhea in the first few days of life is generally caused by *Escherichia coli* and less often by *Clostridium perfringens* type C. Starvation, hypothermia, and diarrhea all can result in weakness. Conversely, weakness can result in starvation and hypothermia, thus creating a cycle that can be fatal to a neonate within hours.

TECHNICIAN NOTE　Starvation and diarrhea are the primary causes of neonatal death on most farms.

Weakness and depression are the most common clinical signs of illness in the neonatal period. Hypothermia and hypoglycemia are the most common causes of weakness and depression, and these disorders often coexist. Neonates are especially susceptible to both conditions. Hypothermia or hypoglycemia, or both, may cause weakness and depression or may be caused by weakness or depression from other diseases. The deadly cycle that can develop between these conditions may lead to rapid mortality. A rectal temperature lower than 100° F warrants immediate treatment; clinical signs of hypothermia begin at approximately 98° F. Affected animals must be kept warm and dry, and they must be given nutritional support. The nutritional needs of the hypoglycemic animal must be provided by supplementing with glucose and perhaps also with electrolytes and other fluids. The route of fluid administration depends on the severity of dehydration and hypoglycemia, as well as practical concerns such as personnel and cost. Subcutaneous fluid therapy is commonly used because of its effectiveness and practicality in animals that cannot be bottle or tube fed (they lack gastrointestinal function).

TECHNICIAN NOTE　A rectal temperature lower than 100° F warrants immediate treatment of hypothermia.

Bottle feeding using a commercial lamb nipple on a bottle works well. The nipple is placed in the lamb's mouth, and the lamb's jaw can be moved to simulate a chewing motion. This often stimulates the nursing reflex. If the neonate is too weak to nurse, tube feeding is required. A small, approximately 8-French (8-F) red rubber urethral tube or a 14- to 18-F infant feeding tube can be attached to a 60-mL catheter-tip syringe and used as an ororumen tube for lambs. Alternatively, commercially available stainless steel lamb probes are available for passage into the esophagus. The lamb is placed in right lateral recumbency, with the head and neck extended. An oral speculum is not required; pressure on the jaw opens the mouth. The tube or probe is inserted into the mouth and is gently advanced to the pharynx. Rather than forcing the tube into the esophagus, it is best to allow the lamb to swallow and advance the tube "with the swallow." If correctly passed, the tube can easily be felt in the esophagus, dorsolateral to the trachea; a small amount of resistance should be felt as the tube is advanced. If the tube is in the trachea, it cannot be palpated, and the lamb likely will cough. When the tube is confirmed to be in the esophagus, the tube is advanced and the dosing syringe is attached. Any liquid given by tube should be warmed, and the fluid should be delivered slowly, either by slowly depressing the syringe plunger or by using gravity flow from the syringe barrel (with the plunger removed).

TECHNICIAN NOTE　Ororumen tubes, if placed correctly, should be readily felt in the esophagus.

Although intensive care medicine is available for treatment of sick lambs just as in other species, the value of a neonatal lamb seldom justifies the expense associated with diagnostic testing, intravenous fluids, respiratory support, plasma transfusions, medications, and other treatments. A practical, economical, "on-the-farm" approach is almost always used.

NUTRITION

Tables 16-5 and 16-6 list dental formulas and a dental eruption table for sheep and goats, respectively. A picture of the dentition can be found in Chapter 12, in the section on

TABLE 16-5	Sheep Dental Formulas	
Deciduous: dental formula: 2(I0/3 C0/1* PM3/3) = 20 total		
Permanent: dental formula: 2(I0/3 C0/1* PM3/3 M3/3) = 32 total		
Eruption	I1	Birth–1 wk
	I2	Birth–1 wk
	I3	Birth–1 wk
	C	1–3 wk
	PM2	Birth–4 wk
	PM3	Birth–4 wk
	PM4	Birth–4 wk
Eruption	I1	12–18 mo
	I2	18–24 mo
	I3	30–36 mo
	C	36–48 mo
	PM2	18–24 mo
	PM3	18–24 mo
	PM4	18–24 mo
	M1	3–4 mo
	M2	8–10 mo
	M3	18–24 mo

*The canine tooth is in line with the incisors and adjacent to them and is shaped like an incisor, thereby giving the false appearance of four incisors. However, it is common practice to refer to the canine tooth as the fourth incisor (14).

TABLE 16-6	Goat Dental Formulas	
Deciduous: 2(I0/3 C0/1* PM3/3) = 20 total		
Permanent: 2(I0/3 C0/1* PM3/3 M 3/3) = 32 total		
Eruption	I1	Birth–2 wk
	I2	Birth–2 wk
	I3	Birth–2 wk
	C	Birth–2 wk
	PM2 (first cheek tooth)	Birth–2 wk
	PM3 (second cheek tooth)	Birth–1 wk
	PM4 (third cheek tooth)	Birth–1 wk
Eruption	I1	1½–2 yr
	I2	2–2½ yr
	I3	3–3½ yr
	C	3½–4 yr
	PM2 (first cheek tooth)	2–2½ yr
	PM3 (second cheek tooth)	1½–2½ yr
	PM4 (third cheek tooth)	2½–3 yr
	M1 (fourth cheek tooth)	5–6 mo
	M2 (fifth cheek tooth)	1–1½ yr
	M3 (sixth cheek tooth)	2–2½ yr

*The canine tooth is in line with the incisors and adjacent to them and is shaped like an incisor, thereby giving the false appearance of four incisors; however, it is common practice to refer to the canine tooth as the fourth incisor (I4).

bovine dentition, because the dentition is the same. Body condition scores for sheep and goats can be seen in Figure 16-33 and Table 16-7.

FEEDING CONSIDERATIONS

Water should be provided *ad libitum* to sheep and goats. Adults generally consume 1 to 1.5 gallons per day. Fat lambs and kids consume approximately 0.5 gallons per day. Sheep are as good as, if not better than, cattle at digesting poor-quality roughage.

Females being bred should not be fat. They should have a slight daily weight gain from weaning to breeding. After mating, females can be maintained on good pasture. During the last 6 to 8 weeks of pregnancy, growth of the fetus is rapid; therefore, nutrition should be an increased gradually. This can be achieved by adding supplemental grain to meet energy requirements.

Lactating animals should be offered high-quality hay and a complete grain ration to maximize milk production. During the winter, a confined animal should be fed a good grain and forage ration with trace mineralized salt added.

Lambs and kids should have access to creep feed at 2 weeks of age. They should be creep fed until pasture becomes available. If pasture is unavailable, they should be finished in a drylot, and feed changes should be gradual. Table 16-8 gives an overview of nutritional requirements in sheep.

MINERALS

Salt should be fed free choice and is needed for general thriftiness. Adults consume approximately 10 g of salt daily.

Calcium is often provided through high-quality roughage. Deficiencies are rare but can be seen with high-grain diets. Deficiencies of calcium can be easily corrected with the addition of limestone to the diet.

Phosphorus availability is influenced by the content in soil. In lactating animals with phosphorus deficiency, milk production declines, bones become fragile, and feed intake is poor. In young animals, deficiencies may result in slow growth and poor appetite. Deficiencies can be corrected by adding phosphorus supplement to the ration. Iodine is important in pregnant animals, and deficiencies can be corrected by feeding stabilized iodized salt.

Cobalt deficiency manifests as anemia, loss of appetite, retarded growth, decreased production, and a rough hair coat.

Sheep require a minimum of 5 mg/kg of dry matter intake of copper. Molybdenum and inorganic sulfates can affect copper absorption. Signs of copper deficiency include anemia, brittle or fragile bones, and loss of wool or hair pigment. A balance of sulfates usually corrects copper deficiencies. Sheep are susceptible to copper toxicity; severe hemorrhagic diarrhea is usually seen with acute toxicity. Chronic toxicity leads to liver and kidney disease, resulting in death.

Selenium levels vary depending on the soil. Selenium supplements are available by injection, oral feeding, or addition of trace mineralized salt. Deficiencies of selenium cause nutritional muscular dystrophy, white muscle disease in lambs, and periodontal disease of the molars. Toxicity results in loss of appetite, loss of hair, sloughing of the hooves, and eventual death.

Higher levels of zinc are required for normal testicular development. High calcium levels increase the need for zinc. Signs of zinc deficiency include slipping of the wool, swelling and lesions around hooves and eyes, excessive salivation, anorexia, wool eating, listlessness, reduced food consumption, reproductive problems, and decreased production.

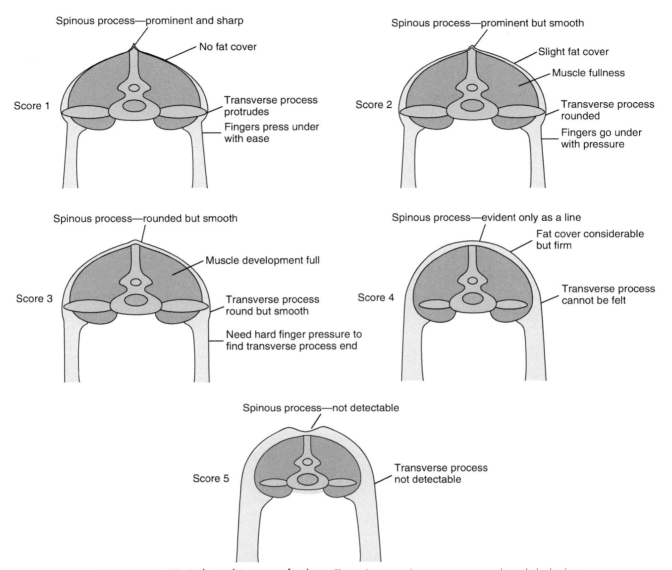

Spinous process—prominent and sharp

No fat cover

Score 1

Transverse process protrudes

Fingers press under with ease

Spinous process—prominent but smooth

Slight fat cover

Muscle fullness

Score 2

Transverse process rounded

Fingers go under with pressure

Spinous process—rounded but smooth

Muscle development full

Score 3

Transverse process round but smooth

Need hard finger pressure to find transverse process end

Spinous process—evident only as a line

Fat cover considerable but firm

Score 4

Transverse process cannot be felt

Spinous process—not detectable

Score 5

Transverse process not detectable

FIGURE 16-33 Body condition scores for sheep. These drawings show a cross-section through the lumbar region and the fat covering (or lack thereof). *Score 1,* Spinous and transverse processes are sharp, and no fat is detectable on the loin area. These animals are emaciated. *Score 2,* Animals are still thin, with prominent spinous and slightly rounded transverse processes. The examiner's fingers can be passed under the edge of the transverse processes. *Score 3,* Animals have smooth, slightly rounded spinous and transverse processes. Slight pressure is required to palpate the transverse process. *Score 4,* These animals are fat. The spinous processes are barely palpable. *Score 5,* These animals are obese, with a midline concavity running over the spinous process. Because these scores are broad, many owners or managers round up to half-scores (e.g., 2.5) if the animal has more fat covering than one score but not quite as much as the next whole-number score. (From Pugh DG, Baird AN: *Sheep and goat medicine,* ed 2, St. Louis, 2012, Saunders.)

TABLE 16-7	Body Condition Scoring System for Goats
SCORE	**APPEARANCE**
0	No subcutaneous tissue seen
1	Dorsal aspect of vertebral column forming a continuous ridge, hollow flank; ribs easily seen Sternal fat easily moved laterally Chondrosternal joints easily palpable No muscle or fat between ribs or bones Transverse processes of lumbar vertebrae easily visualized and articular processes easily palpable
2	Sternal fat moveable but 1 to 2 cm thick Tissue visible between skin and chondrosternal joints Some tissue around transverse processes of lumbar spine, but more difficult to palpate than in score 1 Slight pressure needed to palpate articular processes
3	Dorsal aspect of vertebral column less prominent Sternal fat thick and barely moveable Chondrosternal joints difficult to palpate Lumbar vertebrae with thick tissue covering Articular processes of transverse processes not palpable
4	Sternal fat, costochondral fat, and rib fat continuous Transverse process difficult to palpate Spinous processes not palpable
5	Sternal fat and rib fat bulges between pressed fingers Spinous and transverse processes not palpable

Modified from Santucci PM, Branca A, Napoleone M, et al: Body condition scoring of goats in extensive conditions. In Morand-Fehr P, editor: *Goat nutrition*, Wageningen, Netherlands, 1991, Pudoc.

TABLE 16-8	Nutritional Requirements of Sheep			
AGE	**CRUDE PROTEIN (%)**	**CALCIUM (%)**	**PHOSPHORUS (%)**	**DIGESTIBLE ENERGY (Mcal)**
Weaned or growing	0.35–0.53	4.9–9.4	2.2–4.8	1.3–4.2
Female (110–190 pounds)	0.21–0.33	2–3.9	1.8–3.4	2.4–3.1
Female during gestation or lactation	0.43–0.51	5.6–9.6	4.8–7.8	4–7.5

CASE STUDY

Mr. Brodersen stopped by the clinic today. He is a large sheep breeder in the area. He is looking to increase his lambing crop and has heard about a breed that significantly increases the likelihood of multiple lambs per birth. He cannot remember which breed it is and would like to know. Which breeds of sheep could he be talking about? He currently has about 25% of his flock lambing in the fall. What breed of sheep is he raising that allows him to lamb in the fall?

CASE STUDY

Mr. Torpy is a new breeder of Hampshire sheep in the area. One of his ewes gave birth at about 8:30 this morning. The ewe still has a placenta hanging from the vulva. It is now 5:30 PM. Is this an emergency situation? While he has you on the phone, he asks one more question, "Should I let my ewes eat their placenta?"

SUGGESTED READING

American Finnsheep Breeders Association: <www.finnsheep.org/> (Accessed 12.05.15.)

American Romney Breeders Association: <www.americanromney.org/> (Accessed 12.05.15.)

American Southdown Breeders' Association: <www.southdownsheep.org/> (Accessed 12.05.15.)

Cotswold Sheep Society: <www.cotswoldsheepsociety.co.uk/> (Accessed 12.05.15.)

Gillespie JR, Flanders FB: *Modern livestock and poultry*, ed 8, Clifton Park, NY, 2010, Delmar Cengage Learning.

Hafez ESE, Hafez B, editors: *Reproduction in farm animals*, ed 7, New York, 2000, Wiley-Blackwell.

Hunt E: Neonatal disease and disease management. In Howard JL, Smith RA, editors: *Current veterinary therapy, food animal practice*, ed 4, St. Louis, 2008, Saunders, pp 70–77.

Noakes DE, Parkinson TJ, England GCW: *Arthur's veterinary reproduction and obstetrics*, ed 9, Oxford, 2009, Saunders.

Pugh DG: *Sheep and goat medicine*, St. Louis, 2002, Saunders.

Smith MC, Sherman DM: *Goat medicine*, Baltimore, 1994, Williams & Wilkins.

Smith BP: *Large animal internal medicine*, ed 4, St. Louis, 2008, Mosby.

Spanish Goat Association: <www.spanishgoats.org/> (Accessed 12.05.15.)

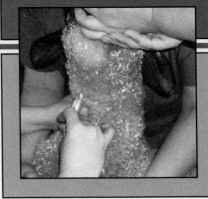

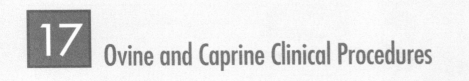

17 Ovine and Caprine Clinical Procedures

LEARNING OBJECTIVES

After completing this chapter, you will be able to

- Set up and prepare the patient for each procedure, perform the procedure (when appropriate), or assist the clinician in performing diagnostic sampling and medication procedures
- Properly insert and maintain an intravenous catheter and monitor the catheter for complications
- Explain the rationale and indications for each of the clinical procedures described
- Set up materials and equipment and prepare the patient as needed for the procedure
- Assist the veterinarian when performing the procedure or perform the procedure when it may be appropriate for a veterinary technician to do so
- Perform or assist necropsy and sample collection procedures and maintain a safe environment during these procedures

KEY TERMS

Balling gun
Cystocentesis
Gluteal muscles

Hoof knives
Intramammary infusion
Lateral cervical muscles

Sigmoid flexure
Trimming shears
Urethral diverticulum

Clinical procedures for sheep and goats are very similar to those for cattle. All the procedures that can be performed in sheep and goats are not necessarily listed in this chapter, but they described for horses and cattle (see Chapters 9 and 13, respectively). All procedures for horses and cattle can be performed in sheep and goats with adjustments for needle sizes and should be followed as they are discussed for those species; however, this chapter outlines necessary alterations and specific procedures relating to small ruminants.

FAMACHA

Haemonchus contortus is a major parasite of sheep and goats. The parasite causes anemia, and the FAMACHA carding system can be used to help in assessing the flock's exposure and in selecting those animals that require treatment. The card contains a variety of colors that are used to evaluate the color of the ocular mucous membranes. The color of the ocular mucous membranes correlates with the level of anemia. The idea is to identify those individuals with the largest number of worms in the abomasum and selectively treat them because 20% of the flock contains 80% of the worms. This approach removes the source of the pasture contaminants and does not cause selective pressures on the worms in the remainder of the flock.

DIAGNOSTIC SAMPLING

VENOUS BLOOD SAMPLING

Equipment for venous blood sampling:
- Alcohol
- 18-, 19-, 20-, 22-gauge (ga) × 1- to 1½-inch needle
- Syringe
- Appropriate collection tubes

Preparation for venous blood collection is the same as described for cattle in Chapter 13. The jugular vein is most often used for venous sampling. In sheep, the jugular vein can be accessed with the animal standing or in the "set-up" rump position (Fig. 17-1).

> **TECHNICIAN NOTE** Sheep often are placed in the "set-up" position for jugular blood draws.

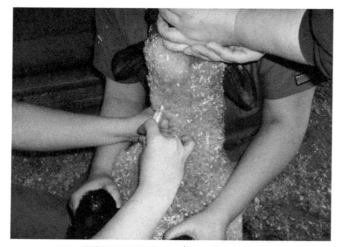

FIGURE 17-1 Jugular venipuncture.

In goats, the standing position is used for jugular venipuncture. For the standing procedure in both goats and sheep, the animal is straddled and squeezed between the handler's legs; it is helpful to back the animal against a solid object. One person can access the vein, but two people can be used if desired.

> **TECHNICIAN NOTE**   Goats are often restrained in a standing position for jugular blood draws.

The cephalic vein on the foreleg or the femoral vein on the hindleg of sheep also can be used. The cephalic vein in sheep can be accessed in the set-up rump position. Lateral recumbency is required for access to the femoral vein.

The cephalic vein on the forearm or the femoral vein on the hindleg of goats also can be used. Goats can remain standing for cephalic vein access. Backing the goat against a solid object is helpful. One person restrains the animal by circling the animal's neck with one arm while the other hand rolls the vein laterally and occludes it. The person drawing the sample needs to hold the distal limb to steady it.

The animal is appropriately restrained. If wool or hair is present, it is parted over and along the selected vein. Alcohol is suitable for disinfecting the skin. An 18-, 19-, 20-, or 22-gauge (ga), 1- to 1½-inch needle is used, depending on the size of the animal; 20-ga is generally preferred. Vacutainer systems also can be used.

Normal values for complete blood count and blood chemistry studies for sheep and goats are listed in Tables 17-1 to 17-4 and in Table A2-3 in Appendix 2.

ABDOMINOCENTESIS

Equipment for abdominocentesis:
- Clippers
- Surgical scrub/alcohol
- 18 ga × 1½-inch needle
- Syringe
- Serum tube/red top tube

TABLE 17-1	Complete Blood Count Normal Values for Sheep

Complete Blood Count

Packed cell volume	24%–50% (average, 38)
Hemoglobin	8–16 g/dL (average, 12)
Red blood cells	$8–16 \times 10^6/\mu L$ (average, 12)
Total protein	6–7.5 g/dL
White blood cells	$4–12 \times 10^3/\mu L$ (average, 8)
Platelets	$2.5–7.5 \times 10^5/\mu L$ (average, 4)
Mean corpuscular volume	23–48 fL (average, 33)
Mean corpuscular hemoglobin	9–13 pg
Mean corpuscular hemoglobin concentration	31–38 g/dL (average, 33.5)
Bone marrow	0.77–1.68:1 myeloid/ erythroid ratio (average, 1.1:1)

Differential, Absolute

Segs	10%–50%
	700–6000 (average, 2400)
Bands	Rare
Lymphocytes	40%–75%
	2000–9000 (average, 5000)
Monocytes	0.6%
	0–750 (average, 200)
Eosinophils	0.1%
	0–1000 (average, 400)
Basophils	0%–3%
	0–300 (average, 50)

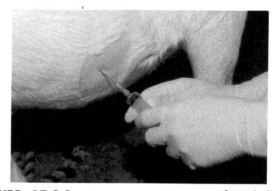

FIGURE 17-2 Percutaneous rumenocentesis performed through the ventral left abdomen. (From Pugh DG: *Sheep and goat medicine*, St. Louis, 2002, Saunders.)

The abdominocentesis procedure for sheep and goats is the same as described for cattle (see Chapter 13), except for the needle size used. The needle used for abdominocentesis in sheep and goats is 1 to 1½ inches long (Fig. 17-2).

> **TECHNICIAN NOTE**   The needle for abdominocentesis should be 1 to 1½ inches long.

TABLE 17-2	Complete Blood Count Normal Values for Goats	
Complete Blood Count		
Packed cell volume	Increased with polycythemia, dehydration, stress, in neonates, and high globulin levels Decreased with anemia, bleeding, overhydration, and in weanlings	22%–38%
Hemoglobin	Increased with polycythemia Decreased with anemia	12.8–17.6 g/dL
Red blood cells	Increased with polycythemia and dehydration Decreased with anemia and overhydration	$11.3–17.5 \times 10^6/\mu L$
Total protein	Increased in dehydration and in lipemic samples Decreased with overhydration	6.5–7 g/dL
White blood cells	Increased with acute local inflammation, toxicity, and bacterial infections Decreased with marrow diseases, radiation, drug therapy, and certain viruses	$4–13 \times 10^3/\mu L$
Platelets	Decreased with radiation and amblyomma infection	$3–6 \times 10^5/\mu L$
Mean corpuscular volume	Increased with vitamin B_{12} and folic acid deficiency Decreased with iron deficiency	16–25 fL
Mean corpuscular hemoglobin	Increased with hemolysis Decreased with iron deficiency	5.2–8 pg
Mean corpuscular hemoglobin concentration	Increased with hemolysis, lipemia, and Heinz bodies	30–36 g/dL
Bone marrow		0.7–1.0:1 myeloid/erythroid ratio
Differential, Absolute		
Segs		30%–48% 1.2–7.2
Bands		Rare
Lymphocytes		50%–70% 2–9
Monocytes		0%–4% 0–0.55
Eosinophils		1%–8% 0.05–0.65
Basophils		0%–1% 0–0.12

RUMEN FLUID COLLECTION

Equipment for rumen fluid collection:
- Clippers
- Surgical scrub and alcohol
- 16- or 18-ga needle
- Syringe
- Serum tube/red top tube

The rumen fluid collection process is performed in the same manner as for cattle (see Chapter 13), except that a 16- or 18-ga needle is used.

URINE COLLECTION

Equipment for urine collection:
- Sterile collection container

Female sheep can sometimes be stimulated to urinate by holding their nostrils and mouth shut for up to 45 seconds (with the animal standing). The hold should be released when the animal indicates discomfort by struggling;

urination usually follows promptly. This maneuver is best performed with two people: one occludes the nostrils, and the other collects the urine specimen.

> *TECHNICIAN NOTE* Holding the ewe's nostrils and mouth shut for up to 45 seconds while the animal is standing can stimulate urination.

Female goats usually must be collected with the "patience" method (wait patiently with a specimen cup for urination to occur); holding the nostrils is seldom effective. Goats often urinate on standing after spending time in recumbency. Placing the animal in a new stall or pen area sometimes encourages urination.

Male goats tend to urinate more frequently during the breeding season as part of their natural mating behavior.

Cystocentesis is possible in the sheep and goats but is seldom performed.

TABLE 17-3	Normal Blood Chemistry Values for Sheep	
Blood urea nitrogen	Increased with kidney disease, azotemia, and uremia	10.3–26 mg/dL
Creatinine	Increased with kidney disease	0.9–2.0 mg/dL
Glucose	Decreased in fatty liver disease Increased with diabetes and stress	44–81.2 mg/dL
Albumin	Increased with dehydration Decreased with brucellosis, chronic liver disease, glomerular disease, hyperglobulinemia, hypertension, malnutrition, and malabsorption	2.7–3.7 g/dL
Total bilirubin	Increased in animals with liver disease, bile duct obstruction, jaundice, or hemolytic anemia	0–0.5 mg/dL
Aspartate aminotransferase	Increased in liver disease or with muscle damage Possibly increased after exercise	49–123.3 µg/L
γ-Glutamyltransferase	Increased with hepatocellular and cholestatic liver disease, hepatocyte necrosis, and cholestasis	19.6–44.1 µg/L
Creatine kinase	Increased with muscle disease	7.7–101 µg/L
Alkaline phosphatase	Increased with liver disease and cholestasis, steroids, and growth	26.9–156.1 µg/L
Lactate dehydrogenase	Increased with hepatocyte damage, muscle damage, and hemolysis	83.1–475.6 µg/L
Sodium	When increased can cause neurologic disorders and hypertension Decreased possibly from *Escherichia coli*, polyuria or polydipsia, weight loss, and anorexia	141.6–159.6 mEq/L
Potassium	Increased possibly from severe metabolic acidosis Decreased possibly from anorexia, increased renal excretion, abomasal stasis, intestinal obstruction, enteritis, and weight loss	4.3–6.3 mEq/L
Chloride	Increased during displaced abomasums	100.8–113 mEq/L
Calcium	Increased with kidney stones, renal failure, and some cancers Decreased in milk fever, renal disease, and bone disease	9.3–11.7 mg/dL
Phosphorus	Increased in renal failure Decreased with osteomalacia, rickets, and tetany	4.0–7.3 mg/dL
Magnesium	Decreased in milk fever, grass tetany, fever, and hypersalivation	2.0–2.7 mg/dL

BLADDER ORURETHRAL CATHETERIZATION
Female Catheterization
Equipment for female catheterization:
- Sterile vaginal speculum
- Sterile lubricant
- 10- to 12-French catheter
- Sterile syringe
- Sterile collection container

A small animal vaginal speculum and light source may be helpful in ewes and allow visualization of the urethral opening.

Adults may be catheterized with a 10-French (10-F) to 12-F catheter. Small females may require slightly smaller-diameter catheters.

TECHNICIAN NOTE   Adults can be catheterized with a 10- to 12-F catheter.

Male Catheterization
The anatomy of the urethra of male ruminants makes bladder catheterization difficult to impossible to perform. All domestic ruminants have an S-shaped curvature of the penis and urethra (*sigmoid flexure*) that often hinders passage of a catheter beyond that point. Yet another anatomical obstruction, the *urethral diverticulum*, is a blind sac near the ischial arch. This usually presents a final roadblock to the catheter tip and keeps it from entering the bladder.

TECHNICIAN NOTE   Male urinary catheters are difficult to place because of the sigmoid flexure and urethral diverticulum.

Extending the penis in many males for urethral catheterization may be difficult. The urethra opens 1 to 2 cm beyond the tip of the glans penis through the urethral process. This narrow structure can be difficult to enter with a catheter and may have to be amputated before a catheter can be introduced into the urethra. Even after successful introduction of a catheter, advancing the catheter into the bladder often is impossible. In sheep and goats, the male can be "set up" and rocked backward slightly on the rump; sedation greatly assists the procedure. The sigmoid flexure can be palpated through the prepuce. The penis is grasped with one hand (through the preputial skin) just caudal to the flexure. The penis is pushed cranially while the other hand retracts the prepuce caudally. This maneuver exteriorizes the glans penis and helps to partially straighten out the S-shaped sigmoid flexure. If desired, the glans can be grasped with a gauze sponge and used to keep the penis extended (Fig. 17-3). The restrainer maintains this position while another person cleans the glans and

TABLE 17-4	Normal Blood Chemistry Values for Goats	
Blood urea nitrogen	Increased with kidney disease, azotemia, and uremia	12.6–25.8 mg/dL
Creatinine	Increased with kidney disease	0.7–1.5 mg/dL
Glucose	Decreased in fatty liver disease Increased with diabetes and stress	48.2–76.0 mg/dL
Albumin	Increased with dehydration Decreased with brucellosis, chronic liver disease, glomerular disease, hyperglobulinemia, hypertension, malnutrition, and malabsorption	2.3–3.6 g/dL
Total bilirubin	Increased in animals with liver disease, bile duct obstruction, jaundice, or hemolytic anemia	0.1–0.2 mg/dL
Aspartate aminotransferase	Increased in liver disease or with muscle damage Possibly increased after exercise	66–230 µg/L
γ-Glutamyltransferase	Increased with hepatocellular and cholestatic liver disease, hepatocyte necrosis, and cholestasis	20–50 µg/L
Creatine kinase	Increased with muscle disease	16.3–47.7 µg/L
Alkaline phosphatase	Increased with liver disease and cholestasis, steroids, and growth	61.3–283.3 µg/L
Lactate dehydrogenase	Increased with hepatocyte damage, muscle damage, and hemolysis	78.5–265.3 µg/L
Sodium	When increased can cause neurologic disorders and hypertension Decreased possibly from *Escherichia coli,* polyuria or polydipsia, weight loss, and anorexia	136.5–151.5 mEq/L
Potassium	Increased possibly from severe metabolic acidosis Decreased possibly from anorexia, increased renal excretion, abomasal stasis, intestinal obstruction, enteritis, and weight loss	3.8–5.7 mEq/L
Chloride	Increased during displaced abomasums	100.3–111.5 mEq/L
Calcium	Increased with kidney stones, renal failure, and some cancers Decreased in milk fever, renal disease, and bone disease	9.0–11.6 mg/dL
Phosphorus	Increased in renal failure Decreased with osteomalacia, rickets, and tetany	3.7–9.7 mg/dL
Magnesium	Decreased in milk fever, grass tetany, fever, and hypersalivation	2.1–2.9 mg/dL

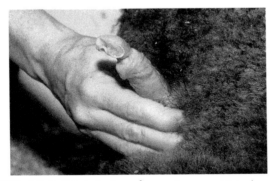

FIGURE 17-3 Exteriorization of a ram's penis. Note the urethral process. (From Pugh DG: *Sheep and goat medicine,* St. Louis, 2002, Saunders.)

performs the urethral catheterization. Extending the penis of young (prepubertal) males may be difficult.

MEDICATION TECHNIQUES

ORAL MEDICATION WITH BALLING GUN

Small ruminants can be backed into a corner or wall and straddled; one hand is used to elevate and restrain the head, and the other hand operates the *balling gun.* The same

precautions established with cattle should be followed for small ruminants.

RUMEN (GASTRIC) INTUBATION

In small ruminants, a block of wood with a circular hole cut in it, a short piece of polyvinyl chloride pipe, or a tape roll can be placed between the lower incisors, and the dental pad can be used as a Frick speculum. A medium foal stomach tube can be used.

> **TECHNICIAN NOTE** A small block of wood with a circular hole, polyvinyl chloride pipe, or a tape role is often used for successful placement of an orogastric tube.

Neonates do not require use of a speculum. Small rubber urinary catheters or infant feeding tubes (10 to 18 F) can be used.

INTRAMUSCULAR INJECTION SITES

Equipment for intramuscular injection:
- 18- to 20-ga × 1-inch needle for adults
- 20- to 22-ga × 1-inch needle for lambs and kids
- Syringe
- Appropriate collection tube

The wool or hair should be parted down to the skin to allow proper cleaning of the injection site. Intramuscular injections should not be performed until the needle has been aspirated to confirm that the needle bevel is not in a blood vessel. An 18- to 20-ga needle should be used for adults and a 20- to 22-ga needle for lambs and kids.

Gluteal Muscles

Equipment for gluteal muscle injection:
- 18- to 20-ga × 1-inch needle for adults
- 20- to 22-ga × 1-inch needle for lambs and kids
- Syringe
- Appropriate collection tube

Sheep and goats have very thin *gluteal muscles,* so these muscles usually are avoided. If the gluteal muscles must be used in these animals, a short (1-inch) needle should be used, and only small quantities of medication (5 mL in goats) should be given.

> **TECHNICIAN NOTE**   Do not inject more than 5 mL per site in small ruminants.

Lateral Cervical Muscles

Equipment for lateral cervical muscle injection:
- 18- to 20-ga × 1-inch needle for adults
- 20- to 22-ga × 1-inch needle for lambs and kids
- Syringe
- Appropriate collection tube

The site containing the *lateral cervical muscles* is the location most commonly used in goats and sheep, especially in meat-producing animals. The needle length should not exceed 1 inch. This location is generally avoided in show goats because of the possibility that a tissue reaction could be mistaken for an abscess of the prescapular lymph node, which mimics the caprine disease caseous lymphadenitis. The landmarks are similar to those described for the horse: a triangular area bounded by the cervical vertebrae ventrally, the shoulder (scapula) caudally, and the nuchal ligament dorsally. Injections should be given well within these boundaries (Fig. 17-4).

Longissimus Muscle

Equipment for longissimus muscle injection:
- 18- to 20-ga × 1-inch needle for adults
- 20- to 22-ga × 1-inch needle for lambs and kids
- Syringe
- Appropriate collection tube

The longissimus muscle lies over the back, along either side of the vertebral column. The lumbar portion of this muscle can be used for injections in goats if the hide is not to be marketed. Injections (of any kind) into any area of the back often devalue the hide as a result of scarring and other blemishes. Only small volumes (<5 mL) should be injected.

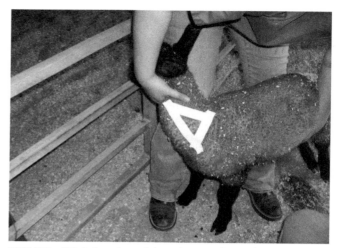

FIGURE 17-4 Location of lateral cervical muscle intramuscular injections.

SUBCUTANEOUS INJECTIONS

Equipment for subcutaneous injection:
- 18- to 22-ga × 1-inch needle
- Syringe
- Appropriate collection tube

An 18- to 22-ga needle should be used for subcutaneous injections in small ruminants. Up to 50 mL can be administered in adult small ruminants. Sheep can be set up for easy access to the axilla and flank fold. The skin should be cleansed with 70% alcohol or other antiseptic. The skin is pinched and elevated to form a "skin tent," and the needle is inserted into the tent, with care taken not to go all the way through the tent. Before injection, the syringe should be aspirated to ensure that it is not within a blood vessel. After injection, the needle is withdrawn, and the tent is released.

INTRAVENOUS CATHETERIZATION

Equipment for intravenous catheterization:
- Clippers
- Surgical scrub and alcohol
- 14- to 18-ga × 2- to 3-inch catheter
- Heparinized saline
- Tape
- Extension set

A 14- to 18-ga needle should be used in small ruminants. Catheters 2 to 3 inches long can be used in small individuals.

INTRAMAMMARY INFUSION

> **TECHNICIAN NOTE**   Equipment for intramammary infusion:

- ⅛-inch infusion tip
- Medication for infusion

TABLE 17-5	California Mastitis Test: Interpretation of Results	
TEST SCORE	**INTERPRETATION IN GOATS**
N	Normal (0–480,000 cells/mL)
T	Normal (0–640,000 cells/mL)
1	Suspicious (240,000–1,440,000 cells/mL)
2	Mastitis (1,080,000–5,850,000 cells/mL)
3	Mastitis (>10,000,000 cells/mL)

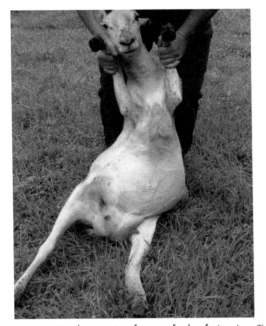

FIGURE 17-5 Simple restraint of a goat for hoof trimming. The handler is pressing the goat against his legs with the arms. The left hand holds the foot while the right hand trims. (From Pugh DG: *Sheep and goat medicine*, ed 2, St. Louis, 2012, Saunders Ltd.)

Mastitis primarily affects dairy goats, but all milk-producing females are susceptible. Bovine cannulas and infusion tips are too large for small ruminants. For *intramammary infusion,* a small ⅛-inch infusion tip is commercially available for these smaller animals. Sterile tomcat catheters can also be used for goats with small teat orifices (Table 17-5).

HOOF TRIMMING

Sheep and goats are some of the easiest large animals to trim because of the minimal restraint needed. Sheep are trimmed in the "set-up" position. *Hoof knives* and *trimming shears* usually are the only equipment needed for sheep.

Goats' hooves usually are trimmed with the animal in the standing position, with the operator standing to the side of the goat and lifting each leg individually (Fig. 17-5). The operator can reach across the back of the goat or stand alongside the goat and pick up the legs in a manner similar to that used for horses. The head of uncooperative goats may need to be tied; an assistant may need to provide additional restraint; or the goats may need to be placed in lateral recumbency, with an assistant providing restraint of the neck and legs. A rump position similar to setting up sheep may be effective in some goats, although they generally resist this position. Hoof knives and trimming shears usually are sufficient for trimming goats' hooves.

> **TECHNICIAN NOTE**   Hoof trimming in sheep and goats is much easier than in horses and cattle because of the need for minimal restraint.

CASE STUDY

Dr. Pinkerton has requested that you collect urine from the sick doe that will be arriving at the clinic in a half hour. What strategies will you use to try and collect this urine? What strategies would you use if it were a sheep?

CASE STUDY

Dr. Welborn is scheduled to perform hoof trims of a herd of goats south of town tomorrow. What equipment and supplies would you want to make sure are stocked in the pickup truck?

SUGGESTED READING

Anderson DR, Rings DM: *Current veterinary therapy: food animal practice,* ed 5, St. Louis, 2008, Saunders.

Bassert JM, McCurnin DM, editors: *McCurnin's clinical textbook for veterinary technicians,* ed 7, St. Louis, 2010, Saunders.

Davis H, Riel DL, Pappagianis M, Miguel K: Diagnostic sampling and therapeutic techniques. In Bassert JM, McCurnin DM, editors: *McCurnin's clinical textbook for veterinary technicians,* 7th ed, St. Louis, 2010, Saunders, pp 585–673.

Cebra ML, Cebra CK: Food animal medicine and surgery. In McCurnin DM, Bassert JM, editors: *Clinical textbook for veterinary technicians,* ed 6, St. Louis, 2010, Saunders, pp 713–768.

Fubini SL, Ducharme NG: *Farm animal surgery,* St. Louis, 2004, Saunders.

Hafez ESE, Hafez B, editors: *Reproduction in farm animals,* ed 7, New York, 2000, Wiley-Blackwell.

Noakes DE, Parkinson RJ, England GCW: *Veterinary reproduction and obstetrics,* ed 9, London, 2009, Saunders.

Pugh DG: *Sheep and goat medicine,* St. Louis, 2002, Saunders.

Sirois M: *Principles and practice of veterinary technology,* ed 3, St. Louis, 2011, Mosby.

Smith BP: *Large animal internal medicine,* ed 4, St. Louis, 2008, Mosby.

Smith MC, Sherman DM: *Goat medicine,* Baltimore, 2009, Williams & Wilkins.

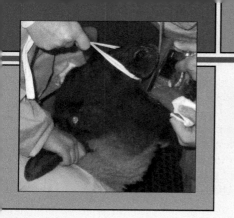

18 Ovine and Caprine Surgical Procedures

OUTLINE

LEARNING OBJECTIVES

When you have completed this chapter, you will be able to

- Display understanding of the basic differences between standing surgical procedures and general anesthesia procedures
- Prepare a sheep or goat for surgery
- Assist and/or perform induction and maintenance of anesthesia
- Provide anesthetic monitoring
- Manage the patient during recovery and immediate postoperative periods
- Display understanding of the basic risks and possible complications associated with anesthesia and surgery, and implement preventive measures when indicated

KEY TERMS

Buck odor
Descenting
Elastrator
Fly strike

Hypoglycemia
Laparotomy
Malacia
Meningitis

Supernumerary teats
Tetanus
Trocar
Urinary calculi

SMALL RUMINANT SURGERY AND ANESTHESIA

Surgical procedures for small ruminants are similar to those for cattle. This chapter outlines the considerations and variations that should be made for small ruminant surgery. The reader should consult Chapter 14 for basic information on ruminant surgery.

PREPARATION FOR STANDING SURGERY

In small ruminants, food is withheld for 12 to 24 hours; it is not necessary to withhold water. Lambs and kids that are consuming solid food material should be fasted for 2 to 4 hours (withhold food only; water is permitted). In very young ruminants, the rumen or reticulum has little function, and the risk of regurgitation is minimal. Fasting of neonates may cause *hypoglycemia* and is not recommended.

> *TECHNICIAN NOTE* Lambs and kids consuming solid food should have only food removed for 2 to 4 hours before surgical procedures.

PAIN MANAGEMENT

For an explanation of drug categories, please see Chapter 10 and Table 18-1.

Sheep and goats especially are more sensitive to lidocaine. Sheep and goats may become toxic with lidocaine administration of 10 mg/kg total dose. For this reason, lidocaine should not be used in concentrations greater than 2%. Especially in goats, dilution to 1% or less solution is advisable; dilution of 2% solution with an equal part of sterile saline achieves a 1% solution. In kids, many clinicians advocate dilution to a maximum 0.5% solution.

> *TECHNICIAN NOTE* Sheep and goats are sensitive to lidocaine.

L Block

Equipment for L block:

- Clippers
- Surgical scrub and alcohol
- 18- to 20-gauge (ga) × 1- to 1½-inch needle

TABLE 18-1	Commonly Used Surgical Drugs				
	DOSE	**CONCENTRATION**	**ROUTE**	**MEAT WITHDRAWAL TIME**	**MILK WITHDRAWL TIME**
Flunixin meglumine	1.1 mg: 2.2 q12–24 hr	50 mg/mL	IV	4 days	36 hr
Phenylbutazone	4 mg/kg q12hr	IV = 200 mg/mL PO: 100-mg tablets 6-g tube 12-g tube	IV or PO		
Ketoprofen	3 mg/kg/day for up to 3 days	100 mg/mL	IV or IM	7 days	24 hr
Meloxicam	0.6 mg/kg q12–24hr	5 mg/mL			
Acetylsalicylic acid (aspirin)	50–100 mg/kg q12hr	240-gr bolus 480-gr bolus	PO	24 hr	24 hr
Xylazine	Sheep: 0.1–0.3 mg/kg IM 0.05–0.1 mg/kg IV Goats: 0.05–0.5 mg/kg IM 0.01–0.5 mg/kg IV	100 mg/mL	IV, IM, SC	Check FARAD; withdrawal varies by dose	Check FARAD; withdrawal varies by dose
Ketamine	1–2 mg/kg	100 mg/mL	IV or IM	3 days	48 hr

FARAD, Food Animal Residue Avoidance Databank; *IM*, intramuscularly; *IV*, intravenously, *PO*, orally, *SC*, subcutaneously.

- Syringe
- Local anesthetic

The L block is still the most common form of local anesthesia in small ruminants and is performed in the same manner as in cattle, except that the needle should be 18- to 20-gauge (ga) × 1 to 1½ inches long.

Paravertebral Block

Equipment for paravertebral block:
- Clippers
- Surgical scrub and alcohol
- 18- to 20-ga × 1½- to 3-inch needle (distal 20-to 22-ga × 1-inch needle)
- Syringe
- Local anesthetic

The paravertebral block is also used in small ruminants, but the needle should be an 18- to 20-ga × 1½- to 3-inch spinal needle. A *trocar* is not needed for the procedure. In goats and sheep, the recommended volume of lidocaine is 2 to 5 mL per site. When the distal paravertebral approach is performed, a 20- to 22-ga × 1-inch needle is used in small ruminants, with 2 to 4 mL of lidocaine administered.

Cornual Nerve Block

Equipment for cornual nerve block:
- Clippers
- Surgical scrub and alcohol
- 22- to 25-ga × 1-inch needle
- Syringe
- Local anesthetic

Goats have a dual nerve supply to each horn; therefore, two sites must be blocked.

> **TECHNICIAN NOTE** Goats have a dual nerve supply to each horn.

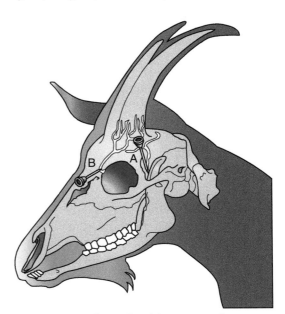

FIGURE 18-1 Anesthesia for dehorning in the goat. Needle placement for desensitizing the cornual branch of the lacrimal nerve. *(A)*. Needle placement for desensitizing the cornual branch of the infratrochlear nerve *(B)*. (Modified from Muir WW 3rd, Hubbell JAE, Bednarski RM, Skarda RT: *Veterinary anesthesia*, ed 4, St. Louis, 2000, Mosby.)

The cornual branch from the lacrimal nerve is blocked just behind the caudal ridge of the supraorbital process, at a depth of approximately 1 to 1.5 cm. A 22- to 23-ga × 1-inch needle is used, and local anesthetic (0.5 to 1 mL for kids, 2 to 4 mL for adults) is deposited.

The cornual branch of the infratrochlear nerve is blocked at the dorsomedial margin of the orbit, at a depth of approximately 0.5 cm. A 22- to 25-ga needle is used, and local anesthetic is deposited (0.5 mL for kids, 1 to 3 mL for adults) (Fig. 18-1).

Sheep are rarely dehorned. The nerve supply is only from the cornual branch of the lacrimal nerve; it is blocked using the same protocol as for blocking the cornual branch of the lacrimal nerve in goats.

INTRAVENOUS REGIONAL ANALGESIA (BIER BLOCK)

Equipment for intravenous regional analgesia:
- Clippers
- Surgical scrub and alcohol
- 22- to 25-ga × 1-inch needle
- Syringe
- Local anesthetic

When intravenous regional analgesia is performed on small ruminants, a 22- to 25-ga needle should be used, and up to 10 mL of anesthetic should be used.

Caudal Epidural Analgesia

Equipment for caudal epidural analgesia:
- Clippers
- Surgical scrub and alcohol
- 18- to 21-ga × 1- to 1½-inch needle
- Syringe
- Local anesthetic

Small ruminants require an 18- to 21-ga × 1- to 1½-inch needle for caudal epidural administration. Because of sensitivity to local anesthetics, the dose should not exceed 0.5 to 1 mL of 2% solution per 50 kg body weight in sheep and goats.

> **TECHNICIAN NOTE**   Cranial epidural techniques are infrequently used in small ruminants.

GENERAL ANESTHESIA

As with cattle, most small ruminant surgical procedures are performed with the animal standing. General anesthesia is required when the technical or anatomical aspects of the procedure or the ability to control pain and motion will exceed the capability of sedative drugs and local anesthesia. The same precautions for cattle should be considered with small ruminants.

Inhalant Gases

In animals weighing less than 150 pounds, facemask induction of anesthesia is possible. Small animal anesthesia machines can be used. Adult sheep and goats may resist face mask induction unless they are sick or sedated. Oxygen (3 to 5 L/minute) is given for 1 to 2 minutes before the anesthetic gas is introduced. Recommended gas concentrations are halothane 3% to 4%, isoflurane 3%, and sevoflurane 4% to 6%. Intubation is performed as soon as depth of anesthesia allows. A long-blade laryngoscope is useful for calves and small ruminants (Fig. 18-2). As with other species, the appropriate size of the endotracheal tube is estimated by palpation of the tracheal diameter through the skin of the neck and usually is 10 to 12 mm in adults. Other commonly used drugs include diazepam and ketamine combinations and propofol in small ruminants.

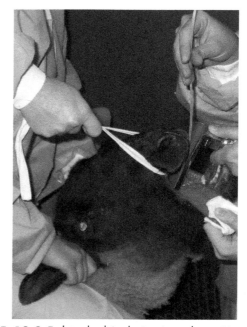

FIGURE 18-2 Endotracheal intubation in a sheep. Note that the head and neck are held in extension to create a straight line from mouth to trachea. An assistant uses gauze strips to open the mouth. A long-blade laryngoscope is used to visualize the larynx and depress the epiglottis. The stylet is placed into the proximal trachea, and then the endotracheal tube is advanced over the stylet and into the trachea. (From Pugh DG: *Sheep and goat medicine,* ed 2, St. Louis, 2012, Saunders.)

While sheep and goats are under general anesthesia, the heart rate should be maintained between 80 and 150 beats/minute (bpm).

> **TECHNICIAN NOTE**   The heart rate under general anesthesia should be maintained between 80 and 150 bpm.

COMMON SURGICAL PROCEDURES

CASTRATION

Routine castration of sheep and goats is usually done in the first week of life. In animals that will be kept long term, such as pets, it is advisable to wait until 5 to 6 months of age. Early castration may retard the full development of the penile urethra, with a resulting narrow urethra that is prone to blockage with urinary calculi. Clients should understand that delayed castration has no effect on the formation of calculi and does not guarantee that obstructions of the urethra will never occur, but it may reduce the incidence of obstructions of the urethra.

> **TECHNICIAN NOTE**   Delaying castration may decrease the likelihood of calculi formation in sheep and goats kept as pets.

Castration of the adult ram and buck has a higher incidence of complications. The mature testicles of these

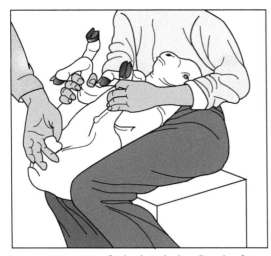

FIGURE 18-3 Restraint of a lamb in the handler's lap for castration and tail docking.

species are quite large for the size of the animal and have a well-developed blood supply; this increases the risk of hemorrhage. These animals should always be sedated for the procedure because the stress of the procedure in a fully awake animal may cause shock and possibly death. Clients should understand the importance of castration before sexual maturity is reached.

> **TECHNICIAN NOTE** Because of the testicular size of adult rams and bucks, these animals should be castrated before sexual maturity.

Restraint is age dependent and also depends on the clinician's preference. Lambs and kids may be restrained on their back in a handler's lap or held upside down by the hindlegs with the body resting against the handler's thighs (Fig. 18-3).

Small ruminants are especially sensitive to *tetanus*. Tetanus prophylaxis from colostrum, tetanus antitoxin, or tetanus toxoid must be provided.

> **TECHNICIAN NOTE** Small ruminants are sensitive to tetanus and should receive tetanus prophylaxis.

Castration Methods
Surgical "Knife" Castration

Sedation and local anesthesia may be used, but when castration is performed when the animal is several days of age, it is common practice to perform the procedure without using either sedation or local anesthesia. Older animals, especially mature males, should be sedated, and the use of local anesthesia should be considered.

> **TECHNICIAN NOTE** Surgical "knife" castration during the first few days of life is often performed without the use of sedation or local anesthesia.

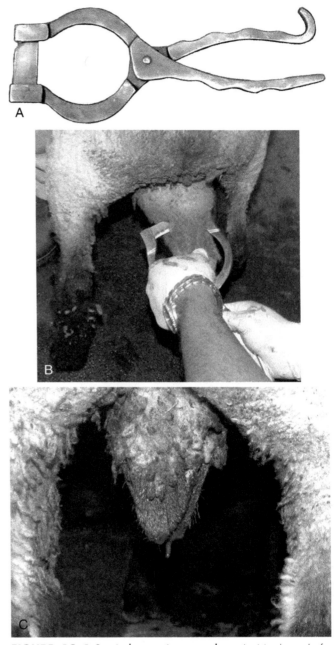

FIGURE 18-4 Surgical castration procedure. **A,** Newberry knife. **B,** The scrotum is grasped with the Newberry knife. **C,** Scrotal flaps after the testes are removed. (From Fubini SL, Ducharme NG: *Farm animal surgery*, St. Louis, 2004, Saunders.)

The scrotum is incised using one of the methods described earlier, and the testicles are exteriorized (Fig. 18-4). The testicles are removed by traction in animals less than 4 months old. Older animals with more development of the spermatic cord require measures to control hemorrhage, by use of an emasculator or by ligation of the cord with suture (Fig. 18-5). The scrotal incisions are left open to heal. Animals should be watched for hemorrhage during the immediate postoperative period and for signs of infection in the following days. Use of insect repellent during fly season is essential to prevent *fly strike* and maggot infestation.

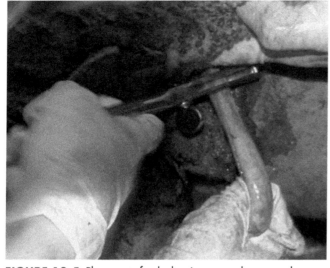

FIGURE 18-5 Placement of a dual-action emasculatome on the spermatic cord. Note the position of the instrument in relation to the testis. (From Fubini SL, Ducharme NG: *Farm animal surgery*, St. Louis, 2004, Saunders.)

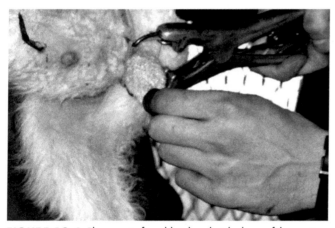

FIGURE 18-6 Placement of a rubber band at the base of the scrotum for the elastrator castration technique. (From Fubini SL, Ducharme NG: *Farm animal surgery*, St. Louis, 2004, Saunders.)

> **TECHNICIAN NOTE** During fly season, it is essential to use insect repellent around the incision site.

Elastrator

The *elastrator* technique is popular among farmers and is technically simple to perform. It is used for animals between 1 and 3 weeks old; after that time, it is considered an inhumane technique because of lingering signs of pain. Necrosis and then sloughing of the entrapped tissues occur in less than 2 weeks (Fig. 18-6). The risk of tetanus, which may occur following the period of necrosis and sloughing, may be more than with other methods. Insect repellent should be used during insect season.

Emasculatome (Burdizzo)

This method is used for older lambs and kids. Anesthesia is rarely used. The emasculatome is applied twice to each

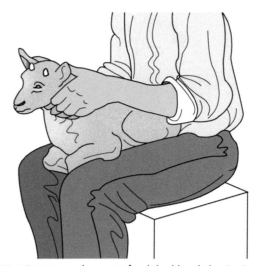

FIGURE 18-7 Manual restraint for disbudding kids. The thumbs are placed behind the kid's ears.

spermatic cord, through the skin, without incisions. Postoperative complications, including discomfort, have led to reduced popularity of this method.

Chemical Castration

The same commercial solution used on calves has been successfully used in lambs and kids, at reduced dosages. Availability of the solution is questionable.

DEHORNING

In the United States, dairy goats cannot be registered or shown if they have horns. Still, some owners desire that horns be left intact on animals kept on range conditions or tethers (for self-defense) or left intact for personal cosmetic preference. Dehorning is a common procedure in goats.

> **TECHNICIAN NOTE** Dehorning of goats is a common procedure.

This fast and almost bloodless method is popular, especially in goat kids. Electric disbudding irons are preferred, but fire-heated irons are still occasionally used in field situations. Clipping the hair from the area is advised, and tetanus prophylaxis should be given.

Kids can be held in the handler's lap with the head held securely (Figs. 18-7 and 18-8). Some form of analgesia is desirable in all species. Local anesthesia using a cornual nerve block is recommended for all patients. Sedation at this age is possible but seldom necessary.

The tip of the disbudding iron is shaped in an open circle. When the iron is sufficiently heated (cherry red color), the tip is centered over the horn bud and is applied with light pressure using a circular "rocking" motion. The goal is to kill the horn corium of the horn bud completely. Afterward, antibiotic powder or ointment should be applied to the area.

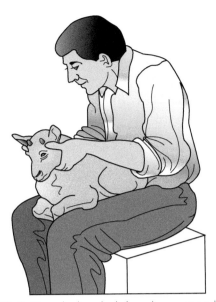

FIGURE 18-8 Once the horn buds have been removed, pressure is applied with the thumbs above the eyes to help control hemorrhage from the cornual artery or placed in a holding or "disbudding" box for the procedure.

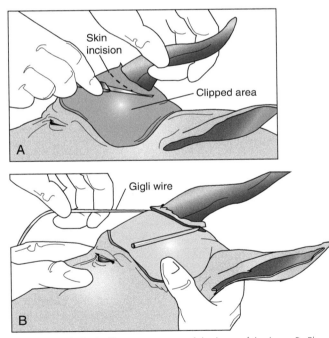

FIGURE 18-9 **A,** Skin incision around the base of the horn. **B,** Placement of Gigli wire saw for dehorning in the goat.

The primary risk of the procedure is overheating the area, possibly resulting in heat-induced *meningitis* and *malacia* (Figs. 18-9 and 18-10).

> **TECHNICIAN NOTE** The primary risks of heat cautery for dehorning are heat-induced meningitis and malacia.

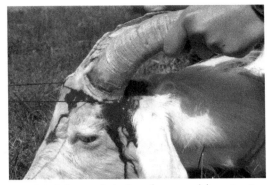

FIGURE 18-10 Removal of a horn from an adult goat, using a Gigli wire. (Courtesy Dr. Mary Smith, Cornell University.)

TAIL AMPUTATION (TAIL DOCKING)

Elective tail amputation (tail docking) is commonly performed in sheep. In sheep, tail docking is performed to reduce the accumulation of feces or diarrhea, which commonly occurs on natural-length tails. The fecal material tends to attract flies, thereby leading to "fly strike" and maggot infestation, which is a potentially devastating condition for the animal. Long tails may interfere with breeding. Tail removal is almost always performed in young lambs between 2 and 3 days to 2 weeks of age. At this young age, pain appears minimal, and local anesthesia is considered optional. Injecting local anesthetic in itself is a painful procedure, sometimes causing as much discomfort as simple removal of the tail. The tail can be removed by several methods:

> **TECHNICIAN NOTE** Tail docking is performed commonly in sheep to decrease the risk of "fly strike."

- Emasculator
- Emasculatome (Burdizzo)
- Heat cautery (electric "hot docker," hot chisel, or similar instrument)
- Sharp excision (scalpel or knife blade)
- Elastrator band (controversial; causes gradual ischemic necrosis)

The lamb is restrained off the ground or in the lap, with the hindquarters facing the clinician. The right legs are held in one hand, and the left legs are held in the other hand (Fig. 18-11). Clipping the hair is not necessary. The skin should be cleaned. The proper level of removal is at the middle to distal extent of the caudal tail fold. Cutting the tail too close to the anus is believed to increase the incidence of rectal prolapse. Healing is complete in 2 to 3 weeks, regardless of the method used, unless complications occur. Hemorrhage and infection are the most common complications but are rare when the procedure is properly performed. Hemorrhage usually is minimal at this early age. Instruments should always be thoroughly cleaned and disinfected between animals. Tetanus prophylaxis should be administered if it has not already been provided.

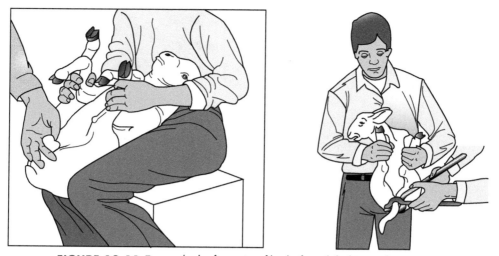

FIGURE 18-11 Two methods of restraint of lambs for tail docking and castration.

CESAREAN SECTION

If cesarean section is needed, the surgical procedure typically is performed through the left flank with the female in right lateral recumbency. The legs can be restrained in extension with cotton ropes or with nylon ropes and padding. Tying the head may be stressful, and having an assistant restrain the head is preferable. The head should not be restrained in an elevated position in case regurgitation occurs. Placing a towel over the eyes is helpful. Local anesthesia is performed with an "inverted L" line block (Fig. 18-12). The flank area is clipped and surgically prepared for the surgical procedure. After the surgeon enters the abdomen and exteriorizes the uterus, sterile towels or *laparotomy* pads are helpful for packing the skin incision to prevent contamination of the abdominal cavity. An assistant (nonsterile) should be available to receive the fetuses and remove them from the surgical area. If they are alive, they are treated as any neonates delivered naturally. Clearing the airways, confirming breathing and pulse, and instituting drying and warming procedures all are necessary. The umbilical cord should be treated with antiseptic. After delivery of the fetuses, the uterus must be sutured closed, and a multilayer suture closure of the abdominal wall is performed. The surgeon determines the use of postoperative antibiotics and antiinflammatory drugs.

> **TECHNICIAN NOTE**   Having the head restrained by an assistant is preferable to tying during a cesarean section.

REMOVAL OF SUPERNUMERARY TEATS

In young kids and lambs, serrated scissors are used to remove the *supernumerary teats* at their base, by cutting in a craniocaudal direction rather than laterally across the udder.

DESCENTING

Intact male goats are infamous for their offensive smell, or *"buck odor."* The odor actually has two sources. First, intact

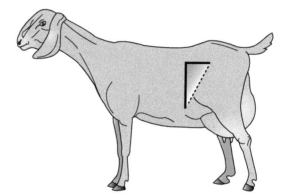

FIGURE 18-12 Cesarean section through a left flank approach in small ruminants. The *dotted line* indicates the surgical incision. The *solid line* indicates the location for the local anesthetic "inverted L" block. (Modified from Pugh DG: *Sheep and goat medicine*, St. Louis, 2002, Saunders.)

male goats urinate on themselves, primarily on their head, beard, and forelegs. This is normal behavior and is especially prominent during the breeding season (fall). The second source of odor is the primary scent glands. One gland is situated at the caudomedial base of each horn (or horn prominences in polled goats) (Fig. 18-13). Other smaller glands are scattered about the neck and shoulder area. The scent glands are responsive to testosterone, which increases during breeding season. The glands secrete a sebaceous material with a fetid odor. Owners frequently complain about the smell and request treatment.

> **TECHNICIAN NOTE**   Male goats often have "buck odor."

Several approaches can be used to reduce and eliminate buck odor. Keeping the hair at the base of the horns clipped and frequently scrubbing the area may reduce, but not eliminate, the odor from the scent glands. Castration

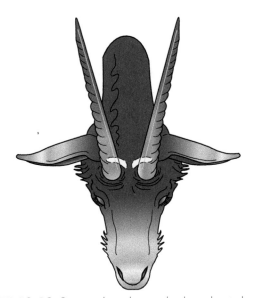

FIGURE 18-13 Crescent-shaped scent glands are located caudome-dial to the base of each horn. (Modified from Dyce KM, Sack WO, Wensing CJG: *Textbook of veterinary anatomy,* ed 4, St. Louis, 2010, Saunders.)

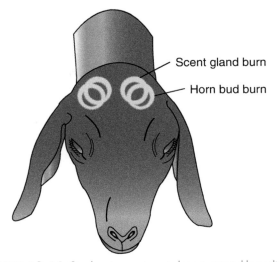

FIGURE 18-14 Overlapping cautery circles are created by a disbud-ding iron, used to disbud and descent kids.

removes the primary sources of testosterone and therefore most of the noticeable odor from the scent glands. However, castration may not completely eliminate the self-urination behavior, especially if castration is performed after maturity. Surgical removal of the scent glands may also be done. It definitively ends the primary scent gland secretions but does not alter the self-urination behavior, if it exists. It is important to provide good client communication because many pet goat owners think that *descenting* is the total answer to buck odor. They must realize that self-urination is not affected by descenting and that only castration may eliminate, with occasional exception, self-urination.

> **TECHNICIAN NOTE** Castration may not completely eliminate self-urination behavior in goats.

Descenting can be done at any age. It is easiest to perform it as a combined procedure with disbudding at an early age. Heat cautery is used to remove the horn buds, as described earlier, and an additional overlapping area just caudomedial to each horn bud is also cauterized (Fig. 18-14). In the adult, the glands are recognized as a small, hairless area with pores, just caudomedial to each horn. They can be removed during the dehorning procedure by extending the skin incisions to include them. They also can be removed at any time without dehorning the goat as a separate procedure performed using sedation and local anesthesia. The glands are identified and removed through surgical incisions. Sutures can be used to close the skin.

Descenting of breeding bucks may have significant effects on breeding behavior. The identifying odor from the glands is used to attract females, and rubbing the top of the head on other animals and surfaces helps to "mark" a male's territory. Breeding females may reject males that lack this scent.

> **TECHNICIAN NOTE** Breeding females may reject males that lack scent glands.

CORRECTION OF ENTROPION

Surgical correction of entropion is best undertaken with the animal anesthetized and placed in lateral recumbency. Using a number 15 scalpel blade, a crescent-shaped flap of skin is removed from the affected eyelid. The flap of skin to be removed is incised 1 to 2 mm distal to the eyelid margin and 3 to 4 mm wider than the affected area. The underlying section of the orbicularis oculi muscle also should be excised. The skin is closed with a simple interrupted suture pattern. Closure should begin in the middle of the incision and proceed to the edges to ensure even skin tension across the suture line. Soft (silk or monofilament nylon), fine (3-0 to 4-0) suture material is suggested. The clinician should take care to tie knots away from the cornea to prevent irritation.

Sutures should be removed in 10 to 14 days. Topical antibiotics should be continued for several days postoperatively or until any corneal ulcers have healed.

CASE STUDY

Mr. Lindsay has called the clinic. When you answer the telephone, Mr. Lindsay asks to make an appointment for his pet male goat. He explains that his goat has an extremely offensive odor that has just developed this spring. What question would you most likely ask him?

CASE STUDY

Dr. Juarez is going to perform a cesarean section on a ewe. The veterinarian asks you to set up for the procedure and tells you the ewe will be here in about a half hour. What supplies will you prepare for the procedure?

SUGGESTED READINGS

Anderson DE, Rings DM: *Current veterinary therapy: food animal practice*, ed 5, St. Louis, 2008, Saunders.

Cebra ML, Cebra CK: Food animal medicine and surgery. In McCurnin DM, Bassert JM, editors: *Clinical textbook for veterinary technicians*, ed 7, St. Louis, 2010, Saunders, pp 713–768.

Fubini SL, Ducharme NG: *Farm animal surgery*, St. Louis, 2004, Saunders.

Hafez ESE, Hafez B, editors: *Reproduction in farm animals*, ed 7, New York, 2000, Wiley-Blackwell.

Muir WW 3rd, Hubbell JAE, Bednarski RM, Skarda RT: *Handbook of veterinary anesthesia*, ed 3, St. Louis, 2006, Mosby.

Noakes DE, Parkinson RJ, England GCW: *Veterinary reproduction and obstetrics*, ed 8, London, 2009, Saunders.

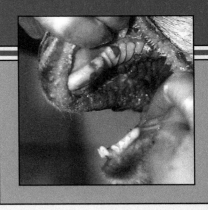

19 | Common Ovine and Caprine Diseases

OUTLINE

OBJECTIVES

After completing this chapter, you will be able to

- Describe and recognize clinical signs associated with specific diseases
- Understand and describe the etiology of the diseases
- Understand and describe common treatments of disease
- Know the common and scientific names of parasites associated with these species
- Know the common vaccinations and their schedules associated with these species

KEY TERMS

Abortion
Blepharospasm
Conjunctiva
Coronary band
Epididymitis
Epiphora

Lochia
Microphthalmia
Opisthotonos
Phthisis bulbi
Prion
Prolapse ring

Retractor bulbi muscle
Serovar
Stillbirth
Tetraplegia

KEY ABBREVIATIONS

AGID: Agar gel immunodiffusion
CAE: Caprine arthritis-encephalitis
EAE: Enzootic abortion in ewes

ELISA: Enzyme-linked immunosorbent assay
OPP: Ovine progressive pneumonia

TSE: Transmissible spongiform encephalopathy

BACTERIAL DISEASES

ANTHRAX

- Etiology: *Bacillus anthracis*
- Gram-positive organism
- Sudden death and septicemia
- Reportable disease
- Vaccine in the presence of an outbreak
  See Chapter 15, on common bovine diseases.

BIG HEAD

- Etiology: *Clostridium novyi, Clostridium sordellii,* or *Clostridium chauvoei*
- Gram-positive organism
- Head and neck edematous swelling

Big head can be caused by the bacteria *Clostridium novyi, Clostridium sordellii,* or *Clostridium chauvoei.* Sheep that are head butting or fighting can cause bruising or laceration of the subcutaneous tissue. The bacteria thrives in this environment, and the animal's face, head, and neck undergo edematous swelling.

The diagnosis is made from clinical signs, and treatment includes antibiotics.

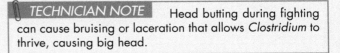

TECHNICIAN NOTE Head butting during fighting can cause bruising or laceration that allows *Clostridium* to thrive, causing big head.

BLACK DISEASE

- Etiology: *C. novyi* type B
- Gram-positive organism
- Necrosis of the liver
- Vaccine available

Black disease is caused by *C. novyi* type B. *C. novyi* is found in soil. Black disease is contracted when the spores of this organism are ingested, which commonly occurs while animals are grazing pastures. As the bacteria replicate, they release toxins that cause necrosis of the liver. The exotoxins produced enter the general circulation, where they cause damage to neurons, vascular endothelium, and other vital cells and tissues that leads to sudden death of the animal.

Clinical black disease consists almost entirely of animals found dead. If the animal is identified as being ill before death, it will be depressed and possibly show signs of respiratory distress and anorexia. Temperature is elevated initially (104° F to 106° F) but declines before death.

The diagnosis of clinical black disease often is made at necropsy. At necropsy, hemorrhage of subcutaneous blood vessels is seen, subendocardial and subepicardial hemorrhages are present, and the kidney and liver show signs of autolysis. Migrating flukes, if present, predispose the flock to black disease, and the liver will have channels and show signs of necrosis. The definitive diagnosis can be accomplished with a Gram stain and culture of the liver lesions at the margins of the liver.

Tetracyclines may prove effective if the disease is diagnosed before death, which is rare. Vaccines to prevent black disease are available. Control of liver fluke infestation is extremely important in the prevention of black disease.

> **TECHNICIAN NOTE**   Control of liver fluke infestation is extremely important in the prevention of black disease.

BLACKLEG

- Etiology: *C. chauvoei*
- Gram-positive rod
- Sudden death and muscle necrosis
- Vaccine available
  See Chapter 15, on common bovine diseases.

BOTULISM

- Etiology: *C. chauvoei*
- Gram-positive rod
- Sudden death and muscle necrosis
- Vaccine available
  See Chapter 11, on common equine diseases.

BRUCELLOSIS

- Etiology: *Brucella ovis, Brucella melitensis*
- Gram-negative rod
- Abortion
- Reportable disease
- Vaccine with limitations

Brucellosis in sheep is caused by *Brucella ovis*. Brucellosis in goats is caused by *Brucella melitensis*. *B. melitensis* may cause *abortion* in sheep. Goats can become infected with *B. abortus* if they are in contact with infected cattle. All these bacteria are gram-negative coccobacillus organisms. The disease is prevalent in the western portions of North America. It rarely causes abortion in sheep but does cause *epididymitis* in rams. In sheep, the disease is spread from ram to ewe and from ewe to ram, but it cannot be spread from ewe to ewe. Rams can pass the organism in their semen. Goats often become infected once they consume contaminated feed or water. Goats shed the disease in their urine, feces, placenta, and milk.

One of the clinical signs that can be seen in sheep is abortion. If the ewe aborts, she will be free of the disease within a few months. If she does not abort, she will give birth to an infected lamb. The placenta is thickened and necrotic on examination. Because ewes rarely abort, the major clinical sign is epididymitis in rams. Clinical signs of goats infected with brucellosis include abortion storms, lameness, mastitis, diarrhea, and depression.

> **TECHNICIAN NOTE**   The major clinical sign of brucellosis in sheep is epididymitis in rams.

The diagnosis is accomplished with the use of agglutination or complement fixation tests.

No treatment exists for brucellosis. Control of the disease usually is accomplished by herd slaughter. To prevent the spread of brucellosis, animals should be serologically tested before they are introduced to the flock. A vaccine is available for sheep, but its ability to prevent the disease is poor. Vaccination of goats is not allowed in the United States. *B. melitensis* and *B. abortus* are considered zoonotic, and precaution should be used when handling potentially infected animals. Only pasteurized milk products should be consumed. *B. melitensis* is the cause of Malta fever in humans.

> **TECHNICIAN NOTE**   *Brucella melitensis* is the cause of Malta fever in humans.

CASEOUS LYMPHADENITIS

- Etiology: *Corynebacterium pseudotuberculosis*
- Gram-positive rod
- Abscessation of lymph nodes

Caseous lymphadenitis is caused by the gram-positive rod *Corynebacterium pseudotuberculosis*. The bacterium infects both goats and sheep and is often found in manure and soil, on the skin, and in infected organs. The organism can gain access into the body through several different methods, including superficial wounds, ingestion, mucous membranes, and inhalation. Indirect infection can occur through contaminated equipment, including bedding, feeders, and clipper blades.

Clinical signs of infection often include dyspnea, tachypnea, cough, and weight loss.

The diagnosis involves culture of the bacteria from a transtracheal wash. Thoracic radiographs may reveal masses in the thoracic cavity. Hepatic abscesses may be found at necropsy (Fig. 19-1). The disease often causes abscessation of the lymph nodes. Identification and removal of sick animals from the herd can help control outbreaks. Sanitation during management practices such as castration, tail docking, and parturition can also help prevent infection. Vaccination is controversial.

CHLAMYDOPHILOSIS

- Etiology: *Chlamydia psittaci*
- Gram-negative coccus
- Abortion
- Reportable disease
- Vaccine available

Chlamydophilosis is also known as enzootic abortion in ewes (EAE). EAE is caused by the bacterium *Chlamydia psittaci*. EAE is one of the most common causes of abortion in North America and is the number one cause of abortion in goats. The bacterium is spread by contact with uterine discharge, the fetus, and the placenta. Rams are another source of infection. Ewes infect rams, and the rams then spread the disease to other ewes in the flock. After aborting, the dam develops a good immune response, and elimination of *Chlamydia* from her uterus usually occurs within 3 months of the abortion, although persistent shedding can occur.

The most common clinical sign of EAE is abortion in the last 2 to 3 weeks of gestation. Lambs can be born weak or stillborn. Chlamydial infections also can produce pneumonia, keratoconjunctivitis, epididymitis, and polyarthritis.

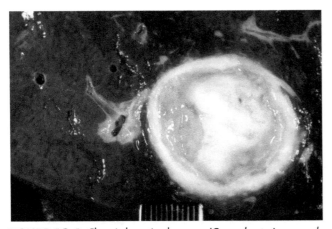

FIGURE 19-1 Chronic hepatic abscesses *(Corynebacterium pseudotuberculosis)* in liver of sheep. Note the thick fibrous capsule and the pale caseous exudate characteristic of pus produced by *C. pseudotuberculosis* in sheep. (Courtesy College of Veterinary Medicine, North Carolina State University. From McGavin MD, Zachary J: *Pathologic basis of veterinary disease,* ed 4, St. Louis, 2006, Mosby.)

The diagnosis is often achieved through the use of *enzyme-linked immunosorbent assay* (ELISA) tests, fluorescent antibody staining, and culture isolation.

Antibiotics can be used during the last few weeks of gestation as a form of treatment. Females that have aborted should be segregated from the herd, and any fetal tissue or placenta from the abortion should be burned or buried. Good feeding practices should be followed to help prevent contamination of the feed and water with *C. psittaci*. Vaccinations are available; however, they most likely will prevent only abortion and not the disease.

CLOSTRIDIUM PERFRINGENS INFECTION

- Etiology: *Clostridium perfringens*
- Gram-positive rod
- Diarrhea
- Vaccine available

Clostridium perfringens is a normal flora of the gastrointestinal (GI) system in sheep. The disease (enterotoxemia, overeating disease) can occur in peracute, acute, and chronic forms. All four types of *C. perfringens* can cause diarrhea in lambs.

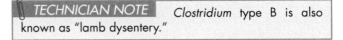

TECHNICIAN NOTE   All four types of *Clostridium perfringens* cause diarrhea in lambs.

Type A

Type A is commonly associated with diarrhea in neonates.

Type B

Types B and C are also known as lamb dysentery. Type B causes acute bloody diarrhea in young lambs and usually has a high mortality rate. Type B creates a severely necrotizing toxin that leaves evidence of mucous ulceration that is seen at necropsy. Treatment usually is unsuccessful. Vaccination is the best form of prevention. In the presence of an outbreak, vaccination of neonates with antiserum immediately after birth may be helpful.

TECHNICIAN NOTE   *Clostridium* type B is also known as "lamb dysentery."

Type C

Goats are most commonly affected by type C. Type C causes diarrhea in young lambs less than 3 weeks old. Type C can also cause diarrhea in adults, and this is commonly referred to as "struck." Type C creates a severely necrotizing toxin that leaves evidence of mucous ulceration that is seen at necropsy. Treatment usually is unsuccessful. Vaccination is the best form of prevention. In the presence of an outbreak, vaccination of neonates with antiserum immediately after birth may be helpful.

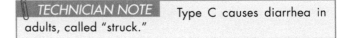

TECHNICIAN NOTE   Type C causes diarrhea in adults, called "struck."

Type D

Type D is usually seen in feedlot lambs that consume high-concentrate diets. It is also known as pulpy kidney disease and overeating disease. The disease often affects the lambs with the highest feed-to-gain ratios and in the best condition. It can be seen in animals with abrupt feed changes. The disease may also be seen in lambs that consume excessive amounts of feed or milk. The disease may manifest with no feeding changes in goats and in vaccinated herds.

Clinical signs include diarrhea, incoordination, excitement, circling, head pressing, convulsions, and sudden death. Sudden death may often occur in sheep without the presence of diarrhea.

The diagnosis before death is often made from clinical signs. At necropsy, samples can be taken and cultured from intestinal fluid. The culture can be uninformative because *C. perfringens* is part of the normal gut flora and often populates quickly after death. Prevention should include vaccination, control of the parasites, and gradual feed changes. Goats rarely die suddenly without the presence of diarrhea.

> **TECHNICIAN NOTE**   *Clostridium* type D usually affects the feedlot lambs on high feed-to-gain ratios and lambs in good condition.

FOOT ROT

- Etiology: *Fusobacterium necrophorum, Dichelobacter nodosus*
- Gram-negative bacillus
- Lameness
- Vaccine available
  See Chapter 15.

JOINT ILL

- Etiology: multiple causes
- Gram-negative bacillus
- Sepsis

Joint ill primarily occurs in kids. It is caused by several bacterial agents, but most are gram-positive agents. Some of the bacteria that cause joint ill include staphylococci, streptococci, *Corynebacterium* species, *Actinomyces,* and coliform bacteria. The bacteria often gain entry to the body through breaks in the skin, the umbilical cord, or the GI or respiratory tract. Predisposing factors include overcrowding and unsanitary conditions.

Clinical signs include warm, painful, swollen joints, lameness, fever, umbilical cord abscessation, and leukocytosis with left shift.

Treatment can be successful if the disease is caught early. Antibiotics and joint flushing can be successful.

> **TECHNICIAN NOTE**   Maintaining sanitary conditions and preventing overcrowding can help reduce the likelihood that kids will contract joint ill.

LEPTOSPIROSIS

- Etiology: *Leptospira* species
- Gram-negative spirochete
- Abortion
- Reportable disease
- Vaccine available
  See Chapter 15.

> **TECHNICIAN NOTE**   Sheep and goats become infected with *Leptospira* through contaminated urine or through water supplies that are contaminated with urine.

LISTERIOSIS

- Etiology: *Listeria monocytogenes*
- Gram-positive coccobacillus
- Neurologic disease and abortion
  Listeriosis is more prevalent in goats than in sheep or cattle (see Chapter 15).

MALIGNANT EDEMA

- Etiology: *Clostridium septicum*
- Gram-positive cocci
- Malaise and edema
- Vaccine available
  See Chapter 15.

PARATUBERCULOSIS (JOHNE DISEASE)

- Etiology: *Mycobacterium avium* subspecies *paratuberculosis*
- Gram-positive organism
- Subclinical to chronic diarrhea and malaise
- Reportable disease
  See Chapter 15 for a discussion of paratuberculosis (Figs. 19-2 and 19-3).

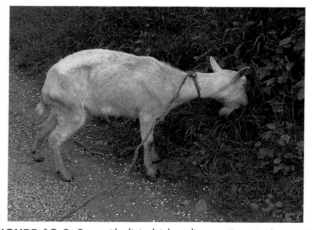

FIGURE 19-2 Goat with clinical Johne disease. (From Anderson DE, Rings DM: *Current veterinary therapy: food animal practice,* ed 5, St. Louis, 2009, Saunders.)

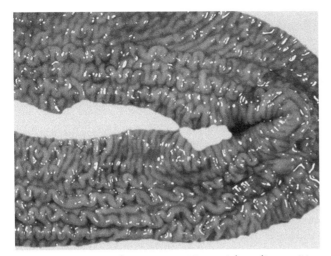

FIGURE 19-3 Granulomatous enteritis, or Johne disease *(Mycobacterium avium* subspecies *paratuberculosis),* in the ileum of a cow. Thickening of the mucosa, which is smooth and shiny (intact) and not ulcerated, is notable. (Courtesy Dr. M.D. McCracken, College of Veterinary Medicine, University of Tennessee; and Noah's Arkive, College of Veterinary Medicine, University of Georgia. From McGavin MD, Zachary J: *Pathologic basis of veterinary disease,* ed 5, St. Louis, 2012, Mosby.)

PINKEYE

- Etiology: *Moraxella bovis*
- Gram-negative organism
- Eye inflammation and irritation
- Vaccine available
  See Chapter 15.

TETANUS

- Etiology: *Clostridium tetani*
- Gram-positive bacillus
- Severe stiffness
- Vaccine available
  Figure 19-4 shows the characteristic appearance of tetanus in a lamb (see also Chapter 11).

TRANSMISSIBLE SPONGIFORM ENCEPHALOPATHIES

- Etiology: prion
- General malaise and neurologic
- Reportable disease
  Transmissible spongiform encephalopathy (TSE) is also known as "scrapie." Scrapie is thought to be caused by a prion. Sheep seem to be more or less sensitive to TSE depending on their genetics. Suffolk sheep are most commonly diagnosed. Sheep and goats are natural reservoirs for scrapie. Transmission of the disease is not fully understood. Sheep are suspected to become infected at birth and often begin displaying clinical signs at approximately 3½ years of age. The infection is thought to be result from contact with infected animals or the environment.

> *TECHNICIAN NOTE*   Suffolk sheep are the most common breed diagnosed with scrapie.

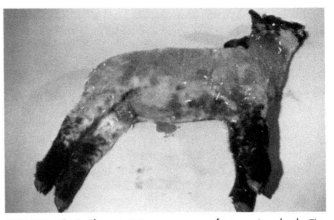

FIGURE 19-4 Characteristic appearance of tetanus in a lamb. This condition developed subsequent to application of an elastrator band to the scrotum. (From Smith BP: *Large animal internal medicine,* ed 5, St. Louis, 2015, Mosby.)

Clinical signs include wool or hair loss, ataxia, weight loss, starring, aggressiveness, floppy ears, tremors, seizures, inability to swallow, and death. The disease is chronic and degenerative.

The diagnosis is accomplished by finding the scrapie prion protein with immunostaining of lymphoid tissue. No treatment exists for scrapie. The disease is considered fatal. The disease is reportable and often results in flock slaughter.

> *TECHNICIAN NOTE*   Scrapie is a reportable disease.

Prevention is being attempted through the Scrapie Flock Certification Program. The program requires flocks to be assessed for 5 years to determine that they do not contain any scrapie-infected sheep. This program has four levels of clearance. When the final level is attained, the producers are able to export and sell sheep both within the United States and internationally without restrictions.

VIBRIOSIS

- Etiology: *Campylobacter jejuni* and *Campylobacter fetus*
- Gram-negative rod
- Abortion
- Vaccine available
  Vibriosis is caused by *Campylobacter jejuni* and *Campylobacter fetus.* The bacteria are gram-negative rods that live in the intestines of sheep, birds, and dogs. In North America, vibriosis is the number one cause of abortion in sheep. Infection occurs through ingestion of the organism by pregnant females.

Clinical signs include late term abortion, *stillbirth,* and weak limbs.

The diagnosis is made from culture of the bacteria.

Antibiotics can be helpful in the event of an outbreak; however, vaccination is the best prevention.

OTHER MICROBIAL DISEASES

TOXOPLASMOSIS

- Etiology: *Toxoplasma gondii*
- Protozoan
- Abortion

Toxoplasma gondii is a protozoan that causes abortion in sheep and goats but only rarely causes abortion in cattle and horses. Infection with *Toxoplasma* results in fetal death and abortion, embryonic death, stillbirth, or birth of weak, nonviable lambs or kids. Placental infection occurs approximately 14 days after ingestion of oocysts. Most abortions take place 1 month before parturition.

The most common evidence of *Toxoplasma* is white, chalky foci of necrosis and calcification up to 2 mm in diameter in cotyledons. Tachyzoites may be found in placenta or other fetal tissues but are not numerous. Several serologic tests, including the modified agglutination test, indirect fluorescent antibody test, Sabin-Feldman dye test, indirect hemagglutination test, and ELISA, reliably detect toxoplasmosis in pleural or amniotic fluid or presuckling serum from nondecomposed fetuses. Aborted tissues may be infectious to humans and should be handled with caution.

> **TECHNICIAN NOTE**   Aborted tissues may be infectious to humans and should be handled with caution.

Ewes or does are often infected by the age of 4 years. They seldom abort from toxoplasmosis in subsequent pregnancies. Prevention should include reducing cat access to sheep areas and equipment, as well as preventing cats from eating placenta and tissue (Tables 19-1 and 19-2).

VIRAL DISEASES

BLUETONGUE

- Etiology: orbivirus
- Abortion
- Reportable disease

Bluetongue is caused by an orbivirus. The disease is noncontagious and affects all ruminants, especially sheep. Although goats are frequently infected with bluetongue in endemic regions, it very rarely causes abortion. The *Culicoides* gnat (or midge) is responsible for transmitting the virus, and cattle are thought to serve as reservoirs.

Sometimes the ewes have ulcerations on the mouth or nose, are lame, and may be febrile. Bluetongue can lead to abortion associated with bluetongue; the abortion usually is seasonal with the life cycle of the gnat. If ewes do not abort, the lambs are commonly born with hydranencephaly.

Diagnosis of bluetongue is accomplished by viral isolation from samples of blood and aborted fetuses. Vaccination against bluetongue is questionable because so many *serovars* *exist*. Prevention of the disease includes insect control.

> **TECHNICIAN NOTE**   Bluetongue commonly causes abortion in sheep.

CAPRINE ARTHRITIS-ENCEPHALITIS

- Etiology: retrovirus
- Pneumonia and neurologic
- Reportable disease

Caprine arthritis-encephalitis (CAE) is caused by a retroviral infection of goats that is similar to ovine progressive pneumonia in sheep. The disease can occur in one of three forms: neurologic, arthritic, and mastitic. It is primarily transmitted from the doe to the kid through colostrum. CAE can be spread by fomites such as needles. Needles should be used only once and then discarded.

> **TECHNICIAN NOTE**   Needles should be used only once and then discarded.

Kids between 1 to 4 months old are often affected with the neurologic form of the disease, but adults occasionally are affected. Clinical signs of the neurologic form of the disease include *tetraplegia*, ataxia, blindness, head tilt, facial paralysis, *opisthotonos*, and generalized paresis. The disease often progresses to its most severe form within 1 to 2 weeks.

The diagnosis of CAE is accomplished with the use of an *agar gel immunodiffusion (AGID)* test for CAE antibodies. Evaluation of cerebrospinal fluid often shows an elevated protein content and mononuclear pleocytosis. At necropsy, perivascular foci and demyelination of the white matter of the brain and spinal cord are often seen.

CAE has no treatment. To prevent the disease, kids should not be fed colostrum from infected dams. If only colostrum from an unknown or infected source is available, it can be heated for 1 hour at 56° C before it is fed to the kid. Surgical equipment should be sterilized to help prevent the spread of CAE. Infected animals should be culled.

CONTAGIOUS ECTHYMA

- Etiology: poxvirus
- Pustular dermatitis

Contagious ecthyma is also known as contagious viral pustular dermatitis, orf, sore mouth, contagious pustular dermatitis, cutaneous pustular dermatitis, and scabby mouth. Transmission is through direct or indirect contact with environmental contaminants. Nursing lambs can spread the infection to ewes.

> **TECHNICIAN NOTE**   Contagious ecthyma has many names, including contagious viral pustular dermatitis, orf, sore mouth, contagious pustular dermatitis, cutaneous pustular dermatitis, and scabby mouth.

During the beginning of a sore mouth infection, papules, pustules, or vesicles become apparent on the skin. Following

TABLE 19-1	Sheep Vaccinations*				
DISEASE OR VACCINATION	**EWES**	**LAMBS**	**FEEDLOT LAMBS**	**RAMS**	**COMMENTS**
Clostridium perfringens type C	4–6 wk before parturition If animals have never been vaccinated, twice 4 wk apart with last dose 4–6 wk before parturition	If born to unvaccinated ewe, at birth and booster in 4–6 wk Lambs from vaccinated ewes should be vaccinated at 12–16 wk and booster given in 4–6 wk	On entering feedlot and booster in 2–4 wk	Annually	
Clostridium perfringens type D	4–6 wk before parturition If animals have never been vaccinated, twice 4 wk apart with last dose 4–6 wk before parturition	If born to unvaccinated ewe, at birth and booster in 4–6 wk Lambs from vaccinated ewes should be vaccinated at 12–16 wk and booster given in 4–6 wk	On entering feedlot and booster in 2–4 wk	Annually	
Clostridium tetani	Can be given during pregnancy with *Clostridium* types C and D	At time of castration and tail docking	Annually	Annually	Often combined with *Clostridium* types C and D
Other clostridial diseases (black disease, blackleg, malignant edema, struck, lamb dysentery, botulism)	4–6 wk before parturition If animals have never been vaccinated, twice 4 wk apart with last dose 4–6 wk before parturition	If born to unvaccinated ewe, at birth and booster in 4–6 wk Lambs from vaccinated ewes should be vaccinated at 12–16 wk and booster given in 4–6 wk	Annually	Annually	Primarily used only in high-risk herds
Leptospirosis					Primarily used only in high-risk herds
Sore mouth	At least 2 mo before parturition and booster every 5–12 mo depending on risk	1–2 days of age and booster every 5–12 mo depending on risk	4 wk before risk and booster every 5–12 mo depending on risk	4 wk before risk and booster every 5–12 mo depending on risk	Live virus Vaccinated sheep can spread the disease for up to 8 wk after vaccination Use in infected herds only Performed by scratching skin in area without wool (inner ear or under tail in adults and inner thigh in young animals) and then brushing on the vaccine Sores will form at application site
Foot rot	4 wk before lambing and booster every 4–6 mo	4 wk of age and booster in 4–8 wk	4 wk before wet or rainy season, booster every 4–6 mo	4 wk before wet or rainy season, booster every 4–6 mo	Vaccinate behind the ear Only reduces infection levels Abscesses not uncommon, discoloration of the wool at the injection site Booster in 4 wk from first time of vaccination

Continued

TABLE 19-1	Sheep Vaccinations*—cont'd				
DISEASE OR VACCINATION	**EWES**	**LAMBS**	**FEEDLOT LAMBS**	**RAMS**	**COMMENTS**
Caseous lymphadenitis	Annually	Annually	Annually	Annually	Primarily used only in high-risk or infected herds Booster in 4 wk after the first dose
Enzootic abortion in ewes (EAE)	4 wk before breeding *Do not use in pregnant ewes*				Primarily used only in high-risk or infected herds
Toxoplasma	4 wk before breeding *Do not use in pregnant ewes* Booster every 2 years				Primarily in only high-risk or infected herds. Vaccine not available in the United States
Vibriosis	Annually, 2 wk before breeding Booster in midpregnancy if first vaccination				Primarily used only in high-risk herds
Brucellosis				Rams test positive if vaccinated	
Rabies					Common in pet sheep and possibly in endemic areas
Escherichia coli	4–6 wk before parturition If animals have never been vaccinated, twice 4 wk apart	If ewes were unvaccinated, oral antibody can be given at birth			Primarily used only if diarrhea in 1- to 2-day-old lambs is a problem

*Vaccination protocols should be designed specific to producers by veterinarians.

TABLE 19-2	Goat Vaccinations*
DISEASE OR VACCINATION	**COMMENTS**
Clostridium perfringens types C and D	Use as in sheep
Clostridium tetani	Use as in sheep
Escherichia coli	Use as in sheep, primarily only in high-risk herds
Foot rot	Use as in sheep
Pasteurella	Use as in sheep, primarily only in high-risk herds
Leptospirosis	Primarily used only in high-risk herds
Caseous lymphadenitis	U.S. Food and Drug Administration does not recommend use of the vaccine in goats
Rabies	Use as in sheep, primarily only in high-risk herds
Enzootic abortion in ewes (EAE)	Use as in sheep, primarily only in high-risk herds; goats are more sensitive

*Vaccination protocols should be designed specific to producers by veterinarians. These vaccines are used off label.

the pustules, thick, brown-to-black crusts form, most often at the corners of the mouth. These lesions may spread to the oral cavity, eyelids, feet, and teats (Fig. 19-5). The lesions typically resolve in 14 to 21 days but may persist in immunocompromised patients. Secondary bacterial infections of the skin are common. Other clinical signs include anorexia, dehydration, malnutrition, and weight loss resulting from the pain associated with the oral lesions. Mastitis is often a secondary bacterial infection caused by lesions on the teats.

Lameness can result from *coronary band* lesions. Rarely, pneumonia and diarrhea develop from lesions in the GI and respiratory systems.

The diagnosis is made based on the clinical signs. Treatment should include therapy for secondary bacterial infections and supportive therapy for dehydrated or malnourished animals.

Prevention should include isolation of all sick animals. Commercial vaccines are available but are not recommended

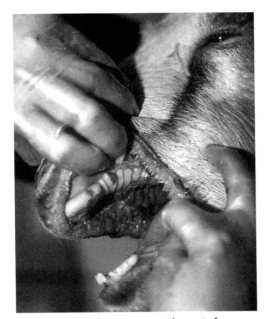

FIGURE 19-5 Goat with contagious ecthyma (orf, sore mouth) has ulcerative and proliferative lesions on the lips and tongue. (From Bassert J, Thomas J, editors: *Clinical textbook for veterinary technicians,* ed 8, St. Louis, 2014, Saunders.)

for disease-free herds. The vaccine is given by scratching the skin, often in an X shape, and brushing the vaccine over the scratch. Because the vaccine is a live virus, the formation of lesions over the injection site is extremely common, and recently vaccinated animals are contagious for up to 8 weeks following vaccination. For adults, the most common location of vaccination is the inner ear or under the tail. In young animals, the vaccine usually is administered on the inner thigh. Contagious ecthyma is highly zoonotic and may produce lesions on the hands or fingers of persons handling infected sheep or goats. Therefore, hygiene is imperative during handling of infected herds and vaccines. In endemic flocks, vaccinating lambs and kids at 2 to 3 days of age may help reduce the severity of a flock outbreak.

> **TECHNICIAN NOTE**   Contagious ecthyma is highly zoonotic.

FOOT AND MOUTH DISEASE

- Etiology: Picornaviridae
- Vesicular disease
- Reportable disease
  See Chapter 15.

OVINE PROGRESSIVE PNEUMONIA

- Etiology: retrovirus
- Pneumonia, mastitis, and encephalitis
  Ovine progressive pneumonia (OPP) is a form of chronic progressive pneumonia caused by a virus from the Retroviridae family. Sheep are most commonly infected through milk and colostrum. Goats are rarely infected with OPP.

Clinical signs include full lung involvement, coughing, bronchial exudates, anorexia, fever, and depression. Encephalitis and mastitis are occasionally seen.

Diagnosis is made from necropsy, which reveals consolidated areas of grayish brown lung tissue as clinical findings. Confirmation of the disease can be accomplished by ELISA, AGID, or virus isolation.

OPP has no treatment. Management of the disease involves testing and culling the flock.

> **TECHNICIAN NOTE**   No treatment exists for ovine progressive pneumonia.

RABIES

- Rhabdovirus
- Neurologic disease
- Reportable disease
- Vaccine available
  See Chapter 11.

NONINFECTIOUS DISEASES

ENTROPION

- Etiology: genetic

Entropion is an inward rolling of the eyelid. This inward rolling of the eyelid causes contact irritation of the cornea and *conjunctiva* by the eyelashes and periocular hair. Entropion is the most common ocular disease in neonatal lambs. From 4% to 80% of a flock may be affected with congenital entropion. Congenital entropion usually is bilateral and usually affects only the lower eyelids. Secondary entropion usually is unilateral and can affect the upper or lower eyelids. Secondary entropion result from trauma, severe dehydration, weight loss, painful ocular conditions that cause contraction of the *retractor bulbi muscle, microphthalmia, phthisis bulbi, blepharospasm,* or old age. Primary entropion (congenital) usually is discovered during the first few days of life, whereas secondary entropion (acquired) can be seen at any age.

Clinical signs include blepharospasm, photophobia, *epiphora,* keratoconjunctivitis, and eye rubbing.

Treatment initially is conservative, with the use of antibiotics and attempts to correct the inward rolling. Antibiotic ointments should be applied at least every 8 to 12 hours. More severe cases may require more frequent administration. Topical 1% atropine can be used in animals with ciliary spasm or severe ocular pain. Nonsurgical eversion using subcutaneous palpebral injection of benzathine or procaine penicillin is attempted. Injection of antibiotics causes local irritation of the eye, with resulting fibrosis that sometimes corrects the problem. Another method is the use of a mosquito hemostat to clamp the eyelid for approximately 30 seconds; this maneuver causes swelling and resultant fibrosis. An additional method involves the placement of skin staples, two or three vertical mattress sutures, or Michel wound clips to evert the eyelid. Surgical corrections are often not attempted until other techniques are unsuccessful.

Because congenital entropion is suspected of being a heritable trait, affected animals should not be used for breeding purposes. Management practices should be taken to reduce housing dust and wind because they predispose animals to entropion.

FREEMARTINISM

- Etiology: male and female twins causing infertility

Goats and sheep rarely give birth to freemartins (see Chapter 15).

HEREDITARY CHONDRODYSPLASIA

- Etiology: genetic

Hereditary chondrodysplasia is also known as "spider lamb syndrome." Spider lamb syndrome is an inherited musculoskeletal condition seen primarily in the Suffolk and Hampshire breeds.

> **TECHNICIAN NOTE**   Hereditary chondrodysplasia is most commonly seen in Suffolk and Hampshire breeds.

Lambs may be born with skeletal defects, or the defects develop at approximately 6 weeks of age (Fig. 19-6). The lambs often have longer legs with angular deviations, shallower bodies, and narrower chests than normal lambs. Other areas that can show evidence of chondrodysplasia are the skull, sternum, appendicular skeleton, and vertebrae (Fig. 19-7). In general, the forelimbs are more severely affected than are the hindlimbs.

Spider lamb syndrome is inherited as an autosomal recessive trait with variable expression. Ewes carrying the gene appear normal, thus making culling of ewes carrying the gene difficult. The locus that causes spider lamb syndrome has been localized to ovine chromosome 6, and deoxyribonucleic acid (DNA) tests may soon allow identification of carrier animals.

METRITIS

- Etiology: multiple causes
- Uterine infection

Metritis, endometritis, and pyometra are not common in sheep and goats but occasionally follow cases of retained placenta or dystocia. Females of these species normally have a brownish-red, thick, nonodorous vaginal discharge for up to 4 weeks after birth; this normal fluid is called *lochia* and requires no treatment. However, the discharge associated with infection is also brownish-red but watery, with a bad odor. Clostridial organisms are sometimes involved in severe cases. Uterine lavage and infusion are more difficult to perform safely in these species, but a 12-French (12-F) to 14-F Foley catheter may be passed through an open cervix with care.

Many clinicians treat uterine infections with hormones such as prostaglandins or oxytocin to cause contraction of the uterus and expulsion of the contents. This is sometimes used as the only treatment in small ruminants (see Chapter 15).

MILK FEVER

- Etiology: decreased calcium
- Down cow
  See Chapter 15.

PREGNANCY TOXEMIA

- Etiology: inadequate caloric intake secondary to multiple fetuses

Pregnancy toxemia is also known as "ketosis" (see Chapter 15).

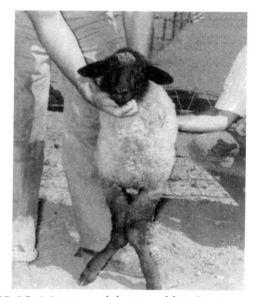

FIGURE 19-6 Rotation and deviation of front legs (carpus valgus) characteristic of spider lamb syndrome in a 16-week-old Suffolk lamb. (From Smith BP: *Large animal internal medicine*, ed 5, St. Louis, 2015, Mosby.)

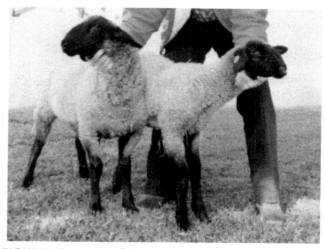

FIGURE 19-7 Twin Suffolk lambs (12 weeks old), with normal lamb (78 lb) on the *left* and lamb with spider syndrome (37 lb) on the *right*. Note the extreme height, narrow chest, scoliosis, kyphosis, and facial deformity of the affected lamb. (From Smith BP: *Large animal internal medicine*, ed 5, St. Louis, 2015, Mosby.)

PROLAPSE

- Etiology: multiple causes
- Organ prolapse

Vaginal Prolapse

Vaginal prolapse is fairly common in ewes, less common in cows, and uncommon in goats (Fig. 19-8). For small ruminants, plastic prolapse retainers are available (Figs. 19-9 and 19-10). Vaginal prolapse can be repaired with a retainer. The retainer has a large spatula arm that is inserted into the vagina and two securing arms with holes that allow them to be sutured to the skin, taped or tied to the wool, or fastened to a body harness. The retainer will not cause injury if delivery occurs while the device is in place. Rubber stents and ropes have also been used to correct vaginal prolapse (Figs. 19-11 and 19-12) (see Chapter 15).

Uterine Prolapse

Dairy cows and ewes are most often affected by uterine prolapse (see Chapter 15).

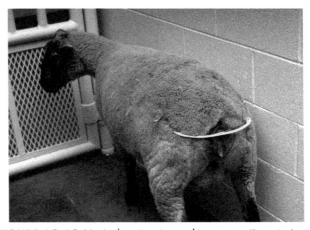

FIGURE 19-10 Vaginal retainer inserted into a ewe. (From Anderson DE, Rings DM: *Current veterinary therapy: food animal practice*, ed 5, St. Louis, 2009, Saunders.)

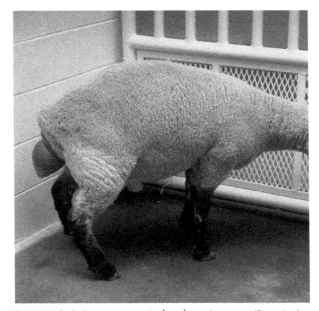

FIGURE 19-8 Prepartum vaginal prolapse in a ewe. (From Anderson DE, Rings DM: *Current veterinary therapy: food animal practice*, ed 5, St. Louis, 2009, Saunders.)

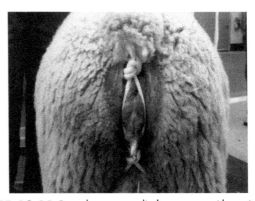

FIGURE 19-11 Rope harness applied to a ewe with vaginal prolapse. (From Anderson DE, Rings DM: *Current veterinary therapy: food animal practice*, ed 5, St. Louis, 2009, Saunders.)

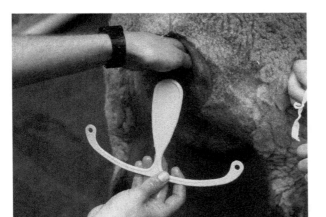

FIGURE 19-9 Vaginal retainer for sheep. (From Anderson DE, Rings DM: *Current veterinary therapy: food animal practice*, ed 5, St. Louis, 2009, Saunders.)

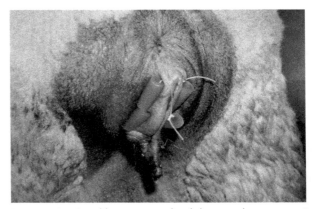

FIGURE 19-12 Rubber stents used with horizontal suture retention of vaginal prolapse. (From Anderson DE, Rings DM: *Current veterinary therapy: food animal practice*, ed 5, St. Louis, 2009, Saunders.)

Rectal Prolapse

In small ruminants, *prolapse rings,* Buhner tape and needle (Fig. 19-13), syringe cases, or plastic tubing can be used as an alternative to surgical amputation (Figs. 19-14 to 19-16). Animals should receive antibiotics postoperatively (see Chapter 15).

> **TECHNICIAN NOTE** In small ruminants, rectal prolapse can be corrected with prolapse rings, syringe cases, or plastic tubing.

RETAINED PLACENTA

- Etiology: failure of placenta to separate

Retained fetal membranes are common in cattle and sheep and are less common in goats (see Chapter 15).

URINARY CALCULI

- Etiology: dietary causes
- Stones in the urinary tract

Urinary calculi are also known as "water belly" and "uro-lithiasis." Urinary tract obstruction is seen most often in male pet sheep and goats, animals being fitted for shows, and feedlot animals. The urethral process of sheep and goats has a small aperture that prevents passage of urinary stones. Goats commonly vocalize when they experience an obstruction (Fig. 19-17). Goats may try to chew their tubes, and Elizabethan collars and belly bandages may be necessary to prevent "self-removal" after surgical repair (see Chapter 15).

> **TECHNICIAN NOTE** Urinary tract obstruction most commonly occurs in pet sheep and goats, animals being fitted for shows, and feedlot animals.

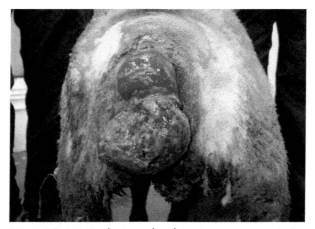

FIGURE 19-14 Grade III rectal prolapse in a ewe. (From Anderson DE, Rings DM: *Current veterinary therapy: food animal practice,* ed 5, St. Louis, 2009, Saunders.)

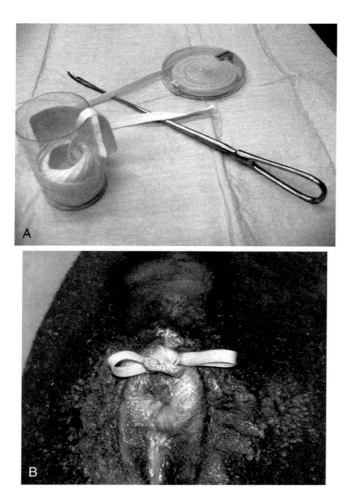

FIGURE 19-13 A, Buhner tape. B, Rectal prolapse with Buhner tape in place. (From Fubini SL, Ducharme NG: *Farm animal surgery,* St. Louis, 2004, Saunders.)

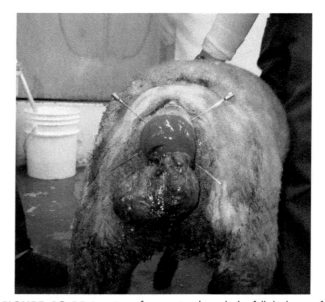

FIGURE 19-15 Insertion of cross-pins through the full thickness of the prolapse such that the pins traverse the lumen of the rectum. (From Anderson DE, Rings DM: *Current veterinary therapy: food animal practice,* ed 5, St. Louis, 2009, Saunders.)

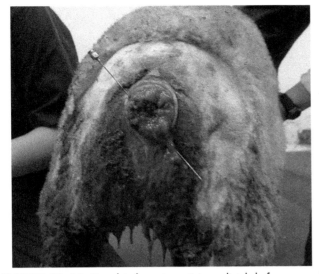

FIGURE 19-16 Completed anastomosis immediately before removal of the final retaining pin. (From Anderson DE, Rings DM: *Current veterinary therapy: food animal practice*, ed 5, St. Louis, 2009, Saunders.)

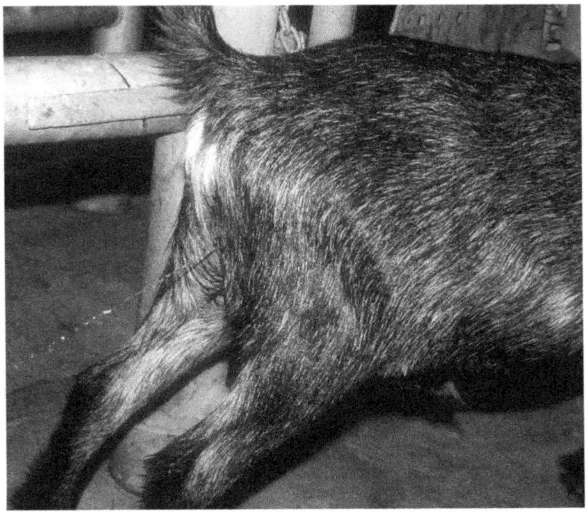

FIGURE 19-17 Urination through a healed perineal urethrostomy in a male goat. (From Bassert J, Thomas J, editors: *Clinical textbook for veterinary technicians*, ed 8, St. Louis, 2014, Saunders.)

FORMULARY

For more information regarding drugs used in sheep and goat medicine, please refer to Appendix 1 in Pugh D: *Sheep and Goat Medicine*, ed 2, St. Louis, 2012, Saunders.

PARASITES

Table 19-3 lists and illustrates common sheep and goat parasites.

TOXINS

Table 19-4 is a list of substances toxic to sheep and goats.

TABLE 19-3	Common Sheep and Goat Parasites			
COMMON NAME AND PHOTOGRAPH	**SCIENTIFIC NAME**	**IMPORTANCE**	**DIAGNOSIS**	**TREATMENT**
Barber's Pole or Wire Worm*: Sheep				
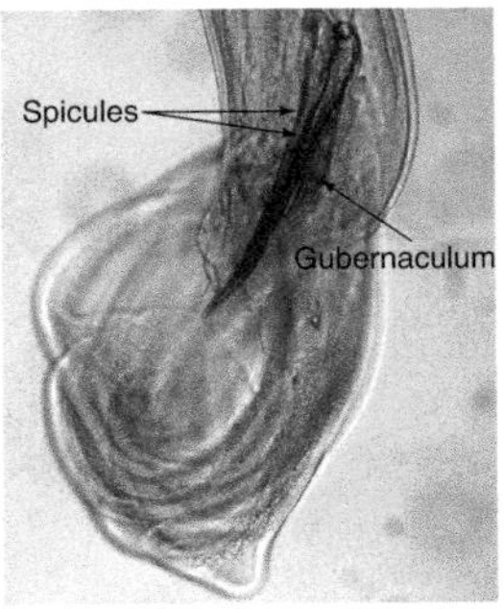	*Haemonchus contortus*	Acute anemia in lambs; bottle jaw, death, chronic weight loss in adults Prepatent period of 17–21 days	Fecal flotation. Eggs do not larvate after 4–5 days of refrigeration Identification at necropsy	Levamisole, ivermectin, albendazole, doramectin, morantel tartrate, moxidectin, eprinomectin, tetramisole

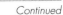

Continued

TABLE 19-3	Common Sheep and Goat Parasites—cont'd

COMMON NAME AND PHOTOGRAPH	SCIENTIFIC NAME	IMPORTANCE	DIAGNOSIS	TREATMENT
Brown Stomach Worm*: Sheep				
	Ostertagia ostertagi	Larval destruction of gastric glands causing severe diarrhea and weight loss Type I: produce eggs Pre-type II: not clinically apparent, and fourth-stage larvae inhibited in gastric glands Type II: eggs often not found in feces	Fecal flotation and identification at necropsy	Fenbendazole, doramectin, eprinomectin, ivermectin, morantel tartrate, moxidectin
Bankrupt Worm or Small Stomach Worm*: Sheep and Goats				
	Trichostrongylus axei	Diarrhea, dehydration, bottle jaw, emaciation in stressed animals Prepatent period of 3 wk	Eggs in fecal flotation and identification at necropsy	Ivermectin, doramectin, eprinomectin, fenbendazole, moxidectin, morantel tartrate
Thin Necked Intestinal Worm†: Sheep and Cattle				
	Nematodirus filicollis, Nematodirus battus, Nematodirus spathiger	*N. battus* especially dangerous Prepatent period of 14–21 days	Fecal flotation and identification at necropsy	Eprinomectin, ivermectin, moxidectin, albendazole, fenbendazole, levamisole, morantel tartrate
Threadworm*: Sheep and Cattle				
	Strongyloides papillosus	Foot rot, diarrhea Prepatent period of 1–2 wk	Eggs in fecal flotation and identification at necropsy	Ivermectin, eprinomectin
Nodular Worm*: Sheep and Goats				
	Oesophagostomum columbianum, Oesophagostomum venulosum	Possible diarrhea Prepatent period of 40 days	Eggs in fecal flotation and identification at necropsy	Moxidectin, morantel tartrate, levamisole, eprinomectin, doramectin

TABLE 19-3	Common Sheep and Goat Parasites—cont'd			
COMMON NAME AND PHOTOGRAPH	**SCIENTIFIC NAME**	**IMPORTANCE**	**DIAGNOSIS**	**TREATMENT**
Hair Worm, Black Scour Worm†: Sheep and Goats	*Trichostrongylus colubriformis*	Diarrhea May cause bottle jaw, decreased weight gain Prepatent period of 3 wk	Eggs in fecal flotation Adults in small intestine at necropsy	Levamisole, morantel tartrate, doramectin, eprinomectin, fenbendazole, moxidectin
Cattle Bankrupt Worm*: Sheep and Goats	*Cooperia punctata, Cooperia pectinata*	Decreased growth, anorexia	Eggs in fecal flotation and identification at necropsy	Doramectin, ivermectin, moxidectin, eprinomectin, albendazole, fenbendazole, levamisole, morantel tartrate
Hookworm*: Sheep	*Bunostomum trigonocephalum*	Weight loss, diarrhea, anemia, death in young animals	Eggs in fecal flotation and identification at necropsy	Ivermectin, moxidectin, doramectin, eprinomectin, fenbendazole
Large-Mouthed Bowel Worm*: Sheep	*Chabertia ovina*	Sometimes anemia Prepatent period of 2 mo	Fecal flotation and identification at necropsy	Albendazole, fenbendazole, ivermectin
Whipworm*: Sheep	*Trichuris ovis*	Extreme infections can cause fatal hemorrhage into cecum Prepatent period of 2 mo	Eggs in fecal flotation and identification at necropsy	Ivermectin, fenbendazole, eprinomectin
Capillary Worm†: Sheep	*Capillaria* spp.	Prepatent period is 6 weeks	Eggs in fecal flotation	Ivermectin, doramectin, eprinomectin, fenbendazole

Continued

TABLE 19-3	Common Sheep and Goat Parasites—cont'd			
COMMON NAME AND PHOTOGRAPH	**SCIENTIFIC NAME**	**IMPORTANCE**	**DIAGNOSIS**	**TREATMENT**
Lungworm*: Sheep *Dictyocaulus filaria* (×250)	*Dictyocaulus filaria*	Respiratory symptoms (e.g., cough, cyanosis, dyspnea) Prepatent period is 4 weeks	Baermann technique for larvae from feces Fecal flotation Adults in lung at necropsy	Ivermectin, doramectin, eprinomectin, moxidectin, levamisole, fenbendazole
Bighorn Sheep Lungworm*: Sheep	*Protostrongylus rufescens, Protostrongylus rushi, Protostrongylus stilesi* (bighorn sheep)	Predisposes sheep to pneumonia Transplacental transmission in bighorn sheep Prepatent period of 5 wk Uncommon in domestic sheep	Eggs in fecal sedimentation Flukes found in liver and bile ducts at necropsy ELISA	Ivermectin, albendazole, fenbendazole
Goat Lungworm†: Goats	*Muellerius capillaris*	Predisposes goats to pneumonia	Baermann technique	Ivermectin, fenbendazole, albendazole
Common Liver Fluke (Fasciolidae)†	*Fasciola hepatica*	Anemia, weight loss, decreased performance, hepatitis, death Prepatent period of 10–12 wk	Eggs in fecal sedimentation Flukes in liver and bile ducts at necropsy ELISA	Clorsulon, nitroxynil, rafoxanide
Tapeworm†: Sheep Trichostrongyle-type egg Monezia egg	*Moniezia expansa*	Prepatent period of 40 days	Proglottids in feces Fecal flotation Adults in small intestine at necropsy	Fenbendazole, albendazole, dichlorophen, lead arsenate, niclosamide
Abdominal Worm†: Sheep and Goats	*Setaria cervi*	May cause cerebral nematodiasis Prepatent period variable	Microfilaria in blood	None

TABLE 19-3	Common Sheep and Goat Parasites—cont'd			
COMMON NAME AND PHOTOGRAPH	**SCIENTIFIC NAME**	**IMPORTANCE**	**DIAGNOSIS**	**TREATMENT**
Fringed Tapeworm†: Sheep	Thysanosoma actinoides	Liver condemnation, weight loss Prepatent period of 1 mo	Proglottids in feces	Fenbendazole, albendazole
Cysticercus Tenuicollis†: Sheep	Taenia hydatigena	Prepatent period in dogs of 51 days	Identification at necropsy	None
Hydatid Cyst*: Sheep	Echinococcus granulosus	Intermediate host and source of infection for carnivores Prepatent period in dogs of 7–9 wk	Identification at necropsy	None
Sheep Cysticercosis*: Sheep	Taenia ovis	Responsible for condemnation, trimming Prepatent period in dogs is 60 days	Identification at necropsy	None
Gid†: Sheep	Taenia multiceps	Causes central nervous system disorder but rare in the United States Prepatent period in dogs of 2–3 mo	Identification at necropsy	None
Sorehead, Filarial Dermatitis: Sheep	Elaeophora schneideri	Commonly found in mule deer in the western United States Causes filarial dermatitis "sorehead," most often in older sheep Prepatent period of 4–5 mo	Identification of microfilariae in skin	None
Sheep Blowflies or Bottle Flies*: Sheep	Lucilia, Phormia, Calliphora	Responsible for strike Life cycle of 10 days	Identification of larvae in rotting wool	Wound treatment, organophosphates

Continued

TABLE 19-3	Common Sheep and Goat Parasites—cont'd			
COMMON NAME AND PHOTOGRAPH	**SCIENTIFIC NAME**	**IMPORTANCE**	**DIAGNOSIS**	**TREATMENT**
Screwworm[†]: Sheep and Goats	*Cochliomyia hominivorax*	Reportable disease in the United States Highly pathogenic, high mortality Maggots penetrate through broken skin Life cycle of 3 wk	Larvae from wounds should be sent to state diagnostic laboratory	Ivermectin, organophosphates
Sheep Nasal Bot Fly[*]: Sheep	*Oestrus ovis*	Dyspnea, nasal discharge	Identification upon necropsy	Ivermectin, *Bacillus thuringiensis* aerosol
Biting Louse[†]: Sheep and Goats	*Bovicola (Damalinia) bovis*	Production losses Most common in fall and winter Usually on neck, brisket, head, and between legs in cattle	Identification eggs, nymphs, adult lice	Pour-on, dips, sprays, dusts, back rubbers, orals, injectables, feed additives
Sucking Lice[*]: Sheep and Goats	*Linognathus pedalis* (sheep foot louse), *Linognathus ovillus* (sheep face and body louse)	Production losses, may cause anemia Life cycle ~4 wk	Identification of eggs, nymphs, adults	Pour-ons, dips, sprays, dusts, back rubbers, orals, injectables, feed additives
Mange Mite or Scab Mite[†]: Sheep and Goats	*Psoroptes* spp.	Reportable disease in some states Dramatic weight loss Life cycle ~3 wk	Skin scrapings	Pour-ons, dips, sprays, dusts, back rubbers, orals, injectables, feed additives
Mange Mite[†]: Sheep	*Sarcoptes scabiei*	Reportable disease in some states Life cycle ~3 wk	Skin scrapings	Pour-ons, dips, sprays, dusts, back rubbers, orals, injectables, feed additives

TABLE 19-3	Common Sheep and Goat Parasites—cont'd			
COMMON NAME AND PHOTOGRAPH	**SCIENTIFIC NAME**	**IMPORTANCE**	**DIAGNOSIS**	**TREATMENT**
Mange Mite†: Sheep and Goats				
	Chorioptes spp.	Reportable disease in cattle in some states Causes tail or foot mange	Skin scrapings	Pour-ons, dips, sprays, dusts, back rubbers, orals, injectables, feed additives
Sheep Ked, Erroneously Called a Sheep Tick†: Sheep				
	Melophagus ovinus	Skin irritation, anemia, weight loss, wool loss Life cycle ~3 mo Adults live ~3 mo	Visual observation	Trichlorphon, fenchlorphos, coumaphos, crotoxyphos, tetrachlorvinphos, phosmet

Data from Bowman DD: *Georgis' parasitology for veterinarians*, ed 10, St. Louis, 2014, Saunders; and Hendrix CM, Robinson E: *Diagnostic parasitology for veterinary technicians*, ed 4, St. Louis, 2012, Saunders.
ELISA, Enzyme-linked immunosorbent assay.
*Figure from Bowman DD: *Georgis' parasitology for veterinarians*, ed 9, St. Louis, 2008, Saunders.
†Figure from Hendrix CM, Robinson E: *Diagnostic parasitology for veterinary technicians*, ed 3, St. Louis, 2006, Mosby.

TABLE 19-4	Common Sheep and Goat Toxins
Copper toxicity	Sever gastritis, lethargy, depression, weakness, rumen stasis, anorexia, dyspnea, thirst, pale mucus membranes, and jaundice
Alkaloids	Liver disease, edema of the abomasum, anorexia, hindleg weakness, knuckling, excessive salivation, pollakiuria, and death
Cyanogenic	Dyspnea, salivation, lacrimation, muscle fasciculation, and death
Photosensitizing agents	Dermatologic signs
Saponins	Vomiting, abdominal pain, diarrhea, convulsions, and death
Tannins	Anorexia, depression, emaciation, ammonia smell to the breath, ocular and nasal discharge, icterus and constimation, liver disease, and death.
Nitrates	Retarded growth, lowered milk production, vitamin A deficiency, goitrogenic effects, abortions, fetotoxicity, and death
Urea	Ruminal tympany, jugular pulses, twitching, tetanic spasms, abnormal central nervous system behavior, and death

CASE STUDY

Mr. Mahony has called the clinic and asked you whether he should vaccinate his herd for orf. What should be your first question to Mr. Mahony? What information would you provide to Mr. Mahony?

CASE STUDY

Ms. Funk has an appointment for a herd of sheep that have multiple scabs around their lips. You are asked to draw blood from each of the sheep. What personal protection, if any, would be wise?

SUGGESTED READING

Anderson DE, Rings DM: *Current veterinary therapy: food animal practice*, ed 5, St. Louis, 2008, Saunders.

Bowman DD: *Georgis' parasitology for veterinarians*, ed 9, St. Louis, 2008, Saunders.

Foreyt WJ: *Veterinary parasitology reference manual*, ed 5, Ames, Iowa, 2007, Iowa State University Press.

Hendrix CM, Robinson E: *Diagnostic parasitology for veterinary technicians*, ed 3, St. Louis, 2006, Mosby.

Kahn CM, Line S: *The Merck veterinary manual*, ed 10, Whitehouse Station, NJ, 2010, Merck & Co.

Pugh DG: *Sheep and goat medicine*, St. Louis, 2002, Saunders.

Radostits O: *Veterinary medicine: a textbook of the diseases of cattle, horses, sheep, pigs and goats*, ed 10, London, 2007, Saunders.

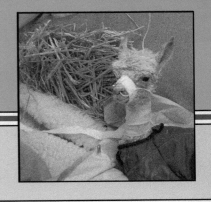

20 Camelid Husbandry

OUTLINE

LEARNING OBJECTIVES

When you have completed this chapter, you will be able to

- Know and understand the zoologic classification of the species
- Know and be able to proficiently use terminology associated with this species
- Know normal physiologic data for the species and be able to identify abnormal data
- Identify and know the uses of common instruments relevant to the species
- Describe prominent anatomical or physiologic properties of the species
- Identify and describe characteristics of common breeds
- Describe normal living environments and husbandry needs of the species
- Understand and describe specific reproductive practices of the species
- Understand specific nutritional requirements of the species

KEY TERMS

Aberrant behavior syndrome
Berserk male syndrome
Cria
Cushed position
Dam

Epitheliochorial
Female
Fighting teeth
Gelding
Malocclusion

Radial immunodiffusion test
South American camelids
Superovulation
Yearling

KEY ABBREVIATION

BMS Berserk male syndrome
FPT Failure of passive transfer

ZOOLOGIC CLASSIFICATION

LLAMA

Kingdom	Animalia
Phylum	Chordata
Class	Mammalia
Order	Artiodactyla
Family	Camelidae
Genus	*Lama*
Species	*Glama*

ALPACA

Kingdom	Animalia
Phylum	Chordata
Class	Mammalia
Order	Artiodactyla
Family	Camelidae
Genus	*Vicugna*
Species	*Pacos*

TERMINOLOGY AND PHYSIOLOGIC DATA

Box 20-1 lists common terminology used to describe the age and breeding status of llamas and alpacas. Table 20-1 lists normal physiologic data for llamas and alpacas.

COMMON CAMELID INSTRUMENTS

Visit the Evolve website to find pictures and descriptions for common camelid instruments.

BOX 20-1	Terminology
Female/dam	Adult female (harem is housed in a group)
Gelding	Castrated male
Cria	Neonate
Yearling	Camelid more than 1 year old but not yet 2 years old

TABLE 20-1	Camelid Physiologic Data
Temperature	99–101.5° F
Pulse rate	60–90 beats/min
Respiratory rate	10–30 breaths/min
Adult weight	Llamas: 280–450 pounds Alpaca: 150–185 pounds

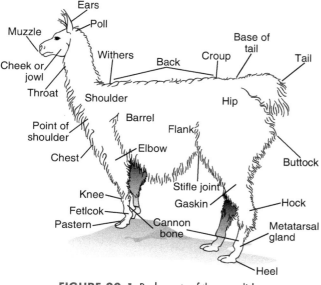

FIGURE 20-1 Body parts of the camelid.

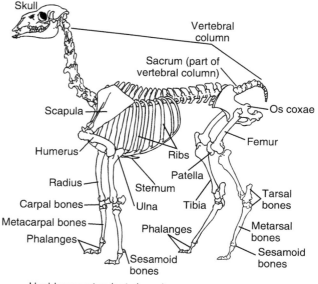

Hyoid apparatus (not shown)

FIGURE 20-2 Skeleton of the camelid.

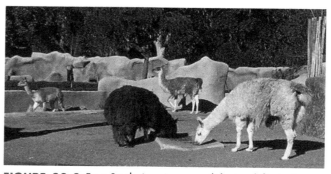

FIGURE 20-3 Four South American camelids: *top left*, vicuña; *top right*, guanaco; *bottom left*, alpaca; *bottom right*, llama. (From Fowler ME: *Zoo and wild animal medicine current therapy*, vol 6, ed 6, St. Louis, 2008, Saunders.)

ANATOMICAL TERMS

Figures 20-1 and 20-2 will help you review the terms for body parts and areas of llamas and alpacas, as well as the names of bones and joints.

CLASSIFICATION

In this section, camelids refers to llamas and alpacas, although the group known as *South American camelids* refers to llamas, alpacas, vicunas, and guanacos.

Alpaca typically are smaller than llamas, but the main difference is within their fibers. Llamas have a dual-fiber coat. Llamas have a fine covering, but it is intermingled with long guard hairs. Alpaca fiber does not contain these long guard hairs. On average, the alpaca stands 34 to 36 inches at the withers (shoulders), whereas the llama stands 42 to 48 inches at the withers (Fig. 20-3).

REPRODUCTION

Breeding information for llamas and alpacas is given in Table 20-2. The normal reproductive course for any large animal species is discussed in Chapter 3. The following reproductive procedures are variations that exist among species.

Live cover is most commonly used in camelids. Camelids are prolific and easily bred because they are induced ovulators (Fig. 20-4). However, much research has been performed on reproductive manipulation within the camelid.

> **TECHNICIAN NOTE**   Live cover is most commonly used in camelids because they are induced ovulators.

SEMEN COLLECTION

Semen collection from camelids can be performed using an artificial vagina or electroejaculation (Figs. 20-5 and 20-6).

TABLE 20-2	Breeding Information
Type of estrous cycle	Polyestrous
Length of spermatogenesis	45–55 days
Length of copulation	20–40 min
Site of semen deposition	Uterus
Ejaculate volume (mL)	2–3
Total sperm (×10⁹)	0.05–0.27
Age of female at puberty	Llama: 6–12 mo Alpaca: 1 yr
Age of male at puberty	Llama: 2–3 yr Alpaca: 2–3 yr
Time of first breeding	2.5–3.5 yr
Estrous cycle frequency	8–12 days
Duration of estrus	4–5 days
Time of ovulation	Induced ovulator Artificial insemination: 24–36 hr after induced ovulation
Optimal time of breeding	Induced ovulator
Maternal recognition of pregnancy in days	8–10 days because of embryo in the left uterine horn
Source of progesterone by days of gestation	Corpus luteum
Type of placenta	Diffuse
Gestation period	335–365 days
Birth weight	Alpaca: 12 pounds Llama: 15 pounds
Litter size	1–2; twinning more common in llama
Weaning age	5–6 mo

Pregnancy detection in days after ovulation

Ultrasound	>16 days
Transrectal palpation	>90 days
Progesterone	>11 days
Estrone sulfate	21–17 days

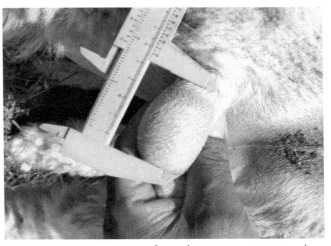

FIGURE 20-5 Measurement of testicular size using a Vernier caliper in camelids. (From Cebra C, Anderson D, Tibary A, et al, editors: *Llama and alpaca care: medicine, surgery, reproduction, nutrition, and herd health,* St. Louis, 2014, Saunders.)

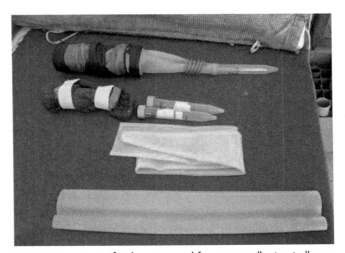

FIGURE 20-6 Artificial vagina used for semen collection in llamas and alpacas. (From Cebra C, Anderson D, Tibary A, et al, editors: *Llama and alpaca care: medicine, surgery, reproduction, nutrition, and herd health,* St. Louis, 2014, Saunders.)

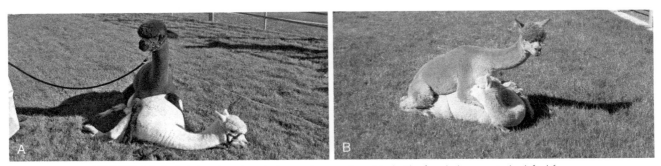

FIGURE 20-4 A, In-hand mating of alpacas in a small paddock. The female has passively shifted from the sternal position to lateral recumbency, with the limbs and neck outstretched. **B,** Pen mating of alpacas in a small paddock. The female is self-auscultating the right flank, a finding suggesting that the male is breeding the right uterine horn. (From Cebra C, Anderson D, Tibary A, et al, editors: *Llama and alpaca care: medicine, surgery, reproduction, nutrition, and herd health,* St. Louis, 2014, Saunders.)

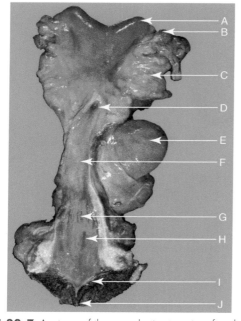

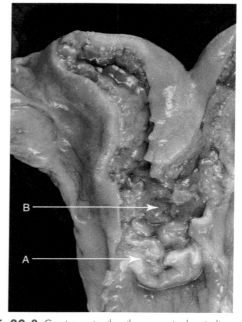

FIGURE 20-7 Anatomy of the reproductive tract in a female alpaca: uterine horn (A), note the absence of clear bifurcation externally; left ovary (B), brad ligament (C), fornix and external os of the cervix (D), urinary bladder (E), vagina (F), vestibule-vaginal sphincter (G), urethral orifice (H), vulvar lip (I), clitoris (J). (From Cebra C, Anderson D, Tibary A, et al, editors: *Llama and alpaca care: medicine, surgery, reproduction, nutrition, and herd health*, St. Louis, 2014, Saunders.)

FIGURE 20-8 Cervix; note the three cervical spiraling rings (A). B, Body of the uterus is very small because of the long septum separating the uterine horns (B). (From Cebra C, Anderson D, Tibary A, et al, editors: *Llama and alpaca care: medicine, surgery, reproduction, nutrition, and herd health*, St. Louis, 2014, Saunders.)

ARTIFICIAL INSEMINATION

Artificial insemination can be performed surgically or transcervically in camelids. Semen should be placed into the left uterine horn (Figs. 20-7 and 20-8). Even though camelids ovulate equally from each uterine horn, much higher conception rates have been achieved from the left horn.

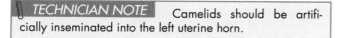

TECHNICIAN NOTE Camelids should be artificially inseminated into the left uterine horn.

EMBRYO TRANSFER

Embryo transfer of camelids begins with *superovulation* of the *female*. The female is then artificially inseminated by the rectopalation route. The embryos are allowed to grow for 72 hours and then are surgically removed. Other methods of embryo transfer involve letting the embryos reach the zygote stage and removing them approximately 7 days after insemination using a flush. After the embryos are collected, they can be placed into the recipient surgically or with an insemination pipette. It is recommended that embryos always be placed into the left uterine horn of the recipient.

CLINICAL SIGNS AND PREPARATION OF IMPENDING PARTURITION

Two to 3 weeks before parturition, camelids show a change in behavior. Udder development is present only sometimes and is a poor indicator of impending parturition. Other signs of impending parturition include elongation of the vulva, lack of interest in eating or grazing, separation from the herd, and increased frequency of urination.

PARTURITION
Stage 1

Stage 1 of delivery is often recognized when the female makes frequent visits to the dung pile and attempts to defecate, with little to no success. The female often lies down and rolls onto her side as labor progresses. She often lies in the *cushed position* (sternal recumbency) with her hindlegs out to the side. She may seem uncomfortable and may even vocalize by humming. Stage 1 should last between 1 and 6 hours (Fig. 20-9).

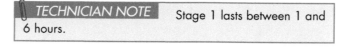

TECHNICIAN NOTE Stage 1 lasts between 1 and 6 hours.

Stage 2

Stage 2 of delivery usually is completed in 20 to 30 minutes and should not take longer than 1 hour. The *cria* should be born in the anterior dorsosacral presentation (Fig. 20-10). Contractions start approximately 10 minutes apart and become progressively closer together. The *dam* often gives birth from a standing position and usually does not lick the cria after birth (Fig. 20-11).

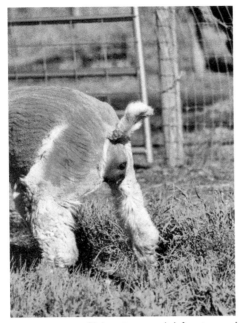

FIGURE 20-9 Stage 1 of labor: increased defecation and urination. (From Cebra C, Anderson D, Tibary A, et al, editors: *Llama and alpaca care: medicine, surgery, reproduction, nutrition, and herd health,* St. Louis, 2014, Saunders.)

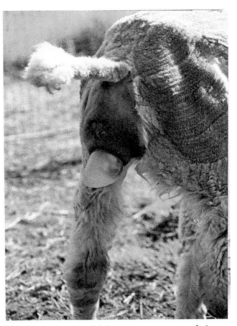

FIGURE 20-11 Stage 2 of labor: appearance of the amniotic sac ("second water bag") and nose of the fetus. (From Cebra C, Anderson D, Tibary A, et al, editors: *Llama and alpaca care: medicine, surgery, reproduction, nutrition, and herd health,* St. Louis, 2014, Saunders.)

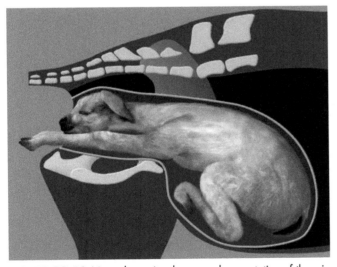

FIGURE 20-10 Normal anterior dorsosacral presentation of the cria at parturition. (Courtesy The Ohio State University, Columbus, Ohio. From Anderson DE, Whitehead CE: *Veterinary clinics of North America food animal practice: alpaca and llama health management,* Philadelphia, 2009, Saunders.)

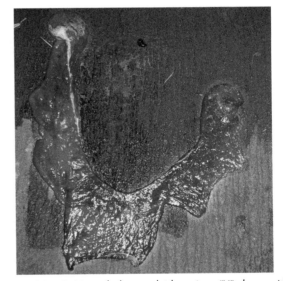

FIGURE 20-12 Normal placenta laid out in a "Y" shape with the chorionic surface exposed. The left uterine horn is obviously larger than the right horn. (From Cebra C, Anderson D, Tibary A, et al, editors: *Llama and alpaca care: medicine, surgery, reproduction, nutrition, and herd health,* St. Louis, 2014, Saunders.)

> **TECHNICIAN NOTE** Stage 2 usually is completed in 20 to 30 minutes and should not last more than 1 hour. Females usually do not lick the cria after birth.

Stage 3

Stage 3 of parturition usually takes place within 1 hour of delivery, and the placenta should be expelled within 4 to 6 hours (Figs. 20-12 and 20-13). If retained placenta is observed, the dam can be treated with oxytocin and prostaglandins. Retained placentas are rare in camelids. Camelids do not eat the placenta.

> **TECHNICIAN NOTE** The placenta usually is passed within 2 hours of delivery but should be expelled within 4 to 6 hours.

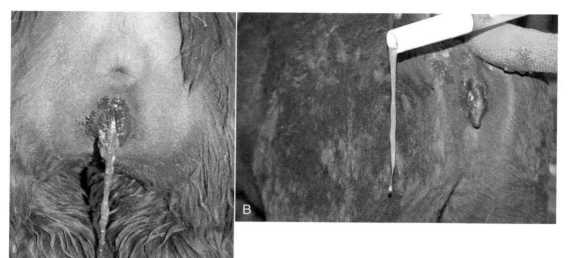

FIGURE 20-13 **A,** Postpartum lochia in alpacas and llamas is very thick and may be confused with partial retention of the placenta by inexperienced individuals. **B,** Lochia may hinder vaginal examination during vaginoscopy. (From Cebra C, Anderson D, Tibary A, et al, editors: *Llama and alpaca care: medicine, surgery, reproduction, nutrition, and herd health,* St. Louis, 2014, Saunders.)

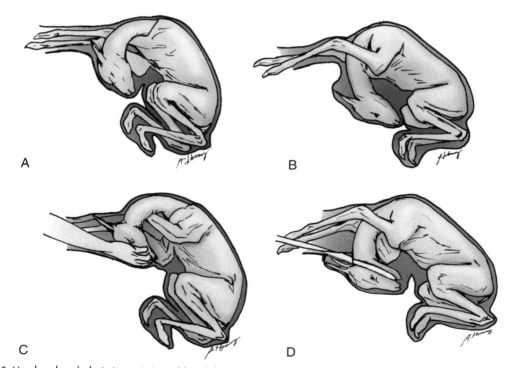

FIGURE 20-14 Head and neck deviations. **A,** Lateral head deviation. **B,** Ventral head and neck deviation. **C,** Correction of lateral head deviation requires elimination of expulsive efforts and relaxation of the uterus. The fetus is repelled, and the operator reaches for the nose, which is cupped in the hand and brought into normal position by slowly pushing against the fetus while extending the neck. **D,** Correction of the ventral neck deviation may proceed in the same manner, but often the nose cannot be reached, so placement of a head snare (or strap) is required. This allows the obstetrician to use the external hand to pull on the fetal head while the other hand is used to repel the fetal body into the uterus and provide space. (From Cebra C, Anderson D, Tibary A, et al, editors: *Llama and alpaca care: medicine, surgery, reproduction, nutrition, and herd health,* St. Louis, 2014, Saunders.)

DYSTOCIA

Dystocia in camelids is uncommon but is corrected as in any other large animal species. The most common causes of dystocia are fetal malpositioning (Figs. 20-14 to 20-16), poor cervical dilation, and uterine torsion. Identification of dystocia in camelids includes identifying a birth that is not complete in 45 minutes of amniotic sac rupture, flexed head or limbs, fetal soles facing dorsally, and forceful straining with no progress within 5 minutes.

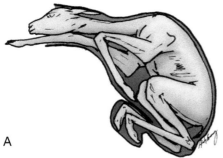
A

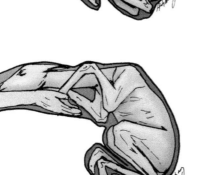
B

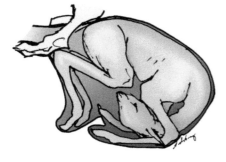
C

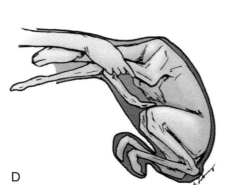
D

FIGURE 20-15 Leg deviations. **A,** Carpal flexion. **B,** Shoulder flexion. **C,** Correction of carpal flexion; the fetus is repelled, and the limb is grasped below the flexed carpus and pushed upward and forward. The foot is cupped in the hand, and the limb is extended. **D,** The first step of the correction of the shoulder flexion is to convert this malposture to carpal flexion by repelling the fetus and grasping the flexed limb below the elbow and bringing it up and toward the birth canal. (From Cebra C, Anderson D, Tibary A, et al, editors: *Llama and alpaca care: medicine, surgery, reproduction, nutrition, and herd health,* St. Louis, 2014, Saunders.)

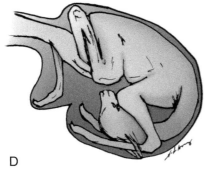
A

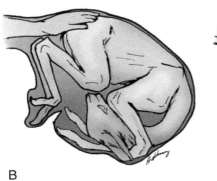
B

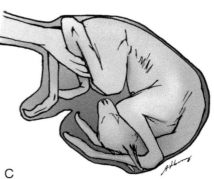
C

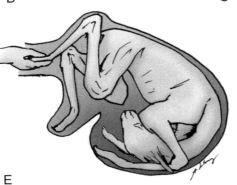
D

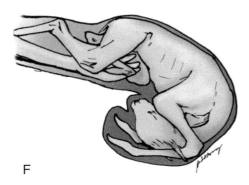
E

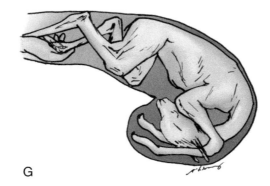
F

G

FIGURE 20-16 Rear leg deviations. **A,** Only the tail and sometimes the hock are palpable. **B,** Fetal repulsion by pressure on the rump. **C,** The hock on one side is located and pulled backward and upward. **D** through **F,** The foot is cupped in the hand, and the whole limb is rotated slightly under the body and extended. **G,** The procedure is repeated on the other side. (From Cebra C, Anderson D, Tibary A, et al, editors: *Llama and alpaca care: medicine, surgery, reproduction, nutrition, and herd health,* St. Louis, 2014, Saunders.)

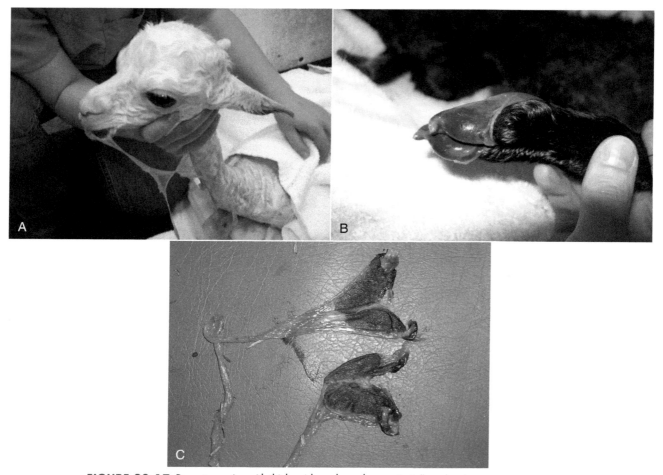

FIGURE 20-17 Premature crias with thick epidermal membrane. **A,** Adhered to the mucocutaneous junctions of the lips. **B,** Adhesions of the epidermal membrane to the foot pad. **C,** Thick epidermal membrane. (From Cebra C, Anderson D, Tibary A, et al, editors: *Llama and alpaca care: medicine, surgery, reproduction, nutrition, and herd health,* St. Louis, 2014, Saunders.)

CAMELID NEONATAL CARE

Once delivery is complete, the following needs of the newborn must be addressed. It is also important to note that crias are born with an epidermal membrane. This membrane is connected to the mucocutaneous junctions and coronary bands. The membrane dries and falls off soon after birth. This membrane is normal and is thought to play a role in preventing dehydration and lubrication during parturition (Fig. 20-17).

> **TECHNICIAN NOTE**   Normal body temperature for a cria is 100° F to 102° F.

Oxygenation and Pulse Assessment

Normal heart rates for crias are between 70 and 100 beats/minute. Respiration should be 20 to 30 breaths/minute.

Temperature Regulation

Normal body temperature for crias is 100° F to 102° F. Cria clothing can be purchased to help keep neonate camelids warm during cold climates. In cold, wet climates, the cria should be kept in a bedded stall. Straw is a good choice of bedding for crias. Heat lamps can be used to help maintain a warm environment.

Care of the Umbilical Cord and Umbilicus

The umbilicus of the cria should be treated with 2% to 3% iodine tincture, although 7% can be used. The umbilical cord usually breaks 2 to 3 inches from the body. Excessive bleeding can be stopped with temporary occlusion, usually for 10 to 15 minutes.

> **TECHNICIAN NOTE**   Suture of the umbilical stump does not allow proper drainage and increases the chances of abscess formation.

Nutrition (Nursing)

Crias normally stand 1 to 2 hours after birth. Ideally, the cria should nurse within 6 to 8 hours of birth. Crias nurse very quickly and spend only a few seconds on each teat, so it is important to pay particular attention to nursing behavior.

If the cria has not nursed within 8 hours, tubing can be performed with the mother's milk stripped from the teats. If camelid milk is unavailable, goat milk can be used as a substitute. Bottle feeding can be performed if loss of the mother occurs. Most crias begin consuming grasses on pasture within 1 to 2 weeks after birth. Crias should not be fed grain before 3 months of age. Feeding gain before 3 months discourages consumption of milk, and crias need the protein supplied in the mother's milk.

> **TECHNICIAN NOTE** Crias should not be fed grain before 3 months of age.

Bonding of Female and Cria

It is important to allow bonding between the female and the cria. When crias are given too much attention by the owner, they may bond to the owner and grow to maturity treating the owner as another camelid in the herd. If camelids treat owners as other camelids, dominant behavior may begin, including knocking people down, biting, and chest butting. If the behavior becomes excessive, it has been called *berserk male syndrome* (BMS). BMS is more common in male cria but can affect female cria. More recently, the term *aberrant behavior syndrome* has been used to describe BMS.

> **TECHNICIAN NOTE** Cria owners should take care to prevent cria from bonding to them instead of the mother.

Passage of Meconium

Depression, straining to defecate, and rolling are indications of retained meconium in crias. The feces should be passed in the first several hours of life. To assist in passage of meconium, a warm, soapy enema can be given. Passage of meconium usually occurs within a few minutes after the enema is administered. Some farms make administration of an enema part of the wellness examination each cria receives.

Adequacy of Passive Transfer of Antibodies

Camelids have a diffuse *epitheliochorial* nature of placentation, which leads to poor passive transfer of antibodies. Failure of passive transfer (FPT) is a common cause of mortality in camelid neonates. Adequate colostrum intake should be 10% to 20% of body weight in 24 hours. If camelid colostrum is not available, cattle, sheep, and goat colostrum can be used. Colostrum can be stored for up to 1 year in the freezer.

> **TECHNICIAN NOTE** Failure of passive transfer is a common cause of mortality in camelid neonates.

If bottle feeding, 10% to 15% of the cria's body weight should be fed over 24 hours. Feedings should be offered every 2 hours. Less frequent, larger feedings tend

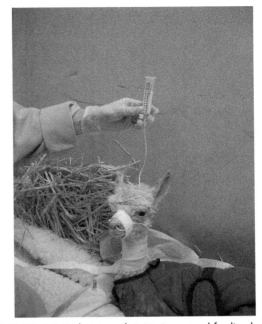

FIGURE 20-18 Technician administering enteral feeding by gravity flow into a nasogastric tube in an alpaca cria. (From Bassert J, Thomas J, editors: *McCurnin's clinical textbook for veterinary technicians*, ed 8, St. Louis, 2014, Saunders.)

to cause acidosis. Every attempt should be made to bottle feed crias; repeated tube feeding may lead to esophagitis (Fig. 20-18).

> **TECHNICIAN NOTE** Every attempt should be made to bottle feed crias; repeated tube feeding may lead to esophagitis.

Low birth weight may indicate FPT. Some clinicians recommend testing the adequacy of passive transfer in crias of low birth weight. The most accurate determination of passive transfer is use of the *radial immunodiffusion test*. The best time to collect samples of blood for determination of adequacy of passive transfer is between 36 hours and 7 days of age. However, earlier often is better.

> **TECHNICIAN NOTE** The best time to test for passive transfer is between 36 hours and 7 days of age.

If crias are not dehydrated, serum protein and globulin concentrations may be helpful in determination of FPT. Serum readings of less than 4.5 g/dL could indicate FPT. Dehydration often correlates with a false-positive result. Commercial sodium sulfate tests are accurate in determining FPT if an end point of 300 mg/dL is used instead of the manufacturer's recommendations.

> **TECHNICIAN NOTE** Dehydration can be correlated with a false-positive result for failure of passive transfer.

Physical Examination of the Cria

The cria should be inspected for birth defects. Several facial deformities may present as congenital defects in crias. The inability to urinate secondary to vulvar deformities is a possibility in crias. Not all congenital defects are hereditary; some are induced by teratogens or viral infections, but once present in animals they still can be passed on to offspring. Therefore, no animal with a defect should be bred.

> **TECHNICIAN NOTE** No camelid with a defect should be bred.

IDENTIFICATION AND CARE OF THE SICK NEONATAL CRIA

Often the first sign of a sick neonatal cria is failure to gain weight or loss of body weight. Another sign of illness is reduced nursing. When a sick cria arrives at the clinic, a prompt physical examination should be performed. The technician should gather a thorough history to evaluate the cria's condition properly. Some of the more common problems associated with crias are hypothermia, FPT, dehydration, hypoglycemia, sepsis, prematurity, and congenital defects.

For crias with FPT, blood testing often reveals leukopenia or leukocytosis, with left shift neutrophilia. These hematologic findings may indicate sepsis. Daily or weekly weighing may increase the likelihood of identifying illness early, which is necessary to increase the probability of successful treatment.

> **TECHNICIAN NOTE** Daily or weekly weighing may increase the likelihood of identifying illness early, which is necessary to increase the probability of successful treatment.

Premature crias have been described as crias born before 335 days of gestation. Clinical signs include unerupted incisors, low birth weight, silky hair coats, floppy ears, and lack of a suckle reflex.

Many crias require the placement of an intravenous catheter for treatment of illness. This procedure is explained further in Chapter 19. On arrival, several tests may be required, including a serum glucose level, packed cell volume, blood gas analysis, complete blood count, and blood chemistry panel.

If oxygen therapy is needed, nasal insufflation tubes such as those for humans can be extremely useful for supplemental supplies of oxygen to the cria; otherwise, masks can be used.

> **TECHNICIAN NOTE** Premature crias are born before 335 days of gestation.

NUTRITION

Table 20-3 lists camelid dental formulas and a dental eruption table. Figure 20-19 shows the teeth of the maxillary and

TABLE 20-3	Camelid Dental Formulas and Dental Eruption Table
Deciduous: I 1/3 C1/1 P2–3/1–2 M0/0 × 2 = 18–22	
Permanent: I 1/3 C1/1 P1–2/1–2 M3/3 × 2 = 28–32	
Incisor 1	2–2.5 yr
Incisor 2	3–3.25 yr
Incisor 3	3.1–6 yr
Canines	2–7 yr (3.5 yr most common)
Premolar 3	3.5–5 yr
Premolar 4	3.5–4 yr
Molar 1	6–9 mo
Molar 2	1.5–2 yr
Molar 3	2.75–3.75 yr

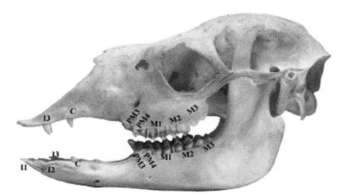

FIGURE 20-19 Skull of a male llama with teeth of the maxillary and mandibular arcades labeled. *C*, Canines; *I*, incisors; *PM*, premolars; *M*, molars. (From Anderson DE, Whitehead CE: *Veterinary clinics of North America food animal practice: alpaca and llama health management*, Philadelphia, 2009, Saunders.)

mandibular arcades, and Figure 20-20 shows body condition scoring for camelids.

DENTAL CARE

Dental problems in camelids often include tooth root abscesses, mandibular osteomyelitis, *malocclusion,* tooth fractures, uneven teeth, tooth overgrowth (Fig. 20-21), worn teeth, and retained deciduous teeth.

Camelids have incomplete rostral arcades with three lower incisors but only one upper incisor per side (Fig. 20-22). The premolars and molars are referred to as cheek teeth and are well established. The cheek teeth function to grind forages. The fourth premolar is almost always present but is smaller than the molars. The third premolar is frequently absent on clinical and radiographic examinations. Llamas and alpacas do not have first and second premolars.

In male llamas and alpacas, the permanent upper incisor and the upper and lower canines are referred to as the *fighting teeth*. Females and castrated males may or may not possess permanent canines. The deciduous canines are small and rarely erupt in females, and they erupt in only approximately

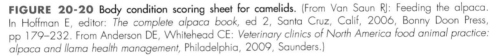

	Score	**Animal Description**	**1** Frontal Profile	**2** Rear Profile	**3** Spinous to Transverse Process	**4** Paralumbar Fossa
Emaciated	1.0	No visible or palpable fat or muscle between skin and bones. Ribs, dorsal spinous and transverse processes, and pelvic bones are individually prominent. Extreme loss of muscle mass.	Prominent "V" Keel	Acutely Inverted "V"	Deep depression	Gaunt, tucked-in fossa
Poor	1.5					
Thin	2.0	Slight cover over bony structure. Ribs, spinous processes still visible and easily palpated as sharp. Less muscle mass loss.	Gradual Flattening of Sternum	Gradual Filling of "V"	Obvious depression	Prominent shelf
Borderline	2.5					
Moderate	3.0	Overall smooth appearance. Slight fat cover over ribs and other bony processes. Ribs and spinous processes can be palpated with slight pressure. No muscle mass loss present	Moderate fat	Moderate fat	Smooth concave curve	Slight shelf
High Moderate	3.5				Smooth slope	
Excess	4.0	Fleshy appearance with visible coverage of fat. Moderate to firm pressure necessary to palpate bony structures under skin			Nearly flat	No shelf
Fat	4.5					Edge barely discernable
Grossly Obese	5.0	Excessive fat cover over entire body with smooth, rounded appearance. Bony prominences cannot be palpated, even with firm pressure. Bulging fat pads visible around tailhead	Sternum Bulging in fat	Inguinal Area Bulging in fat	Rounded	Buried in fat

FIGURE 20-20 Body condition scoring sheet for camelids. (From Van Saun RJ: Feeding the alpaca. In Hoffman E, editor: *The complete alpaca book,* ed 2, Santa Cruz, Calif, 2006, Bonny Doon Press, pp 179–232. From Anderson DE, Whitehead CE: *Veterinary clinics of North America food animal practice: alpaca and llama health management,* Philadelphia, 2009, Saunders.)

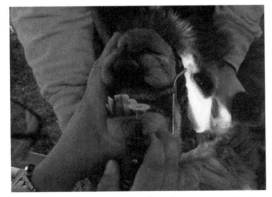

FIGURE 20-21 Alpaca with significantly overgrown incisors being trimmed with a rotary (Dremel)–style tool and diamond cutting plate. Use of a mouth speculum prevents potential injury to the dental pad. (From Anderson DE, Whitehead CE: *Veterinary clinics of North America food animal practice: alpaca and llama health management,* Philadelphia, 2009, Saunders.)

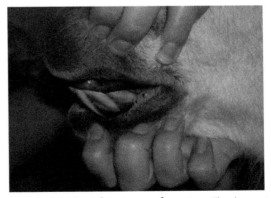

FIGURE 20-22 Normal incisor conformation. The lower incisors meet with the dental pad. Efforts should be made to achieve this incisor height during trimming. (From Anderson DE, Whitehead CE: *Veterinary clinics of North America food animal practice: alpaca and llama health management,* Philadelphia, 2009, Saunders.)

5% of males. They usually are not problematic, and routine floating of teeth is not recommended as in horses.

TECHNICIAN NOTE Routine floating of teeth is not recommended as in horses.

LIFE STAGES OF NUTRITION

Camelids are not classified as ruminants, but they are considered functional ruminants. Just like ruminants, functional ruminants convert roughage to usable nutrients. Camelids are extremely efficient in their ability to convert forages to energy. They do best when they are allowed to graze on pasture freely. Feed consumption is based on a percentage of body weight and is higher in smaller animals and lower in larger animals. Concentrates are rarely needed; if provided, they should be given carefully because obesity is common in overfed camelids.

Protein requirements for camelids are very similar to those in sheep and goats. When crude protein is calculated on a dry matter basis, camelids require 10% crude protein for maintenance and 16% for pregnancy, lactation, and growth.

Water should be provided ad libitum to camelids. Camelids require 9% to 13% of their body weight (kg) in water. When watering camelids in cold weather, it is important to know that camelids will not break through ice to reach a water source. Trail llamas most often drink water during the evening and often refuse to drink during the day. When water is withheld or is unavailable to lactating camelids, they often decrease milk production or stop milk production altogether. In extreme cases of water deprivation, camelids may become hyperthermic. Camelids have oval erythrocytes that can swell up to 240% of their normal size without lysing, whereas round erythrocytes in other animals can swell only up to 150% without lysing.

> *TECHNICIAN NOTE*   Llamas will not break through ice to drink.

MINERALS

The camelid diet should contain no more than 0.3% calcium on a dry matter basis. The calcium-to-phosphorus ratio should be no less than 1.2:1. Camelids are sensitive to copper, and copper toxicity can be a problem. Iron deficiency is thought to be a factor in the failure to thrive syndrome seen in the cria. Zinc deficiency in llamas and alpacas may manifest as dermatitis. All other mineral requirements are similar to those in other ruminants.

> *TECHNICIAN NOTE*   Camelids are sensitive to copper.

CASE STUDY

Mr. Cobb called into the clinic today saying he has a female cria that was born 8 hours ago, and he is sure that she has not been suckling. He would like the veterinarian to come see her and evaluate her status. The veterinarian agrees that the cria has not been suckling. What will the veterinarian most likely ask you to do?

CASE STUDY

Mr. Cobb calls into the clinic again that evening. He informs the veterinarian that the cria still is not suckling. When you explain the situation to the veterinarian, he has you tell Mr. Cobb to continue bottle feeding. What information should you provide to Mr. Cobb concerning milk products, frequency, and bonding?

SUGGESTED READING

Anderson DE, Whitehead CE: *Veterinary clinics of North America food animal practice: alpaca and llama health management*, Philadelphia, 2009, Saunders.

Bassert JM, McCurnin DM: In *McCurnin's clinical textbook for veterinary technicians*, ed 7, St. Louis, 2010, Saunders.

Birutta G: *Storey's guide to raising llamas*, North Adams, Mass, 1997, Versa Press.

Fowler ME: *Medicine and surgery of South American camelids*, ed 2, Ames, Iowa, 1998, Iowa State University Press.

Gerken M, Renieri C: *South American camelids research*, ed 2, Wageningen, Netherlands, 2008, Wageningen Academic Publishers.

Gillespie JR, Flanders FB: *Modern livestock and poultry*, ed 8, Clifton Park, NY, 2010, Delmar Cengage Learning.

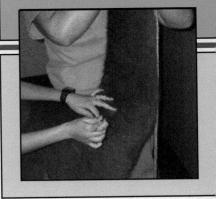

21 | Camelid Clinical Procedures

OUTLINE

LEARNING OBJECTIVES

After completing this chapter, you will be able to

- Set up and prepare the patient for each procedure, perform the procedure (when appropriate), or assist the clinician in performing diagnostic sampling and medication procedures
- Properly insert and maintain an intravenous catheter and monitor the catheter for complications
- Explain the rationale and indications for each of the clinical procedures described
- Set up materials and equipment and prepare the patient as needed for the procedure
- Provide assistance to the veterinarian when performing the procedure or perform the procedure when it may be appropriate for a veterinary technician to do so
- Perform or assist necropsy and sample collection procedures and maintain a safe environment during these procedures

KEY TERMS

Antecubital vein
Costochondral junction

Diverticulum
Dung pile

DIAGNOSTIC SAMPLING

VENOUS BLOOD SAMPLING

Equipment for venous blood sampling:
- Alcohol
- 18- to 20-gauge (ga) × 1½-inch needle
- Syringe
- Appropriate collection tubes

Blood draws for camelids typically are performed in stocks. If stocks are not available, a wall or fence can be used to help decrease movement of the animal. If a wall or fence is used for venous blood sampling, it is important that the camelid be accustomed to a halter.

The hair can be clipped to help gain access to the vein; however, this should be avoided because the wool may take up to 18 months to regrow. The wool should be clipped only with the owner's permission because some animals are used for show purposes.

> **TECHNICIAN NOTE** The owner's permission should be obtained before the wool is clipped because the wool can take up to 18 months to regrow.

Two techniques can be used to draw blood from a camelid: high neck jugular and low neck jugular. Use of the high neck jugular technique decreases the chance of arterial blood collection because the jugular vein is more superficial in this location than in the low venipuncture site.

> **TECHNICIAN NOTE** Use of the high neck jugular technique decreases the chance of arterial blood collection.

High Neck Jugular Technique

The skin in the cervical vertebrae region can be almost ½-inch thick, which can make the procedure more difficult.

However, the more challenging aspect is the location's protection provided by the transverse processes of the cervical vertebrae. To begin drawing blood from the high neck location, place the head of the animal so that the nose is completely perpendicular to the cervical vertebrae. The nose should not be tipped upward or downward. Palpate the sternomandibularis tendon. From this anatomical landmark, draw a line along the tendon, and insert the needle at the location just dorsally and caudally. Insert the needle where the two lines connect.

Distention of the vein is not common and should not be relied on as confirmation of vein location. However, flicking of the vein may lead to waves of blood felt in the occluding fingers. The technician then should insert an 18- to 20-gauge (ga) × 1½-inch-long needle. Digital pressure should be applied following needle withdrawal to help prevent hematoma formation. Hematoma formation is more common in camelids than in other species, especially neonates, so care should be taken to prevent this complication.

> **TECHNICIAN NOTE**   Distention of the vein in a high venipuncture is not common, and the technician should not rely on this as confirmation of vein location. However, flicking of the vein may lead to waves of blood felt in the occluding fingers.

Low Neck Jugular Technique

The low neck jugular venipuncture should be performed with the animal in stocks or performed against a fence or wall if the camelid is accustomed to a halter. To begin, elevate the camelid's head. The anatomical location of interest for this method of collection is the enlarged transverse process of the sixth cervical vertebrae. The jugular vein lies just medial to this process. Care should be taken to avoid the carotid artery, which is also located just medial to the process and can be identified by its pulsating. The technician should begin by occluding the vein. Confirmation of the jugular vein can be made visually by observation of its filling when it is occluded between the fifth and sixth cervical vertebrae (Fig. 21-1). The needle then can be inserted. Use of an 18- to 20-ga × 1½-inch needle is recommended. Table A2-3 in Appendix 2 provides an overview of white blood cell identification.

ARTERIAL BLOOD SAMPLING

Arterial blood sampling can readily be performed from the low neck jugular venipuncture location, which allows for readily palpable pulsing, as in the low neck venipuncture location. Table 21-1 lists normal complete blood count values for llamas, and Table 21-2 lists normal blood chemistry values for llamas.

ABDOMINOCENTESIS

Equipment for abdominocentesis:
- Clippers
- Surgical scrub and alcohol
- Needle, syringe, local anesthetic
- No. 12 scalpel blade
- 14-ga × 3-inch teat cannula
- Serum tube/red top tube

Abdominocentesis can be performed in camelids by placing them in stocks. A 4 × 4-inch area of wool is clipped on the ventral midline just caudal to the umbilicus. This caudal approach decreases the likelihood of entering the omentum. It is extremely important to stay directly on the linea alba because of the significantly thick fat pads lining each side of the linea alba. Insertion into the fat pads will not allow for fluid collection. Another location is the paracostal site (Fig. 21-2). The 4 × 4-inch area should be cleansed with iodine and alcohol, alternating each substance three times as if performing a surgical scrub.

It is common procedure to inject 3 to 5 mL of lidocaine into the needle insertion point at this time. A number 12 scalpel blade is used to make a stab incision. Care should be taken to avoid entering the peritoneal cavity. A 14-ga × 3-inch teat canula is inserted through the stab incision into the peritoneum with one quick thrust. If the sample is available, it can be collected at this time. If unavailable, the cannula can be redirected. If a sample still is unavailable, 10 mL of air can be injected into the abdomen, and negative pressure can be used to attempt collection with a syringe. If the bowel is entered, the collection sample will be green, and an antibiotic should be injected into the site (Figs. 21-3 and 21-4).

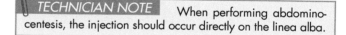

> **TECHNICIAN NOTE**   When performing abdominocentesis, the injection should occur directly on the linea alba.

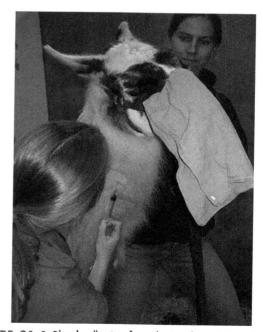

FIGURE 21-1 Blood collection from the jugular vein in a llama. A towel can be draped loosely through the halter on the bridge of the nose to protect personnel from being spat on if the animal objects to the procedure. (From Bassert J, Thomas J, editors: *McCurnin's clinical textbook for veterinary technicians,* ed 8, St. Louis, 2014, Saunders.)

URINE COLLECTION
Voided Urine Sampling
Equipment for voided urine sample:
- Sterile collection container

Free-catch urine samples can be collected by haltering the animal and leading it to the *dung pile*. Early morning collections may prove more effective. Some distance between the handler and the animal may help in the collection process. This can be accomplished by attaching a cup to a long pole (several feet long) and collecting the urine from a distance. Both male and female camelids squat to urinate. Urine can be collected from a lateral and caudal position.

> **TECHNICIAN NOTE** Using a pole several feet long to increase the distance between the handler and the camelid can aid in urine collection.

Bladder or Urethral Catheterization
Equipment for bladder or urethral catheterization:
- Surgical scrub and water
- Sterile gloves
- Sterile lubricating jelly
- 5-French (F) polypropylene or red rubber catheter
- Syringe
- Sterile collection container

Urinary catheterization of females can be accomplished. However, catheterization of male camelids is virtually impossible because of a dorsal recess at the level of the ischial arch. Female catheterization should begin with a thorough cleaning of the vulva with chlorhexidine or dilute iodine and water. The vulvar area then should be dried. The technician should don gloves. The gloves and the lubricating jelly should be sterile. The technician should insert a finger into the vulva and palpate ventrally, locating the external urethral orifice on the floor of the vulva. The technician should insert a 5-French (5-F) polypropylene catheter or red rubber catheter along the dorsal aspect of the orifice. The dorsal approach helps prevent entrance into the *diverticulum* located just ventral and caudal to the urethral orifice. The catheter is advanced approximately 25 cm into the bladder. A syringe then can be attached and urine collected into the syringe. If free-flowing urine is available, it can be collected in a sterile urine collection container.

TABLE 21-1	Normal Values for Complete Blood Count in Llamas	
Complete Blood Count		
Packed cell volume	Increased with polycythemia, dehydration, stress, in neonates, and high globulin levels Decreased with anemia, bleeding, overhydration, and in weanlings	29%–39%
Hemoglobin	Increased with polycythemia Decreased with anemia	12.8–17.6 g/dL
Red blood cells	Increased with polycythemia and dehydration Decreased with anemia and overhydration	$11.3–17.5 \times 10^6/\mu L$
Total protein	Increased in dehydration and in lipemic samples Decreased with overhydration	5.8–7 g/dL
White blood cells	Increased with acute local inflammation, toxicity, and bacterial infections Decreased with marrow diseases, radiation, drug therapy, and certain viruses	$7.5–21.5 \times 10^3/\mu L$
Platelets	Decreased in DIC	$2.4–6.1 \times 10^5/\mu L$
Mean corpuscular volume	Increased with vitamin B_{12} and folic acid deficiency Decreased with iron deficiency	21–28 fL
Mean corpuscular hemoglobin	Increased with hemolysis Decreased with iron deficiency	43.2–46.6 pg
Mean corpuscular hemoglobin concentration	Increased with hemolysis, lipemia, and Heinz bodies	38.9–46.2 g/dL
Bone marrow		0.9–2.9 myeloid/erythroid ratio
Differential, Absolute		
Segs		4.6–16
Bands		0–0.35
Lymphocytes		1–7.5
Monocytes		0.05–0.8
Eosinophils		0–3.3
Basophils		0–0.4

DIC, Disseminated intravascular coagulation.

TABLE 21-2	Normal Blood Chemistry Values in Llamas	
Blood urea nitrogen	Increased with kidney disease, azotemia, and uremia	13–32 mg/dL
Creatinine	Increased with kidney disease	1.5–2.9 mg/dL
Glucose	Decreased in fatty liver disease Increased with diabetes and stress	90–140 mg/dL
Albumin	Increased with dehydration Decreased with brucellosis, chronic liver disease, glomerular disease, hyperglobulinemia, hypertension, malnutrition, and malabsorption	3–5 g/dL
Total bilirubin	Increased in liver disease, bile duct obstruction, jaundice, or hemolytic anemia	0–0.1 mg/dL
Aspartate aminotransferase	Increased in liver disease or with muscle damage Possibly increased after exercise	110–250 μg/L
γ-Glutamyl transferase	Increased with hepatocellular and cholestatic liver disease, hepatocyte necrosis, and cholestasis	5–29 μg/L
Creatine kinase	Increased with muscle disease	30–400 μg/L
Alkaline phosphatase	Increased with liver disease and cholestasis, steroids, and growth	30–780 μg/L
Lactate dehydrogenase	Increased with hepatocyte damage, muscle damage, and hemolysis	50–300 μg/L
Sodium	When increased can cause neurologic disorders and hypertension Decreased possibly from *Escherichia coli*, polyuria or polydipsia, weight loss, and anorexia	147–158 mEq/L
Potassium	Increased possibly from severe metabolic acidosis Decreased possibly from anorexia, increased renal excretion, abomasal stasis, intestinal obstruction, enteritis, and weight loss	4.3–5.6 mEq/L
Chloride	Increased during displaced abomasums	106–118 mEq/L
Calcium	Increased with kidney stones, renal failure, and some cancers Decreased in milk fever, renal disease, and bone disease	7.7–9.4 mg/dL
Phosphorus	Increased in renal failure Decreased with osteomalacia, rickets, and tetany	4.6–9.8 mg/dL
Magnesium	Decreased in milk fever, grass tetany, fever, and hypersalivation	1.5–3 mg/dL

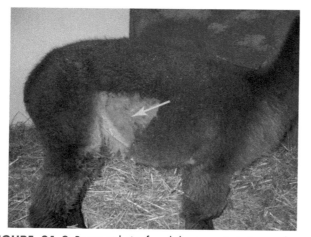

FIGURE 21-2 Paracostal site for abdominocentesis in an alpaca. (From Bassert J, Thomas J, editors: *McCurnin's clinical textbook for veterinary technicians,* ed 8, St. Louis, 2014, Saunders.)

TECHNICIAN NOTE Bladder catheterization of male camelids is virtually impossible as a result of the dorsal recess at the level of the ischial arch.

FECAL COLLECTION

Equipment for fecal collection:
• Glove

Feces for collection can often be readily accessed from the animal's dung pile. Owners can be asked to bring a fresh sample of feces with them when they visit the clinic. If a fresh sample is not available, fecal collection is often performed with use of the dung pile. The animal should be haltered and led to the dung pile. Sometimes this encourages the camelid to defecate. If this method proves ineffective, gentle

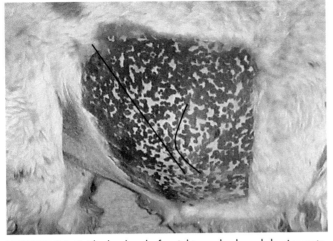

FIGURE 21-3 The landmarks for right paralumbar abdominocentesis. The *black lines* represent the caudal margin of the last rib *(curve)* and the linea semilunaris or aponeurosis of the external abdominal oblique muscle *(straight)*. The *red dot* represents the approximate site for centesis. (From Cebra C, Anderson D, Tibary A, et al, editors: *Llama and alpaca care: medicine, surgery, reproduction, nutrition, and herd health,* St. Louis, 2014, Saunders.)

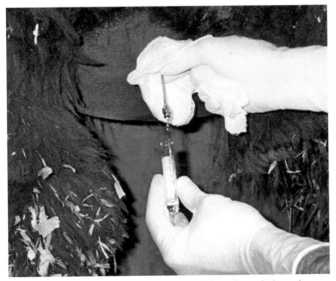

FIGURE 21-4 Obtaining peritoneal fluid from the right lateral site in an alpaca. (From Cebra C, Anderson D, Tibary A, et al, editors: *Llama and alpaca care: medicine, surgery, reproduction, nutrition, and herd health,* St. Louis, 2014, Saunders.)

stimulation of the rectal wall with a lubricated finger can be used to encourage defecation.

> **TECHNICIAN NOTE** Haltering and leading a camelid to the dung pile can encourage defecation.

THORACOCENTESIS

Equipment for thoracocentesis:
- Clippers
- Surgical scrub and alcohol

- 16-ga × 2-inch needle
- Syringe
- Antibiotic ointment
- Iodine

The thoracocentesis procedure in camelids can be performed from the sixth intercostal space. Camelids have 12 ribs, so the sixth intercostal space can be identified by counting from the last rib. At the location of the sixth intercostal space, a 4 × 4-inch area is clipped 1 to 2 inches dorsal to the *costochondral junction.* A surgical scrub is performed. A 16-ga × 2-inch needle is inserted along the cranial border of the seventh rib. The needle is advanced 1 to 1½ inches into the pleural cavity. The insertion point should always be on the cranial border because of the presence of intercostal vessels on the caudal aspect of each rib. The sample can be collected, with use of a 12-mL syringe most often applicable. The needle is removed, and the site is sprayed with iodine. Antibiotic ointment also can be applied.

> **TECHNICIAN NOTE** Camelids have 12 ribs.

> **TECHNICIAN NOTE** When a needle is inserted during thoracocentesis, it should always be placed at the cranial border of the rib because of the presence of intercostal vessels on the caudal aspect of each rib.

LIVER BIOPSY

Equipment for liver biopsy:
- Clippers
- Surgical scrub and alcohol
- Local anesthetic
- 14-ga × 6-inch Tru-cut biopsy needle

The camelid should be restrained in stocks. A 3 × 3-inch area is clipped at the ninth intercostal space approximately 9 to 10 inches from the top of the back on the right side. A surgical preparation should be performed. Approximately 1 mL of lidocaine should be injected over the insertion site. If ultrasound is being used, the exact liver biopsy location can be identified at this time. A 14-ga × 6-inch Tru-cut biopsy needle is inserted and angled toward midline, caudally and slightly ventrally. The diaphragm is immediately adjacent to the chest wall, which is thin. To confirm placement, let go of the needle after placement. Needles that are correctly placed within the diaphragm move cranially and caudally in synchronization with respiration. The needle should be aimed at the contralateral stifle.

MEDICATION TECHNIQUES

ORAL MEDICATIONS
Oral Pastes

Camelids that will be given oral paste are ideally restrained in stocks. If stocks are not available and the animal is handled frequently, oral pastes can be delivered using just a halter. However, if stocks are unavailable and the animal is seldom handled, it can be tied as close to a post as possible. The tube is then placed into the interdental space. The tube is advanced to the caudal aspect of the mouth and inserted. Care should be taken to avoid injecting medication into the cheek pouch for fear of ulceration after prolonged medication contact. The head can be lifted after the procedure to discourage spitting of the medication (Fig. 21-5).

> **TECHNICIAN NOTE** Care should be taken to prevent administration of oral medications into the cheek pouch.

Orogastric Intubation

Orogastric intubation of camelids is performed using the same technique as in cattle (see Chapter 13). Small camelids can be restrained in sternal recumbency with the technician straddling the animal. A small polyvinyl chloride pipe wrapped in tape can be used as an oral speculum. For camelids weighing 10 to 20 pounds, an 18- to 22-F, ¼-inch outside diameter tube can be used. For camelids weighing 65 to 200 pounds, a 30- to 40-F, ½-inch outside diameter tube can be used. For camelids weighing more than 200 pounds, a 40- to 45-F, ½- to ⅝-inch outside diameter tube can be used. Slight flexing of the head may help with tube placement (Fig. 21-6). Camelids may regurgitate during tube placement; if this occurs, the tube should be removed, and the technician should start over.

> **TECHNICIAN NOTE** If camelids regurgitate during placement of an orogastric tube, the tube should be removed, and the technician should start over.

PARENTERAL INJECTION TECHNIQUES

Intramuscular Injections

Equipment for intramuscular injections:
- Alcohol
- 18-ga × 1-inch needle for adults
- 20- to 22-ga × 1-inch needles for crias
- Syringe

The most common locations for intramuscular injections in camelids are the semimembranosus, triceps, semitendinosus (Fig. 21-7), and caudal cervical epaxial muscles (Fig. 21-8). Neck muscles should be avoided in camelids. The camelid should be restrained in stocks if available. However, if the camelid is accustomed to a halter, then injections can be given using halter restraint. The site should be cleansed with alcohol until the 4 × 4 gauze pad used to wipe the area comes away clean. An 18-ga × 1-inch needle should be used for adults, and a 20- to 22-ga × 1-inch needle should be used for crias. The needle should be inserted using one quick motion. The technician should aspirate and then inject. If blood is obtained on

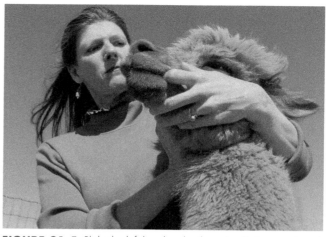

FIGURE 21-5 Slide the left hand under the animal's jaw, and work your index finger well inside the corner of the mouth. (From Cebra C, Anderson D, Tibary A, et al, editors: *Llama and alpaca care: medicine, surgery, reproduction, nutrition, and herd health*, St. Louis, 2014, Saunders.)

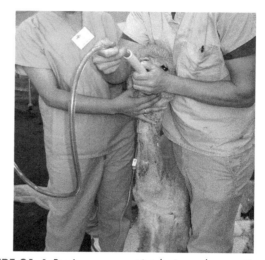

FIGURE 21-6 Passing an orogastric tube in an alpaca patient. (From Bassert J, Thomas J, editors: *McCurnin's clinical textbook for veterinary technicians*, ed 8, St. Louis, 2014, Saunders.)

aspiration, the technician should withdraw the needle, replace it with a new needle, and inject in another location. Multiple injections should be given at least 1 inch apart (Fig. 21-9).

> **TECHNICIAN NOTE** Multiple injections should be given at least 1 inch apart.

Intravenous Injections

Equipment for intravenous injections:
- Alcohol
- 18- to 20-ga × 1½-inch needle for adults
- 20- to 22-ga × 1-inch needles for crias
- Syringe

To perform an intravenous injection in a camelid, restrain the animal in stocks. The location of the injection should be

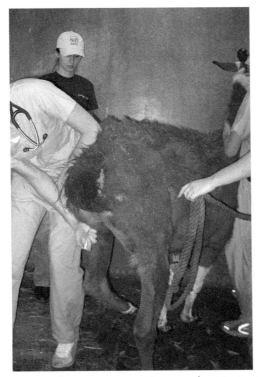

FIGURE 21-7 Llama receiving an intramuscular injection into the semitendinosus muscle. (From Bassert J, Thomas J, editors: *McCurnin's clinical textbook for veterinary technicians*, ed 8, St. Louis, 2014, Saunders.)

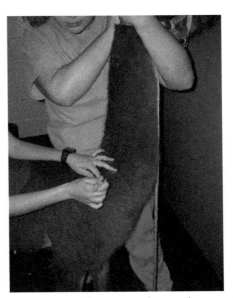

FIGURE 21-8 Intramuscular injection being administered into the caudal cervical epaxial muscles. (From Anderson DE, Whitehead CE: *Veterinary clinics of North America food animal practice: alpaca and llama health management*, Philadelphia, 2009, Saunders.)

the same as for a low neck jugular venipuncture. A 20- to 22-ga × 1-inch needle should be used for crias, and an 18- to 20-ga × 1½-inch needle should be used for adults. The needle should be inserted so that the medication is injected toward the heart. Once the needle is placed, the technician first should confirm by aspiration that the carotid artery has not been entered and then inject. On removal of the needle, digital pressure should be applied to the site for at least 1 minute to decrease the chance of hematoma formation.

> **TECHNICIAN NOTE**   Intravenous injections should be given so that the medication is injected toward the heart.

Subcutaneous Injections

Equipment for subcutaneous injections:
- Alcohol
- 18- to 20-ga × 1-inch needle for adults
- 20- to 22-ga × 1-inch needles for crias
- Syringe

To perform a subcutaneous injection in camelids, the animal should be restrained using a halter or stocks, depending on the extent of previous handling. Injection sites include just cranial to the shoulder and caudal to the elbow (Fig. 21-10). The area should be cleansed with alcohol until the 4 × 4 gauze pad remains clean after wiping. A 20- to 22-ga × 1-inch needle is used for crias, and an 18- to 20-ga × 1-inch needle is used for adults. The skin is tented, and the

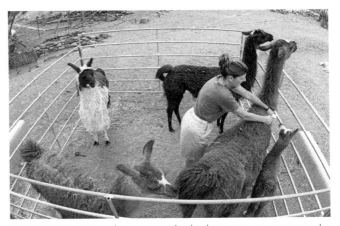

FIGURE 21-9 Reaching across the body to give an intramuscular shot ensures that when the animal moves away from the needle, it moves toward the handler. This means less need for restraint. (From Cebra C, Anderson D, Tibary A, et al, editors: *Llama and alpaca care: medicine, surgery, reproduction, nutrition, and herd health*, St. Louis, 2014, Saunders.)

needle is inserted into the tent. It is common for camelids to kick out during the procedure, so care should be taken to protect other personnel from being kicked and to avoid injecting your hand. The needle should be withdrawn and the site rubbed to ease the pain of injection.

> **TECHNICIAN NOTE**   Camelids often kick out during subcutaneous injections. Care should be taken to avoid being kicked.

Intravenous Catheterization

The procedure for placing intravenous catheters in camelids is similar to that in cattle (see Chapter 13). The camelid should

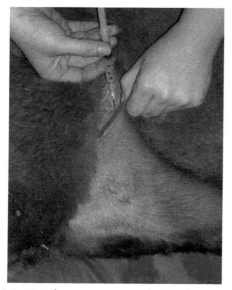

FIGURE 21-10 Subcutaneous injection being administered over the thoracic wall, behind the elbow. (From Anderson DE, Whitehead CE: *Veterinary clinics of North America food animal practice: alpaca and llama health management,* Philadelphia, 2009, Saunders.)

be restrained in stocks and the head secured. The same area used for a low neck jugular venipuncture should be used for catheter placement (Fig. 21-11). A 4 × 4-inch area should be clipped, and surgical preparation should be performed. The right jugular vein seems to be easier to catheterize than the left; however, catheters can be placed in the left jugular vein. Other areas that can be used include the cephalic and *antecubital veins.* The catheter is inserted following the same procedure used in cattle. Another location for placement is the ear artery (Figs. 21-12 and 21-13).

> ⧗ *TECHNICIAN NOTE* When placing intravenous catheters, the technician should wear surgical gloves.

HOOF TRIMMING

Camelids have a toenail around a soft footpad, rather than a hoof. This toenail should be trimmed flush with the soft pad using small, shear-type foot trimming instruments (Fig. 21-14). Most camelids require hoof trimming only once per year, but some may require trimming two to three times per year (Fig. 21-15).

> ⧗ *TECHNICIAN NOTE* Most camelids require hoof trimming only once per year, but some may require trimming two to three times per year.

EUTHANASIA AND NECROPSY

Euthanasia and necropsy of camelids are performed in the same manner as in cattle (see Chapter 13).

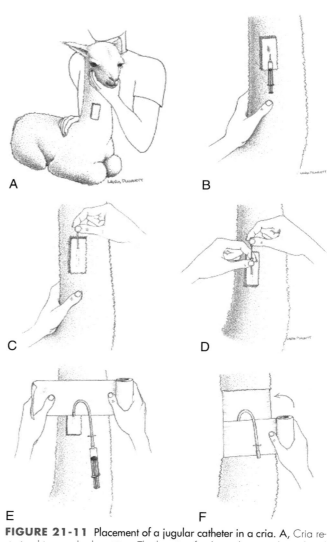

FIGURE 21-11 Placement of a jugular catheter in a cria. **A,** Cria restrained in a cushed position. The location for the catheter is clipped and prepared. **B,** Local anesthetic placement. **C** and **D,** Catheter placement. **E** and **F,** Extension tubing placed and an elastic tape (Elastikon) bandage used for stabilization. (From Anderson DE, Whitehead CE: *Veterinary clinics of North America food animal practice: alpaca and llama health management,* Philadelphia, 2009, Saunders.)

CASE STUDY

Mrs. Zeisler is concerned that her camelid has parasites. You ask her to bring in a sample of feces for evaluation. Mrs. Zeisler asks how she should collect the feces. What do you tell her?

CASE STUDY

Mrs. Luther has a female llama she would like vaccinated. The vaccination is going to be given subcutaneously. You will be performing the vaccination. Just as you are ready to give the injection, you notice that Mrs. Luther is standing just off to the side of the llama's hip. Should you be concerned with this situation? What should you do?

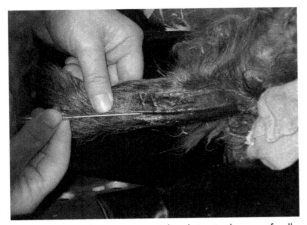

FIGURE 21-12 Placing an arterial catheter in the ear of a llama. (From Bassert J, Thomas J, editors: *McCurnin's clinical textbook for veterinary technicians*, ed 8, St. Louis, 2014, Saunders.)

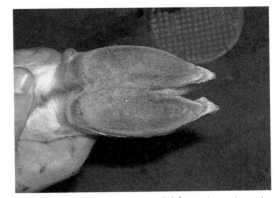

FIGURE 21-14 Well-trimmed camelid foot. The V-shaped nail has been trimmed flush with the weight-bearing surface of the foot. (From Anderson DE, Whitehead CE: *Veterinary clinics of North America food animal practice: alpaca and llama health management*, Philadelphia, 2009, Saunders.)

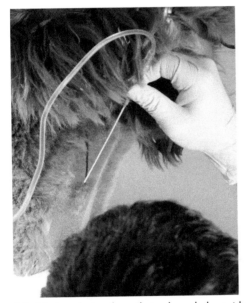

FIGURE 21-13 Introducing the catheter through the guide incision. Note the angle and the catheter being advanced parallel to the course of the vein. (From Cebra C, Anderson D, Tibary A, et al, editors: *Llama and alpaca care: medicine, surgery, reproduction, nutrition, and herd health*, St. Louis, 2014, Saunders.)

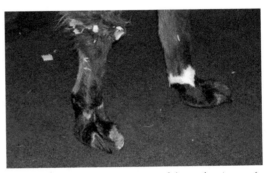

FIGURE 21-15 Llama with deviation of the nails. This conformation generally requires more frequent trimming because of the lack of normal wear. (From Anderson DE, Whitehead CE: *Veterinary clinics of North America food animal practice: alpaca and llama health management*, Philadelphia, 2009, Saunders.)

SUGGESTED READING

Anderson DE, Whitehead CE: *Veterinary clinics of North America food animal practice: alpaca and llama health management*, Philadelphia, 2009, Saunders.

Bassert JM, McCurnin DM, editors: *McCurnin's clinical textbook for veterinary technicians*, ed 7, St. Louis, 2010, Saunders.

Birutta G: *Storey's guide to raising llamas*, North Adams, Mass, 1997, Versa Press.

Fowler ME: *Medicine and surgery of South American camelids*, ed 2, Ames, Iowa, 1998, Iowa State University Press.

Gerken M, Renieri C: *South American camelids research*, ed 8, Wageningen, Netherlands, 2008, Wageningen Academic Publishers.

Gillespie JR, Flanders FB: *Modern livestock and poultry*, ed 8, Clifton Park, NY, 2010, Delmar Cengage Learning.

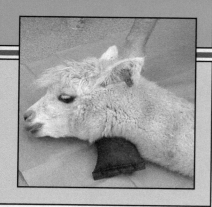

22 Camelid Surgical Procedures

OUTLINE

LEARNING OBJECTIVES

When you finish this chapter, you will be able to

- Understand the basic differences between standing surgical procedures and general anesthesia procedures
- Prepare a patient for surgical procedures
- Assist and/or perform induction and maintenance of anesthesia
- Provide anesthetic monitoring
- Manage the patient during recovery and immediate postoperative periods
- Understand the basic risks and possible complications associated with anesthesia and surgery, and implement preventive measures when indicated

KEY TERMS

Bloat
Double drip

Mean arterial pressure
Packed cell volume

Total protein
Triple drip

PREPARATION FOR SURGERY

FASTING

As with other ruminants, regurgitation can occur during anesthesia. Camelids do not typically *bloat* in lateral recumbency or during anesthesia. Fasting is recommended for patients more than 4 months old. The recommendation is to withhold food for 12 to 18 hours while providing full access to water. Fasting reduces the gastrointestinal (GI) system volume, which reduces pressure on the diaphragm and the potential for passive regurgitation during anesthesia. Fasting of patients less than 4 months old is not recommended because of their limited energy reserves. Younger patients, especially those that are nursing, are at risk for hypoglycemia, so they are often supplemented with dextrose during anesthesia. Technicians should remember that increased body temperature increases the risk for hypoglycemia in younger patients. When hypoglycemia does occur, it usually is not recognized until the recovery period. Struggling with a patient during the preanesthetic period has been shown to increase body temperature and should be avoided.

> **TECHNICIAN NOTE**
> - Fasting is recommended for 12 to 18 hours in camelids older than 4 months. Water should always be provided during this time.
> - Never struggle with surgical patients, especially young patients, because it can increase their risk for hypoglycemia.

GENERAL ANESTHESIA

ANESTHETIC RISKS FOR CAMELID SURGERY

As with other ruminants, camelids produce saliva when they are sedated or anesthetized. The same precautions taken for saliva production in other ruminants should be practiced in camelids. The body of the camelid should be elevated, allowing the head to slope gradually to the operating table or ground (if in a field setting). The head should lie laterally against its resting surface. If the neck must be twisted to rest the head in this position, it is important to avoid major twisting; make the twist gradual from the shoulder to the head. The use of large pads should be avoided because they can limit venous return from the head and cause edema formation.

Nasal edema probably is the most commonly recognized complication of anesthesia in camelid patients. Even though the camelid is able to mouth breathe, nasal edema places unnecessary stress on the animal. All the equipment for endotracheal intubation must be available should respiratory distress occur, especially during the recovery process.

> **TECHNICIAN NOTE** The most common complication of camelid anesthesia is nasal edema.

PREANESTHETIC PREPARATION AND ANESTHETIC MANAGEMENT

Preanesthetic Evaluation

A physical examination should be performed on each camelid patient. The *packed cell volume* and *total protein* should be evaluated preoperatively. If possible, a complete blood cell count and fibrinogen level should be obtained, to provide valuable information before the surgical procedure. It is important to remember to keep the patient calm during the preanesthetic period.

> **TECHNICIAN NOTE** It is important to keep the patient calm during the preanesthetic period.

Preanesthetic Drugs

Anxious or unruly camelid patients experience greater alterations in cardiac output. Using sedatives can help control and alter this response to induction of anesthesia. When camelids are moderately sedated, they tend to lie down in sternal recumbency. If this occurs, induction should begin.

Xylazine is commonly used to reduce anxiety from environment stresses associated with surgical preparation. Other alpha-2 adrenergic agonists (e.g., detomidine, romifidine, and medetomidine) can be used but are more expensive, and the longer duration of action usually is not necessary. Large doses of alpha-2 adrenergic agonists can cause severe respiratory depression. Administration of alpha-2 adrenergic agonists to hyperkalemic patients can result in heart block. Use of alpha-2 adrenergic agonists should be reversed as soon as possible with alpha-2 adrenergic antagonists to minimize GI side effects. Alpha-2 adrenergic antagonists should be given when the animal is able to lift its head from the floor.

Ruminants respond favorably to benzodiazepines when these drugs are used for calming effect. Diazepam is commonly used and is best given intravenously, intramuscularly, or subcutaneously. Intramuscular absorption is variable, and other administration methods are more reliable.

Butorphanol, an opioid agonist–antagonist, is an analgesic drug with sedative effects.

Guaifenesin is a centrally acting muscle relaxant with sedative effects. Guaifenesin concentrations greater than 10% have been known to cause hemolysis in ruminants and should not be used. Concentrations of 5% can be purchased commercially.

> **TECHNICIAN NOTE** Guaifenesin concentrations greater than 10% should not be used in ruminants.

Atropine does not reduce saliva production; it just reduces the aqueous portion (making the mucus thicker). It should not be used in ruminants because it decreases GI motility.

Anesthetic Induction Drugs

Induction of anesthesia in camelids typically uses a combination of sedative and ketamine. In small ruminants, the common combination is diazepam and ketamine. In larger camelids, diazepam and ketamine are infused until the animal becomes weak, and then a bolus of ketamine and diazepam is administered.

Llamas and alpacas that weigh less than 200 kg can be maintained safely with a small animal anesthesia machine. Camelids that weigh more than 200 kg require the use of a large animal anesthetic machine. Small and large animal anesthesia machines use different adapters to connect the endotracheal tubes to the Y-piece. The endotracheal tube size that is appropriate for the patient determines which machine is used because the adapters are different for each machine. Adult alpacas typically require 9- to 10-mm endotracheal tubes. Small animal endotracheal tubes may not always be long enough, but longer 5- to 14-mm silicone endotracheal tubes are available.

> **TECHNICIAN NOTE** Before intubation, technicians should keep the nose of a camelid down to facilitate drainage of saliva and prevent pooling near the larynx.

Small camelids are intubated much like a dog or cat, by using direct visualization. Use of a laryngoscope with a long blade can aid in intubation of camelids. An assistant restrains the camelid while straddling the back and holding the animal in sternal recumbency. The neck is extended, and the mouth is held open by the assistant. Once the camelid loses jaw tone, intubation should be attempted.

> **TECHNICIAN NOTE** Lack of jaw tone and absence of chewing or lingual response are used to indicate the appropriate time of intubation.

A stylet can be used to help with the intubation process. When a stylet is used to intubate, it is important to avoid damaging the mucosal surface of the airway. Regurgitated material is common in the mouth of ruminants and camelids, so care should be taken to ensure that this material does not enter the airway during endotracheal intubation.

In larger camelids, manual intubation is used, similar to the procedure in adult cattle (Figs. 22-1 to 22-4).

> **TECHNICIAN NOTE** Feed material is often found in the mouth on intubation. Care should be taken to avoid introducing this material into the airway.

Surgical procedures in small alpacas and llamas can be performed on a small animal operating table. Larger animals require the use of a foal or large animal operating table. Field surgery requires access to electricity and water. When preparing for surgery in the field, choose a flat, even surface away from fences or buildings. Padding should be used during the surgical procedure to cushion the animal. Arranging the padding into a trough shape makes dorsal recumbency easier to maintain. Most animals are moved from the floor to the operating table by hand, but hoists can be used to move camelids. Hobbles usually are placed on the animal during the surgical procedure.

When the camelid is placed in lateral recumbency, the eye on the downward side should be closed; a towel can be placed under the eye for added protection. Ophthalmic ointment should be placed in the eye. If bodily fluids enter the eye, it should be rinsed before or during recovery.

Maintenance of Anesthesia

Ketamine is the most common injectable anesthetic agent used in camelids. Thiopental is often reserved for use in patients whose depth of anesthesia is too light during inhalation maintenance anesthesia. Because of the cost of Telazol (tiletamine and zolazepam), it is not often used in the livestock industry. *Double-drip* and *triple-drip* combinations seem to provide a more stable plane of anesthesia. Remember that camelids are more resistant to the sedative effect of xylazine than are ruminants.

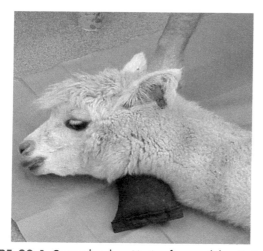

FIGURE 22-1 Correct head positioning for camelid patients in lateral recumbency. (From Cebra C, Anderson D, Tibary A, et al, editors: *Llama and alpaca care: medicine, surgery, reproduction, nutrition, and herd health,* St. Louis, 2014, Saunders.)

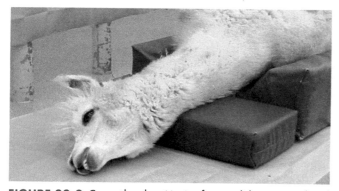

FIGURE 22-2 Correct head positioning for camelid patients in dorsal recumbency. (From Cebra C, Anderson D, Tibary A, et al, editors: *Llama and alpaca care: medicine, surgery, reproduction, nutrition, and herd health,* St. Louis, 2014, Saunders.)

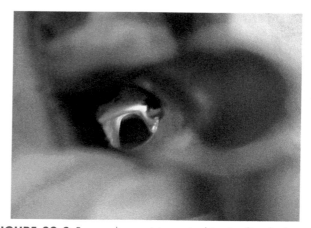

FIGURE 22-3 Proper alignment is required to visualize the larynx. (From Cebra C, Anderson D, Tibary A, et al, editors: *Llama and alpaca care: medicine, surgery, reproduction, nutrition, and herd health,* St. Louis, 2014, Saunders.)

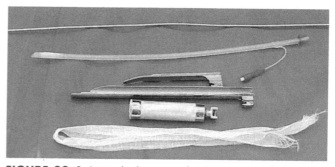

FIGURE 22-4 A ⅛-inch aluminum stylet, Bivona Aire-Cuf silicone endotracheal tube, Miller no. 4 laryngoscope blade, Wisconsin 11-inch laryngoscope blade, laryngoscope handle, and gauze tie. (From Cebra C, Anderson D, Tibary A, et al, editors: *Llama and alpaca care: medicine, surgery, reproduction, nutrition, and herd health,* St. Louis, 2014, Saunders.)

> **TECHNICIAN NOTE** Ketamine is the injectable anesthetic agent most commonly used in camelids.

Depth of Anesthesia

Monitoring the depth of anesthesia is best accomplished using a variety of parameters. Palpebral reflex, eye movement, changes in ventilation, and arterial blood pressure are the most useful parameters.

Monitoring of Anesthesia

During anesthesia, record the heart rate, respiratory rate, arterial blood pressure, and tidal volume every 5 minutes. The occurrence of any problems indicates that these numbers should be recorded and evaluated more often.

Ventilation

The respiratory rate during anesthesia should be 10 to 20 breaths/minute in adults and 15 to 25 in crias. Perhaps because of their high-altitude origins, llamas and alpacas typically exhibit excellent pulmonary gas exchange during anesthesia. Camelids tend to ventilate efficiently during inhalation maintenance anesthesia. The arterial partial pressure of carbon dioxide ($PaCO_2$) typically is 40 to 50 mm Hg. During inhalation maintenance anesthesia, camelid patients generally have end-tidal (ET) CO_2 values of 30 to 40 mm Hg. Applying the expected 10 mm Hg difference produces an estimated $PaCO_2$ of 40 to 50 mm Hg.

> **TECHNICIAN NOTE** Adult camelids should have a respiratory rate of 10 to 30 breaths/minute while they are under anesthesia.

Circulation

In camelids, the ear vein is used to monitor arterial blood pressure. The vein can be cannulated with a 22- or 20-gauge over-the-needle catheter. Blood pressure can also be monitored indirectly using a Doppler microphone and sphygmomanometer or oscillometric monitor. The cuff usually is placed on the forelimb just proximal to the carpus. Mean arterial blood pressure in normal healthy adult camelids is generally 80 to 100 mm Hg at the surgical plane of anesthesia, although crias with a *mean arterial pressure* of 50 mm Hg seem to do fine.

During anesthesia, the heart rate should remain between 40 and 70 beats/minute (bpm) in adults. Crias may have a slightly higher heart rate during anesthesia. Bradycardia is the most common complication of anesthesia. Anticholinergic drugs may be required.

> **TECHNICIAN NOTE** The heart rate should be 40 to 70 bpm in adult anesthetized camelids.

Temperature Regulation

Young animals have trouble maintaining body temperature. A hot water blanket should be placed underneath these patients to reduce the risk for hypothermia.

> **TECHNICIAN NOTE** A hot water blanket can be used to prevent hypothermia in young patients.

Intravenous Fluids

During surgical procedure in camelid patients, a balanced electrolyte solution should be administered at a rate of 10 mL/kg/hour for the first hour and 5 mL/kg/hour for the following hours of surgery and recovery. During cases of hypotension, a single 5 to 10 mL/kg bolus of electrolyte solution can be beneficial, although excess amounts should be avoided because of the risk for edema formation.

Oxygen Supplementation

Camelid patients tend to ventilate efficiently during anesthesia. When ventilation is required, manual ventilation can be performed.

RECOVERY

Camelids usually do not attempt to stand until they are fully awake and functional. Placing the camelid in sternal recumbency helps vent any fermentation gas trapped in the first compartment, although bloat typically does not occur in camelids under anesthesia. Sternal recumbency also allows saliva and any regurgitation material to drain from the oral cavity.

Nasal or laryngeal edema can develop during anesthesia and can produce respiratory distress during recovery. All endotracheal intubation materials should be present during recovery in case the patient requires reintubation.

> **TECHNICIAN NOTE** Nasal edema can develop during anesthesia and result in respiratory distress.

The patient should be extubated once it shows signs of "chewing activity." As with ruminants, camelids should be extubated with the endotracheal cuff inflated. This helps drag saliva and regurgitation material out of the trachea. Because camelids possess sharp teeth, endotracheal tube damage is not uncommon.

> **TECHNICIAN NOTE** Camelids should be extubated with the endotracheal cuff inflated.

For an explanation of drug categories, please see Chapter 10 (Table 22-1).

TABLE 22-1	Drugs Used in Camelid Surgical Procedures					
DRUG	**DOSE**	**CONCENTRATION**	**ROUTE**	**MEAT WITHDRAWAL TIME**	**MILK WITHDRAWAL TIME**
Flunixin meglumine	1.1–2.2 mg q12–24h	50 mg/mL	IV	4 days	36 hr
Phenylbutazone	4 mg/kg q12h	IV: 200 mg/mL PO: 100-mg tablets, 6-g tube, 12-g tube	IV or PO	CANNOT USE IN FOOD ANIMALS >20 MO OLD	
Ketoprofen	3.3 mg/kg q24h	100 mg/mL	IV or IM	4–7 days	
Meloxicam	0.6 mg/kg q12–24h	5 mg/mL			
Acetylsalicylic acid (aspirin)	50–100 mg/kg q12h	240-gr bolus 480-gr bolus	PO	24 hr	24 hr
Xylazine	0.2–1 mg/kg q30min–1h	100 mg/mL	IV, IM, SC		
Detomidine	0.02–0.04 mg/kg q1–2h	10 mg/mL	IV or IM		
Morphine	0.1–0.7 mg/kg q4–6h	0.5–50 g/mL	IV or IM		
Butorphanol	0.01–0.4 mg/kg q2–4h	10 mg/mL	IV, IM, or SC		
Buprenorphine	0.006–0.02 mg/kg q6–8h	0.3 mg/mL	IV, IM, or SC		
Ketamine	1–2 mg/kg q4–6h	100 mg/mL	IV or IM		
Gabapentin	5–20 mg/kg q8–12h	100-mg tablet 300-mg tablet	PO		

IM, Intramuscularly; *IV,* intravenously; *PO,* orally; *SC,* subcutaneously.

COMMON SURGICAL PROCEDURES

CASTRATION

The castration procedure is performed in camelids at approximately 2 years of age. The procedure is performed to help reduce breeding behavior, although it may not always be effective at accomplishing this goal. One of the major debates within the industry is the castration of males before the age of 2 years. Many owners would like to castrate crias at 4 to 6 months of age so that the animals can be sold as pets; however, veterinarians prefer to wait until the musculoskeletal system has matured. Crias gelded before 2 years of age may develop straight hindlimbs that cause undue stress on the joints. They also may develop lateral patellar luxation and degenerative osteoarthritis of the stifle joints.

> **TECHNICIAN NOTE**   It is best to wait until 2 years of age before castrating camelids.

Although all methods of castration used in livestock have been successful in camelids, two procedures have become quite common: the scrotal procedure used in horses and swine and the prescrotal castration procedure similar to that performed in the dog.

Scrotal castration can be done with the animal standing or recumbent. For standing castration, xylazine and butorphanol are commonly used with an epidural technique or a line block along the median raphe. The scrotum is surgically prepared, and an incision is made on either side of the median raphe along the most ventral aspect of the scrotum.

Each testicle is removed with an emasculator or is ligated and removed. Application of insecticide to the area around the incision is advisable during fly season.

Prescrotal castration is performed with the camelid in lateral recumbency. The ventral midline just cranial to the scrotum is surgically prepared. An incision is made on the ventral midline. Each testicle is removed through the incision, ligated, and removed, and the incision is closed. Postoperative care includes confinement of the male to a small pen for approximately 1 to 2 days. The incision should be monitored for bleeding and exudative discharge. Monitoring for regular and normal urination postoperatively is important.

CESAREAN SECTION

Cesarean sections are most commonly performed through a ventral midline laparotomy or paralumbar fossa. When the paralumbar approach is performed, the female should be placed in right lateral recumbency. General anesthesia can be used for cesarean section, but sedation and local anesthesia usually provide more alert cria. An incision is made cranially and ventrally to the tuber coxae and is continued cranially and ventrally toward the costochondral junction. When an incision is made into the uterus, care must be taken to avoid cutting the cria. The lining of the uterus is very thin. The fetuses are removed and treated as any neonate delivered by cesarean section (Fig. 22-5). The uterus is flushed out to remove all blood clots. The uterus is closed, followed by the muscle layers and skin. Antibiotics are administered postoperatively. Removal of the placenta at the time of cesarean section often causes hemorrhage, but the placenta is expected to be passed within 48 to 72 hours of the procedure.

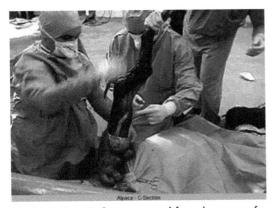

FIGURE 22-5 Live cria being removed from the uterus of an adult alpaca during cesarean section. The female was sedated with butorphanol, received a line block of the flank using lidocaine 2%, and was lying in right lateral recumbency. (Courtesy S. Fernando and David E. Anderson, DVM. From Anderson DE, Whitehead CE: *Veterinary clinics of North America food animal practice: alpaca and llama health management*, Philadelphia, 2009, Saunders.)

SUGGESTED READING

Anderson DE, Whitehead CE: *Veterinary clinics of North America food animal practice: alpaca and llama health management*, Philadelphia, 2009, Saunders.

Bassert J, Thomas J, editors: *McCurnin's clinical textbook for veterinary technicians*, ed 8, St. Louis, 2014, Saunders.

Birutta G: *Storey's guide to raising llamas*, North Adams, Mass, 1997, Versa Press.

Fowler ME: *Medicine and surgery of South American camelids*, ed 2, Ames, Iowa, 1998, Iowa State University Press.

Gerken M, Renieri C: *South American camelids research*, Wageningen, Netherlands, 2008, Academic Publishers.

Gillespie JR, Flanders FB: *Modern livestock and poultry*, ed 8, Clifton Park, NY, 2010, Delmar Cengage Learning.

CASE STUDY

Mr. Baily is currently raising llamas. This year he would like to castrate all his male cria at 6 months of age so that he can market them as pets. What information should you provide to Mr. Baily?

CASE STUDY

You are preparing for a cesarean section on Mr. Brett's female llama. He will be at your clinic with the llama in 20 minutes. Mr. Brett said the female weighed approximately 900 pounds. Which surgery suite will you prepare: the large animal suite or the small animal suite?

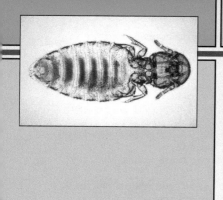

 Common Camelid Diseases

OUTLINE

Bacterial Diseases, *600*
Viral Diseases, *600*
Vaccinations, *600*

Parasites and Toxins, *600*
Case Study, *603*

LEARNING OBJECTIVES

When you have finished this chapter, you will be able to

- Describe and recognize clinical signs associated with specific diseases
- Discuss the etiology of the diseases
- Describe common treatments of disease
- List and discuss the common and scientific names of parasites associated with this species
- List the common vaccinations and their schedules associated with this species

KEY TERMS

Cria
Crypto

Fecal flotation
Jill

Zoonotic

BACTERIAL DISEASES

BLACKLEG

See Chapter 15, on common bovine diseases.

LEPTOSPIROSIS

See Chapter 15.

TETANUS

See Chapter 11 on common equine diseases.

VIRAL DISEASES

BOVINE VIRAL DIARRHEA

See Chapter 15.

RHINOPNEUMONITIS

See Chapter 11.

INFECTIOUS BOVINE RHINOTRACHEITIS

See Chapter 15.

OVINE ENZOOTIC ABORTION

See Chapter 19 on common ovine and caprine diseases.

RABIES

See Chapter 11.

VACCINATIONS

Table 23-1 lists a camelid vaccination regimen.

PARASITES AND TOXINS

Table 23-2 lists common camelid parasites (Figs. 23-1 and 23-2). Table 23-3 contains a list of common toxins and their effects in camelids.

TABLE 23-1	Camelid Vaccinations*		
DISEASE OR VACCINATION	**CRIAS**	**JILLS**	**ADULTS**
Clostridium vaccines	Crias	4 wk before parturition	All adults
Leptospirosis			All adults
Rhinopneumonitis			All adult
Infectious bovine rhinotracheitis			All adults exposed to cattle
Bovine virus diarrhea			All adults exposed to cattle
Ovine enzootic abortion			All adults exposed to sheep
Rabies	Crias at 3–6 mo		All adults in endemic areas

*Vaccination protocols should be designed specific to producers by veterinarians.

TABLE 23-2	Camelid Parasites			
COMMON NAME AND PHOTOGRAPH	**SCIENTIFIC NAME**	**IMPORTANCE**	**DIAGNOSIS**	**TREATMENT**
Biting Lice*	*Damalinia Bovicola* spp.	Often affects llamas during winter Itching and hair loss often seen Life cycle of ~3 wk	Direct observation of hair	Ivermectin, coumaphos, fenvalerate
Sucking Lice	*Microthoracius* spp.	Often affects llamas during winter Itching and hair loss often seen Life cycle of ~3 wk	Direct observation of hair	Ivermectin, coumaphos, fenvalerate
Sarcoptic Mange Mite*	*Sarcoptes scabiei*	Itching and hair loss Life cycle of ~3 wk	Skin scrapings	Ivermectin, doramectin
Meningeal Worm or Brain Worm†	*Parelaphostrongylus tenuis*	Found in white-tailed deer in eastern United States and Canada Causes severe inflammation of central nervous system Snails important in life cycle Death usually occurs 30–60 days after infection	Evaluation of central nervous system fluid Eosinophilia Seen histologically at necropsy in brain and spinal cord	Ivermectin
Strongyles*	*Camelostrongylus, Cooperia, Haemonchus, Oesophagostomum, Ostertagia, Trichostrongylus*		Eggs in fecal flotation	Ivermectin, doramectin, fenbendazole, levamisole, mebendazole, pyrantel pamoate
Whipworm	*Trichuris tenuis*	Prepatent period of 17–36 days	Eggs in fecal flotation	Ivermectin, doramectin, fenbendazole

Continued

TABLE 23-2	Camelid Parasites—cont'd			
COMMON NAME AND PHOTOGRAPH	**SCIENTIFIC NAME**	**IMPORTANCE**	**DIAGNOSIS**	**TREATMENT**
Capillary Worm* 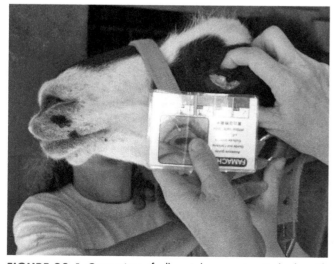	*Capillaria* spp.	Commonly seen at necropsy	Eggs in fecal flotation	Ivermectin, doramectin, fenbendazole
Thin-Necked Intestinal Worm	*Nematodirus battus, Nematodirus helvetianus*	Common in young camelids Prepatent period of 2–3 wk	Eggs in fecal flotation	Ivermectin, doramectin, fenbendazole, levamisole, mebendazole, pyrantel pamoate
Coccidia†	*Eimeria lamae, Eimeria alpacae, Eimeria macusaniensis, Eimeria punoensis*	Common in young camelids Prepatent period, in order: 15–16 days, 16–18 days, 33–34 days, 10 days	Oocysts in fecal flotation	Sulfaguanidine, decoquinate, lasalocid, monensin
Crypto*	*Cryptosporidium* spp.	Diarrhea Prepatent period of 3–7 days Zoonotic	Oocysts in fecal flotation	None

*Figure from Hendrix CM, Robinson E: *Diagnostic parasitology for veterinary technicians*, ed 4, St. Louis, 2012, Mosby.
†Figure from Bowman DD: *Georgis' parasitology for veterinarians*, ed 10, St. Louis, 2014, Saunders.

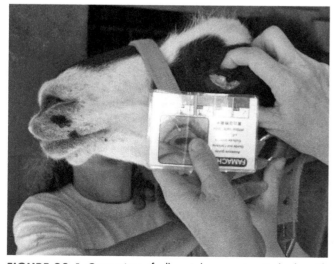

FIGURE 23-1 Comparison of a llama's lower conjunctival color with the color blocks on the FAMACHA card. This llama scored 1 out of 5 (not anemic). (From Cebra C, Anderson D, Tibary A, et al, editors: *Llama and alpaca care: medicine, surgery, reproduction, nutrition, and herd health*, St. Louis, 2014, Saunders.)

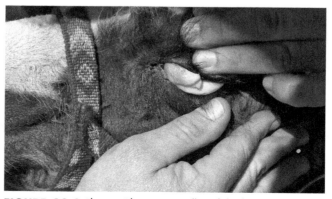

FIGURE 23-2 Llama with extreme pallor of the lower conjunctiva. This animal received a FAMACHA score of 5 out of 5 (very anemic). (From Cebra C, Anderson D, Tibary A, et al, editors: *Llama and alpaca care: medicine, surgery, reproduction, nutrition, and herd health*, St. Louis, 2014, Saunders.)

TABLE 23-3	Common Toxins
COMMON LLAMA AND ALPACA TOXINS	**TOXIC EFFECTS**
Oleander	Azotemia and death
Red maple	Kidney damage
Rhododendron	Gastrointestinal signs, cardiovascular effects, death
Ionophore	Weakness, recumbency, muscle tremors, dyspnea, diarrhea, acute death.
Yew	Cardiotoxicity

CASE STUDY

Mr. Trever has called the clinic and would like to know with what he should be vaccinating his llama herd. What types of questions should you ask Mr. Trever? Your veterinarian strictly adheres to this chapter's recommended vaccine regimen. If Mr. Trever also raises cattle, which vaccinations should he give?

SUGGESTED READING

Anderson DE, Whitehead CE: *Veterinary clinics of North America food animal practice: alpaca and llama health management*, Philadelphia, 2009, Saunders.

Bassert J, Thomas J, editors: *McCurnin's clinical textbook for veterinary technicians*, ed 8, St. Louis, 2014, Saunders.

Birutta G: *Storey's guide to raising llamas*, North Adams, Mass, 1997, Versa Press.

Bowman DD: *Georgis' parasitology for veterinarians*, ed 9, St. Louis, 2008, Saunders.

Foreyt WJ: *Veterinary parasitology reference manual*, ed 5, Ames, Iowa, 2001, Iowa State University Press.

Fowler ME: *Medicine and surgery of South American camelids*, ed 2, Ames, Iowa, 1998, Iowa State University Press.

Gerken M, Renieri C: *South American camelids research*, Wageningen, Netherlands, 2008, Wageningen Academic Publishers.

Gillespie JR, Flanders FB: *Modern livestock and poultry*, ed 8, Clifton Park, NY, 2010, Delmar Cengage Learning.

Hendrix CM, Robinson E: *Diagnostic parasitology for veterinary technicians*, ed 3, St. Louis, 2006, Mosby.

Kahn CM, Line S: *The Merck veterinary manual*, ed 10, Whitehouse Station, NJ, 2010, Merck & Co.

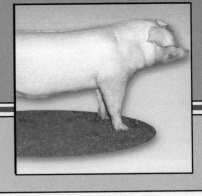

24   Porcine Husbandry

OUTLINE

LEARNING OBJECTIVES

When you finish this chapter, you will be able to

- Know and understand the zoologic classification of the species
- Proficiently use terminology associated with this species
- Describe physiologic data for the species and identify abnormal data
- Identify the common instruments relevant to the species and their uses
- Describe prominent anatomical or physiologic properties of the species
- Identify and describe characteristics of common breeds
- Describe normal production and husbandry needs for the species
- Describe specific reproductive practices of the species
- Discuss specific nutritional requirements of the species

KEY TERMS

Barrow
Boar
Boar effect
Bump weaning
Fall back
Farrowing
Gilt
Heterosis
Heterospermic insemination

Hog
Lordosis
Maternal lines
Oxytocin
Pig
Piglet
Runts
Savaging
Scours

Seed stock breeders
Shoat
Sow
Stag
Stillbirths
Teat order
Terminal lines

PORCINE ZOOLOGIC CLASSIFICATION

Kingdom	Animal
Phylum	Chordata
Class	Mammalia
Order	Artiodactyla
Family	Suidae
Genus	*Sus*
	Vittatus
Species	*Scrofa*

TERMINOLOGY AND PHYSIOLOGIC DATA

Box 24-1 lists common terminology used to describe the age and breeding status of swine. Table 24-1 lists normal physiologic data for swine.

COMMON SWINE INSTRUMENTS

Visit the Evolve website to find pictures and descriptions of common porcine instruments.

BOX 24-1	Terminology
Swine	Refers to the porcine species
Sow	Mature intact female
Boar	Mature intact male
Barrow	Male castrated before puberty
Stag	Male castrated after puberty
Gilt	Immature female, before the birth of her first litter
Farrowing	Act of parturition
Piglet	Very young, small pig, generally from birth to weaning
Shoat	Intact male, before puberty; sometimes used as a synonym for pig
Pig	Young swine of either sex, less than 120 pounds (~4 mo old)
Hog	Large swine, more than 120 pounds, of either sex (commercial swine producers usually prefer this term when referring to any size of swine)

TABLE 24-1	Physiologic Data
Temperature	101–103.5° F
Pulse rate	60–90/min; 200–280/min in newborns
Respiratory rate	10–24/min; up to 50/min in very young swine
Adult weight	Varies by breed

ANATOMICAL TERMS

Figures 24-1 and 24-2 will help you review the terms for body parts and areas of swine as well as the names of bones and joints.

SWINE BREEDS

COMMON SWINE BREEDS

Almost all *hog* producers in the United States use what is termed as "synthetic lines" (lines derived from crossbreeding to increase *heterosis*, which results in offspring that are superior to their parents). However, *seed stock breeders* are a key component of maintaining the breeds used in these synthetic lines.

Breeds can be classified as maternal lines or terminal lines. *Maternal lines* are lines that are used in a crossbreeding program to supply genetic factors that produce more *pigs* per litter, have higher milk production, and typically have a docile temperament. *Terminal lines* are typically used in crossbreeding programs to supply genetic factors that allow for fast growth, produce well-muscled and meaty carcasses, and typically are durable and leaner.

TECHNICIAN NOTE   Swine breeds are classified as maternal lines or terminal lines.

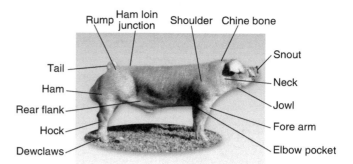

FIGURE 24-1 Body parts of pigs. (Courtesy National Swine Registry, West Lafayette, Ind.)

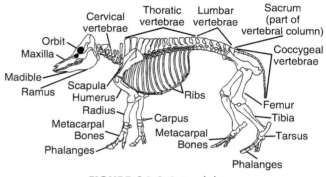

FIGURE 24-2 Swine skeleton.

American Landrace

Color: White
Breed association: American Landrace Association
Website: http://www.nationalswine.com

The American Landrace originated in Denmark. The hog is white. It is long bodied, and the large ears lop forward and down. The Landrace *sow* is noted for its mothering ability. The breed is also known for its large litters and length of side. The breed association is the American Landrace Association. Disqualifications for registry are black hair, erect ears, and the presence of fewer than six teats on a side. This is considered a maternal breed and is mostly used for crossing with other breeds (Fig. 24-3).

Berkshire

Color: Black, with six white points
Breed association: American Berkshire Association
Website: http://www.americanberkshire.com/

The Berkshire originated in England in and around Berkshire and Wiltshire counties. It is a medium-sized hog that produces an acceptable carcass. The animal is black with six white points, four white feet, and some white on the face and the tail. The head is slightly dished, and the ears are erect. The breed association is the American Berkshire Association. Disqualifications for registration are swirls on the back or sides and large amounts of white hair on the body. Selection has placed

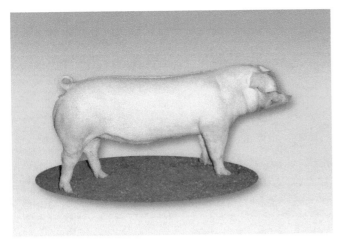

FIGURE 24-3 Landrace gilt. (Courtesy National Swine Registry, West Lafayette, Ind.)

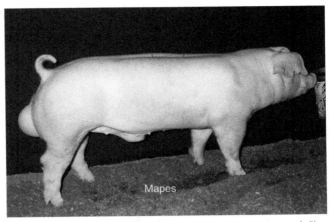

FIGURE 24-5 Chester White boar. (Courtesy Mapes Livestock Photos, Milford Center, Ohio.)

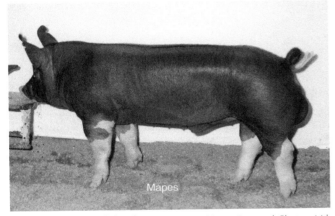

FIGURE 24-4 Berkshire boar. (Courtesy Mapes Livestock Photos, Milford Center, Ohio.)

emphasis on fast and efficient growth, meatiness, and good reproduction. This is considered a terminal breed (Fig. 24-4).

Chester White

Color: White
Breed association: Chest White Swine Record Association
Website: http://www.cpsswine.com/

The Chester White originated in Chester County, Pennsylvania. Producers refer to this breed as "Chesters." The breed is a mixture of Yorkshire, Lincolnshire, Cheshire, and Bedfordshire lines. The color of the breed is white, and the ears droop forward. The breed is noted for its mothering ability. The breed association is the Chester White Swine Record Association. Disqualifications for registry include swirls on the back and sides or any other color than white. This breed is considered a maternal breed (Fig. 24-5).

Duroc

Color: Red

Breed association: United Duroc Swine Registry
Website: http://www.nationalswine.com/

The Duroc breed originated from red hogs raised in New Jersey and New York. The breed was originally called the Duroc-Jersey, but the Jersey was later dropped. The color of the Duroc is red. Shades vary from light to dark, with a medium cherry the preferred shade. The Duroc has ears that droop forward. The breed has good mothering ability, growth rate, and feed conversion. It is one of the most popular breeds of swine in the United States. Swine of this breed can be registered with the United Duroc Swine Registry. Disqualifications for registry include swirls on the back and sides or white hair on the body. This breed is considered a terminal breed (Fig. 24-6).

> **TECHNICIAN NOTE** The Duroc is one of the most popular breeds in the United States.

Hampshire

Color: Black with a white belt
Breed association: The Hampshire Swine Registry
Website: http://www.nationalswine.com/

The Hampshire breed originated in England and was developed in Kentucky. It was previously known as the Thin Rind. The Hampshire is black, with a white belt that encircles the forepart of the body. The forelegs are included in the white belt. The Hampshire has erect ears. The breed is noted for its rustling (foraging) ability, muscle, and carcass leanness. It is a popular breed and is used in many crossbreeding programs. The breed association is the Hampshire Swine Registry. Disqualifications for registry include cryptorchidism, swirls on back or sides, incomplete belt, or white belt more than two thirds back on the body. White is permitted on the hind limbs as long as it does not go above the bottom of the ham or touch the belt. Other disqualifications include white on the head (except on the front of the snout), black front legs, white going above the bottom of

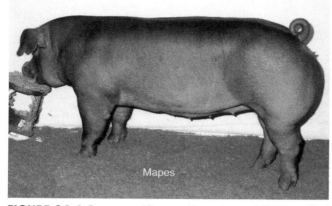

FIGURE 24-6 Duroc sow. (Courtesy Mapes Livestock Photos, Milford Center, Ohio.)

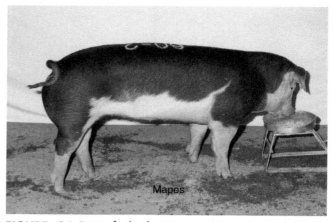

FIGURE 24-8 Hereford gilt. (Courtesy Mapes Livestock Photos, Milford Center, Ohio.)

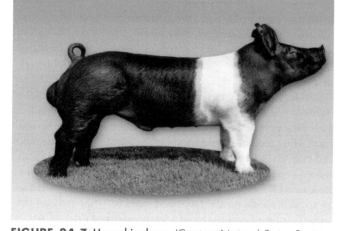

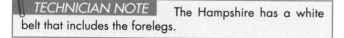

FIGURE 24-7 Hampshire boar. (Courtesy National Swine Registry, West Lafayette, Ind.)

the ham, or white on the belly extending the full length of the body. The Hampshire is considered a terminal breed (Fig. 24-7).

> **TECHNICIAN NOTE**   The Hampshire has a white belt that includes the forelegs.

Hereford

Color: Two thirds red, with some white on the face
Breed association: National Hereford Hog Registry Association
Website: http://www.nationalherefordhogassociation.com/

The Hereford was developed in Missouri, Iowa, and Nebraska. The breed was founded with use of Duroc and Poland China, some influence of Chester White, and Hampshire hogs. The Hereford is red with a white face. The ears are forward and drooping. The breed registry is the National Hereford Hog Registry Association. To be eligible for registry, Hereford hogs must be at least two thirds red and have some white on the face. Herefords are prolific, good mothers, and have good rustling ability. Disqualifications for registry

include no white on the face, less than two thirds of the body red, swirls on the body, or less than two white feet (Fig. 24-8).

Poland China

Color: Black, with six white points
Breed association: Poland China Record Association
Website: http://www.cpsswine.com/

The Poland China originated in the Ohio counties of Butler and Warren. The breed was developed with the use of lines from Russian, Byfield, Big China, Berkshire, and Irish Grazer bloodlines. The Poland China is black with six white points. The white points include the feet, tip of the nose, and the tip of the tail. The Poland China has forward-drooping ears. Poland China is one of the larger breeds of hogs. It is used in many crossbreeding programs. The breed association is the Poland China Record Association. Disqualifications for registry include fewer than six teats on a side, swirls on the upper half of the body, hernia, or cryptorchidism. The absence of any of the white points is not objectionable nor is an occasional splash of white on the body. The Poland China breed is considered a terminal breed (Fig. 24-9).

Spotted Swine

Color: Black and white spotted
Breed association: National Spotted Swine Record
Website: http://www.cpsswine.com/

The Spotted swine was developed in Indiana. Many producers refer to this breed as "Spots." It was created by crossing hogs of Poland China breeding with spotted hogs being grown in the area and later with the use of Gloucester Old Spots. The color of the Spotted breed is black and white. To be eligible for registry, at least 20% but not more than 80% of the body must be either black or white. The body type of the Spotted breed is similar to that of the Poland China. It has forward-drooping ears. Breeders strive to produce a large-framed hog

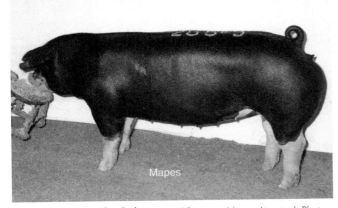

FIGURE 24-9 Poland China sow. (Courtesy Mapes Livestock Photos, Milford Center, Ohio.)

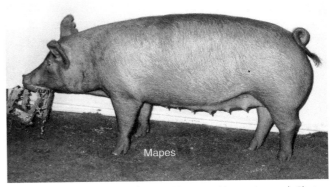

FIGURE 24-11 Tamworth sow. (Courtesy Mapes Livestock Photos, Milford Center, Ohio.)

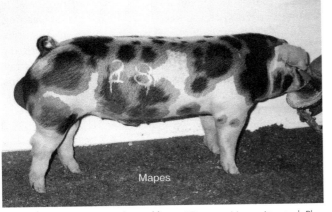

FIGURE 24-10 Spotted Breed boar. (Courtesy Mapes Livestock Photos, Milford Center, Ohio.)

with efficient gains and good muscling. The breed association is the National Spotted Swine Record. Disqualifications for registry include brown or sandy spots, swirls on any part of the body, and cryptorchidism. The breed is considered a terminal breed (Fig. 24-10).

> **TECHNICIAN NOTE** Many producers will refer to Spotted swine as "Spots."

Tamworth

Color: White
Breed association: Tamworth Swine Association
Website: http://www.tamworthswine.org/

The Tamworth hog originated in Ireland. It is one of the oldest of the purebred breeds. The Tamworth is red, with shades varying from light to dark. The ears are erect, and it has a long head and snout. The sows are good mothers and have large litters. The breed is noted for its foraging ability. The breed association is the Tamworth Swine Association. Disqualifications for registry include swirls on the sides and back and inverted teats (Fig. 24-11).

Yorkshire

Color: White
Breed association: American Yorkshire Club
Website: http://www.nationalswine.com/

The Yorkshire hog originated in England, in the county of Yorkshire. The Yorkshire is white. The skin sometimes has black pigmented spots called "freckles." The breed association is the American Yorkshire Club. Hogs with black spots can be registered, but this trait is considered undesirable. The ears are erect, and the face is slightly dished. Yorkshires have large litters, high feed efficiency, rapid growth, good mothering ability, and long carcasses. They are often used in crossbreeding programs. Disqualifications for registry include swirls on the upper third of the body, hair other than white, blind or inverted teats, fewer than six teats on a side, hernia, and cryptorchidism. The breed is considered a maternal breed (Fig. 24-12).

Potbellied Pig

Color: Varies
Breed association: The North American Potbellied Pig Association
Website: http://www.petpigs.com/

The North American Potbellied Pig Association describes the potbellied pig as weighing no more than 95 pounds and having a maximum height of 18 inches. Although some pigs stay small, between 40 and 50 pounds, most pigs weigh closer to 120 pounds. This breed of pig is *not* used for production of meat; it is more commonly kept as a pet. Most potbellied pigs are purchased between 6 and 8 weeks of age and are spayed or neutered within the first few months. Fifty percent of potbellied pigs are abandoned or sent to another home in the first year of life. This occurs because of unrealistic expectations of the owners and their unwillingness or inability to meet the pigs' needs (Fig. 24-13).

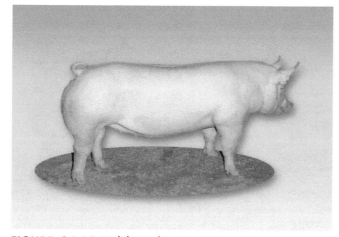

FIGURE 24-12 Yorkshire gilt. (Courtesy National Swine Registry, West Lafayette, Ind.)

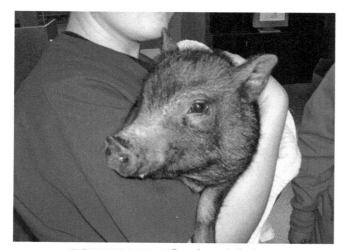

FIGURE 24-13 Wilber, the potbellied pig.

> **TECHNICIAN NOTE**   Fifty percent of potbellied pigs are abandoned or sent to another home in the first year of life.

OTHER BREEDS OF INTEREST

Several breeds are not cornerstones of the industry but are used more for genetic improvement. Some of these breeds include the pietrain because of its high lean-to-fat ratio (Fig. 24-14), as well as Chinese pigs because of their large litter sizes. Several other inbred lines also are available

REPRODUCTION

Table 24-2 lists information about swine reproduction.

HEAT DETECTION

One of the major factors affecting profitability in the swine industry is reproductive efficiency. Producers should strive to wean 22 to 24 pigs per sow per year to meet these

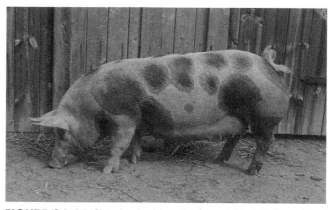

FIGURE 24-14 Pietrain pig. (From Sambraus HH: *A Colour atlas of livestock breeds*, London, 1992, Mosby-Wolfe.)

standards. Theoretically, a sow can average 2.57 litters per year. A producer's goal should be to wean 9 or more *piglets* per litter. Producers try to keep losses from birth to weaning at less than 10% of the piglets born alive. Weaning numbers lower than these standards can affect profitability. Veterinary technicians should be aware that several swine diseases can have devastating effects on swine reproduction. Technicians should be familiar with common reproductive practices, considering their importance to the industry and types of questions that will be fielded in practice.

> **TECHNICIAN NOTE**   Swine producers should strive to wean 21 to 22 pigs per sow per year. This equates to weaning 9 or more piglets per litter and trying to keep death losses to less than 10%.

Gilts typically reach puberty between 5 and 8 months of age. Gilts should be exposed to mature *boars* daily to encourage the *"boar effect"* (stimulating or detecting estrus through the presence of a boar). Daily exposure of gilts to boars will hasten the onset of cyclicity in the female. This procedure is effective because boars have a pheromone-secreting salivary gland that sexually stimulates female pigs.

In sows, the presence of nursing piglets prevents the sow from cycling, and the sow enters estrus 4 to 10 days after its piglets have been weaned. Common signs of estrus in swine include frequent mounting by other sows, restless activity, swelling of the vulva, discharge from the vulva, frequent urination, decreased appetite, occasional loud grunting, and a *lordosis* response during male mounting or when back pressure is applied, resulting in a rigid stance and erect ears.

> **TECHNICIAN NOTE**   Sows enter estrus 4 to 10 days after the piglets are weaned.

Swine ovulation rates are more pronounced at the third estrus after puberty. Ovulation occurs from both ovaries, and 14 to 16 oocytes can be released. Because of the large number of follicles or corpora lutea at any one time, sow ovaries often appear lobulated.

TABLE 24-2 | Breeding Information

Male Reproductive Parameters

Age of male puberty	6–8 mo
Length of spermatogenesis	39 days
Length of copulation	5–20 min
Site of semen deposition	Cervix or uterus
Ejaculate volume (mL)	200–250
Total sperm ($\times 10^{-9}$)	10–100
Motile sperm (%)	60–70
Morphologically normal sperm (%)	70–75
Boar scrotal width multiplied by length	Size (cm)
6–7	4.5 × 7
8–9	5 × 8
10–12	5.5 × 8.5
12–15	6 × 9.5
>15	6.5 × 10

Female Reproductive Parameters

Type of estrus cycle	Polyestrous
Age of female puberty	4–8 mo
Time of first breeding	7–9 mo
Estrous cycle length	18–24 days
Duration of estrus	2–3 days
Time of ovulation	40–46 hr after beginning of estrus
Optimal time of breeding (fresh/frozen)	24–36 hr after onset of estrus 12–24 hr in gilts
Maternal recognition of pregnancy in days	11–12 as a result of estrogen
Source of progesterone by gestation day	Corpus luteum
Type of placenta	Diffuse
Gestation period	114 days (3 mo, 3 wk, 3 days)
Birth weight	4–4.5 pounds
Litter size	8–14
Weaning age	3–6 wk

Earliest time of pregnancy diagnosis in days after ovulation

Ultrasound	>18 days Doppler: >30 days
Transrectal palpation	>21 days
Progesterone	17–20 days
Estrone sulfate	21–27 days
IEPF	1–2 days

IEPF, Immunosuppressive early pregnancy factor.

> **TECHNICIAN NOTE** From 14 to 16 oocytes can be released at each ovulation.

Heat detection in swine is commonly performed by testing for the lordosis response in the presence of a boar twice daily. If the sows or gilts are in estrus, they will begin sniffing each other and make head-to-head contact, followed by mounting attempts by the boar. If live cover is the intended form of breeding, it can be allowed to happen at this time. If artificial insemination is intended, the following protocol should be used.

SEMEN COLLECTION

The glans penis of the boar is shaped like a corkscrew, and the cervix of the female has a corresponding spiral shape. During copulation, the penis enters the cervix with a slight twisting motion to form a locking fit of the two organs. Ejaculation in the boar is stimulated by the firm fit of the glans in the cervix. To effect ejaculation for semen collection in a boar, this stimulation must be simulated. Boars are not as temperature sensitive as males of other species, but they are very pressure sensitive.

> **TECHNICIAN NOTE** The boar has a corkscrew-shaped penis.

Electroejaculation is not recommended. Artificial vaginas of various designs have been used to collect semen from boars, but manual stimulation is more reliable and more commonly used. Boars can be trained to mount a collection dummy, or a sow in estrus can be used. The boar is allowed to mount the sow or dummy. As the penis is extended, the collector diverts the penis to prevent entry into the vagina. The collector wears a lubricated latex glove that has been warmed to body temperature. This hand is wrapped firmly around the glans penis, with the fingers in the corkscrew grooves to simulate the locking fit of the cervix. The body or shaft of the penis should not be touched. The boar will make thrusting motions, which slow somewhat as ejaculation begins. Ejaculation in this species is not rapid, often requiring 3 to 7 minutes to complete the process. The ejaculate is collected in a suitable insulated container at 30° C.

> **TECHNICIAN NOTE** Electroejaculation is not recommended for swine.

Because ejaculation releases large numbers of sperm in this species, the epididymis is quickly depleted of its reserves of sperm. Preferably, semen should be collected every other day. Daily collections, if necessary, should not be done for more than several days, and the boar should receive 2 to 3 days of rest afterward.

Semen Processing

The sperm-rich fraction of semen is filtered from the gel fraction of the ejaculate, evaluated, and diluted with semen extender according to the results of the semen evaluation. A single high-quality ejaculate can provide up to 8 to 10 insemination doses after addition of semen extender. A recommended 1 to 2 billion sperm are used for each insemination dose.

> **TECHNICIAN NOTE** It is recommended that 1 to 2 billion sperm be used for each insemination dose.

Boar semen does not survive current methods of cryopreservation well, although frozen semen can be commercially obtained. Therefore, use of fresh or cooled sperm is preferable. Fresh semen combined with extender is preferred for maximum conception rates.

ARTIFICIAL INSEMINATION

Artificial insemination with fresh or cooled semen is commonly performed in the swine industry. Conception rates are improved if multiple inseminations are performed. The common practice is to inseminate the sow twice, 12 to 24 hours apart, in the middle of the 2 to 3 days of estrus (standing heat). In practice, this means that the first insemination is done 12 hours after detecting standing heat, followed by a second insemination 12 hours after the first. Research has shown increased efficiency of 3 inseminations per estrus while maintaining economic profitability. The insemination dose used in swine varies by technique. Cervical deposition with cooled semen is often 2500 million viable sperm. Cervical deposition with frozen semen is often 6000 million viable sperm. The postcervical insemination dose is often 1000 million cooled viable sperm. Deep uterine insemination doses are 600 million viable sperm when using cooled semen and 1000 million viable sperm when using frozen semen.

It is now fairly common practice to use semen from two boars to inseminate each female. The semen can be mixed together, or each boar can be used for a separate insemination. The rationale is to compensate for possible decreased fertility of one of the boars. Research has confirmed that conception rates are often higher if *"heterospermic insemination"* is practiced.

> **TECHNICIAN NOTE** It is common to mix semen from two boars to inseminate one female.

The presence of a boar nearby is helpful. A spiral-tip insemination pipette (Melrose catheter) or a pipette with a 30-degree angled tip is used to accommodate the shape of the sow's cervix. The pipette is often lubricated; however, care should be taken to avoid the presence of lubricant on the opening of the pipette. Insemination is performed blindly by sliding the pipette cranially along the roof of the vagina until it contacts the cervix ($\approx$8 to 10 inches). If this is not performed correctly, you may have inadvertently entered the urinary bladder, and a backflow of urine may be seen in your pipette. A gentle counterclockwise twisting motion is used to "screw" the catheter in place, and the semen is injected or allowed to flow by gravity slowly into the uterus. To ensure proper placement of the pipette, resistance can be felt by pulling back on the pipette. Once the pipette is in place, the semen container is attached to the pipette, and the semen is flowed in by gravity over 3 to 5 minutes. If backflow is observed, you may be administering the semen too quickly. Rotate the pipette or pull back and reposition, as well as lowering your semen container. Insemination doses average approximately 70 mL (range, 50 to 100 mL). The catheter is removed by twisting it clockwise. During insemination or coitus, *oxytocin* is used to potentiate strong contractions of the cervix of the sow or gilt. The female is often kept in a quiet place for 20 to 30 minutes following insemination. If insemination or live cover is successful, parturition can be expected 114 days later. With good management practices, it is possible to obtain two litters per year from one sow.

CLINICAL SIGNS OF IMPENDING PARTURITION

The gilt or sow needs her best care near the end of the gestation period. Proper timing of good management practices can prevent unnecessary losses. Neonatal piglets are delicate beings. Each lost piglet is lost income, and swine farmers go to great lengths to guarantee a healthy early environment for them.

Sows should be dewormed approximately 10 days before they are due to farrow. Treatment for mange and lice should be performed whenever these parasites become a problem during the gestation period. Sows should be washed thoroughly before they are placed in the farrowing house, and the final rinse should contain a product for treating mange and lice. When farrowing on solid floors, bed lightly with 1 to 2 inches of short-chopped bedding material, such as wood shavings, corn cobs, straw, or stalks. Slotted floors also can be used if available. A dry, warm, draft-free area is necessity for survival of baby pigs. Baby pigs require a temperature of 90° F to 95° F when they are first born. A properly installed, 125-W infrared heat bulb meets this requirement.

> **TECHNICIAN NOTE**
> - Baby pigs require a temperature of 90° F to 95° F when they are first born.
> - Sows should be dewormed approximately 10 days before they are due to farrow.

Sows, conversely, are most comfortable at temperatures of 60° F to 65° F. Observe the sow and litter carefully during farrowing and for the next several days.

Within several days of farrowing, the vulva swells, and the labial mucosa becomes hyperemic. The mammary glands show progressive enlargement in late gestation, but they become especially turgid and warm 1 to 2 days before parturition. Sows usually have milk in their udders 12 to 24 hours before they are due to farrow. The respiratory rate rises several hours before delivery, sometimes as high as 80 breaths/minute. Body temperature changes that signal parturition in other species have not been consistently identified in sows.

PARTURITION

Most sows farrow at night. Signs of approaching parturition include noticeable restlessness within 24 hours of giving birth and building of a "nest" (if bedding material is available). If bedding material is not available, the female will paw at the ground. Sows may lie down for variable periods of time and repeat the cycle of nesting and resting several times.

Vocalization may occur, and sows may become defensive of the nesting area. Within 1 hour of parturition, sows usually lie quietly in lateral recumbency. Sows typically remain in lateral recumbency, but gilts may stand occasionally between deliveries of fetuses. Some paddling of the legs is not unusual. More visible effort is usually required to deliver the first piglet than the others. Only small volumes of fetal fluids are expressed with the fetuses.

> **TECHNICIAN NOTE** Most sows farrow at night.

The normal farrowing interval is approximately 16 minutes; however, intervals of 30 minutes or longer are not unusual and are generally associated with *stillbirths*. The second stage of labor, the completed delivery of *all* fetuses, lasts an average of 3 to 4 hours. All fetal membranes should be delivered in 4 to 6 hours. Monitoring the progress of farrowing at frequent intervals is important to ensure early detection and correction of potential problems, which will prevent loss of piglets. The delivery position of the fetus is not as problematic for swine as it is in other species. Normal delivery, without complication, commonly occurs with both anterior (head-first) and posterior (breech) presentations. The legs typically are flexed alongside the body rather than extended as they are in other species; therefore, it is usual for either a snout or a tail to appear first at the vulva. Up to 45% of fetuses may be delivered in the posterior presentation.

> **TECHNICIAN NOTE** The normal farrowing interval is approximately 16 minutes between piglets.

Stillbirths are common in this species, with an average of 5% to 7% of piglets stillborn. The time interval between the start and finish of parturition directly correlates with the number of stillborn piglets, and it is not surprising that most stillbirths occur in the last third of the litter to be delivered. These latter-born piglets usually originate farther up in the uterine horns and have farther to travel through the birth canal. If the umbilical cord ruptures early, death may result from hypoxia.

> **TECHNICIAN NOTE** From 5% to 7% of piglets are stillbirths.

The third stage of labor is the expulsion of the fetal membranes; it is not a distinct stage of labor as defined in other species. Each piglet is encased in its own fetal membranes, but the membranes of two to three adjacent piglets may be fused together and passed as a unit. The placentas may be passed randomly between the births of piglets or after the last piglet is born. Passage of all fetal membranes should be completed within approximately 4 hours after birth of the last piglet. Retained placentas are uncommon in swine. Females may attempt to eat the placentas as they are passed, so

it is preferable to remove the placentas as they are passed to prevent this activity. Maternal behavior of the sow after giving birth is somewhat different from that in other species. Sows typically are fiercely protective of their young, but occasionally they may kill and eat one or more piglets as they are born; this phenomenon is known as *savaging*. If savaging is observed during farrowing, all piglets should be removed as soon as they are born and kept warm. When farrowing is complete, it usually is safe to return all piglets quietly to the sow. The sow is watched to confirm that she accepts all the piglets by allowing them to nurse. Rarely, tranquilization of the sow is necessary.

Swine are among the few species that do not practice vigorous licking of the newborns. Commonly, the sow stands and urinates after delivering all the fetuses, and then she lies back down and allows the piglets a prolonged time to nurse.

The most common causes of death in the neonatal period are being crushed by the sow, starving from failure to nurse adequately, and chilling (hypothermia). Usually, an attendant is present at the time of farrowing to assist in the delivery and help prevent these problems.

> **TECHNICIAN NOTE** Sows do not practice vigorous licking of their newborns.

If necessary, pharmacologically induced parturition can be used to aid in the birthing process. Prostaglandin administration after 112 days of gestation induces parturition in 20 to 30 hours. Combining a prostaglandin with oxytocin or xylazine will help to improve the precision of the response to prostaglandin administration.

DYSTOCIA

Swine have a low incidence of dystocias, estimated at less than 1% of farrowings. The incidence is higher when litter size is small because the fetuses are generally larger. The most common causes of dystocia are uterine inertia (failure of the myometrium to contract) and obstruction of the birth canal. During parturition, usually a piglet is born every 15 to 20 minutes. When the interval reaches 30 to 45 minutes without delivery of a piglet, the sow should be closely observed. Intervention is advisable after 45 to 60 minutes with no progress.

> **TECHNICIAN NOTE** It is estimated that only 1% of farrowings are classified as dystocias.

Traction in Swine

If the sow is having contractions, the birth canal should be checked for possible blockage. The vulva should be cleaned first. A well-lubricated, gloved hand is introduced into the reproductive tract through the vulva. The hand should be held with the fingers and thumb together in a pointed position to enter the vulva (Fig. 24-15). A slight rotating motion of the hand assists passage into the pelvic inlet. The birth canal is

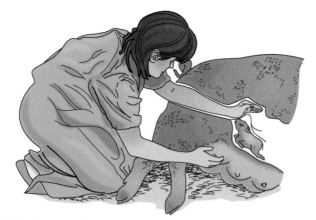

FIGURE 24-15 Dystocia. Vaginal examination. (From Jackson PGG: *Handbook of veterinary obstetrics*, ed 2, Edinburgh, 2004, Saunders.)

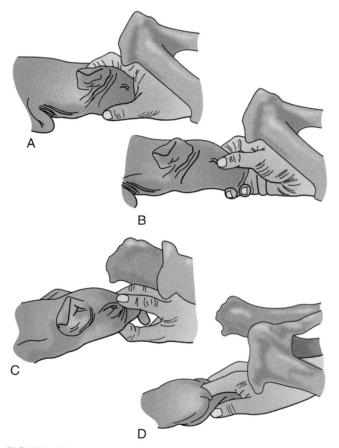

A

B

C

D

FIGURE 24-16 Dystocia. A to D, Fetal delivery and piglet holds. (From Jackson PGG: *Handbook of veterinary obstetrics*, ed 2, Edinburgh, 2004, Saunders.)

searched for fetuses, which may be in a sideways or breech position, or they may be large. Occasionally, two fetuses are entangled. Once an abnormality is detected, repositioning may be necessary. Mild traction then can be placed on the head or limbs to extract the fetus (Fig. 24-16). Various instruments are available to assist in applying traction; lambing snares, pig pullers, forceps, or nylon cord may be helpful. All manipulations should be done carefully to prevent injuring the sow.

Occasionally, a full rectum partially obstructs the sow's pelvic canal. An enema may be necessary to remove fecal material. Uterine inertia may result from exhaustion or hypocalcemia. The sow should be kept comfortably cool and may resume labor after a brief rest. If not, veterinary consultation is advised. Oxytocin injection may help to restore uterine contractions. If not, cesarean section may be the only option to save the sow.

One common problem is determining whether a sow has delivered all her fetuses. The end of parturition usually is signaled by the sow's standing and voiding a large volume of urine, followed by lying down comfortably to allow the litter to nurse. If the question of possible incomplete delivery exists, manual examination of the uterus can be performed. However, it is difficult to reach the full extent of the uterine horns. Transabdominal B-mode ultrasound examination can be used to detect retained fetuses.

> **TECHNICIAN NOTE** A common problem in swine is determining whether a sow has delivered all her fetuses.

NEONATAL CARE

Once delivery is complete, the following needs of the newborn must be addressed.

OXYGENATION

The fetus is often born with its amnion, or the membranes of another fetus, around it. Because the sow does not lick and clean the newborn piglets, the membranes should be immediately removed by hand to prevent any obstruction to breathing. The fingers or a dry cloth can be used to clear the mouth and nostrils. Holding the piglet with the head inclined downward and pumping the hindlegs several times toward the abdomen may clear the lungs; this is a safer alternative to the traditional "slinging" maneuver. Vigorous toweling helps to stimulate breathing.

> **TECHNICIAN NOTE** Holding the piglet slightly inclined and pumping the hindlegs can clear the lungs.

TEMPERATURE REGULATION

Piglets are born with sparse hair cover and therefore are highly susceptible to hypothermia, which can be rapidly fatal. The risk is greatest in the first 2 to 3 days after birth. The newborns should be toweled dry to remove fetal fluids. Farrowing barns typically are kept at an environmental temperature of 80° F to 85° F, and heat lamps or heat pads are used to provide each litter with a warmed area of 90° F to 95° F. Drafts must be prevented.

CARE OF THE UMBILICAL CORD AND UMBILICUS

The fetus may be born with the umbilical cord intact or broken. Intact cords usually are broken naturally as the piglet

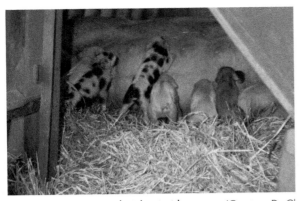

FIGURE 24-17 Sow and piglets inside an arc. (Courtesy D. Chennells. From Jackson PGG, Cockcroft PD: *Handbook of pig medicine*, St. Louis, 2007, Saunders.)

migrates toward the mammary glands to nurse. Intact cords or long cord stumps can be cut or trimmed to a length 4 to 5 cm from the umbilicus. The umbilical stump end should be dipped in 2% povidone–iodine solution or similar antiseptic solution. String or suture material can be used to ligate a bleeding umbilical cord by simply tying the material around the cord.

NUTRITION (NURSING)

Newborn piglets should be active and should reach a teat within 5 minutes of birth. Attempts to nurse should follow and be successful within 30 minutes of birth. Piglets have a preference for the more cranial teats, and they may begin to bite and push each other in competition for these teats. It may be necessary to place some piglets on the more caudal teats to ensure that they all have the opportunity to nurse. A *"teat order"* is established in the first several days after birth, with the larger, stronger piglets tending to dominate the preferred cranial teats, which are easier to access and produce greater volumes of milk (Fig. 24-17). Competition for teats may be deadly for piglets, especially in large litters where some piglets may not obtain enough milk to survive. Dividing large litters by removing several piglets and placing them with sows with smaller litters is a common practice known as *bump weaning*. This practice helps ensure that all piglets have enough to eat. Most often smaller piglets, called *fall backs,* are chosen to be moved onto sows with younger and smaller litters. Sows tolerate the foster mother role well, and piglets are not particular about suckling other sows.

The sow may make a distinctive soft, grunting noise that serves as a nursing call to the newborns. The piglets quickly become responsive to this noise. Most domestic sows nurse while they are recumbent, although standing nursing may be tolerated. On average, the litter nurses once per hour, nearly every hour, for approximately 6 minutes (<1 minute of actual milk ingestion). An average of 24 to 28 g of milk is consumed at each nursing.

Orphaned piglets can be raised on whole cow's milk or commercial sow milk replacer. Sow milk replacer should be mixed and fed according to the instructions. If cow's milk is used, a tablespoon of powdered skim milk can be added

to each pint of milk; do not add sugar or cream. Piglets can be fed by bottle or shallow pan. Pan feeding is most convenient for orphaned litters of multiple piglets. Pans, bottles, and nipples should be clean and sterilized or disinfected. Another good option is to catch milk or colostrum from other sows or gilts and to store it in the freezer in ice cube trays. This allows easy access to small amounts of milk without the need to thaw an entire bag. Orphans should be fed every 2 to 3 hours for the first 2 to 3 days. Milk should be warmed to approximately 100° F. Prestarter or creep feed can be started at 1 week of age.

Runts have been generally defined as weighing less than 2 pounds at birth; they often are among the last pigs of the litter to be born. They seldom thrive because of competition for nursing, and as many as 60% may die without supportive care. Supplemental feeding of runts may increase their survival. Commercial sow milk replacer can be used, and a substitute mixture (1 quart whole cow's milk plus ½ pint half-and-half cream plus one raw egg) has been described. The mixture is warmed and given twice daily (15 to 20 mL per feeding), using a syringe with an attached soft plastic tube placed in the mouth. This mixture is intended to supplement nursing, not replace it. The sow's teat line should be kept clean so that the piglets are less likely to develop *scours*. Scouring leads to poor gains or even death. An anemia prevention program should be in place. Injection or oral iron dextran should be given within the first 3 days of birth. A palatable pig starter diet should be available from 2 weeks of age to weaning.

ADEQUACY OF PASSIVE TRANSFER OF ANTIBODIES

Similar to other domestic species, in swine colostrum ingestion is essential for transferring maternal antibodies to the young. Absorption of antibodies from the gastrointestinal tract diminishes significantly from 12 to 24 hours after birth. Colostrum should be ingested within 12 hours of birth for the best results. Orphan piglets can receive colostrum that has been milked from other sows. Testing for antibody levels in neonates is not routinely done in swine.

Neonatal processing is discussed in Chapter 25.

NUTRITION

Sow body condition scoring is shown in Figure 24-18. Swine dental formulas and dental eruption schedules are listed in Table 24-3, and Figure 24-19 illustrates the permanent dentition of the pig. The protein requirements of swine are given in Table 24-4.

Feed efficiency is the other major factor that affects profitability in the swine industry. Maintaining high feed efficiency is critical for maintaining profitability in today's industry. Many diseases associated with the swine industry can have negative effects on profitability as a result of decreased feed efficiency. Veterinary technicians should be aware of a producer's feed efficiency to gather a proper history during the physical examination.

Pig condition scoring diagram

Score Number	Condition	Description	Shape of Body
5	Overfat	Hips and backbone heavily covered	Bulbous
4	Fat	Hips and backbone cannot be felt	Tending to bulge
3.5	Good condition	Hips and backbone only felt with difficulty	Tube shaped
3	Normal	Hips and backbone only felt with firm pressure	Tube shaped
2.5	Somewhat thin	Hips and backbone felt without firm pressure	Tube shaped but flat (slab) sides
2	Thin	Hips and backbone noticeable and easily felt	Ribs and spine can be felt
1	Emaciated	Hips and backbone visible	Bone structure apparent (ribs and backbone)

Condition scores from left to right, 1, 2, 3, 4, 5

Score: 1. Emaciated
       2. Thin, backbone prominent
       3. Ideal condition during lactation and at weaning, backbone just palpable
       4. Slightly overweight, cannot find the backbone
       5. Body rotund, over fat

Note: The "condition score" and "back fat" correlation does differ between breeds.

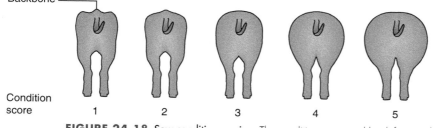

FIGURE 24-18 Sow condition scoring. The condition score and back fat correlation vary among different breeds. (From Jackson PGG, Cockcroft PD: *Handbook of pig medicine*, St. Louis, 2007, Saunders.)

Some pigs grow fast, whereas others grow slowly. The way a pig grows depends on three factors: genetic inheritance, feed, and care. Selecting pigs is important because you cannot grow a productive pig from poor breeding. Proper care means giving your pig a clean, comfortable place to live. It also means deworming and vaccinating the pig. Healthy pigs grow faster than sick pigs. Average daily gain is 1.4 to 1.8 pound/day. It takes approximately 2 to 2.5 pounds of feed to produce 1 pound of pork.

TECHNICIAN NOTE   Average daily gain is 1.4 to 1.8 pound/day; it takes 2 to 2.5 pounds of feed to produce 1 pound of pork.

Technicians should gather information on the diet as well as its components. The major feed component of today's commercial swine producers is corn, processed in several different ways.

Swine are omnivores and as such can accommodate some dietary fiber. Swine diets are most often a combination of purchased or farm-raised feeds such as corn, oats, wheat, barley, and sorghum supplemented with a purchased premix. Swine exhibit a better rate of weight gain when they are given nutritionally balanced feeds.

Grinding feeds increases feed efficiency, but grain that is ground too finely can create digestive problems. Grain should be reduced to a medium-fine particle size. Protein and amino acids are essential for maintenance of growth, gestation, and lactation in swine. Essential amino acids for growing pigs are arginine, histidine, isoleucine, leucine, lysine, methionine, phenylalanine, threonine, tryptophan, and valine. The most important of these are lysine, tryptophan, and threonine. Water should be provided free choice.

TABLE 24-3	Swine Dental Formulas and Dental Eruption Table

Deciduous Dental Formula: 2(I3/3 C1/1 PM3/3) = 28 Total

Permanent Dental Formula: 2(I3/3 C1/1 PM4/4 M3/3) = 44 Total

Deciduous eruption	I1	1–3 wk
	I2	1½–2 mo lower, 2–3 mo upper
	I3	Birth
	C	Birth
	PM2	1–2 mo
	PM3	First month
	PM4	First month
Permanent eruption	I1	12–17 mo
	I2	16–20 mo
	I3	8–10 mo
	C	8–12 mo
	PM1	5 mo
	PM2	12–16 mo
	PM3	12–16 mo
	PM4	12–16 mo
	M1	4–6 mo
	M2	8–12 mo
	M3	18–20 mo

TECHNICIAN NOTE Grinding feeds increases feed efficiency, but grain that is ground too finely can create digestive problems.

FEEDING CONSIDERATIONS BY AGE
Breeding Sows and Litters
Breeding sows are limit fed from breeding up to the last trimester. Sows are fed 4 to 6 pounds of complete ration supplying 6000 to 7000 kcal metabolizable energy (ME). In the last trimester, feed is increased to supply additional energy to the rapidly growing fetuses. Sows are fed a complete ration that supplies 9000 to 10,000 kcal ME per day. The sow should not be overfed because this will directly affect milk production during lactation. To produce healthy pigs, the gestation diets must be adequate in all nutrients. During lactation, energy intake is increased to 15,000 to 20,000 kcal ME per day. Fat can be added to the diet to improve feed palatability and energy density.

Starter or Nursery Diets
Piglets are weaned at 3 to 5 weeks of age and are fed as starters until they weigh 40 to 50 pounds. Starter pigs are fed ad libitum. Starter rations are high in protein (20% to 24%), nutrient dense, supplied as a pellet, and often purchased from a commercial feed supplier because of the feed complexity. Starter ration eventually is changed to a ground feed in the last couple of weeks of the starter program.

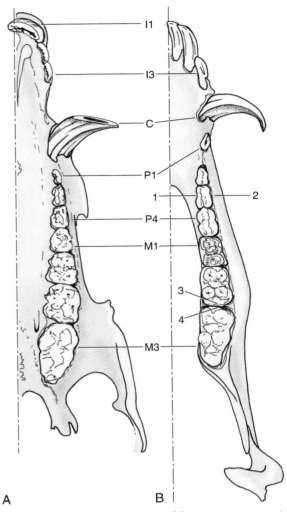

FIGURE 24-19 Permanent dentition of the pig. Upper (**A**) and lower (**B**) jaws. *1,* Lingual surface; *2,* vestibular surface; *3,* distal surface; *4,* mesial surface. (From Dyce KM, Sack WO, Wensing CJG: *Textbook of veterinary anatomy,* ed 4, St. Louis, 2010, Saunders.)

TABLE 24-4	Nutritional Requirements of Swine	
AGE	**CRUDE PROTEIN (%)**	
Weanling (12–20 pounds)	16–20	
Breeding sow	12	
Gilt	13–16	
Lactating sow	17	
Boar	14–16	

TECHNICIAN NOTE Piglets are weaned at 3 to 5 weeks of age and are fed as starters until they weight 40 to 50 pounds.

Growing and Finishing Market Hogs
For today's market hog, higher levels of protein and less energy are fed to develop the leanest animals. Feeds are evaluated based on their amino acid content. Protein sources supplied

in the growing and finishing rations usually are soybean meal, meat, bone meal, and synthetic amino acids. Synthetic amino acids are lysine, methionine, threonine, and tryptophan. Growing and finishing hogs are fed ground cereal grains (corn, wheat, sorghum, and barley), which make up to 85% of a typical ration. Growing and finishing rations are fortified with numerous minerals and vitamins. Calcium and phosphorus should be properly balanced during this period. Housing and space are important aspects in growing and finishing swine. A veterinary technician's role in a swine facility involves herd health and piglet care. The feed supplier with premixes meets nutritional needs and problems and provides rations tailored to individual operations and life stages of the pigs.

Potbellied Pigs

Potbellied pig diets can be commercially purchased. Their diets are generally classified as starter diets, grower diets, breeder diets, or maintenance diets. The maintenance ration usually contains 12% protein, 2% fat, and 12% to 15% fiber. The most common disease of potbellied pigs is obesity. Some commercially available potbellied pig feed has urinary acidifiers to help prevent cystitis, so if this condition seems to be a problem, this specialty ration may be considered. Potbellied pigs should be fed volume according to their body composition. Although potbellied pigs should have a rotund potbelly, they should never have turgid, fat-filled jowls or rolls of fat hanging over the hocks. They should have ribs that can be felt but not seen. Appropriate treats for potbellied pigs include low-fat, low-salt snack food, such as popcorn (air popped without salt or butter), and small amounts of dried or fresh fruit. Water should be provided free choice to prevent cystitis, urolithiasis, and salt poisoning. Pigs spend most of their day sleeping unless they are encouraged to forage for their food, which is a natural behavior in swine.

VITAMINS

When vitamins are provided in swine diets, stabilized vitamin A is commonly used because natural vitamin A is degraded under normal environmental conditions. Vitamin D is necessary for proper bone growth and ossification. Most vitamin D needs are met by exposing hogs to direct sunlight for a short time each day. Sources of vitamin D include irradiated yeast, sun-cured hays, animal sterols, fish oils, and vitamin A and D concentrates. Vitamin E is required by swine of all ages and is interrelated with selenium found in green forage, legume hays, and cereal grains. Vitamin K is necessary for blood clotting to convert fibrinogen to fibrin. Most producers supplement with vitamin K. Thiamine is not of practical importance in the diet, although riboflavin is a requirement of breeding stock and light-weight pigs. Riboflavin is naturally found in green forage, milk by-products, and brewer's yeast. Pantothenic acid is especially important for females and typically is found in crystalline form within premixes. Natural sources include green forage, legume meals, milk products, and brewer's yeast. Choline is essential for normal functioning of the liver and kidneys. Supplementing choline has been shown to increase litter size. It is naturally found in fish solubles, fish meal, and soybean meal. Young pigs require vitamin B_{12} for growth and normal hemopoiesis. Vitamin B_{12} is present in animal, marine, and milk products.

MINERALS

Minerals should include calcium and phosphorus primarily for skeletal growth. They also are important for metabolism and are required for gestation and lactation. These minerals are easily supplied by the use of tankage, meat meal, meat, bone and fish meal, limestone, and oyster shells. Sodium chloride is recommended as 0.25% of the total diet. It is supplied by animal and fish by-products in the diet. Iodine is supplied in the diet for use by the thyroid gland to produce thyroxine and typically is supplied with iodized salt. Iron and copper are necessary for hemoglobin formation and to prevent nutritional anemia. Sow's milk is severely deficient in iron. Feeding lactating sows increased levels of iron does not seem to pass sufficiently high levels to the piglets. Cobalt is present in vitamin B_{12}. Manganese is essential for normal reproduction and growth. Potassium requirements are met in the feedstuffs. Magnesium is essential for growing swine. Zinc in swine nutrition is interrelated with calcium. Supplemented zinc is recommended to prevent parakeratosis. Selenium is interrelated with selenium. Selenium requirements depend on soil condition where crops were grown.

CASE STUDY

Mrs. Holtgrew calls in and says she has a Hereford that is having trouble giving birth. Should you ask what species she is speaking of? Why? If Mrs. Holtgrew is talking about a sow and she tells you the last piglet was born 30 minutes ago, is Mrs. Holtgrew justified in calling the clinic?

CASE STUDY

Mrs. Holtgrew's sow gave birth to 10 piglets; several of them are runts. Mrs. Holtgrew would like you to take care of the runts at the clinic. What requirements will be necessary to keep the piglets at the clinic?

SUGGESTED READING

Bassert JM, McCurnin DM, editors: *McCurnin's clinical textbook for veterinary technicians*, ed 7, St. Louis, 2010, Saunders.

Ensminger ME, Parker RO: *Swine science*, ed 6, Danville, Ill, 2005, Interstate Publishers.

Gillespie JR, Flanders FB: *Modern livestock and poultry*, ed 8, Clifton Park, NY, 2010, Delmar Cengage Learning.

Hafez ESE: *Reproduction in farm animals*, ed 6, Philadelphia, 2000, Lea & Febiger.

Martin LC, Hines RH, Schaake SL, Unruh JA: *Laboratory exercises for animal sciences and industry*, Dubuque, Iowa, 1993. Kendall/Hunt Publishing.

Noakes DE, Parkinson TJ, England GCW: *Veterinary reproduction and obstetrics*, ed 9, London, 2009, Saunders.

Sonsthagen T, Teeple TN: Nursing care of food animals, camelids, and ratites. In Sirois M, editor: *Principles and practice of veterinary technology*, ed 3, St. Louis, 2011, Mosby, pp 585–611.

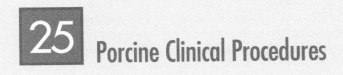

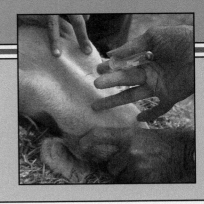

25 Porcine Clinical Procedures

OUTLINE

LEARNING OBJECTIVES

When you have finished this chapter, you will be able to

- Set up and prepare the patient for each procedure, perform the procedure (when appropriate), or assist the clinician in performing diagnostic sampling and medication procedures
- Successfully and safely administer medications by oral, nasal, and parenteral routes
- Properly insert and maintain an intravenous catheter and monitor the catheter for complications
- Explain the rationale and indications for each of the clinical procedures described
- Set up materials and equipment and prepare the patient as needed for the procedure
- Provide assistance to the veterinarian with performing the procedure or perform the procedure when it may be appropriate for a veterinary technician to do so
- Perform or assist with necropsy and sample collection procedures and maintain a safe environment during these procedures

KEY TERMS

Baby pig thumps
Hog snare
Lateral auricular vein

Nasal turbinates
Needle teeth
Needle tooth nippers

Universal ear notching system

DIAGNOSTIC SAMPLING

All diagnostic procedures performed in other species, such as abdominocentesis, arthrocentesis, and transtracheal wash, can be performed in swine. Because of the economic costs associated with some of these tests and the cost of treating serious medical diseases when they occur, these and nonroutine diagnostic tests more likely will be pursued for valuable breeding stock than for production animals. However, routine diagnostic tests such as blood sampling are commonly performed in swine for disease screening.

VENOUS BLOOD SAMPLING

Blood is the material most commonly collected for testing in swine. Swine red blood cells are somewhat fragile; therefore, using appropriately sized needles and avoiding aspiration or injection of blood through needles with unnecessary force

are important. Sites of blood collection should always be cleaned before needle insertion.

> **TECHNICIAN NOTE** Swine red blood cells are somewhat fragile, so using good technique when collecting blood is important.

Several veins are accessible for blood sampling. The site and technique for venipuncture depend on the size of the pig and the method of restraint. The following locations are accessible: lateral auricular vein, coccygeal vein, cranial vena cava, jugular vein, orbital sinus, and cephalic vein.

Lateral Auricular Vein
Equipment needed for lateral auricular venipuncture:
- Alcohol
- 20-gauge (ga) × 1-inch needle

- 18- to 20-ga × 1-inch needle for large adults
- Syringe
- Appropriate collection tubes

The "ear" vein is useful for obtaining small samples of venous blood (<5 mL). It is used for pigs after weaning age (4 to 5 weeks old, 25-pound body weight). A 20-gauge (ga) × 1-inch needle is suitable for most animals. An 18- to 20-ga × 1-inch needle can be used in large adults. Butterfly catheters may be useful. Vacutainers are not recommended at this location because they tend to collapse the vein, especially in small individuals.

> **TECHNICIAN NOTE**   The ear vein can be used to collect less than 5 mL of blood.

The vein runs near the lateral border of the ear pinna and is accessed from the dorsal (haired) side of the pinna (Figs. 25-1 and 25-2). It is easily visualized and can be distended with finger pressure at the base of the lateral surface of the ear, although both hands of the technician can be freed up by using a mechanical method to distend the vein. A rubber band can be placed as a tourniquet around the base of the

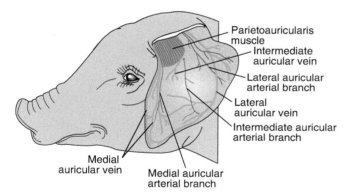

FIGURE 25-1 Left ear showing blood vessels. (Modified from Dyce KM, Sack WO, Wensing CKG: *Textbook of veterinary anatomy*, ed 4, St. Louis, 2010, Saunders.)

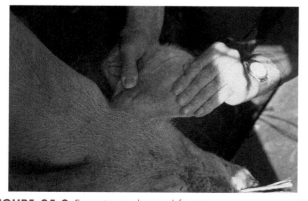

FIGURE 25-2 Ear vein can be used for intravenous injections. It is less useful for blood sampling because it readily collapses when negative pressure is applied. (From Jackson PGG, Cockcroft PD: *Handbook of pig medicine*, Edinburgh, 2007, Saunders.)

ear to distend the vein. Another method uses self-retaining forceps with long, plastic-covered jaws that are placed across the base of the ear to distend the ear vein. This method leaves one hand free to stabilize the tip of the ear while the other hand places the needle and aspirates the blood. The needle should enter the vein at a 45-degree angle to the skin. The ear vein may continue to bleed for several minutes after venipuncture is completed.

Coccygeal Vein

Equipment needed for coccygeal venipuncture:
- Alcohol
- 20-ga × 1-inch needle
- Syringe
- Appropriate collection tubes

The "tail" vein is accessible in animals without docked tails but is infrequently used. It is suitable only for adult swine. A 20-ga × 1-inch needle is used. The coccygeal vein is located on the ventral midline of the tail. The tail is elevated vertically, and the needle is inserted near the base of the tail on the ventral midline, perpendicular or nearly perpendicular to the skin. Small blood volumes (<5 mL) can be obtained.

> **TECHNICIAN NOTE**   The coccygeal vein is not commonly used and is suitable only for adult swine.

Cranial Vena Cava

Equipment needed for cranial vena cava venipuncture:
- Alcohol
- 20-ga × 1½½-inch needle
- Less than 50 pounds: 18- to 20-ga × 1 to 1½-inch needle
- More than 50 pounds: 18- to 20-ga × 2½-inch needle
- Adults: 16- to 17-ga × 4- to 4½-inch needle
- Syringe
- Appropriate collection tubes

The cranial vena cava lies in the thoracic inlet between the first pair of ribs and gives rise to both the right and left jugular veins. Although learning to draw blood from this location is technically more difficult, this location is the most satisfactory for obtaining large blood samples and is suitable for any size animal. The right side of the animal is always used to access the cranial vena cava, to avoid accidental damage to the phrenic nerve. The left phrenic nerve lies in a more vulnerable position, paralleling the left external jugular vein, than does the right phrenic nerve, which is more protected on the right side of the animal. In piglets, a 20-ga × 1½-inch needle can be used. Small pigs up to 50 pounds require an 18- to 20-ga × 1- to 1½-inch needle. Small pigs are placed in dorsal recumbency with the head held firmly still. The front legs are extended and pulled caudally for complete access to the caudal neck and shoulder area. The needle is inserted (syringe attached) on the right side, at the caudal extent of the right jugular furrow, just lateral to the manubrium of the sternum. The needle is directed toward the caudal aspect of the top of the opposite (left) shoulder blade. Slight back-pressure (vacuum) is kept on the syringe. The vena cava is encountered at a depth between ½ and 2 inches, depending on the size of the animal. Blood is easily aspirated when the needle enters the vein.

> | **TECHNICIAN NOTE**   The right side of the animal should always be used to avoid damage to the phrenic nerve.

Larger animals are restrained while they are standing, usually with a *hog snare*. The head should be raised slightly. Alternatively, some farms use a bleeding chute with a head catch. Nonslip footing should be provided. If the pig sits down before or during the procedure, stop the procedure, withdraw the needle, and raise the pig up on all four feet. Sitting alters the anatomical landmarks for the procedure and makes it difficult to perform successfully. An 18- to 20-ga × 2½-inch needle is used for feeder (finisher) pigs weighing more than 50 pounds. In adult swine, a 16- to 17-ga × 4- to 4½-inch needle is needed. The syringe is attached for the procedure. The technician kneels in front of the animal on the right side (facing the body of the pig) or to the side of the right shoulder (facing the neck). The needle is inserted and directed exactly as described earlier (Figs. 25-3 and 25-4). Once the skin has been penetrated, slight backpressure is maintained on the syringe plunger. Blood flows readily when the vein is entered. In adult pigs the vein lies quite deep, up to 4 inches.

Several structures may be encountered accidentally during this procedure. If the needle hits a rib, pull backward slightly and try a different angle. If the needle penetrates the trachea, the syringe will fill with air. If the needle enters the thoracic duct, the syringe will fill with lymph. Punctures of the trachea and thoracic duct rarely are life-threatening; when encountered, they indicate that the needle is angled too far medially. The right vagus nerve, if hit, can damage the function of the parasympathetic nerves to the heart. The right phrenic nerve, if hit, can alter the function of the diaphragm. Cardiac or respiratory signs, or both, may follow and require emergency treatment.

Jugular Vein

Equipment needed for jugular venipuncture:
- Alcohol
- 20-ga × 1½-needles in piglets
- 16-ga × 3- to 3½-inch needles in mature pigs
- Syringes
- Appropriate collection tubes

Because the jugular vein is not as deep a structure as the cranial vena cava, it is a safer structure for access with a needle. However, the jugular veins are not as large in diameter and may be difficult to find and access, especially in large or heavy animals. The jugular vein can be used for sampling animals of any age. Needle size ranges from 20 ga × 1½ inches in piglets to 16 ga × 3 to 3½ inches in mature pigs.

The right jugular vein is preferred, to avoid damaging the phrenic nerve. The jugular vein lies in the jugular furrow and is accessed cranially to the manubrium at the visually

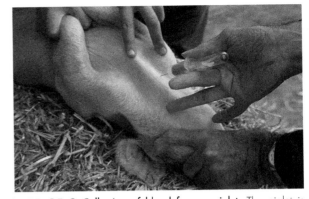

FIGURE 25-3 Collection of blood from a piglet. The piglet is restrained in dorsal recumbency. The Vacutainer needle is inserted into the anterior vena cava between the point of the shoulder and the manubrium of the sternum. (From Jackson PGG, Cockcroft PD: *Handbook of pig medicine*, Edinburgh, 2007, Saunders.)

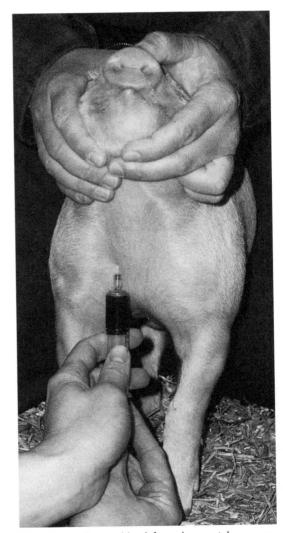

FIGURE 25-4 Collecting blood from the cranial vena cava in a standing pig. The needle is inserted at the caudal extent of the right jugular furrow, lateral to the manubrium. (From Bassert J, Thomas J, editors: *McCurnin's clinical textbook for veterinary technicians*, ed 8, St. Louis, 2014, Saunders.)

deepest point of the jugular furrow. The vein is not distended; this is a blind stick procedure. The needle (with syringe or vacuum attached) is inserted perpendicular to the skin and is directed dorsocaudally and slightly medially. After the skin has been penetrated, slight backpressure should be kept on the syringe.

> **TECHNICIAN NOTE** Jugular vein draws in swine are blind stick procedures.

Orbital Sinus (Medial Canthus of the Eye)
Equipment for orbital sinus puncture:
- Alcohol
- 20-ga × 1-inch needle in piglets
- 16- to 20- ga × 1½-inch needle in mature adults
- Syringe
- Appropriate collection tubes

The venous sinus is located adjacent to the medial canthus of the eye and can be used for venous blood collections in pigs of any age. Approximately 5 to 10 mL of blood can be obtained. Small pigs are restrained in dorsal recumbency, inclined with the head down, and firmly restrained. Larger pigs are restrained standing with a hog snare. Piglets require a 20- to 20-ga × 1-inch needle. Larger pigs require a 16- to 20-ga × 1½-inch needle. The needle is inserted deep to the nictitating membrane (third eyelid) and is advanced at a 45-degree angle toward the opposite jaw. The needle will hit the lacrimal bone. Rotate and slightly withdraw the needle until blood flows from the hub. The needle is then attached. Aspiration should be gentle (Fig. 25-5).

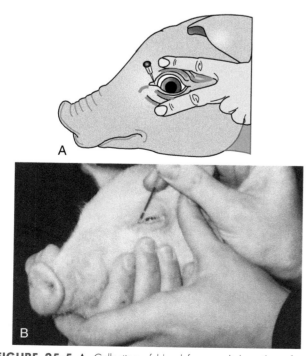

FIGURE 25-5 A, Collection of blood from medial canthus of eye. **B,** Venipuncture of left orbital sinus. Note the firm manual restraint of the head. (B, From Bassert J, Thomas J, editors: *McCurnin's clinical textbook for veterinary technicians,* ed 8, St. Louis, 2014, Saunders.)

Cephalic Vein
Equipment needed for cephalic venipuncture:
- Alcohol
- 20-ga × 1- to 1½-inch needle
- Syringe
- Appropriate collection tubes

The cephalic vein is accessible in small pigs more than 14 weeks old but is not commonly used. It runs along the craniomedial surface of the upper forelimb. The pig is restrained by snout restraint in the standing position. The leg is not lifted off the ground. Distention of the vein is similar to that in small animals and can be achieved by hand or tourniquet. The needle is placed at a 45-degree angle to the skin, in a proximal direction. A 20-ga × 1- to 1½-inch needle is sufficient. Up to 10 mL of blood can be obtained.

Normal complete blood count and blood chemistry values for swine are listed in Tables 25-1 and 25-2, respectively. Table 2A-3 in Appendix 2 shows the morphologic features of white blood cells.

> **TECHNICIAN NOTE** The cephalic vein is not commonly used for blood collection.

URINE COLLECTION
Equipment needed for urine collection:
- Sterile collection container

Voided urine may be collected in swine, although encouraging urination may be difficult. Males should be confined and observed. Once they are quiet, the prepuce can be stroked with a warm, wet towel or soft brush. Titillating the vulva by stroking with the fingers, soft brush, or dry straw can be attempted in females. Adult swine normally urinate two to three times per day.

MEDICATION TECHNIQUES

ORAL MEDICATION
Most oral medications are delivered to groups of pigs in the water or feed. Occasionally, individual pigs must be medicated. The chief dangers to the technician are the sharp teeth and the strong jaws, which must be respected in animals of any age. The hand or fingers should not be placed in the animal's mouth unless a speculum is used to hold the mouth open. In small piglets, the corner of the mouth can be pressed inward with the fingers so that the cheek tissue provides some protection for the finger.

> **TECHNICIAN NOTE**
> - Most oral medications are delivered to groups of pigs in the water or feed.
> - The sharp teeth and strong jaw of swine must be respected.

Oral speculums are available for swine. The pig should first be restrained with a hog snare; this causes the pig to

TABLE 25-1	Complete Blood Count Normal Values for Swine*	
Packed cell volume (%)	Increased with polycythemia, dehydration, stress, in neonates, and with high globulin levels; decreased with anemia, bleeding, overhydration, and in weanlings	32–50 (42)
Hemoglobin (g/dL)	Increased with polycythemia; decreased with anemia	10–16 (13)
Red blood cells ($\times 10^6$/μL)	Increased with polycythemia and dehydration; decreased with anemia, and overhydration	5–8 (6.5)
Total protein (g/dL)	Increased in dehydration and in lipemic samples; decreased with overhydration	5–8 (6.5)
White blood cells ($\times 10^6$/μL)	Increased with acute local inflammation, toxicity, and bacterial infections; decreased with marrow diseases, radiation, drug therapy, and certain viruses	11–22 (16)
Platelets ($\times 10^6$/μL)	Decreased in swine fever, hog cholera, DIC, and endotoxic shock	3.25–7.15 (5.2)
Mean corpuscular volume (fL)	Increased with vitamin B_{12} and folic acid deficiency; decreased with iron deficiency	50–68 (63)
Mean corpuscular hemoglobin (pg)	Increased with hemolysis; decreased with iron deficiency	16.6–22
Mean corpuscular hemoglobin concentration (g/gL)	Increased with hemolysis, lipemia, and Heinz bodies	30–34 (32)
Bone marrow (myeloid-to-erythroid ratio)		1.77 ± 0.52:1
Differential, Absolute		
Segs		28%–47%, 3,000–10,500
Bands		0%–2%
Lymphocytes		39%–62%, 4,300–13,700
Monocytes		2%–30%, 220–2,200
Eosinophils		0.5%–11%, 0–2,500
Basophils		0%–2%, 0–400

DIC, Disseminated intravascular coagulation.
*Average numbers are indicated in parentheses.

TABLE 25-2	Blood Chemistry Normal Values for Swine	
Blood urea nitrogen (mg/dL)	Increased with kidney disease, azotemia, and uremia	8.2–24.6
Creatinine (mg/dL)	Increased with kidney disease	0.8–2.3
Glucose (mg/dL)	Decreased in fatty liver disease, increased with diabetes and stress	66.4–116.1
Albumin (g/dL)	Increased with dehydration. Decreased with brucellosis, chronic liver disease, glomerular disease, hyperglobulinemia, hypertension, malnutrition, and malabsorption	2.3–4
Total bilirubin (mg/dL)	Increased in animals with liver disease, bile duct obstruction, jaundice, or hemolytic anemia	0–0.5
Aspartate aminotransferase (μg/L)	Increased in liver disease or with muscle damage; can be increased after exercise	15.3–55.3
γ-Glutamyl transferase (μg/L)	Increased with hepatocellular and cholestatic liver disease, hepatocyte necrosis, and cholestasis	31–52
Creatinine kinase (μg/L)	Increased with muscle disease	65.7–489.4
Alkaline phosphatase (μg/L)	Increased with liver disease and cholestasis, steroids, and growth	41–176.1
Lactate dehydrogenase (μg/L)	Increased with hepatocyte damage, muscle damage, and hemolysis	159.6–424.7
Sodium (mEq/L)	When increased can cause neurologic disorders and hypertension; decreases can be caused by *Escherichia coli*, polyuria or polydipsia, weight loss, and anorexia	139.2–152.5
Potassium (mEq/L)	Increases can be caused by severe metabolic acidosis; decreases can be caused by anorexia, increased renal excretion, abomasal stasis, intestinal obstruction, enteritis, and weight loss	4.4–6.5
Chloride (mEq/L)	Increased during displaced abomasums	97.1–106.4
Calcium (mg/dL)	Increased with kidney stones, renal failure, and some cancers; decreased in milk fever, renal disease, and bone disease	9.3–11.5
Phosphorus (mg/dL)	Increased in renal failure; decreased with osteomalacia, rickets, and tetany	5.5–9.3
Magnesium (mg/dL)	Decreased in milk fever, grass tetany, fever, and hypersalivation	2.3–3.5

vocalize. The speculum can be placed while the pig's mouth is open. One type of speculum is a simple "hand paddle" style that is inserted into the mouth horizontally and, once behind the canine teeth, is rotated vertically. Medications then can be given by dose syringe or pilling gun, or a stomach tube can be passed through the bars of the speculum (Fig. 25-6).

Piglets are commonly placed in a standing position for oral medication administration. The front legs are elevated, and the piglet's back is placed against the handler's legs for support. A dose syringe or pilling gun can be used to deliver the medication. If the head must be steadied, do not use the ears or throat; rather, place the hands behind the ears or under the jaws (Fig. 25-7).

Very young piglets can be dosed orally using two methods: by mouth and by stomach tube. The piglet can be lifted by the back of the head and neck, and a syringe can be used to deliver small volumes (<5 mL) to the back of the tongue, with care taken to make sure that the piglet swallows the medication. Injecting faster than the piglet can swallow risks aspiration of the liquid into the lungs.

> **TECHNICIAN NOTE**   Injecting faster than the piglet can swallow risks aspiration of the liquid into the lungs.

A flexible, nonkinking rubber tube can be passed into the stomach of a piglet. The length of tubing needed to reach the stomach is estimated by measuring along the pig's body from the mouth to the last rib. The piglet is lifted by the back of the head and neck, and the tube is passed over the back of the tongue to the esophageal entrance. Gentle force usually passes the tube into the esophagus. Piglets usually make swallowing motions as the tube passes down the esophagus, and passage should be easy, with minimal resistance. If the tube is accidentally placed in the trachea, it will pass easily but usually cannot be passed beyond the level of the base of the heart. This distance is less than the estimated distance to the stomach, which is why it is important to obtain this measurement before the procedure. Once the stomach is reached, up to 15 mL can be slowly delivered by a syringe connected to the tube. After injection, kink the tube for removal and remove it slowly. Observe the piglet for 10 minutes after the procedure for discomfort and regurgitation.

> **TECHNICIAN NOTE**   If the tube is placed in the trachea, it will not advance past the level of the base of the heart.

INJECTION TECHNIQUES

Restraint should be appropriate for the size of the animal and the location of the injection. One person can perform some of the procedures in small piglets, but most procedures require two people (one to restrain, one to inject). The skin should always be cleaned before any needle is inserted.

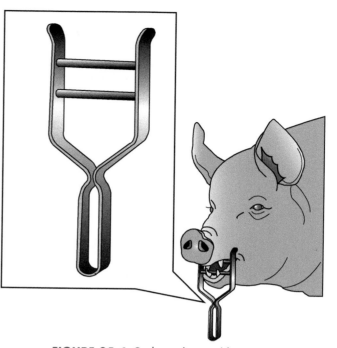

FIGURE 25-6 Oral speculum used for swine.

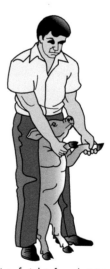

FIGURE 25-7 Restraint of piglets for administration of oral medication.

It is extremely important not to use bent or burred needles. Bent needles could break and remain inside the animal. Burred needles can increase scar tissue and must be cut from the meat at slaughter, thus decreasing the saleable product. All injections should follow the regulations of Pork Quality Assurance (PQA) or the PQA guidelines.

Intravenous Injection and Intravenous Catheterization

Equipment needed for intravenous injection and catheterization:

- Clippers
- Surgical scrub and alcohol
- 18- to 20-ga catheter

- Heparinized saline
- Adhesive tape

Intravenous (IV) injections and solutions for fluid therapy are most often given in the lateral auricular (ear) vein. The cephalic vein can also be used. In small piglets, other veins such as the jugular vein may be used because the ear vein and the cephalic vein at this age are small and difficult to access. Injections should be given slowly. Butterfly catheters (19 to 21 ga) may assist delivery of larger volumes of solutions.

Indwelling IV catheters (18 to 20 ga) can be placed in the *lateral auricular vein* but are difficult to maintain. After placement of a rubber band or forceps to distend the vein, the area over the vein is clipped and aseptically prepared (prepped). The tip of the ear is held for stability, and the catheter is inserted toward the base of the ear. After insertion is completed, the tourniquet is removed, and the catheter is capped and flushed. The hub is secured to the skin of the ear pinna using super glue or a similar adhesive. The pinna is supported by placing roll gauze or roll tape along the inside of the pinna, to form a "strut" for the ear. The pinna is bent around the strut to form a gentle curve. Several strips of 1-inch adhesive tape are used to encircle the ear and secure it to the strut while leaving access to the injection cap and catheter hub.

> **TECHNICIAN NOTE** The hub of the catheter can be secured to the ear pinna with super glue.

Intraperitoneal Injection

Equipment needed for intraperitoneal injection:
- Surgical scrub and alcohol
- Sterile gloves
- 16- to 18-ga × ¾- to 1-inch needle
- Isotonic fluid

Fluid therapy in piglets usually is given intraperitoneally. Fluids given by this route should be isotonic and should always be warmed. The piglet is held by the hindlegs, and the area between the ventral midline and the flank fold is prepared. Sterile gloves should be worn for the injection procedure. A 16- to 18-ga × ¾- to 1-inch needle is sufficient. The needle is inserted approximately halfway between ventral midline and the flank fold and only deep enough to enter the abdominal cavity. The needle should be manually stabilized during the infusion and not allowed to flop around, which could cause severe injury to the internal organs.

> **TECHNICIAN NOTE** Fluids delivered by intraperitoneal injection should be warmed and isotonic.

Intraperitoneal fluids can be given to larger pigs that are restrained in the standing position. After proper aseptic preparation of the skin, the injection is performed through the paralumbar fossa. A 16- to 18-ga × 3-inch needle may be necessary to penetrate the body wall at this location. The needle is stabilized during the infusion.

Intramuscular Injection

Equipment needed for intramuscular injection:
- Piglets: 18- to 20-ga × ⅝- to ½-inch needle
- Nursery pigs: 16- or 18-ga × ¾- to ⅝-inch needle
- Finishing or breeding stock: 14- to 16-ga × 1- to 1½-inch needle
- Syringe

As with meat-producing ruminants, concern for damaging valuable cuts of meat with injections has increased in recent years. The prime cuts of pork come from the hams, loins, and shoulder areas. Therefore, intramuscular (IM) injections are preferably given in the dorsal neck muscle behind the ears. Piglets can be held in one arm and injected with the free hand (Figs. 25-8 and 25-9). When possible, the skin-pinch injection technique is preferred but requires two people: one to restrain the animal and one to perform the injection. The skin adjacent to the injection site is pinched to pull the skin up, and the needle is inserted into the underlying muscle and the injection delivered. After the needle is removed, the skin pinch is released. This provides a natural "Band-Aid" of skin to cover the injection site and may minimize the incidence of injection abscesses.

> **TECHNICIAN NOTE** The prime cuts of meat come from the hams, loins, and shoulder areas. These areas should be avoided when performing intramuscular injections.

An 18- to 20-ga × ⅝- to ½-inch needle is used for IM injection in baby pigs, a 16- or 18-ga × ¾- to ⅝-inch needle is used for nursery pigs, and a 14- to 16-ga × 1- to 1½-inch needle is used for finishing to breeding stock. In animals with a thick layer of subcutaneous fat, the needle should be at least 2 inches long. Injection volume at any single IM site should not exceed 2 mL in piglets or 3 mL in larger pigs.

> **TECHNICIAN NOTE** Never give more than 2 mL per intramuscular injection in piglets or 3 mL in larger pigs.

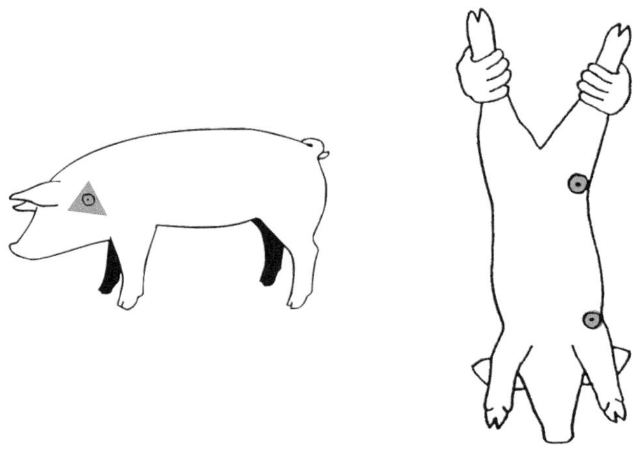

FIGURE 25-8 *Left,* Intramuscular injection site location. *Right,* Subcutaneous injection site locations. (Courtesy the National Pork Board, Des Moines, Iowa.)

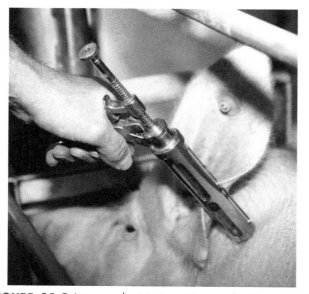

FIGURE 25-9 Intramuscular injection. (Courtesy the National Pork Board, Des Moines, Iowa.)

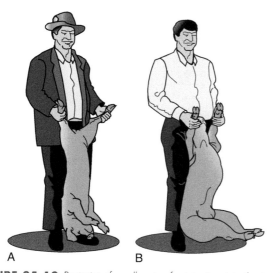

FIGURE 25-10 Restraint of small swine for injection into the inguinal (A) or axillary (B) regions.

Subcutaneous Injection

Equipment needed for subcutaneous injections:
- Piglets: 16- to 18-ga × ½-inch needle
- Finishing: 16-ga ×¾-inch needle
- Breeding stock: 14- to 16-ga × 1-inch needle
- Syringe

Subcutaneous injections can be given at several locations. Injections in small pigs (<50 pounds) are given in the axillary area caudal to the elbow or in the inguinal region in the flank skinfold. The pig is restrained by the legs, using the forelegs for access to the axillary region or the hindlegs for the inguinal region (Fig. 25-10; see also Fig. 25-8). For nursery piglets, a 16- to 18-ga × ½-inch needle is suitable, and 1 to 2 mL can be injected per site.

In larger pigs, restraint is provided with a hog snare. The area of loose skin behind the base of the ear can be used. Finishing hogs should be given subcutaneous injections with a 16-ga × ¾-inch needle, and a 14- to 16-ga × 1-inch needle should be used on breeding stock. Up to 3 mL can be injected per site.

Intranasal Injection
Equipment needed for intranasal injection:
- Needle
- Syringe
- Intranasal cannula

Restraint should place the head in an elevated position. This can be done by elevating the front legs and head in small pigs or by using a hog snare in older pigs. The product is given with a plain syringe or with the syringe and adapter provided with the vaccine or medication. The syringe or adapter is placed inside the nostril and the contents are injected, with the nose kept tilted upward until the injection is complete. It may be helpful to time the injection with the inspiration of the pig. As with other species, sneezing is the usual response after the injection.

> **TECHNICIAN NOTE**   It can be helpful to time the intranasal injection with the inspiration of the pig.

NEONATAL PROCESSING

Several management procedures are commonly performed in the first 1 to 2 days of life. One person, most often a farm worker, usually can perform these procedures. Veterinarians and veterinary technicians may assist in these procedures and can play an important role in teaching farm personnel to perform these procedures correctly and humanely.

> **TECHNICIAN NOTE**   Farm personnel most often perform neonatal processing within the first 1 to 2 days of life.

Because the piglets must be temporarily removed from the sow, personnel should be prepared for possible aggression by the sow in attempts to protect her piglets and for her vocalization and that of the piglets. Some farms have a processing room where the piglets are taken for the procedures, away from the sight and sounds of the sow. Piglets should not be removed from the sow for longer than 1 hour.

> **TECHNICIAN NOTE**   Piglets should not be removed from the sow for longer than 1 hour.

IRON DEXTRAN INJECTION

Equipment needed for iron dextran injection:
- Needle
- Syringe

Deciduous third incisor teeth

Deciduous
canine teeth

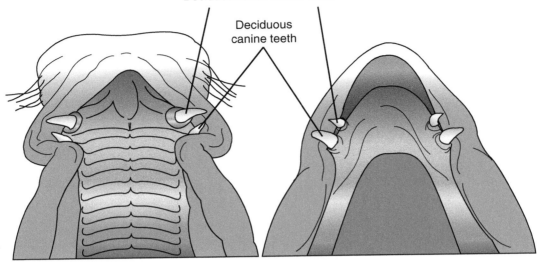

Upper jaw   Lower jaw

FIGURE 25-11 Needle teeth of piglet.

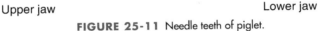

Sow's milk is naturally low in iron, and piglets are born with little iron in their bodies. In a natural setting, pigs acquire iron from eating soil and plants. In confinement rearing, this is not possible, and pigs of all ages are susceptible to anemia. Iron must be supplemented.

The anemia in piglets is referred to as *"baby pig thumps"* because of the extremely high heart rate that can easily be felt over the chest; this condition is accompanied by labored breathing and weakness. Piglets should be provided with a source of iron, usually in the form of injectable iron dextran (150 to 200 mg) given at 1 to 3 days of age. The IM injection should not be given in the ham muscles because permanent staining of the meat may occur. The neck is the preferred site for injection.

> **TECHNICIAN NOTE**
> • Sow's milk is naturally low in iron, and piglets are born with little iron in their bodies, thus making iron supplementation essential.
> • Anemia in piglets is also known as "baby pig thumps."

Continued iron supplementation can be given by a second iron dextran injection in 2 to 3 weeks. Another option is use of oral iron supplements in the creep feed, started at 1 to 2 weeks of age. Iron status can be determined indirectly by measuring the blood hemoglobin concentration; a blood hemoglobin level of 10 mg/dL or higher is considered adequate.

> **TECHNICIAN NOTE** Piglets must have a blood hemoglobin level of 10 mg/dL or higher.

CLIPPING NEEDLE TEETH

Equipment for clipping needle teeth:
• Needle tooth nippers
• Disinfectant

Piglets typically try to nurse almost anything that their snouts come in contact with, including the sow's vulva and other piglets. Piglets also fight each other for nursing position. Unfortunately, piglets are born with eight sharp teeth called *needle teeth*. The needle teeth are actually the deciduous I3 and deciduous canine teeth of each dental arcade (Fig. 25-11). The needle teeth are cut down to reduce injuries to the sow's teats, which are painful and may become infected, and to littermates. Wire cutters (side cutters) can be used to cut the teeth, or commercial *needle tooth nippers* can be used (Fig. 25-12). The nippers should be sharp and not used for other procedures, and they should be disinfected between use in piglets. The piglet is restrained by lifting it by the neck or head. The mouth is opened by placing firm but gentle pressure at the angle of the jaw, with care taken not to injure the jaw. The flat side of the nippers is placed parallel to the gum line so that the distal half to two thirds of each tooth is removed. The cut should be no closer to the gum line than 1 to 2 mm; cutting too short may cut the gums or fracture the tooth roots and thus provide an entrance point for bacteria. The procedure is well tolerated, and no special aftercare is required.

> **TECHNICIAN NOTE**
> • Needle teeth are the deciduous I3 and deciduous canine teeth of each dental arcade.
> • Needle tooth nippers should be disinfected between use in piglets.

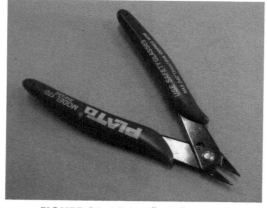

FIGURE 25-12 Needle tooth nippers.

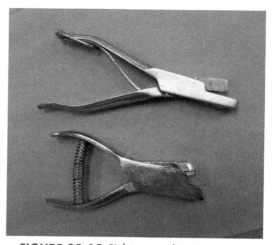

FIGURE 25-13 Piglet ear notching instruments.

TAIL DOCKING

Piglets tend to suck and chew on each other's tails. Tail-biting behavior continues after weaning, even into the feedlot and finishing stages. In addition to causing pain and stress, the open sores may become infected and form abscesses. It is not unusual for the infection to migrate cranially along the spinal nerves of the tail and cause ataxia and even paralysis of the hindlegs. Many feeder pig operations do not accept pigs with tails. To reduce tail biting and its associated complications, tail docking is routinely practiced. Tail docking is preferably performed at 1 to 2 days of age and is tolerated well by neonates. It should not be performed after 2 weeks of age.

> **TECHNICIAN NOTE**   Tail docking is performed because pigs, even adults, will bite each other's tails, thereby causing infection and abscesses that can lead to paralysis.

The piglet is restrained by supporting it under the body and holding it aloft or by holding it between the handler's knees. The tail can be docked with wire (side) cutters or baby pig emasculators. Sharp wire cutter blades tend to result in more bleeding. Using slightly dulled blades or briefly heating the blades to cauterize the blood vessels as the cut is made may be helpful. Emasculators provide a crushing component as the cut is made that helps control bleeding. Emasculators used for tail docking should not be used for castration. The instrument should be cleaned and disinfected between use in piglets. Piglets should be observed for several hours for excessive bleeding and for several days for signs of infection. The level of docking is important because the incidence of rectal prolapse increases if the tail is cut too short. The tail should be docked approximately ½ to 1 inch from the base. The freshly cut stump should be dipped or sprayed with antiseptic solution.

> **TECHNICIAN NOTE**
> - Using slightly dulled blades to perform tail docking can help minimize bleeding.
> - The likelihood of rectal prolapse increases if the tail is cut too short. The tail should be cut ½ inch from the base.

EAR NOTCHING AND TATTOOING

Equipment for ear notching and tattooing:
- Ear notching pliers
- Disinfectant

The most common method for identifying swine is ear notching. This method involves cutting out small, wedge-shaped sections of ear cartilage along the margin of the ear. The wedges do not grow back, and they leave permanent notches that enlarge with the ear as it grows. Special ear notching pliers, or V-notchers, are used to remove the wedges of tissue (Fig. 25-13).

Piglets appear to tolerate the procedure well. The head should be held gently but securely. The notches should be made quickly and firmly to produce a clean cut. Piglets should be observed for excessive bleeding for several hours after the procedure and watched for signs of infection in the following days. Notching pliers should be kept sharp, and they should be cleaned and disinfected between use in piglets.

> **TECHNICIAN NOTE**   Notching pliers should be disinfected between use in piglets.

A standard numbering system (*universal ear notching system*) using standard locations for the ear notches has been developed. However, farmers may use any system recommended by breed associations, or they may design their own. The hog farmer usually numbers each litter sequentially throughout the year. In each litter, each piglet receives an individual number. For example, a litter number of 76 indicates the seventy-sixth litter born during the farrowing season. If nine piglets are in the litter, they are assigned an individual number from 1 to 9. By convention, the litter number is placed in the right ear, and the individual piglet number is placed in the left ear (Fig. 25-14).

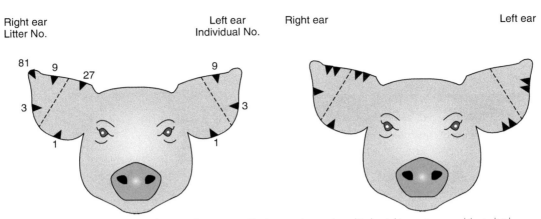

Right ear
Litter No.

Left ear
Individual No.

Right ear

Left ear

FIGURE 25-14 Universal ear notching system. The litter number is placed in the right ear pinna, and the individual pig number is placed in the left ear pinna. The pig on the *right* shows litter number 76, individual pig number 8.

Baby pigs can also be tattooed on the body or ear. Ear tattoos can be placed on the inside or outside of the ear pinna with small ear tattoo pliers. The ear vein should be avoided if possible. Body tattoos can be placed on the shoulder or rump, where they can be easily read. Body tattoos are placed using a commercially available baby pig body tattooer, which basically consists of a short metal handle with a holder on one end for placing the interchangeable number and letter character pins. After the tattoo ink is applied, the pins are pressed directly into the body. Additional ink is rubbed into the holes left by the needles.

EUTHANASIA AND NECROPSY

According to the 2000 Report of the American Veterinary Medical Association (AVMA) Panel on Euthanasia, the following methods of euthanasia are acceptable for swine:
- Barbiturate IV injection
- Carbon dioxide gas, the only chemical used for euthanasia that does not leave residues in tissue
- Potassium chloride (KCl) IV injection in conjunction with general anesthesia, with anesthesia induced first
- Penetrating captive bolt

The following methods are conditionally acceptable:
- Inhalant anesthetic gases (overdose)
- Carbon monoxide
- Chloral hydrate IV injection after sedation
- Gunshot
- Electrocution applied to the head

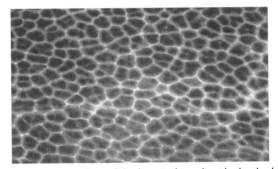

FIGURE 25-15 Surface of the liver (enlarged) with clearly defined hepatic lobules. (From Dyce KM, Sack WO, Wensing CJG: *Textbook of veterinary anatomy*, ed 4, St. Louis, 2010, Saunders.)

- Concussion (blow) to the head; suitable only for animals less than 3 weeks old and must be applied by trained personnel to be humane

The reader should consult the AVMA report for descriptions and details of these methods.

NECROPSY

Necropsy is performed with the animal in left lateral recumbency. The procedure is basically the same as that described for small mammals (dogs, cats).

The technician should be familiar with the normal anatomy of the pig and be aware of several anatomical differences in this species as compared with other large animals, such as horses, cattle, sheep, and goats. The liver of the pig has an unusual appearance that may be mistaken for a pathologic condition. The liver lobules are clearly separated and defined by a high content of fibrous connective tissue (Fig. 25-15). The tonsillar tissue of the pig is diffusely scattered on the lateral pharyngeal walls, rather than being a distinct organ within a tonsillar crypt. The *nasal turbinates* should always be examined for distortion or atrophy, which may indicate atrophic rhinitis. A transverse cut through the snout at the level of the premolars is used to evaluate the turbinates more closely.

> **TECHNICIAN NOTE** The pig's liver lobules are clearly separated and are defined by a high content of fibrous connective tissue.

CASE STUDY

Mr. Schaaf owns approximately 1000 sows among his 3 farrowing barns. He has asked you to come and give an in-service on neonatal pig processing. Lately he has seen an increase in infection after processing. What equipment will you take with you? What will you emphasize to Mr. Schaaf's employees to help reduce the infection rates?

CASE STUDY

Mr. Gentle is farrowing out five sows for his children to use as 4-H projects. Mr. Gentle has called the veterinarian out to perform a physical examination on the piglets. The piglets are approximately 5 days old, and he says they seem to have trouble breathing. He has also noticed they seem to be lethargic and weak. When the veterinarian arrives and holds one of the piglets, she can feel the heartbeat through the chest wall. The veterinarian asks you to draw blood and run a blood hemoglobin test, which reveals a level of 5 mg/dL. The piglet is diagnosed with "baby pig thumps." What methods are available for you to draw the blood? What is actually wrong with the baby pig? What will the doctor most likely prescribe to correct the condition?

SUGGESTED READING

Davis H, Riel DL, Pappagianis M, Miguel K: Diagnostic sampling and therapeutic techniques. In Bassert JM, McCurnin DM, editors: *McCurnin's clinical textbook for veterinary technicians*, ed 7, St. Louis, 2010, Saunders, pp 585–673.

Ensminger ME, Parker RO: *Swine science*, ed 7, Danville, Ill, 2005, Interstate Publishers.

Fubini SL, Ducharme NG: *Farm animal surgery*, St. Louis, 2004, Saunders.

Gillespie JR, Flanders FB: *Modern livestock and poultry*, ed 8, Clifton Park, NY, 2010, Delmar Cengage Learning.

Goswami S: Anatomy and physiology. In Sirois M, editor: *Principles and practice of veterinary technology*, ed 2, St. Louis, 2004, Mosby, pp 77–120.

Hafez ESE: *Reproduction in farm animals*, ed 7, Philadelphia, 2000, Lea & Febiger.

Noakes DE, Parkinson TJ, England GCW: *Veterinary reproduction and obstetrics*, ed 9, London, 2009, Saunders.

Pinto CRF, Eilts BE, Paccamonti DL: Animal reproduction. In Bassert JM, McCurnin DM, editors: *McCurnin's clinical textbook for veterinary technicians*, ed 7, St. Louis, 2010, Saunders, pp 370–399.

Sonsthagen T, Teeple TN: Nursing care of food animals, camelids, and ratites. In Sirois M, editor: *Principles and practice of veterinary technology*, ed 3, St. Louis, 2011, Mosby, pp 585–611.

Turner AS, McIlwraith CW: *Techniques in large animal surgery*, Philadelphia, 1982, Lea & Febiger.

26 Porcine Surgical Procedures

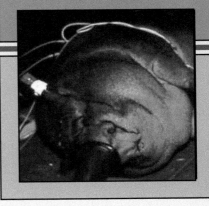

LEARNING OBJECTIVES

After reading this chapter, you will be able to

- Prepare the surgical patient for surgical procedures
- Perform local anesthesia or assist the veterinarian in administering local anesthesia
- Assist or perform induction and maintenance of anesthesia
- Provide anesthetic monitoring
- Manage patient recovery and immediate postoperative care
- Discuss the basic risks and possible complications associated with anesthesia and surgery
- Implement preventive measures when indicated

KEY TERMS

Arytenoid cartilages
Herniorrhaphy
Inguinal hernia
Malignant hyperthermia

Pharyngeal recess
Scrotal hernia
Specific pathogen-free
Stagging

Taint
Tusks
Umbilical hernia

KEY ABBREVIATION

SPF: Specific pathogen-free (piglets)

SWINE SURGERY AND ANESTHESIA

Although the vast array of surgical procedures and technology available for other species is available for swine, economic considerations usually make many procedures impractical except for valuable breeding stock and valued pets.

Standing surgery is an option only for a few minor procedures. Most surgical procedures on swine are performed with the animal in recumbency, using either general anesthesia or a combination of local anesthesia and sedation. As in other species, whenever possible, local anesthesia and sedation are preferred to general anesthesia. Swine face the same risks associated with general anesthesia as other species but with the additional concerns of high body temperatures and the possible development of *malignant hyperthermia* under general anesthesia. Malignant hyperthermia, which is part of the porcine stress syndrome, occurs rarely in swine during inhalation anesthesia.

> **TECHNICIAN NOTE** Malignant hyperthermia is a risk of general anesthesia.

Potbellied pigs can be anesthetized with the techniques used for the other swine breeds. Small animal anesthesia machines and equipment can be used for pigs of this size. Malignant hyperthermia is extremely rare in potbellied pigs.

> **TECHNICIAN NOTE** Malignant hyperthermia is extremely rare in potbellied pigs.

PAIN MANAGEMENT

For an explanation of drug categories, please see Chapter 10 (Table 26-1).

LOCAL ANESTHESIA

Lumbosacral Epidural Anesthesia

Epidural anesthesia in swine is performed at the lumbosacral junction. No other epidural site is readily accessible in this species. The epidural space at this location is fairly large and easy to enter with a needle. Anesthesia administered at this location is considered to be a "cranial epidural," as opposed to the "caudal epidural" frequently used in other large animal species. Epidural procedures are frequently performed for analgesia during cesarean section operations, and the systemic effects on the fetuses are minimal.

The proper site for epidural anesthesia administration must be identified. The lumbosacral junction is just caudal to a line drawn transversely through the animal to connect the crests of the wings of the ilium, where the line bisects the dorsal midline. In small swine, the wings of the ilium are palpable. In large swine, anatomical landmarks must be relied on to locate the site. Large swine are preferably injected when they are in the standing position, standing squarely on all four legs. Looking at the pig from the side, a vertical line is drawn upward from the patella; this line usually identifies the cranial extent of the crest of the ilium. The needle is inserted 1 to 1½ inches caudal to this line, on the dorsal midline (Fig. 26-1).

The animal should be sedated for the procedure, if possible, or restrained with a hog snare, or both. The hair is clipped, and the skin is aseptically prepared. Up to 5 mL of 2% lidocaine is deposited subcutaneously to a depth of 1 to 2 inches to reduce the patient's discomfort and movement during the actual epidural block. A final scrub is applied to the skin.

Sterile gloves should be worn for the procedure. The needle for the epidural block should be an 18- to 20-gauge (ga) spinal needle. A 3-inch-long needle is necessary for small swine, a 4-inch needle for swine weighing more than 100 kg, and a 5- to 7-inch needle for swine weighing 200 kg or more. These needles are easily bent, and some clinicians prefer to use a shorter (1- to 2-inch) 14-ga needle as a protective sleeve trocar for the 18-ga needle. The 14-ga needle is placed first, and then the 18-ga needle is passed through its lumen.

Lidocaine 2% (without epinephrine) is an anesthetic drug commonly used for the block. The dose used depends on the body weight of the patient and the desired effects, ranging from 0.5 to 1 mL/4.5 kg of body weight (maximum, 20 mL). Lower doses provide analgesia caudal to the lumbosacral area, but higher doses can diffuse and produce analgesia as far cranially as the first lumbar vertebra. Anesthesia begins approximately 5 to 10 minutes after injection, reaches a maximum at 20 minutes, and lasts as long as 2 hours.

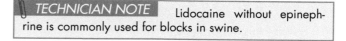

TECHNICIAN NOTE   Lidocaine without epinephrine is commonly used for blocks in swine.

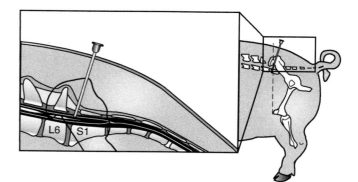

FIGURE 26-1 Location of lumbosacral epidural anesthesia in the pig. L6 is the sixth lumbar vertebra, and S1 is the first sacral vertebra. Note that a vertical line from the patella indicates the crest of the wing of the ilium. The needle is placed just caudally to this line. (Modified from Muir WW 3rd, Hubbell JAE, Bednarski RM, Skarda RT: *Handbook of veterinary anesthesia*, ed 3, St. Louis, 2000, Mosby.)

TABLE 26-1	Drugs Used in Porcine Surgical Procedures			
	DOSE	**CONCENTRATION**	**ROUTE**	**MEAT WITHDRAWAL TIME**
Flunixin meglumine	2.2 mg/kg	50 mg/mL	IM	12 days
Phenylbutazone	4 mg/kg q24h	IV: 200 mg/mL PO: 100-mg tablets 6-g tube 12-g tube	IV	None established; recommended 15 days
Ketoprofen	3 mg/kg/day	100 mg/mL	IV, IM, PO	None established; recommended 7 days
Meloxicam	0.4 mg/kg q24h	5 mg/mL	0.5 mg/mL 7.5- and 15-mg tablets	15 days
Acetylsalicylic acid (aspirin)	10 mg/kg	240-gr bolus 480-gr bolus	PO	24 hr
Xylazine	0.5–3 mg/kg	100 mg/mL	IM	5 days
Ketamine	1–2 mg/kg	100 mg/mL	IV or IM	2 days

IM, Intramuscularly; *IV*, intravenously; *PO*, orally.

Xylazine can also be injected into the lumbosacral epidural space. At a dose of 2 mg/kg (diluted in 5 mL of sterile saline), it produces surgical anesthesia of the body caudal to the umbilicus and paralysis of the hindlegs. The analgesic effects begin within 20 to 30 minutes and may last up to 2 to 3 hours. The dose is important because doses up to 1 mg/kg do not produce surgical anesthesia, and doses 3 mg/kg or greater cause prolonged hindlimb paresis and ataxia that last for 36 hours or more. Lidocaine 2% can be mixed with xylazine to give a more rapid onset of analgesia (5 minutes), which may last as long as 5 hours.

> **TECHNICIAN NOTE** When xylazine is used, it is important to use a dose of 2 mg/kg because lower doses will not work, and higher doses can cause hindlimb paresis for 36 hours or more.

Remember that epidural anesthesia does not desensitize or immobilize the head, neck, or forelimbs of an animal. The animal must be controlled with physical restraint, sedation, or both.

GENERAL ANESTHESIA
Anesthetic Risks for Swine
Before administering anesthesia to swine, the risks of hypoventilation and hyperthermia should be considered.

Swine Are Prone to Hypoventilation
Inadequate ventilation may result in hypoxemia, which may lead to death. Several potential sources of ventilation problems may exist alone or in combination.

Airway Obstruction. Any factor that decreases the cross-sectional area of the upper airways greatly increases the resistance to breathing.
- The larynx of swine is sensitive to physical stimulation. Pressure and touch, even from accumulated saliva, can trigger a laryngospasm.
- The laryngeal lumen of the pig is small in relation to the size of the animal. A pig weighing 100 kg requires an endotracheal tube that would fit a large dog (≈14-mm internal diameter). Flexing the neck partially occludes the laryngeal entrance. Salivation, which is common in anesthetized pigs, can result in accumulations of saliva in the pharynx and laryngeal entrance that actually occlude the larynx.
- Laryngeal edema results readily in swine because of their relatively fragile laryngeal mucosa. The laryngeal mucosa is quite easy to traumatize during endotracheal intubation and responds quickly with swelling. This edema of the larynx causes further narrowing of the already small lumen diameter.

> **TECHNICIAN NOTE** The swine larynx is sensitive to pressure or touch, even from accumulated saliva, which can trigger laryngospasm.

Respiratory Depression. The depressant effects of drugs used for chemical restraint and anesthesia are seen in swine (as in other species).

Limited Expansion of the Chest Wall. Recumbency and anesthetic drug depression may combine to reduce the full expansion of the chest wall. Obesity may magnify this effect.

Swine Are Prone to Hyperthermia Under Anesthesia
Although swine have sweat glands in the skin, the glands do not function efficiently in thermoregulation of the animal. Subcutaneous accumulation of fat contributes to the development of hyperthermia. In addition, swine have a low amount of body surface area for their body size, which inhibits the dissipation of heat. Because of these factors, body temperature tends to rise when swine are anesthetized, and the effects may be increased if anesthesia is performed in a hot environment.

> **TECHNICIAN NOTE** Swine have sweat glands in the skin, but these glands do not function efficiently in thermoregulation of the animal.

Occasionally, malignant hyperthermia develops in genetically predisposed animals. This condition develops rapidly and is difficult to control, and the outcome typically is fatal.

Preanesthetic Preparation and Anesthetic Management
Preanesthetic Evaluation
History and physical examination should be performed, with an emphasis on the respiratory system. Laboratory tests should be appropriate for the length and type of surgical procedure, as well as the physical condition of the patient. A complete blood count is always advisable.

> **TECHNICIAN NOTE** A complete blood count is always advisable before surgical procedures.

Preanesthetic Preparation
Regurgitation may occur when the animal is under anesthesia but is not common. Food is withheld for 6 to 12 hours in adults and 1 to 3 hours in piglets. Water usually is not withdrawn.

Preanesthetic Drugs
Because so few superficial veins other than the ear veins can be accessed, most preanesthetic and injectable anesthetic drugs are given intramuscularly (IM). The location of intramuscular injection can affect the speed and depth of anesthesia. Intramuscular injection into the gluteal, back, or shoulder muscles provides more consistent results than does injections into the neck muscles; however, gluteal injections risk damaging a valuable cut of pork (ham).

The neck muscles have numerous fascial (dense connective tissue) planes; accidental injection into fascia may cause uneven, slow absorption with unreliable results. If the neck muscle is used, the safest site for injection is just caudal to the base of the ear, where less fascia is present in the muscle.

Atropine is sometimes used to control salivation in swine, which can be excessive. Atropine is given at a dosage of 0.044 mg/kg IM.

Induction Drugs

Various anesthetic induction and maintenance regimens are available for swine. Withdrawal times for meat-producing animals should be observed. A quiet induction area is preferred. Restraint in a chute or crate is generally less stressful than other forms of physical restraint (e.g., snout restraint). Some of the techniques in use are listed in Box 26-1.

> **TECHNICIAN NOTE** Withdrawal time for meat-producing animals should be observed.

Endotracheal Intubation

The technician should be aware of several anatomical features that are unique to swine and affect endotracheal intubation. Pigs have a small laryngeal opening and narrow trachea. Endotracheal tube sizes seem small compared with the body weight of the animal. Pigs have a *pharyngeal recess*, which is a blind pouch located dorsal to the esophagus; the endotracheal tube will not advance if it is directed into this location. Visualization of the larynx is difficult because the mouth of the pig does not open widely and the soft palate is long.

> **TECHNICIAN NOTE**
> - Pigs have a small laryngeal opening and a narrow trachea.
> - Pigs have a pharyngeal recess, which is a blind pouch that, if entered, will not allow the endotracheal tube to advance.

To reduce the risk of laryngospasm and the risk of traumatizing the larynx, topical desensitization of the larynx may be performed by spraying it with lidocaine. A soft, small animal urethral catheter can be used to apply the lidocaine on the larynx.

Sternal recumbency with the head and neck extended is the preferred position for intubation. An assistant opens the mouth by using a gauze strip placed around the mandible and another one around the maxilla to pull the mouth jaws apart. Direct visualization with a laryngoscope (long blade) is recommended for endotracheal intubation. Preplacing an endotracheal tube stylet in the laryngeal entrance is helpful, similar to the technique described for small ruminants.

The larynx tends to angle ventrally, and the proximal trachea tends to angle dorsally. Because of the anatomy of the

| **BOX 26-1** | Anesthetic Induction and Maintenance Regimens Available for Swine |

- Telazol (a proprietary combination of tiletamine and zolazepam)/ketamine/xylazine (TKX): All three drugs are mixed together in the Telazol vial and are given intramuscularly (IM). This popular combination provides short-term anesthesia (20 to 30 minutes). It also can be used for stages from induction to inhalant gas maintenance. Endotracheal intubation can be performed with this combination. Repeated injections of the combination can be used to extend the length of general anesthesia. Recovery from anesthesia occurs in 60 to 90 minutes.
- Atropine/acepromazine/ketamine: Atropine and acepromazine are given IM, followed by ketamine IM approximately 20 minutes later. This combination is useful for minor, short procedures. Anesthesia lasts approximately 10 to 15 minutes. Analgesia must be supplemented with local anesthetics for painful procedures.
- Atropine/xylazine/ketamine: Atropine and xylazine are given IM, followed by ketamine IM approximately 10 minutes later. Anesthesia lasts approximately 10 to 15 minutes.
- Xylazine/Telazol: Xylazine is given IM, followed by Telazol IM 5 minutes later. Although analgesia and muscle relaxation are satisfactory, the depth of surgical anesthesia may be light and of short duration. Drowsiness after recovery may be prolonged (up to 24 hours).
- Intratesticular sodium pentobarbital: A technique for anesthesia for castration of large boars has been described. Sodium pentobarbital is injected into each testicle to produce anesthesia in approximately 5 minutes. Removal of the testicles effectively removes the source of the anesthesia.
- Inhalant gases: Mask induction, with or without earlier sedation, can be used in small or heavily sedated swine. Halothane, isoflurane, and sevoflurane all are suitable for use in swine, but halothane is generally avoided because of the risk of inducing malignant hyperthermia in susceptible families of swine.
- Intravenous thiobarbiturates: An intravenous catheter or butterfly administration set can be used in the ear vein to inject thiobarbiturates. This may be the safest choice for anesthesia in pigs from family lines susceptible to malignant hyperthermia.

larynx and proximal trachea, it is suggested to begin placement of the endotracheal tube with the tube curvature angled ventrally until the tip is within the larynx (beyond the *arytenoid cartilages*). After the tip has cleared the larynx, it may be necessary to rotate the tube curvature 180 degrees so that the tube tip points dorsally, to advance the tube. Regurgitation may occur during intubation.

> **TECHNICIAN NOTE** It may be helpful to start intubation with the curve of the tube pointed ventrally and then turn the tube beyond the arytenoid cartilages.

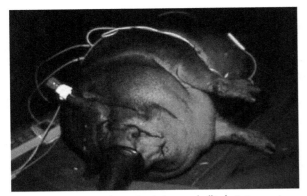

FIGURE 26-2 General anesthesia in a potbellied pig to repair severe bilateral entropion. (From Jackson PGG, Cockcroft PD: *Handbook of pig medicine,* Edinburgh, 2007, Saunders.)

Maintenance of Anesthesia

Anesthesia can be maintained with injectable drugs or inhalant gases. Small animal anesthesia machines can be used for animals up to 140 kg. Slightly larger animals can use a small animal machine if high oxygen gas flow rates (>4 L/minute oxygen) are used (Fig. 26-2).

Halothane, isoflurane, and sevoflurane can be used in swine. Halothane may cause malignant hyperthermia in susceptible individuals and is best avoided, if possible. Isoflurane and sevoflurane are not known to produce hyperthermia. The induction and maintenance concentrations of the anesthetic gases are similar to those used in ruminants.

> **TECHNICIAN NOTE** Halothane may cause malignant hyperthermia in susceptible animals and is best avoided.

Nitrous oxide can be safely used in swine. It is given with oxygen at 40% to 60% of the total inspired gas concentration.

Monitoring Anesthesia

Anesthetic monitoring is similar to that in other large animal species. Differences are listed in Box 26-2.

Fluid Therapy

Fluid therapy with a balanced electrolyte solution can be given intravenously and is recommended for sick or dehydrated patients. The recommended administration rate for stable, anesthetized patients is 10 mL/kg/hour.

> **TECHNICIAN NOTE** The recommended administration rate of fluid therapy for stable, anesthetized patients is 10 mL/kg/hour.

Recovery

Sternal recumbency is preferred for recovery from anesthesia. A cool, quiet environment is desirable. Supplemental oxygen through the endotracheal tube is advisable until the

---

BOX 26-2	Anesthetic Monitoring in Swine

- The auricular artery on the dorsal aspect of the ear pinna can be used for arterial blood gas sampling and for catheterization for direct blood pressure monitoring.
- Heart rate under anesthesia should range from 50 to 150 beats/minute. The auricular and femoral arteries are the best locations for pulse assessment.
- Eye signs may be difficult to interpret in swine and highly depend on the anesthetic drug regimen.
- Hyperthermia is a risk of inhalation anesthesia in swine and must be detected early to have any chance of successful treatment. Rectal temperature should be monitored for hyperthermia. Malignant hyperthermia is recognized by extremely high body temperature (>107° F). Temperatures higher than 103° F are concerning, and measures to cool the animal are advisable. Other clinical signs include muscle rigidity, increased heart rate and respiratory rate, and metabolic acidosis. Note that ketamine tends to increase body temperature.
- Treatment of malignant hyperthermia begins with discontinuing anesthetic gas administration but continuing oxygen delivery; 100% oxygen should be used to flush the anesthetic breathing circuit. Efforts to cool the body by any reasonable means should be instituted immediately. Dantrolene (2.2 mg/kg intravenously), a muscle relaxant, is recommended and is the only specific treatment. Fluids should be given and may include bicarbonate to treat the metabolic acidosis. Corticosteroids may be given to combat shock.

animal is extubated. Smaller tubing then can be placed in a nostril for oxygen delivery until the animal attempts to rise. Extubation is performed when the animal makes strong attempts to swallow and should be done with the cuff deflated. Because hypoventilation is a common problem in swine, the technician should be prepared to assist ventilation, if necessary. Swine are at risk for laryngeal edema and spasm, and tracheostomy materials should be readily available (scalpel handle and number 10 scalpel blade, hemostats, and cuffed tracheostomy tube).

> **TECHNICIAN NOTE** Tracheostomy materials should be readily available during and after surgical procedures.

COMMON SURGICAL PROCEDURES

CASTRATION

In the United States and Canada, intact males cannot be marketed for meat. The primary reason is "boar *taint,*" a distinct, objectionable odor that is released during cooking and produces an unpleasant flavor to the meat. Boar taint begins with the onset of puberty. Castrated males do not produce meat with this odor. If a boar is castrated after sexual maturity (*"stagging"*), the odor will disappear approximately 3 to

4 weeks after castration. Castration may improve feed conversion and make animals easier to handle. All male pigs that are not used for breeding purposes should be castrated by 2 weeks of age. Although castration can be performed at any age, early castration is safer for the animal because of fewer surgical complications and less stress from restraint. Some farm operations castrate on day 1 or 2 after birth.

> **TECHNICIAN NOTE** Early castration is safer for the animal.

Restraint for castration depends on the age and size of the animal. Experienced personnel can hold a neonatal pig with one hand and castrate it with the other hand. Older piglets require one person to hold the animal and another to perform the castration. Piglets up to approximately 50 pounds are held up by the hindlegs, with the back resting against the restrainer so that the restrainer can secure the piglet by squeezing its back and shoulders between the thighs and knees. Alternatively, the piglet can be placed in dorsal recumbency in a clean V-trough with one person holding the front legs and another holding the hindlegs. The surgical room or area should be clean and free of drafts.

Before the surgical procedure is started, the inguinal and scrotal areas are palpated to ensure that both testicles are descended and that inguinal or *scrotal hernias* are not present. A veterinarian should be consulted if abnormalities are detected or suspected. If the animal is palpably normal, the scrotal area is prepared for an aseptic surgical procedure with mild disinfectant solution. The use of lidocaine for local anesthesia is possible. Approximately 2 to 3 mL of lidocaine in a small syringe with a 25-ga needle is used to deposit the anesthetic agent subcutaneously and around the spermatic cord.

> **TECHNICIAN NOTE** The animal should be checked for hernias before the surgical procedure.

A Bard Parker number 3 scalpel handle and number 12 blade are commonly used to castrate piglets. The scrotum is tightened to force the testicles cranially toward the inguinal area (for improved ventral drainage of the incisions postoperatively), and a longitudinal 1-cm incision is made directly over each testicle. The testicles are pushed out through the incisions and are pulled to expose the spermatic cords. The spermatic cords must be severed to remove the testicles. The scalpel blade is used to scrape or "tease" the spermatic cord apart, and this provides more hemostasis than sharply cutting the cord (Fig. 26-3). Alternatively, a piglet emasculator can be used by applying it for approximately 1 minute. The incisions are left open to drain and can be treated with antiseptic spray. Neonatal piglets should be kept warm after the procedure and observed for hemorrhage and infection. Healing requires approximately 5 to 7 days.

Older pigs must be heavily sedated or anesthetized for castration. The animal is restrained in lateral recumbency.

The scrotum is aseptically prepared for the surgical procedure. The testicles usually are removed through two incisions left open to drain, but it is possible to remove them through one incision that is closed with suture (similar to dogs). If the spermatic cords are well developed, they are ligated with suture before an emasculator is used to divide the cord. Hemorrhage, infection, and seroma or hematoma are the most common complications.

> **TECHNICIAN NOTE** The incisions are left open to drain.

Inguinal hernias are fairly common in pigs and have a hereditary origin. The inherited anatomical defect is an abnormally large vaginal ring, which is an entrance to the inguinal canal. The typical hernia occurs when a portion of the intestinal tract enters the inguinal canal. The herniated intestine may go no farther than the inguinal canal, or it may continue into the scrotal sac to form a scrotal hernia. Scrotal hernias are larger and more often noticed, but *inguinal hernias* are not easily seen (Fig. 26-4). The condition may be bilateral. These hernias are often discovered at the time of castration and are problematic for two reasons. First, if castration is performed without correcting the problem first, it is possible to cut into the intestines during the castration procedure. Second, if an animal with an inguinal hernia or scrotal hernia is castrated by a method that leaves the spermatic cord open (not closed with ligatures), the intestines frequently will eviscerate after the castration. This condition usually is fatal for the animal. If an inguinal or scrotal hernia is detected, a veterinarian should be consulted. Surgical treatment by a veterinarian to correct the hernia (inguinal *herniorrhaphy*) and castrate the animal is advised.

Cryptorchidism is common in pigs. Castration should never be performed unless both testicles can be palpated within their scrotal sacs. If cryptorchidism is suspected, a veterinarian should evaluate the animal and perform cryptorchidectomy, if necessary.

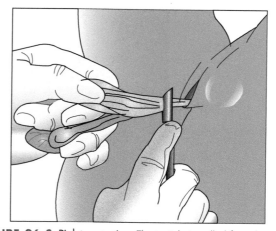

FIGURE 26-3 Piglet castration. The testicle is pulled from the scrotal incision, and a scalpel blade is used to scrape the spermatic cord repeatedly until it severs.

REPAIR OF UMBILICAL HERNIAS

Umbilical herniation occurs when the natural umbilical opening in the abdominal wall fails to close completely after birth and allows contents of the abdomen to protrude through the abdominal wall. The skin and surrounding connective tissue form a "hernia sac," which is a potential space into which abdominal contents may slide in and out. The actual opening in the abdominal wall is referred to as the "hernia ring." The size of the hernia ring determines which abdominal organs or tissues can "herniate." Small defects may allow only omentum to enter the hernia sac, but larger defects may allow portions of the intestinal tract to enter. The greatest risk of a hernia is entrapment of tissue in the hernia sac, with subsequent tissue strangulation, necrosis, and death.

Umbilical hernias are not uncommon in swine. Development of the condition has a hereditary component, but umbilical infections and abscesses may contribute in some cases. Umbilical hernias are not usually recognized until the animal is 9 to 14 weeks of age, when the hernia often is noticeably large. The condition is recognized as a visible enlargement at the umbilicus. The enlargement typically is soft, nonpainful, and fluctuant (uncomplicated hernia) (Figs. 26-5 and 26-6). These animals usually are otherwise healthy in appearance and behavior. It may even be possible to reduce the hernia by gently massaging the hernia sac to force the contents back into the abdomen; however, the hernia usually reappears when the massage is stopped. Hard, painful enlargements usually signal that infection and strangulation of the hernial contents are involved. These animals commonly are febrile, depressed, and possibly in shock if strangulation has occurred.

The condition often can be surgically corrected, but other treatments are frequently used because of the costs of surgical treatment. These animals often are destined for slaughter, and the farmer usually strives to market the pig early, before strangulation of the hernia occurs. If the hernia is large enough to touch the ground or if the skin over the hernia is ulcerated, the pig will be declined for market, and euthanasia is advised. A long-used "home remedy" for umbilical hernias is the hernia clamp. Hernia clamps can be homemade, but aluminum and disposable plastic clamps are commercially available (Fig. 26-7). Before the clamp is used, the contents of the hernia must be completely reduced into the abdomen. With the contents reduced, the skin

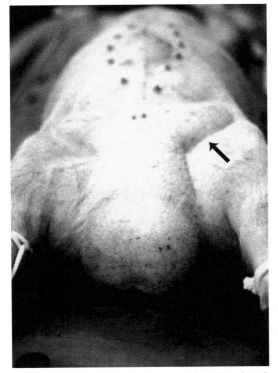

FIGURE 26-4 Pig with a scrotal hernia restrained in dorsal recumbency. Note swelling at the left inguinal area *(arrow)* that continues down into the left scrotal sac. (From Fubini SL, Ducharme NG: *Farm animal surgery,* St. Louis, 2004, Saunders.)

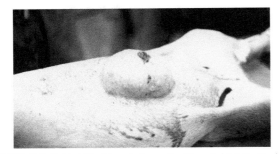

FIGURE 26-5 Umbilical hernia in a pig. (From Fubini SL, Ducharme NG: *Farm animal surgery,* St. Louis, 2004, Saunders.)

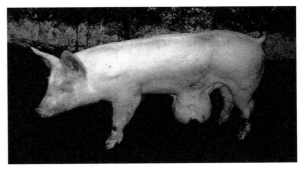

FIGURE 26-6 Umbilical hernia in a weaner. (From Jackson PGG, Cockcroft PD: *Handbook of pig medicine,* Edinburgh, 2007, Saunders.)

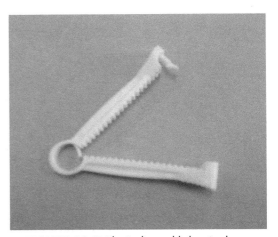

FIGURE 26-7 Plastic disposable hernia clamp.

of the hernia sac is pulled tautly, and the clamp is placed across the base of the sac as close as possible to the abdominal wall. The clamp is designed to prevent reherniation. If left in place long enough, the clamp causes gradual necrosis and death of the skin within its jaws, and the clamp eventually falls off. Ideally, the scar tissue that results will be firm enough to prevent reherniation of abdominal contents. However, the procedure is not without risks. The hernia clamp does nothing to close the actual hernia ring in the abdominal wall, and the hernia may recur. In addition, the necrosis caused by the clamp provides a potential entrance for bacteria such as tetanus. The clamp does not change the deoxyribonucleic acid (DNA) of the animal or the possibility of passing the condition to offspring.

Owners of purebred breeding stock and pet animals are more likely to request surgical correction (herniorrhaphy). General anesthesia is required, and the animal is positioned in dorsal recumbency in a V-trough. The umbilical area is clipped and aseptically prepared. The surgeon replaces the hernia contents, removes the hernia sac, and closes the hernia ring with sutures to restore the abdominal wall. Any strangulated or infected tissue usually is resected (if possible). The skin and subcutaneous tissues are closed. Antibiotics are given for 3 to 5 days. Skin sutures or staples are removed 10 days postoperatively.

> **TECHNICIAN NOTE** Surgical correction of a hernia is called herniorrhaphy.

CESAREAN SECTION

Cesarean section for treatment of dystocia should be performed as early as possible for the best chances of saving the sow and possibly obtaining live piglets. Before the surgical

procedure, physical exhaustion and shock should be treated, and the patient should be stabilized. Fluid support is best obtained by intravenous catheterization of the ear vein. Lactated Ringer's solution or 0.9% saline can be given rapidly at 20 to 40 mL/kg/hour until a response is seen, and then a maintenance rate of 4 mL/kg/hour can be used. Dextrose and calcium solutions can be added to the maintenance fluids. Preoperative antibiotics are commonly given.

> **TECHNICIAN NOTE** Cesarean sections should be done as early as possible for the best chances of obtaining live piglets.

Various anesthetic regimens, patient positions, and incision locations can be used for cesarean section. The clinician determines how best to perform the procedure. Anesthesia for cesarean section depends largely on the physical status of the sow and is selected to have minimal effects on the fetuses. Sedation with local or regional anesthesia (inverted L block or epidural) is commonly used, especially in compromised patients. General anesthesia is another option. The procedure usually is performed with the sow in right or left lateral recumbency, with the legs tied for restraint if necessary. Dorsal recumbency is also possible. The procedure usually is performed through a vertical flank incision, although the Marcenac approach, ventral midline, and paramedian incisions are also used.

The surgical site is clipped and aseptically prepared. If local anesthesia is used, an additional scrub is performed after the anesthetic agent is deposited (Fig. 26-8). Materials for drying, warming, and supporting newborns should be

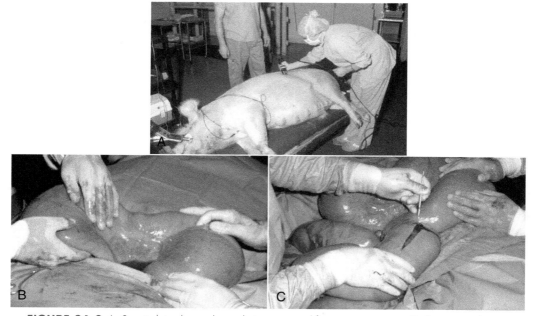

FIGURE 26-8 A, Sow in lateral recumbency being prepared for cesarean section. **B,** One uterine horn is exteriorized. **C,** Longitudinal uterine incision. (From Fubini SL, Ducharme NG: *Farm animal surgery,* St. Louis, 2004, Saunders.)

available in case live fetuses are found. After the surgical procedure, the sow is moved to a clean, dry pen, and the piglets are returned when she recovers. At least a 2-week period of confinement is necessary for healing and recovery.

Cesarean section is also used to deliver *specific pathogen-free* (SPF) piglets. Because these sows typically are healthy, general anesthesia is preferred.

DETUSKING

The permanent canine teeth are referred to as *"tusks."* In females the canine teeth are relatively small, and only occasionally do the tips protrude slightly through the lips. Growth ceases after approximately 2 years of age in females. In males, however, the canine teeth are long and curved, and they grow continuously throughout the life of these pigs. Growth of the mandibular canine teeth is pronounced, and the teeth protrude visibly from the mouth (Fig. 26-9). They are kept sharp by friction against the smaller upper (maxillary) canines. Because pigs use their teeth to fight, tusks are dangerous to humans and to other pigs. Swine owners have two management options for tusks: regular trimming and complete surgical removal.

Tusk trimming, or "detusking," is performed as needed, generally every 10 to 12 months. General anesthesia or heavy sedation can be used. Sedation is combined with a hog snare or snubbing rope on the snout. Snout restraint causes the typical reaction of opening the mouth. While the mouth is open, a Gigli (obstetrical) wire saw can be placed around the

tusk and used to remove the tooth several millimeters above the gum line. At this level, the pulp cavity is not opened. Hoof nippers have also been used but they risk shattering the tooth and exposing the pulp cavity. Trimming all four canines may be necessary in some animals.

> **TECHNICIAN NOTE** Detusking is performed as needed, generally every 10 to 12 months.

Complete surgical removal of the mandibular canine teeth is possible. It can be done electively or for treatment of infections or fractures of a canine tooth. The procedure must be done with the animal under general anesthesia and is technically difficult to perform; it is seldom done as an elective procedure. The tooth roots are long and deeply seated in the mandible. A risk of fracturing the mandible exists during elevation of the extensive tooth root and repulsion of the tooth. Owners should be warned of potential complications.

CASE STUDY

One of your swine producers in the area is talking with Dr. Speece, with whom you work, about producing SPF piglets. What does this mean? What type of equipment would the clinic need to have to meet the producer's needs?

CASE STUDY

You are going to perform a tusk removal on one of the Mr. Kuhl's boars. You are going to place an endotracheal tube for the procedure. What factors should you take into consideration during the intubation process? How will you intubate the boar? What other options does the producer have if he does not want to remove the tusks?

SUGGESTED READING

Fubini SL, Ducharme NG: *Farm animal surgery*, St. Louis, 2004, Saunders.

Gillespie JR, Flanders FB: *Modern livestock and poultry*, ed 8, Clifton Park, NY, 2010, Delmar Cengage Learning.

Muir WW 3rd, Hubbell JAE, Bednarski RM, Skarda RT: *Handbook of veterinary anesthesia*, ed 4, St. Louis, 2007, Mosby.

Thomas JA, Lerche P: Veterinary anesthesia. In Bassert JM, McCurnin DM, editors: *McCurnin's clinical textbook for veterinary technicians*, ed 7, St. Louis, 2010, Saunders, pp 887–939.

Wertz EM, Wagner AE: Anesthesia in pot-bellied pigs, *Comp Contin Ed Pract Vet* 17:369–381, 1995.

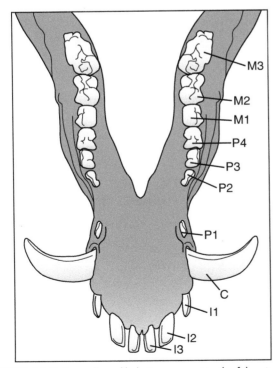

FIGURE 26-9 Lower (mandibular) permanent teeth of the pig. Note the large canine teeth or "tusks" *(C)*. (From Getty R, Sisson S, Grossman JD: *The anatomy of the domestic animals*, ed 5, Philadelphia, 1975, Saunders.)

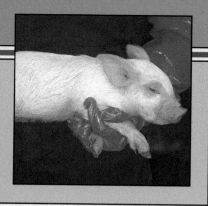

27 Common Porcine Diseases

OUTLINE

LEARNING OBJECTIVES

After reading this chapter, you will be able to

- Describe and recognize clinical signs associated with specific diseases
- Describe the etiology of the diseases
- Describe common treatments of disease
- List the common and scientific names of parasites associated with this species
- List the common vaccinations and their schedules associated with this species

KEY TERMS

Aerobic
All in/all out
Anaerobic
Average daily gain

Bullnose
Diplococci
Facultative
Orchitis

Petechial hemorrhage
Rickettsial
Spondylitis

KEY ABBREVIATIONS

ADG: Average daily gain
APP: *Actinobacillus pleuropneumoniae*
PRRS: Porcine reproductive and respiratory syndrome

PSS: Porcine stress syndrome
SMEDI: Stillbirth, mummification, embryonic death, and
  infertility

BACTERIAL DISEASES

ATROPHIC RHINITIS

- Etiology: *Bordetella bronchiseptica* and *Pasteurella*
- Nasal turbinate atrophy
- Vaccine

Atrophic rhinitis is divided into two forms. The first form, regressive atrophic rhinitis, is caused by *Bordetella bronchiseptica*. It usually is mild and temporary, with little effect on performance (Fig. 27-1). The second form is progressive atrophic rhinitis, caused by toxigenic *Pasteurella multocida*. Progressive atrophic rhinitis typically is severe and permanent, and it affects performance. Although each organism can cause nasal turbinate atrophy (Fig. 27-2) and

nasal distortion independently, clinical signs tend to be more severe when the infection is combined. Although dogs, cats, and rodents can harbor *B. bronchiseptica*, their role in the spread of disease is unknown. Introduction of disease into a herd is usually through infected pigs. The disease can be intensified through overcrowding, mixing and moving of pigs, inadequate ventilation, and other concurrent diseases.

Clinical signs usually appear in animals between 3 and 8 weeks of age and include sneezing, coughing, tear staining at the medial canthus of the eye, blockage or inflammation of the lacrimal duct, epistaxis, decreased performance, and deformation of the upper jaw (Fig. 27-3).

A tentative diagnosis is typically made from the clinical signs and deformation or nasal turbinate atrophy at necropsy.

Nasal turbinate atrophy is best identified during necropsy by examining a transverse section of the snout at the second premolar. Remember, however, it is rare to find even healthy herds with no signs of nasal turbinate atrophy. Culture growth of *P. multocida* is needed for a definitive diagnosis.

Treatment of atrophic rhinitis usually is attempted only when the disease rises to an unacceptable level within the herd.

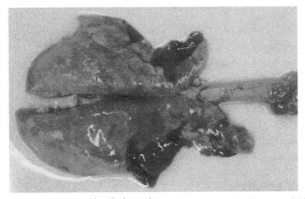

FIGURE 27-1 *Bordetella bronchiseptica* pneumonia. (Courtesy R.W. Blowey. From Jackson PGG, Cockcroft PD: *Handbook of pig medicine,* Edinburgh, 2007, Saunders.)

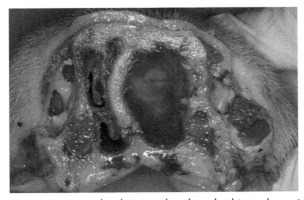

FIGURE 27-2 Atrophic rhinitis, with unilateral turbinate destruction. (From Jackson PGG, Cockcroft PD: *Handbook of pig medicine,* Edinburgh, 2007, Saunders.)

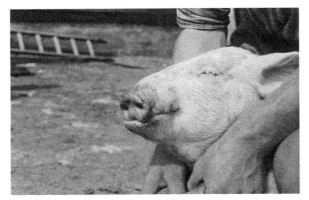

FIGURE 27-3 Atrophic rhinitis, with deviation of the snout. (From Jackson PGG, Cockcroft PD: *Handbook of pig medicine,* Edinburgh, 2007, Saunders.)

Some swine producers periodically measure the degree of turbinate atrophy and apply scores as a form of monitoring the disease. If treatment is indicated, antibiotics such as ceftiofur, sulfonamides, tylosin, and tetracyclines can be administered. Other treatments and preventive measures include vaccination, temporary closure of the herd to introduction of new pigs, better ventilation, improved hygiene practices, purchase of specific pathogen-free stock, segregated early weaning, and use of less dusty feed ingredients.

Atrophic rhinitis should not be confused with necrotic rhinitis ("*bullnose*"). Necrotic rhinitis results in abscesses on the snout as a result of unsanitary conditions.

> **TECHNICIAN NOTE** Atrophic rhinitis should not be confused with necrotic rhinitis ("bullnose").

BRUCELLOSIS

- Etiology: *Brucella abortus*
- Gram-negative rod
- Abortion
- Reportable disease
- Vaccine with limitations

Brucellosis in pigs is caused by the bacterium *Brucella suis.* The most commonly affected animals are breeding stock. Transmission of the disease is spread mainly by ingestion of infected tissues or wastes. Boars can also transmit the disease during service because the organism is found in semen. Suckling pigs can become infected from sows, although this is rare. Clinical signs include bacteremia that persists for 90 days, abortion, *orchitis,* lameness, *spondylitis,* paralysis, metritis, abscesses, and temporary or permanent sterility.

Diagnosis of brucellosis is often made when entire herds are tested using a brucellosis card test. Prevention should include purchase of stock from brucellosis-free herds and isolation for 3 months after purchase or return from fairs or shows. Control of the disease should include testing and slaughter of infected animals.

> **TECHNICIAN NOTE** Producers should buy swine from brucellosis-free herds.

CLOSTRIDIUM PERFRINGENS TYPE C ENTERITIS

- Etiology: *Clostridium perfringens*
- Necrohemorrhagic enteritis
- Vaccine available

Clostridium perfringens causes necrosis of all structural components of the villi. This necrosis produces blood loss into the intestinal wall and lumen (Fig. 27-4). These damaging effects cause necrohemorrhagic enteritis, which commonly leads to hemorrhagic diarrhea (Fig. 27-5), followed by collapse and death in piglets less than 1 to 3 days old. When onset is less acute, the presence of brownish liquid feces develops between 3 and 5 days of age. At necropsy, the small intestine is often dark red and filled with hemorrhagic liquid. In piglets between 3 and 5 days old, gas bubbles in the wall of the jejunum and necrosis of the mucosa within the jejunum and ileum can be seen.

> **TECHNICIAN NOTE**   *Clostridium perfringens* can lead to necrohemorrhagic enteritis.

Diagnosis is often made based on necropsy findings. Treatment is frequently ineffective because the lesions are irreversible once diarrhea has become a clinical sign. Prevention of the disease should include vaccination.

ENTERIC COLIBACILLOSIS

- Etiology: *Escherichia coli*
- Diarrhea

Enteric colibacillosis is caused by *Escherichia coli*. The bacteria colonize in the small intestine of nursing and weanling pigs. Because certain strains of *E. coli* produce enterotoxins that cause fluid and electrolytes to be secreted into the intestinal lumen, diarrhea is a common clinical sign (Fig. 27-6). Other clinical signs include rapid dehydration, acidosis, and death.

A definitive diagnosis can be made by culturing *E. coli* from the small intestine. Treatment typically consists of

antibiotic therapy and correction of fluid and electrolyte imbalances. Prevention should include the use of slatted floors, prevention of chilling, and vaccination of gestating sows.

> **TECHNICIAN NOTE**   Prevention of enteric colibacillosis should include the use of slatted floors, prevention of chilling, and vaccination of gestating sows.

EPERYTHROZOONOSIS

- Etiology: *Eperythrozoon suis*
- Anemia and malaise

Eperythrozoonosis is caused by *Eperythrozoon suis*, a *rickettsial* organism that typically appears as a coccoid organism. The organism is transmitted most commonly by lice (Fig. 27-7). Other forms of transmission are through contaminated needles and surgical instruments. Clinical signs commonly include anemia, fever, pale mucous membranes,

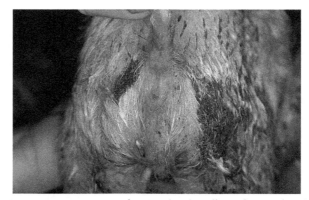

FIGURE 27-6 Perineum of neonatal piglet suffering from *Escherichia coli* enteritis. (From Jackson PGG, Cockcroft PD: *Handbook of pig medicine,* Edinburgh, 2007, Saunders.)

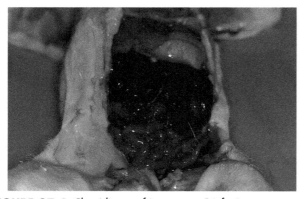

FIGURE 27-4 *Clostridium perfringens* type C infection post mortem. Note the dark small intestine and full stomach. (From Jackson PGG, Cockcroft PD: *Handbook of pig medicine,* Edinburgh, 2007, Saunders.)

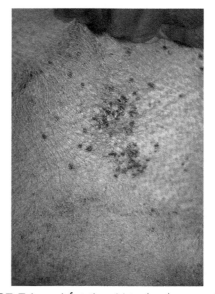

FIGURE 27-7 Louse infestation. Note the dorsoventrally flattened large louse. (From Jackson PGG, Cockcroft PD: *Handbook of pig medicine,* Edinburgh, 2007, Saunders.)

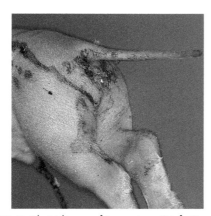

FIGURE 27-5 *Clostridium perfringens* type C infection. Dead piglet showing blood staining around in the anus. (From Jackson PGG, Cockcroft PD: *Handbook of pig medicine,* Edinburgh, 2007, Saunders.)

jaundice, emaciation, staggering or paralysis, neonatal weakness, unthrifty appearances, and reproductive failure.

Diagnosis is typically accomplished by Giemsa-stained peripheral blood smears showing *E. suis* attached to the surface of red blood cells. Treatment typically is accomplished with tetracyclines. Methods of prevention should include use of disposable needles, sterilization of surgical equipment, and control of arthropod parasites.

> **TECHNICIAN NOTE** The use of disposable needles is important to prevent transmission of *Eperythrozoon suis*.

EXUDATIVE EPIDERMITIS

- Etiology: *Staphylococcus hyicus*
- Exudative dermatitis

Exudative epidermitis is also known as greasy pig disease. Infections are caused by *Staphylococcus hyicus*. The bacteria are unable to penetrate the skin and typically gain entry through lacerations on the legs and feet. Carriers tend to be the source of contamination in previously unaffected herds. Younger pigs tend to be more susceptible, but pigs gain immunity to the bacteria as they age. The main source of infection tends to be from sow to piglet during nursing. However, the infection can be spread through older, more immune animals that carry the bacteria. Clinical signs include reddening of the skin, erosions at the coronary band, depression, and anorexia during early stages of the disease. As the disease progresses, the reddened areas of skin turn into brown spots, with production of serum exudates that begin to cover the entire pig. As dirt builds up over the top of the sebum, it becomes black, giving a greasy appearance to the infected animal (Fig. 27-8). In the acute disease, death occurs within 3 to 5 days. Recovery from the disease tends to be time consuming, and decreased growth rates are common.

> **TECHNICIAN NOTE** Exudative epidermitis is also known as greasy pig disease.

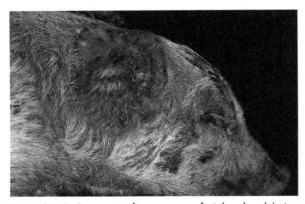

FIGURE 27-8 Greasy pig disease: severe facial and neck lesions in a piglet. (From Jackson PGG, Cockcroft PD: *Handbook of pig medicine*, Edinburgh, 2007, Saunders.)

Treatment of the disease includes administration of antibiotics. Amoxicillin, erythromycin, lincomycin, penicillin, tylosin, ampicillin, trimethoprim-sulfonamide, aminoglycosides, and cephalosporins are effective. High dosages and continued treatment for 7 to 10 days result in the greatest success. Antiseptics applied to the skin of the infected animal also can be beneficial. Efforts to prevent the disease should include disinfection of the farrowing environment and of the sow, clipping of needle teeth in piglets, soft bedding, and efforts to prevent fighting.

GLASSER DISEASE

- Etiology: *Haemophilus parasuis*
- Respiratory disease

Glasser disease is also known as porcine polyserositis and infectious polyarthritis. The disease is thought to be caused by *Haemophilus parasuis* but possibly by *Haemophilus parainfluenzae*. Stress predisposes pigs to the disease. *Mycoplasma hyorhinis* may be the cause in younger pigs. The incubation period is 1 to 5 days.

Clinical signs of the disease include a fever of 104° F to 107° F, depression, difficult breathing, cough, and anorexia. Some pigs develop lameness associated with warm, tender, swollen joints. Pigs are capable of recovery, but chronic cases can lead to pericarditis and congestive heart failure (Fig. 27-9).

A presumptive diagnosis is made based on history and clinical signs. A definitive diagnosis requires culture of the organism from cerebrospinal fluid, cardiac blood, or joints. Antibiotic treatment is usually effective. Prevention should include reducing stress and possibly adding medication to the food or water during times of high stress.

> **TECHNICIAN NOTE** Efforts to reduce stress are always valuable.

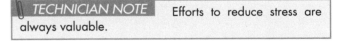

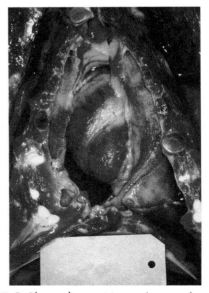

FIGURE 27-9 Glasser disease. Note early signs of pericarditis and pleurisy. (Courtesy W.D. Strachan. From Jackson PGG, Cockcroft PD: *Handbook of pig medicine*, Edinburgh, 2007, Saunders.)

LEPTOSPIROSIS

- Etiology: *Leptospira pomona*
- Abortion
- Reportable disease
- Vaccine available

The two most common bacterial serovars found in swine are *Leptospira pomona* and *Leptospira bratislava*. Other serovars that have been reported in swine *include Leptospira canicola, Leptospira tarassovi, Leptospira muenchen, Leptospira icterohaemorrhagiae,* and *Leptospira grippotyphosa*. In swine, the bacteria are commonly transferred on exposure to infected urine from wildlife or other swine. Clinical signs include abortion 2 to 4 weeks before term, and *SMEDI* (stillbirth, mummification, embryonic death, and infertility). For more information on leptospirosis, see Chapter 15. Treatment and control of leptospirosis includes chlortetracycline and oxytetracycline if given early. Prevention includes annual vaccinations, confinement rearing, rodent control programs, fencing to prevent contact with contaminated water, and purchase of seronegative stock (Fig. 27-10).

> **TECHNICIAN NOTE**   SMEDI (stillbirth, mummification, embryonic death, and infertility) can be a clinical sign of leptospirosis.

MYCOPLASMAL PNEUMONIA

- Etiology: *Mycoplasma hyopneumoniae*
- Respiratory disease

Mycoplasmal pneumonia is also known as enzootic pneumonia and viral pneumonia. It is typically caused by *Mycoplasma hyopneumoniae*. Mycoplasmal pneumonia is chronic but clinically mild. Clinical signs commonly include persistent dry cough, decreased growth rates, decreased feed efficiency, sporadic dyspnea, and a high incidence of lung lesions in slaughtered hogs (Fig. 27-11). Concurrent infections of other mycoplasmas, bacteria, and viruses that can increase the severity of the disease are common. Mortality is high in endemic areas, but morbidity remains low. Pigs of all ages can be affected. Infection usually occurs in the first few weeks of life through contact with the sow or gilt. Young pigs 3 to 5 months old tend to show the highest incidence of lung lesions. As pigs age, regression and recovery from the disease are seen. A high percentage (probably 99%) of commercial swine herds in the United States are believed to be affected.

Diagnosis is commonly made during slaughterhouse examination. Serologic tests can be used, but the results may be difficult to interpret. Treatment is limited. During an initial outbreak, antibiotics such as tylosin, lincomycin, timulin, or tetracyclines can be used to control the severity of clinical signs. Other practices that can limit the effects of the disease are adequate ventilation, reduced crowding, *all in/all out* management, and vaccination.

> **TECHNICIAN NOTE**   All in/all out management should be used to limit the effects of mycoplasmal pneumonia.

PLEUROPNEUMONIA

- Etiology: *Actinobacillus pleuropneumoniae*
- Gram-negative coccobacillus
- Respiratory disease

Pleuropneumonia is caused by *Actinobacillus pleuropneumoniae*, a gram-negative coccobacillus commonly referred to as APP. APP infection is a severe and contagious respiratory disease. The most severe effects are recognized in growing swine up to age 6 months. Onset is sudden, and the disease spreads rapidly in naïve herds. Clinical signs include cyanotic extremities, "thumps" (abdominal breathing), open-mouth breathing with blood-stained frothy nasal and oral discharge, anorexia, reluctance to move, fever up to 107° F, and sudden death. Common clinical signs in adults include abortion and fatal infections.

Once the infection is established in a herd, chronic clinical signs include intermittent coughing and decreased growth rates, which make detection difficult. However, severe internal damage still can be present and exacerbated by transport,

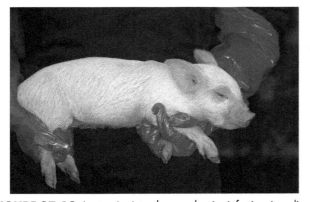

FIGURE 27-10 *Leptospira icterohaemorrhagiae* infection: jaundiced piglet. (From Jackson PGG, Cockcroft PD: *Handbook of pig medicine*, Edinburgh, 2007, Saunders.)

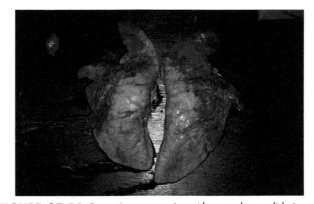

FIGURE 27-11 Enzootic pneumonia, with ventral consolidation of lungs. (Courtesy R.W. Blowey. From Jackson PGG, Cockcroft PD: *Handbook of pig medicine*, Edinburgh, 2007, Saunders.)

overcrowding, and temperature changes, resulting in death. Concurrent infections of *Mycoplasma, Pasteurella,* porcine reproductive and respiratory syndrome (PRRS), and swine influenza also are common. The pneumonia usually is bilateral, with pleurisy and pericarditis commonly seen (Fig. 27-12).

A tentative diagnosis of acute APP infection is made based on the rapid onset, clinical signs, and lesions found at necropsy. A definitive diagnosis can be made by culture but may require growth with *Staphylococcus aureus.*

APP is most commonly spread through nose-to-nose contact. Pigs that have been infected with APP and have recovered often become carriers of the disease. Because of the acute nature of the disease in naïve herds and the significant lack of clinical signs in infected and carrier animals, treatment of the disease poses some difficulty. The first treatment should be a systemic antibiotic because many animals with the disease do not want to eat or drink. Some antibiotic choices are ceftiofur, tetracyclines, synthetic penicillins, tylosin, and sulfonamides. Once animals begin eating and drinking, treatments can be administered in the water or feed. Other suggestions for control include depopulation, early segregated weaning, all in/all out management, improved ventilation, and reduced stocking rates. If the herd is already APP free, new pigs should be purchased from other APP-free herds.

> **TECHNICIAN NOTE** Pigs infected with *Actinobacillus pleuropneumoniae* (APP) that recover often become carriers of the disease.

STREPTOCOCCAL INFECTIONS

- Etiology: *Streptococcus* species
- Gram-positive organism
- Multiple manifestations

Streptococcal infections that commonly infect swine are broken into four groups. The first and most prominent group is group D, followed by groups C, L, and E. *Streptococcus suis* organisms, the bacteria belonging to group D, are gram-positive, *facultative* aerobes that are seen as oval

diplococci or short chains. At least nine serotypes of *S. suis* have been identified. The two most common types present in the United States are type 1 and type 2. Type 7 also is commonly isolated from U.S. herds but is of little clinical significance.

Type 1 from group C randomly affects piglets up to 8 weeks of age (Fig. 27-13). Clinical signs in nursing piglets typically include polyarthritis and meningitis. Type 2 from group C tends to affect large, intensively managed herds, with transmission through carrier pigs or flies. Flies can travel 1 to 2 miles between farms and can carry the infection for up to 5 days. Type 2 commonly affects weaning pigs. Clinical signs of type 2 infection are fatal meningitis, abortion, depression, fever, tremors, incoordination, convulsions, bronchopneumonia, blindness, and deafness. Sudden death can occur from endocarditis or myocarditis.

Necropsy findings for both type 1 and type 2 include reddened patches of skin, enlarged lymph nodes, thickened joint capsules, congestion, edema, excess clear or cloudy cerebrospinal fluid, and bronchopneumonia. A definitive diagnosis depends on isolation and identification of the causative agent. Treatment includes antibiotics in the feed or water (or both) or systemic antibiotic administration. The organism tends to be resistant to tetracyclines and sulfonamides. Penicillins are effective but tend to inactivate in feed. Prevention includes reducing slurry gases, reducing overcrowding, and preventing introductions of carrier pigs.

> **TECHNICIAN NOTE** Penicillins are effective but tend to inactivate in feed.

Streptococcus equisimilis belongs to groups C and L. The bacteria appear as gram-positive elongated cocci in pairs or short chains. They commonly appear in many body locations, including excretions and secretions from normal pig herds. They can be introduced through fomites and typically gain entry to the body after injuries, clipping of needle teeth, docking tails, or floor abrasions. Clinical signs include septicemia, arthritis, and endocarditis. The bacteria can also cause

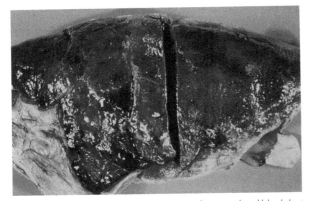

FIGURE 27-12 Pleuropneumonia. Note the raised red-black lesions in the dorsal lung. (From Jackson PGG, Cockcroft PD: *Handbook of pig medicine,* Edinburgh, 2007, Saunders.)

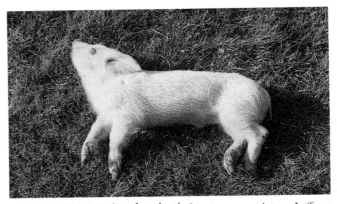

FIGURE 27-13 Piglet infected with *Streptococcus suis* type 1. (From Jackson PGG, Cockcroft PD: *Handbook of pig medicine,* Edinburgh, 2007, Saunders.)

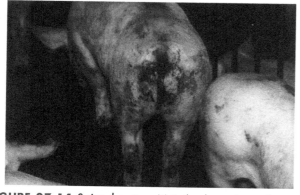

FIGURE 27-14 Swine dysentery. Note the depression and perineal staining with dark, tarry feces. (From Jackson PGG, Cockcroft PD: *Handbook of pig medicine*, Edinburgh, 2007, Saunders.)

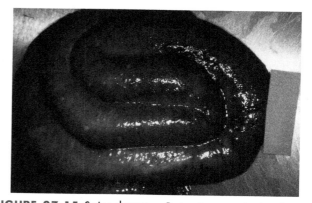

FIGURE 27-15 Swine dysentery. Postmortem examination showing gross appearance of inflamed and discolored spiral colon. (From Jackson PGG, Cockcroft PD: *Handbook of pig medicine*, Edinburgh, 2007, Saunders.)

symptoms such as cutaneous abscesses, mastitis, pneumonia, and ear necrosis.

Diagnosis is often made from the clinical signs, but a definitive diagnosis requires bacterial isolation. Samples are best taken from the reproductive tract and vaginal discharges. Treatment typically involves penicillin and related antibiotics. Prevention includes improved housing conditions, sterilization of equipment, and housing adjustments that minimize abrasions.

Group E streptococcal infections commonly result in jowl abscesses in feeder pigs. Other clinical signs include swelling or abscessation of the cervical lymph nodes. Producers should be concerned about group E streptococcal infections because of the need for carcass trimming and condemnation at slaughter. Diagnosis is made by bacterial isolation. Treatment can include lancing of large abscesses. After infection, antibiotics are of little use. Prevention can include the feeding of antibiotics.

SWINE DYSENTERY

- Etiology: *Brachyspira hyodysenteriae*
- Diarrhea

Swine dysentery is also called bloody scours, vibrionic dysentery, and black scours. Swine dysentery is caused by *Brachyspira hyodysenteriae*, an *anaerobic* spirochete. It commonly infects pigs from 8 to 16 weeks of age. Any age can be affected; however, the disease is not as severe and may be difficult to diagnose in adult swine. Clinical signs typically include anorexia, passage of soft feces, dehydration, weakness, gaunt appearance, and possibly fever. The most common clinical sign is a mucoid diarrhea with flecks of blood and mucus that develops into a watery mucohemorrhagic diarrhea, which eventually turns brown and contains flecks of fibrin and debris (Fig. 27-14). Some pigs die peracutely. At necropsy, lesions on the mucosa of the cecum, spiral colon, and rectum are covered with a layer of transparent to gray mucus (Figs. 27-15 and 27-16). Sows may be carriers of the disease and transmit the disease to piglets through fecal material. Transmission between farms can occur through fecally contaminated fomites, rats, dogs, birds, and flies.

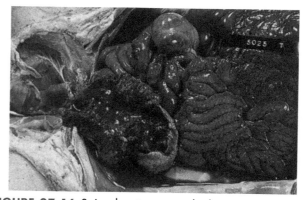

FIGURE 27-16 Swine dysentery: opened colon post mortem. (From Jackson PGG, Cockcroft PD: *Handbook of pig medicine*, Edinburgh, 2007, Saunders.)

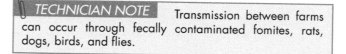

TECHNICIAN NOTE   Transmission between farms can occur through fecally contaminated fomites, rats, dogs, birds, and flies.

A presumptive diagnosis is typically made from clinical signs and necropsy. Definitive diagnosis requires isolation of *S. hyodysenteriae*. Treatment of swine dysentery is typically accomplished with antibiotics in the water. Effective antibiotics include bacitracin, carbadox, lincomycin, nitroimidazoles, timulin, and virginiamycin. Antibiotics should be chosen carefully because drug-resistant strains are prevalent. During the course of treatment, facilities should try to improve sanitary conditions and eliminate rodent populations. Other forms of treatment and control include partial depopulation or total depopulation. Prevention can be accomplished by purchase of specific pathogen-free stock or herds that have been free of dysentery for more than 2 years, as well as by good husbandry practices.

SWINE ERYSIPELAS

- Etiology: *Erysipelothrix rhusiopathiae*
- Dermatitis

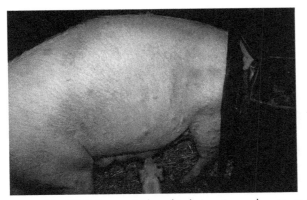

FIGURE 27-17 Swine erysipelas: skin lesions in a subacute case. (From Jackson PGG, Cockcroft PD: *Handbook of pig medicine*, Edinburgh, 2007, Saunders.)

Swine erysipelas is caused by the bacterium *Erysipelothrix rhusiopathiae,* which survives for only for short periods of time in the soil and is commonly passed through carrier pigs. The disease primarily affects growing pigs. The disease occurs in three forms: acute skin form, chronic arthritic form, and endocarditic form. Clinical signs of the acute septicemia form of the disease include fever, lameness, lack of milk production in sows, abortion, skin discoloration leading to lesions, and death. Left untreated, the skin lesions become diamond shaped almost everywhere on the body. They then necrose and separate from the body (Fig. 27-17), commonly starting at the ears and tail. The acute form of the disease is often seen in finishing pigs. Necropsy reveals enlarged lymph nodes, a swollen spleen, and congested lungs.

> **TECHNICIAN NOTE** When skin lesions from swine erysipelas are left untreated, they become diamond shaped.

The chronic arthritic form of the disease can begin as the acute form or may manifest in its arthritic form. This form of the disease produces mild to severe lameness. The joints of the infected animal may become swollen and firm. Because of the severe lameness, decreased growth rates are not uncommon. The endocarditic form of the disease is common in young and adult swine and often results in death from embolism.

Diagnosis of the chronic and endocarditic forms of the disease is commonly made at necropsy. Acute forms of the disease are usually diagnosed based on the clinical signs. Treatment of the disease commonly consists of penicillin. Other effective antibiotics include ceftiofur and tetracycline. The acute form of the disease is often concurrently treated with antiserum. Treatment of chronically infected animals is ineffective, and it is recommended that these animals be removed from the herd.

VIRAL DISEASES

HOG CHOLERA

- Etiology: Flaviviridae
- Neurologic and reproductive disease
- Reportable disease
- Vaccine available

Hog cholera is also known as classic swine fever and swine fever. It is caused by an enveloped virus of the pestivirus group of the family Flaviviridae. Hog cholera belongs to the same group of viruses as bovine viral diarrhea and border disease virus of sheep. Because pigs are susceptible to infection by both of these diseases, it is important to differentiate between hog cholera and the other ruminant pestivirus infections.

Although the United States is free of hog cholera, is extremely important to be aware of the disease because of its devastating effects and potential for epidemic. The main source of infection is through pig-to-pig contact or swine consumption of infected uncooked pig products. The virus can survive if it is kept cold or frozen within meat products. It has been reported that the virus can survive for several years in frozen meat products and even months in chilled meat products. Fomites are another possibility for transmission of disease within endemic areas. Sows that become infected during gestation and recover can give birth to carrier piglets.

Clinical signs of low-virulence strains of acute hog cholera are primarily limited to poor reproductive performance and birth of piglets with neurologic disease. Clinical signs of the severe virulent strains include fever, decreased appetite, constipation, and depression (Fig. 27-18). The incubation period typically is 2 to 6 days, with death occurring 10 to 20 days after infection. Fevers typically persist until the terminal stage of the disease, when dips in temperature below normal are not uncommon. The most common findings at necropsy are inflammation of the blood and lymph vessels and *petechial hemorrhages,* especially in the kidneys, spleen, bladder, lymph nodes, and larynx.

> **TECHNICIAN NOTE** Hog cholera has an incubation period of 2 to 6 days, with death occurring 10 to 20 days after infection.

Diagnosis is made through virologic tests, antigen detection, virus isolation, nucleic acid detection, or serologic testing. Prevention and control of the disease should be achieved through swift reporting of the virus to authorities and actions such as herd slaughter to prevent the spread of disease. Vaccinations for the disease are available.

PORCINE EPIDEMIC DIARRHEA VIRUS

- Etiology: coronavirus
- Diarrhea

Porcine epidemic diarrhea (PED) virus is a transmissible gastroenteritis-like virus that causes diarrhea in a large

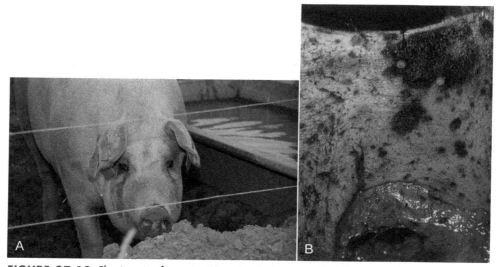

FIGURE 27-18 Classic swine fever. **A,** Gilt ocular discharge and high fever. **B,** Ecchymotic hemorrhages on the skin. (Courtesy J.D. Mackinnon. From Jackson PGG, Cockcroft PD: *Handbook of pig medicine,* Edinburgh, 2007, Saunders.)

proportion of all ages of swine. The virus appeared in the United States in the spring of 2013. PED occurs only in swine.

The disease is spread through fecal-oral contamination of infected pigs for at least 7 days after inoculation. The disease can also be spread by fomites. Whether carrier swine exist is not fully understood.

The virus replicates in the enterocytes on villi of the small intestines and, to a lesser degree, the cryptal cells of both the small intestine and colon. The virus causes necrosis of the enterocytes. The damage leads to diarrhea and subsequent dehydration. At necropsy, the intestine is filled with yellow fluid. Microscopically, the villi are atrophic.

Clinical signs include watery diarrhea. Affected piglets up to 1 week old die of dehydration after 3 to 4 days. Mortality averages approximately 50%. Older piglets recover in approximately 1 week. Feeders, finishers, and adults have diarrhea, depression, anorexia, and abdominal pain. The outbreaks often start in this age group. Within these age groups the morbidity is high, and the affected animals are quite sick, although then tend to recover.

Diagnosis of PED is confirmed with polymerase chain reaction testing on feces or intestines from affected pigs or immunohistochemistry testing on formalin-fixed intestine.

PORCINE PARVOVIRUS INFECTION

- Etiology: parvovirus
- Abortion
- Vaccine available

Porcine parvovirus (PPV) is prevalent in the midwestern United States. Some research suggests that more than 90% of herds are affected.

Clinical signs include mummification of fetuses when sows are infected before 70 days of gestation. Abortions are rare because endometrial tissue is not affected. Most often the only indications that a herd is infected with PPV are increased mummification and stillbirth (Fig. 27-19).

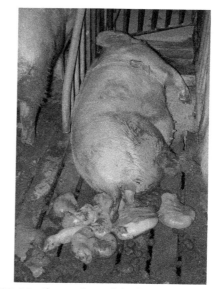

FIGURE 27-19 Abortion litter of dead piglets. (From Jackson PGG, Cockcroft PD: *Handbook of pig medicine,* Edinburgh, 2007, Saunders.)

TECHNICIAN NOTE   Porcine parvovirus is asymptomatic. The only indications of infection are increased stillbirth and mummification.

Diagnosis is accomplished by fluorescent antibody testing of the mummies. The virus has been isolated from boar semen, but its ability to be transmitted in this way is questionable. Prevention should include vaccination.

PORCINE REPRODUCTIVE AND RESPIRATORY SYNDROME

- Etiology: Arteriviridae
- Respiratory and reproductive disease

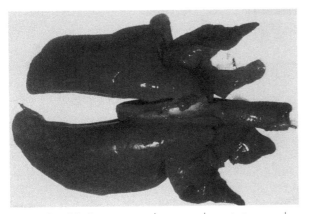

FIGURE 27-20 Porcine reproductive and respiratory syndrome/postweaning multisystemic wasting syndrome. Lungs from a piglet with pneumonia. (Courtesy R.W. Blowey. From Jackson PGG, Cockcroft PD: *Handbook of pig medicine*, Edinburgh, 2007, Saunders.)

- Reportable disease
- Vaccine available

Porcine reproductive and respiratory syndrome is often referred to as PRRS. It was first reported in the United States in 1987. PRRS virus is an enveloped virus that belongs to the Arteriviridae group of viruses. PRRS manifests in two independent stages of production. The first stage typically affects farrowing units, resulting in SMEDI. The second stage affects postweaning piglets with respiratory disease.

PRRS in farrowing units commonly results in SMEDI. Anorexia and agalactia are evident in lactating sows and result in increased preweaning mortality. Nursing piglets often develop thumps and show clinical signs of pneumonia at necropsy. Initial outbreaks of the reproductive form of PRRS can last from 1 to 4 months. Reproductive PRRS loss is extremely high, sometimes as high as 70%.

PRRS in the postweaning pneumonic phase can become chronic, decreasing *average daily gains (ADG)* by 85% and increasing mortality 10% to 25% (Fig. 27-20). Consecutive secondary bacterial infections are common. Other clinical signs include respiratory distress and unthrifty appearance.

> **TECHNICIAN NOTE** Porcine reproductive and respiratory syndrome in the postweaning phase can decrease average daily gains by 85%.

A presumptive diagnosis usually can be made from the clinical signs, but definitive diagnosis requires serologic tests and can be difficult. Currently, effective treatments of PRRS exist. Prevention usually is accomplished by purchase of PRRS-negative animals and by vaccination.

PSEUDORABIES

- Etiology: herpesvirus
- Respiratory and neurologic disease
- Reportable disease
- Vaccine available

Pseudorabies is also known as Aujeszky disease and mad itch. Pseudorabies is caused by an enveloped deoxyribonucleic acid (DNA) herpesvirus. Transmission of the disease occurs from nose to nose, by the fecal-oral route, and from aerosolized virus. Animals that act as dead-end hosts for the virus but can also spread the disease include dogs, cats, and feral animals. Piglets less than 7 days old are highly susceptible, with death losses as high as a 100%. Clinical signs in piglets infected at this age include tremors and paddling. Respiratory disease is the main clinical sign in weaned piglets and is often complicated by secondary bacterial infections. Clinical signs that can affect swine of any age include anorexia and fever. Mortality tends to decrease as the pigs age. Lesions are rarely seen at necropsy; if they are found, most lesions are associated with the respiratory system.

Diagnosis of the disease is made by virus isolation, fluorescent antibody testing, and serologic testing. Organs collected for testing include lung, brain, and spleen. Treatment typically includes treatment of the clinical signs. Control of the disease is accomplished with vaccination, test and cull programs, and segregated weaning. Pseudorabies is a reportable disease.

> **TECHNICIAN NOTE** Pseudorabies is a reportable disease.

SWINE INFLUENZA

- Etiology: orthomyxovirus
- Respiratory disease
- Reportable disease
- Vaccine available

Swine influenza is known also known as hog flu, swine flu, and pig flu. It is an acute, highly contagious respiratory disease. Swine influenza is caused by an orthomyxovirus of the influenza A group. Pigs are the principal hosts of classic swine influenza virus. In North America, outbreaks are commonly seen in the fall or winter. The disease is primarily spread through carrier animals and often enters a herd through the introduction of a carrier animal. The virus can survive in carrier pigs for up to 3 months. Once infection occurs, it spreads rapidly through a herd by pig-to-pig contact and aerosolization. Often the spread of disease can occur within 1 to 3 days.

> **TECHNICIAN NOTE** In North America, outbreaks are commonly seen in the fall or winter.

Clinical signs commonly include fever up to 108° F, depression, difficult breathing, anorexia, and mucous discharge from the eyes and nose. Clinical signs typically last 3 to 7 days. Some economic loss may be seen from fetal mortality and decreased weight gain.

A presumptive diagnosis is made based on the acute nature of the disease and clinical signs. A definitive diagnosis requires virus isolation or demonstration of virus-specific antibodies. Virus isolation samples can be collected from nasal secretions in the febrile phase or from affected lung tissue in the acute stage.

Secondary infections often complicate treatment. Antibiotics can be used to treat secondary bacterial infections, although no effective treatment of swine influenza exists. Prevention includes reducing stress levels, especially those related to overcrowding, reducing dust, vaccination, use of all in/all out management, and strict import regulations. Expectorants can be used to relieve symptoms in severely affected swine.

TRANSMISSIBLE GASTROENTERITIS

- Etiology: coronavirus
- Diarrhea
- Reportable disease
- Vaccine available

Transmissible gastroenteritis is caused by a coronavirus. It affects pigs of all ages. The virus destroys villous epithelial cells of the jejunum and ileum. The incubation period of the virus is 18 hours and is more commonly seen during the winter months. The disease is spread by aerosol and pig-to-pig contact.

> *TECHNICIAN NOTE*   Transmissible gastroenteritis is spread by aerosol and pig-to-pig contact.

Clinical signs in naïve herds include vomiting, osmotic diarrhea, and dehydration. Undigested milk curds in the diarrhea are commonly seen in nursing piglets. Mortality can reach 100% in piglets less than 1 week old. Clinical signs in gestating sows can include abortion, as well as the clinical signs associated with neonates. In endemic herds, pigs often develop the diarrhea a few days after weaning because of passive immunity, although diarrhea can develop during nursing if the immunity was not sufficient to protect the piglets. At necropsy, the stomach may be empty or contain milk curds. The intestine may contain watery fluid, as well as curded milk with a yellow to green appearance.

Diagnosis is often presumptive from clinical signs. Treatment is nonspecific, making prevention extremely important. Prevention includes vaccination, increasing farrowing room temperatures, all in/all out management, and good sanitation.

SWINE VACCINATIONS

Table 27-1 lists the major swine vaccinations.

NONINFECTIOUS DISEASES

ANEMIA

- Genetic: neonatal iron deficiency

Anemia is a regularly diagnosed problem in baby piglets. Clinical signs often manifest between 1 and 2 weeks of age. The signs include difficulty breathing, roughened hair coat, and poor growth. The lack of iron can be corrected by administration of iron intramuscularly or orally. Piglets must be supplemented with iron because of the lack of iron in sow's milk.

MALIGNANT HYPERTHERMIA

- Etiology: genetic

Porcine stress syndrome (PSS) is an inherited disorder that primarily affects the skeletal muscles of susceptible swine. The muscle cells appear to have an impaired ability to regulate calcium flowing in and out of the cell. The responsible gene has become known as the halothane, or *Hal*, gene. It is a single autosomal recessive gene, and susceptible pigs are homozygous for the gene. Three possible clinical manifestations of the genetic condition exist:

1. Pale, soft exudative pork (PSE): Animals with the *Hal* gene produce inferior quality meat that is pale (grayish), soft, and watery, characteristics that devalue the carcass. These changes occur after death of the animal and are caused by an abnormally rapid fall in pH in the muscle cells that damages the cell membrane and allows water to leak freely out of the cells. PSE affects a large percentage of animals that are homozygous for the *Hal* gene, as well as many animals that carry the gene as heterozygotes.
2. Malignant hyperthermia: This is a drug-induced phenomenon characterized by the following: muscle rigidity; tachycardia; tachypnea; metabolic acidosis; and a rapid, extreme, progressive rise in body temperature. Cardiovascular collapse and death usually occur. The condition may be triggered by halothane gas or by some of the neuromuscular blocking agents.

TABLE 27-1	Swine Vaccinations*			
DISEASE OR VACCINATION	**PIGLETS**	**WEANLINGS**	**REPLACEMENT**	**BREEDING STOCK**
Atrophic rhinitis	7–10 days old		Gilts and boars	Sows
Mycoplasma	7–10 days old			Sows
Erysipelas	Before weaning	After weaning	Gilts and boars	Sows
Contagious pleuropneumonia		Weanlings		
Leptospirosis			Gilts and boars	Sows and boars
Parvovirus			Gilts	
Transmissible gastroenteritis			Gilts	Sows
Escherichia coli		Weanlings		Sows
Glasser disease		Weanlings		

*Vaccination protocols are designed by veterinarians specific to producers.

3. PSS: This is an acute manifestation that requires a stressful "trigger" to initiate clinical signs. Physical stressors such as restraint, exertion, fighting, breeding, parturition, veterinary procedures, fighting, transportation, overcrowding, and high environmental temperatures may initiate a sudden attack of dyspnea and open-mouth breathing, elevated body temperature less than 106° F (41.1° C), tail twitching, muscle tremors, and rigidity. As the body temperature rises above 106° F, the terminal stages begin with cyanosis, collapse, and finally death (often within 15 to 20 minutes). PSS may occur at any time of year, but the incidence is much higher during hot and humid weather.

Treatment of malignant hyperthermia and PSS consists of intravenous dantrolene, a muscle relaxant specific for skeletal muscle. However, the condition usually is observed when it is too late for the drug to be effective. Emergency measures to cool the animal should be attempted but seldom are successful. No therapy or prevention is available for PSS.

The condition is seen primarily in heavily muscled but lean individuals. Historically, the prevalence has been higher in the pietrain, Landrace, and Poland China breeds. A simple, highly accurate, inexpensive DNA blood test has been developed to identify the *Hal* gene in homozygous and heterozygous animals. By judicious planned breeding and culling, the incidence of the condition is decreasing and theoretically could be eliminated. In 1997, the National Pork Producers' Council passed a resolution supporting elimination of the *Hal* gene from the U.S. pork population.

Swine in general do not handle heat and humidity well. Efforts should always be made to keep pigs comfortable on hot days. Providing shade, fans, and sprinklers is helpful. Caution should be used if pigs are to be placed in stressful situations on hot days. When tail twitching, open-mouth breathing, and tremors of the rump muscles are seen, the procedure should be stopped, and emergency efforts to cool the pig should be instituted.

PARAKERATOSIS

• Etiology: zinc deficiency

Parakeratosis is a metabolic condition resulting from a deficiency of zinc. The condition is more severe when calcium levels are high in the diet. The main clinical sign associated with parakeratosis is rough, scaly skin (Fig. 27-21). Parakeratosis is prevented and treated by balancing zinc and calcium levels in the diet.

PROLAPSE

• Etiology: varied

Vaginal prolapse usually occurs before parturition (Fig. 27-22). Treatment involves sedation or anesthesia of the sow, cleansing of the prolapsed tissues, and repositioning of the organ. A Buhner retention suture can be used to prevent recurrence. The sow must be closely watched so that the suture can be removed at the onset of labor.

Uterine prolapse occurs during or in the first several days after parturition (Fig. 27-23). Excessive straining is thought to cause the prolapse. Complete prolapse is often accompanied

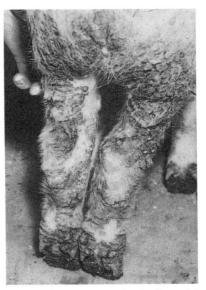

FIGURE 27-21 Parakeratosis. Note the dry, fissured skin on the hindlegs. (From Jackson PGG, Cockcroft PD: *Handbook of pig medicine*, Edinburgh, 2007, Saunders.)

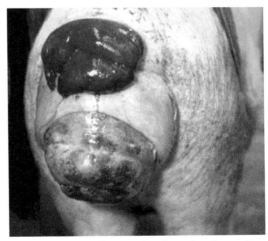

FIGURE 27-22 Sow with vaginal and rectal prolapse. (From Fubini SL, Ducharme NG: *Farm animal surgery*, St. Louis, 2004, Saunders.)

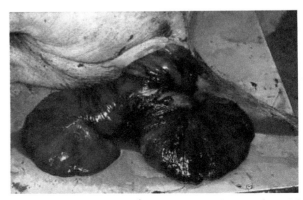

FIGURE 27-23 Uterine prolapse in a sow. (From Jackson PGG, Cockcroft PD: *Handbook of pig medicine*, Edinburgh, 2007, Saunders.)

by hemorrhage and death. Partial prolapses do occur and have a better prognosis for survival. If surgical treatment is to be performed, the sow must first be stabilized and any profuse bleeding stopped. General anesthesia or epidural anesthesia with sedation can be used. The organ is evaluated, cleansed, and replaced if possible. Repositioning is often challenging for the surgeon. Occasionally, a laparotomy incision must be made to assist the replacement. A Buhner retention suture is recommended to prevent recurrence while healing progresses and usually is removed in 7 to 10 days. In extreme cases, amputation of the uterus may be required to salvage the sow for slaughter, which typically is done after the litter is weaned.

RICKETS

- Lack of calcium, phosphorus, or vitamin D

Rickets is caused by a lack of calcium, phosphorus, or vitamin D in the diet. To prevent rickets, it is extremely important that the swine's diet provide the correct ratio of calcium to phosphorus. Clinical signs of rickets include slower than normal growth rates and crocked legs. Prevention and treatment of the disease include proper balances of nutrients in the diet.

PARASITES

Table 27-2 is an overview of the major swine parasites.

TOXINS

Table 27-3 shows common swine toxins.

TABLE 27-2	Swine Parasites			
COMMON NAME/PHOTOGRAPH	**SCIENTIFIC NAME**	**IMPORTANCE**	**DIAGNOSIS**	**TREATMENT**
Mange Mite* 	*Sarcoptes scabiei*	Most common clinical indication: pruritus Life cycle of 3 wk	Skin scrapings	Ivermectin
Hog Louse* 	*Haematopinus suis*	Most common clinical indication: pruritus Life cycle of 3–4 wk	Examination of skin for lice	Amitraz, ivermectin
Roundworm* 	*Ascaris suum*	Reduced weight gain, stunted growth, abdominal breathing, referred to as "thumps" Prepatent period of 8 wk Zoonotic: Contracted through ingestion of larvated eggs	Eggs in fecal flotation Presence of worms in intestine or "milk spots" in liver at necropsy	Ivermectin, fenbendazole, dichlorvos, doramectin, hygromycin, levamisole, piperazine
Whipworm* 	*Trichuris suis*	Diarrhea and unthriftiness Prepatent period of 6 wk	Eggs in fecal flotation Presence of adults in large intestine at necropsy	Ivermectin, dichlorvos, levamisole, fenbendazole, hygromycin

TABLE 27-2	Swine Parasites—cont'd			
COMMON NAME/PHOTOGRAPH	**SCIENTIFIC NAME**	**IMPORTANCE**	**DIAGNOSIS**	**TREATMENT**
Threadworm[†] 	*Strongyloides ransomi*	Severe diarrhea develops between 10 and 14 days of age, with high mortality Prepatent period of 7 days	Fecal flotation Direct observation of mucosal scrapings at necropsy	Ivermectin, fenbendazole, hygromycin, dichlorvos
Coccidia[*] 	*Eimeria* spp.	In piglets, heavy infestations possibly causing significant enterocolitis Prepatent period of 2 wk	Oocysts in fecal flotation Oocysts in intestines seen histologically	Sulfamethazine: piglets Decoquinate: sows
Coccidia[†] 	*Isospora suis*	Common in piglets 6–21 days of age Piglets often stunted; death possible Prepatent period of 2 wk	Oocysts in fecal flotation Oocysts in intestines seen histologically	Sulfamethazine: piglets Decoquinate: sows
Lungworm[†] 	*Metastrongylus* spp.	Coughing, poor growth Prepatent period of 1 mo	Larvated eggs in fecal flotation Adults found in lungs at necropsy	Ivermectin, doramectin, fenbendazole, levamisole
Nodular Worm[†] 	*Oesophagostomum dentatum*	Nodules in gut wall possibly causing enteritis; however, most infections asymptomatic Possible condemnation of intestines at slaughter Prepatent period of 40 days	Eggs in fecal flotation Adults in large intestine at necropsy	Ivermectin, doramectin, levamisole, fenbendazole, pyrantel tartrate, hygromycin, dichlorvos
Stomach Worm[†] 	*Ascarops strongylina*	Dung beetle intermediate host Nonpathogenic unless present in large numbers Prepatent period of 6 wk	Fecal sedimentation shows embryonated ova Adults found in stomach at necropsy	Ivermectin, doramectin, dichlorvos
Swine Kidney Worm[†] 	*Stephanurus dentatus*	Loss of weight Condemnation of organs and tissues affected by migrating larvae Prepatent period of 8–16 mo	Eggs possibly found in urine Adults found in cysts in perirenal fat and pelvis of kidney at necropsy Larvae possibly found in liver	Ivermectin, doramectin

Continued

| TABLE 27-2 | Swine Parasites—cont'd | | | |

COMMON NAME/PHOTOGRAPH	SCIENTIFIC NAME	IMPORTANCE	DIAGNOSIS	TREATMENT
Trichina Worm†				
	Trichinella spiralis	20 days for larvae to be infective Larvae to adults in 4 days Zoonotic: infection through ingestion of raw meat	Antemortem diagnosis in animals rare	No treatment for pigs Do not feed uncooked garbage to pigs; cook all meat to recommended temperatures and for recommended times
Pork Tapeworm				
	Taenia solium	No major pathogenicity to pigs Prepatent period of 2 mo Zoonotic: cause of taeniasis, cysticercosis Infection through ingestion of raw meat	Observation of cysticerci in pigs at necropsy Serologic tests in humans, pigs Eggs in feces of infected humans	No treatment for pigs Prevent pigs from ingesting human feces; cook all meat to recommended temperatures and for recommended times
Balantidium coli†				
	Balantidium coli	Mild to severe enteritis Life cycle of 6–14 days Zoonotic	Clinical signs and large numbers of organisms in fecal flotation or smear Lesions seen at necropsy	Tetracycline

*Figure from Bowman DD: *Georgis' parasitology for veterinarians*, ed 10, St. Louis, 2014, Saunders.
†Figure from Hendrix CM, Robinson E: *Diagnostic parasitology for veterinary technicians*, ed 4, St. Louis, 2012, Mosby.

| TABLE 27-3 | Common Swine Toxins |

TOXIN OR TOXIC CONDITION	CLINICAL SIGNS
Aflatoxicosis	Slow growth, liver disease
Ergotism	Arteriolar vasoconstriction, endothelial cell injury, thrombosis, decreased mammary development, reduced litter size, reduced birth weights, agalactia
Fumonisin	Dyspnea, cyanosis, weakness, death within 4 to 10 days
Trichothecene	Anorexia, salivation, vomiting, paresis, paralysis, seizures, gastrointestinal lesions, skin irritation, necrosis
Ammonia	Reduce growth rate, exacerbation of nasal turbinate lesions
Carbon monoxide	Stillbirths, no lesions, bright red blood
Cocklebur	Depression, hypoglycemia, nausea, incoordination, convulsions, death
Hydrogen sulfide	Death
Pigweed	Trembling, weakness, incoordination, knuckling, rear leg paralysis
Phenyl arsenic	Goose stepping, hindlimb ataxia, limb paresis, blindness, paralysis, gastroenteritis, cutaneous erythema, ataxia, vestibular disturbances, terminal muscular weakness, seizures
Salt	Acute cerebral edema, aimless wandering, blindness, deafness, head pressing, dog sitting, falling, paddling

CASE STUDY

Mrs. Kay owns approximately 300 head of sows in her farrow-to-finish operation. Increased stillbirths are occurring in her farrowing house. When the piglets become growers, she is seeing increases in respiratory disease and death. A veterinarian diagnoses the herd with porcine reproductive and respiratory syndrome (PRRS). Is there a treatment of this disease? What can Mrs. Kay do to prevent this disease?

CASE STUDY

Mr. Parish owns three gilts that his children will be showing at the county fair. The gilts have developed diamond-shaped lesions on their backs. A veterinarian diagnoses the gilts with swine erysipelas. What antibiotics did the veterinarian most likely prescribe for the gilts?

SUGGESTED READING

Anderson DE, Rings M: *Current veterinary therapy: food animal practice*, ed 5, St. Louis, 2008, Saunders.

Bowman DD: *Georgis' parasitology for veterinarians*, ed 9, St. Louis, 2009, Saunders.

Foreyt WJ: *Veterinary parasitology reference manual*, ed 5, Ames, Iowa, 2007, Iowa State University Press.

Gillespie JR, Flanders F: *Modern livestock and poultry*, ed 8, Clifton Park, NY, 2010, Delmar Cengage Learning.

Hendrix CM, Robinson E: *Diagnostic parasitology for veterinary technicians*, ed 3, St. Louis, 2006, Mosby.

Jackson PGG, Cockcroft PD: *Handbook of pig medicine*, Edinburgh, 2007, Saunders.

Kahn CM, Line S: *The Merck veterinary manual*, ed 10, Whitehouse Station, NJ, 2010, Merck & Co.

Radostits O, Gay C, Hinchcliff KW, et al.: *Veterinary medicine: a textbook of the diseases of cattle, horses, sheep, pigs and goats*, ed 10, Oxford, 2008, Saunders.

Smith BP: *Large animal internal medicine*, ed 4, St. Louis, 2009, Mosby.

Glossary

Layperson's terms are included. Terminology varies depending on geographic location, species and breed of animal, and age of the person using the term.

AAEP American Association of Equine Practitioners.

A-mode Type of display mode in which the cathode ray tube displays one axis representing the time required for the return of the echo and the other corresponds to the strength of the echo.

Aberrant behavior syndrome Psychological condition suffered by human-raised llamas and alpacas that can cause them to exhibit dangerously aggressive behavior toward humans. Also known as berserk male syndrome.

Abomasum Fourth compartment of the ruminant stomach. An elongated sac comparable in structure and function to the stomach of nonruminants. It lies in the right half of the abdominal cavity, largely on the abdominal floor, except in late pregnancy, when it is pushed cranially by the enlarging uterus and may be lifted from the abdominal floor.

Abortion Premature expulsion from the uterus of the products of conception, either an embryo or a nonviable fetus.

Abscess Localized collection of pus in a cavity formed by the disintegration of tissue. Most abscesses are formed by invasion of tissues by bacteria, but some are caused by fungi, protozoa, or even helminths, and others are sterile. The effects of abscesses are determined by their location, the pressure they exert on nearby organs, and the degree of toxemia they create from their bacterial content and the amount of tissue they destroy.

Accessory sex gland Any gland, other than the gonad, associated with the genital tract, such as the ampulla of the ductus deferens and the bulbourethral, prostate, and vesicular glands of the male.

Ad libitum Feeding an animal as much as it will eat. Free feed.

Aerobic With air.

AGID Agar gel immunodiffusion. Technique that involves evaluation of the precipitin reaction in a clear gel, seen when an antigen placed in a hole in the agarose diffuses evenly into the medium.

Agroceryosis Starvation; deprived of adequate food.

All in/all out System of hog production in which pigs are managed by grouping them into farrowing, nursery, and growing or finishing groups. Each group is housed in a different facility, which is thoroughly cleaned and disinfected when the group moves out. Used to control many swine diseases.

Alleyway Narrow passageway.

Ambulatory practice Type of veterinary practice in which the veterinarian goes to the animal instead of the animal coming to the veterinarian. Also called farm call and field service.

Anaerobic Without air.

Anaphylactic shock Type I hypersensitivity reaction.

Angel berries Warts.

Ankle band Form of identification worn on the ankle.

Anorexia Lack or loss of appetite for food.

Antecubital vein Also known as the cephalic vein.

Antemortem Before death.

Antibiotic Chemical substance having the capacity, in dilute solution, to kill or inhibit growth of microorganisms. Antibiotic that is sufficiently nontoxic to the host is used as chemotherapeutic agent to treat infectious disease of humans, animals, and plants. Term originally was restricted to substances produced by microorganisms but has been extended to include synthetic and semisynthetic compounds of similar chemical activity.

Antioxidant Preventing or delaying oxidation.

Antitoxin Purified antiserum from animals (usually horses) immunized by injections of a toxin or toxoid, administered as a passive immunizing agent to neutralize a specific bacterial toxin (e.g., botulinus, tetanus, diphtheria).

Artificial insemination Implantation of live spermatozoa into the genital tract of the female. The diluted or otherwise treated semen usually is deposited in the body of the uterus because of the higher fertility rate obtained, but insemination into the uterine cervix or even the vagina may be practiced. Insemination usually is carried out through the vagina, but transperitoneal insemination may be used in animals whose anatomy precludes a satisfactory vaginal approach.

Arytenoid cartilages Pair of small, three-sided pyramids that form part of the larynx to which the vocal cords are attached.

Ash Incombustible, inorganic residue remaining after any process of incineration.

Ataxia Failure of muscular coordination; irregularity of muscular action.

Atlantooccipital space Location of cerebrospinal fluid collection.

Atresia ani Absence or closure of the anus or rectum.

Atresia coli Absence or closure of the colon. This developmental abnormality in cattle is lethal without surgical correction.

Atresia recti Absence or closure of the rectum.

Atrophy Wasting away; diminution in the size of a cell, tissue, organ, or part.

Auger Piece of equipment used in agriculture to move grain from trucks and grain carts into grain storage bins (from where it is later removed by gravity chutes at the bottom). A grain auger may be powered by the following: an electric motor; a tractor, through the power takeoff; or sometimes an internal combustion engine mounted on the auger. The helical flighting rotates inside a long metal tube that moves the grain upward.

Auscultation Act of listening for sounds within the body, chiefly to ascertain the condition of the lungs, heart, pleura, abdomen, and other organs.

Average daily gain (ADG) Average amount of weight gained in 1 day.

B-mode Type of ultrasound display mode in which the position of a spot on the cathode ray tube display corresponds to the time elapsed (and thus to the position of the echogenic surface), and the brightness of the spot corresponds to the strength of the echo. Movement of the transducer produces a sweep of the ultrasound beam and a tomographic scan of a cross-section of the body.

Baby pig thumps Respiratory distress in a baby pig.

Back stop Metal bar within an alleyway that, once an animal moves past it within the alleyway, swings out to prevent the animal from backing up.

Backgrounding Growing and feeding of calves from weaning until they are ready to enter the feedlot.

Bad flap Horse with laryngeal hemiplegia.

Bag Udder.

Bagging up Enlargement of the udder with milk before parturition.

Ball Give a tablet or bolus per os.

Balling gun Piece of equipment used in cattle to administer oral medications.

Ballottement Palpation by pressing both fists firmly into the left paralumbar fossa.

Bandage bow Tendon or ligament damage to the distal limb from an improperly fitting bandage.

Bandy legged Horse that is pigeon-toed on the hindlegs; the points of the hocks turn outward.

Bang's disease Brucellosis (*Brucella abortus*) in cattle; named for Danish veterinarian Fredrick Bang, who discovered the bacterium in 1897.

Bangtail Horse with the tail hairs cut off horizontally at the level of the hocks.

Barren mare Mare that has never conceived or carried a foal to term.

Barrow Castrated male of the porcine species.

Bat Jockey's whip.

Beans Rounded, firm accumulations of smegma in the urethral recess of the glans penis of the horse.

Beard Long hair that grows off the mandible of the jaw in goats.

Belly tap Abdominocentesis.

Berserk male syndrome See Aberrant behavior syndrome.

Bight Loop or bent part of a rope, as distinguished from the ends.

Bike Two-wheeled cart pulled by harness racing horses.

Bile Fluid secreted by the liver and drained into the small intestine through the bile ducts. Important constituents are conjugated bile salts, cholesterol, phospholipids, bilirubin diglucuronide, and electrolytes. Bile is alkaline because of its bicarbonate content, is golden brown to greenish yellow, and has a bitter taste. After it is secreted by the liver, bile is concentrated in the gallbladder. Bile formation depends on active secretion by hepatic cells into the bile canaliculi. Excretion of bile salts by hepatic cells and secretion of bicarbonate-rich fluid by ductular cells in response to secretin are the major factors that normally determine the volume of secretion. Conjugated bile salts and phospholipids normally dissolve cholesterol in a mixed micellar solution. In the upper small intestine, bile is partly responsible for alkalinizing the intestinal contents, and conjugated bile salts play an essential role in fat absorption by dissolving the products of fat digestion (fatty acids and monoglycerides) in water-soluble micelles. Also called gall.

Billy Intact male goat.

Biosecurity Security from transmission of infectious diseases, parasites, and pests.

Bishoping Altering the natural characteristics of the incisor teeth of a horse with files, drills, hot irons, or silver nitrate to make the horse appear younger than it really is. This fraudulent practice is used to pass older animals off as being younger, thus enhancing the possibility of a sale.

Black baldy Black bovine with solid white face.

Black brockle face Black bovine with blotchy white face.

Black teeth Another name for the needle teeth of piglets.

Bladder marsupialization Treatment for obstructive urolithiasis in male goats.

Bleeder Horse with exercise-induced pulmonary hemorrhage (EIPH); bleeding occurs in the small airways of the lungs during hard exercise. In a small percentage, bleeding may be severe enough that blood from the lungs appears at the nostrils following hard exercise.

Blemish Any defect that does not affect the intended use of an animal.

Blepharospasm Tonic spasm of the orbicularis oculi muscle that produces more or less complete closure of the eyelids.

Blind quarter/blind half A quarter or half of a mammary gland that is not producing milk when the other quarters are lactating.

Blind spavin Hock lameness in the horse, without physical or radiographic evidence. Usually considered an early stage of bone spavin. Also called occult spavin.

Blind teat A quarter obviously full of milk that cannot be expressed from the teat orifice, and a teat cannula cannot be passed up into the teat cistern. May occur by blockage from infection, trauma, or congenital defect.

Blister A strong chemical vesicant, historically applied to the skin over a leg injury in hopes of stimulating healing and preventing reinjury. A form of counterirritation.

Bloat Medical condition in which the stomach becomes overstretched by excessive gas content.

Blunt eye hook Instrument used during fetotomy.

Boar Intact male of the porcine species.

Boar effect Effect that causes a sow to display signs of estrus or to come into estrus when in the presence of a boar.

Bog spavin Effusion of the tibiotarsal joint of the hock.

Bone spavin A form of hock (tarsus) lameness in the horse caused by arthritis of the distal intertarsal or tarsometatarsal joints. Also called jack spavin.

Borborygmi Rumbling noises caused by propulsion of gas through the intestines.

Bottom line The dam's side of a pedigree.

Bovine Of or pertaining to the subfamily Bovinae, which includes cattle, buffalo, and kudus.

Bowed tendon Inflammation of a tendon; usually refers specifically to tendinitis of the superficial or deep digital flexor tendons of the lower leg of the horse.

Bradycardia Slowness of the heartbeat.

Breaking water Rupture of the chorioallantoic membrane with release of chorioallantoic fluid; signals the onset of the second stage of labor.

Breeder's stitch Additional heave gauze suture placed across the most ventral aspect of the suture line in the Caslick surgical procedure.

Breeding season Parts of the year during which animals mate. This season may be artificially arranged by humans. Animals that are not controlled are more sexually active during certain periods of the year.

Breeze In racehorse training, a workout at less than maximal speed.

Broken mouth Aged ruminant that has lost some, but not all, of its incisors.

Broken penis Hematoma of the penis.

Buck Intact male goat.

Buck kid Intact male neonate goat.

Buck odor Smell associated with bucks during the breeding season.

Bucked shins Inflammation of the periosteum (periostitis) on the dorsal aspect of the third metacarpal bone, often with swelling and lameness; it is a repetitive bone stress injury, most commonly seen in young horses in the early phases of race training.

Bull Intact male bovine.

Bull calf Young male bovine.

Buller Nymphomaniac cow that mounts other cattle or a steer that allows other steers to mount.

Bullnose Suppuration, necrosis, and swelling of the nose of a pig as a result of infection by *Fusobacterium necrophorum* that enters through a wound. Also known as necrotic rhinitis.

Bummer lamb Orphan lamb being raised by hand or by a foster ewe; it is "bumming" milk from other sources.

Bump weaning Method of moving piglets from one mother to another.

Bunches Subcutaneous abscesses.

Burro Synonym for a donkey (*Equus asinus)*; term used more commonly in the western United States.

Bussled pig Pig with a scrotal hernia.

By Referring to the male parent of an animal. Compare "out of."

By-product Secondary or incidental product, as in a process of manufacture.

Calf Young bovine of either sex.

Calf bed out Prolapsed uterus.

Calf crop Number or percentage of calves produced within a herd in a given year divided by the number of cows and heifers exposed to breeding.

Calf jack Mechanical device used as a pulley system on bovines with dystocia.

Calves Young of the domestic cow or other bovine animal.

Calving Act of parturition in the bovine species.

Camelid Any member of the alpaca and llama family Camelidae.

Capillary refill time Test used to estimate hydration and blood circulation in animals.

Capped elbow Inflammation of the olecranon bursa, over the point of the elbow.

Capped hock Inflammation of the calcaneal bursa, over the point of the hock.

Caps Deciduous cheek teeth of the horse. They normally are shed when the permanent teeth erupt but occasionally are retained and require removal.

Carbonaceous Concentrates with larger volumes of carbon. Examples are corn, oats, sorghum, barley, rye, and wheat.

Cardia Part of the stomach immediately adjacent to and surrounding the cardiac opening where the esophagus connects to the stomach. Contains the cardiac glands but no parietal cells or chief cells. Also called pars cardiaca gastris and cardiac part of stomach.

Cashmere Soft down or winter undercoat of fiber produced by most breeds of goats, except the Angora.

Caslick surgery Surgical procedure performed to treat pneumovagina and prevent contamination of the vagina.

Cast in stall Animal that is positioned awkwardly in a stall or pen and cannot rise to its feet.

Casting Technique of using a rope or a special harness designed to make an animal fall to the ground or onto a specially prepared area. Used for large animals, especially horses and cattle.

Catch Indicates successful conception after breeding.

Cattle prod Device that can be applied to the rear end of cattle to encourage them to forward movement as a result of a small electrical shock. It should be used only when other methods have failed.

Caudal epidural Analgesic placed into the first intercoccygeal space.

Caveson Noseband on a bridle.

Cecum Blind pouch.

Celiotomy Laparotomy.

Central sulcus of the frog Depression on the palmar and plantar aspect of the frog itself.

Cesarean section Birth of a fetus accomplished by performing a surgical incision through the maternal abdomen and uterus.

Chain shank Leather lead with a short section of chain at the proximal end. It can be placed over the horse's nose, through the mouth, or across the upper gum for greater control.

Challenge feeding Feeding livestock to promote increased weight gain.

Cheek teeth The premolars and molars.

Chemical marking patch Chemical patch that changes color when pressure is applied. Used to detect heat in livestock.

Chemical restraint Use of pharmaceuticals to alter an animal's mental or physical abilities.

Chest tap Thoracocentesis.

Chestnuts Small, horny callus on the inner surface of a horse's leg.

Chevon Goat meat.

Chewing cud Process that includes regurgitation, remastication, ensalivation, and reswallowing. Regurgitation of fluid reticular contents occurs as a result of a positive lowering of intrathoracic pressure, the arrival of a ruminal contraction at the cardial sphincter at the appropriate time, relaxation of the cardia, and reverse peristalsis in the lower esophagus. The regurgitus is compressed at the back of the tongue, and the fluid is immediately reswallowed. The solid material is chewed for about a minute and reswallowed. The cycle is then ready to recommence. Rumination requires a positive approach by the cow and is easily disrupted by fright or food.

Choke Obstruction of the esophagus.

Chorionic gonadotropin Hormone that promotes secretion of progesterone by the corpus luteum. Its presence in the urine is an indication of pregnancy.

Chute Open set of bars with two doors at the front and back often used for cattle restraint.

Chyme Semifluid, homogeneous, creamy, or gruel-like material produced by digestion of food in the stomach. Also called chymus.

Claw Division into four tubes of the milking unit.

Claws Digits on a cloven hoof.

Clean up (a female) Examine and lavage the uterus after giving birth, or treat uterine infection.

Clinical mastitis Visible signs of disease in the milk or the affected quarter.

Clip Amount of wool shorn in one season.

Coccoid Resembling a globe.

Cod Scrotum of a steer.

Cold shoeing Fitting and shaping a horseshoe without use of heat.

Cold-backed Horse that resents tightening of the girth or cinch during placement of the saddle.

Coldblood Horse without Arabian blood or other "desert breeds" in the pedigree; horses descended from the colder climate of Europe. Generally refers to the draft horse breeds and some pony breeds of European descent.

Colostrum Thin, yellow, milky fluid secreted by the mammary gland before or after parturition. Contains up to 20% protein, predominant among which are immunoglobulins, representing the antibodies found in maternal blood. Contains more minerals and less fat and carbohydrate than doe's milk. Also contains many colostrum corpuscles and usually coagulates on boiling because of the large amount of lactalbumin.

Commercial farming Production of agricultural products on a large scale.

Commodity Secondary or incidental product, as in a process of manufacture.

Compartment syndrome Syndrome in which muscles that are contained in an aponeurotic sheath may be subject to serious ischemia caused by an increase in muscle size as a result of vigorous muscular activity.

Complement fixation test Immunologic medical test used to detect the presence of either a specific antibody or a specific antigen in a patient's serum. Widely used to diagnose infections, particularly with microbes that are not easily detected by culture methods, and rheumatic diseases.

Conjunctiva Clear mucous membrane consisting of cells and underlying basement membrane that covers the sclera (white part of eye) and lines the inside of the eyelids.

Connecting air Portion of the milking unit that creates the vacuum.

Contagious case Capable of being transmitted from animal to animal.

Contagious mastitis Type of mastitis that can be spread directly from cow to cow, usually at milking time (through milking machines or contaminated hands or towels).

Coon-footed Horse with a long pastern, long toe, and low heel.

Corded leg Damaged tendons or ligaments of the leg that result from an improperly applied or maintained bandage.

Corded vein Thickened vein, often secondary to thrombus formation.

Corded-up Myositis of the hindquarters with stiffness of the hindlimbs; otherwise known as tying-up or tied-up.

Corkscrew claw An elongated claw that grows with rotation around its long axis, thus producing a rolled-under appearance; usually affects the lateral claw on the hindfeet of cattle.

Corns Bruising of a horse's hoof in the area of the bars.

Coronary band Band at the top of the hoof where the hoof meets the skin.

Cosmetic dehorning Use of a surgical incision to remove a horn below the integument.

Costochondral junction Location at which the rib bone and rib cartilage meet.

Covering a mare Natural breeding or "servicing" of a female horse.

Cow Female bovine.

Cow-hocked Horse with the points of the hocks turned inward (medially) instead of facing directly behind the horse.

Creep feeding Feeding creep or sweet feed to neonates.

Cria Neonate camelid.

Cribbing Aerophagia; vice of horses where the horse swallows air through the mouth, usually while grasping a solid object with its incisors; it produces a distinct audible noise.

Crippled orchid Mispronunciation of "cryptorchid."

Crossbreeding Hybridization. Mating of organisms of different strains or species (e.g., mating animals of different breeds). Practiced extensively in farm animals to capitalize on advantages conferred by hybrid vigor.

Crutching Shearing the wool from the perineal region of sheep.

Cryopreservation Maintenance of the viability of excised tissue or organs by storing at very low temperatures.

Crypto Layperson's abbreviation for *Cryptosporidium.*

Cryptorchidectomy Excision of an undescended testis.

Curb Inflammation of the plantar ligament, on the caudal aspect of the calcaneus. Horses with sickle hocks are predisposed to developing curbs and are referred to as "curby." Cow-hocked horses are also predisposed.

Cured Dried in the sun (grasses).

Cushed position Sternal recumbency.

Cut Castrate.

Cutdown Creation of an incision. Usually the incision used for direct tracheal intubation.

Cyanosis Bluish discoloration, especially of the skin and mucous membranes, resulting from excessive concentration of deoxyhemoglobin in the blood.

Cystic ovary Ovary containing multiple small follicular cysts filled with yellow or blood-stained thin serous fluid.

Cystotomy Surgical incision of urinary bladder. Also called vesicotomy.

Dam Female camelid.

Dancing pig disease Congenital tremor syndrome (myoclonia congenita) of piglets. Characterized by severe muscle tremors when awake; disappears when asleep.

Decubital ulcer Ulcer acquired over a bony prominence as a result of lying down.

Dehorning Removal of horns.

Dental pad Firm ridge that replaces incisors in the maxilla of ruminants.

Descenting Removal of the scent glands.

Dewlap Hanging fold of skin under the neck of animals, especially some breeds of cattle and goats.

Diamond skin disease Swine erysipelas (*Erysipelothrix rhusiopathiae*); produces discolored diamond-shaped blotches of the skin over the back area.

Diestrus In female mammals that have estrous cycles, a period of sexual quiescence between metestrus and the next proestrus. Represents the phase of the mature corpus luteum.

Digestible energy (DE) Proportion of potential energy in a feed that actually is digested.

Dingleberries Dried accumulations of feces on the hair, wool, or skin.

Diplococci Round bacteria (cocci) that typically occur in pairs of two joined cells.

Direct blood pressure measurement Arterial blood pressure measurement.

Direct tracheal intubation Placement of endotracheal tube directly into the trachea.

Dirty mare Mare with a uterine infection.

Dishrag foal Limp, very weak, or comatose foal.

Distemper (equine) Strangles in horses (*Streptococcus equi*); an upper respiratory disease characterized by purulent nasal discharge and abscessed lymph nodes in the head and throat region.

Diverticulum Herniation through the muscular wall of a tubular organ.

Doe Female goat.

Doe kid Female neonate goat.

Double drip Drug combination consisting of two drugs administered for anesthesia.

Draft horse One of the heavy breeds of horse, developed originally for farm or heavy freight work. Average weight: 1500 to 2200 pounds.

Drench Administer liquids or liquid medications by mouth.

Drops Newborn lambs.

Dry Not lactating.

Dry matter Measurement of the mass of something completely dried.

Drylot Type of pen in which the main feed source is not grass.

Dummy Animal with abnormal mentation or stuporous behavior; does not respond to normal stimuli.

Dung pile Common area used by camelids for defecation.

Dyspnea Labored or difficult breathing.

Dystocia Abnormal or difficult birth.

Ear notching Permanent form of identification in which pieces of skin in the form of notches are removed from quarters of the ear.

Easy keeper Animal that maintains its bodyweight or gains weight on less feed than other animals in similar conditions.

Ecchymotic hemorrhages Hemorrhagic spots, larger than petechiae, in the skin or mucous membrane that form nonelevated, rounded or irregular, blue or purplish patches.

Elastrator Tool used to cut off blood supply to the testicles, thus leading to castration.

Electroejaculation Induction of ejaculation by delivery of a gradually increasing electrical current through a probe inserted into the rectum. Technique originally used in veterinary medicine and now also used in humans for collection of sperm for insemination from men with spinal cord injuries and other conditions that prevent ejaculation.

Electroejaculator Device consisting of a rectal probe, a power control system that gives stepwise control over the current applied, and a stimulator control that permits variation within the steps. Probes vary in construction, and a good design directs stimulation at the relevant nerves, thereby reducing stimulation of the back and hindlimbs.

Electronic identification tag (EID) Electronic form of identification.

ELISA Enzyme-linked immunosorbent assay. Biochemical technique used mainly in immunology to detect the presence of an antibody or an antigen in a sample. Also known as enzyme immunoassay (EIA).

Embryo transfer Placement of an embryo (fertilized egg) into the uterus for implantation.

End of a rope Short end of the rope or the end that can be freely moved about.

Energy feeds Livestock feed containing less than 20% crude protein. Most grains are energy feeds.

Environmental mastitis Type of mastitis contracted through environmental contamination of bedding, soil, standing water, or feces, for example.

Ependymal Pertaining to or composed of ependyma, the membrane lining the canal of the spinal cord and the ventricles of the brain.

Epididymitis Inflammation of the epididymis.

Epiphora Abnormal overflow of tears down the cheek, mainly from stricture of the lacrimal passages.

Epistaxis Hemorrhage from the nose. Also called nosebleed or nasal hemorrhage.

Epitheliochorial Type of placenta in which the chorion is apposed to the uterine epithelium but does not erode it.

Ergot Seed of the bulrush millet, *Pennisetum typhoides,* which may be infested with *Claviceps fusiformis.*

Eructation Casting up of wind from the stomach through the mouth. Also called belching.

Eruption bumps Firm, temporary enlargements along the ventral border of the mandible, corresponding with eruption of permanent cheek teeth in horses 2 to 4 years old. Caused by remodeling of the mandible to accommodate the developing roots of the cheek teeth; as the teeth erupt and advance, the bone remodels and removes the "bumps."

Estimated progeny differences (EPD) Estimated breeding values give an estimate of the average transmitting ability of the parent. EPDs are useful in comparing or ranking individuals within a breed for traits of interest.

Estrus Recurrent, restricted period of sexual receptivity in female mammals, other than human females, marked by an intense sexual urge.

Estrus synchronization Practice of using hormones to alter the reproductive cycle of females so that they all are in the same phase of estrus at the same time.

Ewe Female sheep.

Ewe lamb Female neonate sheep.

Ewe-necked Horse with a neck that has a slightly concave topline (like a ewe) when viewed from the side; the neck appears to attach low on the chest.

Exciter ram Vasectomized ram that is turned out with a flock of ewes just before breeding season, to help "bring out" females with silent estrous cycles.

Extender Liquid diluent mixed with semen to preserve its fertilizing ability.

External genitalia Reproductive organs outside of the body.

External preputial ring Rim of the external orifice of the prepuce proper, the internal prepuce, on the penis of the horse.

Extralabel drug use Use of an approved drug in a manner that is not in accordance with the approved labeling yet meets the conditions set forth by the Animal Medicinal Drug Use Clarification Act of 1994 and U.S. Food and Drug Administration regulations

Facing Clipping the wool from the face and eyes of a sheep to prevent wool blindness.

Facultative Capable of using or not using air.

Fall back Baby piglet that is bump weaned because it is falling behind in development.

False rig Castrated male horse that exhibits persistent stallion-like behavior.

Far side Right side of a horse; also known as off side.

Farm call Type of veterinary practice in which the veterinarian goes to the animal instead of the animal coming to the veterinarian. Also called ambulatory practice and field service.

Farrier Person who trims and shoes horse's hooves; preferred term to blacksmith. May complete certification courses and examinations administered by the American Farriers Association (AFA).

Farrow to finish Operation that raises hogs from birth to slaughter weight.

Farrowing Act of parturition in the porcine species.

Feathering Long hair on the distal limbs of horses, often draft horses.

Fecal flotation Technique for floating eggs in fecal material to test for parasite infestation.

Feed additive Pharmaceutical or nutritional substance that is not natural feedstuff and is added to made-up and stored feeds for various purposes, chiefly to control infectious disease or promote growth. Improper use may cause poisoning in subject animals or undesirable residues in food for human consumption produced by the animals. Use of additives in this way is strictly controlled by legislation in most countries, some of which require a veterinarian's prescription to comply with local poison laws.

Feedstuff Materials of nutritional value fed to animals.

Fetlock Metacarpophalangeal joint.

Fetotomy Dissection of a dead fetus in utero. Applicable particularly to cows because of the size of the uterus and the opportunity to introduce instruments to the full depth of the fetus.

Field service Type of veterinary practice in which the veterinarian goes to the animal instead of the animal coming to the veterinarian. Also called ambulatory practice and farm calls.

Fighting teeth Very sharp, daggerlike teeth, on the upper and lower jaws, developed by the male llama on maturity. Total of six teeth.

Fistulous withers Chronic suppurative inflammation of the supraspinous bursa in horses that is caused by infection.

Flanking A method of throwing a calf to the ground by reaching across its back, grabbing the skinfold of the flank, and using that skinfold to lift the animal off its feet.

Flaps Arytenoid cartilages.

Fleece rot Dermatitis of sheep caused by prolonged wetness of the skin; open sores develop, and exudates form crusts and mat the wool.

Flounder Common mispronunciation of "founder."

Flushing Nutritional practice, in ruminants and swine, of increasing a female's intake of protein or carbohydrates, or both, just before breeding, to improve ovulation and conception rates.

Fly strike Excessive fly bites often found on tips of the ears.

Foley catheter Flexible (usually latex) tube that is passed through the urethra during urinary catheterization and into the bladder to drain urine.

Fomite Any inanimate object or substance capable of carrying and hence transferring infectious organisms (e.g., germs, parasites) from one individual to another.

Food Animal Residue Avoidance Databank (FARAD) Convenient source of information about withdrawal times for drugs.

Foot bath Used in the control of foot rot in sheep and cattle. Made of concrete or metal, but preferably not metal because of the corrosive nature of copper sulfate solution. Deep enough to accommodate a 4-inch depth of solution, wide enough so that animals can stand comfortably on all four hooves, with a side fence to ensure that they do actually stand in the bath, and long enough to accommodate 5 to 10 animals. Animals need to stand in the solution for approximately 10 minutes. Solutions used include copper sulfate or formalin. For dairy cattle, the foot bath may be located at the entrance to the milking parlor so that cows walk through the foot bath twice each day.

Foot rot Contagious degenerative infection of the feet of hoofed animals.

Forage Another name for roughage.

Forceps Two-bladed instrument with a handle for compressing or grasping tissues in surgical operations and for handling sterile dressings, for example.

Founder Chronic laminitis, with displacement of P3 from its normal position within the hoof. Clients often use the term to refer to any case of laminitis, acute or chronic.

Free stall barn Loose housing system in which stalls are provided for cows.

Freeze branding Branding animals by depigmentation of the hair coat with supercooled instruments. A carefully gauged degree of cold application causes selective destruction of the pigment-producing cells (melanocytes).

Freeze firing Practice of applying liquid nitrogen to the skin overlying an injured tendon, ligament, or bone. Used on the legs of horses with the belief that healing of the treated injury will be faster and of better quality. A form of counterirritation.

Fresh Recently calved.

Freshening Calving.

Frick speculum Piece of equipment used to assist in placing a gastric tube in ruminants.

Full mouth Ruminant or horse with all permanent teeth present.

Furlong ⅛ mile = 740 ft = 201.17 m.

Gall Saddle or girth sore in horses.

Gallbladder Pear-shaped reservoir for bile attached to the visceral surface or between lobes of the liver in all domestic animal species except horses. Serves as a storage place for bile. The gallbladder may be subject to disorders such as inflammation and formation of gallstones.

Gangrenous mastitis Severe mastitis that results in destruction of the affected quarter, with necrosis and sloughing. Severe *Staphylococcus* infections and wounds that allow *Clostridium* species to become established may result in gangrenous mastitis.

Gare Long, noncrimped wool fibers that are unsuitable for spinning or dyeing.

Garget Mastitis.

Gaskin Region of a horse's hind leg between the hock and stifle.

Gastric lipase Group of enzymes that catalyze hydrolysis of fats into glycerol and fatty acids.

Gelding Castrated male horse or camelid.

Genetic principles Use of genetic knowledge. An example is mendelian genetics.

Genetics Science of heredity, dealing with resemblances and differences of related organisms resulting from interaction of their genes and the environment.

Genital tubercle Eminence in the embryo that develops into the clitoris or penis.

Get The offspring of a male animal; progeny.

Gill flirt Mare with a rectovaginal tear; usually results from laceration of the vaginal roof and rectal floor by the hoof of the fetus during delivery.

Gilt Female of the porcine species that has not had a litter.

Girth Heavy rope or leather strap that holds the saddle on a horse by circling the thorax.

Glans penis Distal, free end of the penis. Has a rich supply of sensory nerve endings.

Glass eye Blue iris.

Glucose Aldohexose ($C_6H_{12}O_6$) that occurs naturally as the D-form and is found as a free monosaccharide in fruits and other plants and in the normal blood of all animals; also is combined in glucosides and disaccharides, oligosaccharides, and polysaccharides. It is an end product of carbohydrate metabolism and the chief source of energy for living organisms; its use is controlled by insulin. Excess glucose is converted to glycogen, stored in the liver and muscles for use as needed, and then converted to fat and stored as adipose tissue. See also Hyperglycemia and Hypoglycemia. Called dextrose in pharmaceutical use.

Gluteal Pertaining to the buttocks.

Gomer Male that has been surgically prepared to ensure that it cannot mate or is not fertile. In cattle and sheep, a vasectomized animal or a castrate injected with testosterone is used.

Gomer bull Teaser bull, surgically prepared by vasectomy or penile deviation to prevent impregnation of females. Gomer bulls are used to detect females in standing heat.

Grade Animal without documentable lineage.

Grading up Animal of inferior breeding and quality is bred to one of much superior standing.

Gram negative Characteristic of bacteria that do not retain crystal violet dye in the Gram staining protocol.

Gram positive Characteristic of bacteria that stain dark blue or violet by the Gram staining protocol.

Grass staggers Hypomagnesemia of ruminants.

Grass tetany Hypomagnesemia of ruminants.

Gravel Purulent material or abscess in the hoof that migrates proximally and ruptures and drains at the coronary band.

Grease heel Moist exudative dermatitis of the pastern or fetlock region in the horse, generally from excessive moisture. Also known as scratches.

Green Inexperienced animal (or human).

Gummer Animal with no teeth or ruminant with no incisors; a sign of aging.

Half hitch Knot or hitch made by forming a bight and passing the end of the rope around the standing part and through the bight.

Halter Rope or strap with a head stall for leading or restraining horses or cattle.

Hand Measurement of equine height; equal to 4 inches.

Hand mating Mating in which the female detected to be in estrus is handheld while she is mated or is let into a paddock or pen with a male, where she is the only female. Mating is observed and can be guaranteed to have occurred. Allows accurate recording of the day and genetics of breeding, as opposed to pen mating.

Hard keeper Animal that requires more feed to maintain its bodyweight than other animals kept under similar conditions.

Hard milker Teat with constriction at the teat orifice that makes it difficult, but not impossible, to express milk; often affects all teats.

Hardware Metallic foreign bodies in the reticulum of ruminants; they may puncture the wall of the reticulum and penetrate the diaphragm and pericardium, thus causing hardware disease (traumatic reticuloperitonitis).

Harem Mating scheme in which multiple females are bred with one male. Can also imply a group of female camelids.

Hay flake A small section of a hay bale. During the baling process, the baling machine divides the bale into small, regular, pressed portions. On average, one flake is 2 to 4 inches wide and weighs approximately 3 to 4 pounds. Also known as a wafer.

Head shy Animal that is sensitive to movements around the head and often tries to avoid contact in the head area.

Heat detection In most natural mating situations, the male is the best possible detector. In artificial breeding or hand mating, the need to pick cows that are in heat is of paramount importance. Techniques include use of infertile teasers combined with heat mount detectors, tail paint, or chin ball or siresine harnesses. In dairy herds it is usual practice to dispense with the teasers and depend on other cows to pick out and mount the cows that are in heat.

Heat mount detector Device used to detect when livestock are in heat.

Heaves Equine respiratory condition characterized by difficult, labored breathing with a marked abdominal component on expiration. May lead to hypertrophy of abdominal muscle (external abdominal oblique muscle) and formation of a noticeable ridge of musculature ("heave line") from the flank forward to the elbow. Caused by chronic airway disease, usually from a chronic hypersensitivity response to environmental allergens such as dust, mold, and grasses. Sometimes incorrectly referred to as asthma.

Heifer Female bovine before she has had her first calf.

Heifer calf Young female bovine.

Hemal process Prominence from a bone.

Hematoma Localized collection of blood, usually clotted, in an organ, space, or tissue, usually resulting from a break in the wall of a blood vessel.

Hemostasis Arrest of bleeding, either by physiologic properties of vasoconstriction and coagulation or by surgical means or interruption of blood flow through a vessel or to a part.

Herd A group of animals kept or living together.

Herniorrhaphy Surgical procedure for correcting a hernia. Also known as hernioplasty or hernia repair.

Heterosis Increase in growth, size, fecundity, function, yield, or other characteristics in hybrids over those of the parents.

Heterospermic insemination Mixing sperm for insemination from more than one male.

High flanker Testicle retained near the body wall, "high" in the inguinal area, and not descended into the scrotum.

High trough fever Starvation; lack of adequate nutrition.

Hinny Hybrid resulting from crossing a stallion (*Equus caballus*) with a jennet (*Equus asinus*); a rare type of mule.

Hitch To fasten or tie, especially temporarily, by means of a hook, rope, strap, or tether.

Hog Pig that weighs more than 120 pounds.

Hog snare Instrument used in swine to restrain the animal by holding the maxilla.

Hogget Young sheep between weaning and the first shearing.

Hoof block Piece of equipment that can be used to help cattle with claw problems. It is placed on the good claw.

Hoof knife Instrument used to remove excess hoof wall.

Hook bone Hip bone; tuber coxae.

Horn button Small horn from which a horn grows.

Horned Term used to describe cattle that are naturally born with horns.

Hot branding Method of identification in which heat is used to scar the skin with a specific mark.

Hot zone Area within a clinic where equipment may enter but cannot leave until it has been disinfected. The area is considered contaminated. Often used with contagious cases.

Hotblood Horse with a pedigree tracing primarily to the "desert breeds" of Northern Africa and the Mediterranean. Includes the Arabian, the Barb, and breeds primarily descended from them, such as Thoroughbred, Standardbred, Quarter horse, and Tennessee Walking horse.

Hothouse lambs Lambs born out of season in the fall or early winter so that they can be marketed between Christmas and May, a time of peak ethnic demand for lamb meat.

Hulet rod Hollow plastic palpation rod.

Hydraulic Operated by, moved by, or using water or other liquids in motion.

Hyperemic Animal with increased blood in part because of local or general relaxation of the arterioles.

Hyperglycemia Abnormally increased glucose in the blood, such as in diabetes mellitus.

Hypoglycemia Abnormally diminished concentration of glucose in the blood.

Iceberg concept Concept stating that in some diseases, clinically sick animals represent only the tip of the iceberg and that many more animals are ill but are not displaying clinical signs.

Ileus Intestinal obstruction with a nonmechanical cause, such as paralysis and failure of peristalsis.

Inbreeding Breeding of closely related individuals.

Incubation period Time elapsed between exposure to a pathogenic organism, a chemical, or radiation and when symptoms and signs are first apparent.

Indirect contact Disease spread by indirect contact means. Animals themselves did not come in contact with each other.

Individual breeding Mating of two animals, unobserved.

Inguinal hernia Usually a sac formed by the lining of the abdominal cavity (peritoneum).

Injection site lesion Lesion created from an injection.

Insurance examination Examination required by an insurance company for a horse to receive coverage.

Intramammary infusion Infusion of medication into the teat canal.

Jack 1. Male donkey (*Equus asinus*). 2. One of the two tendons of insertion of the cranial tibial muscle of the horse; the tendon inserts on the medial aspect of the hock and is sometimes cut as a treatment for bone spavin.

Jack spavin Bone spavin.

Jennet Female donkey (*Equus asinus*); also called a jenny.

Jill Female camelid.

Jog cart Two-wheeled exercise cart pulled by harness racing horses.

Joint ill Joint infection.

Joint tap Arthrocentesis.

Jug Lambing pen where a ewe and her lambs are kept for several days.

Jugging Administering a solution of various components (e.g., electrolytes, amino acids, vitamins, hormones, carbohydrates) intravenously through the jugular vein. Usually given to horses before a race or other sporting event in the hopes of improving performance.

Kid Neonate goat.

Kidding Act of parturition in goats.

Knocked-down hip Fracture of the point of the hip (tuber coxae), with displacement of the fractured fragment, which usually displaces ventrally.

Knot Interlacing, twining, looping (e.g., of a cord or rope), drawn tight into a knob or lump, for fastening, binding, or connecting two cords together or a cord to something else.

Lamb Young sheep.

Lambing Act of parturition in sheep.

Lambing snare Instrument used to help manipulate a lamb from the birth canal during dystocia.

Lameness Pain in the limbs that does not allow for natural movement.

Laparotomy Surgical incision into the abdominal cavity.

Lateral auricular vein Vein of the ear.

Lateral cervical muscles Muscles along each side of the neck.

Lateral sulci of the frog Depressions on the medial and lateral sides of the frog.

Lead rope Rope often with a clasp to attach to a horse's halter. Used for leading.

Legume Plant of the family Leguminoseae that carries its seeds in a pod that splits along its seams. Many legumes have nitrogen-fixing bacteria in nodules on the roots that can transform nitrogen in the air into a form (NH_3) that can be used by plants. Peanuts, soybeans, clovers, and alfalfa are common legumes used in agriculture.

Light horse Average riding horse.

Line breeding Form of inbreeding directed toward keeping the offspring closely related to a superior ancestor.

Lipase Triacylglycerol lipase. Any enzyme that hydrolytically cleaves a fatty acid anion from a triglyceride or phospholipid.

Lithotripsy Crushing of urinary calculus or gallstone within the body, followed at once by washing out of the fragments. Formerly done surgically but now can be done by various noninvasive methods.

Live cover Natural practice of a male naturally mating a female.

Lochia Vaginal discharge that takes place during the first week or two after parturition.

Loop Portion of a cord (e.g., ribbon) that is folded or doubled on itself to leave an opening between the parts.

Lordosis Characteristic standing response seen in some animals during estrus. Stance that will allow a male to mount.

Loss of use insurance Insurance that states specifically the intended use of the horse and may reimburse the owner if the horse cannot perform its intended use because of illness or injury.

Lumbosacral space Space in the sacrum.

Lunge (longe) Method of exercising horses in a circle. An approximately 30-foot rope or lead ("lunge line") is attached to the horse's head, and the horse is asked to walk, trot, or canter in circles around the handler. Used to train, exercise, and examine horses.

Lunger Animal with a chronic respiratory disease.

Luteal phase Phase after estrus until pregnancy or luteolysis.

Mad itch Pseudorabies; a herpesvirus disease of swine with respiratory, nervous, and reproductive signs. Ruminants may occasionally be affected.

Magpies Cattle with evidence of Holstein breeding (black and white coloring).

Maiden Horse that has never won a race.

Maiden mare Female horse that has never become pregnant.

Maintenance nutrient requirements In terms of animal nutrition, the amount and quality of the diet required to maintain an adult animal without providing additional nutriment for production, reproduction, or weight gain.

Malacia Morbid softening or softness of a part or tissue.

Malignant hyperthermia (MH) Rare, life-threatening condition triggered by exposure to certain drugs used for general anesthesia (specifically all volatile anesthetics), nearly all gas anesthetics, and the neuromuscular blocking agent succinylcholine. Also known as malignant hyperthermia syndrome (MHS) or malignant hyperpyrexia resulting from anesthesia.

Malocclusion Malposition and contact of the maxillary and mandibular teeth that interfere with highest efficiency during the excursive movements of the jaw essential for mastication.

Marbling Small streaks of fat found within the muscle.

Marcenac approach Abdominal surgical approach.

Mare Female horse.

Marking White area of hair on the face and legs of horses.

Mastitis Inflammation of the mammary gland.

Maternal line Breed of swine that has stronger maternal characteristics.

Mathematician Lame animal ("puts down 3 and carries 1").

Mean arterial pressure Average blood pressure.

Meconium Dark green mucilaginous material in the intestine of the full-term fetus. Consists of mixture of the secretions of the liver, intestinal glands, and some amniotic fluid.

Meningitis Inflammation of the meninges.

Metaestrus In female mammals that have estrous cycles, the period of subsiding follicular function or rest following estrus.

Microphthalmia Developmental disorder of the eye that causes eyes to be small.

Milk fat Fat content in milk.

Milk replacer Powdered milk that can be fed to neonatal animals.

Milk ring test Special form of agglutination test performed on pooled milk of many cows, usually entire herds, for detection of herds containing individuals infected with bovine brucellosis.

Milk teeth Deciduous (baby) teeth.

Milk tube Portion of the milking unit that carries the milk to the bulk tank.

Milking unit Part of the milking machine that attaches to the udder.

Milkshaking Procedure of giving a solution of bicarbonate, carbohydrates, and other additives to a horse by nasogastric tube, before a race or other athletic event, to reduce fatigue and improve performance during the event. This is an illegal practice in most racing jurisdictions.

Miniature horse Horse that is smaller than a pony.

Modified ruminant Animal that is not a true ruminant but has a similar digestive system (e.g., a camelid).

Monday morning disease Exertional rhabdomyolysis syndrome of horses. The name originated in draft horses that were exercised Monday through Saturday and then rested on Sunday; occasionally, on the following Monday morning, the animal was stiff and reluctant to move and had palpable hardening of the rump muscles (especially the gluteals).

Moon blindness Periodic ophthalmia (recurrent anterior uveitis) in horses.

Morbidity Portion of animals that become sick.

Mortality Portion of animals that die.

Mortality insurance Insurance that covers the value of the horse in case of death. Insurance company pays the owner the estimated worth of the horse if it dies, although exclusions may exist for certain causes of death.

Mother up Process of a dam bonding with its newborn or reuniting with it after a brief separation.

Mouthing Aging an animal by its teeth.

Mucopurulent Containing both mucus and pus.

Mule Hybrid resulting from crossing a mare (*Equus caballus*) with a jack (*Equus asinus*).

Muley cattle Polled (hornless) cattle.

Mutation In genetics, a permanent transmissible change in the genetic material, usually in a single gene. Term sometimes used to include gross alterations in chromosomal structure.

Myiasis Condition caused by infestation of the body by fly maggots.

Myoglobinurea Oxygen-transporting pigment of muscle, a type of hemoprotein resembling a single subunit of hemoglobin, composed of one globin polypeptide chain and one heme group (containing one iron atom). Combines with oxygen released by erythrocytes, stores it, and transports it to the mitochondria of muscle cells, where it generates energy by combustion of glucose to carbon dioxide and water.

Nanny Female goat.

Nasal turbinate In anatomy, a nasal concha (or turbinate) is a long, narrow, curled bone shelf (shaped like an elongated seashell) that protrudes into the breathing passage of the nose.

Nasogastric intubation Intubation into the stomach or intestine to remove gastric or intestinal contents for relief or prevention of distension, obtain a specimen for analysis, or introduce drugs, medication, food, or nutrients. A rubber or plastic nasogastric tube is introduced through the nose and into the stomach.

National Animal Identification System (NAIS) Government-run program in the United States intended to extend government animal health.

National Farm Identification and Records System National animal identification and traceability system. Database certified by the United States Department of Agriculture as an official animal tracking database (ATD).

Navel ill Infection of the umbilicus in young animals.

Near side Left side of a horse, from which they are handled.

Needle teeth Deciduous upper and lower third incisors (I3) and deciduous canine teeth in the newborn piglet. Routinely clipped to remove the sharp tips, to prevent damage to sow's teats and to other piglets.

Needle tooth nippers Instrument used to trim needle teeth in piglets.

Nerved Horse that has had surgical posterior digital neurectomy for treatment of chronic pain in the heel region of the hoof.

Net energy (NE) Metabolizable energy less energy used in specific dynamic action response.

Neurologic examination Examination of the neurologic function of an animal.

Nonambulatory Unable to stand up.

Nonruminant Animal that is not a ruminant.

Nose band Part of the halter that passes over the bridge of the nose.

Nose hose Nasogastric tube.

Nose lead Scissorlike instrument with blades that curve toward each other and are fitted with a knob on each of their ends. The tool is inserted into the nostrils with the blades opened, is positioned on either side of the septum, and then is closed tight. The end of the nasal septum is grasped between the ends of the tongs. It provides fair restraint for a cow having a minor procedure (e.g., intravenous injection).

Nose ring Metal ring that can be placed through the nasal septum as a form of restraint, sometimes used in bulls.

NPO (nulla per os) Nothing by mouth.

NSAID Nonsteroidal antiinflammatory drug.

Nursery Building in a swine operation where weaned piglets are kept.

Nutrient Chemical element or compound that aids in the support of life.

Offal The organs (viscera) removed from a carcass at slaughter.

Omasum Third and smallest compartment of the forestomach of the ruminant. Connects with the reticulum through the reticulo-omasal orifice and with the abomasum through the omaso-abomasal orifice. Also called the "bible" because of its many, tightly packed leaves.

Omphalophlebitis Inflammation of the umbilical veins.

On one line Harness-racing horse carrying its head preferentially to one side, usually in response to lameness, especially of a hindlimb (will usually carry its head toward the side with the hindlimb lameness).

On one shaft Hindlimb lameness in harness-racing horses often causes the horse to carry its hindquarters to the opposite side of the lameness, sometimes touching the shaft ("on the shaft") of the sulky or jog cart.

Open Not pregnant.

Open knees   Incomplete ossification of the distal radial physis (growth plate), as confirmed by a radiograph. When ossification is complete (closed knees), it is an indication of skeletal maturity. Many trainers will not place a young animal in hard training until a radiograph confirms that the knees have "closed."

Open up a mare   Release the scar tissue formed by the Caslick surgical procedure, before parturition, so the mare's vulva is not torn during delivery of the foal.

Opisthotonos   Form of spasm consisting of extreme hyperextension of the body. The head and heels are bent backward, and the body is bowed forward.

Orchidectomy   Excision of one or both testes. Common procedure in animal husbandry as a promoter of growth. May be necessary when a testis is seriously diseased or injured. Also known as castration in farm parlance, caponizing for birds, gelding for horses, and as part of the term mark for lambs.

Orchitis   Inflammation of a testis, marked by pain, swelling, and a feeling of weight, often accompanying epididymitis.

Order buyer   Person who buys feeder cattle on order for cattle feeders.

Original   A cryptorchid horse.

Ororumen   Method of placing a tube through the mouth to the rumen.

OSHA   Occupational Safety and Health Administration.

Osselets   Chronic inflammation of the fetlock joint and joint capsule, noticed primarily as thickening of the dorsal aspect of the fetlock. Referred to as green osselets in the acute stage of inflammation, before the joint capsule has thickened.

Out of   Mothered by; referring to the female parent of an animal. Compare "By."

Out of Oklahoma, by truck   Horse of questionable breeding. Also, a stolen horse.

Outcrossing   Practice of introducing unrelated genetic material into a breeding line.

Overo   Color pattern in Paint horses in which the white usually does not cross the back of the horse between its withers and its tail. Generally, at least one and often all four legs are dark. Generally, the white is irregular and is scattered or splashy. Head markings are distinctive, often bald faced, apron faced, or bonnet faced.

Oxytocin   Nonapeptide secreted by magnocellular neurons of hypothalamus and stored as a posterior pituitary hormone along with vasopressin. Promotes uterine contractions and milk ejection and contributes to the second stage of labor.

Packed cell volume   Portion of whole blood volume occupied by erythrocytes (red blood cells).

Paired serum sample   Serum samples taken about 1 week or so apart, depending on the disease, and tested for antibody levels.

Palpation gate   Gate near the rear of a working chute that opens to allow access to the rear of the animal. Often used for palpation of cattle.

Pancreatic amylase   Enzyme that breaks down starch into sugar.

Pancreatic juice   Fluid secreted into the duodenum by the pancreas. Important for breaking down starches, proteins, and fats.

Panel tag   Tag placed in the ear as a form of identification.

Paralysis   Loss or impairment of motor function in part because of a lesion of the neural or muscular mechanism.

Paraphimosis   Inability to retract the penis back into the prepuce, usually from excessive swelling of prepuce or penis.

Parrot mouth   Brachygnathia; overbite; the incisors fail to meet and occlude properly.

Parturition   Birth.

Pasture   Pen in which grass is the main feed source. Usually much larger than a drylot.

Pasture plant   Plant naturally found in a pasture.

Patent ductus arteriosus   Continuous "machinery murmur" over the left heart base.

Patent urachus   Condition in which the urachus does not close and remains patent after birth.

Pen mating   In species other than pigs, form of mating that is synonymous with hand mating (see Hand mating). In swine, the boar is placed in a pen with a group of sows for breeding. Not all sows may be bred, and the day of breeding may not be known.

Penile paralysis   Inability to retract the penis into the prepuce as a result of nerve or muscle (retractor penis muscle) disease.

Pepsin   Proteolytic enzyme that is the principal digestive component of gastric juice. Acts as a catalyst in the chemical breakdown of protein to form a mixture of polypeptides. Formed from pepsinogen in the presence of acid or, autocatalytically, in the presence of pepsin itself. Has milk clotting action similar to that of rennin and thereby facilitates digestion of milk protein.

Performance record   Record maintained about an animal's performance.

Perineum   Region and associated structures occupying the pelvic outlet and beneath the pelvic diaphragm. Bounded anteriorly by the pubic symphysis, anterolaterally by the ischiopubic rami and ischial tuberosities, posterolaterally by the sacrotuberous ligaments, and posteriorly by the coccyx. The deep limit is inferior surface of pelvic diaphragm, and the superficial limit is the skin. Region between the thighs, bounded in the male by the scrotum and anus and in the female by the vulva and anus, containing the roots of the external genitalia.

Persistent corpus luteum   Corpus luteum that does not lyse.

Petechiae   Minute, pinpoint, nonraised, perfectly round, purplish red spots caused by intradermal or submucous hemorrhage that later turn blue or yellow.

Petechial hemorrhages   Tiny pinpoint red marks that are an important sign of asphyxia caused by some external means of obstructing the airways.

Phantom   Mounting dummy used in equine semen collection.

Pharyngeal recess   Area dorsal and caudal to the orifice of the auditory tube in the pharynx of the ruminant.

Phenothiazine tranquilizers   Term also used to denote a group of major tranquilizers resembling phenothiazine in molecular structure.

Phimosis   Inability to extend the penis from the prepuce, usually from excessive swelling of the prepuce, which prevents the penis from exiting.

Phthisis bulbi   Shrunken, nonfunctional eye that results from severe ocular disease.

Physical examination   Examination of an animal's overall health.

Physical restraint   Methods applied to an animal with or without the use of special equipment.

Picking   Practice of cleaning a stall in which only the wet or dirty bedding is removed (picked out).

Pig   Animal of the genus *Sus*.

Pig mouth   Prognathia; underbite of the incisors. Also known as sow mouth, monkey mouth.

Pig pullers   Instrument used to help manipulate a piglet from the birth canal during dystocia.

Piggy   Sow due to farrow soon.

Piglet   Neonate of the porcine species.

Pin bone   Ischiatic tuberosity.

Pin firing Thermocautery applied to the skin over an injured tendon, bone, or joint in hopes of stimulating faster and higher-quality healing. It is applied with a heated "firing iron" in a regular pattern across the skin that leaves small, focal scars. Used historically. Any beneficial effects are now attributed to the period of rest that was prescribed after the firing was performed, rather than to the firing itself. A form of counterirritation.

Pizzle Penis of a male ruminant. Sometimes used to indicate only the urethral process of the ruminant penis.

Placentome Attachment of ruminant placenta.

Pneumothorax Accumulation of air or gas in the pleural space. Three types are traumatic, primary spontaneous, and secondary spontaneous. Formerly sometimes induced for treatment of pulmonary tuberculosis.

Pneumovagina Involuntary aspiration of air into the vagina so that the vagina is chronically distended.

Point of balance At the shoulder. the point on an animal's body that can be used for movement. Moving in front of the point of balance, toward the head, makes the animal back up. Moving past the point of balance, toward the rear, makes the animal go forward.

Points Black hair on horses. Most commonly the ears, mane, tail, and lower legs.

Poll Top of the head; the occiput.

Polled Term used to describe cattle that are naturally born without horns.

Polydipsia Excessive fluid intake.

Polymerase chain reaction (PCR) Amplification of a specific DNA sequence (target or template sequence) present in a complex mixture by adding two or more short oligonucleotides (also called primers) that are specific for the terminal or outer limits of the template sequence. The template-primers mixture is subjected to repeated cycles of heating to separate (melt) the double-stranded DNA and cooling in the presence of nucleotides and DNA polymerase such that the template sequence is copied at each cycle. Thermostable polymerases such as those obtained from a hot springs bacterium *Thermus aquaticus*, commonly termed "Taq polymerase," are used. At the end of 20 to 30 such cycles, the amplified target sequence, which may have been present in as few as a single copy in the original mixture, can be readily detected, for example, by electrophoresis and ethidium bromide staining in an agarose gel.

Polyuria Excessive urine excretion.

Pony Small horse.

Popped a splint Term describing acute inflammation and swelling of the periosteum of a splint bone (metacarpal [MC2 or 4] or metatarsal [MT2 or 4]) in the horse or the ligament that attaches the splint bone to the adjacent cannon bone.

Popped knee Carpitis; synovitis and capsulitis of one or more carpal joints.

Postanesthetic myopathy Condition in which a horse is unable to rise after a period of recumbency with general anesthesia. If it does rise, it shows severe tremor, weakness, and easy falling. Serum muscle enzyme levels indicate gross muscle damage, and both forelimbs and hindlimbs are affected.

Posting Placing a post behind an animal while in a working chute to prevent it from backing up.

Postmortem After death.

Pouches Guttural pouches of the horse.

Poultice Soft, moist, mass with the consistency of cooked cereal that is spread between layers of muslin, linen, gauze, or towels and applied hot to an area to create moist local heat or counterirritation.

Premises registration Portion of the National Animal Identification System in which farmers or ranchers register with the government the properties where they keep their animals.

Prepuce Invagination of skin that covers the free portion of the penis in the nonerect state. The invagination is double in horses. Also called pizzle in cattle.

Prepurchase examination Examination conducted before completing the sale of an animal. Common procedure in equine practice. A seller and a buyer are identified, and the veterinarian performing the examination is presumed to be working in the buyer's best interest (the veterinarian is paid by the buyer). Like the insurance examination, the prepurchase examination is dictated by the intended use of the horse and its estimated value. It may be a simple physical examination or an in-depth examination including biopsies, blood samples, endoscopy, electrocardiogram or echocardiogram, and diagnostic imaging.

Priapism Prolonged erection unrelated to sexual desire, usually secondary to failure of the blood to exit the erectile tissue of the glans penis. Swelling of the prepuce and penis develops within hours and results in paraphimosis in addition to priapism.

Prion Protein infectious agent.

Proestrus In female mammals that have estrous cycles, the period of heightened follicular activity preceding estrus.

Prolapse ring Ring used to treat a prolapse.

Proteinaceous Concentrates with higher levels of protein. Examples are urea, biuret, diammonium phosphate, monoammonium phosphate, ammonium sulfate, soybean meal, cottonseed meal, linseed meal, sunflower meal, and safflower meal.

Proud cut Stallion-like behavior in a horse that has been castrated. Often (incorrectly) blamed on "incomplete" castration that failed to remove all the epididymis or spermatic cord; however, neither of these tissues produces testosterone.

Proud flesh Exuberant granulation (scar) tissue; usually affects healing wounds on the legs of horses.

Pruritus Unpleasant cutaneous sensation that provokes the desire to rub or scratch the skin to obtain relief. Also called itching.

PTO Power takeoff.

Pulse deficit Difference between heart rate and pulse rate in atrial fibrillation that results from failure of some of ventricular contractions to produce peripheral pulse waves of sufficient magnitude to be detected by palpation.

Pure breeding Mating two animals of the same breed. Most often both are registered with the same association.

Purpuric hemorrhage Large hemorrhage.

Pyrexia Fever.

Quality grade Composite evaluation of factors that affect palatability of meat (tenderness, juiciness, flavor). Factors include the following: carcass maturity; firmness, texture, and color of the lean; and amount and distribution of marbling within the lean. Beef carcass quality grading is based on (1) degree of marbling and (2) degree of maturity.

Quidding Dropping feed while chewing; often indicates poor mastication from dental abnormalities.

Radial immunodiffusion test Technique for quantitating soluble proteins that involves placing the solution to be measured into a well cut into an agar or agarose gel containing antiserum specific for the protein. As the solution to be measured diffuses out of the well, it complexes with the antiserum and forms a ring, the size of which is proportional to the quantity of soluble protein in the well. Commonly abbreviated SRID (single radial immunodiffusion test). Also known as the Mancini method.

Ram Intact male sheep.

Ram lamb Intact male neonate sheep.

Ramp trailer Horse or livestock trailer with a ramp in the back that allows the animal to walk up to gain access to the trailer.

Ranting Behavior of an agitated boar; nervousness, frothing at the mouth, and chomping.

Ration Diet formulated for livestock.

Recumbent Lying down.

Red nose Infectious bovine rhinotracheitis (IBR) of cattle; produces noticeable hyperemia of the nasal mucosa. Highly contagious herpesvirus respiratory disease.

Reefing Circumcision, sometimes necessary to treat lesions or malignant diseases of the glans penis.

Renin Proteolytic enzyme secreted by the kidneys. Catalyzes formation of angiotensin and thus affects blood pressure.

Restraint Term used to imply control of an animal. May be necessary for medical and nonmedical procedures.

Retained placenta Placenta that is not expelled after parturition.

Reticulum Smallest, most cranial section of the compound stomach of ruminants, lined with mucous membrane folded into a hexagonal pattern. Communicates cranially with esophagus and caudally with rumen. Also called honeycomb.

Retractor bulbi muscle Muscle of the eye.

Retractor penis muscle Elastic, bandlike muscle that pulls the nonerect penis of animals with a sigmoid flexure back into its S-shaped configuration.

Rickettsia Genus of nonmotile, gram-negative, non–spore-forming, highly pleomorphic bacteria that can manifest as cocci.

Ridgling Cryptorchid horse or other animal.

Rig Cryptorchid horse. Also known as a false rig.

Ringing Placing nose rings in bulls (for handling and restraint) or in swine (to prevent rooting by pigs housed on dirt or pasture).

Roached mane Practice of clipping away the entire mane or clipping the mane so short that it stands erect.

Roarer Horse that makes a respiratory noise (stertor) during exercise; usually refers to a horse affected with laryngeal hemiplegia or paralysis that makes a characteristic "roaring" noise during inspiration.

Rose Bengal test Fluorescein compound used as a pink dye in a liver function test and as a coloring agent in feed. Also used in the eye to stain necrotic tissue and devitalized cells of the cornea in keratoconjunctivitis sicca. Animals injected with the dye are temporarily photosensitive. Old-fashioned field plate test for brucellosis in serum; dye was used to mark the antigen and make its clumping visible. Suitable only as a screening test for brucellosis.

Roughage Feed containing more than 18% crude fiber when dry. Examples are hay, silage, and pasture.

Rumen First stomach of a ruminant. Consists of a huge sac lined by a mucous membrane, with several subdivisions, where partially chewed food is stored before rumination. Also called paunch.

Rumenocentesis Method used to collect rumen fluid.

Ruminant Any of the suborder Ruminantia (order Artiodactyla). Hoofed mammal that has four stomachs (rumen, reticulum, omasum, and abomasum) through which food passes in digestion. Includes cattle, sheep, goats, deer, and antelopes.

Rumination In ruminants, the casting up of food (called cud) out of the rumen and chewing of it a second time. Also called cudding.

Rundowns A type of equine leg bandage.

Runt Piglet that is smaller than its littermates.

Rupture Hernia.

Salivary amylase Enzyme that breaks starch down into sugar.

Salivary maltase Enzyme that breaks down the disaccharide maltose.

Savaging The act of a sow killing and eating one or more piglets as they are born.

Scissor claw Excessive growth of one or both claws on a ruminant's foot such that they overlap like scissors.

Scope (e.g., throat, joint) Use an endoscope or arthroscope.

Scours Diarrhea.

Scratches Moist exudative dermatitis of the lower legs of horses, especially on the back of the pastern. Lesions (open sores, scabs, cracking of the skin) are painful and often accompanied by regional swelling and lameness. Usually caused by excessive moisture conditions (mud, wet pasture, wet bedding) around the horse's lower legs and feet. Also known as grease heel or mud fever.

Scrotal hernia Inguinal hernia that has passed into the scrotum.

Scur Loosely attached horns.

Seed stock breeder Producer who raises livestock as replacement breeding stock.

Seedy toe Separation of the hoof wall and sole at the white line of the toe in horses with chronic laminitis; characterized by a widened, weak white line that often allows infection to develop in the lamina of the front of the hoof.

Semen straw Plastic straw used to hold frozen semen.

Serology Originally, the study of in vitro reactions of immune sera (e.g., precipitin, agglutination, complement fixation reactions). Now the term refers to the use of such reactions to measure serum antibody titers in infectious disease (serologic tests), the clinical correlations of the antibody titer (the "serology" of a disease), and the use of serologic reactions to detect antigens.

Serovar Taxonomic subdivision of bacteria based on the kinds and combinations of constituent antigens present in the cell, or a formula expressing the antigenic analysis on which such a subdivision is based.

Service Breeding of a female by a male.

Settled Successfully bred and conceived.

Sew up/stitch up a mare Perform the Caslick surgical procedure.

Sheath Common term for prepuce.

Shipping fever Acute respiratory disease that affects animals after transportation; may involve several factors, especially stress.

Shoat Neonate of the porcine species.

Shoe boil Olecranon bursitis in the horse; most often caused by repeated hitting of the elbow with the hoof during motion or trauma from lying down in sternal recumbency (also known as capped elbow).

Shower-in, shower-out Method of disease control on swine farms. Personnel entering the facility must remove all clothing, shower completely, and dress in clean clothing. The process is repeated before leaving the facility.

Shying Unexpected movement of an animal away from a source of pain or fear.

Sickle-hocked Conformation fault of the horse; the hocks appear to have too much angulation (flexion) when viewed from the side.

Sidewinder Male that has been surgically prepared to ensure that it cannot mate or is not fertile. The penis is surgically diverted to the side of the linea alba. In cattle and sheep, a vasectomized animal or a castrate injected with testosterone is used.

Sigmoid flexure Part of the male reproductive system that helps to extend the penis from the sheath for the purpose of copulation.

Sinker Horse with laminitis, in which distal displacement of the distal phalanx (P3) has occurred. P3 may actually protrude from the bottom of the hoof.

Sinocentesis Taping into the sinus.

Sitfast Necrosis that often extends into the fatty tissue of the crest of the neck in draft horses, from trauma caused by the harness collar.

Skin scald Burning of the skin.

Skin turgor Test used to estimate hydration in an animal.

Slant-load trailer Horse trailer in which the animals stand at an angle with partitions separating the horses.

Slipped Aborted.

Slipper foot Claw that is flat and curls upward to form a square end.

Sliver Strand of loose, untwisted fiber produced in carding.

SMEDI Stillbirth, mummification, embryonic death, and infertility.

Smegma Type of secretion of sebaceous glands, found chiefly beneath the prepuce. Consists principally of desquamated epithelial cells and sometimes has a cheesy consistency.

Smooth mouth Old animal with teeth worn nearly to the gumline.

Snots Nasal discharge.

Sorting Process of going through a herd and separating animals into groups.

Sour Horse with a bad attitude or apparent boredom; may resist certain circumstances or perform without enthusiasm, such as in a riding ring (ring sour) or on a racetrack (track sour). May occur when the animal's daily schedule has little variation.

South American camelid *Lama* is the modern genus name for two South American camelids, the wild guanaco and the domesticated llama. This genus is closely allied to the wild vicuña and domesticated alpaca of the genus *Vicugna*.

Sow Female of the porcine species.

Specific pathogen-free (SPF) Term used to guarantee that an animal is free from particular pathogens.

Spirochete Spiral bacterium.

Splint Inflammation or exostosis of the small metacarpal (MC2 or 4) or metatarsal (MT2 or 4) bones in the horse.

Split tail A female animal.

Spondylitis Inflammation of the vertebra.

Sporocyst Protective case or cyst in which sporozoites develop and from which they are transferred to different hosts.

Springer First-calf heifer in the latter stages of gestation.

Squeeze Application of pressure to the sides of a bovine in a working chute by bringing in the sides of a chute.

Stag Male of the porcine species that was castrated after it reached puberty.

Stagging Male pig castrated after it has reached maturity.

Stallion Intact male horse.

Stanchion Simple head catch that usually has a horizontal single bar on the sides and an open rear area.

Standing heat Stage of estrus in which the cow stands to be mounted by other cows or by the bull.

Standing part of a rope Longer end of the rope or the end attached to the animal.

Steer Castrated male bovine.

Step-up trailer Horse or livestock trailer that requires the animal to step up in order to walk into the trailer.

Stifled Horse with upward fixation of the patella.

Stillbirth Delivery of a dead neonate.

Stock trailer Trailer with gates that allow an animal to move throughout one portion of the trailer.

Stocking up Enlargement (swelling) of the legs with subcutaneous edema; common in the distal limbs of horses.

Stocks 1. Open set of bars with two doors at the front and back often used for horse restraint; similar to a working chute. 2. Green portion of the plant, not the seed (e.g., corn stalks, which are left over after the corn has been combined).

Streak canal Short, small-caliber duct at the tip of the teat that communicates to the exterior.

Street nail surgery Surgical treatment of a navicular bursa or bone infection usually resulting from a deep puncture wound to the caudal aspect of the bottom of the hoof.

Stringy Horse with stringhalt, an involuntary hyperflexion of the hock when the horse is in motion that produces a characteristic jerking of the hindleg toward the abdomen.

Stripping Practice of cleaning a stall in which all the bedding is removed.

Subarachnoid space Area between the arachnoid and the pia mater.

Subclinical mastitis Mastitis without visible signs of disease. Causes the greatest economic loss to dairy farmers because of lowered production. Requires special diagnostic testing of the milk to diagnose.

Subcutaneous emphysema Air in the tissue.

Subpalpebral lavage An ophthalmic treatment placed through one or two incisions in the upper or lower eyelid. Narrow rubber tubing is placed through the eyelid to open directly in the conjunctival sac, away from the cornea.

Suburethral diverticulum Lies below the opening of the urethra of the cow.

Suint The perspiration of sheep; the contents are water soluble.

Sulky Two-wheeled racing cart pulled by harness racing horses.

Summer sore Open skin lesion complicated by the presence of the larvae of *Habronema* species; habronemiasis.

Sunken anus Depressed anus usually seen in mares.

Supernumerary teats Irregular number of teats.

Superovulation Extraordinary acceleration of ovulation that produces a greater than normal number of oocytes, usually as a result of administration of exogenous gonadotropins.

Surgical insurance Insurance that covers the specific costs of surgical treatment and hospitalization, with some limitations, similar to human health insurance policies.

Suspension cup See Claw.

Suspensory ligament Modified interosseous muscle of the horse that arises from the palmar carpal ligament behind the knee (or hock in hindlimb) and suspends the pair of sesamoid bones behind the fetlock. Distal continuation of the ligament is composed of the cruciate, oblique, and straight sesamoid ligaments and the pair of extensor branches that unite with the common digital extensor tendon.

Sweat Wrap designed to reduce fluid buildup in the lower legs.

Sweeney Injury to the suprascapular nerve in horses, usually from blunt trauma to the front of the shoulder or scapula region, or chronic trauma from harness collars. Produces a characteristic gait with lateral instability of the shoulder joint.

Sweet itch   Pruritic skin disease of horses, caused by hypersensitivity to the bites of *Culicoides* species.

Switch   "Fake" tail used in horses by harvesting tail hairs from other horses of similar color and binding them together at one end; the switch is taped or braided into the recipient horse's natural tail to make it appear fuller or longer.

Switch   Distal part of the bovine tail that bears longer hairs than the body of the tail.

Synchronization   Use of hormones to cause all livestock to come into estrus at the same time.

Tack   The equipment worn by a horse for riding (e.g., saddle, bridle, martingale).

Tagging   Shearing the wool from the perineal area and udder of a ewe, before lambing. Also, shearing the perineal area before shearing, or in animals with diarrhea.

Tail gate   Rear gate on a working chute.

Tail jack   Method of restraint in which the tail of a bovine is brought dorsally over the back of the animal.

Tailing   Restraint technique used in cattle in which the butt of the tail is grasped with both hands and raised vertically as far as it will go without breaking. While the tail is in this position, the animal is unlikely to kick and then only lightly.

Taint   Offensive odor or taste, often from cooking boar meat.

Tankage   Material made from heat-digested animal abattoir residues without gut contents, hide, horn, and hoof. Material is concentrated and dried and possesses a high biologic value protein content of 60%.

Teased in   Positive response to teasing; female is in heat.

Teaser   Animal used to tease sexually but not impregnate the members of the opposite sex. Usually male; it may be surgically prepared to ensure that it cannot mate or is not fertile. In cattle and sheep, a vasectomized animal or a castrate injected with testosterone is used. In horses, an entire or cryptorchid is used but at a distance so that no act of mating can take place.

Teasing   Method of observing signs of estrus in a female horse by exposing her to limited physical or visual contact with a male horse. Used to assess readiness for breeding of the female.

Teat cup assembly   Portion of the milking unit that contains the steel shell and liner.

Teat order   Social hierarchy established within a litter of nursing piglets.

Teg   A 2-year-old sheep.

Temporary marking paint   Form of identification in which the animal is drawn on with temporary nontoxic paint.

Terminal line   Breed of swine that has stronger meat characteristics.

Tetanus   Infection of the nervous system by the potentially deadly bacterium *Clostridium tetani* (*C. tetani*).

Tetraplegia   Quadriplegia.

Thermal neutral zone   Endotherm's temperature tolerance range.

Three-titter   Cow with a nonfunctional teat.

Thrombocytopenia   Decrease in number of platelets, as occurs in thrombocytopenic purpura.

Thrombophlebitis   Inflammation of a vein (phlebitis) associated with thrombus formation (thrombosis).

Throw   1. In the restraint of horses and cows, to cast them. 2. When tying a knot, the action of making a loop and passing it (as if throwing a lariat) around an object, which may be a cow's tail or, more commonly, the suture material, which has already been placed to commence a knot.

Tie-back   Equine surgical procedure to treat laryngeal hemiplegia by suturing the affected arytenoid cartilage in an abducted position, away from the lumen of the larynx. Also known as roaring surgery.

Tipping horns   Cutting off the tip of the horns.

Titillating   Stimulation of the vulvar region to stimulate urination in cattle.

Tobiano   Color pattern in Paint horses in which the dark color usually covers one or both flanks. Generally, all four legs are white, at least below the hocks and knees. The spots are usually regular and distinct as ovals or round patterns that extend down over the neck and chest, thus giving the appearance of a shield. Head markings are like those of a solid-colored horse: solid, or with a blaze, strip, star, or snip. Horse may be either predominantly dark or white. The tail is often two colors.

Tongue tie   Practice of tying a horse's tongue in position by circling the tongue and mandible one to two times with roll gauze or string. Done to prevent dorsal displacement of the soft palate during a race by preventing caudal movement of the tongue during swallowing; it is placed just before a race and removed as soon as the race is over. Also called a tie down.

Total digestible nutrients (TDN)   Outmoded method of expressing the energy value of a feed. Estimated as follows:

$$\% \, \text{TDN} = \frac{\text{DCP} + \text{DCF} + \text{DNFE} + (\text{DEF} \times 2.25)}{\text{Feed consumed} \times 100}$$

where DCP is digestible crude protein, DCF is digestible crude fat, DNFE is digestible nitrogen-free extract, and DEE is digestible ether extract. One pound of TDN equals 2000 kcal of digestible energy.

Total protein   Total serum protein test that measures the total amount of protein in the blood.

Tovero   Color pattern in Paint horses in which the dark pigmentation around the ears may expand to cover the forehead or eyes. One or both eyes are blue. Dark pigmentation around the mouth may extend up the sides of the face and form spots. Chest spots come in varying sizes and may extend up the neck. Flank spots range in size and often are accompanied by smaller spots that extend forward across the barrel, up over the loin. Spots of varying sizes occur at the base of the tail.

Traces   Long straps, usually leather, that attach a horse's harness to the shafts of a two- or four-wheeled cart, buggy, or wagon; the traces provide the connection and traction for pulling the vehicle.

Traction   Act of drawing or exerting a pulling force, as along the long axis of a structure.

Trailer   Portion of the branch of a horseshoe that extends caudally behind the hoof; used to correct abnormal landing of the hind hooves in some horses. Difficult to use successfully on front hooves because trailers are likely to be stepped on with the toes of the hind feet, thus pulling off the shoe.

Transducer   Device used in ultrasonography. Contains a piezoelectric crystal that can translate mechanical energy into electrical signals or electrical signals into mechanical energy.

Trephining   Surgical intervention with a trephine.

Trimming shears   Scissorlike clippers used to trim wool.

Triple drip   Drug combination consisting of three drugs administered for anesthesia.

Trocar   Penlike object with a sharp end used to relieve excess gas in the event of bloat.

Trots   Diarrhea.

Trypsin Serine endopeptidase that catalyzes cleavage of peptide bonds on the carboxyl side of either arginine or lysine. Secreted by the pancreas as the proenzyme trypsinogen and converted to the active form in the small intestine by enteropeptidase. Active enzyme catalyzes cleavage and activation of additional trypsinogen and other pancreatic proenzymes important to protein digestion.

Tub Area before the chute where animals can be crowded and encouraged to move up the alleyway. Also known as a crowding pen.

Tuber coxae Bony prominence on the dorsal aspect of the hip.

Tucked-up Standing with the back rounded and having a seemingly compact abdomen (resembling a greyhound); often indicates abdominal discomfort or, less frequently, musculoskeletal pain.

Tup Ram.

Turbinate Delicate scroll-like bone that occupies the nasal chambers and supports the nasal mucous membrane. Dorsal conchae belong to the ethmoturbinate part of the ethmoid bone.

Tusks Canine teeth.

Twin lamb disease Pregnancy ketosis in sheep.

Twitches Restraint method in which pressure is applied to an area of the horse as a distraction.

Two-horse trailer Horse trailer that will hold only two horses.

Tying-up General term for stiffness and reluctance to move the hindlimbs, usually with palpable hardening of the gluteal muscles. Caused by exertional rhabdomyolysis syndrome, a condition with several clinical manifestations and probably a multifactorial origin.

Umbilical hernia Outward bulging (protrusion) of the abdominal lining or part of the abdominal organs through the area around the naval.

Universal ear notching system System of ear notches that correspond to numbers used to identify swine.

Unsoundness Any defect that prevents an animal from achieving its intended use.

Urethral diverticulum Condition in which a variably sized "pocket" or outpouching forms next to the urethra. Because it most often connects to the urethra, this outpouching repeatedly becomes filled with urine during the act of urination, thus causing symptoms.

Urethrostomy Surgical formation of a permanent opening of the urethra at the perineal surface.

Urethrotomy Incision of the urethra, usually for relief of a stricture.

Urinary calculi Urinary stones.

Urine scald Scalding of the perineal area, and sometimes the hindlegs, by urine. May be the result of urinary incontinence or the animal's inability to assume normal posture when urinating (i.e., from paresis or paralysis of hindlimbs). In rabbits it is caused by poor cage accommodation and frequent wetting of the area with urine. Secondary infection of the dermatitis is common.

USDA United States Department of Agriculture. Conducts research to discover, test, and implement improved genetic evaluation techniques for economically important traits.

Uterine inertia Insufficiently strong or poorly coordinated uterine contractions during labor.

Vaccination Introduction of vaccine into the body for the purpose of inducing immunity. Originally used to describe the injection of smallpox vaccine, the term has come to mean any immunizing procedure in which vaccine is injected.

Valgus Bent or twisted outward. Denotes a deformity in which the angulation of the part is away from the midline of the body. The term is an adjective and should be used only in connection with the noun it describes, such as talipes valgus, genu valgum, and coxa valga. The meanings of valgus and varus are often reversed, so that genu valgum is knock-knee, not bowleg.

Varus Bent or twisted inward. Denoting a deformity in which the angulation of the part is toward the midline of the body. The term varus is an adjective and should be used only in connection with the noun it describes, such as talipes varus, genu varum, and coxa vara. The meanings of varus and valgus are often reversed, so that genu varum is bowleg, not knock-knee.

Vasectomized Having undergone removal of the ductus deferentes (vasa deferentes) by surgical means.

Vernacular disease Mispronunciation of "navicular disease."

Vertical integration Process in which several steps in the production or distribution of a product or service are controlled by a single company or entity to increase that company's or entity's power in the marketplace.

Vice Objectionable or bad habit, often detrimental to the animal or destructive to its environment. Higher incidence in animals kept in confinement.

Viral antigen Viral molecule recognized by the immune system.

Viral nucleic acid detection Method of detecting viral nucleic acids.

Virus isolation Gold standard test used to diagnose viral infections. The virus is isolated in embryos inside chicken eggs. A series of tests follows to identify, for example, H and N subtypes of the avian influenza virus specifically.

Vulva External genital organs in the female.

Warmblood Group of middle-weight horse types and breeds, primarily originating in Europe, registered with organizations. Characterized by open studbook policy, studbook selection, and the aim of breeding for equestrian sport.

Water belly Ruptured bladder or urethra, with accumulation of urine in the subcutaneous tissues around the prepuce and ventral abdomen; seen with obstructive urolithiasis of ruminants.

Wattle Projection of skin hanging from the chin or throat, especially in poultry and some breeds of goats.

Wave mouth An undulating occlusal surface of the cheek teeth (premolars and molars).

Waxing Accumulation of soft, dried colostrum at the teat ends in mares that often signals parturition within 24 to 48 hours.

Wether Castrated male sheep.

Wether lamb Castrated male neonatal sheep.

Whirl bone Greater trochanter of the femur.

White muscle disease Disease caused by selenium or vitamin E deficiency.

Wilgil Male pseudohermaphrodite sheep.

Wind puff Effusion of a joint, not accompanied by lameness.

Windsucker Female horse that involuntarily aspirates air through the lips of the vulva (pneumovagina); may sometimes produce a noise as air enters and exits the vagina, especially at speeds faster than a walk.

Windsucker Horse that cribs (aerophagia).

Windswept Foal born with bilateral angular limb deformities, with a valgus deformity in limb and a varus deformity in the same joint in the opposite limb; presumed to be caused by malposition in the uterus. Seen most often in the hocks.

Withdrawal time   Length of time needed for a drug to be eliminated from animal tissue or products after it is no longer used.

Wobbler   Horse with ataxia of the front or back legs, usually as a result of a compressive spinal cord lesion in the neck region, although other spinal cord diseases can cause similar signs.

Wolf tooth   First premolars of the horse; small, rudimentary teeth that do not always erupt in every horse. They are often removed to prevent interference with the bit. Mandibular wolf teeth are very uncommon.

Wool blindness   Extreme growth of wool around the eyes that limits or prevents vision.

Working chute   Device used to restrain large animals, especially cattle and horses. A small stall into which the animal is encouraged to walk. The animal's head is fixed (in cattle by a head bail), and the back of the chute is closed. The animal then can be examined or treated. The quality of the chute depends on its freedom from injury to the animal and the operator and the accessibility of the animal for the procedures to be conducted. Speed of throughput is an important consideration when large numbers are to be handled in repetitive treatments, and quick-release gates are an essential part of the unit.

Wry neck   Torticollis (twisted neck); may be congenital or secondary to other conditions.

Wry nose   Severe congenital defect characterized by a lateral deviation of the nasal septum; appears as a twisted nose and muzzle.

Yean   Give birth, in sheep and goats.

Yearling   Animal that is more than 1 year old but less than 2 years old.

Yearling doe   Female goat more than 1 year old but less than 2 years old.

Yearling ewe   Female sheep more than 1 year old but less than 2 years old.

Yeld mare   Mare that does not produce or raise a foal during the season.

Yellowhammer   Cattle showing evidence of Jersey blood.

Yield grade   Measurements of cattle and lamb carcass cutability categorized into numeric categories, with 1 being the leanest and having the highest percentage of boneless, closely trimmed retail cuts.

Zoonotic   Diseases and parasites that may be transmitted between humans and animals.

Index

Page numbers followed by *f* indicate figure, by *t* table, and by *b* box.